Stahl's Essential Psychopharmacology

Prescriber's Guide

SIXTH EDITION

With the range of psychotropic drugs expanding and the usages of existing medications diversifying, we are pleased to present this very latest edition of what has become the indispensable formulary in psychopharmacology.

This new edition features seven new compounds as well as information about several new formulations of existing drugs. In addition, many important new indications are covered for existing drugs, as are updates to the profiles of the entire content and collection, including expansion of the sections on long-acting injectable formulations of antipsychotics.

With its easy-to-use, template-driven navigation system, *The Prescriber's Guide* combines evidence-based data with clinically informed advice to support everyone prescribing in the field of mental health.

Stephen M. Stahl is Adjunct Professor of Psychiatry at the University of California, San Diego, and Honorary Visiting Senior Fellow in Psychiatry at the University of Cambridge, UK. He has conducted various research projects awarded by the National Institute of Mental Health, Veterans Affairs, and the pharmaceutical industry. Author of more than 500 articles and chapters, Dr Stahl is also the author of the bestseller *Stahl's Essential Psychopharmacology*.

Stahl's Essential Psychopharmacology

Prescriber's Guide

SIXTH EDITION

Stephen M. Stahl

University of California at San Diego,
San Diego, California

Editorial assistant
Meghan M. Grady

With illustrations by
Nancy Muntner

CAMBRIDGE
UNIVERSITY PRESS

CAMBRIDGE
UNIVERSITY PRESS

University Printing House, Cambridge CB2 8BS, United Kingdom

One Liberty Plaza, 20th Floor, New York, NY 10006, USA

477 Williamstown Road, Port Melbourne, VIC 3207, Australia

314-321, 3rd Floor, Plot 3, Splendor Forum, Jasola District Centre, New Delhi – 110025, India

79 Anson Road, #06-04/06, Singapore 079906

Cambridge University Press is part of the University of Cambridge.

It furthers the University's mission by disseminating knowledge in the pursuit of education, learning, and research at the highest international levels of excellence.

www.cambridge.org
Information on this title: www.cambridge.org/9781316618134

First published 2005
Revised and updated edition published 2006
Third edition published 2009
Fourth edition published 2011
Fifth edition published 2014
Sixth edition published 2017
Reprinted 2018

Printed in the United Kingdom by Clays, St Ives plc

A catalog record for this publication is available from the British Library.

ISBN 978-1-316-61813-4 Paperback
ISBN 978-1-108-40488-4 Spiral

Additional resources for this publication at www.stahlonline.org

Contents

Introduction

This *Guide* is intended to complement *Stahl's Essential Psychopharmacology*. *Stahl's Essential Psychopharmacology* emphasizes mechanisms of action and how psychotropic drugs work upon receptors and enzymes in the brain. This *Guide* gives practical information on how to use these drugs in clinical practice.

It would be impossible to include all available information about any drug in a single work, and no attempt is made here to be comprehensive. The purpose of this *Guide* is instead to integrate the art of clinical practice with the science of psychopharmacology. That means including only essential facts in order to keep things short. Unfortunately that also means excluding less critical facts as well as extraneous information, which may nevertheless be useful to the reader but would make the book too long and dilute the most important information. In deciding what to include and what to omit, the author has drawn upon common sense and 30 years of clinical experience with patients. He has also consulted with many experienced clinicians and analyzed the evidence from controlled clinical trials and regulatory filings with government agencies.

In order to meet the needs of the clinician and to facilitate future updates of this *Guide*, the opinions of readers are sincerely solicited. Feedback can be emailed to feedback@neiglobal.com. Specifically, are the best and most essential psychotropic drugs included here? Do you find any factual errors? Are there agreements or disagreements with any of the opinions expressed here? Are there suggestions for any additional tips or pearls for future editions? Any and all suggestions and comments are welcomed.

All of the selected drugs are presented in the same design format in order to facilitate rapid access to information. Specifically, each drug is broken down into five sections, each designated by a unique color background: ■ therapeutics, ■ side effects, ■ dosing and use, ■ special populations, and ■ the art of psychopharmacology, followed by key references.

Therapeutics covers the brand names in major countries; the class of drug; what it is commonly prescribed and approved for by the United States Food and Drug Administration (FDA); how the drug works; how long it takes to work; what to do if it works or if it doesn't work; the best augmenting combinations for partial response or treatment resistance; and the tests (if any) that are required.

Side effects explains how the drug causes side effects; gives a list of notable, life-threatening, or dangerous side effects; gives a specific rating for weight gain or sedation; and gives advice about how to handle side effects, including best augmenting agents for side effects.

Dosing and use gives the usual dosing range; dosage forms; how to dose and dosing tips; symptoms of overdose; long-term use; if habit forming, how to stop; pharmacokinetics; drug interactions; when not to use; and other warnings or precautions.

Special populations gives specific information about any possible renal, hepatic, and cardiac impairments, and any precautions to be taken for treating the elderly, children, adolescents, and pregnant and breast-feeding women.

The art of psychopharmacology gives the author's opinions on issues such as the potential advantages and disadvantages of any one drug, the primary target symptoms, and clinical pearls to get the best out of a drug.

In addition, drugs for which switching between medications can be complicated have a special section called The Art of Switching, which includes clinical pearls and graphical representations to help guide the switching process.

There is a list of icons used in this *Guide* following this Introduction and at the back of the *Guide* are several indices. The first is an index by drug name, giving both generic names (uncapitalized) and trade names (capitalized and followed by the generic name in parentheses). The second is an index of common uses for the generic drugs included in the *Guide* and is organized by disorder/symptom. Agents that are approved by the FDA for a particular use are shown in bold. The third index is organized by drug class and lists all the agents that fall within each particular class. In addition to these indices there is a list of abbreviations.

Readers are encouraged to consult standard references[1] and comprehensive psychiatry and pharmacology textbooks for more in-depth information. They are also reminded that the art of psychopharmacology section is the author's opinion.

It is strongly advised that readers familiarize themselves with the standard use of these drugs before attempting any of the more exotic uses discussed, such as unusual drug combinations and doses. Reading about both drugs before augmenting one with the other is also strongly recommended. Today's psychopharmacologist should also regularly track blood pressure, weight, and body mass index for most of his or her patients. The dutiful clinician will also check out the drug interactions of non-central nervous system (CNS) drugs with those that act in the CNS, including any prescribed by other clinicians.

Certain drugs may be for experts only and might include clozapine, thioridazine, pimozide, nefazodone, mesoridazine, and monoamine oxidase (MAO) inhibitors, among others. Off-label uses not approved by the FDA and inadequately studied doses or combinations of drugs may also be for the expert only, who can weigh risks and benefits in the presence of sometimes vague and conflicting evidence. Pregnant or nursing women, or people with two or more psychiatric illnesses, substance abuse, and/or a concomitant medical illness may be suitable patients for the expert only. Controlled substances also require expertise. Use your best judgment as to your level of expertise and realize that we are all learning in this rapidly advancing field. The practice of medicine is often not so much a science as it is an art. It is important to stay within the standards of medical care for the field, and also within your personal comfort zone, while trying to help extremely ill and often difficult patients with medicines that can sometimes transform their lives and relieve their suffering.

Finally, this book is intended to be genuinely helpful for practitioners of psychopharmacology by providing them with the mixture of facts and opinions selected by the author. Ultimately, prescribing choices are the reader's responsibility. Every effort has been made in preparing this book to provide accurate and up-to-date information in accord with accepted standards and practice at the time of publication. Nevertheless, the psychopharmacology field is evolving rapidly and the author and publisher make no warranties that the information contained herein is totally free from error, not least because clinical standards are constantly changing through research and regulation. Furthermore, the author and publisher disclaim any responsibility for the

[1] For example, *Physician's Desk Reference* and *Martindale: The Complete Drug Reference.*

continued currency of this information and disclaim all liability for any and all damages, including direct or consequential damages, resulting from the use of information contained in this book. Doctors recommending and patients using these drugs are strongly advised to pay careful attention to, and consult information provided by, the manufacturer.

List of icons

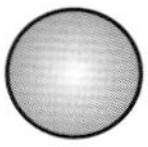
alcohol dependence treatment

alpha adrenergic blocker

alpha 2 agonist

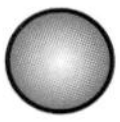
anticonvulsant

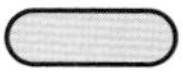
antihistamine

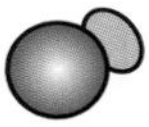
antiparkinson/anticholinergic

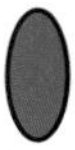
benzodiazepine

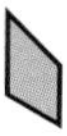
beta blocker

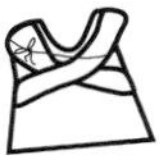
cholinesterase inhibitor

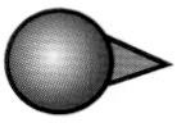
conventional antipsychotic

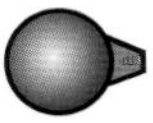
dopamine stabilizer

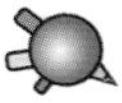
flibanserin

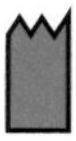
lithium

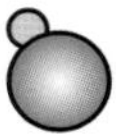
lorcaserin

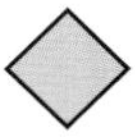
medical food

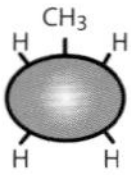

l-methylfolate

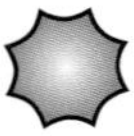

modafinil (wake-promoter)

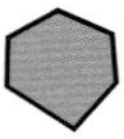

monoamine oxidase inhibitor

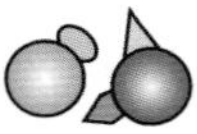

naltrexone-bupropion

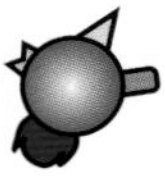

nefazodone (serotonin antagonist/reuptake inhibitor)

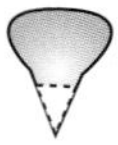

nicotinic partial agonist

N-methyl-D-aspartate antagonist

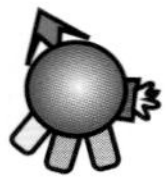

noradrenergic and specific serotonergic antidepressant

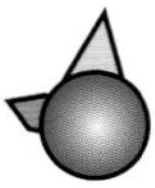

norepinephrine and dopamine reuptake inhibitor

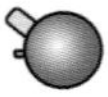

pimavanserin

sedative-hypnotic

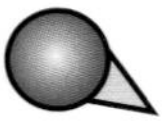

selective norepinephrine reuptake inhibitor

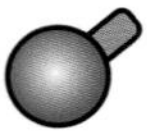

selective serotonin reuptake inhibitor

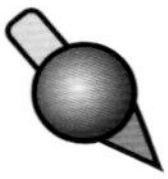

serotonin-dopamine antagonist

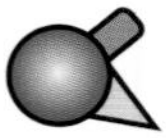

serotonin and norepinephrine reuptake inhibitor

serotonin 1A partial agonist

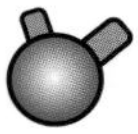

serotonin partial agonist reuptake inhibitor

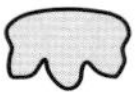

sodium oxybate

stimulant

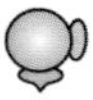

suvorexant

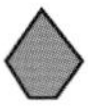

tasimelteon

thyroid hormone

topiramate/phentermine

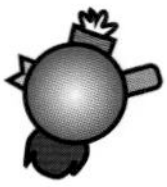

trazodone (serotonin antagonist/reuptake inhibitor)

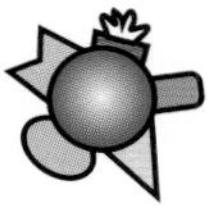

tricyclic/tetracyclic antidepressant

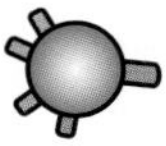

vortioxetine

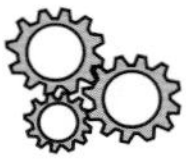

How the drug works, mechanism of action

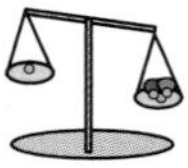

Best augmenting agents to add for partial response or treatment resistance

Life-threatening or dangerous side effects

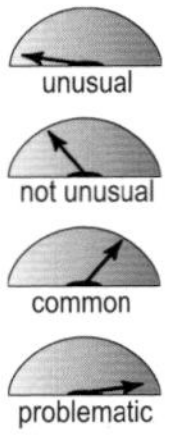

Weight Gain: Degrees of weight gain associated with the drug, with unusual signifying that weight gain has been reported but is not expected; not unusual signifying that weight gain occurs in a significant minority; common signifying that many experience weight gain and/or it can be significant in amount; and problematic signifying that weight gain occurs frequently, can be significant in amount, and may be a health problem in some patients

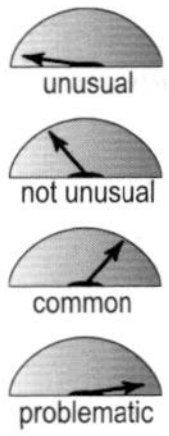

Sedation: Degrees of sedation associated with the drug, with unusual signifying that sedation has been reported but is not expected; not unusual signifying that sedation occurs in a significant minority; common signifying that many experience sedation and/or it can be significant in amount; and problematic signifying that sedation occurs frequently, can be significant in amount, and may be a health problem in some patients

Tips for dosing based on the clinical expertise of the author

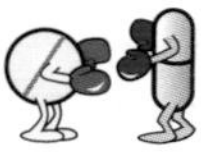

Drug interactions that may occur

Warnings and precautions regarding use of the drug

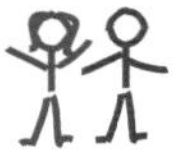

Dosing and other information specific to children and adolescents

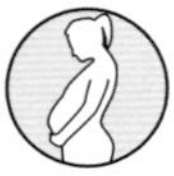

Information regarding use of the drug during pregnancy

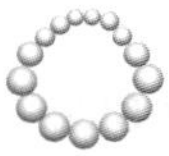

Clinical pearls of information based on the clinical expertise of the author

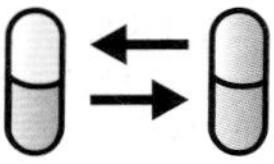

The art of switching

Suggested reading

THERAPEUTICS

Brands • Campral
see index for additional brand names

Generic? Not in USA

Class
- Neuroscience-based Nomenclature: glutamate multi-modal (Glu-MM)
- Alcohol dependence treatment

Commonly Prescribed for
(bold for FDA approved)
- **Maintenance of alcohol abstinence**

How the Drug Works
- Theoretically reduces excitatory glutamate neurotransmission and increases inhibitory gamma-aminobutyric acid (GABA) neurotransmission
- Binds to and blocks certain glutamate receptors, including metabotropic glutamate receptors
- Because withdrawal of alcohol following chronic administration can lead to excessive glutamate activity and deficient GABA activity, acamprosate can act as "artificial alcohol" to mitigate these effects

How Long Until It Works
- Has demonstrated efficacy in trials lasting between 13 and 52 weeks

If It Works
- Increases abstinence from alcohol

If It Doesn't Work
- Evaluate for and address contributing factors
- Consider switching to another agent
- Consider augmenting with naltrexone

Best Augmenting Combos for Partial Response or Treatment Resistance
- Naltrexone
- Augmentation therapy may be more effective than monotherapy
- Augmentation with behavioral, educational, and/or supportive therapy in groups or as an individual is probably key to successful treatment

Tests
- None for healthy individuals

SIDE EFFECTS

How Drug Causes Side Effects
- Theoretically, behavioral side effects due to changes in neurotransmitter concentrations at receptors in parts of the brain and body other than those that cause therapeutic actions
- Gastrointestinal side effects may be related to large doses of a drug that is an amino acid derivative, increasing osmotic absorption in the gastrointestinal tract

Notable Side Effects
- Diarrhea, nausea
- Anxiety, depression

Life-Threatening or Dangerous Side Effects
- Suicidal ideation and behavior (suicidality)

Weight Gain
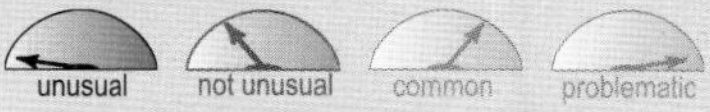

- Reported but not expected

Sedation
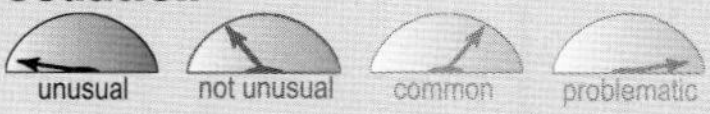

- Reported but not expected

What to Do About Side Effects
- Wait
- Adjust dose
- If side effects persist, discontinue use

Best Augmenting Agents for Side Effects
- Dose reduction or switching to another agent may be more effective since most side effects cannot be improved with an augmenting agent

DOSING AND USE

Usual Dosage Range
- 666 mg three times daily (>60 kg)
- 666 mg two times daily (<60 kg)

Dosage Forms
- Tablet 333 mg

How to Dose
- Patient should begin treatment as soon as possible after achieving abstinence
- Recommended dose is 666 mg three times daily; titration is not required

Dosing Tips
- Providing educational materials and counseling in combination with acamprosate treatment can increase the chances of success
- Patients should be advised to continue treatment even if relapse occurs and to disclose any renewed drinking
- Although absorption of acamprosate is not affected by food, it may aid adherence if patients who regularly eat three meals per day take each dose with a meal
- Adherence with three times daily dosing can be a problem; having patient focus on frequent oral dosing of drug rather than frequent drinking may be helpful in some patients

Overdose
- Limited available data; diarrhea

Long-Term Use
- Has been studied in trials up to 1 year

Habit Forming
- No

How to Stop
- Taper not necessary

Pharmacokinetics
- Terminal half-life 20–33 hours
- Excreted unchanged via the kidneys

Drug Interactions
- Does not inhibit hepatic enzymes, and thus is unlikely to affect plasma concentrations of drugs metabolized by those enzymes
- Is not hepatically metabolized and thus is unlikely to be affected by drugs that induce or inhibit hepatic enzymes
- Concomitant administration with naltrexone may increase plasma levels of acamprosate, but this does not appear to be clinically significant and dose adjustment is not recommended

Other Warnings/ Precautions
- Monitor patients for emergence of depressed mood or suicidal ideation and behavior (suicidality)
- Use cautiously in individuals with known psychiatric illness

Do Not Use
- If patient has severe renal impairment
- If there is a proven allergy to acamprosate

SPECIAL POPULATIONS

Renal Impairment
- For moderate impairment, recommended dose is 333 mg three times daily
- Contraindicated in severe impairment

Hepatic Impairment
- Dose adjustment not generally necessary

Cardiac Impairment
- Limited data available

Elderly
- Some patients may tolerate lower doses better
- Consider monitoring renal function

Children and Adolescents
- Safety and efficacy have not been established

Pregnancy
- Effective June 30, 2015, the US FDA requires changes to the content and format of pregnancy and lactation information in prescription drug labels, including the elimination of the pregnancy letter categories; the Pregnancy and Lactation

Labeling Rule (PLLR or final rule) applies only to prescription drugs and will be phased in gradually for drugs approved on or after June 30, 2001
- Controlled studies have not been conducted in pregnant women
- In animal studies, acamprosate demonstrated teratogenicity in doses approximately equal to the human dose (rat studies) and in doses approximately 3 times the human dose (rabbit studies)
- Pregnant women needing to stop drinking may consider behavioral therapy before pharmacotherapy
- Not generally recommended for use during pregnancy, especially during first trimester

Breast Feeding
- Unknown if acamprosate is secreted in human breast milk, but all psychotropics assumed to be secreted in breast milk
- Recommended either to discontinue drug or bottle feed

THE ART OF PSYCHOPHARMACOLOGY

Potential Advantages
- Individuals who have recently abstained from alcohol
- For the chronic daily drinker

Potential Disadvantages
- Individuals who are not abstinent at time of treatment initiation
- For binge drinkers

Primary Target Symptoms
- Alcohol dependence

Pearls
- Because acamprosate serves as "artificial alcohol," it may be less effective in situations in which the individual has not yet abstained from alcohol or suffers a relapse
- Thus acamprosate may be a preferred treatment if the goal is complete abstinence, but may not be preferred if the goal is reduced-risk drinking

Suggested Reading

Anton RF, O'Malley SS, Ciraulo DA, et al. Combined pharmacotherapies and behavioral interventions for alcohol dependence: the COMBINE study: a randomized controlled trial. JAMA 2006;295(17):2003–17.

Kranzler HR, Gage A. Acamprosate efficacy in alcohol-dependent patients: summary of results from three pivotal trials. Am J Addictions 2008; 17:70–6.

Rosner S, Leucht P, Soyka M. Acamprosate supports abstinence, naltrexone prevents excessive drinking: evidence from a met-analysis with unreported outcomes. J Psychopharmacol 2008;22:11–23.

THERAPEUTICS

Brands • Valdoxan
see index for additional brand names

Generic? No

Class
- Neuroscience-based Nomenclature: melatonin multi-modal (Mel-MM)
- Agonist at melatonergic 1 and melatonergic 2 receptors
- Antagonist at 5HT2C receptors

Commonly Prescribed for
(bold for FDA approved)
- Depression
- Generalized anxiety disorder

How the Drug Works
- Actions at both melatonergic and 5HT2C receptors may be synergistic and increase norepinephrine and dopamine neurotransmission in the prefrontal cortex; may resynchronize circadian rhythms that are disturbed in depression
- No influence on extracellular levels of serotonin

How Long Until It Works
- Daytime functioning, anhedonia, and sleep can improve from the first week of treatment
- Onset of full therapeutic actions in depression is usually not immediate, but often delayed 2–4 weeks
- May continue to work for many years to prevent relapse of symptoms

If It Works
- The goal of treatment is complete remission of current symptoms as well as prevention of future relapses
- Treatment most often reduces or even eliminates symptoms, but not a cure since symptoms can recur after medicine is stopped
- Continue treatment until all symptoms are gone (remission)
- Once symptoms gone, continue treating for 1 year for the first episode of depression
- For second and subsequent episodes of depression, treatment may need to be indefinite

If It Doesn't Work
- Many patients have only a partial response where some symptoms are improved but others persist (especially insomnia, fatigue, and problems concentrating)
- Other patients may be nonresponders, sometimes called treatment-resistant or treatment-refractory
- Consider increasing dose as early as 2 weeks after initiating treatment if response is insufficient (decision on dose increase has to be balanced with a higher risk of transaminase elevation; any dose increase should be made on an individual patient benefit/risk basis and with strict respect of liver function tests monitoring)
- Consider switching to another agent or adding an appropriate augmenting agent
- Consider psychotherapy
- Consider evaluation for another diagnosis or for a comorbid condition (e.g., medical illness, substance abuse, etc.)
- Some patients may experience apparent lack of consistent efficacy due to activation of latent or underlying bipolar disorder, and require antidepressant discontinuation and a switch to a mood stabilizer

Best Augmenting Combos for Partial Response or Treatment Resistance
- SSRIs (excluding fluvoxamine), SNRIs, bupropion, reboxetine, atomoxetine (use combinations of antidepressant with caution as this may activate bipolar disorder and suicidal ideation)
- Modafinil, especially for fatigue, sleepiness, and lack of concentration
- Mood stabilizers or atypical antipsychotics for bipolar depression, psychotic depression, or treatment-resistant depression
- Benzodiazepines

Tests
- Liver function tests before initiation of treatment and then at 3 weeks, 6 weeks, 12 weeks, 24 weeks, and thereafter when clinically indicated
- When increasing the dose, liver function tests should be performed at the same frequency as when initiating treatment
- Liver function tests should be repeated within 48 hours in any patient who develops raised transaminases

SIDE EFFECTS

How Drug Causes Side Effects
- Adverse reactions usually mild to moderate and occur within the first 2 weeks of treatment
- Actions at melatonergic receptors and at 5HT2C receptors could contibute to the side effects described below

Notable Side Effects
- Nausea and dizziness are most common
- Other adverse reactions are somnolence, fatigue, insomnia, headache, anxiety, diarrhea, constipation, upper abdominal pain, vomiting, hyperhidrosis
- Increase of transaminase levels

Life-Threatening or Dangerous Side Effects
✻ Rare hepatitis, hepatic failure
- Theoretically rare induction of mania (class warning)
- Rare activation of suicidal ideation and behavior (suicidality) (short-term studies did not show an increase in the risk of suicidality with antidepressants compared to placebo beyond age 24) (class warning)

Weight Gain
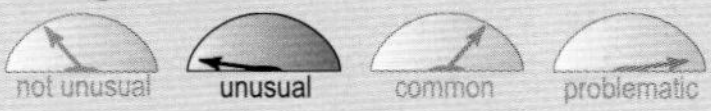

- Occurs in significant minority
- In clinical studies, weight changes were similar to those in placebo
- Cases of weight decrease have been reported

Sedation (Somnolence)
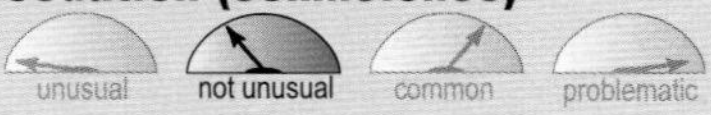

- Occurs in significant minority
- Generally transient
- May be more likely to cause fatigue than sedation

What to Do About Side Effects
- Wait
- Wait
- Stop if transaminase levels reach 3 times the upper limit of normal
- Switch to another drug

Best Augmenting Agents for Side Effects
- Often best to try another antidepressant monotherapy prior to resorting to augmentation strategies to treat side effects
- Many side effects are time-dependent (i.e., they start immediately upon dosing and upon each dose increase, but go away with time)
- Many side effects cannot be improved with an augmenting agent
- Therotically activation and agitation may represent the induction of a bipolar state, especially a mixed dysphoric bipolar II condition sometimes associated with suicidal ideation, and require the addition of lithium, a mood stabilizer or an atypical antipsychotic, and/or discontinuation of agomelatine (class warning)

DOSING AND USE

Usual Dosage Range
- 25–50 mg/day at bedtime

Dosage Forms
- Tablet 25 mg

How to Dose
- Initial 25 mg/day at bedtime; after 2 weeks can increase to 50 mg/day at bedtime

Dosing Tips
- If intolerable anxiety, insomnia, agitation, akathisia, or activation occur either upon dosing initiation or discontinuation, consider the possibility of activated bipolar disorder and switch to a mood stabilizer or an atypical antipsychotic

Overdose
- Drowsiness and epigastralgia; fatigue, agitation, anxiety, tension, dizziness, cyanosis, or malaise have also been reported

Long-Term Use
- Treatment up to 12 months has been found to decrease rate of relapse

Habit Forming
- No

How to Stop
- No need to taper dose

Pharmacokinetics
- Half-life 1–2 hours
- Metabolized primarily by CYP450 1A2

Drug Interactions
- Use of agomelatine with potent CYP450 1A2 inhibitors (e.g., fluvoxamine) is contraindicated
- Tramadol increases the risk of seizures in patients taking an antidepressant (class warning)

Other Warnings/ Precautions
- Use with caution in patients with hepatic injury risk factors, such as obesity/ overweight/non-alcoholic fatty liver disease, diabetes, patients who drink large quantities of alcohol and/or have alcohol use disorder, or who take medication associated with risk of hepatic injury. Doctors should ask their patients if they have ever had liver problems.
- If symptoms or signs of potential liver injury (dark urine, light-colored stools, yellow skin/eyes, pain in upper right belly, sustained new-onset and unexplained fatigue) are present, agomelatine should be discontinued immediately
- Use caution in patients with pre-treatment elevated transaminases (> the upper limit of the normal range and <3 times the upper limit of the normal range)
- Discontinue treatment if serum transaminases increase to 3 times the upper limit of normal; liver function tests should be performed regularly until serum transaminases return to normal
- Agomelatine should be administered at bedtime
- Use with caution in patients with bipolar disorder unless treated with concomitant mood-stabilizing agent
- When treating children off label (an unapproved use), carefully weigh the risks and benefits of pharmacological treatment against the risks and benefits of nontreatment with antidepressants and make sure to document this in the patient's chart
- Warn patients and their caregivers about the possibility of activating side effects and advise them to report such symptoms immediately
- Monitor patients for activation of suicidal ideation, especially children and adolescents

Do Not Use
- If patient has hepatic impairment
- If patient has transaminase levels >3 times the upper limit of normal
- If patient is taking a potent CYP450 1A2 inhibitor (e.g., fluvoxamine, ciprofloxacin)
- If patient is taking an MAO inhibitor (MAOI)
- If patient has galactose intolerance, Lapp lactase deficiency, or glucose-galactose malabsorption
- If there is a proven allergy to agomelatine

SPECIAL POPULATIONS

Renal Impairment
- Drug should be used with caution

Hepatic Impairment
- Contraindicated

Cardiac Impairment
- Dose adjustment not necessary

Elderly
- Efficacy and safety have been established (<75 years old)
- Dose adjustment not necessary
- Should not be used in patients age 75 years and older
- Should not be used in elderly patients with dementia

Children and Adolescents
- Carefully weigh the risks and benefits of pharmacological treatment against the risks and benefits of nontreatment with antidepressants and make sure to document this in the patient's chart
- Monitor patients face-to-face regularly, particularly during the first several weeks of treatment
- Safety and efficacy have not been established and it is not recommended

Pregnancy
- Controlled studies have not been conducted in pregnant women
- Not generally recommended for use during pregnancy, especially during first trimester

- Must weigh the risk of treatment (first trimester fetal development, third trimester newborn delivery) to the child against the risk of no treatment (recurrence of depression, maternal health, infant bonding) to the mother and child
- For many patients this may mean continuing treatment during pregnancy

Breast Feeding
- Unknown if agomelatine is secreted in human breast milk, but all psychotropics assumed to be secreted in breast milk
- Therefore, breast feeding or drug needs to be discontinued
- Immediate postpartum period is a high-risk time for depression, especially in women who have had prior depressive episodes, so drug may need to be reinstituted late in the third trimester or shortly after childbirth to prevent a recurrence during the postpartum period

THE ART OF PSYCHOPHARMACOLOGY

Potential Advantages
- Patients with lack of energy, anhedonia, anxious comorbidity, and sleep-wake disturbances
- Patients particularly concerned about sexual side effects or weight gain

Potential Disadvantages
- Patients with hepatic impairment

Primary Target Symptoms
- Depressed mood, anhedonia
- Functioning
- Anxiety within depression

Pearls
- Agomelatine represents a novel approach to depression through a novel pharmacologic profile, agonist at melatonergic MT1 / MT2 receptors and antagonist at 5HT2C receptors acting synergistically
- This synergy provides agomelatine with a distinctive efficacy profile, different from conventional antidepressants with potentially an early and continuous improvement over time
- Agomelatine improves anhedonia early in treatment
- Improves anxiety in major depressive disorder
- May be fewer withdrawals/discontinuations for adverse events than with other antidepressants
- No significant effect on cardiac parameters such as blood pressure and heart rate
- Some data suggest that agomelatine may be specially efficacious in achieving functional remission
- Agomelatine may improve sleep quality by promoting proper maintenance of circadian rhythms underlying a normal sleep-wake cycle

Suggested Reading

DeBodinat C, Guardiola-Lemaitre B, Mocaer E, et al. Agomelatine, the first melatonergic antidepressant: discovery, characterization, and development. Nat Rev Drug Discov 2010;9:628–42.

Goodwin GM, Emsley R, Rembry S, Rouillon F. Agomelatine prevents relapse in patients with major depressive disorder without evidence of a discontinuation syndrome: a 24-week randomized, double-blind, placebo-controlled trial. J Clin Psychiatry 2009;70:1128–37.

Kennedy SH, Avedisova A, Belaïdi C, Picarel-Blanchot F, de Bodinat C. Sustained efficacy of agomelatine 10 mg, 25 mg, and 25–50 mg on depressive symptoms and functional outcomes in patients with major depressive disorder. A placebo-controlled study over 6 months. Neuropsychopharmacol 2016;26(2):378–89.

Khoo AL, Zhou HJ, Teng M, et al. Network meta-analysis and cost-effectiveness analysis of new generation antidepressants. CNS Drugs 2015;29(8):695–712.

Martinotti G, Sepede G, Gambi F, et al. Agomelatine versus venlafaxine XR in the treatment of anhedonia in major depressive disorder: a pilot study. J Clin Psychopharmacol 2012;32(4):487–91.

Racagni G, Riva MA, Molteni R, et al. Mode of action of agomelatine: synergy between melatonergic and 5-HT2C receptors. World J Biol Psychiatry 2011;12(8):574–87.

Stahl SM, Fava M, Trivedi M, et al. Agomelatine in the treatment of major depressive disorder. An 8 week, multicenter, randomized, placebo-controlled trial. J Clin Psychiatry 2010;71(5):616–26.

Stahl SM. Mechanism of action of agomelatine: a novel antidepressant exploiting synergy between monoaminergic and melatonergic properties. CNS Spectrums 2014;19:207–12.

Stein DJ, Picarel-Blanchot F, Kennedy SH. Efficacy of the novel antidepressant agomelatine on anxiety symptoms in major depression. Hum Psychopharmacol 2013;28(2):151–9.

Taylor D, Sparshatt A, Varma S, Olofinjana O. Antidepressant efficacy of agomelatine: meta-analysis of published and unpublished studies. BMJ 2014;348: g2496.

THERAPEUTICS

Brands • Xanax, Xanax XR

see index for additional brand names

Generic? Yes

Class

- Neuroscience-based Nomenclature: GABA positive allosteric modulator (GABA-PAM)
- Benzodiazepine (anxiolytic)

Commonly Prescribed for

(bold for FDA approved)

- **Generalized anxiety disorder (IR)**
- **Panic disorder (IR and XR)**
- Other anxiety disorders
- Anxiety associated with depression
- Premenstrual dysphoric disorder
- Irritable bowel syndrome and other somatic symptoms associated with anxiety disorders
- Insomnia
- Acute mania (adjunctive)
- Acute psychosis (adjunctive)
- Catatonia

How the Drug Works

- Binds to benzodiazepine receptors at the GABA-A ligand-gated chloride channel complex
- Enhances the inhibitory effects of GABA
- Boosts chloride conductance through GABA-regulated channels
- Inhibits neuronal activity presumably in amygdala-centered fear circuits to provide therapeutic benefits in anxiety disorders

How Long Until It Works

- Some immediate relief with first dosing is common; can take several weeks with daily dosing for maximal therapeutic benefit

If It Works

- For short-term symptoms of anxiety – after a few weeks, discontinue use or use on an "as-needed" basis
- For chronic anxiety disorders, the goal of treatment is complete remission of symptoms as well as prevention of future relapses
- For chronic anxiety disorders, treatment most often reduces or even eliminates symptoms, but not a cure since symptoms can recur after medicine stopped
- For long-term symptoms of anxiety, consider switching to an SSRI or SNRI for long-term maintenance
- If long-term maintenance with a benzodiazepine is necessary, continue treatment for 6 months after symptoms resolve, and then taper dose slowly
- If symptoms reemerge, consider treatment with an SSRI or SNRI, or consider restarting the benzodiazepine; sometimes benzodiazepines have to be used in combination with SSRIs or SNRIs for best results

If It Doesn't Work

- Consider switching to another agent or adding an appropriate augmenting agent
- Consider psychotherapy, especially cognitive behavioral psychotherapy
- Consider presence of concomitant substance abuse
- Consider presence of alprazolam abuse
- Consider another diagnosis, such as a comorbid medical condition

Best Augmenting Combos for Partial Response or Treatment Resistance

- Benzodiazepines are frequently used as augmenting agents for antipsychotics and mood stabilizers in the treatment of psychotic and bipolar disorders
- Benzodiazepines are frequently used as augmenting agents for SSRIs and SNRIs in the treatment of anxiety disorders
- Not generally rational to combine with other benzodiazepines
- Caution if using as an anxiolytic concomitantly with other sedative hypnotics for sleep
- Could consider augmenting alprazolam with either gabapentin or pregabalin for treatment of anxiety disorders

Tests

- In patients with seizure disorders, concomitant medical illness, and/or those with multiple concomitant long-term medications, periodic liver tests and blood counts may be prudent

SIDE EFFECTS

How Drug Causes Side Effects

- Same mechanism for side effects as for therapeutic effects – namely due to excessive actions at benzodiazepine receptors

- Long-term adaptations in benzodiazepine receptors may explain the development of dependence, tolerance, and withdrawal
- Side effects are generally immediate, but immediate side effects often disappear in time

Notable Side Effects

✻ Sedation, fatigue, depression
✻ Dizziness, ataxia, slurred speech, weakness
✻ Forgetfulness, confusion
✻ Hyperexcitability, nervousness
- Rare hallucinations, mania
- Rare hypotension
- Hypersalivation, dry mouth

Life-Threatening or Dangerous Side Effects

- Respiratory depression, especially when taken with CNS depressants in overdose
- Rare hepatic dysfunction, renal dysfunction, blood dyscrasias

Weight Gain

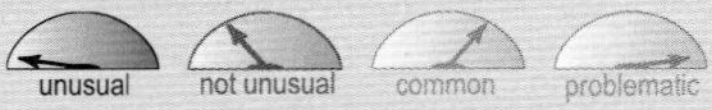

- Reported but not expected

Sedation

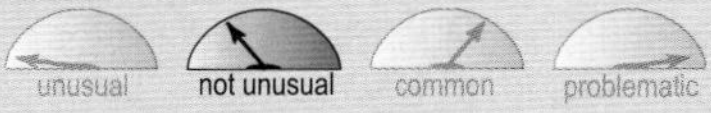

- Occurs in significant minority
- Especially at initiation of treatment or when dose increases
- Tolerance often develops over time

What to Do About Side Effects

- Wait
- Wait
- Wait
- Lower the dose
- Switch to alprazolam XR
- Take largest dose at bedtime to avoid sedative effects during the day
- Switch to another agent
- Administer flumazenil if side effects are severe or life-threatening

Best Augmenting Agents for Side Effects

- Many side effects cannot be improved with an augmenting agent

DOSING AND USE

Usual Dosage Range

- Anxiety: alprazolam IR: 1–4 mg/day
- Panic: alprazolam IR: 5–6 mg/day
- Panic: alprazolam XR: 3–6 mg/day

Dosage Forms

- Alprazolam IR tablet 0.25 mg scored, 0.4 mg (Japan), 0.5 mg scored, 0.8 mg (Japan), 1 mg scored, 2 mg multiscored
- Alprazolam IR orally disintegrating tablet 0.25 mg, 0.5 mg, 1 mg, 2 mg
- Alprazolam IR solution, concentrate 1 mg/mL
- Alprazolam XR (extended-release) tablet 0.5 mg, 1 mg, 2 mg, 3 mg

How to Dose

- For anxiety, alprazolam IR should be started at 0.75–1.5 mg/day divided into 3 doses; increase dose every 3–4 days until desired efficacy is reached; maximum dose generally 4 mg/day
- For panic, alprazolam IR should be started at 1.5 mg/day divided into 3 doses; increase 1 mg or less every 3–4 days until desired efficacy is reached, increasing by smaller amounts for dosage over 4 mg/day; may require as much as 10 mg/day for desired efficacy in difficult cases
- For panic, alprazolam XR should be started at 0.5–1 mg/day once daily in the morning; dose may be increased by 1 mg/day every 3–4 days until desired efficacy is reached; maximum dose generally 10 mg/day

Dosing Tips

- Use lowest possible effective dose for the shortest possible period of time (a benzodiazepine-sparing strategy)
- Assess need for continued treatment regularly
- Risk of dependence may increase with dose and duration of treatment
- For interdose symptoms of anxiety, can either increase dose or maintain same total daily dose but divide into more frequent doses, or give as extended-release formulation
- Can also use an as-needed occasional "top up" dose for interdose anxiety
- Because panic disorder can require doses higher than 4 mg/day, the risk

of dependence may be greater in these patients
- Some severely ill patients may require 8 mg/day or more
- Extended-release formulation only needs to be taken once or twice daily
- Do not break or chew XR tablets as this will alter controlled-release properties
- Frequency of dosing in practice is often greater than predicted from half-life, as duration of biological activity is often shorter than pharmacokinetic terminal half-life
- Alprazolam and alprazolam XR generally dosed about one tenth the dosage of diazepam

✻ Alprazolam and alprazolam XR generally dosed about twice the dosage of clonazepam

Overdose
- Fatalities have been reported both in monotherapy and in conjunction with alcohol; sedation, confusion, poor coordination, diminished reflexes, coma

Long-Term Use
- Risk of dependence, particularly for treatment periods longer than 12 weeks and especially in patients with past or current polysubstance abuse

Habit Forming
- Alprazolam is a Schedule IV drug
- Patients may develop dependence and/or tolerance with long-term use

How to Stop
- Seizures may rarely occur on withdrawal, especially if withdrawal is abrupt; greater risk for doses above 4 mg and in those with additional risks for seizures, including those with a history of seizures
- Taper by 0.5 mg every 3 days to reduce chances of withdrawal effects
- For difficult to taper cases, consider reducing dose much more slowly after reaching 3 mg/day, perhaps by as little as 0.25 mg per week or less (not for XR)
- For other patients with severe problems discontinuing a benzodiazepine, dosing may need to be tapered over many months (i.e., reduce dose by 1% every 3 days by crushing tablet and suspending or dissolving in 100 mL of fruit juice and then disposing of 1 mL while drinking the rest; 3–7 days later, dispose of 2 mL, and so on). This is both a form of very slow biological tapering and a form of behavioral desensitization. Not for XR
- Be sure to differentiate reemergence of symptoms requiring reinstitution of treatment from withdrawal symptoms
- Benzodiazepine-dependent anxiety patients and insulin-dependent diabetics are not addicted to their medications. When benzodiazepine-dependent patients stop their medication, disease symptoms can reemerge, disease symptoms can worsen (rebound), and/or withdrawal symptoms can emerge

Pharmacokinetics
- Metabolized by CYP450 3A4
- Inactive metabolites
- Elimination half-life 12–15 hours
- Food does not affect absorption

Drug Interactions
- Increased depressive effects when taken with other CNS depressants (see Warnings below)
- Inhibitors of CYP450 3A, such as nefazodone, fluvoxamine, fluoxetine, and even grapefruit juice, may decrease clearance of alprazolam and thereby raise alprazolam plasma levels and enhance sedative side effects; alprazolam dose may need to be lowered
- Thus, azole antifungal agents (such as ketoconazole and itraconazole), macrolide antibiotics, and protease inhibitors may also raise alprazolam plasma levels
- Inducers of CYP450 3A, such as carbamazepine, may increase clearance of alprazolam and lower alprazolam plasma levels and possibly reduce therapeutic effects

Other Warnings/ Precautions
- Boxed warning regarding the increased risk of CNS depressant effects when benzodiazepines and opioid medications are used together, including specifically the risk of slowed or difficulty breathing and death
- If alternatives to the combined use of benzodiazepines and opioids are not available, clinicians should limit the dosage and duration of each drug to the minimum

possible while still achieving therapeutic efficacy
- Patients and their caregivers should be warned to seek medical attention if unusual dizziness, lightheadedness, sedation, slowed or difficulty breathing, or unresponsiveness occur
- Dosage changes should be made in collaboration with prescriber
- Use with caution in patients with pulmonary disease; rare reports of death after initiation of benzodiazepines in patients with severe pulmonary impairment
- History of drug or alcohol abuse often creates greater risk for dependency
- Hypomania and mania have occurred in depressed patients taking alprazolam
- Use only with extreme caution if patient has obstructive sleep apnea
- Some depressed patients may experience a worsening of suicidal ideation
- Some patients may exhibit abnormal thinking or behavioral changes similar to those caused by other CNS depressants (i.e., either depressant actions or disinhibiting actions)

Do Not Use
- If patient has angle-closure glaucoma
- If patient is taking ketoconazole or itraconazole (azole antifungal agents)
- If there is a proven allergy to alprazolam or any benzodiazepine

SPECIAL POPULATIONS

Renal Impairment
- Drug should be used with caution

Hepatic Impairment
- Should begin with lower starting dose (0.5–0.75 mg/day in 2 or 3 divided doses)

Cardiac Impairment
- Benzodiazepines have been used to treat anxiety associated with acute myocardial infarction

Elderly
- Should begin with lower starting dose (0.5–0.75 mg/day in 2 or 3 divided doses) and be monitored closely

Children and Adolescents
- Safety and efficacy not established but often used, especially short-term and at the lower end of the dosing scale
- Long-term effects of alprazolam in children/adolescents are unknown
- Should generally receive lower doses and be more closely monitored

Pregnancy
- Effective June 30, 2015, the US FDA requires changes to the content and format of pregnancy and lactation information in prescription drug labels, including the elimination of the pregnancy letter categories; the Pregnancy and Lactation Labeling Rule (PLLR or final rule) applies only to prescription drugs and will be phased in gradually for drugs approved on or after June 30, 2001
- Possible increased risk of birth defects when benzodiazepines taken during pregnancy
- Because of the potential risks, alprazolam is not generally recommended as treatment for anxiety during pregnancy, especially during the first trimester
- Drug should be tapered if discontinued
- Infants whose mothers received a benzodiazepine late in pregnancy may experience withdrawal effects
- Neonatal flaccidity has been reported in infants whose mothers took a benzodiazepine during pregnancy
- Seizures, even mild seizures, may cause harm to the embryo/fetus

Breast Feeding
- Some drug is found in mother's breast milk
- ✻ Recommended either to discontinue drug or bottle feed
- Effects on infant have been observed and include feeding difficulties, sedation, and weight loss

THE ART OF PSYCHOPHARMACOLOGY

Potential Advantages

- Rapid onset of action
- Less sedation than some other benzodiazepines
- Availability of an XR formulation with longer duration of action

Potential Disadvantages

- Euphoria may lead to abuse
- Abuse especially risky in past or present substance abusers

Primary Target Symptoms

- Panic attacks
- Anxiety

Pearls

* One of the most popular benzodiazepines for anxiety, especially among primary care physicians and psychiatrists
- Is a very useful adjunct to SSRIs and SNRIs in the treatment of numerous anxiety disorders
- Not effective for treating psychosis as a monotherapy, but can be used as an adjunct to antipsychotics
- Not effective for treating bipolar disorder as a monotherapy, but can be used as an adjunct to mood stabilizers and antipsychotics
- May both cause depression and treat depression in different patients
- Risk of seizure is greatest during the first 3 days after discontinuation of alprazolam, especially in those with prior seizures, head injuries, or withdrawal from drugs of abuse
- Clinical duration of action may be shorter than plasma half-life, leading to dosing more frequently than 2–3 times daily in some patients, especially for immediate-release alprazolam
- Adding fluvoxamine, fluoxetine, or nefazodone can increase alprazolam levels and make the patient very sleepy unless the alprazolam dose is lowered by half or more
- When using to treat insomnia, remember that insomnia may be a symptom of some other primary disorder itself, and thus warrant evaluation for comorbid psychiatric and/or medical conditions

* Alprazolam XR may be less sedating than immediate-release alprazolam
* Alprazolam XR may be dosed less frequently than immediate-release alprazolam, and lead to less interdose breakthrough symptoms and less "clock-watching" in anxious patients
- Slower rises in plasma drug levels for alprazolam XR have the potential to reduce euphoria/abuse liability, but this has not been proven
- Slower falls in plasma drug levels for alprazolam XR have the potential to facilitate drug discontinuation by reducing withdrawal symptoms, but this has not been proven

* Alprozolam XR generally has longer biological duration of action than clonazepam
* If clonazepam can be considered a "long-acting alprazolam-like anxiolytic," then alprazolam XR can be considered "an even longer-acting clonazepam-like anxiolytic" with the potential of improved tolerability features in terms of less euphoria, abuse, dependence, and withdrawal problems, but this has not been proven
- Though not systematically studied, benzodiazepines have been used effectively to treat catatonia and are the initial recommended treatment

Suggested Reading

DeVane CL, Ware MR, Lydiard RB. Pharmacokinetics, pharmacodynamics, and treatment issues of benzodiazepines: alprazolam, adinazolam, and clonazepam. Psychopharmacol Bull 1991;27:463–73.

Greenblatt DJ, Wright CE. Clinical pharmacokinetics of alprazolam. Therapeutic implications. Clin Pharmacokinet 1993; 24:453–71.

Jonas JM, Cohon MS. A comparison of the safety and efficacy of alprazolam versus other agents in the treatment of anxiety, panic, and depression: a review of the literature. J Clin Psychiatry 1993;54(Suppl):S25–45.

Klein E. The role of extended-release benzodiazepines in the treatment of anxiety: a risk-benefit evaluation with a focus on extended-release alprazolam. J Clin Psychiatry 2002;63(Suppl 14):S27–33.

Speigel DA. Efficacy studies of alprazolam in panic disorder. Psychopharmacol Bull 1998; 34:191–5.

van Marwijk H, Allick G, Wegman F, Bax A, Riphagen II. Alprazolam for depression. Cochrane Database Syst Rev 2012; 7:CD007139.

THERAPEUTICS

Brands • Solian

see index for additional brand names

Generic? No

Class

- Neuroscience-based Nomenclature: dopamine receptor antagonist (D-RAn)
- Atypical antipsychotic (benzamide; possibly a dopamine stabilizer and dopamine partial agonist)

Commonly Prescribed for

(bold for FDA approved)

- Schizophrenia, acute and chronic (outside of USA, especially Europe)
- Dysthymia

How the Drug Works

- Theoretically blocks presynaptic dopamine 2 receptors at low doses
- Theoretically blocks postsynaptic dopamine 2 receptors at higher doses

✻ May be a partial agonist at dopamine 2 receptors, which would theoretically reduce dopamine output when dopamine concentrations are high and increase dopamine output when dopamine concentrations are low

- Blocks dopamine 3 receptors, which may contribute to its clinical actions

✻ Unlike other atypical antipsychotics, amisulpride does not have potent actions at serotonin 2A or serotonin 1A receptors

✻ Does have antagonist actions at serotonin 7 receptors and serotonin 2B receptors, which may contribute to antidepressant effects

How Long Until It Works

- Psychotic symptoms can improve within 1 week, but it may take several weeks for full effect on behavior as well as on cognition and affective stabilization
- Classically recommended to wait at least 4–6 weeks to determine efficacy of drug, but in practice some patients require up to 16–20 weeks to show a good response, especially on cognitive symptoms

If It Works

- Most often reduces positive symptoms in schizophrenia but does not eliminate them
- Can improve negative symptoms, as well as aggressive, cognitive, and affective symptoms in schizophrenia
- Most schizophrenic patients do not have a total remission of symptoms but rather a reduction of symptoms by about a third
- Perhaps 5–15% of schizophrenic patients can experience an overall improvement of greater than 50–60%, especially when receiving stable treatment for more than a year
- Such patients are considered super-responders or "awakeners" since they may be well enough to be employed, live independently, and sustain long-term relationships
- Continue treatment until reaching a plateau of improvement
- After reaching a satisfactory plateau, continue treatment for at least a year after first episode of psychosis
- For second and subsequent episodes of psychosis, treatment may need to be indefinite
- Even for first episodes of psychosis, it may be preferable to continue treatment indefinitely to avoid subsequent episodes

If It Doesn't Work

- Try one of the other first-line atypical antipsychotics (risperidone, olanzapine, quetiapine, ziprasidone, aripiprazole, paliperidone, asenapine, iloperidone, lurasidone)
- If two or more antipsychotic monotherapies do not work, consider clozapine
- Some patients may require treatment with a conventional antipsychotic
- If no atypical antipsychotic is effective, consider higher doses or augmentation with valproate or lamotrigine
- Consider noncompliance and switch to another antipsychotic with fewer side effects or to an antipsychotic that can be given by depot injection
- Consider initiating rehabilitation and psychotherapy such as cognitive remediation
- Consider presence of concomitant drug abuse

Best Augmenting Combos for Partial Response or Treatment Resistance

- Valproic acid (valproate, divalproex, divalproex ER)
- Augmentation of amisulpride has not been systematically studied

- Other mood-stabilizing anticonvulsants (carbamazepine, oxcarbazepine, lamotrigine)
- Lithium
- Benzodiazepines

Tests

✻ Although risk of diabetes and dyslipidemia with amisulpride has not been systematically studied, monitoring as for all other atypical antipsychotics is suggested

Before starting an atypical antipsychotic

✻ Weigh all patients and track BMI during treatment

- Get baseline personal and family history of diabetes, obesity, dyslipidemia, hypertension, and cardiovascular disease
- Get waistline circumference (at umbilicus), blood pressure, fasting plasma glucose, and fasting lipid profile
- Determine if patient is
  - overweight (BMI 25.0–29.9)
  - obese (BMI ≥30)
  - has pre-diabetes (fasting plasma glucose 100–125 mg/dL)
  - has diabetes (fasting plasma glucose >126 mg/dL)
  - has hypertension (BP >140/90 mm Hg)
  - has dyslipidemia (increased total cholesterol, LDL cholesterol, and triglycerides; decreased HDL cholesterol)
- Treat or refer such patients for treatment, including nutrition and weight management, physical activity counseling, smoking cessation, and medical management

Monitoring after starting an atypical antipsychotic

✻ BMI monthly for 3 months, then quarterly

- Consider monitoring fasting triglycerides monthly for several months in patients at high risk for metabolic complications and when initiating or switching antipsychotics
- Blood pressure, fasting plasma glucose, fasting lipids within 3 months and then annually, but earlier and more frequently for patients with diabetes or who have gained >5% initial weight
- Treat or refer for treatment and consider switching to another atypical antipsychotic for patients who become overweight, obese, pre-diabetic, diabetic, hypertensive, or dyslipidemic while receiving an atypical antipsychotic

✻ Even in patients without known diabetes, be vigilant for the rare but life-threatening onset of diabetic ketoacidosis, which always requires immediate treatment by monitoring for the rapid onset of polyuria, polydipsia, weight loss, nausea, vomiting, dehydration, rapid respiration, weakness and clouding of sensorium, even coma

- EKGs may be useful for selected patients (e.g., those with personal or family history of QTc prolongation; cardiac arrhythmia; recent myocardial infarction; uncompensated heart failure; or taking agents that prolong QTc interval such as pimozide, thioridazine, selected antiarrhythmics, moxifloxacin, sparfloxacin, etc.)
- Patients at risk for electrolyte disturbances (e.g., patients on diuretic therapy) should have baseline and periodic serum potassium and magnesium measurements
- Patients with low white blood cell count (WBC) or history of drug-induced leucopenia/neutropenia should have complete blood count (CBC) monitored frequently during the first few months and amisulpride should be discontinued at the first sign of decline of WBC in the absence of other causative factors

SIDE EFFECTS

How Drug Causes Side Effects

- By blocking dopamine 2 receptors in the striatum, it can cause motor side effects, especially at high doses
- By blocking dopamine 2 receptors in the pituitary, it can cause elevations in prolactin
- Mechanism of weight gain and possible increased incidence of diabetes and dyslipidemia with atypical antipsychotics is unknown

Notable Side Effects

✻ Extrapyramidal symptoms

✻ Galactorrhea, amenorrhea

✻ Atypical antipsychotics may increase the risk for diabetes and dyslipidemia, although the specific risks associated with amisulpride are unknown

- Insomnia, sedation, agitation, anxiety
- Constipation, weight gain
- Rare tardive dyskinesia

Life-Threatening or Dangerous Side Effects

- Rare neuroleptic malignant syndrome
- Rare seizures
- Dose-dependent QTc prolongation
- Increased risk of death and cerebrovascular events in elderly patients with dementia-related psychosis

Weight Gain

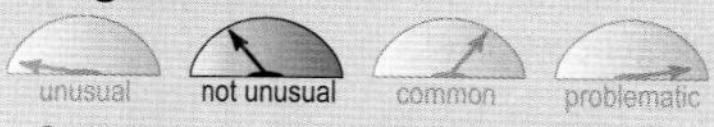

- Occurs in significant minority

Sedation

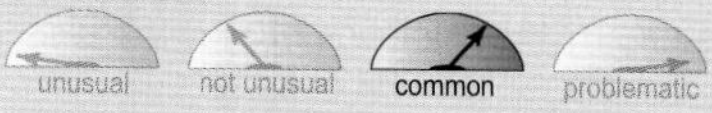

- Many experience and/or can be significant in amount, especially at high doses

What to Do About Side Effects

- Wait
- Wait
- Wait
- Lower the dose
- For motor symptoms, add an anticholinergic agent
- Take more of the dose at bedtime to help reduce daytime sedation
- Weight loss, exercise programs, and medical management for high BMIs, diabetes, dyslipidemia
- Switch to another atypical antipsychotic

Best Augmenting Agents for Side Effects

- Benztropine or trihexyphenidyl for motor side effects
- Many side effects cannot be improved with an augmenting agent

DOSING AND USE

Usual Dosage Range

- Schizophrenia: 400–800 mg/day in 2 doses
- Negative symptoms only: 50–300 mg/day
- Dysthymia: 50 mg/day

Dosage Forms

- Different formulations may be available in different markets
- Tablet 50 mg, 100 mg, 200 mg, 400 mg
- Oral solution 100 mg/mL

How to Dose

- Initial 400–800 mg/day in 2 doses; daily doses above 400 mg should be divided in 2; maximum generally 1200 mg/day
- See also the Switching section below, after Pearls

Dosing Tips

✻ Efficacy for negative symptoms in schizophrenia may be achieved at lower doses, while efficacy for positive symptoms may require higher doses

- Patients receiving low doses may only need to take the drug once daily

✻ For dysthymia and depression, use only low doses

✻ Dose-dependent QTc prolongation, so use with caution, especially at higher doses (>800 mg/day)

✻ Amisulpride may accumulate in patients with renal insufficiency, requiring lower dosing or switching to another antipsychotic to avoid QTc prolongation in these patients

- Treatment should be suspended if absolute neutrophil count falls below 1,000/mm^3

Overdose

- Sedation, coma, hypotension, extrapyramidal symptoms

Long-Term Use

- Amisulpride is used for both acute and chronic schizophrenia treatment

Habit Forming

- No

How to Stop

- See Switching section of individual agents for how to stop amisulpride
- Rapid discontinuation may lead to rebound psychosis and worsening of symptoms

Pharmacokinetics

- Elimination half-life approximately 12 hours
- Excreted largely unchanged

Drug Interactions

- Can decrease the effects of levodopa, dopamine agonists
- Can increase the effects of antihypertensive drugs

- CNS effects may be increased if used with a CNS depressant
- May enhance QTc prolongation of other drugs capable of prolonging QTc interval
- Since amisulpride is only weakly metabolized, few drug interactions that could raise amisulpride plasma levels are expected

Other Warnings/ Precautions

- Use cautiously in patients with alcohol withdrawal or convulsive disorders because of possible lowering of seizure threshold
- If signs of neuroleptic malignant syndrome develop, treatment should be immediately discontinued
- Because amisulpride may dose-dependently prolong QTc interval, use with caution in patients who have bradycardia or who are taking drugs that can induce bradycardia (e.g., beta blockers, calcium channel blockers, clonidine, digitalis)
- Because amisulpride may dose-dependently prolong QTc interval, use with caution in patients who have hypokalemia and/or hypomagnesemia or who are taking drugs that can induce hypokalemia and/or magnesemia (e.g., diuretics, stimulant laxatives, intravenous amphotericin B, glucocorticoids, tetracosactide)
- Use only with caution if at all in Parkinson's disease or Lewy body dementia, especially at high doses

Do Not Use

- If patient has pheochromocytoma
- If patient has prolactin-dependent tumor
- If patient is pregnant or nursing
- If patient is taking agents capable of significantly prolonging QTc interval (e.g., pimozide; thioridazine; selected antiarrhythmics such as quinidine, disopyramide, amiodarone, and sotalol; selected antibiotics such as moxifloxacin and sparfloxacin)
- If there is a history of QTc prolongation or cardiac arrhythmia, recent acute myocardial infarction, uncompensated heart failure
- If patient is taking cisapride, intravenous erythromycin, or pentamidine
- In children
- If there is a proven allergy to amisulpride

SPECIAL POPULATIONS

Renal Impairment

- Use with caution; drug may accumulate
- Amisulpride is eliminated by the renal route; in cases of severe renal insufficiency, the dose should be decreased and intermittent treatment or switching to another antipsychotic should be considered

Hepatic Impairment

- Use with caution, but dose adjustment not generally necessary

Cardiac Impairment

- Amisulpride produces a dose-dependent prolongation of QTc interval, which may be enhanced by the existence of bradycardia, hypokalemia, congenital or acquired long QTc interval, which should be evaluated prior to administering amisulpride
- Use with caution if treating concomitantly with a medication likely to produce prolonged bradycardia, hypokalemia, slowing of intracardiac conduction, or prolongation of the QTc interval
- Avoid amisulpride in patients with a known history of QTc prolongation, recent acute myocardial infarction, and uncompensated heart failure

Elderly

- Some patients may be more susceptible to sedative and hypotensive effects
- Although atypical antipsychotics are commonly used for behavioral disturbances in dementia, no agent has been approved for treatment of elderly patients with dementia-related psychosis
- Elderly patients with dementia-related psychosis treated with atypical antipsychotics are at an increased risk of death compared to placebo, and also have an increased risk of cerebrovascular events

Children and Adolescents

- Efficacy and safety not established under age 18

Pregnancy

- Although animal studies have not shown teratogenic effect, amisulpride is not recommended for use during pregnancy

- There is a risk of abnormal muscle movements and withdrawal symptoms in newborns whose mothers took an antipsychotic during the third trimester; symptoms may include agitation, abnormally increased or decreased muscle tone, tremor, sleepiness, severe difficulty breathing, and difficulty feeding
- Psychotic symptoms may worsen during pregnancy and some form of treatment may be necessary

Breast Feeding

- Unknown if amisulpride is secreted in human breast milk, but all psychotropics assumed to be secreted in breast milk

✻ Recommended either to discontinue drug or bottle feed

THE ART OF PSYCHOPHARMACOLOGY

Potential Advantages

- Not as clearly associated with weight gain as some other atypical antipsychotics
- For patients who are responsive to low-dose activation effects that reduce negative symptoms and depression

Potential Disadvantages

- Patients who have difficulty being compliant with twice daily dosing
- Patients for whom elevated prolactin may not be desired (e.g., possibly pregnant patients; pubescent girls with amenorrhea; postmenopausal women with low estrogen who do not take estrogen replacement therapy)
- Patients with severe renal impairment

Primary Target Symptoms

- Positive symptoms of psychosis
- Negative symptoms of psychosis
- Depressive symptoms

Pearls

✻ Efficacy has been particularly well demonstrated in patients with predominantly negative symptoms

✻ The increase in prolactin caused by amisulpride may cause menstruation to stop

- Some treatment-resistant patients with inadequate responses to clozapine may benefit from amisulpride augmentation of clozapine
- Risks of diabetes and dyslipidemia not well studied, but does not seem to cause as much weight gain as some other atypical antipsychotics
- Has atypical antipsychotic properties (i.e., antipsychotic action without a high incidence of extrapyramidal symptoms), especially at low doses, but not a serotonin dopamine antagonist
- Mediates its atypical antipsychotic properties via novel actions on dopamine receptors, perhaps dopamine stabilizing partial agonist actions on dopamine 2 receptors
- May be more of a dopamine 2 antagonist than aripiprazole, but less of a dopamine 2 antagonist than other atypical or conventional antipsychotics
- Low-dose activating actions may be beneficial for negative symptoms in schizophrenia
- Very low doses may be useful in dysthymia
- Compared to sulpiride, amisulpride has better oral bioavailability and more potency, thus allowing lower dosing, less weight gain, and fewer extrapyramidal symptoms
- Compared to other atypical antipsychotics with potent serotonin 2A antagonism, amisulpride may have more extrapyramidal symptoms and prolactin elevation, but may still be classified as an atypical antipsychotic, particularly at low doses
- Patients have very similar antipsychotic responses to any conventional antipsychotic, which is different from atypical antipsychotics where antipsychotic responses of individual patients can occasionally vary greatly from one atypical antipsychotic to another
- Patients with inadequate responses to atypical antipsychotics may benefit from determination of plasma drug levels and, if low, a dosage increase even beyond the usual prescribing limits
- Patients with inadequate responses to atypical antipsychotics may also benefit from a trial of augmentation with a

conventional antipsychotic or switching to a conventional antipsychotic
- However, long-term polypharmacy with a combination of a conventional antipsychotic with an atypical antipsychotic may combine their side effects without clearly augmenting the efficacy of either
- For treatment-resistant patients, especially those with impulsivity, aggression, violence, and self-harm, long-term polypharmacy with 2 atypical antipsychotics or with 1 atypical antipsychotic and 1 conventional antipsychotic may be useful or even necessary while closely monitoring
- In such cases, it may be beneficial to combine 1 depot antipsychotic with 1 oral antipsychotic
- Although a frequent practice by some prescribers, adding two conventional antipsychotics together has little rationale and may reduce tolerability without clearly enhancing efficacy

THE ART OF SWITCHING

Switching from Oral Antipsychotics to Amisulpride

- It is advisable to begin amisulpride at an intermediate dose and build the dose rapidly over 3–7 days
- Clinical experience has shown that asenapine, quetiapine, and olanzapine should be tapered off slowly over a period of 3–4 weeks, to allow patients to readapt to the withdrawal of blocking cholinergic, histaminergic, and alpha-1 receptors
- Clozapine should always be tapered off slowly, over a period of 4 weeks or more

* Benzodiazepine or anticholinergic medication can be administered during cross-titration to help alleviate side effects such as insomnia, agitation, and/or psychosis

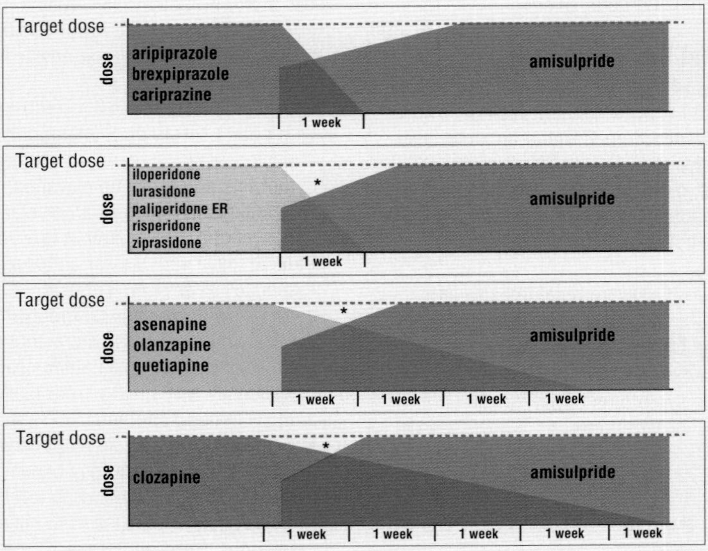

Suggested Reading

Burns T, Bale R. Clinical advantages of amisulpride in the treatment of acute schizophrenia. J Int Med Res 2001;29(6): 451–66.

Curran MP, Perry CM. Spotlight on amisulpride in schizophrenia. CNS Drugs 2002;16(3): 207–11.

Komossa K, Rummel-Kluge C, Hunder H, et al. Amisulpride versus other atypical antipsychotics for schizophrenia. Cochrane Database Syst Rev 2010;(1):CD006624.

Leucht S, Pitschel-Walz G, Engel RR, Kissling W. Amisulpride, an unusual "atypical" antipsychotic: a meta-analysis of randomized controlled trials. Am J Psychiatry 2002;159 (2):180–90.

THERAPEUTICS

Brands • Elavil

see index for additional brand names

Generic? Yes

Class

- Neuroscience-based Nomenclature: serotonin, norepinephrine multi-modal (SN-MM)
- Tricyclic antidepressant (TCA)
- Serotonin and norepinephrine/noradrenaline reuptake inhibitor

Commonly Prescribed for

(bold for FDA approved)

- **Depression**
- **Endogenous depression**
- ✻ Neuropathic pain/chronic pain
- ✻ Fibromyalgia
- ✻ Headache
- ✻ Low back pain/neck pain
- Anxiety
- Insomnia
- Treatment-resistant depression

How the Drug Works

- Boosts neurotransmitters serotonin and norepinephrine/noradrenaline
- Blocks serotonin reuptake pump (serotonin transporter), presumably increasing serotonergic neurotransmission
- Blocks norepinephrine reuptake pump (norepinephrine transporter), presumably increasing noradrenergic neurotransmission
- Presumably desensitizes both serotonin 1A receptors and beta adrenergic receptors
- Since dopamine is inactivated by norepinephrine reuptake in frontal cortex, which largely lacks dopamine transporters, amitriptyline can increase dopamine neurotransmission in this part of the brain

How Long Until It Works

- May have immediate effects in treating insomnia or anxiety
- Onset of therapeutic actions usually not immediate, but often delayed 2–4 weeks
- If it is not working within 6–8 weeks for depression, it may require a dosage increase or it may not work at all
- May continue to work for many years to prevent relapse of symptoms

If It Works

- The goal of treatment of depression is complete remission of current symptoms as well as prevention of future relapses
- The goal of treatment of chronic pain conditions such as neuropathic pain, fibromyalgia, headaches, low back pain, and neck pain is to reduce symptoms as much as possible, especially in combination with other treatments
- Treatment of depression most often reduces or even eliminates symptoms, but not a cure since symptoms can recur after medicine stopped
- Treatment of chronic pain conditions such as neuropathic pain, fibromyalgia, headache, low back pain, and neck pain may reduce symptoms, but rarely eliminates them completely, and is not a cure since symptoms can recur after medicine is stopped
- Continue treatment of depression until all symptoms are gone (remission)
- Once symptoms of depression are gone, continue treating for 1 year for the first episode of depression
- For second and subsequent episodes of depression, treatment may need to be indefinite
- Use in anxiety disorders and chronic pain conditions such as neuropathic pain, fibromyalgia, headache, low back pain, and neck pain may also need to be indefinite, but long-term treatment is not well studied in these conditions

If It Doesn't Work

- Many depressed patients have only a partial response where some symptoms are improved but others persist (especially insomnia, fatigue, and problems concentrating)
- Other depressed patients may be nonresponders, sometimes called treatment-resistant or treatment-refractory
- Consider increasing dose, switching to another agent or adding an appropriate augmenting agent
- Consider psychotherapy
- Consider evaluation for another diagnosis or for a comorbid condition (e.g., medical illness, substance abuse, etc.)

- Some patients may experience apparent lack of consistent efficacy due to activation of latent or underlying bipolar disorder, and require antidepressant discontinuation and a switch to a mood stabilizer

Best Augmenting Combos for Partial Response or Treatment Resistance

- Lithium, buspirone, thyroid hormone (for depression)
- Gabapentin, tiagabine, other anticonvulsants, even opiates if done by experts while monitoring carefully in difficult cases (for chronic pain)

Tests

- Baseline ECG is recommended for patients over age 50

❋ Since tricyclic and tetracyclic antidepressants are frequently associated with weight gain, before starting treatment, weigh all patients and determine if the patient is already overweight (BMI 25.0–29.9) or obese (BMI ≥30)

- Before giving a drug that can cause weight gain to an overweight or obese patient, consider determining whether the patient already has pre-diabetes (fasting plasma glucose 100–125 mg/dL), diabetes (fasting plasma glucose >126 mg/dL), or dyslipidemia (increased total cholesterol, LDL cholesterol and triglycerides; decreased HDL cholesterol), and treat or refer such patients for treatment, including nutrition and weight management, physical activity counseling, smoking cessation, and medical management

❋ Monitor weight and BMI during treatment

❋ While giving a drug to a patient who has gained >5% of initial weight, consider evaluating for the presence of pre-diabetes, diabetes, or dyslipidemia, or consider switching to a different antidepressant

- EKGs may be useful for selected patients (e.g., those with personal or family history of QTc prolongation; cardiac arrhythmia; recent myocardial infarction; uncompensated heart failure; or taking agents that prolong QTc interval such as pimozide, thioridazine, selected antiarrhythmics, moxifloxacin, sparfloxacin, etc.)
- Patients at risk for electrolyte disturbances (e.g., patients on diuretic therapy) should have baseline and periodic serum potassium and magnesium measurements

SIDE EFFECTS

How Drug Causes Side Effects

- Anticholinergic activity may explain sedative effects, dry mouth, constipation, and blurred vision
- Sedative effects and weight gain may be due to antihistamine properties
- Blockade of alpha adrenergic 1 receptors may explain dizziness, sedation, and hypotension
- Cardiac arrhythmias and seizures, especially in overdose, may be caused by blockade of ion channels

Notable Side Effects

- Blurred vision, constipation, urinary retention, increased appetite, dry mouth, nausea, diarrhea, heartburn, unusual taste in mouth, weight gain
- Fatigue, weakness, dizziness, sedation, headache, anxiety, nervousness, restlessness
- Sexual dysfunction (impotence, change in libido)
- Sweating, rash, itching

Life-Threatening or Dangerous Side Effects

- Paralytic ileus, hyperthermia (TCAs + anticholinergic agents)
- Lowered seizure threshold and rare seizures
- Orthostatic hypotension, sudden death, arrhythmias, tachycardia
- QTc prolongation
- Hepatic failure, extrapyramidal symptoms
- Increased intraocular pressure
- Rare induction of mania
- Rare activation of suicidal ideation and behavior (suicidality) (short-term studies did not show an increase in the risk of suicidality with antidepressants compared to placebo beyond age 24)

Weight Gain

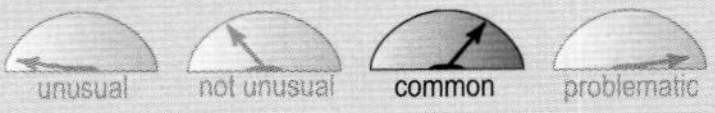

- Many experience and/or can be significant in amount
- Can increase appetite and carbohydrate craving

Sedation

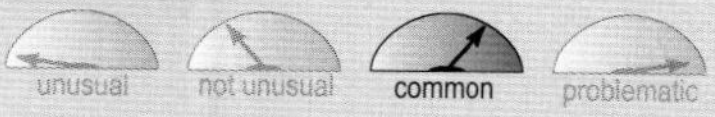

- Many experience and/or can be significant in amount
- Tolerance to sedative effects may develop with long-term use

What to Do About Side Effects

- Wait
- Wait
- Wait
- Lower the dose
- Switch to an SSRI or newer antidepressant

Best Augmenting Agents for Side Effects

- Many side effects cannot be improved with an augmenting agent

DOSING AND USE

Usual Dosage Range

- 50–150 mg/day

Dosage Forms

- Capsule 25 mg, 50 mg, 100 mg

How to Dose

- Initial 25 mg/day at bedtime; increase by 25 mg every 3–7 days
- 75 mg/day in divided doses; increase to 150 mg/day; maximum 300 mg/day

Dosing Tips

- If given in a single dose, should generally be administered at bedtime because of its sedative properties
- If given in split doses, largest dose should generally be given at bedtime because of its sedative properties
- If patients experience nightmares, split dose and do not give large dose at bedtime
- Patients treated for chronic pain may only require lower doses
- If intolerable anxiety, insomnia, agitation, akathisia, or activation occur either upon dosing initiation or discontinuation, consider the possibility of activated bipolar disorder, and switch to a mood stabilizer or an atypical antipsychotic

Overdose

- Death may occur; CNS depression, convulsions, cardiac dysrhythmias, severe hypotension, EKG changes, coma

Long-Term Use

- Safe

Habit Forming

- No

How to Stop

- Taper to avoid withdrawal effects
- Even with gradual dose reduction, some withdrawal symptoms may appear within the first 2 weeks
- Many patients tolerate 50% dose reduction for 3 days, then another 50% reduction for 3 days, then discontinuation
- If withdrawal symptoms emerge during discontinuation, raise dose to stop symptoms and then restart withdrawal much more slowly

Pharmacokinetics

- Substrate for CYP450 2D6 and 1A2
- Plasma half-life 10–28 hours
- Metabolized to an active metabolite, nortriptyline, which is predominantly a norepinephrine reuptake inhibitor, by demethylation via CYP450 1A2
- Food does not affect absorption

Drug Interactions

- Tramadol increases the risk of seizures in patients taking TCAs
- Use of TCAs with anticholinergic drugs may result in paralytic ileus or hyperthermia
- Fluoxetine, paroxetine, bupropion, duloxetine, and other CYP450 2D6 inhibitors may increase TCA concentrations
- Fluvoxamine, a CYP450 1A2 inhibitor, can decrease the conversion of amitriptyline to nortriptyline and increase amitriptyline plasma concentrations
- Cimetidine may increase plasma concentrations of TCAs and cause anticholinergic symptoms
- Phenothiazines or haloperidol may raise TCA blood concentrations
- May alter effects of antihypertensive drugs; may inhibit hypotensive effects of clonidine
- Use of TCAs with sympathomimetic agents may increase sympathetic activity

- Methylphenidate may inhibit metabolism of TCAs
- Activation and agitation, especially following switching or adding antidepressants, may represent the induction of a bipolar state, especially a mixed dysphoric bipolar II condition sometimes associated with suicidal ideation, and require the addition of lithium, a mood stabilizer or an atypical antipsychotic, and/or discontinuation of amitriptyline

Other Warnings/ Precautions

- Add or initiate other antidepressants with caution for up to 2 weeks after discontinuing amitriptyline
- Generally, do not use with MAOIs, including 14 days after MAOIs are stopped; do not start an MAOI for at least 5 half-lives (5 to 7 days for most drugs) after discontinuing amitriptyline, but see Pearls
- Use with caution in patients with history of seizures, urinary retention, angle-closure glaucoma, hyperthyroidism
- TCAs can increase QTc interval, especially at toxic doses, which can be attained not only by overdose but also by combining with drugs that inhibit TCA metabolism via CYP450 2D6, potentially causing torsade de pointes-type arrhythmia or sudden death
- Because TCAs can prolong QTc interval, use with caution in patients who have bradycardia or who are taking drugs that can induce bradycardia (e.g., beta blockers, calcium channel blockers, clonidine, digitalis)
- Because TCAs can prolong QTc interval, use with caution in patients who have hypokalemia and/or hypomagnesemia, or who are taking drugs that can induce hypokalemia and/or magnesemia (e.g., diuretics, stimulant laxatives, intravenous amphotericin B, glucocorticoids, tetracosactide)
- When treating children, carefully weigh the risks and benefits of pharmacological treatment against the risks and benefits of nontreatment with antidepressants and make sure to document this in the patient's chart
- Distribute the brochures provided by the FDA and the drug companies
- Warn patients and their caregivers about the possibility of activating side effects and advise them to report such symptoms immediately
- Monitor patients for activation of suicidal ideation, especially children and adolescents

Do Not Use

- If patient is recovering from myocardial infarction
- If patient is taking agents capable of significantly prolonging QTc interval (e.g., pimozide, thioridazine, selected antiarrhythmics, moxifloxacin, sparfloxacin)
- If there is a history of QTc prolongation or cardiac arrhythmia, recent acute myocardial infarction, uncompensated heart failure
- If patient is taking drugs that inhibit TCA metabolism, including CYP450 2D6 inhibitors, except by an expert
- If there is reduced CYP450 2D6 function, such as patients who are poor 2D6 metabolizers, except by an expert and at low doses
- If there is a proven allergy to amitriptyline or nortriptyline

SPECIAL POPULATIONS

Renal Impairment

- Use with caution; may need to lower dose

Hepatic Impairment

- Use with caution; may need to lower dose

Cardiac Impairment

- Baseline ECG is recommended
- TCAs have been reported to cause arrhythmias, prolongation of conduction time, orthostatic hypotension, sinus tachycardia, and heart failure, especially in the diseased heart
- Myocardial infarction and stroke have been reported with TCAs
- TCAs produce QTc prolongation, which may be enhanced by the existence of bradycardia, hypokalemia, congenital or acquired long QTc interval, which should be evaluated prior to administering amitriptyline
- Use with caution if treating concomitantly with a medication likely to produce prolonged bradycardia, hypokalemia,

slowing of intracardiac conduction, or prolongation of the QTc interval

- Avoid TCAs in patients with a known history of QTc prolongation, recent acute myocardial infarction, and uncompensated heart failure
- TCAs may cause a sustained increase in heart rate in patients with ischemic heart disease and may worsen (decrease) heart rate variability, an independent risk of mortality in cardiac populations
- Since SSRIs may improve (increase) heart rate variability in patients following a myocardial infarct and may improve survival as well as mood in patients with acute angina or following a myocardial infarction, these are more appropriate agents for cardiac population than tricyclic/ tetracyclic antidepressants

✽ Risk/benefit ratio may not justify use of TCAs in cardiac impairment

Elderly

- Baseline ECG is recommended for patients over age 50
- May be more sensitive to anticholinergic, cardiovascular, hypotensive, and sedative effects
- Initial dose 50 mg/day; increase gradually up to 100 mg/day
- Reduction in the risk of suicidality with antidepressants compared to placebo in adults age 65 and older

Children and Adolescents

- Carefully weigh the risks and benefits of pharmacological treatment against the risks and benefits of nontreatment with antidepressants and make sure to document this in the patient's chart
- Use with caution, observing for activation of known or unknown bipolar disorder and/ or suicidal ideation, and inform parents or guardians of this risk so they can help observe child or adolescent patients
- Monitor patients face-to-face regularly, particularly during the first several weeks of treatment
- Not generally recommended for use under age 12
- Several studies show lack of efficacy of TCAs for depression
- May be used to treat enuresis or hyperactive/impulsive behaviors
- Some cases of sudden death have occurred in children taking TCAs
- Adolescents: initial dose 50 mg/day; increase gradually up to 100 mg/day

Pregnancy

- Effective June 30, 2015, the US FDA requires changes to the content and format of pregnancy and lactation information in prescription drug labels, including the elimination of the pregnancy letter categories; the Pregnancy and Lactation Labeling Rule (PLLR or final rule) applies only to prescription drugs and will be phased in gradually for drugs approved on or after June 30, 2001
- Controlled studies have not been conducted in pregnant women
- Crosses the placenta
- Adverse effects have been reported in infants whose mothers took a TCA (lethargy, withdrawal symptoms, fetal malformations)
- Must weigh the risk of treatment (first trimester fetal development, third trimester newborn delivery) to the child against the risk of no treatment (recurrence of depression, maternal health, infant bonding) to the mother and child
- For many patients this may mean continuing treatment during pregnancy

Breast Feeding

- Some drug is found in mother's breast milk

✽ Recommended either to discontinue drug or bottle feed

- Immediate postpartum period is a high-risk time for depression, especially in women who have had prior depressive episodes, so drug may need to be reinstituted late in the third trimester or shortly after childbirth to prevent a recurrence during the postpartum period
- Must weigh benefits of breast feeding with risks and benefits of antidepressant treatment versus nontreatment to both the infant and the mother
- For many patients this may mean continuing treatment during breast feeding

THE ART OF PSYCHOPHARMACOLOGY

Potential Advantages
- Patients with insomnia
- Severe or treatment-resistant depression
- Patients with a wide variety of chronic pain syndromes

Potential Disadvantages
- Pediatric and geriatric patients
- Patients concerned with weight gain
- Cardiac patients

Primary Target Symptoms
- Depressed mood
- Symptoms of anxiety
- Somatic symptoms
- Chronic pain
- Insomnia

Pearls
- Was once one of the most widely prescribed agents for depression
- Remains one of the most favored TCAs for treating headache and a wide variety of chronic pain syndromes, including neuropathic pain, fibromyalgia, migraine, neck pain, and low back pain
- ✻ Preference of some prescribers for amitriptyline over other tricyclic/tetracyclic antidepressants for the treatment of chronic pain syndromes is based more upon art and anecdote rather than controlled clinical trials, since many TCAs/tetracylics may be effective for chronic pain syndromes
- TCAs are no longer generally considered a first-line treatment option for depression because of their side effect profile
- ✻ Amitriptyline has been shown to be effective in primary insomnia
- TCAs may aggravate psychotic symptoms
- Alcohol should be avoided because of additive CNS effects
- Underweight patients may be more susceptible to adverse cardiovascular effects
- Children, patients with inadequate hydration, and patients with cardiac disease may be more susceptible to TCA-induced cardiotoxicity than healthy adults
- For the expert only: although generally prohibited, a heroic but potentially dangerous treatment for severely treatment-resistant patients is to give a tricyclic/tetracyclic antidepressant other than clomipramine simultaneously with an MAOI for patients who fail to respond to numerous other antidepressants
- If this option is elected, start the MAOI with the tricyclic/tetracyclic antidepressant simultaneously at low doses after appropriate drug washout, then alternately increase doses of these agents every few days to a week as tolerated
- Although very strict dietary and concomitant drug restrictions must be observed to prevent hypertensive crises and serotonin syndrome, the most common side effects of MAOI/tricyclic or tetracyclic combinations may be weight gain and orthostatic hypotension
- Patients on TCAs should be aware that they may experience symptoms such as photosensitivity or blue-green urine
- SSRIs may be more effective than TCAs in women, and TCAs may be more effective than SSRIs in men
- Since tricyclic/tetracyclic antidepressants are substrates for CYP450 2D6, and 7% of the population (especially Caucasians) may have a genetic variant leading to reduced activity of 2D6, such patients may not safely tolerate normal doses of tricyclic/tetracyclic antidepressants and may require dose reduction
- Phenotypic testing may be necessary to detect this genetic variant prior to dosing with a tricyclic/tetracyclic antidepressant, especially in vulnerable populations such as children, elderly, cardiac populations, and those on concomitant medications
- Patients who seem to have extraordinarily severe side effects at normal or low doses may have this phenotypic CYP450 2D6 variant and require low doses or switching to another antidepressant not metabolized by 2D6

Suggested Reading

Guaiana G, Barbui C, Hotopf M. Amitriptyline for depression. Cochrane Database Syst Rev 2007;(3):CD004186.

Hauser W, Petzke F, Uceyler N, Sommer C. Comparative efficacy and acceptability of amitriptyline, duloxetine and milnacipran in fibromyalgia syndrome: a systematic review with meta-analysis. Rheumatology (Oxford) 2011;50(3):532–43.

Torrente Castells E, Vazquez Delgado E, Gay Escoda C. Use of amitriptyline for the treatment of chronic tension-type headache. Review of the literature. Med Oral Patol Oral Cir Bucal 2008;13(9):E567–72.

AMOXAPINE

THERAPEUTICS

Brands • Asendin

see index for additional brand names

Generic? Yes

Class

- Neuroscience-based Nomenclature: norepinephrine, serotonin reuptake inhibitor (SN-RI)
- Tricyclic antidepressant (TCA), sometimes classified as a tetracyclic antidepressant
- Norepinephrine/noradrenaline reuptake inhibitor
- Serotonin 2A antagonist
- Parent drug and especially an active metabolite are dopamine 2 antagonists

Commonly Prescribed for

(bold for FDA approved)

- **Neurotic or reactive depressive disorder**
- **Endogenous and psychotic depressions**
- **Depression accompanied by anxiety or agitation**
- Depressive phase of bipolar disorder
- Anxiety
- Insomnia
- Neuropathic pain/chronic pain
- Treatment-resistant depression

How the Drug Works

- Boosts neurotransmitter norepinephrine/noradrenaline
- Blocks norepinephrine reuptake pump (norepinephrine transporter), presumably increasing noradrenergic neurotransmission
- Since dopamine is inactivated by norepinephrine reuptake in frontal cortex, which largely lacks dopamine transporters, amoxapine can thus increase dopamine neurotransmission in this part of the brain
- A more potent inhibitor of norepinephrine reuptake pump than serotonin reuptake pump (serotonin transporter)
- At high doses may also boost neurotransmitter serotonin and presumably increase serotonergic neurotransmission
- Blocks dopamine 2 receptors, reducing positive symptoms of psychosis

How Long Until It Works

- Onset of therapeutic actions usually not immediate, but often delayed 2–4 weeks
- If it is not working within 6–8 weeks for depression, it may require a dosage increase or it may not work at all
- May continue to work for many years to prevent relapse of symptoms

If It Works

- The goal of treatment is complete remission of current symptoms as well as prevention of future relapses
- Treatment most often reduces or even eliminates symptoms, but not a cure since symptoms can recur after medicine stopped
- Continue treatment until all symptoms are gone (remission)
- Once symptoms gone, continue treating for 1 year for the first episode of depression
- For second and subsequent episodes of depression, treatment may need to be indefinite
- Use in anxiety disorders may also need to be indefinite

If It Doesn't Work

- Many patients have only a partial response where some symptoms are improved but others persist (especially insomnia, fatigue, and problems concentrating)
- Other patients may be nonresponders, sometimes called treatment-resistant or treatment-refractory
- Consider increasing dose, switching to another agent or adding an appropriate augmenting agent
- Consider psychotherapy
- Consider evaluation for another diagnosis or for a comorbid condition (e.g., medical illness, substance abuse, etc.)
- Some patients may experience apparent lack of consistent efficacy due to activation of latent or underlying bipolar disorder, and require antidepressant discontinuation and a switch to a mood stabilizer

Best Augmenting Combos for Partial Response or Treatment Resistance

- Lithium, buspirone, thyroid hormone

Tests

- Baseline ECG is recommended for patients over age 50

* Since tricyclic and tetracyclic antidepressants are frequently associated with weight gain, before starting treatment, weigh all patients and determine if the patient is already overweight (BMI 25.0–29.9) or obese (BMI ≥30)
- Before giving a drug that can cause weight gain to an overweight or obese patient, consider determining whether the patient already has pre-diabetes (fasting plasma glucose 100–125 mg/dL), diabetes (fasting plasma glucose >126 mg/dL), or dyslipidemia (increased total cholesterol, LDL cholesterol and triglycerides; decreased HDL cholesterol), and treat or refer such patients for treatment, including nutrition and weight management, physical activity counseling, smoking cessation, and medical management

* Monitor weight and BMI during treatment
* While giving a drug to a patient who has gained >5% of initial weight, consider evaluating for the presence of pre-diabetes, diabetes, or dyslipidemia, or consider switching to a different antidepressant
- EKGs may be useful for selected patients (e.g., those with personal or family history of QTc prolongation; cardiac arrhythmia; recent myocardial infarction; uncompensated heart failure; or taking agents that prolong QTc interval such as pimozide, thioridazine, selected antiarrhythmics, moxifloxacin, sparfloxacin, etc.)
- Patients at risk for electrolyte disturbances (e.g., patients on diuretic therapy) should have baseline and periodic serum potassium and magnesium measurements

SIDE EFFECTS

How Drug Causes Side Effects
- Anticholinergic activity may explain sedative effects, dry mouth, constipation, and blurred vision
- Sedative effects and weight gain may be due to antihistamine properties
- Blockade of alpha adrenergic 1 receptors may explain dizziness, sedation, and hypotension
- Cardiac arrhythmias and seizures, especially in overdose, may be caused by blockade of ion channels

Notable Side Effects
- Blurred vision, constipation, urinary retention, increased appetite, dry mouth, nausea, diarrhea, heartburn, unusual taste in mouth, weight gain
- Fatigue, weakness, dizziness, sedation, headache, anxiety, nervousness, restlessness
- Sexual dysfunction, sweating

* Can cause extrapyramidal symptoms, akathisia, and theoretically, tardive dyskinesia

Life-Threatening or Dangerous Side Effects
- Paralytic ileus, hyperthermia (TCAs/tetracyclics + anticholinergic agents)
- Lowered seizure threshold and rare seizures
- Orthostatic hypotension, sudden death, arrhythmias, tachycardia
- QTc prolongation
- Hepatic failure, extrapyramidal symptoms
- Increased intraocular pressure
- Rare induction of mania
- Rare activation of suicidal ideation and behavior (suicidality) (short-term studies did not show an increase in the risk of suicidality with antidepressants compared to placebo beyond age 24)

Weight Gain
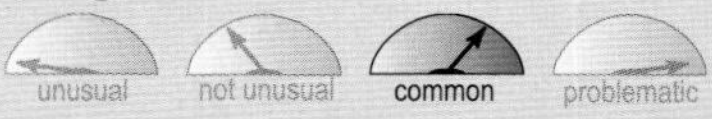

- Many experience and/or can be significant in amount
- Can increase appetite and carbohydrate craving

Sedation
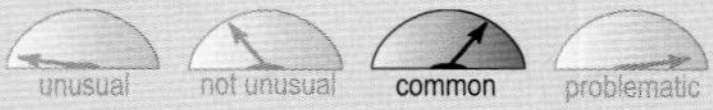

- Many experience and/or can be significant in amount
- Tolerance to sedative effect may develop with long-term use

What to Do About Side Effects
- Wait
- Wait
- Wait
- Lower the dose
- Switch to an SSRI or newer antidepressant

Best Augmenting Agents for Side Effects

- Many side effects cannot be improved with an augmenting agent
- May use anticholinergics for extrapyramidal symptoms, or switch to another antidepressant

DOSING AND USE

Usual Dosage Range

- 200–300 mg/day

Dosage Forms

- Tablets 25 mg, 50 mg, 100 mg, 150 mg

How to Dose

- Initial 25 mg 2–3 times/day; increase gradually to 100 mg 2–3 times/day or a single dose at bedtime; maximum 400 mg/day (may dose up to 600 mg/day in inpatients)

Dosing Tips

- If given in a single dose, should generally be administered at bedtime because of its sedative properties
- If given in split doses, largest dose should generally be given at bedtime because of its sedative properties
- If patients experience nightmares, split dose and do not give large dose at bedtime
- If intolerable anxiety, insomnia, agitation, akathisia, or activation occur either upon dosing initiation or discontinuation, consider the possibility of activated bipolar disorder, and switch to a mood stabilizer or an atypical antipsychotic

Overdose

- Death may occur; convulsions, cardiac dysrhythmias, severe hypotension, CNS depression, coma, changes in EKG

Long-Term Use

- Generally safe
- Some patients may develop withdrawal dyskinesias when discontinuing amoxapine after long-term use

Habit Forming

- Some patients may develop tolerance

How to Stop

- Taper to avoid withdrawal effects
- Even with gradual dose reduction some withdrawal symptoms may appear within the first 2 weeks
- Many patients tolerate 50% dose reduction for 3 days, then another 50% reduction for 3 days, then discontinuation
- If withdrawal symptoms emerge during discontinuation, raise dose to stop symptoms and then restart withdrawal much more slowly

Pharmacokinetics

- Substrate for CYP450 2D6
- Half-life of parent drug approximately 8 hours

✻ 7- and 8-hydroxymetabolites are active and possess serotonin 2A and dopamine 2 antagonist properties, similar to atypical antipsychotics

✻ Amoxapine is the *N*-desmethyl metabolite of the conventional antipsychotic loxapine

- Half-life of the active metabolites approximately 24 hours

Drug Interactions

- Tramadol increases the risk of seizures in patients taking TCAs
- Use of TCAs/tetracyclics with anticholinergic drugs may result in paralytic ileus or hyperthermia
- Fluoxetine, paroxetine, bupropion, duloxetine, and other CYP450 2D6 inhibitors may increase TCA/tetracyclic concentrations
- Cimetidine may increase plasma concentrations of TCAs/tetracyclics and cause anticholinergic symptoms
- Phenothiazines or haloperidol may raise TCA/tetracyclic blood concentrations
- May alter effects of antihypertensive drugs; may inhibit hypotensive effects of clonidine
- Use of TCAs/tetracyclics with sympathomimetic agents may increase sympathetic activity
- Methylphenidate may inhibit metabolism of TCAs/tetracyclics
- Activation and agitation, especially following switching or adding antidepressants, may represent the induction of a bipolar state, especially a mixed dysphoric bipolar II condition sometimes associated with suicidal

ideation, and require the addition of lithium, a mood stabilizer or an atypical antipsychotic, and/or discontinuation of amoxapine

Other Warnings/ Precautions

- Add or initiate other antidepressants with caution for up to 2 weeks after discontinuing amoxapine
- Generally, do not use with MAOIs, including 14 days after MAOIs are stopped; do not start an MAOI for at least 5 half-lives (5 to 7 days for most drugs) after discontinuing amoxapine, but see Pearls
- Use with caution in patients with history of seizure, urinary retention, angle-closure glaucoma, hyperthyroidism
- TCAs/tetracyclics can increase QTc interval, especially at toxic doses, which can be attained not only by overdose but also by combining with drugs that inhibit its metabolism via CYP450 2D6, potentially causing torsade de pointes-type arrhythmia or sudden death
- Because TCAs/tetracyclics can prolong QTc interval, use with caution in patients who have bradycardia or who are taking drugs that can induce bradycardia (e.g., beta blockers, calcium channel blockers, clonidine, digitalis)
- Because TCAs/tetracyclics can prolong QTc interval, use with caution in patients who have hypokalemia and/ or hypomagnesemia, or who are taking drugs that can induce hypokalemia and/ or magnesemia (e.g., diuretics, stimulant laxatives, intravenous amphotericin B, glucocorticoids, tetracosactide)
- When treating children, carefully weigh the risks and benefits of pharmacological treatment against the risks and benefits of nontreatment with antidepressants and make sure to document this in the patient's chart
- Distribute the brochures provided by the FDA and the drug companies
- Warn patients and their caregivers about the possibility of activating side effects and advise them to report such symptoms immediately
- Monitor patients for activation of suicidal ideation, especially children and adolescents

Do Not Use

- If patient is recovering from myocardial infarction
- If patient is taking agents capable of significantly prolonging QTc interval (e.g., pimozide, thioridazine, selected antiarrhythmics, moxifloxacin, sparfloxacin)
- If there is a history of QTc prolongation or cardiac arrhythmia, recent acute myocardial infarction, uncompensated heart failure
- If patient is taking drugs that inhibit TCA/ tetracyclic metabolism, including CYP450 2D6 inhibitors, except by an expert
- If there is reduced CYP450 2D6 function, such as patients who are poor 2D6 metabolizers, except by an expert and at low doses
- If there is a proven allergy to amoxapine or loxapine

SPECIAL POPULATIONS

Renal Impairment

- Use with caution – may require lower than usual adult dose

Hepatic Impairment

- Use with caution – may require lower than usual adult dose

Cardiac Impairment

- Baseline ECG is recommended
- TCAs/tetracyclics have been reported to cause arrhythmias, prolongation of conduction time, orthostatic hypotension, sinus tachycardia, and heart failure, especially in the diseased heart
- Myocardial infarction and stroke have been reported with TCAs/tetracyclics
- TCAs/tetracyclics produce QTc prolongation, which may be enhanced by the existence of bradycardia, hypokalemia, congenital or acquired long QTc interval, which should be evaluated prior to administering amoxapine
- Use with caution if treating concomitantly with a medication likely to produce prolonged bradycardia, hypokalemia, slowing of intracardiac conduction, or prolongation of the QTc interval
- Avoid TCAs/tetracyclics in patients with a known history of QTc prolongation, recent acute myocardial infarction, and uncompensated heart failure

- TCAs/tetracyclics may cause a sustained increase in heart rate in patients with ischemic heart disease and may worsen (decrease) heart rate variability, an independent risk of mortality in cardiac populations
- Since SSRIs may improve (increase) heart rate variability in patients following a myocardial infarct and may improve survival as well as mood in patients with acute angina or following a myocardial infarction, these are more appropriate agents for cardiac population than tricyclic/tetracyclic antidepressants

✻ Risk/benefit ratio may not justify use of TCAs/tetracyclics in cardiac impairment

Elderly

- Baseline ECG is recommended for patients over age 50
- May be more sensitive to anticholinergic, cardiovascular, hypotensive, and sedative effects
- Initial dose 25 mg/day at bedtime; increase by 25 mg/day each week; maximum dose 300 mg/day

Children and Adolescents

- Carefully weigh the risks and benefits of pharmacological treatment against the risks and benefits of nontreatment with antidepressants and make sure to document this in the patient's chart
- Use with caution, observing for activation of known or unknown bipolar disorder and/or suicidal ideation, and inform parents or guardians of this risk so they can help observe child or adolescent patients
- Monitor patients face-to-face regularly, particularly during the first several weeks of treatment
- Not generally recommended for use under age 16
- Several studies show lack of efficacy of TCAs/tetracyclics for depression
- May be used to treat enuresis or hyperactive/impulsive behaviors
- Some cases of sudden death have occurred in children taking TCAs/tetracyclics
- Adolescents: initial 25–50 mg/day; increase gradually to 100 mg/day in divided doses or single dose at bedtime

Pregnancy

- Controlled studies have not been conducted in pregnant women
- Some animal studies show adverse effects
- Amoxapine crosses the placenta
- Adverse effects have been reported in infants whose mothers took a TCA (lethargy, withdrawal symptoms, fetal malformations)
- Evaluate for treatment with an antidepressant with a better risk/benefit ratio

Breast Feeding

- Some drug is found in mother's breast milk

✻ Recommended either to discontinue drug or bottle feed

- Immediate postpartum period is a high-risk time for depression, especially in women who have had prior depressive episodes, so drug may need to be reinstituted late in the third trimester or shortly after childbirth to prevent a recurrence during the postpartum period
- Evaluate for treatment with an antidepressant with a better risk/benefit ratio

THE ART OF PSYCHOPHARMACOLOGY

Potential Advantages

- Severe or treatment-resistant depression
- Treatment-resistant psychotic depression

Potential Disadvantages

- Pediatric and geriatric patients
- Patients concerned with weight gain
- Cardiac patients
- Patients with Parkinson's disease or tardive dyskinesia

Primary Target Symptoms

- Depressed mood

Pearls

- Tricyclic/tetracyclic antidepressants are no longer generally considered a first-line treatment option for depression because of their side effect profile
- Tricyclic/tetracyclic antidepressants continue to be useful for severe or treatment-resistant depression

✻ Because of potential extrapyramidal symptoms, akathisia, and theoretical risk of tardive dyskinesia, first consider other TCAs/tetracyclics for long-term use in general and for treatment of chronic patients
- TCAs may aggravate psychotic symptoms
- Alcohol should be avoided because of additive CNS effects
- Underweight patients may be more susceptible to adverse cardiovascular effects
- Children, patients with inadequate hydration, and patients with cardiac disease may be more susceptible to TCA-induced cardiotoxicity than healthy adults
- For the expert only: although generally prohibited, a heroic but potentially dangerous treatment for severely treatment-resistant patients is to give a tricyclic/tetracyclic antidepressant other than clomipramine simultaneously with an MAOIs for patients who fail to respond to numerous other antidepressants
- Use of MAOIs with clomipramine is always prohibited because of the risk of serotonin syndrome and death
- Amoxapine may be the preferred trycyclic/tetracyclic antidepressant to combine with an MAOI in heroic cases due to its theoretically protective 5HT2A antagonist properties
- If this option is elected, start the MAOI with the tricyclic/tetracyclic antidepressant simultaneously at low doses after appropriate drug washout, then alternately increase doses of these agents every few days to a week as tolerated
- Although very strict dietary and concomitant drug restrictions must be observed to prevent hypertensive crises and serotonin syndrome, the most common side effects of MAOI/tricyclic or tetracyclic combinations may be weight gain and orthostatic hypotension
- Patients on TCAs/tetracyclics should be aware that they may experience symptoms such as photosensitivity or blue-green urine
- SSRIs may be more effective than TCAs/tetracyclics in women, and TCAs/tetracyclics may be more effective than SSRIs in men

✻ May cause some motor effects, possibly due to effects on dopamine receptors

✻ Amoxapine may have a faster onset of action than some other antidepressants

✻ May be pharmacologically similar to an atypical antipsychotic in some patients

✻ At high doses, patients who form high concentrations of active metabolites may have akathisia, extrapyramidal symptoms, and possibly develop tardive dyskinesia

✻ Structurally and pharmacologically related to the antipsychotic loxapine
- Since tricyclic/tetracyclic antidepressants are substrates for CYP450 2D6, and 7% of the population (especially Caucasians) may have a genetic variant leading to reduced activity of 2D6, such patients may not safely tolerate normal doses of tricyclic/tetracyclic antidepressants and may require dose reduction
- Phenotypic testing may be necessary to detect this genetic variant prior to dosing with a tricyclic/tetracyclic antidepressant, especially in vulnerable populations such as children, elderly, cardiac populations, and those on concomitant medications
- Patients who seem to have extraordinarily severe side effects at normal or low doses may have this phenotypic CYP450 2D6 variant and require low doses or switching to another antidepressant not metabolized by 2D6

Suggested Reading

Anderson IM. Meta-analytical studies on new antidepressants. Br Med Bull 2001; 57:161–78.

Anderson IM. Selective serotonin reuptake inhibitors versus tricyclic antidepressants: a meta-analysis of efficacy and tolerability. J Aff Disorders 2000;58:19–36.

Hayes PE, Kristoff CA. Adverse reactions to five new antidepressants. Clin Pharm 1986; 5:471–80.

Jue SG, Dawson GW, Brogden RN. Amoxapine: a review of its pharmacology and efficacy in depressed states. Drugs 1982;24:1–23.

THERAPEUTICS

Brands
- Dexedrine
- Dexedrine Spansules
- Zenzedi
- ProCentra

see index for additional brand names

Generic? Yes

Class
- Neuroscience-based Nomenclature: dopamine, norepinephrine reuptake inhibitor and releaser (DN-RIRe)
- Stimulant

Commonly Prescribed for
(bold for FDA approved)
- **Attention deficit hyperactivity disorder (ADHD) (ages 6 and older or 3 and older depending on formulation)**
- **Narcolepsy (ages 12 and older or 6 and older depending on formulation)**
- Treatment-resistant depression

How the Drug Works
* Increases norepinephrine and especially dopamine actions by blocking their reuptake and facilitating their release
- Enhancement of dopamine and norepinephrine actions in certain brain regions may improve attention, concentration, executive function, and wakefulness (e.g., dorsolateral prefrontal cortex)
- Enhancement of dopamine actions in other brain regions (e.g., basal ganglia) may improve hyperactivity
- Enhancement of dopamine and norepinephrine in yet other brain regions (e.g., medial prefrontal cortex, hypothalamus) may improve depression, fatigue, and sleepiness

How Long Until It Works
- Some immediate effects can be seen with first dosing
- Can take several weeks to attain maximum therapeutic benefit

If It Works (for ADHD)
- The goal of treatment of ADHD is reduction of symptoms of inattentiveness, motor hyperactivity, and/or impulsiveness that disrupt social, school, and/or occupational functioning
- Continue treatment until all symptoms are under control or improvement is stable and then continue treatment indefinitely as long as improvement persists
- Reevaluate the need for treatment periodically
- Treatment for ADHD begun in childhood may need to be continued into adolescence and adulthood if continued benefit is documented

If It Doesn't Work (for ADHD)
- Consider adjusting dose or switching to another formulation of d-amphetamine or to another agent
- Consider behavioral therapy
- Consider the presence of noncompliance and counsel patient and parents
- Consider evaluation for another diagnosis or for a comorbid condition (e.g., bipolar disorder, substance abuse, medical illness, etc.)

* Some ADHD patients and some depressed patients may experience lack of consistent efficacy due to activation of latent or underlying bipolar disorder, and require either augmenting with a mood stabilizer or switching to a mood stabilizer

Best Augmenting Combos for Partial Response or Treatment Resistance
* Best to attempt other monotherapies prior to augmenting
- For the expert, can combine immediate-release formulation with a sustained-release formulation of d-amphetamine for ADHD
- For the expert, can combine with modafinil or atomoxetine for ADHD
- For the expert, can occasionally combine with atypical antipsychotics in highly treatment-resistant cases of bipolar disorder or ADHD
- For the expert, can combine with antidepressants to boost antidepressant efficacy in highly treatment-resistant cases of depression while carefully monitoring patient

Tests
- Before treatment, assess for presence of cardiac disease (history, family history, physical exam)
- Blood pressure should be monitored regularly
- In children, monitor weight and height

SIDE EFFECTS

How Drug Causes Side Effects
- Increases in norepinephrine peripherally can cause autonomic side effects, including tremor, tachycardia, hypertension, and cardiac arrhythmias
- Increases in norepinephrine and dopamine centrally can cause CNS side effects such as insomnia, agitation, psychosis, and substance abuse

Notable Side Effects
✻ Insomnia, headache, exacerbation of tics, nervousness, irritability, overstimulation, tremor, dizziness
- Anorexia, nausea, dry mouth, constipation, diarrhea, weight loss
- Can temporarily slow normal growth in children (controversial)
- Sexual dysfunction long-term (impotence, libido changes) but can also improve sexual dysfunction short-term

Life-Threatening or Dangerous Side Effects
- Psychotic episodes, especially with parenteral abuse
- Seizures
- Palpitations, tachycardia, hypertension
- Rare activation of hypomania, mania, or suicidal ideation (controversial)
- Cardiovascular adverse effects, sudden death in patients with preexisting cardiac structural abnormalities

Weight Gain
unusual | not unusual | common | problematic
- Reported but not expected
- Some patients may experience weight loss

Sedation
unusual | not unusual | common | problematic
- Reported but not expected
- Activation much more common than sedation

What to Do About Side Effects
- Wait
- Adjust dose
- Switch to a long-acting stimulant
- Switch to another agent
- For insomnia, avoid dosing in afternoon/evening

Best Augmenting Agents for Side Effects
- Beta blockers for peripheral autonomic side effects
- Dose reduction or switching to another agent may be more effective since most side effects cannot be improved with an augmenting agent

DOSING AND USE

Usual Dosage Range
- Narcolepsy: 5–60 mg/day (divided doses for tablet, once daily morning dose for Spansule capsule)
- ADHD: 5–40 mg/day (divided doses for tablet, once daily morning dose for Spansule capsule)

Dosage Forms
- Immediate-release tablet 2.5 mg, 5 mg, 7.5 mg, 10 mg, 15 mg, 20 mg, 30 mg
- Extended-release capsule 5 mg, 10 mg, 15 mg
- Immediate-release oral solution 5 mg/5 mL

How to Dose
- Narcolepsy, ages 12 and older (Spansule capsule or tablet): initial 10 mg/day; can increase by 10 mg each week; give first dose on waking; tablet is administered in divided doses
- Narcolepsy, ages 6 to 12 (tablet IR): initial 5 mg/day; can increase by 5 mg each week; administered in divided doses
- ADHD, ages 6 and older (Spansule capsule or tablet): initial 5 mg/day; can increase by 5 mg each week; give first dose on waking
- ADHD, ages 3 to 5 (tablet IR): Initial 2.5 mg/day; can increase by 2.5 mg each week; administered in divided doses

Dosing Tips
- Clinical duration of action often differs from pharmacokinetic half-life

✻ Immediate-release dextroamphetamine has 3–6 hour duration of clinical action

✻ Sustained-release dextroamphetamine (Dexedrine Spansule) has up to 8-hour duration of clinical action

- Tablets contain tartrazine, which may cause allergic reactions, particularly in patients allergic to aspirin
- Dexedrine Spansules are controlled-release and should therefore not be chewed but rather should only be swallowed whole

✽ Controlled-release delivery of dextroamphetamine may be sufficiently long in duration to allow elimination of lunchtime dosing in many but not all patients

✽ This innovation can be an important practical element in stimulant utilization, eliminating the hassle and pragmatic difficulties of lunchtime dosing at school, including storage problems, potential diversion, and the need for a medical professional to supervise dosing away from home

- Avoid dosing late in the day because of the risk of insomnia

✽ May be possible to dose only during the school week for some ADHD patients

- Off-label uses are dosed the same as for ADHD

✽ May be able to give drug holidays over the summer in order to reassess therapeutic utility and effects on growth and to allow catch-up from any growth suppression as well as to assess any other side effects and the need to reinstitute stimulant treatment for the next school term

- Side effects are generally dose-related
- Taking with food may delay peak actions for 2–3 hours

Overdose

- Rarely fatal; panic, hyperreflexia, rhabdomyolysis, rapid respiration, confusion, coma, hallucination, convulsion, arrhythmia, change in blood pressure, circulatory collapse

Long-Term Use

- Often used long-term for ADHD when ongoing monitoring documents continued efficacy
- Dependence and/or abuse may develop
- Tolerance to therapeutic effects may develop in some patients
- Long-term stimulant use may be associated with growth suppression in children (controversial)
- Periodic monitoring of weight, blood pressure, CBC, platelet counts, and liver function may be prudent

Habit Forming

- High abuse potential, Schedule II drug
- Patients may develop tolerance, psychological dependence

How to Stop

- Taper to avoid withdrawal effects
- Withdrawal following chronic therapeutic use may unmask symptoms of the underlying disorder and may require follow-up and reinstitution of treatment
- Careful supervision is required during withdrawal from abusive use since severe depression may occur

Pharmacokinetics

- Half-life approximately 10–12 hours

Drug Interactions

- May affect blood pressure and should be used cautiously with agents used to control blood pressure
- Gastrointestinal acidifying agents (guanethidine, reserpine, glutamic acid, ascorbic acid, fruit juices, etc.) and urinary acidifying agents (ammonium chloride, sodium phosphate, etc.) lower amphetamine plasma levels, so such agents can be useful to administer after an overdose but may also lower therapeutic efficacy of amphetamines
- Gastrointestinal alkalinizing agents (sodium bicarbonate, etc.) and urinary alkalinizing agents (acetazolamide, some thiazides) increase amphetamine plasma levels and potentiate amphetamine's actions
- Desipramine and protryptiline can cause striking and sustained increases in brain concentrations of d-amphetamine and may also add to d-amphetamine's cardiovascular effects
- Theoretically, other agents with norepinephrine reuptake blocking properties, such as venlafaxine, duloxetine, atomoxetine, milnacipran, and reboxetine, could also add to amphetamine's CNS and cardiovascular effects
- Amphetamines may counteract the sedative effects of antihistamines
- Haloperidol, chlorpromazine, and lithium may inhibit stimulatory effects of amphetamines
- Theoretically, atypical antipsychotics should also inhibit stimulatory effects of amphetamines

- Theoretically, amphetamines could inhibit the antipsychotic actions of antipsychotics
- Theoretically, amphetamines could inhibit the mood-stabilizing actions of atypical antipsychotics in some patients
- Combinations of amphetamines with mood stabilizers (lithium, anticonvulsants, atypical antipsychotics) is generally something for experts only, when monitoring patients closely and when other options fail
- Absorption of phenobarbital, phenytoin, and ethosuximide is delayed by amphetamines
- Amphetamines inhibit adrenergic blockers and enhance adrenergic effects of norepinephrine
- Amphetamines may antagonize hypotensive effects of veratrum alkaloids and other antihypertensives
- Amphetamines increase the analgesic effects of meperidine
- Amphetamines contribute to excessive CNS stimulation if used with large doses of propoxyphene
- Amphetamines can raise plasma corticosteroid levels
- MAOIs slow absorption of amphetamines and thus potentiate their actions, which can cause headache, hypertension, and rarely hypertensive crisis and malignant hyperthermia, sometimes with fatal results
- Use with MAOIs, including within 14 days of MAOI use, is not advised, but this can sometimes be considered by experts who monitor depressed patients closely when other treatment options for depression fail

Other Warnings/ Precautions

- Use with caution in patients with any degree of hypertension, hyperthyroidism, or history of drug abuse
- Children who are not growing or gaining weight should stop treatment, at least temporarily
- May worsen motor and phonic tics
- May worsen symptoms of thought disorder and behavioral disturbance in psychotic patients
- Stimulants have a high potential for abuse and must be used with caution in anyone with a current or past history of substance abuse or alcoholism or in emotionally unstable patients
- Administration of stimulants for prolonged periods of time should be avoided whenever possible or done only with close monitoring, as it may lead to marked tolerance and drug dependence, including psychological dependence with varying degrees of abnormal behavior
- Particular attention should be paid to the possibility of subjects obtaining stimulants for nontherapeutic use or distribution to others and the drugs should in general be prescribed sparingly with documentation of appropriate use
- Usual dosing has been associated with sudden death in children with structural cardiac abnormalities
- Not an appropriate first-line treatment for depression or for normal fatigue
- May lower the seizure threshold
- Emergence or worsening of activation and agitation may represent the induction of a bipolar state, especially a mixed dysphoric bipolar II condition sometimes associated with suicidal ideation, and require the addition of a mood stabilizer and/or discontinuation of d-amphetamine

Do Not Use

- If patient has extreme anxiety or agitation
- If patient has motor tics or Tourette's sydrome or if there is a family history of Tourette's, unless administered by an expert in cases when the potential benefits for ADHD outweigh the risks of worsening tics
- Should generally not be administered with an MAOI, including within 14 days of MAOI use, except in heroic circumstances and by an expert
- If patient has arteriosclerosis, cardiovascular disease, or severe hypertension
- If patient has glaucoma
- If patient has structural cardiac abnormalities
- If there is a proven allergy to any sympathomimetic agent

SPECIAL POPULATIONS

Renal Impairment

- No dose adjustment necessary

Hepatic Impairment

- Use with caution

Cardiac Impairment
- Use with caution, particularly in patients with recent myocardial infarction or other conditions that could be negatively affected by increased blood pressure
- Do not use in patients with structural cardiac abnormalities

Elderly
- Some patients may tolerate lower doses better

Children and Adolescents
- Safety and efficacy not established in children under age 3
- Use in young children should be reserved for the expert
- d-amphetamine may worsen symptoms of behavioral disturbance and thought disorder in psychotic children
- d-amphetamine has acute effects on growth hormone; long-term effects are unknown but weight and height should be monitored during long-term treatment
- Narcolepsy: ages 6–12: initial 5 mg/day; increase by 5 mg each week
- ADHD: ages 3–5: initial 2.5 mg/day; increase by 2.5 mg each week
- Sudden death in children and adolescents with serious heart problems has been reported
- American Heart Association recommends EKG prior to initiating stimulant treatment in children, although not all experts agree

Pregnancy
- Effective June 30, 2015, the US FDA requires changes to the content and format of pregnancy and lactation information in prescription drug labels, including the elimination of the pregnancy letter categories; the Pregnancy and Lactation Labeling Rule (PLLR or final rule) applies only to prescription drugs and will be phased in gradually for drugs approved on or after June 30, 2001
- Controlled studies have not been conducted in pregnant women
- There is a greater risk of premature birth and low birth weight in infants whose mothers take d-amphetamine during pregnancy
- Infants whose mothers take d-amphetamine during pregnancy may experience withdrawal symptoms
- In animal studies, d-amphetamine caused delayed skeletal ossification and decreased postweaning weight gain in rats; no major malformations occurred in rat or rabbit studies
- Use in women of childbearing potential requires weighing potential benefits to the mother against potential risks to the fetus

✽ For ADHD patients, d-amphetamine should generally be discontinued before anticipated pregnancies

Breast Feeding
- Some drug is found in mother's breast milk

✽ Recommended either to discontinue drug or bottle feed

- If infant shows signs of irritability, drug may need to be discontinued

THE ART OF PSYCHOPHARMACOLOGY

Potential Advantages
- May work in ADHD patients unresponsive to other stimulants
- Established long-term efficacy of immediate-release and Spansule formulations

Potential Disadvantages
- Patients with current or past substance abuse
- Patients with current or past bipolar disorder or psychosis

Primary Target Symptoms
- Concentration, attention span
- Motor hyperactivity
- Impulsiveness
- Physical and mental fatigue
- Daytime sleepiness
- Depression

Pearls
✽ May be useful for treatment of depressive symptoms in medically ill elderly patients

✽ May be useful for treatment of post-stroke depression

✽ A classical augmentation strategy for treatment-refractory depression

* Specifically, may be useful for treatment of cognitive dysfunction and fatigue as residual symptoms of major depressive disorder unresponsive to multiple prior treatments
* May also be useful for the treatment of cognitive impairment, depressive symptoms, and severe fatigue in patients with HIV infection and in cancer patients
- Can be used to potentiate opioid analgesia and reduce sedation, particularly in end-of-life management
- Some patients respond to or tolerate d-amphetamin better than methylphenidate and vice versa
- Some patients may benefit from an occasional addition of 5–10 mg of immediate-release d-amphetamine to their daily base of sustained-release Dexedrine Spansules
* Despite warnings, can be a useful adjunct to MAOIs for heroic treatment of highly refractory mood disorders when monitored with vigilance
* Can reverse sexual dysfunction caused by psychiatric illness and by some drugs such as SSRIs, including decreased libido, erectile dysfunction, delayed ejaculation, and anorgasmia
- Atypical antipsychotics may be useful in treating stimulant or psychotic consequences of overdose
- Taking with food may delay peak actions for 2–3 hours
- Half-life and duration of clinical action tend to be shorter in younger children
- Drug abuse may actually be lower in ADHD adolescents treated with stimulants than in ADHD adolescents who are not treated

Suggested Reading

Fry JM. Treatment modalities for narcolepsy. Neurology 1998;50(2 Suppl 1):S43–8.

Greenhill LL, Pliszka S, Dulcan MK, et al. Practice parameter for the use of stimulant medications in the treatment of children, adolescents, and adults. J Am Acad Child Adolesc Psychiatry 2002;41 (2):S26–49.

Jadad AR, Boyle M, Cunningham C, Kim M, Schachar R. Treatment of attention-deficit/hyperactivity disorder. Evid Rep Technol Assess (Summ) 1999;(11):i–viii, 1–341.

Stiefel G, Besag FM. Cardiovascular effects of methylphenidate, amphetamines, and atomoxetine in the treatment of attention-deficit hyperactivity disorder. Drug Saf 2010;33(10):821–42.

Vinson DC. Therapy for attention-deficit hyperactivity disorder. Arch Fam Med 1994;3:445–51.

Wender PH, Wolf LE, Wasserstein J. Adults with ADHD. An overview. Ann N Y Acad Sci 2001;931:1–16.

AMPHETAMINE (D,L)

THERAPEUTICS

Brands
- Adderall
- Adderall XR
- Evekeo
- Adzenys-XR-ODT
- Dyanavel XR

see index for additional brand names

Generic? Yes

Class
- Neuroscience-based Nomenclature: dopamine, norepinephrine reuptake inhibitor and releaser (DN-RIRe)
- Stimulant

Commonly Prescribed for
(bold for FDA approved)
- **Attention deficit hyperactivity disorder (ADHD) in children ages 3–12 (Adderall, Evekeo)**
- **Attention deficit hyperactivity disorder (ADHD) in children ages 6–17 (Adderall XR, Evekeo, Dyanavel XR, Adzenys XR-ODT) and in adults (Adderall XR, Evekeo, Adzenys XR-ODT)**
- **Narcolepsy (Adderall, Evekeo)**
- **Exogenous obesity (Evekeo)**
- Treatment-resistant depression

How the Drug Works
* Increases norepinephrine and especially dopamine actions by blocking their reuptake and facilitating their release
- Enhancement of dopamine and norepinephrine actions in certain brain regions (e.g., dorsolateral prefrontal cortex) may improve attention, concentration, executive function, and wakefulness
- Enhancement of dopamine actions in other brain regions (e.g., basal ganglia) may improve hyperactivity
- Enhancement of dopamine and norepinephrine in yet other brain regions (e.g., medial prefrontal cortex, hypothalamus) may improve depression, fatigue, and sleepiness

How Long Until It Works
- Some immediate effects can be seen with first dosing
- Can take several weeks to attain maximum therapeutic benefit

If It Works (for ADHD)
- The goal of treatment of ADHD is reduction of symptoms of inattentiveness, motor hyperactivity, and/or impulsiveness that disrupt social, school, and/or occupational functioning
- Continue treatment until all symptoms are under control or improvement is stable and then continue treatment indefinitely as long as improvement persists
- Reevaluate the need for treatment periodically
- Treatment for ADHD begun in childhood may need to be continued into adolescence and adulthood if continued benefit is documented

If It Doesn't Work (for ADHD)
- Consider adjusting dose or switching to another formulation of d,l-amphetamine or to another agent
- Consider behavioral therapy
- Consider the presence of noncompliance and counsel patient and parents
- Consider evaluation for another diagnosis or for a comorbid condition (e.g., bipolar disorder, substance abuse, medical illness, etc.)

* Some ADHD patients and some depressed patients may experience lack of consistent efficacy due to activation of latent or underlying bipolar disorder, and require either augmenting with a mood stabilizer or switching to a mood stabilizer

Best Augmenting Combos for Partial Response or Treatment Resistance
- Best to attempt other monotherapies prior to augmenting
- For the expert, can combine immediate-release formulation with a sustained-release formulation of d,l-amphetamine for ADHD
- For the expert, can combine with modafinil or atomoxetine for ADHD
- For the expert, can occasionally combine with atypical antipsychotics in highly treatment-resistant cases of bipolar disorder or ADHD
- For the expert, can combine with antidepressants to boost antidepressant efficacy in highly treatment-resistant cases of depression while carefully monitoring patient

Tests
- Before treatment, assess for presence of cardiac disease (history, family history, physical exam)
- Blood pressure should be monitored regularly
- In children, monitor weight and height

SIDE EFFECTS

How Drug Causes Side Effects
- Increases in norepinephrine peripherally can cause autonomic side effects, including tremor, tachycardia, hypertension, and cardiac arrhythmias
- Increases in norepinephrine and dopamine centrally can cause CNS side effects such as insomnia, agitation, psychosis, and substance abuse

Notable Side Effects
- ✻ Insomnia, headache, exacerbation of tics, nervousness, irritability, overstimulation, tremor, dizziness
- Anorexia, nausea, dry mouth, constipation, diarrhea, weight loss
- Can temporarily slow normal growth in children (controversial)
- Sexual dysfunction long-term (impotence, libido changes) but can also improve sexual dysfunction short-term

Life-Threatening or Dangerous Side Effects
- Psychotic episodes, especially with parenteral abuse
- Seizures
- Palpitations, tachycardia, hypertension
- Rare activation of hypomania, mania, or suicidal ideation (controversial)
- Cardiovascular adverse effects, sudden death in patients with preexisting cardiac structural abnormalities

Weight Gain
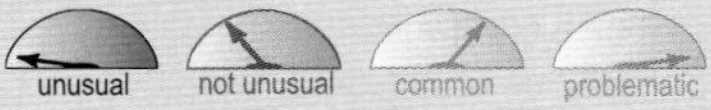

- Reported but not expected
- Some patients may experience weight loss

Sedation
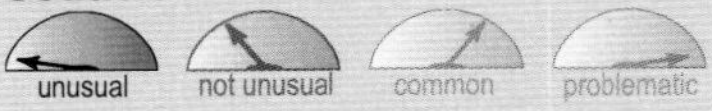

- Reported but not expected
- Activation much more common than sedation

What to Do About Side Effects
- Wait
- Adjust dose
- Switch to a long-acting stimulant
- Switch to another agent
- For insomnia, avoid dosing in afternoon/evening

Best Augmenting Agents for Side Effects
- Beta blockers for peripheral autonomic side effects
- Dose reduction or switching to another agent may be more effective since most side effects cannot be improved with an augmenting agent

DOSING AND USE

Usual Dosage Range
- Narcolepsy: 5–60 mg/day in divided doses
- ADHD: 5–40 mg/day (divided doses for immediate-release tablet, once daily morning dose for extended-release tablet)
- Exogenous obesity: 30 mg/day in divided doses

Dosage Forms
- Immediate-release Adderall tablet 5 mg double-scored, 7.5 mg double-scored, 10 mg double-scored, 12.5 mg double-scored, 15 mg double-scored, 20 mg double-scored, 30 mg double-scored
- Immediate-release Evekeo tablet 5 mg scored, 10 mg double-scored
- Extended-release orally disintegrating tablet (Adzenys XR-ODT) 3.1 mg, 6.3 mg, 9.4 mg, 12.5 mg, 15.7 mg, 18.8 mg
- Extended-release tablet (Adderal XR) 5 mg, 10 mg, 15 mg, 20 mg, 25 mg, 30 mg
- Extended-release oral suspension (Dynavel XR) 2.5 mg/mL

How to Dose

- Immediate-release Adderall or Evekeo in ADHD (ages 6 and older): initial 5 mg once or twice per day; can increase by 5 mg each week; maximum dose generally 40 mg/day; split daily dose with first dose on waking and every 4–6 hours thereafter
- Immediate-release Evekeo in ADHD (ages 3 to 5): initial 2.5 mg/day; can increase by 2.5 mg each week; administered in divided doses
- Immediate-release Adderall or Evekeo in narcolepsy (ages 12 and older): initial 10 mg/day; can increase by 10 mg each week; split daily dose with first dose on waking and every 4–6 hours thereafter
- Immediate-release Evekeo in narcolepsy (ages 6 to 12): initial 5 mg/day; can increase by 5 mg each week; administered in divided doses
- Extended-release tablet in ADHD: initial 10 mg/day in the morning; can increase by 5–10 mg/day at weekly intervals; maximum dose generally 30 mg/day
- Immediate-release Evekeo in exogenous obesity (ages 12 and older): usual daily dose 30 mg; taken in divided doses of 5–10 mg, 30–60 minutes before meals

Dosing Tips

- Clinical duration of action often differs from pharmacokinetic half-life

✻ Immediate-release d,l-amphetamine has 3–6 hour duration of clinical action

✻ Extended-release d,l-amphetamine has up to 8-hour duration of clinical action

- Adderall XR is controlled-release and should therefore not be chewed but rather should only be swallowed whole
- Extended-release oral suspension (Dyanavel XR) and extended-release orally disintegraint tablet (Adzenys XR-ODT) should not be substituted for other amphetamine products on a mg-per-mg basis due to differing amphetamine base compositions and pharmacokinetic profiles

✻ Controlled-release delivery of d,l-amphetamine is sufficiently long in duration to allow elimination of lunchtime dosing

✻ This innovation can be an important practical element in stimulant utilization, eliminating the hassle and pragmatic difficulties of lunchtime dosing at school, including storage problems, potential diversion, and the need for a medical professional to supervise dosing away from home

- Avoid dosing late in the day because of the risk of insomnia
- May be possible to dose only during the school week for some ADHD patients
- Off-label uses are dosed the same as for ADHD

✻ May be able to give drug holidays over the summer in order to reassess therapeutic utility and effects on growth and to allow catch-up from any growth suppression as well as to assess any other side effects and the need to reinstitute stimulant treatment for the next school term

- Side effects are generally dose-related
- Taking with food may delay peak actions for 2–3 hours

Overdose

- Rarely fatal; panic, hyperreflexia, rhabdomyolysis, rapid respiration, confusion, coma, hallucinations, convulsions, arrhythmia, change in blood pressure, circulatory collapse

Long-Term Use

- Often used long-term for ADHD when ongoing monitoring documents continued efficacy
- Dependence and/or abuse may develop
- Tolerance to therapeutic effects may develop in some patients
- Long-term stimulant use may be associated with growth suppression in children (controversial)
- Periodic monitoring of weight, blood pressure, CBC, platelet counts, and liver function may be prudent

Habit Forming

- High abuse potential, Schedule II drug
- Patients may develop tolerance, psychological dependence

How to Stop

- Taper to avoid withdrawal effects
- Withdrawal following chronic therapeutic use may unmask symptoms of the underlying disorder and may require follow-up and reinstitution of treatment

- Careful supervision is required during withdrawal from abusive use since severe depression may occur

Pharmacokinetics

- Adderall and Adderall XR are a mixture of d-amphetamine and l-amphetamine salts in the ratio of 3:1
- A single dose of Adderall XR 20 mg gives drug levels of both d-amphetamine and l-amphetamine comparable to Adderall immediate-release 20 mg administered in 2 divided doses 4 hours apart
- In adults, half-life for d-amphetamine is 10 hours and for l-amphetamine is 13 hours
- For children ages 6–12, half-life for d-amphetamine is 9 hours and for l-amphetamine is 11 hours

Drug Interactions

- May affect blood pressure and should be used cautiously with agents used to control blood pressure
- Gastrointestinal acidifying agents (guanethidine, reserpine, glutamic acid, ascorbic acid, fruit juices, etc.) and urinary acidifying agents (ammonium chloride, sodium phosphate, etc.) lower amphetamine plasma levels, so such agents can be useful to administer after an overdose but may also lower therapeutic efficacy of amphetamines
- Gastrointestinal alkalinizing agents (sodium bicarbonate, etc.) and urinary alkalinizing agents (acetazolamide, some thiazides) increase amphetamine plasma levels and potentiate amphetamine's actions
- Desipramine and protryptiline can cause striking and sustained increases in brain concentrations of amphetamine and may also add to amphetamine's cardiovascular effects
- Theoretically, other agents with norepinephrine reuptake blocking properties, such as venlafaxine, duloxetine, atomoxetine, milnacipran, and reboxetine, could also add to amphetamine's CNS and cardiovascular effects
- Amphetamines may counteract the sedative effects of antihistamines
- Haloperidol, chlorpromazine, and lithium may inhibit stimulatory effects of amphetamines
- Theoretically, atypical antipsychotics should also inhibit stimulatory effects of amphetamines
- Theoretically, amphetamines could inhibit the antipsychotic actions of antipsychotics
- Theoretically, amphetamines could inhibit the mood-stabilizing actions of atypical antipsychotics in some patients
- Combinations of amphetamines with mood stabilizers (lithium, anticonvulsants, atypical antipsychotics) is generally something for experts only, when monitoring patients closely and when other options fail
- Absorption of phenobarbital, phenytoin, and ethosuximide is delayed by amphetamines
- Amphetamines inhibit adrenergic blockers and enhance adrenergic effects of norepinephrine
- Amphetamines may antagonize hypotensive effects of veratrum alkaloids and other antihypertensives
- Amphetamines increase the analgesic effects of meperidine
- Amphetamines contribute to excessive CNS stimulation if used with large doses of propoxyphene
- Amphetamines can raise plasma corticosteroid levels
- MAOIs slow absorption of amphetamines and thus potentiate their actions, which can cause headache, hypertension, and rarely hypertensive crisis and malignant hyperthermia, sometimes with fatal results
- Use with MAOIs, including within 14 days of MAOI use, is not advised, but this can sometimes be considered by experts who monitor depressed patients closely when other treatment options for depression fail

Other Warnings/ Precautions

- Use with caution in patients with any degree of hypertension, hyperthyroidism, or history of drug abuse
- Children who are not growing or gaining weight should stop treatment, at least temporarily
- May worsen motor and phonic tics

- May worsen symptoms of thought disorder and behavioral disturbance in psychotic patients
- Stimulants have a high potential for abuse and must be used with caution in anyone with a current or past history of substance abuse or alcoholism or in emotionally unstable patients
- Administration of stimulants for prolonged periods of time should be avoided whenever possible or done only with close monitoring, as it may lead to marked tolerance and drug dependence, including psychological dependence with varying degrees of abnormal behavior
- Particular attention should be paid to the possibility of subjects obtaining stimulants for nontherapeutic use or distribution to others and the drugs should in general be prescribed sparingly with documentation of appropriate use
- Usual dosing has been associated with sudden death in children with structural cardiac abnormalities
- Not an appropriate first-line treatment for depression or for normal fatigue
- May lower the seizure threshold
- Emergence or worsening of activation and agitation may represent the induction of a bipolar state, especially a mixed dysphoric bipolar II condition sometimes associated with suicidal ideation, and require the addition of a mood stabilizer and/or discontinuation of d,l-amphetamine

Do Not Use

- If patient has extreme anxiety or agitation
- If patient has motor tics or Tourette's sydrome or if there is a family history of Tourette's, unless administered by an expert in cases when the potential benefits for ADHD outweigh the risks of worsening tics
- Should generally not be administered with an MAOI, including within 14 days of MAOI use, except in heroic circumstances and by an expert
- If patient has arteriosclerosis, cardiovascular disease, or severe hypertension
- If patient has glaucoma
- If patient has structural cardiac abnormalities
- If there is a proven allergy to any sympathomimetic agent

SPECIAL POPULATIONS

Renal Impairment

- No dose adjustment necessary

Hepatic Impairment

- No dose adjustment necessary

Cardiac Impairment

- Use with caution, particularly in patients with recent myocardial infarction or other conditions that could be negatively affected by increased blood pressure
- Do not use in patients with structural cardiac abnormalities

Elderly

- Some patients may tolerate lower doses better

Children and Adolescents

- Safety and efficacy not established under age 3
- Use in young children should be reserved for the expert
- d,l-amphetamine may worsen symptoms of behavioral disturbance and thought disorder in psychotic children
- d,l-amphetamine has acute effects on growth hormone; long-term effects are unknown but weight and height should be monitored during long-term treatment
- ADHD: ages 3–5: initial 2.5 mg/day; can increase by 2.5 mg each week
- Narcolepsy: ages 6–12: initial 5 mg/day; increase by 5 mg each week
- Sudden death in children and adolescents with serious heart problems has been reported
- American Heart Association recommends EKG prior to initiating stimulant treatment in children, although not all experts agree

Pregnancy

- Effective June 30, 2015, the US FDA requires changes to the content and format of pregnancy and lactation information in prescription drug labels, including the elimination of the pregnancy letter categories; the Pregnancy and Lactation Labeling Rule (PLLR or final rule) applies only to prescription drugs and will be

phased in gradually for drugs approved on or after June 30, 2001
- Controlled studies have not been conducted in pregnant women
- Infants whose mothers take d,l-amphetamine during pregnancy may experience withdrawal symptoms
- In rat and rabbit studies, amphetamine D,L did not affect embryofetal development or survival throughout organogenesis at doses of approximately one and a half and eight times the maximum recommended human dose of 30 mg/day (child)
- In animal studies, D-amphetamine caused delayed skeletal ossification and decreased post-weaning weight gain in rats; no major malformations occurred in rat or rabbit studies
- Use in women of childbearing potential requires weighing potential benefits to the mother against potential risks to the fetus

✻ For ADHD patients, d,l-amphetamine should generally be discontinued before anticipated pregnancies

Breast Feeding
- Some drug is found in mother's breast milk

✻ Recommended either to discontinue drug or bottle feed
- If infant shows signs of irritability, drug may need to be discontinued

THE ART OF PSYCHOPHARMACOLOGY

Potential Advantages
- May work in ADHD patients unresponsive to other stimulants, including pure d-amphetamine sulfate
- New sustained-release option

Potential Disadvantages
- Patients with current or past substance abuse
- Patients with current or past bipolar disorder or psychosis

Primary Target Symptoms
- Concentration, attention span
- Motor hyperactivity
- Impulsiveness
- Physical and mental fatigue
- Daytime sleepiness
- Depression

Pearls

✻ May be useful for treatment of depressive symptoms in medically ill elderly patients

✻ May be useful for treatment of post-stroke depression

✻ A classical augmentation strategy for treatment-refractory depression

✻ Specifically, may be useful for treatment of cognitive dysfunction and fatigue as residual symptoms of major depressive disorder unresponsive to multiple prior treatments

✻ May also be useful for the treatment of cognitive impairment, depressive symptoms, and severe fatigue in patients with HIV infection and in cancer patients
- Can be used to potentiate opioid analgesia and reduce sedation, particularly in end-of-life management

✻ Despite warnings, can be a useful adjunct to MAOIs for heroic treatment of highly refractory mood disorders when monitored with vigilance

✻ Can reverse sexual dysfunction caused by psychiatric illness and by some drugs such as SSRIs, including decreased libido, erectile dysfunction, delayed ejaculation, and anorgasmia
- Atypical antipsychotics may be useful in treating stimulant or psychotic consequences of overdose
- Taking with food may delay peak actions for 2–3 hours
- Half-life and duration of clinical action tend to be shorter in younger children
- Drug abuse may actually be lower in ADHD adolescents treated with stimulants than in ADHD adolescents who are not treated
- Some patients respond to or tolerate d,l-amphetamine better than methylphenidate and vice versa

✻ Adderall and Adderall XR are a mixture of d-amphetamine and l-amphetamine salts in the ratio of 3:1

✻ Specifically, Adderall and Adderall XR combine 1 part dextro-amphetamine saccharate, 1 part dextro-amphetamine sulfate, 1 part d,l-amphetamine aspartate, and 1 part d,l-amphetamine sulfate

- ✻ This mixture of salts may have a different pharmacologic profile, including mechanism of therapeutic action and duration of action, compared to pure dextro-amphetamine, which is given as the sulfate salt
- ✻ Specifically, d-amphetamine may have more profound action on dopamine than norepinephrine whereas l-amphetamine may have a more balanced action on both dopamine and norepinephrine
- ✻ Theoretically, this could lead to relatively more noradrenergic actions of the Adderall mixture of amphetamine salts than that of pure dextro-amphetamine sulfate, but this is unproven and of no clear clinical significance
- Nevertheless, some patients may respond to or tolerate Adderall/Adderall XR differently than they do pure dextro-amphetamine sulfate
- Adderall XR capsules also contain 2 types of drug-containing beads designed to give a double-pulsed delivery of amphetamines to prolong their release

Suggested Reading

Fry JM. Treatment modalities for narcolepsy. Neurology 1998;50(2 Suppl 1):S43–8.

Greenhill LL, Pliszka S, Dulcan MK, et al. Practice parameter for the use of stimulant medications in the treatment of children, adolescents, and adults. J Am Acad Child Adolesc Psychiatry 2002;41 (2 Suppl):S26–49.

Jadad AR, Boyle M, Cunningham C, Kim M, Schachar R. Treatment of attention-deficit/hyperactivity disorder. Evid Rep Technol Assess (Summ)1999;(11):i–viii,1–341.

Stiefel G, Besag FM. Cardiovascular effects of methylphenidate, amphetamines, and atomoxetine in the treatment of attention-deficit hyperactivity disorder. Drug Saf 2010;33(10):821–42.

Vinson DC. Therapy for attention-deficit hyperactivity disorder. Arch Fam Med 1994;3:445–51.

Wender PH, Wolf LE, Wasserstein J. Adults with ADHD. An overview. Ann NY Acad Sci 2001;931:1–16.

ARIPIPRAZOLE

THERAPEUTICS

Brands
- Abilify
- Abilify Maintena
- Aristada

see index for additional brand names

Generic? Yes

Class

- Neuroscience-based Nomenclature: dopamine, serotonin receptor partial agonist (DS-RPA)
- Dopamine partial agonist (dopamine stabilizer, atypical antipsychotic, third-generation antipsychotic; sometimes included as a second-generation antipsychotic; also a mood stabilizer)

Commonly Prescribed for

(bold for FDA approved)

- **Schizophrenia (ages 13 and older) (Abilify, Abilify Maintena, Aristada)**
- **Maintaining stability in schizophrenia**
- **Acute mania/mixed mania (ages 10 and older; monotherapy and adjunct)**
- **Bipolar maintenance (monotherapy and adjunct)**
- **Depression (adjunct)**
- **Autism-related irritability in children ages 6 to 17**
- **Tourette's disorder in children ages 6 to 18**
- **Acute agitation associated with schizophrenia or bipolar disorder (IM)**
- Bipolar depression
- Other psychotic disorders
- Behavioral disturbances in dementias
- Behavioral disturbances in children and adolescents
- Disorders associated with problems with impulse control

How the Drug Works

✽ Partial agonism at dopamine 2 receptors
- Theoretically reduces dopamine output when dopamine concentrations are high, thus improving positive symptoms and mediating antipsychotic actions
- Theoretically increases dopamine output when dopamine concentrations are low, thus improving cognitive, negative, and mood symptoms
- Actions at dopamine 3 receptors could theoretically contribute to aripiprazole's efficacy
- Partial agonism at 5HT1A receptors may be relevant at clinical doses
- Blockade of serotonin type 2A receptors may contribute at clinical doses to cause enhancement of dopamine release in certain brain regions, thus reducing motor side effects and possibly improving cognitive and affective symptoms
- Blockade of serotonin type 2C and 7 receptors as well as partial agonist actions at 5HT1A receptors may contribute to antidepressant actions

How Long Until It Works

- Psychotic and manic symptoms can improve within 1 week, but it may take several weeks for full effect on behavior as well as on cognition and affective stabilization
- Classically recommended to wait at least 4–6 weeks to determine efficacy of drug, but in practice some patients require up to 16–20 weeks to show a good response, especially on cognitive symptoms

If It Works

- Most often reduces positive symptoms in schizophrenia but does not eliminate them
- Can improve negative symptoms, as well as aggressive, cognitive, and affective symptoms in schizophrenia
- Most schizophrenic patients do not have a total remission of symptoms but rather a reduction of symptoms by about a third
- Perhaps 5–15% of schizophrenic patients can experience an overall improvement of greater than 50–60%, especially when receiving stable treatment for more than a year
- Such patients are considered super-responders or "awakeners" since they may be well enough to be employed, live independently, and sustain long-term relationships
- Many bipolar patients may experience a reduction of symptoms by half or more
- Continue treatment until reaching a plateau of improvement
- After reaching a satisfactory plateau, continue treatment for at least a year after first episode of psychosis

- For second and subsequent episodes of psychosis, treatment may need to be indefinite
- Even for first episodes of psychosis, it may be preferable to continue treatment indefinitely to avoid subsequent episodes
- Treatment may not only reduce mania but also prevent recurrences of mania in bipolar disorder

If It Doesn't Work

- Try one of the other atypical antipsychotics (risperidone, olanzapine, quetiapine, ziprasidone, paliperidone, amisulpride, asenapine, iloperidone, lurasidone)
- If two or more antipsychotic monotherapies do not work, consider clozapine
- Some patients may require treatment with a conventional antipsychotic
- If no first-line atypical antipsychotic is effective, consider higher doses or augmentation with valproate or lamotrigine
- Consider noncompliance and switch to another antipsychotic with fewer side effects or to an antipsychotic that can be given by depot injection
- Consider initiating rehabilitation and psychotherapy such as cognitive remediation
- Consider presence of concomitant drug abuse

Best Augmenting Combos for Partial Response or Treatment Resistance

- Valproic acid (valproate, divalproex, divalproex ER)
- Other mood-stabilizing anticonvulsants (carbamazepine, oxcarbazepine, lamotrigine)
- Lithium
- Benzodiazepines

Tests

Before starting an atypical antipsychotic

✽ Weigh all patients and track BMI during treatment

- Get baseline personal and family history of diabetes, obesity, dyslipidemia, hypertension, and cardiovascular disease

✽ Get waist circumference (at umbilicus), blood pressure, fasting plasma glucose, and fasting lipid profile

- Determine if the patient is
  - overweight (BMI 25.0–29.9)
  - obese (BMI ≥30)
  - has pre-diabetes (fasting plasma glucose 100–125 mg/dL)
  - has diabetes (fasting plasma glucose >126 mg/dL)
  - has hypertension (BP >140/90 mm Hg)
  - has dyslipidemia (increased total cholesterol, LDL cholesterol, and triglycerides; decreased HDL cholesterol)
- Treat or refer such patients for treatment, including nutrition and weight management, physical activity counseling, smoking cessation, and medical management

Monitoring after starting an atypical antipsychotic

✽ BMI monthly for 3 months, then quarterly

✽ Consider monitoring fasting triglycerides monthly for several months in patients at high risk for metabolic complications and when initiating or switching antipsychotics

✽ Blood pressure, fasting plasma glucose, fasting lipids within 3 months and then annually, but earlier and more frequently for patients with diabetes or who have gained >5% of initial weight

- Treat or refer for treatment and consider switching to another atypical antipsychotic for patients who become overweight, obese, pre-diabetic, diabetic, hypertensive, or dyslipidemic while receiving an atypical antipsychotic

✽ Even in patients without known diabetes, be vigilant for the rare but life-threatening onset of diabetic ketoacidosis, which always requires immediate treatment, by monitoring for the rapid onset of polyuria, polydipsia, weight loss, nausea, vomiting, dehydration, rapid respiration, weakness and clouding of sensorium, even coma

- Patients with low white blood cell count (WBC) or history of drug-induced leucopenia/neutropenia should have complete blood count (CBC) monitored frequently during the first few months and aripiprazole should be discontinued at the first sign of decline of WBC in the absence of other causative factors

SIDE EFFECTS

How Drug Causes Side Effects

- By blocking alpha 1 adrenergic receptors, it can cause dizziness, sedation, and hypotension
- Partial agonist actions at dopamine 2 receptors in the striatum can cause motor side effects, such as akathisia
- Partial agonist actions at dopamine 2 receptors can also cause nausea, occasional vomiting, and activating side effects

✻ Mechanism of any possible weight gain is unknown; weight gain is not common with aripiprazole and may thus have a different mechanism from atypical antipsychotics for which weight gain is common or problematic

✻ Mechanism of any possible increased incidence of diabetes or dyslipidemia is unknown; early experience suggests these complications are not clearly associated with aripiprazole and if present may therefore have a different mechanism from that of atypical antipsychotics associated with an increased incidence of diabetes and dyslipidemia

Notable Side Effects

✻ Dizziness, insomnia, akathisia, activation

✻ Nausea, vomiting

- Orthostatic hypotension, occasionally during initial dosing
- Constipation
- Headache, asthenia, sedation
- Theoretical risk of tardive dyskinesia

Life-Threatening or Dangerous Side Effects

- Rare impulse control problems
- Rare neuroleptic malignant syndrome (much reduced risk compared to conventional antipsychotics)
- Rare seizures
- Increased risk of death and cerebrovascular events in elderly patients with dementia-related psychosis

Weight Gain

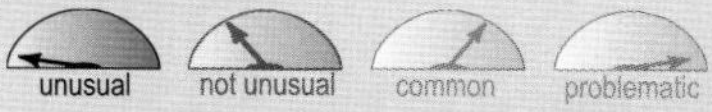

- Reported in a few patients, especially those with low BMIs, but not expected
- Less frequent and less severe than for most other antipsychotics
- May be more risk of weight gain in children than in adults

Sedation

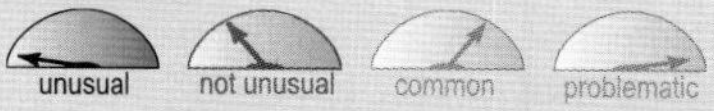

- Reported in a few patients but not expected
- May be less than for some other antipsychotics, but never say never
- Can be activating

What to Do About Side Effects

- Wait
- Wait
- Wait
- Reduce the dose
- Anticholinergics or a low dose benzodiazepine or a beta blocker may reduce akathisia when present
- Weight loss, exercise programs, and medical management for high BMIs, diabetes, dyslipidemia
- Switch to another atypical antipsychotic

Best Augmenting Agents for Side Effects

- Benztropine or trihexyphenidyl for motor side effects and akathisia
- Many side effects cannot be improved with an augmenting agent

DOSING AND USE

Usual Dosage Range

- 15–30 mg/day for schizophrenia and mania
- 2–10 mg/day for augmenting SSRIs/SNRIs in depression
- 5–15 mg/day for autism
- 5–20 mg/day for Tourette's disorder
- 300–400 mg/4 weeks (LAI Maintena; see Aripiprazole Depot Formulations after Pearls for dosing and use)
- 441 mg, 662 mg, or 882 mg administered monthly or 882 mg administered every 6 weeks (LAI Aristada; see Aripiprazole Depot Formulations after Pearls for dosing and use)

Dosage Forms

- Tablet 2 mg, 5 mg, 10 mg, 15 mg, 20 mg, 30 mg
- Orally disintegrating tablet 10 mg, 15 mg

- Oral solution 1 mg/mL
- Injection 9.75 mg/1.3 mL
- Depot (Maintena) 300 mg, 400 mg
- Depot (Aristada) 441 mg, 662 mg, 882 mg

How to Dose – Oral and Acute IM

- Schizophrenia, mania: initial approved recommendation is 10–15 mg/day; maximum approved dose 30 mg/day
- Depression (adjunct): initial dose 2–5 mg/day; can increase by 5 mg/day at intervals of no less than 1 week; maximum dose 15 mg/day
- Autism: initial dose 2 mg/day; can increase by 5 mg/day at intervals of no less than 1 week; maximum dose 15 mg/day
- Tourette's disorder (patients weighing less than 50 kg): initial dose 2 mg/day; after 2 days increase to 5 mg/day; after 1 additional week can increase to 10 mg/day if needed
- Tourette's disorder (patients weighing more than 50 kg): initial dose 2 mg/day; after 2 days increase to 5 mg/day; after 5 additional days can increase to 10 mg/day; can increase by 5 mg/day at intervals of no less than 1 week; maximum dose 20 mg/day
- Agitation: 9.75 mg/1.3 ml; maximun 30 mg/day
- Depot: must initiate oral aripiprazole first; after tolerability is established can administer initial injection along with an overlapping 14-day (Maintena) or 21-day (Aristada) dosing of oral aripiprazole; initial and maintenance doses are described under dosing tips below
- Oral solution: solution doses can be substituted for tablet doses on a mg-per-mg basis up to 25 mg; patients receiving 30-mg tablet should receive 25-mg solution

Dosing Tips – Oral

✻ **For some, less may be more:** frequently, patients not acutely psychotic may need to be dosed lower (e.g., 2.5–10 mg/day) in order to avoid akathisia and activation and for maximum tolerability
- **For others, more may be more:** rarely, patients may need to be dosed higher than 30 mg/day for optimum efficacy
- Consider administering 1–5 mg as the oral solution for children and adolescents, as well as for adults very sensitive to side effects

✻ Although studies suggest patients switching to aripiprazole from another antipsychotic can do well with rapid switch or with cross-titration, clinical experience suggests many patients may do best by adding either an intermediate or full dose of aripiprazole to the maintenance dose of the first antipsychotic for at least several days and possibly as long as 3 or 4 weeks prior to slow down-titration of the first antipsychotic. See also the Switching section below, after Pearls
- Rather than raise the dose above these levels in acutely agitated patients requiring acute antipsychotic actions, consider augmentation with a benzodiazepine or conventional antipsychotic, either orally or intramuscularly
- Rather than raise the dose above these levels in partial responders, consider augmentation with a mood-stabilizing anticonvulsant, such as valproate or lamotrigine
- Children and elderly should generally be dosed at the lower end of the dosage spectrum
- Due to its very long half-life, aripiprazole will take longer to reach steady state when initiating dosing, and longer to wash out when stopping dosing, than other atypical antipsychotics
- Treatment should be suspended if absolute neutrophil count falls below 1,000/mm^3

Overdose

- No fatalities have been reported; sedation, vomiting

Long-Term Use

- Approved to delay relapse in long-term treatment of schizophrenia
- Approved for long-term maintenance in bipolar disorder
- Often used for long-term maintenance in various behavioral disorders

Habit Forming

- No

How to Stop

- See Switching section of individual agents for how to stop aripiprazole

- Rapid discontinuation could theoretically lead to rebound psychosis and worsening of symptoms, but less likely with aripiprazole due to its long half-life

Pharmacokinetics
- Metabolized primarily by CYP450 2D6 and CYP450 3A4
- Mean elimination half-life 75 hours (aripiprazole) and 94 hours (major metabolite dehydro-aripiprazole)
- Food does not affect absorption

Drug Interactions
- Ketaconazole and possibly other CYP450 3A4 inhibitors such as nefazodone, fluvoxamine, and fluoxetine may increase plasma levels of aripiprazole
- Carbamazepine and possibly other inducers of CYP450 3A4 may decrease plasma levels of aripiprazole
- Quinidine and possibly other inhibitors of CYP450 2D6 such as paroxetine, fluoxetine, and duloxetine may increase plasma levels of aripiprazole
- Aripiprazole may enhance the effects of antihypertensive drugs
- Aripiprazole may antagonize levodopa, dopamine agonists

Other Warnings/ Precautions
- There have been reports of problems with impulse control in patients taking aripiprazole, including compulsive gambling, shopping, binge eating, and sexual activity; use caution when prescribing to patients at high risk for impulse-control problems (e.g., patients with bipolar disorder, impulsive personality, obsessive-compulsive disorder, substance use disorders) and monitor all patients for emergence of these symptoms; dose should be lowered or discontinued if impulse-control problems manifest
- Use with caution in patients with conditions that predispose to hypotension (dehydration, overheating)
- Dysphagia has been associated with antipsychotic use, and aripiprazole should be used cautiously in patients at risk for aspiration pneumonia

Do Not Use
- If there is a proven allergy to aripiprazole

SPECIAL POPULATIONS

Renal Impairment
- Dose adjustment not necessary

Hepatic Impairment
- Dose adjustment not necessary

Cardiac Impairment
- Use in patients with cardiac impairment has not been studied, so use with caution because of risk of orthostatic hypotension

Elderly
- Dose adjustment generally not necessary, but some elderly patients may tolerate lower doses better
- Although atypical antipsychotics are commonly used for behavioral disturbances in dementia, no agent has been approved for treatment of elderly patients with dementia-related psychosis
- Elderly patients with dementia-related psychosis treated with atypical antipsychotics are at an increased risk of death compared to placebo, and also have an increased risk of cerebrovascular events

Children and Adolescents
- Approved for use in schizophrenia (ages 13 and older), manic/mixed episodes (ages 10 and older), irritability associated with autism (ages 6–17), and treatment of Tourette's disorder (ages 6–18)
- Clinical experience and early data suggest aripiprazole may be safe and effective for behavioral disturbances in children and adolescents, especially at lower doses
- Children and adolescents using aripiprazole may need to be monitored more often than adults and may tolerate lower doses better
- May be more risk of weight gain in children than in adults

Pregnancy

- Effective June 30, 2015, the US FDA requires changes to the content and format of pregnancy and lactation information in prescription drug labels, including the elimination of the pregnancy letter categories; the Pregnancy and Lactation Labeling Rule (PLLR or final rule) applies only to prescription drugs and will be phased in gradually for drugs approved on or after June 30, 2001
- Controlled studies have not been conducted in pregnant women
- There is a risk of abnormal muscle movements and withdrawal symptoms in newborns whose mothers took an antipsychotic during the third trimester; symptoms may include agitation, abnormally increased or decreased muscle tone, tremor, sleepiness, severe difficulty breathing, and difficulty feeding
- In animal studies, aripiprazole demonstrated developmental toxicity, including possible teratogenic effects, at doses higher than the maximum recommended human dose
- Psychotic symptoms may worsen during pregnancy and some form of treatment may be necessary
- Aripiprazole may be preferable to anticonvulsant mood stabilizers if treatment is required during pregnancy
- National Pregnancy Registry for Atypical Antipsychotics: 1-866-961-2388 or http://womensmentalhealth.org/clinical-and-research-programs/pregnancyregistry/

Breast Feeding

- Some drug is found in mother's breast milk
- ✻ Recommended either to discontinue drug or bottle feed
- Infants of women who choose to breast feed while on aripiprazole should be monitored for possible adverse effects

THE ART OF PSYCHOPHARMACOLOGY

Potential Advantages

- Some cases of psychosis and bipolar disorder refractory to treatment with other antipsychotics
- ✻ Patients concerned about gaining weight and patients who are already obese or overweight
- ✻ Patients with diabetes
- ✻ Patients with dyslipidemia (especially elevated triglycerides)
- Patients requiring rapid onset of antipsychotic action without dosage titration
- ✻ Patients who wish to avoid sedation

Potential Disadvantages

- Patients in whom sedation is desired
- May be more difficult to dose for children, elderly, or "off-label" uses

Primary Target Symptoms

- Positive symptoms of psychosis
- Negative symptoms of psychosis
- Cognitive symptoms
- Unstable mood and depression
- Aggressive symptoms

Pearls

- ✻ Approved as an adjunct treatment for depression (e.g., to SSRIs, SNRIs)
- May work better in 2–10 mg/day range than at higher doses for augmenting SSRIs/SNRIs in treatment-resistant unipolar depression
- Frequently used for bipolar depression as augmenting agent to lithium, valproate and/or lamotrigine
- ✻ Well accepted in clinical practice when wanting to avoid weight gain because less weight gain than most other antipsychotics
- ✻ Well accepted in clinical practice when wanting to avoid sedation because less sedation than most other antipsychotics at all doses
- ✻ Can even be activating, which can be reduced by lowering the dose or starting at a lower dose
- If sedation is desired, a benzodiazepine can be added short-term at the initiation of treatment until symptoms of agitation and insomnia are stabilized or intermittently as needed
- ✻ May not have diabetes or dyslipidemia risk, but monitoring is still indicated
- Anecdotal reports of utility in treatment-resistant cases of psychosis

- Has a very favorable tolerability profile in clinical practice
- Favorable tolerability profile leading to "off-label" uses for many indications other than schizophrenia (e.g., bipolar II disorder, including hypomanic, mixed, rapid cycling, and depressed phases; treatment-resistant depression; anxiety disorders)
- A short-acting intramuscular formulation is available as well as long-acting depot
- Lacks D1 antagonist, anticholinergic, and antihistamine properties, which may explain relative lack of sedation or cognitive side effects in most patients
- High affinity of aripiprazole for D2 receptors means that combining with other D2 antagonist antipsychotics could reverse their actions and thus often makes sense not to combine with other antipsychotics
- An exception to this is in case of hyperprolactinemia or galactorrhea, when administration of even low dose (1–5 mg) can reverse the hyperprolactinemia/galactorrhea of other antipsychotics, also proving that aripiprazole interferes with the D2 actions of other antipsychotics
- Abilify Maintena (depot) may be particularly well suited to early-onset psychosis/first-episode psychosis to reduce rehospitalizations and to enhance adherence with relatively low side effect burden

DEPOT FORMULATIONS

	Monohydrate (Maintena)	Lauroxil (Aristada)
Vehicle	Water	Water
Tmax	6.5–7.1 days	44.1–50.0 days
T1/2 with multiple dosing	29.9–46.5 days	29.2–34.9 days
Time to reach steady state		4 monthly injections
Able to be loaded	No	No
Dosing schedule (maintenance)	4 weeks	4–6 weeks
Injection site	Intramuscular gluteal	Intramuscular injection in deltoid (441 mg dose only) or gluteal (441, 662, or 882 mg)
Needle gauge	21	20 or 21
Dosage forms	300 mg, 400 mg	441 mg, 662 mg, 882 mg
Injection volume	200 mg/mL; range 0.8 mL (160 mg)–2 mL (400 mg)	441 mg/1.6 mL; 662 mg/2.4 mL; 882 mg/3.2 mL

Usual Dosage Range

- 300–400 mg/4 weeks (monohydrate Maintena)
- 441 mg, 662 mg, or 882 mg administered monthly or 882 mg administered every 6 weeks (lauroxil Aristada)

How to Dose

- Not recommended for patients who have not first demonstrated tolerability to oral aripiprazole (in clinical trials, 2 oral or short-acting IM doses are generally used to establish tolerability)
- Loading is not possible, necessitating oral coverage for 14 days (Maintena) or 21 days (Aristada)
- Conversion from oral to Maintena: administer initial 400 mg injection along with an overlapping 14-day dosing of oral aripiprazole
- Conversion from oral to Aristada: administer initial injection (441 mg, 662 mg, or 882 mg) along with an overlapping 21-day dosing of oral aripiprazole

Dosing Tips

- With LAIs, the absorption rate constant is slower than the elimination rate constant, thus resulting in "flip-flop" kinetics—i.e., time to steady-state is a function of absorption rate, while concentration at steady-state is a function of elimination rate
- The rate-limiting step for plasma drug levels for LAIs is not drug metabolism, but rather slow absorption from the injection site
- In general, 5 half-lives of any medication are needed to achieve 97% of steady-state levels
- The long half-lives of depot antipsychotics mean that one must either adequately load the dose (if possible) or provide oral supplementation
- The failure to adequately load the dose leads either to prolonged cross-titration from oral antipsychotic or to sub-therapeutic antipsychotic plasma levels for weeks or months in patients who are not receiving (or adhering to) oral supplementation
- Because plasma antipsychotic levels increase gradually over time, dose requirements may ultimately decrease from initial; obtaining periodic plasma levels can be beneficial to prevent unnecessary plasma level creep
- The time to get a blood level for patients receiving LAI is the morning of the day they will receive their next injection
- Advantages: refrigeration not required; option of 6-week injections with Aristada
- Disadvantages: both formulations require oral coverage
- Downward dose adjustment is needed for poor CYP450 2D6 metabolizers and patients taking strong CYP450 2D6 or 3A4 inhibitors; avoid use with strong CYP450 3A4 inducers, as this can lead to sub-therapeutic plasma levels

Maintena			
	Adjusted dose for patients taking 400 mg	Adjusted dose for patients taking 300 mg	
Poor 2D6 metabolizers	300 mg	N/A	
Patients taking strong 2D6 OR 3A4 inhibitors	300 mg	200 mg	
Poor 2D6 metabolizers taking concomitant 3A4 inhibitors	200 mg	N/A	
Patients taking 2D6 AND 3A4 inhibitors	200 mg	160 mg	
Patients taking 3A4 inducers	Avoid	Avoid	
Aristada			
	Adjusted dose for patients taking 441 mg	Adjusted dose for patients taking 662 mg	Adjusted dose for patients taking 882 mg
Poor 2D6 metabolizers	N/A	N/A	N/A
Patients taking strong 2D6 OR 3A4 inhibitors	N/A	441 mg	662 mg
Poor 2D6 metabolizers taking concomitant 3A4 inhibitors	N/A	441 mg	441 mg
Patients taking 2D6 AND 3A4 inhibitors	N/A	Avoid	Avoid
Patients taking 3A4 inducers	662 mg	N/A	N/A

Switching from Oral Antipsychotics to Aripiprazole Depot Formulations

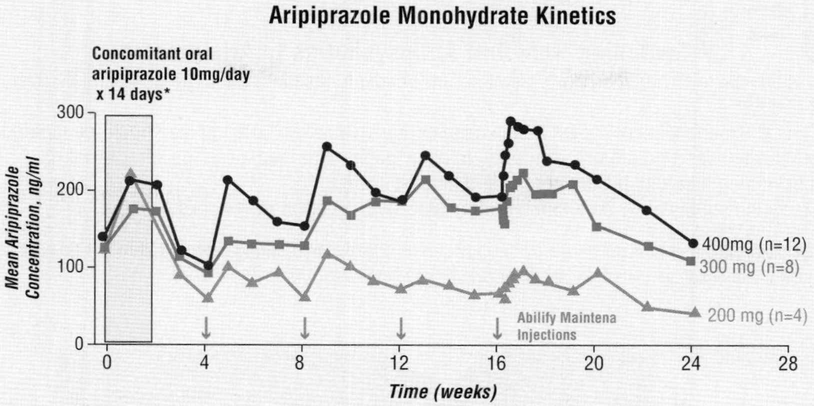

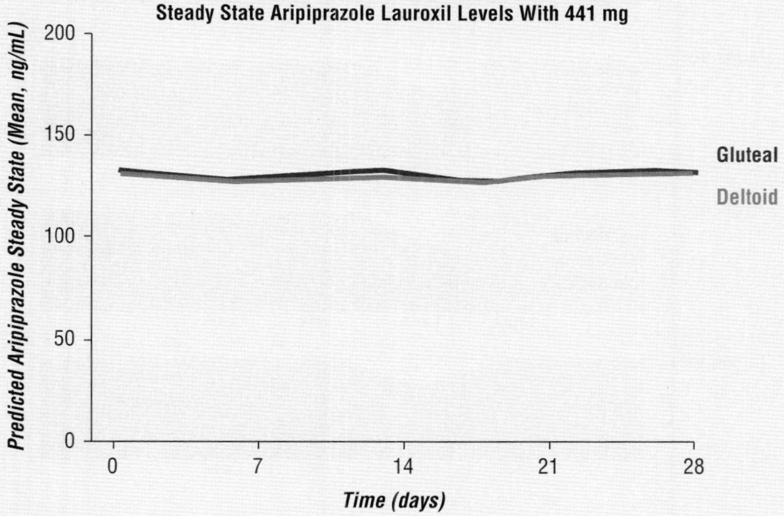

- Discontinuation of oral antipsychotic can begin following oral coverage of 14 days (Maintena) or 21 days (Aristada)
- How to discontinue oral formulations
  - Down-titration is not required for: amisulpride, aripiprazole, brexpiprazole, cariprazine, paliperidone ER
  - 1-week down-titration is required for: iloperidone, lurasidone, risperidone, ziprasidone
  - 3–4-week down-titration is required for: asenapine, olanzapine, quetiapine
  - 4+-week down-titration is required for: clozapine
  - For patients taking benzodiazepine or anticholinergic medication, this can be continued during cross-titration to help alleviate side effects such as insomnia, agitation, and/or psychosis. Once the patient is stable on LAI, these can be tapered one at a time as appropriate.

THE ART OF SWITCHING

Switching from Oral Antipsychotics to Aripiprazole

- It is advisable to begin aripiprazole at an intermediate dose and build the dose rapidly over 3–7 days
- Clinical experience has shown that asenapine, quetiapine, and olanzapine should be tapered off slowly over a period of 3–4 weeks, to allow patients to readapt to the withdrawal of blocking cholinergic, histaminergic, and alpha-1 receptors
- Clozapine should always be tapered off slowly, over a period of 4 weeks or more

* Benzodiazepine or anticholinergic medication can be administered during cross-titration to help alleviate side effects such as insomnia, agitation, and/or psychosis

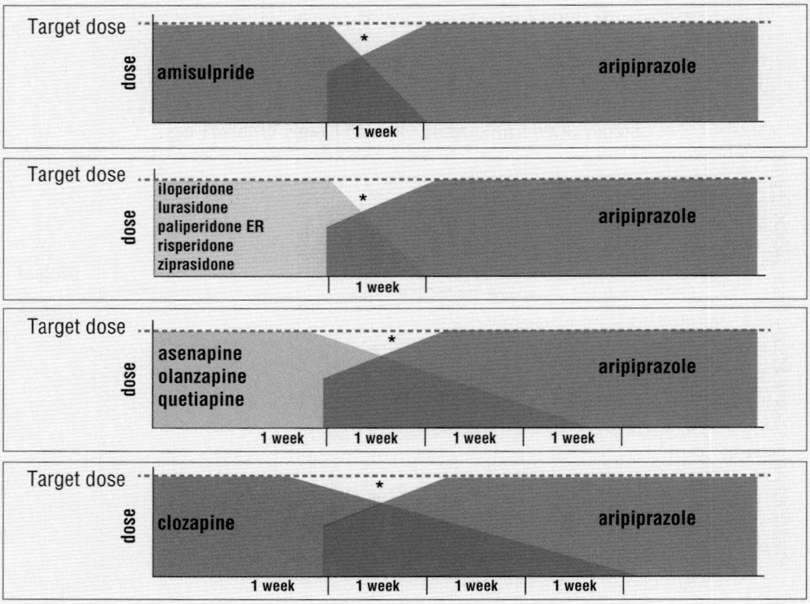

Suggested Reading

Andrezina R, Josiassen RC, Marcus RN, et al. Intramuscular aripiprazole for the treatment of acute agitation in patients with schizophrenia or schizoaffective disorder: a double-blind, placebo-controlled comparison with intramuscular haloperidol. Psychopharmacology 2006;188(3):281–92.

Citrome L. Adjunctive aripiprazole, olanzapine, or quetiapine for major depressive disorder: an analysis of number needed to treat, number needed to harm, and likelihood to be helped or harmed. Postgrad Med 2010;122(4):39–48.

El-Sayeh HG, Morganti C. Aripiprazole for schizophrenia. Cochrane Database Syst Rev 2006;2:CD004578.

Kane JM, Sanchez R, Perry PP, et al. Aripiprazole intramuscular depot as maintenance treatment in patients with schizophrenia: a 52-week, multicenter, randomized, double-blind, placebo-controlled study. J Clin Psychiatry 2012;73(5):617–24.

Marcus RN, McQuade RD, Carson WH, et al. The efficacy and safety of aripiprazole as adjunctive therapy in major depressive disorder: a second multicenter, randomized, double-blind, placebo-controlled study. J Clin Psychopharmacol 2008;28(2):156–65.

Nasrallah HA. Atypical antipsychotic-induced metabolic side effects: insights from receptor-binding profiles. Mol Psychiatry 2008;13(1):27–35.

Smith LA, Cornelius V, Warnock A, Tacchi MJ, Taylor D. Pharmacological interventions for acute bipolar mania: a systematic review of randomized placebo-controlled trials. Bipolar Disord 2007;9(6):551–60.

THERAPEUTICS

Brands • Nuvigil

see index for additional brand names

Generic? Yes

Class

- Neuroscience-based Nomenclature: dopamine reuptake inhibitor (D-RI)
- Wake-promoting

Commonly Prescribed for

(bold for FDA approved)

- **Reducing excessive sleepiness in patients with narcolepsy and shift work sleep disorder**
- **Reducing excessive sleepiness in patients with obstructive sleep apnea/ hypopnea syndrome (OSAHS) (adjunct to standard treatment for underlying airway obstruction)**
- Attention deficit hyperactivity disorder (ADHD)
- Fatigue and sleepiness in depression
- Fatigue in multiple sclerosis
- Bipolar depression

How the Drug Works

- Unknown, but clearly different from classical stimulants such as methylphenidate and amphetamine
- Binds to and requires the presence of the dopamine transporter; also requires the presence of alpha adrenergic receptors
- Hypothetically acts as an inhibitor of the dopamine transporter
- Increases neuronal activity selectively in the hypothalamus

✻ Presumably enhances activity in hypothalamic wakefulness center (TMN, tuberomammillary nucleus) within the hypothalamic sleep-wake switch by an unknown mechanism

✻ Activates tuberomammillary nucleus neurons that release histamine

✻ Activates other hypothalamic neurons that release orexin/hypocretin

How Long Until It Works

- Can immediately reduce daytime sleepiness and improve cognitive task performance within 2 hours of first dosing
- Can take several days to optimize dosing and clinical improvement

If It Works

✻ Improves daytime sleepiness and may improve attention as well as fatigue

✻ Does not generally prevent one from falling asleep when needed

- May not completely normalize wakefulness
- Treat until improvement stabilizes and then continue treatment indefinitely as long as improvement persists (studies support at least 12 weeks of treatment)

If It Doesn't Work

✻ Change dose; some patients may do better with an increased dose but some may actually do better with a decreased dose

- Augment or consider an alternative treatment for daytime sleepiness, fatigue, or ADHD

Best Augmenting Combos for Partial Response or Treatment Resistance

✻ Armodafinil is itself an adjunct to standard treatments for OSAHS; if continuous positive airway pressure (CPAP) is the treatment of choice, a maximal effort to treat first with CPAP should be made prior to initiating armodafinil and CPAP should be continued after initiation of armodafinil

✻ Armodafinil is itself an augmenting therapy to antidepressants for residual sleepiness and fatigue in major depressive disorder

✻ Armodafinil is itself an augmenting therapy to mood stabilizers for bipolar depression

- Best to attempt another monotherapy prior to augmenting with other drugs in the treatment of sleepiness associated with sleep disorders or problems concentrating in ADHD
- Combination of armodafinil with stimulants such as methylphenidate or amphetamine or with atomoxetine for ADHD has not been systematically studied
- However, such combinations may be useful options for experts, with close monitoring, when numerous monotherapies for sleepiness or ADHD have failed

Tests
- None for healthy individuals

SIDE EFFECTS

How Drug Causes Side Effects
- Unknown
- CNS side effects presumably due to excessive CNS actions on various neurotransmitter systems

Notable Side Effects
* Headache
- Anxiety, dizziness, insomnia
- Dry mouth, diarrhea, nausea

Life-Threatening or Dangerous Side Effects
- Transient EKG ischemic changes in patients with mitral valve prolapse or left ventricular hypertrophy have been reported (rare)
- Rare activation of (hypo)mania, anxiety, hallucinations, or suicidal ideation
- Rare severe dermatologic reactions (Stevens-Johnson syndrome and others)
- Angioedema, anaphylactoid reactions, and multi-organ hypersensitivity reactions have been reported

Weight Gain
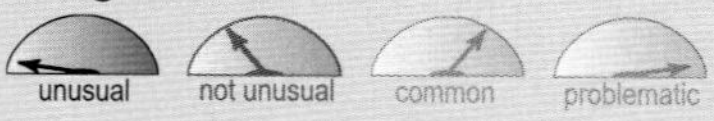

- Reported but not expected

Sedation
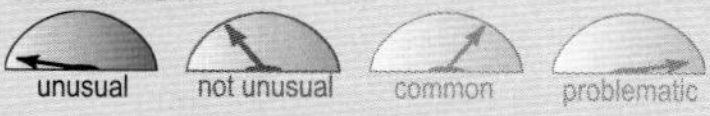

- Reported but not expected
- Patients are usually awakened and some may be activated

What to Do About Side Effects
- Wait
- Lower the dose
- For activation or insomnia, do not give in the evening
- If unacceptable side effects persist, discontinue use
- For life-threatening or dangerous side effects, discountinue immediately (e.g., at first sign of a drug-related rash)

Best Augmenting Agents for Side Effects
- Many side effects cannot be improved with an augmenting agent

DOSING AND USE

Usual Dosage Range
- 150–250 mg/day

Dosage Forms
- Tablet 50 mg, 150 mg, 250 mg

How to Dose
- Titration up or down only necessary if not optimally efficacious at the standard starting dose of 150 mg once a day
- For OSA and narcolepsy, give as a single dose in the morning
- For shift work sleep disorder, give as a single dose 1 hour prior to the start of the work shift

Dosing Tips
* For sleepiness, more may be more: higher doses may be better than lower doses in patients with daytime sleepiness in sleep disorders
* For problems concentrating and fatigue, less may be more: lower doses may be paradoxically better than higher in some patients
- At high doses, may slightly induce its own metabolism, possibly by actions of inducing CYP450 3A4
- Dose may creep upward in some patients with long-term treatment due to autoinduction; drug holiday may restore efficacy at original dose
- Pharmacokinetics and clinical experience suggest armodafinil has longer duration of action than racemic modafinil, generally requiring only once daily administration

Overdose
- Agitation, insomnia, increase in hemodynamic parameters
- Postmarketing experience includes CNS symptoms, such as restlessness, disorientation, confusion, excitation, and hallucinations; digestive changes, such as

nausea and diarrhea; and cardiovascular changes, such as tachycardia, bradycardia, hypertension, and chest pain

Long-Term Use
- The need for continued treatment should be reevaluated periodically

Habit Forming
- Schedule IV; may have some potential for abuse but unusual in clinical practice

How to Stop
- Taper not necessary; patients may have sleepiness on discontinuation

Pharmacokinetics
- Metabolized by the liver
- Elimination half-life approximately 15 hours
- Inhibits CYP450 2C19
- Induces CYP450 3A4 (and slightly 1A2)

Drug Interactions
- May increase plasma levels of drugs metabolized by CYP450 2C19 (e.g., diazepam, phenytoin, propranolol)
- May decrease plasma levels of CYP450 3A4 substrates such as ethinyl estradiol and triazolam
- Due to induction of CYP450 3A4, effectiveness of steroidal contraceptives may be reduced by armodafinil, including 1 month after discontinuation
- Inducers or inhibitors of CYP450 3A4 may affect levels of armodafinil (e.g., carbamazepine may lower modafinil plasma levels; fluvoxamine and fluoxetine may raise armodafinil plasma levels)
- Armodafinil may slightly reduce its own levels by autoinduction of CYP450 3A4
- Patients on armodafinil and warfarin should have prothrombin times monitored
- Methylphenidate and dextroamphetamine may delay absorption of armodafinil by an hour

✻ However, coadministration with methylphenidate or dextroamphetamine does not significantly change the pharmacokinetics of armodafinil or either stimulant

- Interaction studies with MAOIs have not been performed, but MAOIs can be given with armodafinil by experts with cautious monitoring

Other Warnings/ Precautions
- Patients with history of drug abuse should be monitored closely
- Armodafinil may cause CNS effects similar to those caused by other CNS agents (e.g., changes in mood and, theoretically, activation of psychosis, mania, or suicidal ideation)
- Armodafinil should be used in patients with sleep disorders that have been completely evaluated for narcolepsy, OSAHS, and shift work sleep disorder
- In OSAHS patients for whom CPAP is the treatment of choice, a maximal effort to treat first with CPAP should be made prior to initiating armodafinil, and then CPAP should be continued after initiating armodafinil
- The effectiveness of steroidal contraceptives may be reduced when used with armodafinil and for 1 month after discontinuation of armodafinil
- Armodafinil is not a replacement for sleep

Do Not Use
- If there is a proven allergy to armodafinil or modafinil

SPECIAL POPULATIONS

Renal Impairment
- Use with caution

Hepatic Impairment
- Reduce dose in severely impaired patients

Cardiac Impairment
- Use with caution
- Not recommended for use in patients with a history of left ventricular hypertrophy, ischemic EKG changes, chest pain, arrhythmias, or recent myocardial infarction

Elderly
- Limited experience in patients over 65
- Clearance of armodafinil may be reduced in elderly patients

Children and Adolescents

- Safety and efficacy have not been established
- Can be used cautiously by experts for children and adolescents

Pregnancy

- Effective June 30, 2015, the US FDA requires changes to the content and format of pregnancy and lactation information in prescription drug labels, including the elimination of the pregnancy letter categories; the Pregnancy and Lactation Labeling Rule (PLLR or final rule) applies only to prescription drugs and will be phased in gradually for drugs approved on or after June 30, 2001
- Controlled studies have not been conducted in pregnant women
- Intrauterine growth restriction and spontaneous abortion have been reported with armodafinil and modafinil
- In animal studies, developmental toxicity was observed at clinically relevant plasma exposures
- Use in women of childbearing potential requires weighing potential benefits to the mother against potential risks to the fetus

✻ Generally, armodafinil should be discontinued prior to anticipated pregnancies

Breast Feeding

- Unknown if armodafinil is secreted in human breast milk, but all psychotropics assumed to be secreted in breast milk

✻ Recommended either to discontinue drug or bottle feed

THE ART OF PSYCHOPHARMACOLOGY

Potential Advantages

- Selective for areas of brain involved in sleep/wake promotion
- Less activating and less abuse potential than stimulants

Potential Disadvantages

- May not work as well as stimulants in some patients

Primary Target Symptoms

- Sleepiness
- Concentration
- Physical and mental fatigue

Pearls

- Armodafinil is the longer-lasting R enantiomer of racemic modafinil
- Armodafinil maintains high plasma concentrations later in the day than does modafinil on a mg-to-mg basis, which could theoretically result in improved wakefulness throughout the day with armodafinil compared to modafinil

✻ Armodafinil is not a replacement for sleep

✻ The treatment for sleep deprivation is sleep, not armodafinil

- Controlled studies suggest armodafinil improves attention in OSAHS and shift work sleep disorder, but controlled studies of attention have not been performed in ADHD or major depressive disorder
- Controlled studies of racemic modafinil in ADHD suggest improvement in attention

✻ May be useful to treat fatigue in patients with depression as well as other disorders, such as multiple sclerosis, myotonic dystrophy, HIV/AIDS

- May be useful in treating sleepiness associated with opioid analgesia, particularly in end-of-life management
- Subjective sensation associated with armodafinil is usually one of normal wakefulness, not of stimulation, although jitteriness can rarely occur

✻ Compared to traditional stimulants, armodafinil has a novel mechanism of action, novel therapeutic uses, and less abuse potential

- Alpha 1 antagonists such as prazosin may block the therapeutic actions of armodafinil
- Some controlled trials suggest efficacy in bipolar depression as an adjunct to atypical antipsychotics

Suggested Reading

Darwish M, Kirby M, Hellriegel ET, Robertson P Jr. Armodafinil and modafinil have substantially different pharmacokinetic profiles despite having the same terminal half-lives: analysis of data from three randomized, single-dose, pharmacokinetic studies. Clin Drug Investig 2009;29(9):613–23.

Darwish M, Kirby M, Hellriegel ET, Robertson Jr P. Interaction profile of armodafinil with medications metabolized by cytochrome P450 enzymes 1A2, 3A4, and 2C19 in healthy subjects. Clin Pharmacokinet 2008;47(1): 61–74.

Garnock-Jones KP, Dhillon S, Scott LJ. Armodafinil. CNS Drugs 2009;23(9):793–803.

THERAPEUTICS

Brands • SAPHRIS

see index for additional brand names

Generic? No

Class

- Neuroscience-based Nomenclature: dopamine, serotonin, norepinephrine receptor antagonist (DSN-RAn)
- Atypical antipsychotic (serotonin-dopamine antagonist; second generation antipsychotics; also a mood stabilizer)

Commonly Prescribed for

(bold for FDA approved)

- **Schizophrenia, acute and maintenance (adults)**
- **Acute mania/mixed mania, monotherapy (ages 10 to 17 and in adults)**
- **Acute mania/mixed mania, adjunct to lithium or valproate (adults)**
- Other psychotic disorders
- Bipolar maintenance
- Bipolar depression
- Treatment-resistant depression
- Behavioral disturbances in dementia
- Behavioral disturbances in children and adolescents
- Disorders associated with problems with impulse control

How the Drug Works

- Blocks dopamine 2 receptors, reducing positive symptoms of psychosis and stabilizing affective symptoms
- Blocks serotonin 2A receptors, causing enhancement of dopamine release in certain brain regions and thus reducing motor side effects and possibly improving cognitive and affective symptoms

✻ Serotonin 2C, serotonin 7, and alpha 2 antagonist properties may contribute to antidepressant actions

How Long Until It Works

- Psychotic symptoms can improve within 1 week, but it may take several weeks for full effect on behavior as well as on cognition
- Classically recommended to wait at least 4–6 weeks to determine efficacy of drug, but in practice some patients may require up to 16–20 weeks to show a good response, especially on cognitive symptoms

If It Works

- Most often reduces positive symptoms but does not eliminate them
- Can improve negative symptoms, as well as aggressive, cognitive, and affective symptoms in schizophrenia
- Most schizophrenia patients do not have a total remission of symptoms but rather a reduction of symptoms by about a third
- Perhaps 5–15% of schizophrenia patients can experience an overall improvement of greater than 50–60%, especially when receiving stable treatment for more than a year
- Such patients are considered super-responders or "awakeners" since they may be well enough to be employed, live independently, and sustain long-term relationships
- Many bipolar patients may experience a reduction of symptoms by half or more
- Continue treatment until reaching a plateau of improvement
- After reaching a satisfactory plateau, continue treatment for at least a year after first episode of psychosis
- For second and subsequent episodes of psychosis, treatment may need to be indefinite
- Even for first episodes of psychosis, it may be preferable to continue treatment
- Treatment may not only reduce mania but also prevent recurrences of mania in bipolar disorder

If It Doesn't Work

- Try one of the other atypical antipsychotics (risperidone, olanzapine, quetiapine, ziprasidone, aripiprazole, paliperidone, iloperidone, amisulpride, lurasidone)
- If 2 or more antipsychotic monotherapies do not work, consider clozapine
- Some patients may require treatment with a conventional antipsychotic
- If no first-line atypical antipsychotic is effective, consider higher doses or augmentation with valproate or lamotrigine
- Consider noncompliance and switch to another antipsychotic with fewer side effects or to an antipsychotic that can be given by depot injection

- Consider initiating rehabilitation and psychotherapy such as cognitive remediation
- Consider presence of concomitant drug abuse

Best Augmenting Combos for Partial Response or Treatment Resistance

- Valproic acid (valproate, divalproex, divalproex ER)
- Other mood-stabilizing anticonvulsants (carbamazepine, oxcarbazepine, lamotrigine)
- Lithium
- Benzodiazepines

Tests

Before starting an a typical antipsychotic

* Weigh all patients and track BMI during treatment
- Get baseline personal and family history of diabetes, obesity, dyslipidemia, hypertension, and cardiovascular disease
* Get waist circumference (at umbilicus), blood pressure, fasting plasma glucose, and fasting lipid profile
- Determine if the patient is
  - overweight (BMI 25.0–29.9)
  - obese (BMI >30)
  - has pre-diabetes (fasting plasma glucose 100–125 mg/dL)
  - has diabetes (fasting plasma glucose >126 mg/dL)
  - has hypertension (BP >140/90 mm Hg)
  - has dyslipidemia (increased total cholesterol, LDL cholesterol, and triglycerides; decreased HDL cholesterol)
- Treat or refer such patients for treatment, including nutrition and weight management, physical activity counseling, smoking cessation, and medical management

Monitoring after starting an atypical antipsychotic

* BMI monthly for 3 months, then quarterly
* Consider monitoring fasting triglycerides monthly for several months in patients at high risk for metabolic complications and when initiating or switching antipsychotics
* Blood pressure, fasting plasma glucose, fasting lipids within 3 months and then annually, but earlier and more frequently for patients with diabetes or who have gained >5% of initial weight
- Treat or refer for treatment and consider switching to another atypical antipsychotic for patients who become overweight, obese, pre-diabetic, diabetic, hypertensive, or dyslipidemic while receiving an atypical antipsychotic
* Even in patients without known diabetes, be vigilant for the rare but life-threatening onset of diabetic ketoacidosis, which always requires immediate treatment, by monitoring for the rapid onset of polyuria, polydipsia, weight loss, nausea, vomiting, dehydration, rapid respiration, weakness and clouding of sensorium, even coma
- Patients with low white blood cell count (WBC) or history of drug-induced leucopenia/neutropenia should have complete blood count (CBC) monitored frequently during the first few months and asenapine should be discontinued at the first sign of decline in WBC in the absence of other causative factors

SIDE EFFECTS

How Drug Causes Side Effects

- By blocking alpha 1 adrenergic receptors, it can cause dizziness, sedation, and hypotension
- By blocking dopamine 2 receptors in the striatum, it can cause motor side effects
- By blocking dopamine 2 receptors in the pituitary, it can theoretically cause elevations in prolactin
- Mechanism of weight gain and increased incidence of diabetes and dyslipidemia with atypical antipsychotics is unknown

Notable Side Effects

* Sedation, dizziness
- Oral hypoesthesia
- Application site reactions: oral ulcers, blisters, peeling/sloughing, inflammation
* Extrapyramidal symptoms, akathisia
* May increase risk for diabetes and dyslipidemia
- Rare tardive dyskinesia (much reduced risk compared to conventional antipsychotics)
- Orthostatic hypotension

Life-Threatening or Dangerous Side Effects

- Type 1 hypersensitivity reactions (anaphylaxis, angioedema, low blood pressure, rapid heart rate, swollen tongue, difficulty breathing, wheezing, rash)

- Hyperglycemia, in some cases extreme and associated with ketoacidosis or hyperosmolar coma or death, has been reported in patients taking atypical antipsychotics
- Increased risk of death and cerebrovascular events in elderly patients with dementia-related psychosis
- Rare neuroleptic malignant syndrome (much reduced risk compared to conventional antipsychotics)
- Rare seizures

Weight Gain

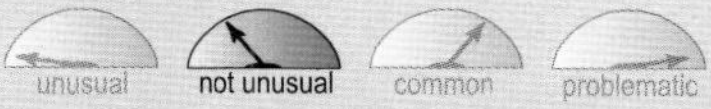

- Occurs in a significant minority
- May be less than for some antipsychotics, more than for others

Sedation

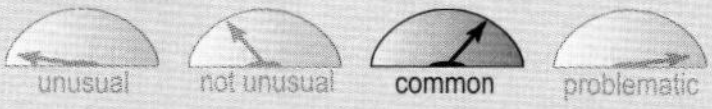

- Many experience and/or can be significant in amount

What to Do About Side Effects

- Wait
- Wait
- Wait
- Anticholinergics may reduce motor side effects when present
- Weight loss, exercise programs, and medical management for high BMIs, diabetes, dyslipidemia
- Switch to another atypical antipsychotic

Best Augmenting Agents for Side Effects

- Benztropine or trihexyphenidyl for motor side effects
- Many side effects cannot be improved with an augmenting agent

DOSING AND USE

Usual Dosage Range

- 10–20 mg/day in 2 divided doses for schizophrenia
- 10–20 mg/day in 2 divided doses for bipolar mania

Dosage Forms

- Sublingual tablet 2.5 mg, 5 mg, 10 mg

How to Dose

- Must be administered sublingually; patients may not eat or drink for 10 minutes following administration
- Schizophrenia: initial 10 mg/day in 2 divided doses; maximum dose generally 20 mg/day in 2 divided doses; limited experience with once daily administration
- Bipolar mania (adults, monotherapy): initial 20 mg/day in 2 divided doses; can reduce dose to 10 mg/day in 2 divided doses if there are adverse effects
- Bipolar mania (adults, adjunct): initial 10 mg/day in 2 divided doses; can increase to 20 mg/day in 2 divided doses
- Bipolar mania (children, monotherapy): initial 5 mg/day in 2 divided doses; after 3 days can increase to 10 mg/day in 2 divided doses; after 3 more days can increase to 20 mg/day in 2 divided doses
- Pediatric patients may be more sensitive to dystonia with initial dosing if the recommended titration schedule is not followed

Dosing Tips

- Asenapine is not absorbed after swallowing (less than 2% bioavailable orally) and thus must be administered sublingually (35% bioavailable), as swallowing would render asenapine inactive
- Patients should be instructed to place the tablet under the tongue and allow it to dissolve completely, which will occur in seconds; tablet should not be divided, crushed, chewed, or swallowed
- Patients may not eat or drink for 10 minutes following sublingual administration so that the drug in the oral cavity can be absorbed locally and not washed into the stomach (where it would not be absorbed)
- Once daily use seems theoretically possible because the half-life of asenapine is 13–39 hours, but this has not been extensively studied and may be limited by the need to expose the limited sublingual surface area to a limited amount of sublingual drug dosage
- Some patients may respond to doses greater than 20 mg/day but no single administration should be greater than 10 mg, thus necessitating 3 or 4 separate daily doses

- Due to rapid onset of action, can be used as a rapid acting "prn" or "as needed" dose for agitation or transient worsening of psychosis or mania instead of an injection
- Treatment should be suspended if absolute neutrophil count falls below 1,000/mm^3

Overdose
- Agitation, confusion

Long-Term Use
- Not studied, but long-term maintenance treatment is often necessary for schizophrenia and bipolar disorder

Habit Forming
- No

How to Stop
- Down-titration, over 2–4 weeks when possible, especially when simultaneously beginning a new antipsychotic while switching (i.e., cross-titration)
- Rapid discontinuation could theoretically lead to rebound psychosis and worsening of symptoms

Pharmacokinetics
- Half-life 13–39 hours
- Inhibits CYP450 2D6
- Substrate for CYP450 1A2
- Optimal bioavailability is with sublingual administration (~35%); if food or liquid is consumed within 10 minutes of administration bioavailability decreases to 28%; bioavailability decreases to 2% if swallowed

Drug Interactions
- May increase effects of antihypertensive agents
- May antagonize levodopa, dopamine agonists
- CYP450 1A2 inhibitors (e.g., fluvoxamine) can raise asenapine levels
- Via CYP450 2D6 inhibition, asenapine could theoretically interfere with the analgesic effects of codeine, and increase the plasma levels of some beta blockers and of atomoxetine
- Via CYP450 2D6 inhibition, asenapine could theoretically increase concentrations of thioridazine and cause dangerous cardiac arrhythmias

Other Warnings/ Precautions
- Use with caution in patients with conditions that predispose to hypotension (dehydration, overheating)
- Dysphagia has been associated with antipsychotic use, and asenapine should be used cautiously in patients at risk for aspiration pneumonia

Do Not Use
- If there is a proven allergy to asenapine

SPECIAL POPULATIONS

Renal Impairment
- Dose adjustment not generally necessary

Hepatic Impairment
- No dose adjustment necessary for mild to moderate impairment
- Not recommended for patients with severe hepatic impairment

Cardiac Impairment
- Drug should be used with caution because of risk of orthostatic hypotension

Elderly
- Some patients may tolerate lower doses better
- Although atypical antipsychotics are commonly used for behavioral disturbances in dementia, no agent has been approved for treatment of elderly patients with dementia-related psychosis
- Elderly patients with dementia-related psychosis treated with atypical antipsychotics are at an increased risk of death compared to placebo, and also have an increased risk of cerebrovascular events

Children and Adolescents
- Approved to treat acute manic/mixed episodes of bipolar I disorder in children ages 10 and older
- Children and adolescents using asenapine may need to be monitored more often than adults

Pregnancy

- Effective June 30, 2015, the US FDA requires changes to the content and format of pregnancy and lactation information in prescription drug labels, including the elimination of the pregnancy letter categories; the Pregnancy and Lactation Labeling Rule (PLLR or final rule) applies only to prescription drugs and will be phased in gradually for drugs approved on or after June 30, 2001
- Controlled studies have not been conducted in pregnant women
- There is a risk of abnormal muscle movements and withdrawal symptoms in newborns whose mothers took an antipsychotic during the third trimester; symptoms may include agitation, abnormally increased or decreased muscle tone, tremor, sleepiness, severe difficulty breathing, and difficulty feeding
- In animal studies, asenapine increased post-implantation loss and decreased pup weight and survival at doses similar to or less than recommended clinical doses; there was no increase in the incidence of structural abnormalities
- Psychotic symptoms may worsen during pregnancy and some form of treatment may be necessary
- Asenapine may be preferable to anticonvulsant mood stabilizers if treatment is required during pregnancy
- National Pregnancy Registry for Atypical Antipsychotics: 1-866-961-2388 or http://womensmentalhealth.org/clinical-and-research-programs/pregnancyregistry/

Breast Feeding

- Unknown if asenapine is secreted in human breast milk, but all psychotropics assumed to be secreted in breast milk
- ✻ Recommended either to discontinue drug or bottle feed
- Infants of women who choose to breast feed while on asenapine should be monitored for possible adverse effects

THE ART OF PSYCHOPHARMACOLOGY

Potential Advantages

- Patients requiring rapid onset of antipsychotic action without dosage titration

Potential Disadvantages

- Patients who are less likely to be adherent

Primary Target Symptoms

- Positive symptoms of psychosis
- Negative symptoms of psychosis
- Cognitive symptoms
- Unstable mood (both depression and mania)
- Aggressive symptoms

Pearls

- Asenapine's chemical structure is related to the antidepressant mirtazapine and it shares many of the same pharmacologic binding properties of mirtazapine plus many others
- Not approved for depression, but binding properties suggest potential use in treatment-resistant and bipolar depression
- Sublingual administration may require prescribing asenapine to reliable, adherent patients, or those who have someone who can supervise drug administration
- Patients with inadequate responses to atypical antipsychotics may benefit from determination of plasma drug levels and, if low, a dosage increase even beyond the usual prescribing limits
- Patients with inadequate responses to atypical antipsychotics may also benefit from a trial of augmentation with a conventional antipsychotic or switching to a conventional antipsychotic
- However, long-term polypharmacy with a combination of a conventional antipsychotic with an atypical antipsychotic may combine their side effects without clearly augmenting the efficacy of either
- For treatment-resistant patients, especially those with impulsivity, aggression, violence, and self-harm, long-term polypharmacy with 2 atypical antipsychotics or with 1 atypical antipsychotic and 1 conventional

antipsychotic may be useful or even necessary while closely monitoring
- In such cases, it may be beneficial to combine 1 depot antipsychotic with 1 oral antipsychotic
- Although a frequent practice by some prescribers, adding 2 conventional antipsychotics together has little rationale and may reduce tolerability without clearly enhancing efficacy

THE ART OF SWITCHING

Switching from Oral Antipsychotics to Asenapine

- With aripiprazole, amisulpride, and paliperidone ER, immediate stop is possible; begin asenapine at middle dose
- With risperidone, ziprasidone, iloperidone, and luasidone: begin asenapine gradually, titrating over at least 2 weeks to allow patients to become tolerant to the sedating effect

* May need to taper clozapine slowly over 4 weeks or longer

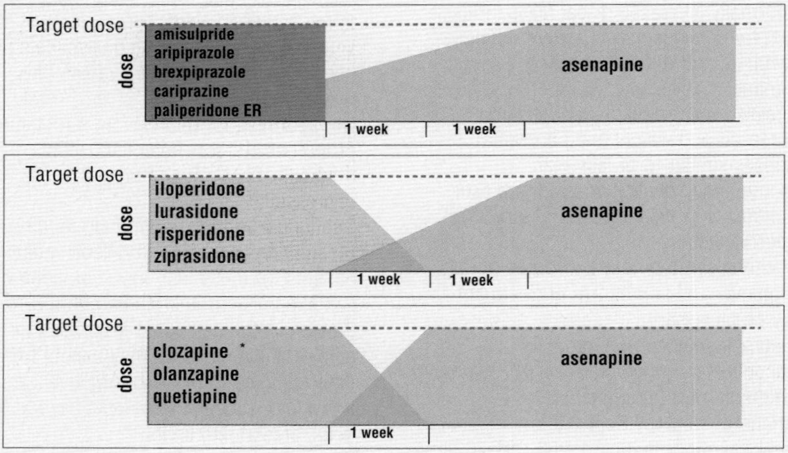

Suggested Reading

Citrome L. Asenapine for schizophrenia and bipolar disorder: a review of the efficacy and safety profile for this newly approved sublingually absorbed second-generation antipsychotic. Int J Clin Pract 2009;63(12):1762–84.

Shahid M, Walker GB, Zorn SH, Wong EH. Asenapine: a novel psychopharmacologic agent with a unique human receptor signature. J Psychopharmacol 2009;23(1):65–73.

Tarazi F, Stahl SM. Iloperidone, asenapine and lurasidone: a primer on their current status. Exp Opin Pharmacother 2012;13(13):1911–22.

THERAPEUTICS

Brands • Strattera

see index for additional brand names

Generic? Yes

Class

- Neuroscience-based Nomenclature: norepinephrine reuptake inhibitor (N-RI)
- Selective norepinephrine reuptake inhibitor (NRI)

Commonly Prescribed for

(bold for FDA approved)

- **Attention deficit hyperactivity disorder (ADHD) in adults and children over 6**
- Treatment-resistant depression

How the Drug Works

- Boosts neurotransmitter norepinephrine/ noradrenaline and may also increase dopamine in profrontal cortex
- Blocks norepinephrine reuptake pumps, also known as norepinephrine transporters
- Presumably this increases noradrenergic neurotransmission
- Since dopamine is inactivated by norepinephrine reuptake in frontal cortex, which largely lacks dopamine transporters, atomoxetine can also increase dopamine neurotransmission in this part of the brain

How Long Until It Works

✻ Onset of therapeutic actions in ADHD can be seen as early as the first day of dosing
- Therapeutic actions may continue to improve for 8–12 weeks
- If it is not working within 6–8 weeks, it may not work at all

If It Works

- The goal of treatment of ADHD is reduction of symptoms of inattentiveness, motor hyperactivity, and/or impulsiveness that disrupt social, school, and/or occupational functioning
- Continue treatment until all symptoms are under control or improvement is stable and then continue treatment indefinitely as long as improvement persists
- Reevaluate the need for treatment periodically
- Treatment for ADHD begun in childhood may need to be continued into adolescence and adulthood if continued benefit is documented

If It Doesn't Work

- Consider adjusting dose or switching to another agent
- Consider behavioral therapy
- Consider the presence of noncompliance and counsel patient and parents
- Consider evaluation for another diagnosis or for a comorbid condition (e.g., bipolar disorder, substance abuse, medical illness, etc.)
- Some patients may experience apparent lack of consistent efficacy due to activation of latent or underlying bipolar disorder, and require atomoxetine discontinuation and a switch to a mood stabilizer

Best Augmenting Combos for Partial Response or Treatment Resistance

✻ Best to attempt other monotherapies prior to augmenting
- SSRIs, SNRIs, or mirtazapine for treatment-resistant depression (use combinations of antidepressants with atomoxetine with caution as this may theoretically activate bipolar disorder and suicidal ideation)
- Mood stabilizers or atypical antipsychotics for comorbid bipolar disorder
- For the expert, can combine with modafinil, methylphenidate, or amphetamine for ADHD

Tests

- None recommended for healthy patients
- May be prudent to monitor blood pressure and pulse when initiating treatment and until dosage increments have stabilized

SIDE EFFECTS

How Drug Causes Side Effects

- Norepinephrine increases in parts of the brain and body and at receptors other than those that cause therapeutic actions (e.g., unwanted actions of norepinephrine on acetylcholine release causing decreased appetite, increased heart rate and blood pressure, dry mouth, urinary retention, etc.)

- Most side effects are immediate but often go away with time
- Lack of enhancing dopamine activity in limbic areas theoretically explains atomoxetine's lack of abuse potential

Notable Side Effects

✻ Sedation, fatigue (particularly in children)
✻ Decreased appetite
✻ Rare priapism
- Increased heart rate (6–9 beats/min)
- Increased blood pressure (2–4 mm Hg)
- Insomnia, dizziness, anxiety, agitation, aggression, irritability
- Dry mouth, constipation, nausea, vomiting, abdominal pain, dyspepsia
- Urinary hesitancy, urinary retention (older men)
- Dysmenorrhea, sweating
- Sexual dysfunction (men: decreased libido, erectile disturbance, impotence, ejaculatory dysfunction, abnormal orgasm; women: decreased libido, abnormal orgasm)

Life-Threatening or Dangerous Side Effects

- Increased heart rate and hypertension
- Orthostatic hypotension
- Severe liver damage (rare)
- Hypomania and, theoretically, rare induction of mania
- Rare activation of suicidal ideation and behavior (suicidality) (short-term studies did not show an increase in the risk of suicidality with antidepressants compared to placebo beyond age 24)

Weight Gain

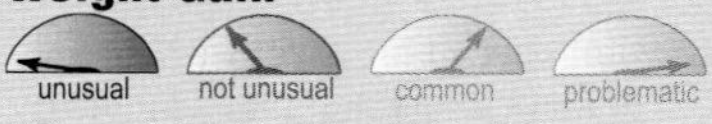

- Reported but not expected
- Patients may experience weight loss

Sedation

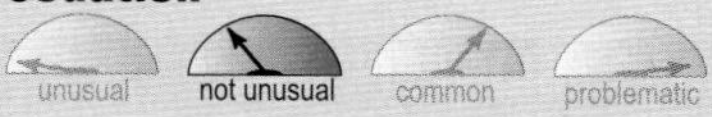

- Occurs in significant minority, particularly in children

What to Do About Side Effects

- Wait
- Wait
- Wait
- Lower the dose
- If giving once daily, can change to split dose twice daily
- If atomoxetine is sedating, take at night to reduce daytime drowsiness
- In a few weeks, switch or add other drugs

Best Augmenting Agents for Side Effects

- For urinary hesitancy, give an alpha 1 blocker such as tamsulosin
- Often best to try another monotherapy prior to resorting to augmentation strategies to treat side effects
- Many side effects are dose-dependent (i.e., they increase as dose increases, or they reemerge until tolerance redevelops)
- Many side effects are time-dependent (i.e., they start immediately upon dosing and upon each dose increase, but go away with time)
- Activation and agitation may represent the induction of a bipolar state, especially a mixed dysphoric bipolar II condition sometimes associated with suicidal ideation, and require the addition of lithium, a mood stabilizer or an atypical antipsychotic, and/or discontinuation of atomoxetine

DOSING AND USE

Usual Dosage Range

- 0.5–1.2 mg/kg/day in children up to 70 kg; 40–100 mg/day in adults

Dosage Forms

- Capsule 10 mg, 18 mg, 25 mg, 40 mg, 60 mg, 80 mg, 100 mg

How to Dose

- For children 70 kg or less: initial dose 0.5 mg/kg per day; after 7 days can increase to 1.2 mg/kg per day either once in the morning or divided; maximum dose 1.4 mg/kg per day or 100 mg/day, whichever is less
- For adults and children over 70 kg: initial dose 40 mg/day; after 7 days can increase to 80 mg/day once in the morning or divided; after 2–4 weeks can increase to 100 mg/day if necessary; maximum daily dose 100 mg

Dosing Tips

- Can be given once a day in the morning
- ✻ Efficacy with once daily dosing despite a half-life of 5 hours suggests therapeutic effects persist beyond direct pharmacologic effects, unlike stimulants whose effects are generally closely correlated with plasma drug levels
- Once daily dosing may increase gastrointestinal side effects
- Lower starting dose allows detection of those patients who may be especially sensitive to side effects such as tachycardia and increased blood pressure
- Patients especially sensitive to the side effects of atomoxetine may include those individuals deficient in the enzyme that metabolizes atomoxetine, CYP450 2D6 (i.e., 7% of Caucasians and 2% of African Americans)
- In such individuals, drug should be titrated slowly to tolerability and effectiveness
- Other individuals may require up to 1.8 mg/kg total daily dose

Overdose

- No fatalities have been reported as monotherapy; sedation, agitation, hyperactivity, abnormal behavior, gastrointestinal symptoms

Long-Term Use

- Safe

Habit Forming

- No

How to Stop

- Taper not necessary

Pharmacokinetics

- Metabolized by CYP450 2D6
- Half-life approximately 5 hours
- Food does not affect absorption

Drug Interactions

- Tramadol increases the risk of seizures in patients taking an antidepressant
- Plasma concentrations of atomoxetine may be increased by drugs that inhibit CYP450 2D6 (e.g., paroxetine, fluoxetine), so atomoxetine dose may need to be reduced if coadministered
- Coadministration of atomoxetine and oral or IV albuterol may lead to increases in heart rate and blood pressure
- Coadministration with methylphenidate does not increase cardiovascular side effects beyond those seen with methylphenidate alone
- Use with caution with MAOIs, including 14 days after MAOIs are stopped (for the expert)

Other Warnings/ Precautions

- Growth (height and weight) should be monitored during treatment with atomoxetine; for patients who are not growing or gaining weight satisfactorily, interruption of treatment should be considered
- Use with caution in patients with hypertension, tachycardia, cardiovascular disease, or cerebrovascular disease
- Use with caution in patients with bipolar disorder
- Use with caution in patients with urinary retention, benign prostatic hypertrophy
- Rare reports of hepatotoxicity; although causality has not been established, atomoxetine should be discontinued in patients who develop jaundice or other evidence of significant liver dysfunction
- Use with caution with antihypertensive drugs
- Increased risk of sudden death has been reported in children with structural cardiac abnormalities or other serious heart conditions
- When treating children, carefully weigh the risks and benefits of pharmacological treatment against the risks and benefits of nontreatment and make sure to document this in the patient's chart
- Distribute the brochures provided by the FDA and the drug companies
- Warn patients and their caregivers about the possibility of activating side effects and advise them to report such symptoms immediately
- Monitor patients for activation of suicidal ideation, especially children and adolescents

Do Not Use

- If patient is taking an MAOI (except as noted under drug interactions)

- If patient has pheochromocytoma or history of pheochromocytoma
- If patient has a severe cardiovascular disorder that might deteriorate with clinically important increases in heart rate and blood pressure
- If patient has angle-closure glaucoma
- If there is a proven allergy to atomoxetine

SPECIAL POPULATIONS

Renal Impairment
- Dose adjustment not generally necessary

Hepatic Impairment
- For patients with moderate liver impairment, dose should be reduced to 50% of normal dose
- For patients with severe liver impairment, dose should be reduced to 25% of normal dose

Cardiac Impairment
- Use with caution because atomoxetine can increase heart rate and blood pressure
- Do not use in patients with structural cardiac abnormalities

Elderly
- Some patients may tolerate lower doses better
- Reduction in the risk of suicidality with antidepressants compared to placebo in adults age 65 and older

Children and Adolescents
- Approved to treat ADHD in children over age 6
- Recommended target dose is 1.2 mg/kg per day
- Do not use in children with structural cardiac abnormalities or other serious cardiac problems
- Carefully weigh the risks and benefits of pharmacological treatment against the risks and benefits of nontreatment and make sure to document this in the patient's chart
- Monitor patients face-to-face regularly, particularly during the first several weeks of treatment
- Use with caution, observing for activation of known or unknown bipolar disorder and/or suicidal ideation, and inform parents or guardians of this risk so they can help observe child or adolescent patients

Pregnancy
- Effective June 30, 2015, the US FDA requires changes to the content and format of pregnancy and lactation information in prescription drug labels, including the elimination of the pregnancy letter categories; the Pregnancy and Lactation Labeling Rule (PLLR or final rule) applies only to prescription drugs and will be phased in gradually for drugs approved on or after June 30, 2001
- Controlled studies have not been conducted in pregnant women
- Some animal studies have shown adverse effects
- Use in women of childbearing potential requires weighing potential benefits to the mother against potential risks to the fetus

✻ For women of childbearing potential, atomoxetine should generally be discontinued before anticipated pregnancies

Breast Feeding
- Unknown if atomoxetine is secreted in human breast milk, but all psychotropics assumed to be secreted in breast milk

✻ Recommend either to discontinue drug or bottle feed

THE ART OF PSYCHOPHARMACOLOGY

Potential Advantages
- No known abuse potential

Potential Disadvantages
- May not act as rapidly as stimulants when initiating treatment in some patients

Primary Target Symptoms
- Concentration, attention span
- Motor hyperactivity
- Depressed mood

Pearls

- ✻ Unlike other agents approved for ADHD, atomoxetine does not have abuse potential and is not a scheduled substance
- ✻ Despite its name as a selective norepinephrine reuptake inhibitor, atomoxetine enhances both dopamine and norepinephrine in frontal cortex, presumably accounting for its therapeutic actions on attention and concentration
- Since dopamine is inactivated by norepinephrine reuptake in frontal cortex, which largely lacks dopamine transporters, atomoxetine can increase dopamine as well as norepinephrine in this part of the brain, presumably causing therapeutic actions in ADHD
- Since dopamine is inactivated by dopamine reuptake in nucleus accumbens, which largely lacks norepinephrine transporters, atomoxetine does not increase dopamine in this part of the brain, presumably explaining why atomoxetine lacks abuse potential
- Atomoxetine's known mechanism of action as a selective norepinephrine reuptake inhibitor suggests its efficacy as an antidepressant
- Pro-noradrenergic actions may be theoretically useful for the treatment of chronic pain
- Atomoxetine's mechanism of action and its potential antidepressant actions suggest it has the potential to destabilize latent or undiagnosed bipolar disorder, similar to the known actions of proven antidepressants
- Thus, administer with caution to ADHD patients who may also have bipolar disorder
- Unlike stimulants, atomoxetine may not exacerbate tics in Tourette's syndrome patients with comorbid ADHD
- Urinary retention in men over 50 with borderline urine flow has been observed with other agents with potent norepinephrine reuptake blocking properties (e.g., reboxetine, milnacipran), so administer atomoxetine with caution to these patients
- Atomoxetine was originally called tomoxetine but the name was changed to avoid potential confusion with tamoxifen, which might lead to errors in drug dispensing

Suggested Reading

Garnock-Jones KP, Keating GM. Atomoxetine: a review of its use in attention-deficit hyperactivity disorder in children and adolescents. Paediatr Drugs 2009;11(3):203–26.

Kelsey D, Sumner C, Casat C, et al. Once daily atomoxetine treatment for children with attention deficit hyperactivity behavior including an assessment of evening and morning behavior: a double-blind, placebo-controlled trial. Pediatrics 2004;114:el–8.

Michelson D, Adler LL, Spencer T, et al. Atomoxetine in adults with ADHD: two randomized, placebo-controlled studies. Biol Psychiatry 2003;53(2):112–20.

Michelson D, Buitelaar JK, Danckaerts M, et al. Relapse prevention in pediatric patients with ADHD treated with atomoxetine: a randomized, double-blind, placebo-controlled study. J Am Acad Child Adolesc Psychiatry 2004;43(7): 896–904.

Stiefel G, Besag FM. Cardiovascular effects of methylphenidate, amphetamines, and atomoxetine in the treatment of attention-deficit hyperactivity disorder. Drug Saf 2010;33(10):821–42.

BENZTROPINE

THERAPEUTICS

Brands • Cogentin

see index for additional brand names

Generic? Yes

Class
- Antiparkinson agent; anticholinergic

Commonly Prescribed for
(bold for FDA approved)
- **Extrapyramidal disorders**
- **Parkinsonism**
- Acute dystonic reactions
- Idiopathic generalized dystonia
- Focal dystonias
- Dopa-responsive dystonia

How the Drug Works
- Diminishes the excess acetylcholine activity caused by removal of dopamine inhibition when dopamine receptors are blocked
- May also inhibit the reuptake and storage of dopamine at central dopamine receptors, prolonging dopamine action

How Long Until It Works
- For extrapyramidal disorders and parkinsonism, onset of action can be within minutes or hours

If It Works
- Reduces motor side effects
- Does not lessen the ability of antipsychotics to cause tardive dyskinesia

If It Doesn't Work
- Consider switching to trihexyphenidyl, diphenhydramine, or a benzodiazepine
- Disorders that develop after prolonged antipsychotic use may not respond to treatment
- Consider discontinuing the agent that precipitated the EPS

Best Augmenting Combos for Partial Response or Treatment Resistance
- If ineffective, switch to another agent rather than augment
- Benztropine is itself an augmenting agent to antipsychotics

Tests
- None for healthy individuals

SIDE EFFECTS

How Drug Causes Side Effects
- Prevents the action of acetylcholine on muscarinic receptors

Notable Side Effects
- Dry mouth, blurred vision, diplopia
- Confusion, hallucinations
- Constipation, nausea, vomiting
- Dilation of colon/paralytic ileus/bowel obstruction
- Erectile dysfunction

Life-Threatening or Dangerous Side Effects
- Angle-closure glaucoma
- Heat stroke, especially in elderly patients
- Tachycardia, cardiac arrhythmias, hypotension
- Urinary retention
- Anticholinergic agents such as benztropine can exacerbate or unmask tardive dyskinesia

Weight Gain

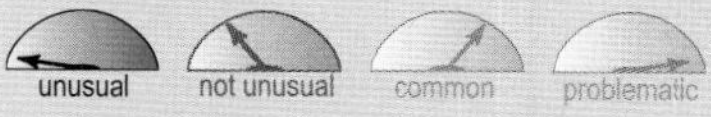

- Reported but not expected

Sedation

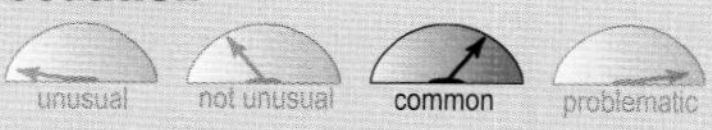

- Many experience and/or can be significant in amount

What to Do About Side Effects
- For confusion or hallucinations, discontinue use
- For sedation, lower the dose and/or take the entire dose at night
- For dry mouth, chew gum or drink water
- For urinary retention, obtain a urological evaluation; may need to discontinue use

Best Augmenting Agents for Side Effects
- Many side effects cannot be improved with an augmenting agent

DOSING AND USE

Usual Dosage Range
- Extrapyramidal disorders: 2–8 mg/day
- Parkinsonism: 0.5–6 mg/day

Dosage Forms
- Tablet 0.5 mg, 1 mg, 2 mg
- Injection 1 mg/mL

How to Dose
- Extrapyramidal disorders: 1–4 mg once or twice daily; can be given orally or parenterally
- Parkinsonism (oral): initial 0.5 mg once daily; increase by 0.5 mg at 5–6 day intervals until desired efficacy is reached

Dosing Tips
- If drug-induced EPS occur soon after initiation of a neuroleptic drug, they are likely to be transient; thus, attempt to withdraw benztropine after 1–2 weeks to determine if still needed
- Patients may take benztropine once daily at night to improve sleep and allow for earlier rising in the morning
- Taking benztropine with meals can reduce side effects
- Intramuscular and intravenous dosing are equally effective and fast acting

Overdose
- Circulatory collapse, cardiac arrest, respiratory depression or arrest, psychosis, shock, coma, seizure, ataxia, combativeness, anhidrosis and hyperthermia, fever, dysphagia, decreased bowel sounds, sluggish pupils

Long-Term Use
- Safe
- Effectiveness may decrease over time (years), and side effects such as sedation and cognitive impairment may worsen

Habit Forming
- No

How to Stop
- Taper not necessary

Pharmacokinetics
- Half-life 36 hours, although greatest effect lasts about 6–8 hours
- Metabolism is not well understood

Drug Interactions
- Use with amantadine may increase side effects
- Benztropine and all other anticholinergic agents may increase serum levels and effects of digoxin
- Can lower concentration of haloperidol and other phenothiazines, causing worsening of schizophrenia symptoms
- Can decrease gastric motility, resulting in increased gastric deactivation of levodopa and reduction in efficacy

Other Warnings/ Precautions
- Use with caution in hot weather, as benztropine may increase susceptibility to heat stroke
- Anticholinergic agents have additive effects when used with drugs of abuse such as cannabinoids, barbiturates, opioids, and alcohol

Do Not Use
- In patients with glaucoma, particularly angle-closure glaucoma
- In patients with pyloric or duodenal obstruction, stenosing peptic ulcers, prostate hypertrophy or bladder neck obstructions, achalasia, or megacolon
- If there is a proven allergy to benztropine

SPECIAL POPULATIONS

Renal Impairment
- No known effects, but use with caution

Hepatic Impairment
- No known effects, but use with caution

Cardiac Impairment
- Use with caution in patients with known arrhythmias, especially tachycardia

Elderly
- Use with caution
- Elderly patients may be more susceptible to side effects

Children and Adolescents

- Do not use in children ages 3 and younger
- Generalized dystonias may respond to anticholinergic treatment, and young patients usually tolerate the medication better than the elderly
- Usual dose is 0.05 mg/kg once or twice daily

Pregnancy

- Effective June 30, 2015, the US FDA requires changes to the content and format of pregnancy and lactation information in prescription drug labels, including the elimination of the pregnancy letter categories; the Pregnancy and Lactation Labeling Rule (PLLR or final rule) applies only to prescription drugs and will be phased in gradually for drugs approved on or after June 30, 2001
- Controlled studies have not been conducted in pregnant women

Breast Feeding

- Unknown if benztropine is secreted in human breast milk, but all psychotropics assumed to be secreted in breast milk

✻ Recommended either to discontinue drug or bottle feed unless the potential benefit to the mother justifies the potential risk to the child

- Infants of women who choose to breast feed while on benztropine should be monitored for possible adverse effects

THE ART OF PSYCHOPHARMACOLOGY

Potential Advantages

- Extrapyramidal disorders related to antipsychotic use, particularly in acute setting

Potential Disadvantages

- Patients with long-standing extrapyramidal disorders may not respond to treatment
- Generalized dystonias (less established as treatment than trihexyphenidyl)

Primary Target Symptoms

- Tremor, akinesia, rigidity, drooling

Pearls

- First-line agent for extrapyramidal disorders related to antipsychotic use
- Useful adjunct in younger Parkinson's patients with tremor, but trihexiphenidyl is more commonly used
- Useful in the treatment of post-encephalitic Parkinson's disease and for extrapyramidal reactions, other than tardive dyskinesias
- Post-encephalitic Parkinson's patients usually tolerate higher doses better than idiopathic Parkinson's patients
- Generalized dystonias are more likely to benefit from anticholinergic therapy than focal dystonias; trihexyphenidyl is used more commonly than benztropine
- Sedation limits use, especially in older patients
- Patients with cognitive impairment may do poorly
- Can cause cognitive side effects with chronic use, so periodic trials of discontinuation may be useful to justify continuous use, especially in institutional settings when used as an adjunct to antipsychotics
- Can be abused in institutional or correctional settings
- Commonly used in an oral or intramuscular formulation as needed with concomitant antipsychotics to reduce or prevent EPS

Suggested Reading

Brocks DR. Anticholinergic drugs used in Parkinson's disease: an overlooked class of drugs from a pharmacokinetic perspective. J Pharm Pharm Sci 1999;2(2):39–46.

Colosimo C, Gori MC, Inghilleri M. Postencephalitic tremor and delayed-onset parkinsonism. Parkinsonism Relat Disord 1999;5(3):123–4.

Costa J, Espírito-Santo C, Borges A, et al. Botulinum toxin type A versus anticholinergics for cervical dystonia. Cochrane Database Syst Rev 2005;(1):CD004312.

Hai NT, Kim J, Park ES, Chi SC. Formulation and biopharmaceutical evaluation of transdermal patch containing benztropine. Int J Pharm 2008;357(1–2):55–60.

BLONANSERIN

THERAPEUTICS

Brands • Lonasen
see index for additional brand names

Generic? No

Class

- Atypical antipsychotic (serotonin dopamine antagonist; second-generation antipsychotic; also a potential mood stabilizer)

Commonly Prescribed for

(bold for FDA approved)

- Schizophrenia
- Acute mania/mixed mania
- Other psychotic disorders
- Bipolar maintenance
- Bipolar depression
- Treatment-resistant depression
- Behavioral disturbances in dementia
- Behavioral disturbances in children and adolescents
- Disorders associated with problems with impulse control

How the Drug Works

- Blocks dopamine 2 receptors, reducing positive symptoms of psychosis and stabilizing affective symptoms
- Blocks serotonin 2A receptors, causing enhancement of dopamine release in certain brain regions and thus reducing motor side effects and possibly improving cognition and affective symptoms
- Actions at dopamine 3 receptors could theoretically contribute to blonanserin's efficacy

How Long Until It Works

- Psychotic symptoms can improve within 1 week, but it may take several weeks for full effect on behavior as well as on cognition
- Classically recommended to wait at least 4–6 weeks to determine efficacy of drug, but in practice some patients may require up to 16–20 weeks to show a good response, especially on cognitive impairment and functional outcome

If It Works

- Most often reduces positive symptoms but does not eliminate them
- Can improve negative symptoms, as well as aggressive, cognitive, and affective symptoms in schizophrenia
- Most schizophrenia patients do not have a total remission of symptoms but rather a reduction of symptoms by about a third
- Perhaps 5–15% of schizophrenia patients can experience an overall improvement of greater than 50–60%, especially when receiving stable treatment for more than a year
- Such patients are considered super-responders or "awakeners" since they may be well enough to be employed, live independently, and sustain long-term relationships
- Continue treatment until reaching a plateau of improvement
- After reaching a satisfactory plateau, continue treatment for at least a year after first episode of psychosis
- For second and subsequent episodes of psychosis, treatment may need to be indefinite
- Even for first episodes of psychosis, it may be preferable to continue treatment

If It Doesn't Work

- Try one of the other atypical antipsychotics (risperidone, olanzapine, quetiapine, ziprasidone, aripiprazole, paliperidone, asenapine, iloperidone, lurasidone, amisulpride)
- If 2 or more antipsychotic monotherapies do not work, consider clozapine
- Some patients may require treatment with a conventional antipsychotic
- If no first-line atypical antipsychotic is effective, consider higher doses or augmentation with valproate or lamotrigine
- Consider noncompliance and switch to another antipsychotic with fewer side effects or to an antipsychotic that can be given by depot injection
- Consider initiating rehabilitation and psychotherapy such as cognitive remediation
- Consider presence of concomitant drug abuse

Best Augmenting Combos for Partial Response or Treatment Resistance

- Valproic acid (valproate, divalproex, divalproex ER)
- Mood stabilizing anticonvulsants (carbamazepine, oxcarbazepine, lamotrigine)
- Lithium
- Benzodiazepines

Tests

Before starting any atypical antipsychotic

✻ Weigh all patients and track BMI during treatment
- Get baseline personal and family history of diabetes, obesity, dyslipidemia, hypertension, and cardiovascular disease

✻ Get waist circumference (at umbilicus), blood pressure, fasting plasma glucose, and fasting lipid profile
- Determine if the patient is
  - overweight (BMI 25.0–29.9)
  - obese (BMI >30)
  - has pre-diabetes (fasting plasma glucose 100–125 mg/dl)
  - has diabetes (fasting plasma glucose >126 mg/dl)
  - has hypertension (BP >140/90 mm Hg)
  - has dyslipidemia (increased total cholesterol, LDL cholesterol, and triglycerides; decreased HDL cholesterol)
- Treat or refer such patients for treatment, including nutrition and weight management, physical activity counseling, smoking cessation, and medical management

Monitoring after starting any atypical antipsychotic

✻ BMI monthly for 3 months, then quarterly

✻ Consider monitoring fasting triglycerides monthly for several months in patients at high risk for metabolic complications and when initiating or switching antipsychotics

✻ Blood pressure, fasting plasma glucose, fasting lipids within 3 months and then annually, but earlier and more frequently for patients with diabetes or who have gained >5% of initial weight
- Treat or refer for treatment and consider switching to another atypical antipsychotic for patients who become overweight, obese, pre-diabetic, diabetic, hypertensive, or dyslipidemic while receiving an atypical antipsychotic

✻ Even in patients without known diabetes, be vigilant for the rare but life-threatening onset of diabetic ketoacidosis, which always requires immediate treatment, by monitoring for the rapid onset of polyuria, polydipsia, weight loss, nausea, vomiting, dehydration, rapid respiration, weakness and clouding of sensorium, even coma
- Patients with low white blood cell count (WBC) or history of drug-induced leucopenia/neutropenia should have complete blood count (CBC) monitored frequently during the first few months, and blonanserin should be discontinued at the first sign of decline in WBC in the absence of other causative factors

SIDE EFFECTS

How Drug Causes Side Effects

- By blocking dopamine 2 receptors in the striatum, it can cause motor side effects
- By blocking dopamine 2 receptors in the pituitary, it can cause elevations in prolactin
- Mechanism of weight gain and increased incidence of diabetes and dyslipidemia with atypical antipsychotics is unknown

Notable Side Effects

- Akathisia, EPS
- Insomnia, anxiety, sedation
- Urinary retention
- Theoretical risk of tardive dyskinesia

Life-Threatening or Dangerous Side Effects

- Hyperglycemia, in some cases extreme and associated with ketoacidosis or hyperosmolar coma or death, has been reported in patients taking atypical antipsychotics
- Increased risk of death and cerebrovascular events in elderly patients with dementia-related psychosis
- Rare neuroleptic malignant syndrome (much reduced risk compared to conventional antipsychotics)
- Rare seizures

Weight Gain

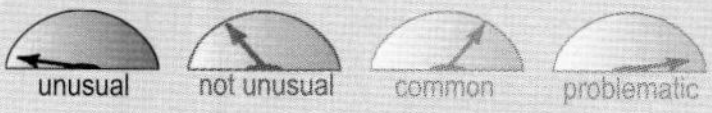

- Reported but not expected

Sedation

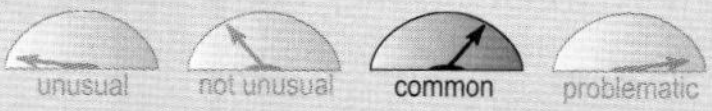

- Many experience and/or can be significant in amount

What to Do About Side Effects

- Wait
- Wait
- Wait
- Anticholinergics may reduce motor side effects when present
- Weight loss, exercise programs, and medical management for high BMIs, diabetes, dyslipidemia
- Switch to another atypical antipsychotic

Best Augmenting Agents for Side Effects

- Benztropine or trihexyphenidyl for motor side effects
- Beta blockers or benzodiazepines may reduce akathisia when present
- Many side effects cannot be improved with an augmenting agent

DOSING AND USE

Usual Dosage Range

- 8–16 mg/day divided in 2 doses

Dosage Forms

- Tablet 2 mg, 4 mg, 8 mg
- Powder 20 mg per 1 g powder

How to Dose

- Initial 8 mg/day divided in 2 doses; maintenance dose 8–16 mg/day divided in 2 doses; maximum dose 24 mg/day
- Blonanserin should be taken after a meal, as maximum concentrations are increased in the fed state; however, because the increase in systemic exposure continues until at least 4 hours after food intake, blonanserin can be taken before bedtime

Dosing Tips

- Start with twice daily dosing; once stabilized, some patients do well with 1 dose given at night

Overdose

- Limited data

Long-Term Use

- Not extensively studied past 56 weeks, but long-term maintenance treatment is often necessary for schizophrenia
- Should periodically reevaluate long-term usefulness in individual patients, but treatment may need to continue for many years in patients with schizophrenia

Habit Forming

- No

How to Stop

- Down-titration, especially when simultaneously beginning a new antipsychotic while switching (i.e., cross-titration)
- Rapid discontinuation could theoretically lead to rebound psychosis and worsening of symptoms

Pharmacokinetics

- Elimination half-life 10–16 hours after single dose
- Metabolized by CYP450 3A4

Drug Interactions

- CYP450 3A4 inducers, such as carbamazepine, can lower the plasma levels of blonanserin
- CYP450 3A4 inhibitors, such as ketoconazole, nefazodone, fluvoxamine, and fluoxetine, can increase plasma levels of blonanserin
- May increase effects of antihypertensive agents
- May antagonize levodopa, dopamine agonists

Other Warnings/ Precautions

- Use with caution in patients with conditions that predispose to hypotension (dehydration, overheating)
- Dysphagia has been associated with antipsychotic use, and blonanserin should be used cautiously in patients at risk for aspiration pneumonia

Do Not Use

- In conjunction with adrenaline/epinephrine
- If patient is taking ketoconazole
- If there is a proven allergy to blonanserin

SPECIAL POPULATIONS

Renal Impairment

- Not studied

Hepatic Impairment

- Use with caution; may need to lower dose

Cardiac Impairment

- Use in patients with cardiac impairment has not been studied, so use with caution

Elderly

- Some patients may tolerate lower doses better
- Although atypical antipsychotics are commonly used for behavioral disturbances in dementia, no agent has been approved for treatment of elderly patients with dementia-related psychosis
- Elderly patients with dementia-related psychosis treated with atypical antipsychotics are at an increased risk of death compared to placebo and also have an increased risk of cerebrovascular events

Children and Adolescents

- Safety and efficacy have not been established
- Children and adolescents using blonanserin may need to be monitored more often than adults

Pregnancy

- Controlled studies have not been conducted in pregnant women
- Psychotic symptoms may worsen during pregnancy, and some form of treatment may be necessary

Breast Feeding

- Unknown if blonanserin is secreted in human breast milk, but all psychotropics assumed to be secreted in breast milk
- ✻ Recommended either to discontinue drug or bottle feed unless the potential benefit to the mother justifies the potential risk to the child
- Infants of women who choose to breast feed while on blonanserin should be monitored for possible adverse effects

THE ART OF PSYCHOPHARMACOLOGY

Potential Advantages

- May be useful when other antipsychotics have failed to provide adequate response or have not been tolerated

Potential Disadvantages

- Patients who require once daily dosing from the initiation of treatment
- Patients who require intramuscular administration

Primary Target Symptoms

- Positive symptoms of psychosis
- Negative symptoms of psychosis
- Cognitive symptoms
- Unstable mood (both depression and mania)
- Aggressive symptoms

Pearls

- Relatively selective binding profile
- Not approved for mania, but almost all atypical antipsychotics approved for acute treatment of schizophrenia have proven effective in the acute treatment of mania as well

Suggested Reading

Deeks ED, Keating GM. Blonanserin. A review of its use in the management of schizophrenia. CNS Drugs 2010;24(1):65–84.

Hida H, Mouri A, Mori K, et al. Blonanserin ameliorates phencyclidine-induced visual-recognition memory deficits: the complex mechanism of blonanserin action involving D3-5-HT2A and D1-NMDA receptors in the mPFC. Neuropsychopharmacology 2015;40(3):601–13.

Kishi T, Matsuda Y, Nakamura H, Iwata N. Blonanserin for schizophrenia: a systematic review and meta-analysis of double-blind, randomized, controlled trials. J Psychiatr Res 2013;47(2):149–54.

Yang J, Bahk WM, Cho HS, et al. Efficacy and tolerability of blonanserin in the patients with schizophrenia: a randomized, double-blind, risperidone-compared trial. Clin Neuropharmacol 2010;33(4):169–75.

THERAPEUTICS

Brands • Rexulti

see index for additional brand names

Generic? No

Class

- Dopamine partial agonist (dopamine stabilizer, atypical antipsychotic, third-generation antipsychotic; sometimes included as a second-generation antipsychotic; also a potential mood stabilizer)

Commonly Prescribed for

(bold for FDA approved)

- **Schizophrenia**
- **Treatment-resistant depression (adjunct)**
- Acute mania/mixed mania
- Other psychotic disorders
- Bipolar maintenance
- Bipolar depression
- Behavioral disturbances in dementia
- Behavioral disturbances in children and adolescents
- Disorders associated with problems with impulse control

How the Drug Works

* Partial agonism at dopamine 2 receptors
- Theoretically reduces dopamine output when dopamine concentrations are high, thus improving positive symptoms and mediating antipsychotic actions
- Theoretically increases dopamine output when dopamine concentrations are low, thus improving cognitive, negative, and mood symptoms
- Partial agonist at 5HT1A receptors, which may be beneficial for mood, anxiety, and cognition in a number of disorders
- Blockade of serotonin type 2A receptors may contribute at clinical doses to cause enhancement of dopamine release in certain brain regions, thus reducing motor side effects and possibly improving cognitive and affective symptoms
- Blockade of alpha 1B receptors may reduce motor side effects such as akathisia
- Blockade of alpha 2C receptors may contribute to antidepressant actions
- Actions at dopamine 3 receptors could theoretically contribute to brexpiprazole's efficacy
- Blocks serotonin 7 receptors, which may be beneficial for mood, cognitive impairment, and negative symptoms in schizophrenia, and also in bipolar disorder and major depressive disorder

How Long Until It Works

- Psychotic symptoms can improve within 1 week, but it may take several weeks for full effect on behavior as well as on cognition
- For psychosis, classically recommended to wait at least 4–6 weeks to determine efficacy of drug, but in practice some patients may require up to 16–20 weeks to show a good response, especially on cognitive impairment and functional outcome
- For depression, onset of therapeutic actions usually not immediate, but often delayed 2–4 weeks

If It Works (for Schizophrenia)

- Most often reduces positive symptoms but does not eliminate them
- Can improve negative symptoms, as well as aggressive, cognitive, and affective symptoms in schizophrenia
- Most schizophrenia patients do not have a total remission of symptoms but rather a reduction of symptoms by about a third
- Perhaps 5–15% of schizophrenia patients can experience an overall improvement of greater than 50–60%, especially when receiving stable treatment for more than a year
- Such patients are considered super-responders or "awakeners" since they may be well enough to be employed, live independently, and sustain long-term relationships
- Continue treatment until reaching a plateau of improvement
- After reaching a satisfactory plateau, continue treatment for at least a year after first episode of psychosis
- For second and subsequent episodes of psychosis, treatment may need to be indefinite
- Even for first episodes of psychosis, it may be preferable to continue treatment

If It Works (for Depression)

- The goal of treatment is complete remission of current symptoms as well as prevention of future relapses
- Treatment most often reduces or even eliminates symptoms, but not a cure since symptoms can recur after medicine stopped
- Continue treatment until all symptoms are gone (remission) or significantly reduced
- Once symptoms are gone, continue treating for 1 year for the first episode of depression
- For second and subsequent episodes of depression, treatment may need to be indefinite

If It Doesn't Work (for Schizophrenia)

- Try one of the other atypical antipsychotics
- If 2 or more antipsychotic monotherapies do not work, consider clozapine
- Some patients may require treatment with a conventional antipsychotic
- If no first-line atypical antipsychotic is effective, consider higher doses or augmentation with valproate or lamotrigine
- Consider noncompliance and switch to another antipsychotic with fewer side effects or to an antipsychotic that can be given by depot injection
- Consider initiating rehabilitation and psychotherapy
- Consider presence of concomitant drug abuse

If It Doesn't Work (for Depression)

- Some patients may be nonresponders, sometimes called treatment-resistant or treatment-refractory
- Some patients who have an initial response may relapse even though they continue treatment, sometimes called "poop-out"
- Consider psychotherapy
- Consider evaluation for another diagnosis or for a comorbid condition (e.g., medical illness, substance abuse, etc.)
- Some patients may experience apparent lack of consistent efficacy due to activation of latent or underlying bipolar disorder

Best Augmenting Combos for Partial Response or Treatment Resistance

- For depression, brexpiprazole is itself an augmenting agent
- Valproic acid (valproate, divalproex, divalproex ER)
- Mood stabilizing anticonvulsants (carbamazepine, oxcarbazepine, lamotrigine)
- Lithium
- Benzodiazepines

Tests

Before starting any atypical antipsychotic

❋ Weigh all patients and track BMI during treatment

- Get baseline personal and family history of diabetes, obesity, dyslipidemia, hypertension, and cardiovascular disease

❋ Get waist circumference (at umbilicus), blood pressure, fasting plasma glucose, and fasting lipid profile

- Determine if the patient is
  - overweight (BMI 25.0–29.9)
  - obese (BMI ≥30)
  - has pre-diabetes (fasting plasma glucose 100–125 mg/dL)
  - has diabetes (fasting plasma glucose ≥126 mg/dL)
  - has hypertension (BP >140/90 mmHg)
  - has dyslipidemia (increased total cholesterol, LDL cholesterol, and triglycerides; decreased HDL cholesterol)
- Treat or refer such patients for treatment, including nutrition and weight management, physical activity counseling, smoking cessation, and medical management

Monitoring after starting any atypical antipsychotic

❋ BMI monthly for 3 months, then quarterly

❋ Consider monitoring fasting triglycerides monthly for several months in patients at high risk for metabolic complications and when initiating or switching antipsychotics

❋ Blood pressure, fasting plasma glucose, fasting lipids within 3 months and then annually, but earlier and more frequently for patients with diabetes or who have gained >5% of initial weight

- Treat or refer for treatment and consider switching to another atypical antipsychotic for patients who become overweight, obese, pre-diabetic, diabetic, hypertensive, or dyslipidemic while receiving an atypical antipsychotic

* Even in patients without known diabetes, be vigilant for the rare but life-threatening onset of diabetic ketoacidosis, which always requires immediate treatment, by monitoring for the rapid onset of polyuria, polydipsia, weight loss, nausea, vomiting, dehydration, rapid respiration, weakness and clouding of sensorium, even coma

- Patients with low white blood cell count (WBC) or history of drug-induced leukopenia/neutropenia should have complete blood count (CBC) monitored frequently during the first few months and brexpiprazole should be discontinued at the first sign of decline in WBC in the absence of other causative factors

SIDE EFFECTS

How Drug Causes Side Effects

- By blocking alpha 1 adrenergic receptors, it can cause dizziness, sedation, and hypotension
- Partial agonist actions at dopamine 2 receptors in the striatum can cause motor side effects, such as akathisia
- Partial agonist actions at dopamine 2 receptors and 5HT1A receptors can also cause nausea, occasional vomiting, and activating side effects
- Mechanism of weight gain and increased incidence of diabetes and dyslipidemia with atypical antipsychotics is unknown

Notable Side Effects

- Weight gain
- Akathisia (dose dependent), restlessness (dose dependent), anxiety
- Sedation, headache
- Theoretical risk of tardive dyskinesia

Life-Threatening or Dangerous Side Effects

- Hyperglycemia, in some cases extreme and associated with ketoacidosis or hyperosmolar coma or death, has been reported in patients taking atypical antipsychotics
- Increased risk of death and cerebrovascular events in elderly patients with dementia-related psychosis
- Rare neuroleptic malignant syndrome (much reduced risk compared to conventional antipsychotics)
- Rare seizures

Weight Gain

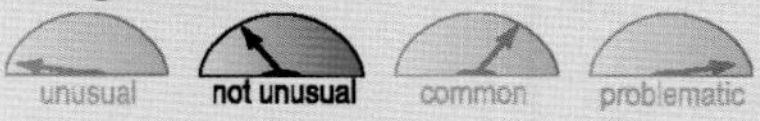

- Occurs in a significant minority

Sedation

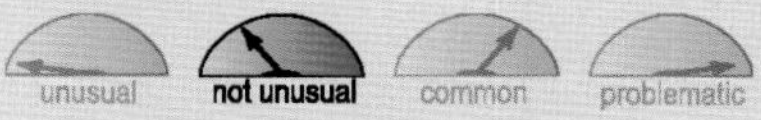

- Occurs in a significant minority

What to Do About Side Effects

- Wait
- Wait
- Wait
- Anticholinergics may reduce motor side effects when present
- Weight loss, exercise programs, and medical management for high BMIs, diabetes, dyslipidemia
- Switch to another atypical antipsychotic

Best Augmenting Agents for Side Effects

- Benztropine or trihexyphenidyl for motor side effects
- Beta blockers or sometimes benzodiazepines for akathisia
- Many side effects cannot be improved with an augmenting agent

DOSING AND USE

Usual Dosage Range

- Schizophrenia: 2–4 mg once daily
- Depression: 2 mg once daily

Dosage Forms

- Tablet 0.25 mg, 0.5 mg, 1 mg, 2 mg, 3 mg, 4 mg

How to Dose

- Schizophrenia: Initial 1 mg once daily for days 1–4; increase to 2 mg once daily for

days 5–7; increase to 4 mg once daily on day 8; maximum dose 4 mg once daily
- Depression: Initial 0.5–1 mg once daily; increase in weekly intervals up to 1 mg once daily and then up to 2 mg once daily; maximum dose 3 mg once daily

Dosing Tips
- Can be taken with or without food

Overdose
- Limited experience

Long-Term Use
- Safety and efficacy demonstrated in schizophrenia in a maintenance study lasting over 1 year
- Should periodically reevaluate long-term usefulness in individual patients, but treatment may need to continue for many years in patients with schizophrenia or treatment-resistant depression

Habit Forming
- No

How to Stop
- Because clinical experience is lacking, down-titration may be prudent, especially when simultaneously beginning a new antipsychotic while switching (i.e., cross-titration)
- However, the long half-life suggests that it may be possible to stop brexpiprazole abruptly
- The method for stopping brexpiprazole can vary depending on which agent is being switched to; see switching guidelines of individual agents for how to stop brexpiprazole
- Rapid discontinuation could theoretically lead to rebound psychosis and worsening of symptoms, but less likely with brexpiprazole due to its long half-life

Pharmacokinetics
- Mean half-life 91 hours (brexpiprazole) and 86 hours (major metabolite DM-3411)
- Metabolized primarily by CYP450 2D6 and CYP450 3A4

Drug Interactions
- In patients receiving a strong/moderate CYP450 3A4 inhibitor (e.g., ketaconazole), brexpiprazole should be administered at half the usual dose
- In patients receiving a strong CYP450 3A4 inducer (e.g., carbamazepine), brexpiprazole should be administered at double the usual dose
- In patients with schizophrenia who are receiving a strong/moderate CYP450 2D6 inhibitor (e.g., quinidine) or who are known CYP450 2D6 poor metabolizers, brexpiprazole should be administered at half the usual dose
- However, clinical trials in major depressive disorder took into account the potential concomitant administration of strong CYP450 2D6 inhibitors (e.g., paroxetine, fluoxetine), so the dose of brexpiprazole does not need to be adjusted in these cases
- In patients receiving both a strong/moderate CYP3A4 inhibitor and a strong/moderate CYP450 2D6 inhibitor, brexpiprazole should be administered at one quarter the usual dose
- In patients receiving a strong/moderate CYP3A4 inhibitor who are known CYP450 2D6 poor metabolizers, brexpiprazole should be administered at one quarter the usual dose
- May increase effects of antihypertensive agents
- May antagonize levodopa, dopamine agonists

Other Warnings/ Precautions
- Use with caution in patients with conditions that predispose to hypotension (dehydration, overheating)
- Dysphagia has been associated with antipsychotic use, and brexpiprazole should be used cautiously in patients at risk for aspiration pneumonia

Do Not Use
- If there is a proven allergy to brexpiprazole

SPECIAL POPULATIONS

Renal Impairment
- Moderate, severe, or end-stage: maximum recommended dose for depression is 2 mg once daily and for schizophrenia is 3 mg once daily

Hepatic Impairment
- Moderate to severe: maximum recommended dose for depression is 2 mg once daily and for schizophrenia is 3 mg once daily

Cardiac Impairment
- Use in patients with cardiac impairment has not been studied, so use with caution

Elderly
- Some elderly patients may tolerate lower doses better
- Although atypical antipsychotics are commonly used for behavioral disturbances in dementia, no agent has been approved for treatment of elderly patients with dementia-related psychosis
- Elderly patients with dementia-related psychosis treated with atypical antipsychotics are at an increased risk of death compared to placebo, and also have an increased risk of cerebrovascular events

Children and Adolescents
- Safety and efficacy have not been established
- Children and adolescents using brexpiprazole may need to be monitored more often than adults

Pregnancy
- Effective June 30, 2015, the US FDA requires changes to the content and format of pregnancy and lactation information in prescription drug labels, including the elimination of the pregnancy letter categories; the Pregnancy and Lactation Labeling Rule (PLLR or final rule) applies only to prescription drugs and will be phased in gradually for drugs approved on or after June 30, 2001
- Controlled studies have not been conducted in pregnant women
- In animal studies, brexpiprazole did not demonstrate teratogenicity
- There is a risk of abnormal muscle movements and withdrawal symptoms in newborns whose mothers took an antipsychotic during the third trimester; symptoms may include agitation, abnormally increased or decreased muscle tone, tremor, sleepiness, severe difficulty breathing, and difficulty feeding
- Psychotic symptoms may worsen during pregnancy and some form of treatment may be necessary
- Brexpiprazole may be preferable to anticonvulsant mood stabilizers if treatment is required during pregnancy
- National Pregnancy Registry for Atypical Antipsychotics: 1-866-961-2388 or http://womensmentalhealth.org/clinical-and-research-programs/pregnancyregistry/

Breast Feeding
- Unknown if brexpiprazole is secreted in human breast milk, but all psychotropics assumed to be secreted in breast milk

* Recommended either to discontinue drug or bottle feed unless the potential benefit to the mother justifies the potential risk to the child

- Infants of women who choose to breast feed while on brexpiprazole should be monitored for possible adverse effects

THE ART OF PSYCHOPHARMACOLOGY

Potential Advantages
- For patients who do not tolerate aripiprazole

Potential Disadvantages
- Expensive

Primary Target Symptoms
- Positive symptoms of psychosis
- Negative symptoms of psychosis
- Cognitive symptoms
- Unstable mood and depression
- Aggressive symptoms

Pearls
- Approved as an adjunct treatment for depression

- Animal data suggest that brexpiprazole may improve cognitive impairment in schizophrenia
- Brexpiprazole is also being studied in clinical trials in attention deficit hyperactivity disorder, post-traumatic stress disorder, and agitation associated with Alzheimer dementia
- Not approved for mania, but almost all atypical antipsychotics approved for acute treatment of schizophrenia have proven effective in the acute treatment of mania as well
- Pharmacological differences from aripiprazole suggest less akathisia with brexpiprazole, but no head-to-head trials
- Compared to aripiprazole, brexpiprazole has more potent binding of several receptor sites relative to dopamine 2 receptor binding, namely 5HT1A, 5HT2A, and alpha 1 receptors; however, the clinical significance of these differences is still under investigation

THE ART OF SWITCHING

Switching from Oral Antipsychotics to Brexpiprazole

- It is advisable to begin brexpiprazole at an intermediate dose and build the dose rapidly over 3–7 days
- Clinical experience has shown that asenapine, quetiapine, and olanzapine should be tapered off slowly over a period of 3–4 weeks, to allow patients to readapt to the withdrawal of blocking cholinergic, histaminergic, and alpha 1 receptors
- Clozapine should always be tapered off slowly, over a period of 4 weeks or more

* Benzodiazepine or anticholinergic medication can be administered during cross-titration to help alleviate side effects such as insomnia, agitation, and/or psychosis

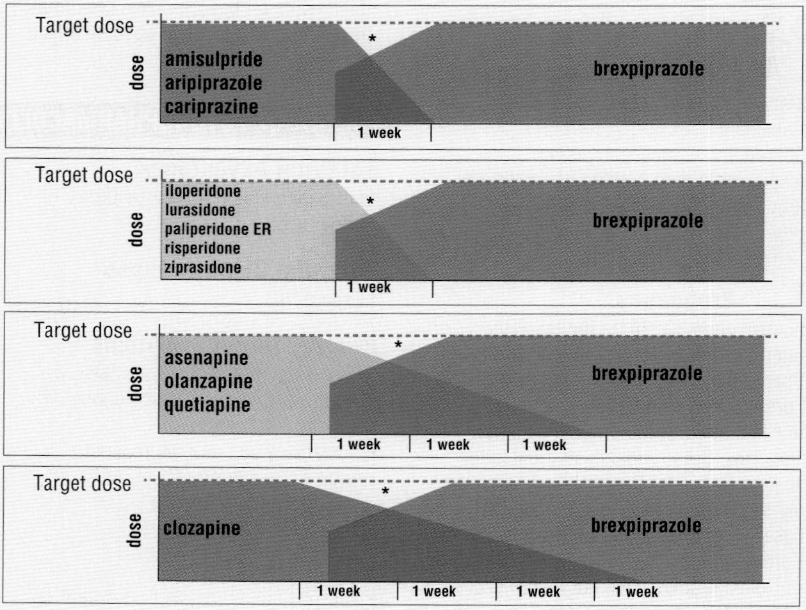

Suggested Reading

Correll Cu, Skuban A, Ouyang J, et al. Efficacy and safety of brexpiprazole for the treatment of acute schizophrenia: a 6-week randomized, double-blind, placebo-controlled trial. Am J Psychiatry 2015;172(9):870–80.

Kane JM, Skuban A, Ouyang J, et al. A multicenter, randomized, double-blind, controlled phase 3 trial of fixed-dose brexpiprazole for the treatment of adults with acute schizophrenia. Schizophr Res 2015;164(1–3):127–35.

Maeda K, Lerdrup L, Sugino H, et al. Brexpiprazole II: antipsychotic-like and procognitive effects of a novel serotonin-dopamine activity modulator. J Pharmacol Exp Ther 2014;350(3):605–14.

Oosterhof CA, El Mansari M, Blier P. Acute effects of brexpiprazole on serotonin, dopamine, and norepinephrine systems: an in vivo electrophysiologic characterization. J Pharmacol Exp Ther 2014;351(3):585–95.

THERAPEUTICS

Brands • Suboxone (with naloxone)
• Probuphine (implant)

see index for additional brand names

Generic? Yes (not for buprenorphine with naloxone or implant)

Class

• mu opioid receptor partial agonist

Commonly Prescribed for (sublingual)

(bold for FDA approved)

- **Maintenance treatment of opioid dependence**
- **Maintenance treatment of opioid dependence in patients who have achieved and sustained prolonged clinical stability on low-to-moderate doses (no more than 8 mg) of a transmucosal buprenorphine-containing product (implant)**

How the Drug Works

- Binds with strong affinity to the mu opioid receptor, preventing exogenous opioids from binding there and thus preventing the pleasurable effects of opioid consumption
- Because buprenorphine is a partial agonist, it can cause immediate withdrawal in a patient currently taking opioids (i.e., reduces receptor stimulation in the presence of a full agonist) but can relieve withdrawal if a patient is already experiencing it (i.e., increases receptor stimulation in the absence of a full agonist)
- Buprenorphine is also an antagonist at the kappa opioid receptor
- In combination with naloxone: naloxone is a mu opioid receptor antagonist and can therefore block the effects of buprenorphine; however, because naloxone has poor sublingual bioavailability, it does not interfere with buprenorphine's effects when used properly. Naloxone does have good parenteral bioavailability; thus, if one tries to administer the buprenorphine/naloxone formulation intravenously, naloxone will prevent any rewarding effects from buprenorphine.

How Long Until It Works

- Effects on withdrawal can be immediate
- Effects on reducing opioid use disorder/dependence can take many months of treatment

If It Works

- Reduces cravings, decreases opioid consumption
- Reduces effects of opioid withdrawal
- Diminishes rewarding effects of opioid consumption

If It Doesn't Work

- Evaluate for and address contributing factors
- Consider switching to another agent
- If patients receiving the implant feel a need for supplemental dosing, they should be evaluated and transmucosal buprenorphine should be considered

Best Augmenting Combos for Partial Response or Treatment Resistance

- Augmentation with behavioral, educational, and/or supportive therapy in groups or as an individual is probably key to successful treatment
- Buprenorphine can be prescribed in combination with naloxone (Suboxone) to decrease the potential for abuse or diversion

Tests

- Liver function tests at baseline and during treatment

SIDE EFFECTS

How Drug Causes Side Effects

- Binding at mu opioid receptors

Notable Side Effects

- Headache, constipation, nausea
- Oral hypoesthesia, glossodynia
- Orthostatic hypotension
- Implant specific: insertion site pain, pruritis, erythema

Life-Threatening or Dangerous Side Effects

- Respiratory depression
- Hepatotoxicity

Weight Gain

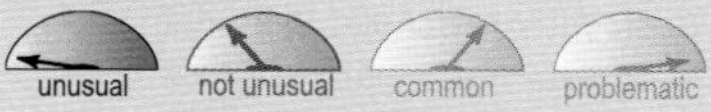

- Reported but not expected

Sedation

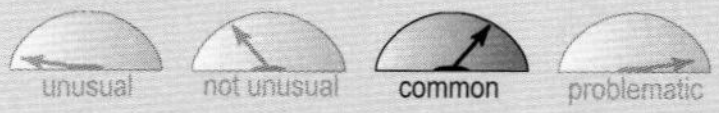

- Many experience and/or can be significant in amount

What to Do About Side Effects

- Wait
- Reduce dose
- Switch to another agent

Best Augmenting Agents for Side Effects

- Dose reduction or switching to another agent may be more effective since most side effects cannot be improved with an augmenting agent

DOSING AND USE

Usual Dosage Range

- Sublingual: 8–32 mg/day
- Implant: 4 implants intended to be in place for 6 months

Dosage Forms

- Sublingual tablet 2 mg, 8 mg
- Sublingual tablet (with naloxone) 2 mg/ 0.5 mg, 8 mg/ 2 mg
- Sublingual film (with naloxone) 2 mg/ 0.5 mg, 4 mg/1 mg, 8 mg/2 mg, 12 mg/3 mg
- Each implant is 26 mm in length and 2.5 mm diameter and contains 74.2 mg of buprenorphine (equivalent to 80 mg of buprenorphine hydrochloride)

How to Dose – Sublingual

- Patients must be in a mild withdrawal state prior to starting buprenorphine

Initiation (7 days)			
	Day 1	Day 2	Days 3–7
Buprenorphine	8 mg	12 or 16 mg	Increase in increments of 4 mg; maximum 32 mg
Buprenorphine/ naloxone	8 mg/2 mg	12 mg/3 mg or 16 mg/4 mg	Increase in increments of 4 mg/1 mg; maximum 32 mg/8 mg

- Observe patient for at least 2 hours with initial dose, then have 1–2 visits in first week
- Achieve the lowest dose that eliminates withdrawal symptoms and illicit opioid use
- Stabilization (up to 2 months) and maintenance dose is generally 8–24 mg (8 mg/2 mg up to 24 mg/6 mg for buprenorphine/naloxone)
- During stabilization patients should be seen once per week
- During maintenance patients should be seen biweekly or monthly

Dosing Tips – Sublingual

- Buprenorphine must be administered sublingually, as swallowing reduces its bioavailability
- Patients should be instructed to place the sublingual formulation under the tongue and allow it to dissolve completely; the formulation should not be divided, crushed, chewed, or swallowed
- Can be dosed less often than once daily; one should double the dose for each additional 24-hour interval
- Buprenorphine alone is often used to initiate treatment, while buprenorphine/ naloxone is preferred for stabilization and maintenance treatment
- Only buprenorphine with naloxone should be used for unsupervised administration, unless the patient has a proven allergy to naloxone
- Can be distributed through clinicians' offices by those who obtain a DEA DATA 2000 waiver
- Patients being switched between the 2 sublingual formulations (tablet and film) should be started on the same dose as the previously administered product; however, because the sublingual film has greater bioavailability than the sublingual tablet, patients must be monitored for over-medication (when switching from tablet to film) or under-medication (when switching from film to tablet); dose adjustment may be necessary

How to Dose – Implant

- Patient must have achieved and sustained prolonged clinical stability on transmucosal buprenorphine

- Four implants are inserted subdermally in the inner side of the upper arm for 6 months of treatment and are removed by the end of the sixth month

Dosing Tips – Implant
- Implants must be inserted and removed by trained healthcare providers who are certified in the Probuphine REMS program; information is available at http://www.probuphinerems.com or 1-844-859-6341
- Patients must currently be on a maintenance dose of 8 mg/day or less of transmucosal buprenorphine and should not be transitioned to a lower dose for the sole purpose of transitioning to the implant
- Patients should be on a stable transmucosal buprenorphine dose (8 mg/day or less) for 3 months or longer without any need for supplemental dosing or adjustments
- Examine the insertion site 1 week after implant insertion for signs of infection or other problems
- Patients should not receive prescriptions for transmucosal buprenorphine for as-needed use; patients who feel a need for supplemental dosing should be evaluated and alternative treatment should be considered
- For continued treatment, new implants may be inserted subdermally in an area of the inner side of either upper arm that has not been previously used at the time of removal
- If new implants are not inserted on the same day as removal, then patients should be maintained on their previous dosage of transmucosal buprenorphine
- After one insertion in each arm, most patients should be transitioned back to transmucosal buprenorphine if continued treatment is desired, as there is no experience with re-insertion into previously used administration sites or insertion into sites other than the upper arm

Overdose
- Can be fatal (less common than with methadone); respiratory depression, sedation, constricted pupils, bradycardia, hypotension, coma

Long-Term Use
- Maintenance treatment may be required; typical maintenance period is up to 2 years but may need to be indefinite

Habit Forming
- Buprenorphine is a Schedule III drug
- Can cause physical dependence

How to Stop
- Patients may experience a mild withdrawal syndrome if buprenorphine is stopped abruptly
- Taper to avoid withdrawal effects

Pharmacokinetics
- Metabolized by CYP450 3A4
- Elimination half-life of sublingual buprenorphine is 24–42 hours
- Elimination half-life of naloxone is 2–12 hours
- Implant: Tmax is 12 hours; time to steady state is 4 weeks

Drug Interactions
- Increased depressive effects, particularly respiratory depression, have occurred when taken with other CNS depressants; consider dose reduction of either or both when taken concomitantly
- Plasma concentrations of buprenorphine may be increased by drugs that inhibit CYP450 3A4, so buprenorphine dose may need to be reduced if coadministered
- Patients taking a CYP450 3A4 inhibitor who transfer to the implant should be monitored to ensure that plasma buprenorphine levels are adequate
- If a CYP450 3A4 inhibitor is initiated in a patient with the implant, the patient should be monitored for signs of over-medication
- If a CYP450 3A4 inhibitor is discontinued in a patient with the implant, the patient should be monitored for signs of withdrawal
- Plasma concentrations of buprenorphine may be reduced by drugs that induce CYP450 3A4, so buprenorphine dose may need to be increased if coadministered
- Patients taking a CYP450 3A4 inducer who transfer to the implant should be monitored to ensure that plasma buprenorphine levels are not excessive

- If a CYP450 3A4 inducer is initiated in a patient with the implant, patients should be monitored for signs of withdrawal
- If a CYP450 3A4 inducer is discontinued in a patient with the implant, patients should be monitored for signs of over-medication

Other Warnings/ Precautions

- Although the risk is lower, buprenorphine can be abused in a manner similar to other opioids
- Parenteral misuse of buprenorphine/ naloxone may result in marked opioid withdrawal syndrome
- To prevent withdrawal in patients dependent on opioids, patients must be in a mild withdrawal state prior to initiating treatment
- Attempts by patients to overcome blockade of opioid receptors by taking large amounts of exogenous opioids could lead to opioid intoxication or even fatal overdose
- Use with caution in patients with compromised respiratory function
- Risk of respiratory depression is increased with concomitant use of CNS depressants, particularly with parenteral administration
- Can cause severe, possibly fatal respiratory depression in children who are accidentally exposed to it
- Withdrawal symptoms can occur when switching from methadone to buprenorphine
- Buprenorphine may elevate cerebrospinal fluid pressure and should be used with caution in patients with head injury, intracranial lesions, and other circumstances when cerebrospinal pressure may be increased
- Buprenorphine may increase intracholedochal pressure and should be administered with caution to patients with dysfunction of the biliary tract
- Use with caution in debilitated patients and those with myxedema or hypothyroidism, adrenal cortical insufficiency (e.g., Addison's disease); CNS depression or coma; toxic psychoses; prostatic hypertrophy or urethral stricture; acute alcoholism; delirium tremens; or kyphoscoliosis
- Use the implant with caution in patients with a history of keloid formation, connective tissue disease, or history of recurrent methicillin-resistant *Staphylococens aureus* (MRSA) infections
- Rare nerve damage and migration resulting in embolism and death may occur due to improper insertion of the implant in the upper arm; local migration, protrusion, and expulsion can also occur as a result of improper or incomplete insertion; protrusion and expulsion may occur as a result of infection
- In the event that an implant is expelled, the patient should store it in a plastic bag out of reach of children and bring it to their healthcare provider to ensure that the entire implant was expelled
- The prescribing healthcare provider will need to monitor the patient until the implant is replaced

Do Not Use

- As an analgesic
- If the patient is naive to opioid use
- If there is a proven allergy to buprenorphine
- If patient has severe hepatic impairment (buprenorphine/naloxone combinations only)
- If there is a proven allergy to naloxone (buprenorphine/naloxone combinations only)

SPECIAL POPULATIONS

Renal Impairment

- Dose adjustment not necessary

Hepatic Impairment

- In patients with moderate to severe impairment, plasma levels of buprenorphine can be higher and half-life can be longer; thus, these patients should be monitored for signs and symptoms of toxicity or overdose
- For severe impairment, the dose should be reduced
- Because dose adjustment is not possible with the implant, it is not recommended for use in patients with moderate to severe hepatic impairment
- Hepatic impairment results in reduced clearance of naloxone, so patients with severe impairment should not take buprenorphine/naloxone combinations; caution is warranted for patients with moderate impairment

Cardiac Impairment
- Use with caution

Elderly
- Use with caution
- Some patients may tolerate lower doses better

Children and Adolescents
- Safety and efficacy have not been established

Pregnancy
- Effective June 30, 2015, the US FDA requires changes to the content and format of pregnancy and lactation information in prescription drug labels, including the elimination of the pregnancy letter categories; the Pregnancy and Lactation Labeling Rule (PLLR or final rule) applies only to prescription drugs and will be phased in gradually for drugs approved on or after June 30, 2001
- Controlled studies have not been conducted in pregnant women
- Buprenorphine may be preferable to methadone in pregnant women
- Neonatal withdrawal has been reported following use of buprenorphine during pregnancy
- In animal studies, adverse events have been observed at clinically relevant doses; no clear teratogenic effects were seen
- Not generally recommended for use during pregnancy, especially during first trimester

Breast Feeding
- Some drug is found in mother's breast milk
- ✻ Recommended either to discontinue drug or bottle feed

THE ART OF PSYCHOPHARMACOLOGY

Potential Advantages
- Patients with mild to moderate physical dependence

Potential Disadvantages
- Patients unable to tolerate mild withdrawal symptoms

Primary Target Symptoms
- Opioid dependence

Pearls
- Considered a "take home" medication that generally has less stigma and better adherence than methadone
- Relatively convenient to administer, with flexible dosing and ease of discontinuation

Suggested Reading

Bonhomme J, Shim RS, Gooden R, Tyus D, Rust G. Opioid addiction and abuse in primary care practice: a comparison of methadone and buprenorphine as treatment options. J Natl Med Assoc 2012;104(7–8):342–50.

Jones HE, Finnegan LP, Kaltenbach K. Methadone and buprenorphine for the management of opioid dependence in pregnancy. Drugs 2012;72(6):747–57.

Kraus ML, Alford DP, Kotz MM, et al. Statement of the American Society of Addiction Medicine Consensus Panel on the use of buprenorphine in office-based treatment of opioid addiction. J Addict Med 2011;5(4):254–63.

Yokell MA, Zaller ND, Green TC, Rich JD. Buprenorphine and buprenorphine/naloxone diversion, misuse, and illicit use: an international review. Curr Drug Abuse Rev 2011;4(1):28–41.

THERAPEUTICS

Brands
- Wellbutrin, Wellbutrin SR, Wellbutrin XL
- Zyban
- Aplenzin

Generic? Yes

Class
- Neuroscience-based Nomenclature: dopamine reuptake inhibitor and releaser (D-RIRe)
- NDRI (norepinephrine dopamine reuptake inhibitor); antidepressant; smoking cessation treatment

Commonly Prescribed for
(bold for FDA approved)
- **Major depressive disorder (bupropion, bupropion SR, and bupropion XL)**
- **Seasonal affective disorder (bupropion XL)**
- **Nicotine addiction (bupropion SR)**
- Bipolar depression
- Attention deficit /hyperactivity disorder (ADHD)
- Sexual dysfunction

How the Drug Works
- Boosts neurotransmitters norepinephrine/noradrenaline and dopamine
- Blocks norepinephrine reuptake pump (norepinephrine transporter), presumably increasing norepinephrine neurotransmission
- Since dopamine is inactivated by norepinephrine reuptake in frontal cortex, which largely lacks dopamine transporters, bupropion can increase dopamine neurotransmission in this part of the brain
- Blocks dopamine reuptake pump (dopamine transporter), presumably increasing dopaminergic neurotransmission

How Long Until It Works
- Onset of therapeutic actions usually not immediate, but often delayed 2–4 weeks
- If it is not working within 6–8 weeks for depression, it may require a dosage increase or it may not work at all
- May continue to work for many years to prevent relapse of symptoms

If It Works
- The goal of treatment of depression is complete remission of current symptoms as well as prevention of future relapses
- Treatment of depression most often reduces or even eliminates symptoms, but is not a cure since symptoms can recur after medicine stopped
- Continue treatment of depression until all symptoms are gone (remission)
- Once symptoms of depression are gone, continue treating for 1 year for the first episode of depression
- For second and subsequent episodes of depression, treatment may need to be indefinite
- Treatment for nicotine addiction should consist of a single treatment for 6 weeks

If It Doesn't Work
- Many patients have only a partial response where some symptoms are improved but others persist (especially insomnia, fatigue, and problems concentrating)
- Other patients may be nonresponders, sometimes called treatment-resistant or treatment-refractory
- Some patients who have an initial response may relapse even though they continue treatment, sometimes called "poop-out"
- Consider increasing dose, switching to another agent or adding an appropriate augmenting agent
- Consider psychotherapy
- Consider evaluation for another diagnosis or for a comorbid condition (e.g., medical illness, substance abuse, etc.)
- Some patients may experience apparent lack of consistent efficacy due to activation of latent or underlying bipolar disorder, and require antidepressant discontinuation and a switch to a mood stabilizer, although this may be a less frequent problem with bupropion than with other antidepressants

Best Augmenting Combos for Partial Response or Treatment Resistance
- Trazodone for residual insomnia
- Benzodiazepines for residual anxiety

✻ Can be added to SSRIs to reverse SSRI-induced sexual dysfunction, SSRI-induced apathy (use combinations of antidepressants with caution as this may activate bipolar disorder and suicidal ideation)

✽ Can be added to SSRIs to treat partial responders

✽ Often used as an augmenting agent to mood stabilizers and/or atypical antipsychotics in bipolar depression

- Mood stabilizers or atypical antipsychotics can also be added to bupropion for psychotic depression or treatment-resistant depression
- Hypnotics for insomnia
- Mirtazapine, modafinil, atomoxetine (add with caution and at lower doses since bupropion could theoretically raise atomoxetine levels) both for residual symptoms of depression and attention deficit disorder

Tests

- Recommended to assess blood pressure at baseline and periodically during treatment

SIDE EFFECTS

How Drug Causes Side Effects

- Side effects are probably caused in part by actions of norepinephrine and dopamine in brain areas with undesired effects (e.g., insomnia, tremor, agitation, headache, dizziness)
- Side effects are probably also caused in part by actions of norepinephrine in the periphery with undesired effects (e.g., sympathetic and parasympathetic effects such as dry mouth, constipation, nausea, anorexia, sweating)
- Most side effects are immediate but often go away with time

Notable Side Effects

- Dry mouth, constipation, nausea, weight loss, anorexia, myalgia
- Insomnia, dizziness, headache, agitation, anxiety, tremor, abdominal pain, tinnitus
- Sweating, rash
- Hypertension

Life-Threatening or Dangerous Side Effects

- Rare seizures (higher incidence for immediate-release than for sustained-release; risk increases with doses above the recommended maximums; risk increases for patients with predisposing factors)
- Anaphylactoid/anaphylactic reactions and Stevens-Johnson syndrome have been reported
- Hypomania (more likely in bipolar patients but perhaps less common than with some other antidepressants)
- Rare induction of mania
- Rare activation of suicidal ideation and behavior (suicidality) (short-term studies did not show an increase in the risk of suicidality with antidepressants compared to placebo beyond age 24)

Weight Gain

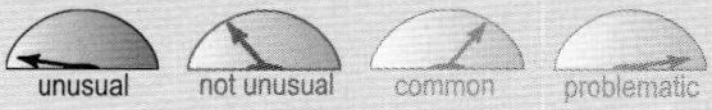

- Reported but not expected

✽ Patients may experience weight loss

Sedation

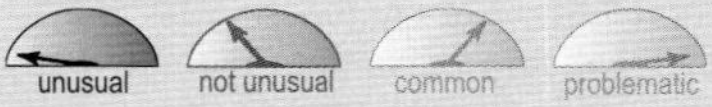

- Reported but not expected

What to Do About Side Effects

- Wait
- Wait
- Wait
- Keep dose as low as possible
- Take no later than mid-afternoon to avoid insomnia
- Switch to another drug

Best Augmenting Agents for Side Effects

- Often best to try another antidepressant monotherapy prior to resorting to augmentation strategies to treat side effects
- Trazodone or a hypnotic for drug-induced insomnia
- Mirtazapine for insomnia, agitation, and gastrointestinal side effects
- Benzodiazepines or buspirone for drug-induced anxiety, agitation
- Many side effects are dose-dependent (i.e., they increase as dose increases, or they reemerge until tolerance redevelops)
- Many side effects are time-dependent (i.e., they start immediately upon dosing and upon each dose increase, but go away with time)
- Activation and agitation may represent the induction of a bipolar state, especially

a mixed dysphoric bipolar II condition sometimes associated with suicidal ideation, and require the addition of lithium, a mood stabilizer or an atypical antipsychotic, and/or discontinuation of bupropion

DOSING AND USE

Usual Dosage Range

- Bupropion: 225–450 mg in 3 divided doses (maximum single dose 150 mg)
- Bupropion SR: 200–450 mg in 2 divided doses (maximum single dose 200 mg)
- Bupropion XL: 150–450 mg once daily (maximum single dose 450 mg)
- Bupropion hydrobromide: 174–522 mg once daily (maximum single dose 522 mg)

Dosage Forms

- Bupropion: tablet 75 mg, 100 mg
- Bupropion SR (sustained-release): tablet 100 mg, 150 mg, 200 mg
- Bupropion XL (extended-release): tablet 150 mg, 300 mg, 450 mg
- Bupropion hydrobromide (extended-release): tablet 174 mg, 378 mg, 522 mg

How to Dose

- Depression: for bupropion immediate-release, dosing should be in divided doses, starting at 75 mg twice daily, increasing to 100 mg twice daily, then to 100 mg 3 times daily; maximum dose 450 mg per day
- Depression: for bupropion SR, initial dose 100 mg twice a day, increase to 150 mg twice a day after at least 3 days; wait 4 weeks or longer to ensure drug effects before increasing dose; maximum dose 400 mg total per day
- Depression: for bupropion XL, initial dose 150 mg once daily in the morning; can increase to 300 mg once daily after 4 days; maximum single dose 450 mg once daily
- Depression: for bupropion hydrobromide, initial dose 174 mg once daily in the morning; can increase to 522 mg administered as a single dose
- Nicotine addiction [for bupropion SR]: initial dose 150 mg/day once a day, increase to 150 mg twice a day after at least 3 days; maximum dose 300 mg/day; bupropion treatment should begin 1–2 weeks before smoking is discontinued

Dosing Tips

- XL formulation has replaced immediate release and SR formulations as the preferred option
- XL is best dosed once a day, whereas SR is best dosed twice daily, and immediate release is best dosed 3 times daily
- Dosing higher than 450 mg/day (400 mg/day SR) increases seizure risk
- Patients who do not respond to 450 mg/day should discontinue use or get blood levels of bupropion and its major active metabolite 6-hydroxy-bupropion
- If levels of parent drug and active metabolite are low despite dosing at 450 mg/day, experts can prudently increase dosing beyond the therapeutic range while monitoring closely, informing the patient of the potential risk of seizures and weighing risk/benefit ratios in difficult-to-treat patients
- When used for bipolar depression, it is usually as an augmenting agent to mood stabilizers, lithium, and/or atypical antipsychotics
- For smoking cessation, may be used in conjunction with nicotine replacement therapy
- Do not break or chew SR or XL tablets as this will alter controlled-release properties
- The more anxious and agitated the patient, the lower the starting dose, the slower the titration, and the more likely the need for a concomitant agent such as trazodone or a benzodiazepine
- If intolerable anxiety, insomnia, agitation, akathisia, or activation occur either upon dosing initiation or discontinuation, consider the possibility of activated bipolar disorder and switch to a mood stabilizer or an atypical antipsychotic

Overdose

- Rarely lethal; seizures, cardiac disturbances, hallucinations, loss of consciousness

Long-Term Use

- For smoking cessation, treatment for up to 6 months has been found effective
- For depression, treatment up to 1 year has been found to decrease rate of relapse

Habit Forming
- No
- Can be abused by individuals who crush and then snort or inject it

How to Stop
- Tapering is prudent to avoid withdrawal effects, but no well-documented tolerance, dependence, or withdrawal reactions

Pharmacokinetics
- Inhibits CYP450 2D6
- Parent half-life 10–14 hours
- Metabolite half-life 20–27 hours
- Food does not affect absorption

Drug Interactions
- Tramadol increases the risk of seizures in patients taking an antidepressant
- Can increase TCA levels; use with caution with TCAs or when switching from a TCA to bupropion
- Use with caution with MAOIs, including 14 days after MAOIs are stopped (for the expert)
- There is increased risk of hypertensive reaction if bupropion is used in conjunction with MAOIs or other drugs that increase norepinephrine
- There may be an increased risk of hypertension if bupropion is combined with nicotine replacement therapy
- Via CYP450 2D6 inhibition, bupropion could theoretically interfere with the analgesic actions of codeine, and increase the plasma levels of some beta blockers and of atomoxetine
- Via CYP450 2D6 inhibition, bupropion could theoretically increase concentrations of thioridazine and cause dangerous cardiac arrhythmias

Other Warnings/ Precautions
- Use cautiously with other drugs that increase seizure risk (TCAs, lithium, phenothiazines, thioxanthenes, some antipsychotics)
- Bupropion should be used with caution in patients taking levodopa or amantadine, as these agents can potentially enhance dopamine neurotransmission and be activating
- Do not use if patient has severe insomnia
- Use with caution in patients with bipolar disorder unless treated with concomitant mood-stabilizing agent
- When treating children, carefully weigh the risks and benefits of pharmacological treatment against the risks and benefits of nontreatment and make sure to document this in the patient's chart
- Distribute the brochures provided by the FDA and the drug companies
- Warn patients and their caregivers about the possibility of activating side effects and advise them to report such symptoms immediately
- Monitor patients for activation of suicidal ideation, especially children and adolescents
- Discontinuing smoking may lead to pharmacokinetic or pharmacodynamic changes in other drugs the patient is taking, which could potentially require dose adjustment

Do Not Use
- Zyban or Aplenzin in combination with each other or with any formulation of Wellbutrin
- If patient has history of seizures
- If patient is anorexic or bulimic, either currently or in the past, but see Pearls
- If patient is abruptly discontinuing alcohol, sedative use, or anticonvulsant medication
- If patient has had recent head injury
- If patient has a nervous system tumor
- If patient is taking an MAOI (except as noted under Drug Interactions)
- If patient is taking thioridazine
- If there is a proven allergy to bupropion

SPECIAL POPULATIONS

Renal Impairment
- Lower initial dose, perhaps give less frequently
- Drug concentration may be increased
- Patient should be monitored closely

Hepatic Impairment
- Lower initial dose, perhaps give less frequently
- Patient should be monitored closely

- In severe hepatic cirrhosis, bupropion XL should be administered at no more than 150 mg every other day

Cardiac Impairment

- Limited available data
- Evidence of rise in supine blood pressure
- Use with caution

Elderly

- Some patients may tolerate lower doses better
- Reduction in the risk of suicidality with antidepressants compared to placebo in adults age 65 and older

Children and Adolescents

- Carefully weigh the risks and benefits of pharmacological treatment against the risks and benefits of nontreatment with antidepressants and make sure to document this in the patient's chart
- Monitor patients face-to-face regularly, particularly during the first several weeks of treatment
- Use with caution, observing for activation of known or unknown bipolar disorder and/or suicidal ideation, and inform parents or guardians of this risk so they can help observe child or adolescent patients
- Safety and efficacy have not been established
- May be used for ADHD in children or adolescents
- May be used for smoking cessation in adolescents
- Preliminary research suggests efficacy in comorbid depression and ADHD
- Dosage may follow adult pattern for adolescents
- Children may require lower doses initially, with a maximum dose of 300 mg/day

Pregnancy

- Effective June 30, 2015, the US FDA requires changes to the content and format of pregnancy and lactation information in prescription drug labels, including the elimination of the pregnancy letter categories; the Pregnancy and Lactation Labeling Rule (PLLR or final rule) applies only to prescription drugs and will be phased in gradually for drugs approved on or after June 30, 2001
- Controlled studies have not been conducted in pregnant women
- Epidemiological studies do not indicate increased risk of congenital malformations overall or of cardiovascular malformations
- In animal studies, no clear evidence of teratogenicity has been observed; however, slightly increased incidences of fetal malformations and skeletal variations were observed in rabbit studies at doses approximately equal to and greater than the maximum recommended human doses, and greater and decreased fetal weights were observed in rat studies at doses greater than the maximum recommended human doses
- Pregnant women wishing to stop smoking may consider behavioral therapy before pharmacotherapy
- Not generally recommended for use during pregnancy, especially during first trimester
- Must weigh the risk of treatment (first trimester fetal development, third trimester newborn delivery) to the child against the risk of no treatment (recurrence of depression, maternal health, infant bonding) to the mother and child
- For many patients this may mean continuing treatment during pregnancy

Breast Feeding

- Some drug is found in mother's breast milk
- If child becomes irritable or sedated, breast feeding or drug may need to be discontinued
- Immediate postpartum period is a high-risk time for depression, especially in women who have had prior depressive episodes, so drug may need to be reinstituted late in the third trimester or shortly after childbirth to prevent a recurrence during the postpartum period
- Must weigh benefits of breast feeding with risks and benefits of antidepressant treatment versus nontreatment to both the infant and the mother
- For many patients, this may mean continuing treatment during breast feeding

THE ART OF PSYCHOPHARMACOLOGY

Potential Advantages
- Retarded depression
- Atypical depression
- Bipolar depression
- Patients concerned about sexual dysfunction
- Patients concerned about weight gain

Potential Disadvantages
- Patients experiencing weight loss associated with their depression
- Patients who are excessively activated

Primary Target Symptoms
- Depressed mood
- Sleep disturbance, especially hypersomnia
- Cravings associated with nicotine withdrawal
- Cognitive functioning

Pearls
✽ May be effective if SSRIs have failed or for SSRI "poop-out"
- Less likely to produce hypomania than some other antidepressants

✽ May improve cognitive slowing/ pseudodementia

✽ Reduces hypersomnia and fatigue
- Approved to help reduce craving during smoking cessation
- Anecdotal use in attention deficit disorder
- May cause sexual dysfunction only infrequently
- May exacerbate tics
- Bupropion may not be as effective in anxiety disorders as many other antidepressants
- Prohibition for use in eating disorders due to increased risk of seizures is related to past observations when bupropion immediate-release was dosed at especially high levels to low body weight patients with active anorexia nervosa
- Current practice suggests that patients of normal BMI without additional risk factors for seizures can benefit from bupropion, especially if given prudent doses of the XL formulation; such treatment should be administered by experts, and patients should be monitored closely and informed of the potential risks
- Recently approved hydrobromide salt formulation of bupropion may facilitate high dosing for difficult-to-treat patients, as it allows administration of single-pill doses up to 450 mg equivalency to bupropion hydrochloride salt (522 mg tablet), unlike bupropion hydrochloride controlled-release formulations for which the biggest dose in a single pill is 300 mg
- As bromide salts have anticonvulsant properties, hydrobromide salts of bupropion could theoretically reduce risk of seizures, but this has not been proven
- The active enantiomer of the principal active metabolite [(+)-6-hydroxy-bupropion] is in clinical development as a novel antidepressant
- The combination of bupropion and naltrexone has demonstrated efficacy as a treatment for obesity and is currently being evaluated in a long-term study to assess the cardiovascular health outcomes of this treatment
- Phase II trials of the combination of bupropion and zonisamide for the treatment of obesity have been completed

Suggested Reading

Clayton AH. Extended-release bupropion: an antidepressant with a broad spectrum of therapeutic activity? Expert Opin Pharmacother 2007;8(4):457–66.

Ferry L, Johnston JA. Efficacy and safety of bupropion SR for smoking cessation: data from clinical trials and five years of postmarketing experience. Int J Clin Pract 2003;57(3):224–30.

Foley KF, DeSanty KP, Kast RE. Bupropion: pharmacology and therapeutic applications. Expert Rev Neurother 2006;6(9):1249–65.

Jefferson JW, Pradko JF, Muir KT. Bupropion for major depressive disorder: pharmacokinetic and formulation considerations. Clin Ther 2005;27(11):1685–95.

Papakostas GI, Nutt DJ, Hallett LA, et al. Resolution of sleepiness and fatigue in major depressive disorder: a comparison of bupropion and the selective serotonin reuptake inhibitors. Biol Psychiatry 2006;60(12):1350–5.

BUSPIRONE

THERAPEUTICS

Brands • BuSpar

see index for additional brand names

Generic? Yes

Class

- Neuroscience-based Nomenclature: serotonin receptor partial agonist (S-RPA)
- Anxiolytic (azapirone; serotonin 1A partial agonist; serotonin stabilizer)

Commonly Prescribed for

(bold for FDA approved)

- **Management of anxiety disorders**
- **Short-term treatment of symptoms of anxiety**
- Mixed anxiety and depression
- Treatment-resistant depression (adjunctive)

How the Drug Works

- Binds to serotonin type 1A receptors
- Partial agonist actions postsynaptically may theoretically diminish serotonergic activity and contribute to anxiolytic actions
- Partial agonist actions at presynaptic somatodendritic serotonin autoreceptors may theoretically enhance serotonergic activity and contribute to antidepressant actions

How Long Until It Works

- Generally takes within 2–4 weeks to achieve efficacy
- If it is not working within 6–8 weeks, it may require a dosage increase or it may not work at all

If It Works

- The goal of treatment is complete remission of symptoms as well as prevention of future relapses
- Treatment most often reduces or even eliminates symptoms, but not a cure since symptoms can recur after medicine stopped
- Chronic anxiety disorders may require long-term maintenance with buspirone to control symptoms

If It Doesn't Work

- Consider switching to another agent (a benzodiazepine or antidepressant)

Best Augmenting Combos for Partial Response or Treatment Resistance

- Sedative hypnotic for insomnia
- Buspirone is often given as an augmenting agent to SSRIs or SNRIs

Tests

- None for healthy individuals

SIDE EFFECTS

How Drug Causes Side Effects

- Serotonin partial agonist actions in parts of the brain and body and at receptors other than those that cause therapeutic actions

Notable Side Effects

- ✻ Dizziness, headache, nervousness, sedation, excitement
- Nausea
- Restlessness

Life-Threatening or Dangerous Side Effects

- Rare cardiac symptoms

Weight Gain

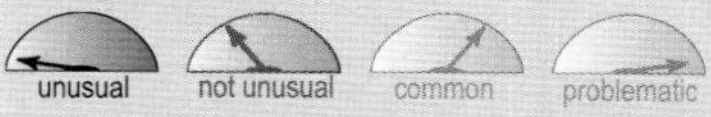

- Reported but not expected

Sedation

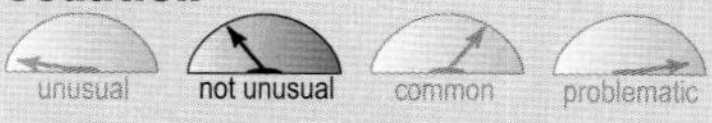

- Occurs in significant minority

What to Do About Side Effects

- Wait
- Wait
- Wait
- Lower the dose
- Give total daily dose divided into 3, 4, or more doses
- Switch to another agent

Best Augmenting Agents for Side Effects

- Many side effects cannot be improved with an augmenting agent

DOSING AND USE

Usual Dosage Range
- 20–30 mg/day

Dosage Forms
- Tablet 5 mg scored, 10 mg scored, 15 mg multiscored, 30 mg multiscored

How to Dose
- Initial 15 mg twice a day; increase in 5 mg/day increments every 2–3 days until desired efficacy is reached; maximum dose generally 60 mg/day

Dosing Tips
- Requires dosing 2–3 times a day for full effect
- Absorption is affected by food, so administration with or without food should be consistent

Overdose
- No deaths reported in monotherapy; sedation, dizziness, small pupils, nausea, vomiting

Long-Term Use
- Limited data suggest that it is safe

Habit Forming
- No

How to Stop
- Taper generally not necessary

Pharmacokinetics
- Metabolized primarily by CYP450 3A4
- Elimination half-life approximately 2–3 hours
- Absorption is affected by food

Drug Interactions
- Use with caution with MAOIs, including 14 days after MAOIs are stopped (for the expert)
- CYP450 3A4 inhibitors (e.g., fluxotine, fluvoxamine, nefazodone) may reduce clearance of buspirone and raise its plasma levels, so the dose of buspirone may need to be lowered when given concomitantly with these agents
- CYP450 3A4 inducers (e.g., carbamazepine) may increase clearance of buspirone, so the dose of buspirone may need to be raised
- Buspirone may increase plasma concentrations of haloperidol
- Buspirone may raise levels of nordiazepam, the active metabolite of diazepam, which may result in increased symptoms of dizziness, headache, or nausea

Other Warnings/ Precautions
- None

Do Not Use
- If patient is taking an MAOI (except as noted under Drug Interactions)
- If there is a proven allergy to buspirone

SPECIAL POPULATIONS

Renal Impairment
- Use with caution
- Not recommended for patients with severe renal impairment

Hepatic Impairment
- Use with caution
- Not recommended for patients with severe hepatic impairment

Cardiac Impairment
- Buspirone has been used to treat hostility in patients with cardiac impairment

Elderly
- Some patients may tolerate lower doses better

Children and Adolescents
- Studies in children age 6–17 do not show significant reduction in anxiety symptoms in generalized anxiety disorder (GAD)
- Safety profile in children encourages use

Pregnancy
- Effective June 30, 2015, the US FDA requires changes to the content and format of pregnancy and lactation information in prescription drug labels, including the elimination of the pregnancy letter

categories; the Pregnancy and Lactation Labeling Rule (PLLR or final rule) applies only to prescription drugs and will be phased in gradually for drugs approved on or after June 30, 2001
- Controlled studies have not been conducted in pregnant women
- Animal studies have not shown adverse effects
- Not generally recommended in pregnancy, but may be safer than some other options

Breast Feeding
- Some drug is found in mother's breast milk
- Trace amounts may be present in nursing children whose mothers are on buspirone
- If child becomes irritable or sedated, breast feeding or drug may need to be discontinued

THE ART OF PSYCHOPHARMACOLOGY

Potential Advantages
- Safety profile
- Lack of dependence, withdrawal
- Lack of sexual dysfunction or weight gain

Potential Disadvantages
- Takes 4 weeks for results, whereas benzodiazepines have immediate effects

Primary Target Symptoms
- Anxiety

Pearls
- * Buspirone does not appear to cause dependence and shows virtually no withdrawal symptoms
- May have less severe side effects than benzodiazepines
- * Buspirone generally lacks sexual dysfunction
- Buspirone may reduce sexual dysfunction associated with GAD and with serotonergic antidepressants
- Sedative effects may be more likely at doses above 20 mg/day
- May have less anxiolytic efficacy than benzodiazepines for some patients
- Buspirone is generally reserved as an augmenting agent to treat anxiety

Suggested Reading

Apter JT, Allen LA. Buspirone: future directions. J Clin Psychopharmacol 1999;19:86–93.

Mahmood I, Sahaiwalla C. Clinical pharmacokinetics and pharmacodynamics of buspirone, an anxiolytic drug. Clin Pharmacokinet 1999;36:277–87.

Pecknold JC. A risk-benefit assessment of buspirone in the treatment of anxiety disorders. Drug Saf 1997;16:118–32.

Sramek JJ, Hong WW, Hamid S, Nape B, Cutler NR. Meta-analysis of the safety and tolerability of two dose regimens of buspirone in patients with persistent anxiety. Depress Anxiety 1999;9:131–4.

THERAPEUTICS

Brands • Axona

see index for additional brand names

Generic? No

Class
- Medical food
- Cognitive enhancer

Commonly Prescribed for
(bold for FDA approved)
- **Dietary management of metabolic processes associated with Alzheimer disease (mild to moderate)**
- Mild cognitive impairment

How the Drug Works
- Induces hyperketonemia and provides an alternative energy substrate to glucose in the brain
- Caprylidene is processed in the gut, resulting in medium chain fatty acids that pass to the liver and undergo obligate oxidation, ultimately being formed into ketone bodies (acetoacetate and beta-hydroxybutyric acid (BHB))
- Ketone bodies cross the blood-brain barrier and are taken up by neurons and enter the mitochondria, where they increase mitochondrial efficiency
- Ketone bodies also generate ATP and increase pools of acetyl-CoA and acetylcholine

How Long Until It Works
- May begin working immediately

If It Works
- May improve or stabilize memory and cognitive function, but does not reverse the degenerative process

If It Doesn't Work
- Consider a cholinesterase inhibitor or memantine

Best Augmenting Combos for Partial Response or Treatment Resistance
- Cholinesterase inhibitors or memantine

Tests
- None for healthy individuals
- Triglyceride levels should be monitored periodically for individuals who meet multiple criteria for metabolic syndrome (i.e., elevated waist circumference, elevated triglycerides, high blood pressure, reduced fasting HDL, and/or elevated fasting glucose)

SIDE EFFECTS

How Drug Causes Side Effects
- Caprylidene is processed in the gut, which may contribute to gastrointestinal side effects

Notable Side Effects
- Diarrhea, flatulence, dyspepsia
- Nausea, headache

Life-Threatening or Dangerous Side Effects
- None reported

Weight Gain
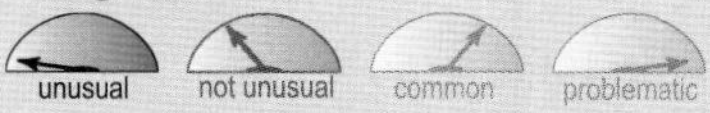

- Reported but not expected
- Some patients may experience weight loss

Sedation
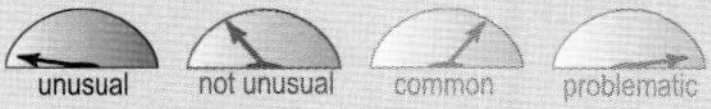

- Reported but not expected

What to Do About Side Effects
- Take it with food
- Sip it slowly over approximately 30 minutes
- Consider lowering the dose

Best Augmenting Agents for Side Effects
- Many side effects cannot be improved with an augmenting agent
- Over-the-counter simethicone, antacids, or antidiarrheals

DOSING AND USE

Usual Dosage Range
- 40 grams/day

Dosage Forms
- Powder 40 grams/packet

How to Dose
- One 40-gram packet of caprylidene should be fully mixed with 4–8 ounces of liquid; dosing should occur shortly after a meal (preferably breakfast or lunch)

Dosing Tips
- Each 40-gram packet of caprylidene powder contains 20 grams of medium-chain triglycerides (MCTs)
- Gastrointestinal side effects are reduced if caprylidene is taken with food and/or sipped slowly over approximately 30 minutes
- Some patients may require a lower starting dose in order to improve tolerability

Overdose
- No fatalities have been reported; diarrhea, sometimes severe

Long-Term Use
- Not studied
- Drug may lose effectiveness as the course of Alzheimer disease progresses

Habit Forming
- No

How to Stop
- Taper not necessary

Pharmacokinetics
- Absorbed in the gut; metabolized in the liver
- Crosses the blood-brain barrier

Drug Interactions
- None reported

Other Warnings/ Precautions
- Use with caution in patients with known hypersensitivity to palm or coconut oil
- Use with caution in patients at risk for ketoacidosis (e.g., alcoholics, patients with poorly controlled diabetes)
- Use with caution in patients with a history of gastrointestinal inflammatory conditions

Do Not Use
- If there is a proven allergy to caprylidene, milk, or soy

SPECIAL POPULATIONS

Renal Impairment
- Not studied

Hepatic Impairment
- Not studied

Cardiac Impairment
- Not studied

Elderly
- Dose adjustment not necessary

Children and Adolescents
- Safety and efficacy have not been established

Pregnancy
- Controlled studies have not been conducted in pregnant women
- Animal studies have not shown teratogenic effects

Breast Feeding
- Unknown if caprylidene is secreted in human breast milk

THE ART OF PSYCHOPHARMACOLOGY

Potential Advantages
- Patients with residual memory problems on Alzheimer treatment

Potential Disadvantages
- Patients with gastrointestinal disorders

Primary Target Symptoms
- Memory loss in Alzheimer disease

- Memory loss in mild cognitive impairment

Pearls

- Dramatic reversal of symptoms of Alzheimer disease is not generally seen with caprylidene
- * Perhaps only 50% of Alzheimer patients are diagnosed, and only 50% of those diagnosed are treated, and then only for 200 days in a disease that lasts 7–10 years
- Must evaluate lack of efficacy and loss of efficacy over months, not weeks
- Patients who complain themselves of memory problems may have depression, whereas patients whose spouses or children complain of the patient's memory problems may have Alzheimer disease
- Treat the patient but ask the caregiver about efficacy
- What you see may depend upon how early you treat
- The first symptoms of Alzheimer disease are generally mood changes; thus, Alzheimer disease may initially be diagnosed as depression
- Women may experience cognitive symptoms in perimenopause as a result of hormonal changes that are not a sign of dementia or Alzheimer disease
- If treatment with antidepressants fails to improve apathy and depressed mood in the elderly, it is possible that this represents early Alzheimer disease
- Delay in progression in Alzheimer disease is not evidence of disease-modifying actions of caprylidene
- The most prominent side effects of caprylidene are gastrointestinal effects, which are usually mild and transient
- Weight loss can be a problem in Alzheimer patients with debilitation and muscle wasting

Suggested Reading

Henderson ST. Ketone bodies as therapeutic for Alzheimer's disease. Neurotherapeutics 2008;5(3):470–80.

Traul KA, Driedger A, Ingle DL, Nakhasi D. Review of the toxicoogic properties of medium-chain triglycerides. Food Chem Toxicol 2000;38:79–98.

THERAPEUTICS

Brands
- Tegretol
- Carbatrol
- Equetro

see index for additional brand names

Generic? Yes (not for extended-release formulation)

Class

- Neuroscience-based Nomenclature: glutamate, voltage-gated sodium and calcium channel blocker (Glu-CB)
- Anticonvulsant, antineuralgic for chronic pain, voltage-sensitive sodium channel antagonist

Commonly Prescribed for

(bold for FDA approved)

- **Partial seizures with complex symptomatology**
- **Generalized tonic-clonic seizures (grand mal)**
- **Mixed seizure patterns**
- **Pain associated with true trigeminal neuralgia**
- **Acute mania/mixed mania (Equetro)**
- Glossopharyngeal neuralgia
- Bipolar depression
- Bipolar maintenance
- Psychosis, schizophrenia (adjunctive)

How the Drug Works

- ✱ Acts as a use-dependent blocker of voltage-sensitive sodium channels
- ✱ Interacts with the open channel conformation of voltage-sensitive sodium channels
- ✱ Interacts at a specific site of the alpha pore-forming subunit of voltage-sensitive sodium channels
- Inhibits release of glutamate

How Long Until It Works

- For acute mania, effects should occur within a few weeks
- May take several weeks to months to optimize an effect on mood stabilization
- Should reduce seizures by 2 weeks

If It Works

- The goal of treatment is complete remission of symptoms (e.g., seizures, mania, pain)
- Continue treatment until all symptoms are gone or until improvement is stable and then continue treating indefinitely as long as improvement persists
- Continue treatment indefinitely to avoid recurrence of mania and seizures
- Treatment of chronic neuropathic pain most often reduces but does not eliminate pain and is not a cure since symptoms usually recur after medicine stopped

If It Doesn't Work (for bipolar disorder)

- ✱ Many patients have only a partial response where some symptoms are improved but others persist or continue to wax and wane without stabilization of mood
- Other patients may be nonresponders, sometimes called treatment-resistant or treatment-refractory
- Consider increasing dose, switching to another agent or adding an appropriate augmenting agent
- Consider adding psychotherapy
- Consider biofeedback or hypnosis for pain
- For bipolar disorder, consider the presence of noncompliance and counsel patient
- Switch to another mood stabilizer with fewer side effects or to extended-release carbamazepine
- Consider evaluation for another diagnosis or for a comorbid condition (e.g., medical illness, substance abuse, etc.)

Best Augmenting Combos for Partial Response or Treatment Resistance

- Lithium
- Atypical antipsychotics (especially risperidone, olanzapine, quetiapine, ziprasidone, and aripiprazole)
- Valproate (carbamazepine can decrease valproate levels)
- Lamotrigine (carbamazepine can decrease lamotrigine levels)
- ✱ Antidepressants (with caution because antidepressants can destabilize mood in some patients, including induction of rapid cycling or suicidal ideation; in particular consider bupropion; also SSRIs, SNRIs, others; generally avoid TCAs, MAOIs)

Tests

- ✻ Before starting: blood count, liver, kidney, and thyroid function tests
- During treatment: blood count every 2–4 weeks for 2 months, then every 3–6 months throughout treatment
- During treatment: liver, kidney, and thyroid function tests every 6–12 months
- Consider monitoring sodium levels because of possibility of hyponatremia
- ✻ Before starting: individuals with ancestry across broad areas of Asia should consider screening for the presence of the HLA-B*1502 allele; those with HLA-B*1502 should not be treated with carbamazepine

SIDE EFFECTS

How Drug Causes Side Effects

- CNS side effects theoretically due to excessive actions at voltage-sensitive sodium channels
- Major metabolite (carbamazepine-10, 11 epoxide) may be the cause of many side effects
- Mild anticholinergic effects may contribute to sedation, blurred vision

Notable Side Effects

- ✻ Sedation, dizziness, confusion, unsteadiness, headache
- ✻ Nausea, vomiting, diarrhea
- Blurred vision
- ✻ Benign leukopenia (transient; in up to 10%)
- ✻ Rash

Life-Threatening or Dangerous Side Effects

- ✻ Rare aplastic anemia, agranulocytosis (unusual bleeding or bruising, mouth sores, infections, fever, sore throat)
- ✻ Rare severe dermatologic reactions (purpura, Stevens-Johnson syndrome)
- Rare cardiac problems
- Rare induction of psychosis or mania
- ✻ SIADH (syndrome of inappropriate antidiuretic hormone secretion) with hyponatremia
- Increased frequency of generalized convulsions (in patients with atypical absence seizures)
- Rare activation of suicidal ideation and behavior (suicidality)

Weight Gain

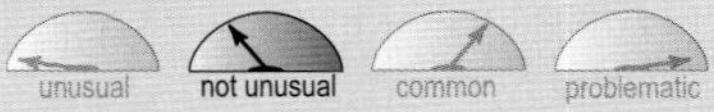

- Occurs in significant minority

Sedation

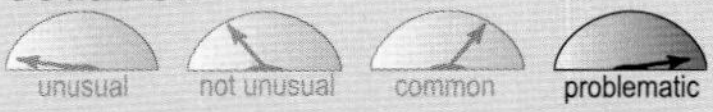

- Frequent and can be significant in amount
- Some patients may not tolerate it
- Dose-related
- Can wear off with time, but commonly does not wear off at high doses
- CNS side effects significantly lower with controlled-release formulation (e.g., Equetro, Carbatrol)

What to Do About Side Effects

- Wait
- Wait
- Wait
- Take with food or split dose to avoid gastrointestinal effects
- Extended-release carbamazepine can be sprinkled on soft food
- Take at night to reduce daytime sedation
- Switch to another agent or to extended-release carbamazepine

Best Augmenting Agents for Side Effects

- Many side effects cannot be improved with an augmenting agent

DOSING AND USE

Usual Dosage Range

- 400–1,200 mg/day
- Under age 6: 10–20 mg/kg per day

Dosage Forms

- Tablet 100 mg chewable, 200 mg chewable, 200 mg
- Extended-release tablet 100 mg, 200 mg, 400 mg
- Extended-release capsule 100 mg, 200 mg, 300 mg
- Oral suspension 100 mg/5mL (450 mL)

How to Dose

- For bipolar disorder and seizures (ages 13 and older): initial 200 mg twice daily (tablet) or 1 teaspoon (100 mg) 4 times a day (suspension); each week increase by up to 200 mg/day in divided doses (2 doses for extended-release formulation, 3–4 doses for other tablets); maximum dose generally 1,200 mg/day for adults and 1,000 mg/day for children under age 15; maintenance dose generally 800–1,200 mg/day for adults; some patients may require up to 1,600 mg/day
- Seizures (under age 13): see Children and Adolescents
- Trigeminal neuralgia: initial 100 mg twice daily (tablet) or 0.5 teaspoon (50 mg) 4 times a day; each week increase by up to 200 mg/day in divided doses (100 mg every 12 hours for tablet formulations, 50 mg 4 times a day for suspension formulation); maximum dose generally 1,200 mg/day
- Lower initial dose and slower titration should be used for carbamazepine suspension

Dosing Tips

- Higher peak levels occur with the suspension formulation than with the same dose of the tablet formulation, so suspension should generally be started at a lower dose and titrated slowly
- Take carbamazepine with food to avoid gastrointestinal effects

✽ Slow dose titration may delay onset of therapeutic action but enhance tolerability to sedating side effects

- Controlled-release formulations (e.g., Equetro, Carbatrol) can significantly reduce sedation and other CNS side effects
- Should titrate slowly in the presence of other sedating agents, such as other anticonvulsants, in order to best tolerate additive sedative side effects

✽ Can sometimes minimize the impact of carbamazepine upon the bone marrow by dosing slowly and monitoring closely when initiating treatment; initial trend to leukopenia/neutropenia may reverse with continued conservative dosing over time and allow subsequent dosage increases with careful monitoring

✽ Carbamazepine often requires a dosage adjustment upward with time, as the drug induces its own metabolism, thus lowering its own plasma levels over the first several weeks to months of treatment

- Do not break or chew carbamazepine extended-release tablets as this will alter controlled-release properties

Overdose

- Can be fatal (lowest known fatal dose in adults is 3.2 g, in adolescents is 4 g, and in children is 1.6 g); nausea, vomiting, involuntary movements, irregular heartbeat, urinary retention, trouble breathing, sedation, coma

Long-Term Use

- May lower sex drive
- Monitoring of liver, kidney, thyroid functions, blood counts and sodium may be required

Habit Forming

- No

How to Stop

- Taper; may need to adjust dosage of concurrent medications as carbamazepine is being discontinued

✽ Rapid discontinuation may increase the risk of relapse in bipolar disorder

- Epilepsy patients may seize upon withdrawal, especially if withdrawal is abrupt
- Discontinuation symptoms uncommon

Pharmacokinetics

- Metabolized in the liver, primarily by CYP450 3A4
- Renally excreted
- Active metabolite (carbamazepine-10,11 epoxide)
- Initial half-life 26–65 hours (35–40 hours for extended-release formulation); half-life 12–17 hours with repeated doses
- Half-life of active metabolite is approximately 34 hours

✽ Is not only a substrate for CYP450 3A4, but also an inducer of CYP450 3A4

✽ Thus, carbamazepine induces its own metabolism, often requiring an upward dosage adjustment

- Is also an inducer of CYP450 2C9 and weakly of 1A2 and 2C19
- Food does not affect absorption

Drug Interactions

- Enzyme-inducing antiepileptic drugs (carbamazepine itself as well as phenobarbital, phenytoin, and primidone) may increase the clearance of carbamazepine and lower its plasma levels
- CYP450 3A4 inducers, such as carbamazepine itself, can lower the plasma levels of carbamazepine
- CYP450 3A4 inhibitors, such as nefazodone, fluvoxamine, and fluoxetine, can increase plasma levels of carbamazepine
- Carbamazepine can increase plasma levels of clomipramine, phenytoin, primidone
- Carbamazepine can decrease plasma levels of acetaminophen, clozapine, benzodiazepines, dicumarol, doxycycline, theophylline, warfarin, and haloperidol as well as other anticonvulsants such as phensuximide, methsuximide, ethosuximide, phenytoin, tiagabine, topiramate, lamotrigine, and valproate
- Carbamazepine can decrease plasma levels of hormonal contraceptives and adversely affect their efficacy
- Combined use of carbamazepine with other anticonvulsants may lead to altered thyroid function
- Combined use of carbamazepine and lithium may increase risk of neurotoxic effects
- Depressive effects are increased by other CNS depressants (alcohol, MAOIs, other anticonvulsants, etc.)
- Combined use of carbamazepine suspension with liquid formulations of chlorpromazine has been shown to result in excretion of an orange rubbery precipitate; because of this, combined use of carbamazepine suspension with any liquid medicine is not recommended

Other Warnings/ Precautions

✻ Patients should be monitored carefully for signs of unusual bleeding or bruising, mouth sores, infections, fever, or sore throat, as the risk of aplastic anemia and agranulocytosis with carbamazepine use is 5–8 times greater than in the general population (risk in the untreated general population is 6 patients per 1 million per year for agranulocytosis and 2 patients per 1 million per year for aplastic anemia)

- Because carbamazepine has a tricyclic chemical structure, use with caution with MAOIs, including 14 days after MAOIs are stopped (for the expert)
- May exacerbate angle-closure glaucoma
- Because carbamazepine can lower plasma levels of hormonal contraceptives, it may also reduce their effectiveness
- May need to restrict fluid intake because of risk of developing syndrome of inappropriate antidiuretic hormone secretion, hyponatremia and its complications
- Use with caution in patients with mixed seizure disorders that include atypical absence seizures because carbamazepine has been associated with increased frequency of generalized convulsions in such patients
- Individuals with the HLA-B*1502 allele are at increased risk of developing Stevens-Johnson syndrome and toxic epidermal necrolysis
- Warn patients and their caregivers about the possibility of activation of suicidal ideation and advise them to report such side effects immediately

Do Not Use

- If patient has history of bone marrow suppression
- If patient tests positive for the HLA-B*1502 allele
- If there is a proven allergy to any tricyclic compound
- If there is a proven allergy to carbamazepine
- Suspension: in patients with hereditary problems with fructose intolerance

SPECIAL POPULATIONS

Renal Impairment

- Carbamazepine is renally secreted, so the dose may need to be lowered

Hepatic Impairment

- Drug should be used with caution
- Rare cases of hepatic failure have occurred

Cardiac Impairment

- Drug should be used with caution

Elderly

- Some patients may tolerate lower doses better
- Elderly patients may be more susceptible to adverse effects

Children and Adolescents

- Approved use for epilepsy; therapeutic range of total carbamazepine in plasma is considered the same for children and adults
- Ages 6–12: initial dose 100 mg twice daily (tablets) or 0.5 teaspoon (50 mg) 4 times a day (suspension); each week increase by up to 100 mg/day in divided doses (2 doses for extended-release formulation, 3–4 doses for all other formulations); maximum dose generally 1,000 mg/day; maintenance dose generally 400–800 mg/day
- Ages 5 and younger: initial 10–20 mg/kg per day in divided doses (2–3 doses for tablet formulations, 4 doses for suspension); increase weekly as needed; maximum dose generally 35 mg/kg/day

Pregnancy

- Effective June 30, 2015, the US FDA requires changes to the content and format of pregnancy and lactation information in prescription drug labels, including the elimination of the pregnancy letter categories; the Pregnancy and Lactation Labeling Rule (PLLR or final rule) applies only to prescription drugs and will be phased in gradually for drugs approved on or after June 30, 2001

✻ Use during first trimester may raise risk of neural tube defects (e.g., spina bifida) or other congenital anomalies

- Use in women of childbearing potential requires weighing potential benefits to the mother against the risks to the fetus

✻ If drug is continued, perform tests to detect birth defects

✻ If drug is continued, start on folate 1 mg/day early in pregnancy to reduce risk of neural tube defects

- Antiepileptic Drug Pregnancy Registry: (888) 233–2334
- Use of anticonvulsants in combination may cause a higher prevalence of teratogenic effects than anticonvulsant monotherapy
- Taper drug if discontinuing
- Seizures, even mild seizures, may cause harm to the embryo/fetus

✻ For bipolar patients, carbamazepine should generally be discontinued before anticipated pregnancies

- Recurrent bipolar illness during pregnancy can be quite disruptive
- For bipolar patients, given the risk of relapse in the postpartum period, some form of mood stabilizer treatment may need to be restarted immediately after delivery if patient is unmedicated during pregnancy

✻ Atypical antipsychotics may be preferable to lithium or anticonvulsants such as carbamazepine if treatment of bipolar disorder is required during pregnancy

- Bipolar symptoms may recur or worsen during pregnancy and some form of treatment may be necessary

Breast Feeding

- Some drug is found in mother's breast milk

✻ Recommended either to discontinue drug or bottle feed

- If drug is continued while breast feeding, infant should be monitored for possible adverse effects, including hematological effects
- If infant shows signs of irritability or sedation, drug may need to be discontinued
- Some cases of neonatal seizures, respiratory depression, vomiting, and diarrhea have been reported in infants whose mothers received carbamazepine during pregnancy

✻ Bipolar disorder may recur during the postpartum period, particularly if there is a history of prior postpartum episodes of either depression or psychosis

- Relapse rates may be lower in women who receive prophylactic treatment for postpartum episodes of bipolar disorder
- Atypical antipsychotics and anticonvulsants such as valproate may be safer than carbamazepine during the postpartum period when breast feeding

THE ART OF PSYCHOPHARMACOLOGY

Potential Advantages
- Treatment-resistant bipolar and psychotic disorders

Potential Disadvantages
- Patients who do not wish to or cannot comply with blood testing and close monitoring
- Patients who cannot tolerate sedation
- Pregnant patients

Primary Target Symptoms
- Incidence of seizures
- Unstable mood, especially mania
- Pain

Pearls
- Carbamazepine was the first anticonvulsant widely used for the treatment of bipolar disorder and is now formally approved for acute mania and mixed mania

* An extended-release formulation has better evidence of efficacy and improved tolerability in bipolar disorder than does immediate-release carbamazepine
- Dosage frequency as well as sedation, diplopia, confusion, and ataxia may be reduced with extended-release carbamazepine
- Risk of serious side effects is greatest in the first few months of treatment
- Common side effects such as sedation often abate after a few months

* May be effective in patients who fail to respond to lithium or other mood stabilizers
- May be effective for the depressed phase of bipolar disorder and for maintenance in bipolar disorder
- Can be complicated to use with concomitant medications

Suggested Reading

Leucht S, McGrath J, White P, Kissling W. Carbamazepine for schizophrenia and schizoaffective psychoses. Cochrane Database Syst Rev 2002;(3):CD001258.

Marson AG, Williamson PR, Hutton JL, Clough HE, Chadwick DW. Carbamazepine versus valproate monotherapy for epilepsy. Cochrane Database Syst Rev 2000;(3):CD001030.

Smith LA, Cornelius V, Warnock A, Tacchi MJ, Taylor D. Pharmacological interventions for acute bipolar mania: a systematic review of randomized placebo-controlled trials. Bipolar Disord 2007;9(6):551–60.

Weisler RH, Kalali AH, Ketter TA. A multicenter, randomized, double-blind, placebo-controlled trial of extended-release carbamazepine capsules as monotherapy for bipolar disorder patients with manic or mixed episodes. J Clin Psychiatry 2004;65:478–84.

THERAPEUTICS

Brands
• Vraylar

see index for additional brand names

Generic?
No

Class
- Neuroscience-based Nomenclature: dopamine, serotonin, norepinephrine receptor antagonist (DSN-Ran)
- Dopamine partial agonist (dopamine stabilizer, atypical antipsychotic, third-generation antipsychotic; sometimes included as a second-generation antipsychotic; also a potential mood stabilizer)

Commonly Prescribed for
(bold for FDA approved)
- **Schizophrenia**
- **Acute mania/mixed mania**
- Other psychotic disorders
- Bipolar maintenance
- Bipolar depression
- Treatment-resistant depression
- Behavioral disturbances in dementia
- Behavioral disturbances in children and adolescents
- Disorders associated with problems with impulse control

How the Drug Works
✻ Partial agonism at dopamine 2 receptors
- Theoretically reduces dopamine output when dopamine concentrations are high, thus improving positive symptoms and mediating antipsychotic actions
- Theoretically increases dopamine output when dopamine concentrations are low, thus improving cognitive, negative, and mood symptoms
- Preferentially binds to dopamine 3 over dopamine 2 receptors at low doses; the clinical significance is unknown but could theoretically contribute to cariprazine's efficacy for negative symptoms. D3 partial agonism could theoretically be useful for treating cognition, mood, emotions, and reward/substance use
- Cariprazine also has high affinity for the serotonin 1A (partial agonist) and 2B (antagonist) receptors
- Cariprazine has moderate affinity for serotonin 2A receptors (antagonist)

How Long Until It Works
- Psychotic and manic symptoms can improve within 1 week, but it may take several weeks for full effect on behavior as well as on cognition
- Classically recommended to wait at least 4–6 weeks to determine full antipsychotic efficacy of drug, but in practice some patients may require up to 16–20 weeks to show a good response, especially on cognitive impairment and functional outcome

If It Works
- Most often reduces positive symptoms but does not eliminate them
- May reduce and eliminate acute manic symptoms
- Can improve negative symptoms, as well as aggressive, cognitive, and affective symptoms in schizophrenia
- Most schizophrenia patients do not have a total remission of symptoms but rather a reduction of symptoms by about a third
- Perhaps 5–15% of schizophrenia patients can experience an overall improvement of greater than 50–60%, especially when receiving stable treatment for more than a year
- Such patients are considered super-responders or "awakeners" since they may be well enough to be employed, live independently, and sustain long-term relationships
- Continue treatment until reaching a plateau of improvement
- After reaching a satisfactory plateau, continue treatment for at least a year after first episode of psychosis
- For second and subsequent episodes of psychosis, treatment may need to be indefinite
- Even for first episodes of psychosis, it may be preferable to continue treatment

If It Doesn't Work
- Try one of the other atypical antipsychotics
- If 2 or more antipsychotic monotherapies do not work, consider clozapine
- Some patients may require treatment with a conventional antipsychotic
- If no first-line atypical antipsychotic is effective for schizophrenia, consider higher

doses or augmentation with valproate or lamotrigine
- Consider lithium and anticonvulsant mood stabilizers for mania
- Consider noncompliance and switch to another antipsychotic with fewer side effects or to an antipsychotic that can be given by depot injection
- Consider initiating rehabilitation and psychotherapy
- Consider presence of concomitant drug abuse

Best Augmenting Combos for Partial Response or Treatment Resistance
- Valproic acid (valproate, divalproex, divalproex ER)
- Lamotrigine
- Lithium
- Benzodiazepines

Tests
Before starting any atypical antipsychotic

✽ Weigh all patients and track BMI during treatment
- Get baseline personal and family history of diabetes, obesity, dyslipidemia, hypertension, and cardiovascular disease

✽ Get waist circumference (at umbilicus), blood pressure, fasting plasma glucose, and fasting lipid profile
- Determine if the patient is
  - overweight (BMI 25.0–29.9)
  - obese (BMI >30)
  - has pre-diabetes (fasting plasma glucose 100–125 mg/dL)
  - has diabetes (fasting plasma glucose >126 mg/dL)
  - has hypertension (BP >140/90 mmHg)
  - has dyslipidemia (increased total cholesterol, LDL cholesterol, and triglycerides; decreased HDL cholesterol)
- Treat or refer such patients for treatment, including nutrition and weight management, physical activity counseling, smoking cessation, and medical management

Monitoring after starting any atypical antipsychotic

✽ BMI monthly for 3 months, then quarterly

✽ Consider monitoring fasting triglycerides monthly for several months in patients at high risk for metabolic complications and when initiating or switching antipsychotics

✽ Blood pressure, fasting plasma glucose, fasting lipids within 3 months and then annually, but earlier and more frequently for patients with diabetes or who have gained >5% of initial weight
- Treat or refer for treatment and consider switching to another atypical antipsychotic for patients who become overweight, obese, pre-diabetic, diabetic, hypertensive, or dyslipidemic while receiving an atypical antipsychotic

✽ Even in patients without known diabetes, be vigilant for the rare but life-threatening onset of diabetic ketoacidosis, which always requires immediate treatment, by monitoring for the rapid onset of polyuria, polydipsia, weight loss, nausea, vomiting, dehydration, rapid respiration, weakness and clouding of sensorium, even coma
- Patients with low white blood cell count (WBC) or history of drug-induced leukopenia/neutropenia should have complete blood count (CBC) monitored frequently during the first few months and cariprazine should be discontinued at the first sign of decline in WBC in the absence of other causative factors

SIDE EFFECTS

How Drug Causes Side Effects
- Partial agonist actions at dopamine 2 receptors in the striatum can cause motor side effects, such as akathisia (occasionally)
- Partial agonist actions at dopamine 2 receptors can also cause nausea, occasional vomiting, and activating side effects
- Mechanism of weight gain and increased incidence of diabetes and dyslipidemia with atypical antipsychotics is unknown

Notable Side Effects
- Akathisia, extrapyramidal symptoms, restlessness
- Gastrointestinal distress
- Sedation
- Theoretical risk of tardive dyskinesia

Life-Threatening or Dangerous Side Effects

- Hyperglycemia, in some cases extreme and associated with ketoacidosis or hyperosmolar coma or death, has been reported in patients taking atypical antipsychotics
- Increased risk of death and cerebrovascular events in elderly patients with dementia-related psychosis
- Rare neuroleptic malignant syndrome (much reduced risk compared to conventional antipsychotics)
- Rare seizures

Weight Gain

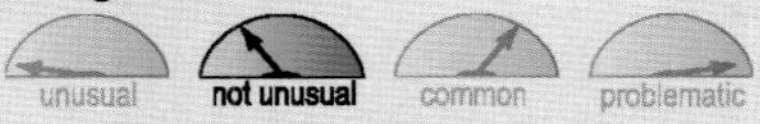

- Occurs in significant minority

Sedation

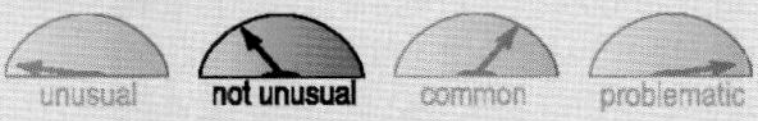

- Occurs in significant minority

What to Do About Side Effects

- Wait
- Wait
- Wait
- Anticholinergics or a low-dose benzodiazepine or a beta blocker may reduce akathisia effects when present
- Weight loss, exercise programs, and medical management for high BMIs, diabetes, dyslipidemia
- Switch to another atypical antipsychotic

Best Augmenting Agents for Side Effects

- Beta blockers or sometimes benzodiazepines for akathisia
- Benztropine or trihexyphenidyl for motor side effects
- Many side effects cannot be improved with an augmenting agent

DOSING AND USE

Usual Dosage Range

- Schizophrenia: 1.5–6 mg once daily
- Bipolar mania: 3–6 mg once daily

Dosage Forms

- Capsule 1.5 mg, 3 mg, 4.5 mg, 6 mg

How to Dose

- Schizophrenia: initial 1.5 mg once daily; can increase to 3 mg once daily on day 2; can increase in 1.5–3 mg increments to reach therapeutic dose (recommended dose 1.5–6 mg once daily)
- Bipolar mania: initial 1.5 mg once daily; can increase to 3 mg once daily on day 2; can increase in 1.5–3 mg increments to reach therapeutic dose (recommended dose 3–6 mg once daily)

Dosing Tips

- Because of its long half-life, and the especially long half-life of one of its active metabolites, monitor for adverse effects and response for several weeks after starting cariprazine and with each dosage change; also washout of active drug will take several weeks
- Because of its long half-life, missing a few doses may not be as detrimental compared to other antipsychotics
- Can be taken with or without food

Overdose

- Limited experience

Long-Term Use

- Not extensively studied, but long-term maintenance treatment is often necessary for schizophrenia and bipolar mania
- Should periodically reevaluate long-term usefulness in individual patients, but treatment may need to continue for many years in patients with schizophrenia

Habit Forming

- No

How to Stop

- Because clinical experience is lacking, down-titration may be prudent, especially when simultaneously beginning a new antipsychotic while switching (i.e., cross-titration)
- However, the long half-lives of cariprazine and its two active metabolites suggest that it may be possible to stop cariprazine abruptly

- The method for stopping cariprazine can vary depending on which agent is being switched to; see switching guidelines of individual agents for how to stop cariprazine
- Rapid discontinuation could theoretically lead to rebound psychosis and worsening of symptoms, but less likely with cariprazine due to its long half-life

Pharmacokinetics

- Metabolized by CYP450 3A4 into two long-lasting active metabolites
- Based on time to reach steady state, half-life for cariprazine is 2–4 days and for one of its active metabolites, didesmethyl cariprazine (DDCAR), is 1–3 weeks

Drug Interactions

- Initiating a strong CYP450 3A4 inhibitor in patients on a stable dose of cariprazine: reduce the current dose of cariprazine by half (for patients taking 4.5 mg, reduce to either 1.5 mg or 3 mg once daily; for patients taking 1.5 mg once daily, reduce to 1.5 mg every other day)
- Initiating cariprazine in patients taking a strong CYP450 3A4 inhibitor: administer 1.5 mg on day 1; do not dose on day 2; administer 1.5 mg on day 3 and on day 4; maximum dose 3 mg once daily
- Concomitant use of cariprazine and a CYP450 3A4 inducer is not recommended
- May increase effects of antihypertensive agents
- May antagonize levodopa, dopamine agonists

Other Warnings/ Precautions

- Use with caution in patients with conditions that predispose to hypotension (dehydration, overheating)
- Dysphagia has been associated with antipsychotic use, and cariprazine should be used cautiously in patients at risk for aspiration pneumonia

Do Not Use

- If there is a proven allergy to cariprazine

SPECIAL POPULATIONS

Renal Impairment

- Mild to moderate impairment (creatinine clearance <30 mL/minute): no dose adjustment necessary
- Severe or end-stage: not recommended

Hepatic Impairment

- Mild to moderate impairment (Child-Pugh score between 5 and 9): no dose adjustment necessary
- Severe: not recommended

Cardiac Impairment

- Use in patients with cardiac impairment has not been studied, so use with caution

Elderly

- Some elderly patients may tolerate lower doses better
- Although atypical antipsychotics are commonly used for behavioral disturbances in dementia, no agent has been approved for treatment of elderly patients with dementia-related psychosis
- Elderly patients with dementia-related psychosis treated with atypical antipsychotics are at an increased risk of death compared to placebo, and also have an increased risk of cerebrovascular events

Children and Adolescents

- Safety and efficacy have not been established
- Children and adolescents using cariprazine may need to be monitored more often than adults

Pregnancy

- Effective June 30, 2015, the US FDA requires changes to the content and format of pregnancy and lactation information in prescription drug labels, including the elimination of the pregnancy letter categories; the Pregnancy and Lactation Labeling Rule (PLLR or final rule) applies only to prescription drugs and will be phased in gradually for drugs approved on or after June 30, 2001
- Controlled studies have not been conducted in pregnant women

- In rats, administration of cariprazine during organogenesis caused malformations, lower pup survival, and developmental delays at exposures less than the human exposure at maximum recommended human dose (6 mg/day); cariprazine was not teratogenic in rabbits at doses up to 4.6 times the maximum recommended human dose
- There is a risk of abnormal muscle movements and withdrawal symptoms in newborns whose mothers took an antipsychotic during the third trimester; symptoms may include agitation, abnormally increased or decreased muscle tone, tremor, sleepiness, severe difficulty breathing, and difficulty feeding
- Psychotic symptoms may worsen during pregnancy and some form of treatment may be necessary
- National Pregnancy Registry for Atypical Antipsychotics: 1-866-961-2388 or http://womensmentalhealth.org/clinical-and-research-programs/pregnancyregistry/

Breast Feeding

- Unknown if cariprazine is secreted in human breast milk, but all psychotropics assumed to be secreted in breast milk
- ✻ Recommended either to discontinue drug or bottle feed unless the potential benefit to the mother justifies the potential risk to the child
- Infants of women who choose to breast feed while on cariprazine should be monitored for possible adverse effects

THE ART OF PSYCHOPHARMACOLOGY

Potential Advantages

- For patients who do not tolerate aripiprazole or brexpiprazole
- Possibly negative symptoms in schizophrenia

Potential Disadvantages

- Expensive

Primary Target Symptoms

- Positive symptoms of psychosis
- Negative symptoms of psychosis
- Symptoms of acute mania/mixed mania
- Cognitive symptoms
- Unstable mood (both depression and mania)
- Aggressive symptoms

Pearls

- Cariprazine is metabolized into a very long-lasting active metabolite; it is therefore possible that adverse events could appear several weeks after initiation of cariprazine due to accumulation of cariprazine and major metabolites over time
- It is also possible that cariprazine or its very long-lasting active metabolites could be developed as an "oral depot" namely, a very long-lasting oral formulation for weekly or even monthly oral administration
- Based on short-term clinical trials, cariprazine appears to have a favorable metabolic profile, with changes in triglycerides, fasting glucose, and cholesterol similar to placebo; however, it may cause a small amount of dose-dependent weight gain
- Cariprazine is also being studied for the treatment of bipolar depression and as an adjunct for treatment-resistant unipolar depression
- D3-preferring (over D2) actions represent a novel pharmacologic profile among antipsychotics, especially at lower doses; clinical advantages of this profile remain to be determined but animal models suggest that targeting D3 receptors may have advantages for mood, negative symptoms, and substance abuse
- All antipsychotics bind to the D3 receptor in vitro, but only cariprazine has affinity for the D3 receptor greater than dopamine itself, so it is the only antipsychotic with functional D3 partial agonism in vivo in the living human brain

THE ART OF SWITCHING

Switching from Oral Antipsychotics to Cariprazine

- It is advisable to begin cariprazine at an intermediate dose and build the dose rapidly over 3–7 days
- Clinical experience has shown that asenapine, quetiapine, and olanzapine should be tapered off slowly over a period of 3–4 weeks, to allow patients to readapt to the withdrawal of blocking cholinergic, histaminergic, and alpha 1 receptors
- Clozapine should always be tapered off slowly, over a period of 4 weeks or more

* Benzodiazepine or anticholinergic medication can be administered during cross-titration to help alleviate side effects such as insomnia, agitation, and/or psychosis

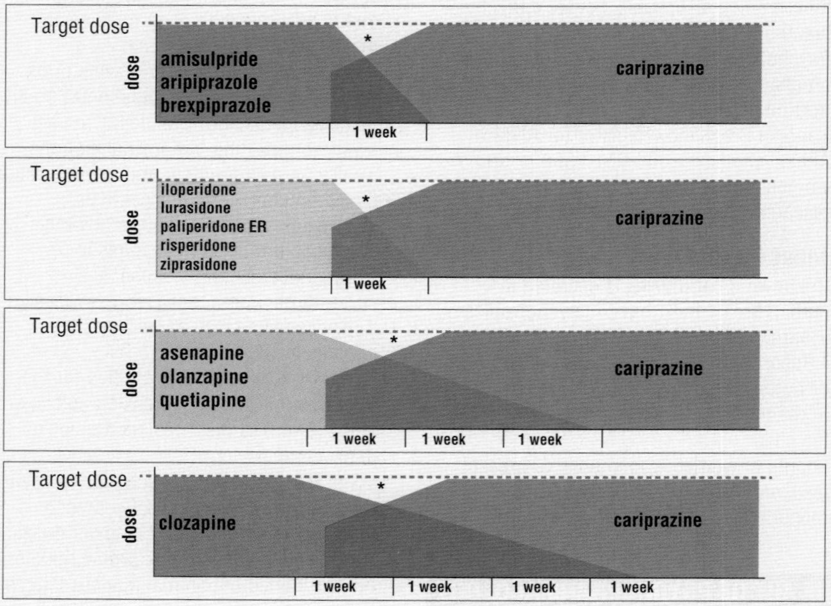

Suggested Reading

Choi YK, Adham N, Kiss B, Gyertyán I, Tarazi FI. Long-term effects of cariprazine exposure on dopamine receptor subtypes. CNS Spectr 2014;19(3):268–77.

Citrome L. Cariprazine in schizophrenia: clinical efficacy, tolerability, and place in therapy. Adv Ther 2013;30(2):114–26.

Vieta E, Durgam S, Lu K, et al. Effect of cariprazine across the symptoms of mania in bipolar I disorder: Analyses of pooled data from phase II/III trials. Eur Neuropsychopharmacol 2015;25(11):1882–91.

CHLORDIAZEPOXIDE

THERAPEUTICS

Brands • Limbitrol
• Librium
• Librax

see index for additional brand names

Generic? Yes

Class
• Neuroscience-based Nomenclature: GABA positive allosteric modulator (GABA-PAM)
• Benzodiazepine (anxiolytic)

Commonly Prescribed for
(bold for FDA approved)
• **Anxiety disorders**
• **Symptoms of anxiety**
• **Preoperative apprehension and anxiety**
• **Withdrawal symptoms of acute alcoholism**
• Catatonia

How the Drug Works
• Binds to benzodiazepine receptors at the GABA-A ligand-gated chloride channel complex
• Enhances the inhibitory effects of GABA
• Boosts chloride conductance through GABA-regulated channels
• Inhibits neuronal activity presumably in amygdala-centered fear circuits to provide therapeutic benefits in anxiety disorders

How Long Until It Works
• Some immediate relief with first dosing is common; can take several weeks with daily dosing for maximal therapeutic benefit

If It Works
• For short-term symptoms of anxiety – after a few weeks, discontinue use or use on an "as-needed" basis
• For chronic anxiety disorders, the goal of treatment is complete remission of symptoms as well as prevention of future relapses
• For chronic anxiety disorders, treatment most often reduces or even eliminates symptoms, but not a cure since symptoms can recur after medicine stopped
• For long-term symptoms of anxiety, consider switching to an SSRI or SNRI for long-term maintenance
• If long-term maintenance with a benzodiazepine is necessary, continue treatment for 6 months after symptoms resolve, and then taper dose slowly
• If symptoms reemerge, consider treatment with an SSRI or SNRI, or consider restarting the benzodiazepine; sometimes benzodiazepines have to be used in combination with SSRIs or SNRIs for best results

If It Doesn't Work
• Consider switching to another agent or adding an appropriate augmenting agent
• Consider psychotherapy, especially cognitive behavioral psychotherapy
• Consider presence of concomitant substance abuse
• Consider presence of chlordiazepoxide abuse
• Consider another diagnosis, such as a comorbid medical condition

Best Augmenting Combos for Partial Response or Treatment Resistance
• Benzodiazepines are frequently used as augmenting agents for antipsychotics and mood stabilizers in the treatment of psychotic and bipolar disorders
• Benzodiazepines are frequently used as augmenting agents for SSRIs and SNRIs in the treatment of anxiety disorders
• Not generally rational to combine with other benzodiazepines
• Caution if using as an anxiolytic concomitantly with other sedative hypnotics for sleep

Tests
• In patients with seizure disorders, concomitant medical illness, and/or those with multiple concomitant long-term medications, periodic liver tests and blood counts may be prudent

SIDE EFFECTS

How Drug Causes Side Effects
• Same mechanism for side effects as for therapeutic effects – namely due to excessive actions at benzodiazepine receptors

- Long-term adaptations in benzodiazepine receptors may explain the development of dependence, tolerance, and withdrawal
- Side effects are generally immediate, but immediate side effects often disappear in time

Notable Side Effects

✻ Sedation, fatigue, depression
✻ Dizziness, ataxia, slurred speech, weakness
✻ Forgetfulness, confusion
✻ Hyper-excitability, nervousness
✻ Pain at injection site
- Rare hallucinations, mania
- Rare hypotension
- Hypersalivation, dry mouth

Life-Threatening or Dangerous Side Effects

- Respiratory depression, especially when taken with CNS depressants in overdose
- Rare hepatic dysfunction, renal dysfunction, blood dyscrasias

Weight Gain

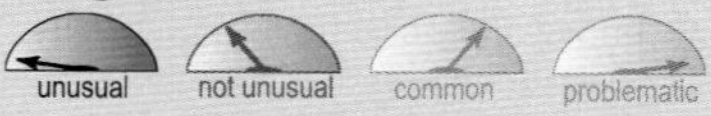

- Reported but not expected

Sedation

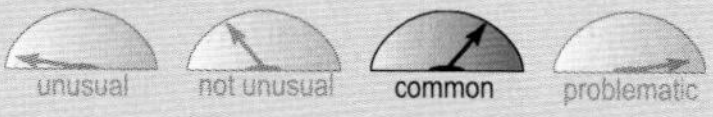

- Many experience and/or can be significant in amount
- Especially at initiation of treatment or when dose increases
- Tolerance often develops over time

What to Do About Side Effects

- Wait
- Wait
- Wait
- Lower the dose
- Take largest dose at bedtime to avoid sedative effects during the day
- Switch to another agent
- Administer flumazenil if side effects are severe or life-threatening

Best Augmenting Agents for Side Effects

- Many side effects cannot be improved with an augmenting agent

DOSING AND USE

Usual Dosage Range

- Oral: mild to moderate anxiety: 15–40 mg/day in 3–4 doses
- Oral: severe anxiety: 60–100 mg/day in 3–4 doses

Dosage Forms

- Capsule 5 mg, 10 mg, 25 mg
- Injectable 100 mg/5 mL

How to Dose

- Injectable: acute/severe anxiety: initial 50–100 mg; 25–50 mg 3–4 times/day if necessary
- Injectable: alcohol withdrawal: initial 50–100 mg; repeat after 2 hours if necessary
- Injectable: preoperative: 50–100 mg 1 hour before surgery
- Patients who receive injectable chlordiazepoxide should be observed for up to 3 hours

Dosing Tips

✻ One of the few benzodiazepines available in an injectable formulation
- Chlordiazepoxide injection is intended for acute use; patients who require longer treatment should be switched to the oral formulation
- Use lowest possible effective dose for the shortest possible period of time (a benzodiazepine-sparing strategy)
- Assess need for continued treatment regularly
- Risk of dependence may increase with dose and duration of treatment
- For interdose symptoms of anxiety, can either increase dose or maintain same total daily dose but divide into more frequent doses
- Can also use an as-needed occasional “top up” dose for interdose anxiety
- Because anxiety disorders can require higher doses, the risk of dependence may be greater in these patients
- Some severely ill patients may require doses higher than the generally recommended maximum dose
- Frequency of dosing in practice is often greater than predicted from half-life, as duration of biological activity is often

shorter than pharmacokinetic terminal half-life

Overdose
- Fatalities can occur; hypotension, tiredness, ataxia, confusion, coma

Long-Term Use
- Evidence of efficacy for up to 16 weeks
- Risk of dependence, particularly for treatment periods longer than 12 weeks, and especially in patients with past or current polysubstance abuse

Habit Forming
- Chlordiazepoxide is a Schedule IV drug
- Patients may develop dependence and/or tolerance with long-term use

How to Stop
- Patients with history of seizure may seize upon withdrawal, especially if withdrawal is abrupt
- Taper by 10 mg every 3 days to reduce chances of withdrawal effects
- For difficult to taper patients, consider reducing dose much more slowly after reaching 20 mg/day, perhaps by as little as 5 mg per week or less
- For other patients with severe problems discontinuing a benzodiazepine, dosing may need to be tapered over many months (i.e., reduce dose by 1% every 3 days by crushing tablet and suspending or dissolving in 100 mL of fruit juice and then disposing of 1 mL while drinking the rest; 3–7 days later, dispose of 2 mL, and so on). This is both a form of very slow biological tapering and a form of behavioral desensitization
- Be sure to differentiate reemergence of symptoms requiring reinstitution of treatment from withdrawal symptoms
- Benzodiazepine-dependent anxiety patients and insulin-dependent diabetics are not addicted to their medications. When benzodiazepine-dependent patients stop their medication, disease symptoms can reemerge, disease symptoms can worsen (rebound), and/or withdrawal symptoms can emerge

Pharmacokinetics
- Elimination half-life 24–48 hours

Drug Interactions
- Increased depressive effects when taken with other CNS depressants (see Warnings below)

Other Warnings/ Precautions
- Boxed warning regarding the increased risk of CNS depressant effects when benzodiazepines and opioid medications are used together, including specifically the risk of slowed or difficulty breathing and death
- If alternatives to the combined use of benzodiazepines and opioids are not available, clinicians should limit the dosage and duration of each drug to the minimum possible while still achieving therapeutic efficacy
- Patients and their caregivers should be warned to seek medical attention if unusual dizziness, lightheadedness, sedation, slowed or difficulty breathing, or unresponsiveness occur
- Dosage changes should be made in collaboration with prescriber
- Use with caution in patients with pulmonary disease; rare reports of death after initiation of benzodiazepines in patients with severe pulmonary impairment
- History of drug or alcohol abuse often creates greater risk for dependency
- Some depressed patients may experience a worsening of suicidal ideation
- Some patients may exhibit abnormal thinking or behavioral changes similar to those caused by other CNS depressants (i.e., either depressant actions or disinhibiting actions)

Do Not Use
- If patient has angle-closure glaucoma
- If there is a proven allergy to chlordiazepoxide or any benzodiazepine

SPECIAL POPULATIONS

Renal Impairment
- Oral: initial 10–20 mg/day in 2–4 doses; increase as needed
- Injectable: 25–50 mg

Hepatic Impairment

- Oral: initial 10–20 mg/day in 2–4 doses; increase as needed
- Injectable: 25–50 mg

Cardiac Impairment

- Benzodiazepines have been used to treat anxiety associated with acute myocardial infarction

Elderly

- Oral: initial 10–20 mg/day in 2–4 doses; increase as needed
- Injectable: 25–50 mg
- Elderly patients may be more sensitive to sedative effects

Children and Adolescents

- Oral: Not recommended for use in children under age 6
- Oral: initial 10–20 mg/day in 2–4 doses; may increase to 20–30 mg/day in 2–3 doses if ineffective
- Injectable: Not recommended for use in children under age 12
- Injectable: 25–50 mg
- Hyperactive children should be monitored for paradoxical effects
- Long-term effects of chlordiazepoxide in children/adolescents are unknown
- Should generally receive lower doses and be more closely monitored

Pregnancy

- Effective June 30, 2015, the US FDA requires changes to the content and format of pregnancy and lactation information in prescription drug labels, including the elimination of the pregnancy letter categories; the Pregnancy and Lactation Labeling Rule (PLLR or final rule) applies only to prescription drugs and will be phased in gradually for drugs approved on or after June 30, 2001
- Possible increased risk of birth defects when benzodiazepines taken during pregnancy
- Because of the potential risks, chlordiazepoxide is not generally recommended as treatment for anxiety during pregnancy, especially during the first trimester
- Drug should be tapered if discontinued
- Infants whose mothers received a benzodiazepine late in pregnancy may experience withdrawal effects
- Neonatal flaccidity has been reported in infants whose mothers took a benzodiazepine during pregnancy
- Seizures, even mild seizures, may cause harm to the embryo/fetus

Breast Feeding

- Unknown if chlordiazepoxide is secreted in human breast milk, but all psychotropics assumed to be secreted in breast milk
- ✻ Recommended either to discontinue drug or bottle feed
- Effects of benzodiazepines on nursing infants have been reported and include feeding difficulties, sedation, and weight loss

THE ART OF PSYCHOPHARMACOLOGY

Potential Advantages

- Rapid onset of action

Potential Disadvantages

- Euphoria may lead to abuse
- Abuse especially risky in past or present substance abusers

Primary Target Symptoms

- Panic attacks
- Anxiety

Pearls

- Can be a useful adjunct to SSRIs and SNRIs in the treatment of numerous anxiety disorders, but not used as frequently as some other benzodiazepines
- Not effective for treating psychosis as a monotherapy, but can be used as an adjunct to antipsychotics
- Not effective for treating bipolar disorder as a monotherapy, but can be used as an adjunct to mood stabilizers and antipsychotics
- Can both cause depression and treat depression in different patients
- When using to treat insomnia, remember that insomnia may be a symptom of some

other primary disorder itself, and thus warrant evaluation for comorbid psychiatric and/or medical conditions

* Remains a viable treatment option for alcohol withdrawal

- Though not systematically studied, benzodiazepines have been used effectively to treat catatonia and are the initial recommended treatment

Suggested Reading

Baskin SI, Esdale A. Is chlordiazepoxide the rational choice among benzodiazepines? Pharmacotherapy 1982;2:110–19.

Erstad BL, Cotugno CL. Management of alcohol withdrawal. Am J Health Syst Pharm 1995;52:697–709.

Fraser AD. Use and abuse of the benzodiazepines. Ther Drug Monit 1998;20:481–9.

Murray JB. Effects of valium and librium on human psychomotor and cognitive functions. Genet Psychol Monogr 1984;109(2D Half):167–97.

CHLORPROMAZINE

THERAPEUTICS

Brands • Thorazine

see index for additional brand names

Generic? Yes

Class

- Neuroscience-based Nomenclature: dopamine and serotonin receptor antagonist (DS-RAn)
- Conventional antipsychotic (neuroleptic, phenothiazine, dopamine 2 antagonist, antiemetic)

Commonly Prescribed for

(bold for FDA approved)

- **Schizophrenia**
- **Nausea, vomiting**
- **Restlessness and apprehension before surgery**
- **Acute intermittent porphyria**
- **Manifestations of manic type of manic-depressive illness**
- **Tetanus (adjunct)**
- **Intractable hiccups**
- **Combativeness and/or explosive hyperexcitable behavior (in children)**
- **Hyperactive children who show excessive motor activity with accompanying conduct disorders consisting of some or all of the following symptoms: impulsivity, difficulty sustaining attention, aggressivity, mood lability, and poor frustration tolerance**
- **Psychosis**
- Bipolar disorder

How the Drug Works

- Blocks dopamine 2 receptors, reducing positive symptoms of psychosis and improving other behaviors
- Combination of dopamine D2, histamine H1, and cholinergic M1 blockade in the vomiting center may reduce nausea and vomiting

How Long Until It Works

- Psychotic symptoms can improve within 1 week, but it may take several weeks for full effect on behavior
- Actions on nausea and vomiting are immediate

If It Works

- Most often reduces positive symptoms in schizophrenia but does not eliminate them
- Most schizophrenic patients do not have a total remission of symptoms but rather a reduction of symptoms by about a third
- Continue treatment in schizophrenia until reaching a plateau of improvement
- After reaching a satisfactory plateau, continue treatment for at least a year after first episode of psychosis in schizophrenia
- For second and subsequent episodes of psychosis in schizophrenia, treatment may need to be indefinite
- Reduces symptoms of acute psychotic mania but not proven as a mood stabilizer or as an effective maintenance treatment in bipolar disorder
- After reducing acute psychotic symptoms in mania, switch to a mood stabilizer and/or an atypical antipsychotic for mood stabilization and maintenance

If It Doesn't Work

- Consider trying one of the first-line atypical antipsychotics (risperidone, olanzapine, quetiapine, ziprasidone, aripiprazole, paliperidone, amisulpride, asenapine, iloperidone, lurasidone)
- Consider trying another conventional antipsychotic
- If 2 or more antipsychotic monotherapies do not work, consider clozapine

Best Augmenting Combos for Partial Response or Treatment Resistance

- Augmentation of conventional antipsychotics has not been systematically studied
- Addition of a mood-stabilizing anticonvulsant such as valproate, carbamazepine, or lamotrigine may be helpful in both schizophrenia and bipolar mania
- Augmentation with lithium in bipolar mania may be helpful
- Addition of a benzodiazepine, especially short-term for agitation

Tests

✻ Since conventional antipsychotics are frequently associated with weight gain, before starting treatment, weigh all patients and determine if the patient is already overweight (BMI 25.0–29.9) or obese (BMI ≥30)

- Before giving a drug that can cause weight gain to an overweight or obese patient, consider determining whether the patient already has pre-diabetes (fasting plasma glucose 100–125 mg/dL), diabetes (fasting plasma glucose >126 mg/dL), or dyslipidemia (increased total cholesterol, LDL cholesterol and triglycerides; decreased HDL cholesterol), and treat or refer such patients for treatment, including nutrition and weight management, physical activity counseling, smoking cessation, and medical management

✱ Monitor weight and BMI during treatment

✱ Consider monitoring fasting triglycerides monthly for several months in patients at high risk for metabolic complications and when initiating or switching antipsychotics

✱ While giving a drug to a patient who has gained >5% of initial weight, consider evaluating for the presence of pre-diabetes, diabetes, or dyslipidemia, or consider switching to a different antipsychotic

- Should check blood pressure in the elderly before starting and for the first few weeks of treatment
- Monitoring elevated prolactin levels of dubious clinical benefit
- Phenothiazines may cause false positive phenylketonuria results
- Patients with low white blood cell count (WBC) or history of drug-induced leucopenia/neutropenia should have complete blood count (CBC) monitored frequently during the first few months and chlorpromazine should be discontinued at the first sign of decline of WBC in the absence of other causative factors

SIDE EFFECTS

How Drug Causes Side Effects

- By blocking dopamine 2 receptors in the striatum, it can cause motor side effects
- By blocking dopamine 2 receptors in the pituitary, it can cause elevations in prolactin
- By blocking dopamine 2 receptors excessively in the mesocortical and mesolimbic dopamine pathways, especially at high doses, it can cause worsening of negative and cognitive symptoms (neuroleptic-induced deficit syndrome)
- Anticholinergic actions may cause sedation, blurred vision, constipation, dry mouth
- Antihistaminic actions may cause sedation, weight gain
- By blocking alpha 1 adrenergic receptors, it can cause dizziness, sedation, and hypotension
- Mechanism of weight gain and any possible increased incidence of diabetes or dyslipidemia with conventional antipsychotics is unknown

Notable Side Effects

✱ Neuroleptic-induced deficit syndrome

✱ Akathisia

✱ Priapism

✱ Extrapyramidal symptoms, parkinsonism, tardive dyskinesia

✱ Galactorrhea, amenorrhea

- Dizziness, sedation, impaired memory
- Dry mouth, constipation, urinary retention, blurred vision
- Decreased sweating
- Sexual dysfunction
- Hypotension, tachycardia, syncope
- Weight gain

Life-Threatening or Dangerous Side Effects

- Rare neuroleptic malignant syndrome
- Rare jaundice, agranulocytosis
- Rare seizures
- Increased risk of death and cerebrovascular events in elderly patients with dementia-related psychosis

Weight Gain

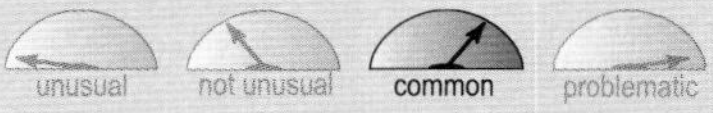

- Many experience and/or can be significant in amount

Sedation

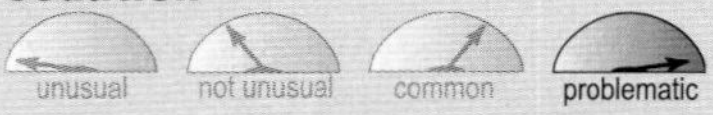

- Tolerance to sedation can develop over time

What to Do About Side Effects

- Wait
- Wait
- Wait
- For motor symptoms, add an anticholinergic agent
- Reduce the dose
- For sedation, give at night

- Switch to an atypical antipsychotic
- Weight loss, exercise programs, and medical management for high BMIs, diabetes dyslipidemia

Best Augmenting Agents for Side Effects

- Benztropine or trihexyphenidyl for motor side effects
- Sometimes amantadine can be helpful for motor side effects
- Benzodiazepines may be helpful for akathisia
- Many side effects cannot be improved with an augmenting agent

DOSING AND USE

Usual Dosage Range

- 200–800 mg/day

Dosage Forms

- Tablet 10 mg, 25 mg, 50 mg, 100 mg, 200 mg
- Capsule 30 mg, 75 mg, 150 mg
- Ampul 25 mg/mL; 1 mL, 2 mL
- Vial 25 mg/mL; 10 mL
- Liquid 10 mg/5 mL
- Suppository 25 mg, 100 mg

How to Dose

- Psychosis: increase dose until symptoms are controlled; after 2 weeks reduce to lowest effective dose
- Psychosis (intramuscular): varies by severity of symptoms and inpatient/outpatient status

Dosing Tips

- Low doses may have more sedative actions than antipsychotic actions
- Low doses have been used to provide short-term relief of daytime agitation and anxiety and to enhance sedative hypnotic actions in nonpsychotic patients, but other treatment options such as atypical antipsychotics are now preferred
- Higher doses may induce or worsen negative symptoms of schizophrenia
- Ampuls and vials contain sulfites that may cause allergic reactions, particularly in patients with asthma
- One of the few antipsychotics available as a suppository
- Treatment should be suspended if absolute neutrophil count falls below 1,000/mm^3

Overdose

- Extrapyramidal symptoms, sedation, hypotension, coma, respiratory depression

Long-Term Use

- Some side effects may be irreversible (e.g., tardive dyskinesia)

Habit Forming

- No

How to Stop

- Slow down-titration of oral formulation (over 6–8 weeks), especially when simultaneously beginning a new antipsychotic while switching (i.e., cross-titration)
- Rapid oral discontinuation may lead to rebound psychosis and worsening of symptoms
- If antiparkinson agents are being used, they should be continued for a few weeks after chlorpromazine is discontinued

Pharmacokinetics

- Half-life approximately 8–33 hours

Drug Interactions

- May decrease the effects of levodopa, dopamine agonists
- May increase the effects of antihypertensive drugs except for guanethidine, whose antihypertensive actions chlorpromazine may antagonize
- Additive effects may occur if used with CNS depressants
- Some pressor agents (e.g., epinephrine) may interact with chlorpromazine to lower blood pressure
- Alcohol and diuretics may increase the risk of hypotension
- Reduces effects of anticoagulants
- May reduce phenytoin metabolism and increase phenytoin levels
- Plasma levels of chlorpromazine and propranolol may increase if used concomitantly
- Some patients taking a neuroleptic and lithium have developed an encephalopathic

syndrome similar to neuroleptic malignant syndrome

Other Warnings/ Precautions

- If signs of neuroleptic malignant syndrome develop, treatment should be immediately discontinued
- Use cautiously in patients with alcohol withdrawal or convulsive disorders because of possible lowering of seizure threshold
- Use with caution in patients with respiratory disorders, glaucoma, or urinary retention
- Avoid extreme heat exposure
- Avoid undue exposure to sunlight
- Antiemetic effect of chlorpromazine may mask signs of other disorders or overdose; suppression of cough reflex may cause asphyxia
- Use only with caution if at all in Parkinson's disease or Lewy body dementia

Do Not Use

- If patient is in a comatose state
- If patient is taking metrizamide or large doses of CNS depressants
- If there is a proven allergy to chlorpromazine
- If there is a known sensitivity to any phenothiazine

SPECIAL POPULATIONS

Renal Impairment

- Use with caution

Hepatic Impairment

- Use with caution

Cardiac Impairment

- Cardiovascular toxicity can occur, especially orthostatic hypotension

Elderly

- Lower doses should be used and patient should be monitored closely
- Often do not tolerate sedating actions of chlorpromazine
- Although conventional antipsychotics are commonly used for behavioral disturbances in dementia, no agent has been approved for treatment of elderly patients with dementia-related psychosis
- Elderly patients with dementia-related psychosis treated with antipsychotics are at an increased risk of death compared to placebo, and also have an increased risk of cerebrovascular events

Children and Adolescents

- Can be used cautiously in children or adolescents over age 1 with severe behavioral problems
- Oral – 0.25 mg/lb every 4–6 hours as needed; rectal – 0.5 mg/lb every 6–8 hours as needed; IM – 0.25 mg/lb every 6–8 hours as needed; maximum 40 mg/day (under 5), 75 mg/day (5–12)
- Do not use if patient shows signs of Reye's syndrome
- Generally consider second-line after atypical antipsychotics

Pregnancy

- Effective June 30, 2015, the US FDA requires changes to the content and format of pregnancy and lactation information in prescription drug labels, including the elimination of the pregnancy letter categories; the Pregnancy and Lactation Labeling Rule (PLLR or final rule) applies only to prescription drugs and will be phased in gradually for drugs approved on or after June 30, 2001
- Controlled studies have not been conducted in pregnant women
- There is a risk of abnormal muscle movements and withdrawal symptoms in newborns whose mothers took an antipsychotic during the third trimester; symptoms may include agitation, abnormally increased or decreased muscle tone, tremor, sleepiness, severe difficulty breathing, and difficulty feeding
- Reports of extrapyramidal symptoms, jaundice, hyperreflexia, hyporeflexia in infants whose mothers took a phenothiazine during pregnancy
- Chlorpromazine should generally not be used during the first trimester
- Chlorpromazine should be used during pregnancy only if clearly needed

- Psychotic symptoms may worsen during pregnancy and some form of treatment may be necessary
- Atypical antipsychotics may be preferable to conventional antipsychotics or anticonvulsant mood stabilizers if treatment is required during pregnancy

Breast Feeding
- Some drug is found in mother's breast milk
- Effects on infant have been observed (dystonia, tardive dyskinesia, sedation)
- ✽ Recommended either to discontinue drug or bottle feed

THE ART OF PSYCHOPHARMACOLOGY

Potential Advantages
- Intramuscular formulation for emergency use
- Patients who require sedation for behavioral control

Potential Disadvantages
- Patients with tardive dyskinesia
- Children
- Elderly
- Patients who wish to avoid sedation

Primary Target Symptoms
- Positive symptoms of psychosis
- Motor and autonomic hyperactivity
- Violent or aggressive behavior

Pearls
- Chlorpromazine is one of the earliest classical conventional antipsychotics
- Chlorpromazine has a broad spectrum of efficacy, but risk of tardive dyskinesia and the availability of alternative treatments make its utilization outside of psychosis a short-term and second-line treatment option
- Chlorpromazine is a low-potency phenothiazine
- Sedative actions of low-potency phenothiazines are an important aspect of their therapeutic actions in some patients and side effect profile in others
- Low-potency phenothiazines like chlorpromazine have a greater risk of cardiovascular side effects
- Patients have very similar antipsychotic responses to any conventional antipsychotic, which is different from atypical antipsychotics where antipsychotic responses of individual patients can occasionally vary greatly from one atypical antipsychotic to another
- Patients with inadequate responses to atypical antipsychotics may benefit from a trial of augmentation with a conventional antipsychotic such as chlorpromazine or from switching to a conventional antipsychotic such as chlorpromazine
- However, long-term polypharmacy with a combination of a conventional antipsychotic such as chlorpromazine with an atypical antipsychotic may combine their side effects without clearly augmenting the efficacy of either
- For treatment-resistant patients, especially those with impulsivity, aggression, violence, and self-harm, long-term polypharmacy with 2 atypical antipsychotics or with 1 atypical antipsychotic and 1 conventional antipsychotic may be useful or even necessary while closely monitoring
- In such cases, it may be beneficial to combine 1 depot antipsychotic with 1 oral antipsychotic

Suggested Reading

Adams CE, Awad G, Rathbone J, Thornley B. Chlorpromazine versus placebo for schizophrenia. Cochrane Database Syst Rev 2007;18(2):CD000284.

Ahmed U, Jones H, Adams CE. Chlorpromazine for psychosis induced aggression or agitation. Cochrane Database Syst Rev 2010;14(4):CD007445.

Almerie MQ, Alkhateeb H, Essali A, Matar HE, Rezk E. Cessation of medication for people with schizophrenia already stable on chlorpromazine. Cochrane Database Syst Rev 2007;24(1):CD006329.

Leucht C, Kitzmantel M, Chua L, Kane J, Leucht S. Haloperidol versus chlorpromazine for schizophrenia. Cochrane Database Syst Rev 2008;23(1):CD004278.

Liu X, De Haan S. Chlorpromazine dose for people with schizophrenia. Cochrane Database Syst Rev 2009;15(2):CD007778.

THERAPEUTICS

Brands • Celexa

see index for additional brand names

Generic? Yes

Class

- Neuroscience-based Nomenclature: serotonin reuptake inhibitor (S-RI)
- SSRI (selective serotonin reuptake inhibitor); often classified as an antidepressant, but it is not just an antidepressant

Commonly Prescribed for

(bold for FDA approved)

- **Depression**
- Premenstrual dysphoric disorder (PMDD)
- Obsessive-compulsive disorder (OCD)
- Panic disorder
- Generalized anxiety disorder (GAD)
- Posttraumatic stress disorder (PTSD)
- Social anxiety disorder (social phobia)

How the Drug Works

- Boosts neurotransmitter serotonin
- Blocks serotonin reuptake pump (serotonin transporter)
- Desensitizes serotonin receptors, especially serotonin 1A autoreceptors
- Presumably increases serotonergic neurotransmission

✻ Citalopram also has mild antagonist actions at H1 histamine receptors

✻ Citalopram's inactive R enantiomer may interfere with the therapeutic actions of the active S enantiomer at serotonin reuptake pumps

How Long Until It Works

- Onset of therapeutic actions usually not immediate, but often delayed 2–4 weeks
- If it is not working within 6–8 weeks, it may require a dosage increase or it may not work at all
- May continue to work for many years to prevent relapse of symptoms

If It Works

- The goal of treatment is complete remission of current symptoms as well as prevention of future relapses
- Treatment most often reduces or even eliminates symptoms, but not a cure since symptoms can recur after medicine stopped
- Continue treatment until all symptoms are gone (remission) or significantly reduced (e.g., OCD, PTSD)
- Once symptoms are gone, continue treating for 1 year for the first episode of depression
- For second and subsequent episodes of depression, treatment may need to be indefinite
- Use in anxiety disorders may also need to be indefinite

If It Doesn't Work

- Many patients have only a partial response where some symptoms are improved but others persist (especially insomnia, fatigue, and problems concentrating in depression)
- Other patients may be nonresponders, sometimes called treatment-resistant or treatment-refractory
- Some patients who have an initial response may relapse even though they continue treatment, sometimes called "poop-out"
- Consider increasing dose, switching to another agent or adding an appropriate augmenting agent
- Consider psychotherapy
- Consider evaluation for another diagnosis or for a comorbid condition (e.g., medical illness, substance abuse, etc.)
- Some patients may experience apparent lack of consistent efficacy due to activation of latent or underlying bipolar disorder, and require antidepressant discontinuation and a switch to a mood stabilizer

Best Augmenting Combos for Partial Response or Treatment Resistance

- Trazodone, especially for insomnia
- Bupropion, mirtazapine, reboxetine, or atomoxetine (add with caution and at lower doses since citalopram could theoretically raise atomoxetine levels); use combinations of antidepressants with caution as this may activate bipolar disorder and suicidal ideation
- Modafinil, especially for fatigue, sleepiness, and lack of concentration
- Mood stabilizers or atypical antipsychotics for bipolar depression, psychotic depression, treatment-resistant depression, or treatment-resistant anxiety disorders

- Benzodiazepines
- If all else fails for anxiety disorders, consider gabapentin or tiagabine
- Hypnotics for insomnia
- Classically, lithium, buspirone, or thyroid hormone

Tests
- None for healthy individuals

SIDE EFFECTS

How Drug Causes Side Effects
- Theoretically due to increases in serotonin concentrations at serotonin receptors in parts of the brain and body other than those that cause therapeutic actions (e.g., unwanted actions of serotonin in sleep centers causing insomnia, unwanted actions of serotonin in the gut causing diarrhea, etc.)
- Increasing serotonin can cause diminished dopamine release and might contribute to emotional flattening, cognitive slowing, and apathy in some patients
- Most side effects are immediate but often go away with time, in contrast to most therapeutic effects which are delayed and are enhanced over time

* Citalopram's unique mild antihistamine properties may contribute to sedation and fatigue in some patients

Notable Side Effects
- Sexual dysfunction (dose-dependent; men: delayed ejaculation, erectile dysfunction; men and women: decreased sexual desire, anorgasmia)
- Gastrointestinal (decreased appetite, nausea, diarrhea, constipation, dry mouth)
- Mostly CNS (dose-dependent insomnia but also sedation, agitation, tremors, headache, dizziness)
- Activation (short-term; patients with diagnosed or undiagnosed bipolar or psychotic disorders may be more vulnerable to CNS-activating actions of SSRIs)
- Sweating (dose-dependent)
- Bruising and rare bleeding
- Rare hyponatremia (mostly in elderly patients and generally reversible on discontinuation of citalopram)
- SIADH (syndrome of inappropriate antidiuretic hormone secretion)

Life-Threatening or Dangerous Side Effects
- Rare seizures
- Rare induction of mania
- Rare activation of suicidal ideation and behavior (suicidality) (short-term studies did not show an increase in the risk of suicidality with antidepressants compared to placebo beyond age 24)

Weight Gain
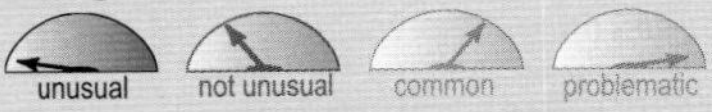

- Reported but not expected
- Citalopram has been associated with both weight gain and weight loss in various studies, but is relatively weight neutral overall

Sedation
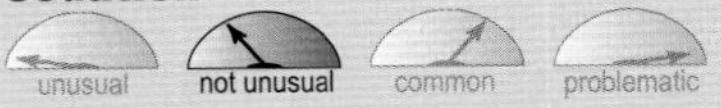

- Occurs in significant minority

What to Do About Side Effects
- Wait
- Wait
- Wait
- Take in the morning if nighttime insomnia
- Take at night if daytime sedation
- In a few weeks, switch to another agent or add other drugs

Best Augmenting Agents for Side Effects
- Often best to try another SSRI or another antidepressant monotherapy prior to resorting to augmentation strategies to treat side effects
- Trazodone or a hypnotic for insomnia
- Bupropion, sildenafil, vardenafil, or tadalafil for sexual dysfunction
- Bupropion for emotional flattening, cognitive slowing, or apathy
- Mirtazapine for insomnia, agitation, and gastrointestinal side effects
- Benzodiazepines for jitteriness and anxiety, especially at initiation of treatment and especially for anxious patients
- Many side effects are dose-dependent (i.e., they increase as dose increases, or they reemerge until tolerance redevelops)

- Many side effects are time-dependent (i.e., they start immediately upon dosing and upon each dose increase, but go away with time)
- Activation and agitation may represent the induction of a bipolar state, especially a mixed dysphoric bipolar II condition sometimes associated with suicidal ideation, and require the addition of lithium, a mood stabilizer or an atypical antipsychotic, and/or discontinuation of citalopram

DOSING AND USE

Usual Dosage Range
- 20–40 mg/day

Dosage Forms
- Tablets 10 mg, 20 mg scored, 40 mg scored
- Orally disintegrating tablet 10 mg, 20 mg, 40 mg
- Capsule 10 mg, 20 mg, 40 mg

How to Dose
- Initial 20 mg/day; increase by 20 mg/day after 1 or more weeks; maximum 40 mg/day; single dose administration, morning or evening

Dosing Tips
- Citalopram should no longer be prescribed at doses greater than 40 mg/day because if can cause abnormal changes in the electrical activity of the heart
- Some controversy with FDA dosage limit of 40 mg/day, and higher doses may be prescribed by experts
- Tablets are scored, so to save costs, give 10 mg as half of 20-mg tablet or 20 mg as half of 40-mg tablet, since the tablets cost about the same in many markets
- Many patients respond better to 40 mg than to 20 mg
- Given once daily, any time of day when best tolerated by the individual
- If intolerable anxiety, insomnia, agitation, akathisia, or activation occur either upon dosing initiation or discontinuation, consider the possibility of activated bipolar disorder and switch to a mood stabilizer or an atypical antipsychotic

Overdose
- Rare fatalities have been reported with citalopram overdose, both alone and in combination with other drugs
- Vomiting, sedation, heart rhythm disturbances, dizziness, sweating, nausea, tremor
- Rarely amnesia, confusion, coma, convulsions

Long-Term Use
- Safe

Habit Forming
- No

How to Stop
- Taper not usually necessary
- However, tapering to avoid potential withdrawal reactions generally prudent
- Many patients tolerate 50% dose reduction for 3 days, then another 50% reduction for 3 days, then discontinuation
- If withdrawal symptoms emerge during discontinuation, raise dose to stop symptoms and then restart withdrawal much more slowly

Pharmacokinetics
- Parent drug has 23–45 hour half-life
- Weak inhibitor of CYP450 2D6
- Metabolized by CYP450 3A4 and 2C19

Drug Interactions
- Tramadol increases the risk of seizures in patients taking an antidepressant
- Can increase TCA levels; use with caution with TCAs
- Can cause a fatal "serotonin syndrome" when combined with MAOIs, so do not use with MAOIs or at least for 14 days after MAOIs are stopped
- Do not start an MAOI for at least 5 half-lives (5 to 7 days for most drugs) after discontinuing citalopram
- May displace highly protein bound drugs (e.g., warfarin)
- Can rarely cause weakness, hyperreflexia, and incoordination when combined with

sumatriptan or possibly other triptans, requiring careful monitoring of patient
- Possible increased risk of bleeding especially when combined with anticoagulants (e.g., warfarin, NSAIDs)
- NSAIDs may impair effectiveness of SSRIs
- Should not be dosed above 20 mg/day in patients taking a CYP450 2C19 inhibitor (e.g., cimetidine) due to risk of QT prolongation
- Via CYP450 2D6 inhibition, citalopram could theoretically interfere with the analgesic actions of codeine, and increase the plasma levels of some beta blockers and of atomoxetine
- Via CYP450 2D6 inhibition, citalopram could theoretically increase concentrations of thioridazine and cause dangerous cardiac arrhythmias

Other Warnings/ Precautions

- Use with caution in patients with history of seizures
- Use with caution in patients with bipolar disorder unless treated with concomitant mood-stabilizing agent
- When treating children, carefully weigh the risks and benefits of pharmacological treatment against the risks and benefits of nontreatment with antidepressants and make sure to document this in the patient's chart
- Distribute the brochures provided by the FDA and the drug companies
- Warn patients and their caregivers about the possibility of activating side effects and advise them to report such symptoms immediately
- Monitor patients for activation of suicidal ideation, especially children and adolescents

Do Not Use

- If patient is taking an MAOI
- If patient is taking thioridazine or pimozide
- If there is a proven allergy to citalopram or escitalopram

SPECIAL POPULATIONS

Renal Impairment

- No dose adjustment for mild to moderate impairment
- Use cautiously in patients with severe impairment

Hepatic Impairment

- Should not be used at doses greater than 20 mg/day
- May need to dose cautiously at the lower end of the dose range in some patients for maximal tolerability

Cardiac Impairment

- May cause abnormal changes in the electrical activity of the heart at doses greater than 40 mg/day
- Treating depression with SSRIs in patients with acute angina or following myocardial infarction may reduce cardiac events and improve survival as well as mood

Elderly

- Doses greater than 20 mg/day should not be used in patients over age 60 years
- May need to dose at the lower end of the dose range in some patients for maximal tolerability
- Risk of SIADH with SSRIs is higher in the elderly
- Citalopram may be an especially well-tolerated SSRI in the elderly
- Reduction in the risk of suicidality with antidepressants compared to placebo in adults age 65 and older

Children and Adolescents

- Carefully weigh the risks and benefits of pharmacological treatment against the risks and benefits of nontreatment with antidepressants and make sure to document this in the patient's chart
- Monitor patients face-to-face regularly, particularly during the first several weeks of treatment
- Use with caution, observing for activation of known or unknown bipolar disorder and/or suicidal ideation, and inform parents or guardians of this risk so they can help observe child or adolescent patients

- Not specifically approved, but preliminary data suggest citalopram is safe and effective in children and adolescents with OCD and with depression

Pregnancy

- Effective June 30, 2015, the US FDA requires changes to the content and format of pregnancy and lactation information in prescription drug labels, including the elimination of the pregnancy letter categories; the Pregnancy and Lactation Labeling Rule (PLLR or final rule) applies only to prescription drugs and will be phased in gradually for drugs approved on or after June 30, 2001
- Controlled studies have not been conducted in pregnant women
- Not generally recommended for use during pregnancy, especially during first trimester
- Nonetheless, continuous treatment during pregnancy may be necessary and has not been proven to be harmful to the fetus
- At delivery there may be more bleeding in the mother and transient irritability or sedation in the newborn
- Must weigh the risk of treatment (first trimester fetal development, third trimester newborn delivery) to the child against the risk of no treatment (recurrence of depression, maternal health, infant bonding) to the mother and child
- For many patients, this may mean continuing treatment during pregnancy
- Exposure to SSRIs early in pregnancy may be associated with increased risk of septal heart defects (absolute risk is small)
- SSRI use beyond the 20th week of pregnancy may be associated with increased risk of pulmonary hypertension in newborns, although this is not proven
- Exposure to SSRIs late in pregnancy may be associated with increased risk of gestational hypertension and preeclampsia
- Neonates exposed to SSRIs or SNRIs late in the third trimester have developed complications requiring prolonged hospitalization, respiratory support, and tube feeding; reported symptoms are consistent with either a direct toxic effect of SSRIs and SNRIs or, possibly, a drug discontinuation syndrome, and include respiratory distress, cyanosis, apnea, seizures, temperature instability, feeding difficulty, vomiting, hypoglycemia, hypotonia, hypertonia, hyperreflexia, tremor, jitteriness, irritability, and constant crying

Breast Feeding

- Some drug is found in mother's breast milk
- Trace amounts may be present in nursing children whose mothers are on citalopram
- If child becomes irritable or sedated, breast feeding or drug may need to be discontinued
- Immediate postpartum period is a high-risk time for depression, especially in women who have had prior depressive episodes, so drug may need to be reinstituted late in the third trimester or shortly after childbirth to prevent a recurrence during the postpartum period
- Must weigh benefits of breast feeding with risks and benefits of antidepressant treatment versus nontreatment to both the infant and the mother
- For many patients, this may mean continuing treatment during breast feeding

THE ART OF PSYCHOPHARMACOLOGY

Potential Advantages

- Elderly patients
- Patients excessively activated or sedated by other SSRIs

Potential Disadvantages

- May require dosage titration to attain optimal efficacy
- Can be sedating in some patients

Primary Target Symptoms

- Depressed mood
- Anxiety
- Panic attacks, avoidant behavior, reexperiencing, hyperarousal
- Sleep disturbance, both insomnia and hypersomnia

Pearls

* May be more tolerable than some other antidepressants
- May have less sexual dysfunction than some other SSRIs

- May be especially well tolerated in the elderly
- ✻ May be less well tolerated than escitalopram
- Documentation of efficacy in anxiety disorders is less comprehensive than for escitalopram and other SSRIs
- Can cause cognitive and affective "flattening"
- Some evidence suggests that citalopram treatment during only the luteal phase may be more effective than continuous treatment for patients with PMDD
- SSRIs may be less effective in women over 50, especially if they are not taking estrogen
- SSRIs may be useful for hot flushes in perimenopausal women
- Nonresponse to citalopram in elderly may require consideration of mild cognitive impairment or Alzheimer disease

Suggested Reading

Cipriani A, Purgato M, Furukawa TA, et al. Citalopram versus other anti-depressive agents for depression. Cochrane Database Syst Rev 2012;11(7):CD006534.

Rush AJ, Trivedi MH, Wisniewski SR. Acute and longer-term outcomes in depressed outpatients requiring one or several treatment steps: a STAR*D report. Am J Psychiatry 2006;163(11):1905–17.

Vieweg WV, Hasnain M, Howland RH, et al. Citalopram, QTc interval prolongation, and torsade de pointes. How should we apply the recent FDA ruling? Am J Med 2012;125(9):859–68.

CLOMIPRAMINE

THERAPEUTICS

Brands • Anafranil
see index for additional brand names

Generic? Yes

Class
- Neuroscience-based Nomenclature: serotonin reuptake inhibitor (SRI)
- Tricyclic antidepressant (TCA)
- Parent drug is a potent serotonin reuptake inhibitor
- Active metabolite is a potent norepinephrine/noradrenaline reuptake inhibitor

Commonly Prescribed for
(bold for FDA approved)
✱ **Obsessive-compulsive disorder**
- Depression

✱ Severe and treatment-resistant depression
✱ Cataplexy syndrome
- Anxiety
- Insomnia
- Neuropathic pain/chronic pain

How the Drug Works
- Boosts neurotransmitters serotonin and norepinephrine/noradrenaline
- Blocks serotonin reuptake pump (serotonin transporter), presumably increasing serotonergic neurotransmission
- Blocks norepinephrine reuptake pump (norepinephrine transporter), presumably increasing noradrenergic neurotransmission
- Presumably desensitizes both serotonin 1A receptors and beta adrenergic receptors
- Since dopamine is inactivated by norepinephrine reuptake in frontal cortex, which largely lacks dopamine transporters, clomipramine can increase dopamine neurotransmission in this part of the brain

How Long Until It Works
- May have immediate effects in treating insomnia or anxiety
- Onset of therapeutic actions in depression usually not immediate, but often delayed 2 to 4 weeks
- Onset of therapeutic action in OCD can be delayed 6 to 12 weeks
- If it is not working for depression within 6 to 8 weeks, it may require a dosage increase or it may not work at all
- If it is not working for OCD within 12 weeks, it may not work at all
- May continue to work for many years to prevent relapse of symptoms

If It Works
- The goal of treatment of depression is complete remission of current symptoms as well as prevention of future relapses
- Treatment most often reduces or even eliminates symptoms, but not a cure since symptoms can recur after medicine stopped
- Although the goal of treatment of OCD is also complete remission of symptoms, this may be less likely than in depression
- The goal of treatment of chronic neuropathic pain is to reduce symptoms as much as possible, especially in combination with other treatments
- Continue treatment of depression until all symptoms are gone (remission)
- Once symptoms of depression are gone, continue treating for 1 year for the first episode of depression
- For second and subsequent episodes of depression, treatment may need to be indefinite
- Use in OCD may also need to be indefinite, starting from the time of initial treatment
- Use in other anxiety disorders and chronic pain may also need to be indefinite, but long-term treatment is not well studied in these conditions

If It Doesn't Work
- Many patients have only a partial response where some symptoms are improved but others persist (especially insomnia, fatigue, and problems concentrating)
- Other patients may be nonresponders, sometimes called treatment-resistant or treatment-refractory
- Consider increasing dose, switching to another agent or adding an appropriate augmenting agent
- Consider psychotherapy, especially behavioral therapy in OCD
- Consider evaluation for another diagnosis or for a comorbid condition (e.g., medical illness, substance abuse, etc.)
- Some patients may experience apparent lack of consistent efficacy due to activation

of latent or underlying bipolar disorder, and require antidepressant discontinuation and a switch to a mood stabilizer

Best Augmenting Combos for Partial Response or Treatment Resistance

- Lithium, buspirone, hormone (for depression and OCD)
- For the expert: consider cautious addition of fluvoxamine for treatment-resistant OCD
- Thyroid hormone (for depression)
- Atypical antipsychotics (for OCD)

Tests

- Baseline ECG is recommended for patients over age 50

✻ Monitoring of plasma drug levels is potentially available at specialty laboratories for the expert

✻ Since tricyclic and tetracyclic antidepressants are frequently associated with weight gain, before starting treatment, weigh all patients and determine if the patient is already overweight (BMI 25.0–29.9) or obese (BMI ≥30)

- Before giving a drug that can cause weight gain to an overweight or obese patient, consider determining whether the patient already has pre-diabetes (fasting plasma glucose 100–125 mg/dL), diabetes (fasting plasma glucose >126 mg/dL), or dyslipidemia (increased total cholesterol, LDL cholesterol and triglycerides; decreased HDL cholesterol), and treat or refer such patients for treatment, including nutrition and weight management, physical activity counseling, smoking cessation, and medical management

✻ Weight and BMI during treatment

✻ While giving a drug to a patient who has gained >5% of initial weight, consider evaluating for the presence of pre-diabetes, diabetes, or dyslipidemia, or consider switching to a different antidepressant

- EKGs may be useful for selected patients (e.g., those with personal or family history of QTc prolongation; cardiac arrhythmia; recent myocardial infarction; uncompensated heart failure; or taking agents that prolong QTc interval such as pimozide, thioridazine, selected antiarrhythmics, moxifloxacin, sparfloxacin, etc.)
- Patients at risk for electrolyte disturbances (e.g., patients on diuretic therapy) should have baseline and periodic serum potassium and magnesium measurements

SIDE EFFECTS

How Drug Causes Side Effects

- Anticholinergic activity may explain sedative effects, dry mouth, constipation, and blurred vision
- Sedative effects and weight gain may be due to antihistamine properties
- Blockade of alpha adrenergic 1 receptors may explain dizziness, sedation, and hypotension
- Cardiac arrhythmias and seizures, especially in overdose, may be caused by blockade of ion channels

Notable Side Effects

- Blurred vision, constipation, urinary retention, increased appetite, dry mouth, nausea, diarrhea, heartburn, unusual taste in mouth, weight gain
- Fatigue, weakness, dizziness, sedation, headache, anxiety, nervousness, restlessness
- Sexual dysfunction, sweating

Life-Threatening or Dangerous Side Effects

- Paralytic ileus, hyperthermia (TCAs + anticholinergic agents)
- Lowered seizure threshold and rare seizures
- Orthostatic hypotension, sudden death, arrhythmias, tachycardia
- QTc prolongation
- Hepatic failure, extrapyramidal symptoms
- Increased intraocular pressure
- Rare induction of mania
- Rare activation of suicidal ideation and behavior (suicidality) (short-term studies did not show an increase in the risk of suicidality with antidepressants compared to placebo beyond age 24)

Weight Gain

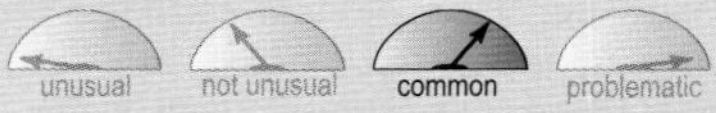

- Many experience and/or can be significant in amount
- Can increase appetite and carbohydrate craving

Sedation

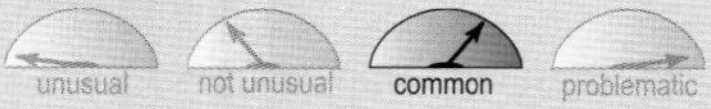

- Many experience and/or can be significant in amount
- Tolerance to sedative effect may develop with long-term use

What to Do About Side Effects

- Wait
- Wait
- Wait
- Lower the dose
- Switch to an SSRI or newer antidepressant

Best Augmenting Agents for Side Effects

- Many side effects cannot be improved with an augmenting agent

DOSING AND USE

Usual Dosage Range

- 100–200 mg/day

Dosage Forms

- Capsule 25 mg, 50 mg, 75 mg

How to Dose

- Initial 25 mg/day; increase over 2 weeks to 100 mg/day; maximum dose generally 250 mg/day

Dosing Tips

- If given in a single dose, should generally be administered at bedtime because of its sedative properties
- If given in split doses, largest dose should generally be given at bedtime because of its sedative properties
- If patients experience nightmares, split dose and do not give large dose at bedtime
- Patients treated for chronic pain may only require lower doses

✻ Patients treated for OCD may often require doses at the high end of the range (e.g., 200–250 mg/day)

- Risk of seizure increases with dose, especially with clomipramine at doses above 250 mg/day

✻ Dose of 300 mg may be associated with up to 7/1,000 incidence of seizures, a generally unacceptable risk

- If intolerable anxiety, insomnia, agitation, akathisia, or activation occur either upon dosing initiation or discontinuation, consider the possibility of activated bipolar disorder, and switch to a mood stabilizer or an atypical antipsychotic

Overdose

- Death may occur; convulsions, cardiac dysrhythmias, severe hypotension, CNS depression, coma, changes in EKG

Long-Term Use

- Limited data but appears to be efficacious and safe long-term

Habit Forming

- No

How to Stop

- Taper to avoid withdrawal effects
- Even with gradual dose reduction some withdrawal symptoms may appear within the first 2 weeks
- Many patients tolerate 50% dose reduction for 3 days, then another 50% reduction for 3 days, then discontinuation
- If withdrawal symptoms emerge during discontinuation, raise dose to stop symptoms and then restart withdrawal much more slowly

Pharmacokinetics

- Substrate for CYP450 2D6 and 1A2
- Metabolized to an active metabolite, desmethyl-clomipramine, a predominantly norepinephrine reuptake inhibitor, by demethylation via CYP450 1A2
- Inhibits CYP450 2D6
- Half-life approximately 17–28 hours
- Food does not affect absorption

Drug Interactions

- Tramadol increases the risk of seizures in patients taking TCAs
- Can cause a fatal "serotonin syndrome" when combined with MAOIs, so do not use with MAOI or at least for 14 days after MAOIs are stopped

- Do not start an MAOI for at least 5 half-lives (5 to 7 days for most drugs) after discontinuing clomipramine
- Use of TCAs with anticholinergic drugs may result in paralytic ileus or hyperthermia
- Fluoxetine, paroxetine, bupropion, duloxetine, and other CYP450 2D6 inhibitors may increase TCA concentrations
- Fluvoxamine, a CYP450 1A2 inhibitor, can decrease the conversion of clomipramine to desmethyl-clomipramine, and increase clomipramine plasma concentrations
- Cimetidine may increase plasma concentrations of TCAs and cause anticholinergic symptoms
- Phenothiazines or haloperidol may raise TCA blood concentrations
- May alter effects of antihypertensive drugs
- Use of TCAs with sympathomimetic agents may increase sympathetic activity
- TCAs may inhibit hypotensive effects of clonidine
- Methylphenidate may inhibit metabolism of TCAs
- Activation and agitation, especially following switching or adding antidepressants, may represent the induction of a bipolar state, especially a mixed dysphoric bipolar II condition sometimes associated with suicidal ideation, and require the addition of lithium, a mood stabilizer or an atypical antipsychotic, and/or discontinuation of clomipramine

Other Warnings/ Precautions

- Add or initiate other antidepressants with caution for up to 2 weeks after discontinuing clomipramine
- Use with caution in patients with history of seizures, urinary retention, angle-closure glaucoma, hyperthyroidism
- TCAs can increase QTc interval, especially at toxic doses, which can be attained not only by overdose but also by combining with drugs that inhibit TCA metabolism via CYP450 2D6, potentially causing torsade de pointes-type arrhythmia or sudden death
- Because TCAs can prolong QTc interval, use with caution in patients who have bradycardia or who are taking drugs that can induce bradycardia (e.g., beta blockers, calcium channel blockers, clonidine, digitalis)
- Because TCAs can prolong QTc interval, use with caution in patients who have hypokalemia and/or hypomagnesemia or who are taking drugs that can induce hypokalemia and/or magnesemia (e.g., diuretics, stimulant laxatives, intravenous amphotericin B, glucocorticoids, tetracosactide)
- When treating children, carefully weigh the risks and benefits of pharmacological treatment against the risks and benefits of nontreatment with antidepressants and make sure to document this in the patient's chart
- Distribute the brochures provided by the FDA and the drug companies
- Warn patients and their caregivers about the possibility of activating side effects and advise them to report such symptoms immediately
- Monitor patients for activation of suicidal ideation, especially children and adolescents

Do Not Use

- If patient is taking an MAOI
- If patient is recovering from myocardial infarction
- If patient is taking agents capable of significantly prolonging QTc interval (e.g., pimozide, thioridazine, selected antiarrhythmics, moxifloxacin, sparfloxacin)
- If there is a history of QTc prolongation or cardiac arrhythmia, recent acute myocardial infarction, uncompensated heart failure
- If patient is taking drugs that inhibit TCA metabolism, including CYP450 2D6 inhibitors, except by an expert
- If there is reduced CYP450 2D6 function, such as patients who are poor 2D6 metabolizers, except by an expert and at low doses
- If there is a proven allergy to clomipramine

SPECIAL POPULATIONS

Renal Impairment

- Use with caution

Hepatic Impairment

- Use with caution

Cardiac Impairment

- Baseline ECG is recommended
- TCAs have been reported to cause arrhythmias, prolongation of conduction time, orthostatic hypotension, sinus tachycardia, and heart failure, especially in the diseased heart
- Myocardial infarction and stroke have been reported with TCAs
- TCAs produce QTc prolongation, which may be enhanced by the existence of bradycardia, hypokalemia, congenital or acquired long QTc interval, which should be evaluated prior to administering clomipramine
- Use with caution if treating concomitantly with a medication likely to produce prolonged bradycardia, hypokalemia, slowing of intracardiac conduction, or prolongation of the QTc interval
- Avoid TCAs in patients with a known history of QTc prolongation, recent acute myocardial infarction, and uncompensated heart failure
- TCAs may cause a sustained increase in heart rate in patients with ischemic heart disease and may worsen (decrease) heart rate variability, an independent risk of mortality in cardiac populations
- Since SSRIs may improve (increase) heart rate variability in patients following a myocardial infarct and may improve survival as well as mood in patients with acute angina or following a myocardial infarction, these are more appropriate agents for cardiac population than tricyclic/tetracyclic antidepressants

✻ Risk/benefit ratio may not justify use of TCAs in cardiac impairment

Elderly

- Baseline ECG is recommended for patients over age 50
- May be more sensitive to anticholinergic, cardiovascular, hypotensive, and sedative effects
- Dose may need to be lower than usual adult dose, at least initially
- Reduction in the risk of suicidality with antidepressants compared to placebo in adults age 65 and older

Children and Adolescents

- Carefully weigh the risks and benefits of pharmacological treatment against the risks and benefits of nontreatment with antidepressants and make sure to document this in the patient's chart
- Monitor patients face-to-face regularly, particularly during the first several weeks of treatment
- Use with caution, observing for activation of known or unknown bipolar disorder and/or suicidal ideation, and inform parents or guardians of this risk so they can help observe child or adolescent patients
- Not recommended for use in children under age 10
- Several studies show lack of efficacy of TCAs for depression
- May be used to treat enuresis or hyperactive/impulsive behaviors
- Effective for OCD in children
- Some cases of sudden death have occurred in children taking TCAs
- Dose in children/adolescents should be titrated to a maximum of 100 mg/day or 3 mg/kg per day after 2 weeks, after which dose can then be titrated up to a maximum of 200 mg/day or 3 mg/kg per day

Pregnancy

- Effective June 30, 2015, the US FDA requires changes to the content and format of pregnancy and lactation information in prescription drug labels, including the elimination of the pregnancy letter categories; the Pregnancy and Lactation Labeling Rule (PLLR or final rule) applies only to prescription drugs and will be phased in gradually for drugs approved on or after June 30, 2001
- Controlled studies have not been conducted in pregnant women
- Clomipramine crosses the placenta
- Adverse effects have been reported in infants whose mothers took a TCA (lethargy, withdrawal symptoms, fetal malformations)
- Must weigh the risk of treatment (first trimester fetal development, third trimester newborn delivery) to the child against the risk of no treatment (recurrence of

depression, worsening of OCD, maternal health, infant bonding) to the mother and child
- For many patients this may mean continuing treatment during pregnancy

Breast Feeding
- Some drug is found in mother's breast milk
- ✻ Recommended either to discontinue drug or bottle feed
- Immediate postpartum period is a high-risk time for depression and worsening of OCD, especially in women who have had prior depressive episodes or OCD symptoms, so drug may need to be reinstituted late in the third trimester or shortly after childbirth to prevent a recurrence or exacerbation during the postpartum period
- Must weigh benefits of breast feeding with risks and benefits of antidepressant treatment versus nontreatment to both the infant and the mother
- For many patients this may mean continuing treatment during breast feeding

THE ART OF PSYCHOPHARMACOLOGY

Potential Advantages
- Patients with insomnia
- Severe or treatment-resistant depression
- Patients with comorbid OCD and depression
- Patients with cataplexy

Potential Disadvantages
- Pediatric and geriatric patients
- Patients concerned with weight gain
- Cardiac patients
- Patients with seizure disorders

Primary Target Symptoms
- Depressed mood
- Obsessive thoughts
- Compulsive behaviors

Pearls
- ✻ The only TCA with proven efficacy in OCD
- Normally, clomipramine (CMI), a potent serotonin reuptake blocker, at steady state is metabolized extensively to its active metabolite desmethyl-clomipramine (de-CMI), a potent nonadrenaline reuptake blocker, by the enzyme CYP450 1A2
- Thus, at steady state, plasma drug activity is generally more noradrenergic (with higher de-CMI levels) than serotonergic (with lower parent CMI levels)
- Addition of the SSRI and CYP450 1A2 inhibitor fluvoxamine blocks this conversion and results in higher CMI levels than de-CMI levels
- For the expert only: addition of the SSRI fluvoxamine to CMI in treatment-resistant OCD can powerfully enhance serotonergic activity, not only due to the inherent additive pharmacodynamic serotonergic activity of fluvoxamine added to CMI, but also due to a favorable pharmacokinetic interaction inhibiting CYP450 1A2 and thus converting CMI's metabolism to a more powerful serotonergic portfolio of parent drug
- ✻ One of the most favored TCAs for treating severe depression
- TCAs are no longer generally considered a first-line treatment option for depression because of their side effect profile
- TCAs continue to be useful for severe or treatment-resistant depression
- TCAs are often a first-line treatment option for chronic pain
- ✻ Unique among TCAs, clomipramine has a potentially fatal interaction with MAOIs in addition to the danger of hypertension characteristic of all MAOI-TCA combinations
- ✻ A potentially fatal serotonin syndrome with high fever, seizures, and coma, analogous to that caused by SSRIs and MAOIs, can occur with clomipramine and SSRIs, presumably due to clomipramine's potent serotonin reuptake blocking properties
- TCAs may aggravate psychotic symptoms
- Alcohol should be avoided because of additive CNS effects
- Underweight patients may be more susceptible to adverse cardiovascular effects
- Children, patients with inadequate hydration, and patients with cardiac disease may be more susceptible to TCA-induced cardiotoxicity than healthy adults

- Patients on TCAs should be aware that they may experience symptoms such as photosensitivity or blue-green urine
- SSRIs may be more effective than TCAs in women, and TCAs may be more effective than SSRIs in men
- Since tricyclic/tetracyclic antidepressants are substrates for CYP450 2D6, and 7% of the population (especially Caucasians) may have a genetic variant leading to reduced activity of 2D6, such patients may not safely tolerate normal doses of tricyclic/tetracyclic antidepressants and may require dose reduction
- Phenotypic testing may be necessary to detect this genetic variant prior to dosing with a tricyclic/tetracyclic antidepressant, especially in vulnerable populations such as children, elderly, cardiac populations, and those on concomitant medications
- Patients who seem to have extraordinarily severe side effects at normal or low doses may have this phenotypic CYP450 2D6 variant and require low doses or switching to another antidepressant not metabolized by 2D6

Suggested Reading

Anderson IM. Meta-analytical studies on new antidepressants. Br Med Bull 2001;57:161–78.

Anderson IM. Selective serotonin reuptake inhibitors versus tricyclic antidepressants: a meta-analysis of efficacy and tolerability. J Aff Disorders 2000;58:19–36.

Cox BJ, Swinson RP, Morrison B, Lee PS. Clomipramine, fluoxetine, and behavior therapy in the treatment of obsessive-compulsive disorder: a meta-analysis. J Behav Ther Exp Psychiatry 1993;24:149–53.

Feinberg M. Clomipramine for obsessive-compulsive disorder. Am Fam Physician 1991;43:1735–8.

THERAPEUTICS

Brands • Klonopin

see index for additional brand names

Generic? Yes

Class

- Neuroscience-based Nomenclature: GABA positive allosteric modulator (GABA-PAM)
- Benzodiazepine (anxiolytic, anticonvulsant)

Commonly Prescribed for

(bold for FDA approved)

- **Panic disorder, with or without agoraphobia**
- **Lennox-Gastaut syndrome (petit mal variant)**
- **Akinetic seizure**
- **Myoclonic seizure**
- **Absence seizure (petit mal)**
- Atonic seizures
- Other seizure disorders
- Other anxiety disorders
- Acute mania (adjunctive)
- Acute psychosis (adjunctive)
- Insomnia
- Catatonia

How the Drug Works

- Binds to benzodiazepine receptors at the GABA-A ligand-gated chloride channel complex
- Enhances the inhibitory effects of GABA
- Boosts chloride conductance through GABA-regulated channels
- Inhibits neuronal activity presumably in amygdala-centered fear circuits to provide therapeutic benefits in anxiety disorders
- Inhibitory actions in cerebral cortex may provide therapeutic benefits in seizure disorders

How Long Until It Works

- Some immediate relief with first dosing is common; can take several weeks with daily dosing for maximal therapeutic benefit

If It Works

- For short-term symptoms of anxiety – after a few weeks, discontinue use or use on an "as-needed" basis
- For chronic anxiety disorders, the goal of treatment is complete remission of symptoms as well as prevention of future relapses
- For chronic anxiety disorders, treatment most often reduces or even eliminates symptoms, but not a cure since symptoms can recur after medicine stopped
- For long-term symptoms of anxiety, consider switching to an SSRI or SNRI for long-term maintenance
- If long-term maintenance with a benzodiazepine is necessary, continue treatment for 6 months after symptoms resolve, and then taper dose slowly
- If symptoms reemerge, consider treatment with an SSRI or SNRI, or consider restarting the benzodiazepine; sometimes benzodiazepines have to be used in combination with SSRIs or SNRIs for best results
- For long-term treatment of seizure disorders, development of tolerance dose escalation and loss of efficacy necessitating adding or switching to other anticonvulsants is not uncommon

If It Doesn't Work

- Consider switching to another agent or adding an appropriate augmenting agent
- Consider psychotherapy, especially cognitive behavioral psychotherapy
- Consider presence of concomitant substance abuse
- Consider presence of clonazepam abuse
- Consider another diagnosis such as a comorbid medical condition

Best Augmenting Combos for Partial Response or Treatment Resistance

- Benzodiazepines are frequently used as augmenting agents for antipsychotics and mood stabilizers in the treatment of psychotic and bipolar disorders
- Benzodiazepines are frequently used as augmenting agents for SSRIs and SNRIs in the treatment of anxiety disorders
- Not generally rational to combine with other benzodiazepines
- Caution if using as an anxiolytic concomitantly with other sedative hypnotics for sleep
- Clonazepam is commonly combined with other anticonvulsants for the treatment of seizure disorders

Tests
- In patients with seizure disorders, concomitant medical illness, and/or those with multiple concomitant long-term medications, periodic liver tests and blood counts may be prudent

SIDE EFFECTS

How Drug Causes Side Effects
- Same mechanism for side effects as for therapeutic effects – namely due to excessive actions at benzodiazepine receptors
- Long-term adaptations in benzodiazepine receptors may explain the development of dependence, tolerance, and withdrawal
- Side effects are generally immediate, but immediate side effects often disappear in time

Notable Side Effects
✽ Sedation, fatigue, depression
✽ Dizziness, ataxia, slurred speech, weakness
✽ Forgetfulness, confusion
✽ Hyperexcitability, nervousness
- Rare hallucinations, mania
- Rare hypotension
- Hypersalivation, dry mouth

Life-Threatening or Dangerous Side Effects
- Respiratory depression, especially when taken with CNS depressants in overdose
- Rare hepatic dysfunction, renal dysfunction, blood dyscrasias
- Grand mal seizures

Weight Gain
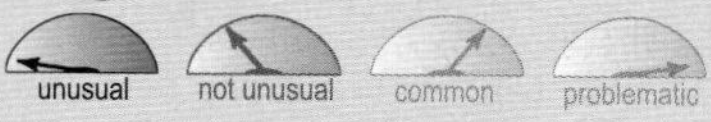

- Reported but not expected

Sedation
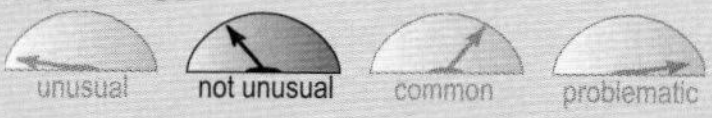

- Occurs in significant minority
- Especially at initiation of treatment or when dose increases
- Tolerance often develops over time

What to Do About Side Effects
- Wait
- Wait
- Wait
- Lower the dose
- Take largest dose at bedtime to avoid sedative effects during the day
- Switch to another agent
- Administer flumazenil if side effects are severe or life-threatening

Best Augmenting Agents for Side Effects
- Many side effects cannot be improved with an augmenting agent

DOSING AND USE

Usual Dosage Range
- Seizures: dependent on individual response of patient, up to 20 mg/day
- Panic: 0.5–2 mg/day either as divided doses or once at bedtime

Dosage Forms
- Tablet 0.5 mg scored, 1 mg, 2 mg
- Disintegrating (wafer): 0.125 mg, 0.25 mg, 0.5 mg, 1 mg, 2 mg

How to Dose
- Seizures – 1.5 mg divided into 3 doses, raise by 0.5 mg every 3 days until desired effect is reached; divide into 3 even doses or else give largest dose at bedtime; maximum dose generally 20 mg/day
- Panic – 1 mg/day; start at 0.25 mg divided into 2 doses, raise to 1 mg after 3 days; dose either twice daily or once at bedtime; maximum dose generally 4 mg/day

Dosing Tips
- For anxiety disorders, use lowest possible effective dose for the shortest possible period of time (a benzodiazepine sparing strategy)
- Assess need for continuous treatment regularly
- Risk of dependence may increase with dose and duration of treatment
- For interdose symptoms of anxiety, can either increase dose or maintain same daily dose but divide into more frequent doses

- Can also use an as-needed occasional "top-up" dose for interdose anxiety
- Because seizure disorder can require doses much higher than 2 mg/day, the risk of dependence may be greater in these patients
- Because panic disorder can require doses somewhat higher than 2 mg/day, the risk of dependence may be greater in these patients than in anxiety patients maintained at lower doses
- Some severely ill seizure patients may require more than 20 mg/day
- Some severely ill panic patients may require 4 mg/day or more
- Frequency of dosing in practice is often greater than predicted from half-life, as duration of biological activity is often shorter than pharmacokinetic terminal half-life

✽ Clonazepam is generally dosed half the dosage of alprazolam

- Escalation of dose may be necessary if tolerance develops in seizure disorders
- Escalation of dose usually not necessary in anxiety disorders, as tolerance to clonazepam does not generally develop in the treatment of anxiety disorders

✽ Available as an oral disintegrating wafer

Overdose

- Rarely fatal in monotherapy; sedation, confusion, coma, diminished reflexes

Long-Term Use

- May lose efficacy for seizures; dose increase may restore efficacy
- Risk of dependence, particularly for treatment periods longer than 12 weeks and especially in patients with past or current polysubstance abuse

Habit Forming

- Clonazepam is a Schedule IV drug
- Patients may develop dependence and/or tolerance with long-term use

How to Stop

- Patients with history of seizures may seize upon withdrawal, especially if withdrawal is abrupt
- Taper by 0.25 mg every 3 days to reduce chances of withdrawal effects
- For difficult to taper cases, consider reducing dose much more slowly after reaching 1.5 mg/day, perhaps by as little as 0.125 mg per week or less
- For other patients with severe problems discontinuing a benzodiazepine, dosing may need to be tapered over many months (i.e., reduce dose by 1% every 3 days by crushing tablet and suspending or dissolving in 100 mL of fruit juice and then disposing of 1 mL while drinking the rest; 3–7 days later, dispose of 2 mL, and so on). This is both a form of very slow biological tapering and a form of behavioral desensitization
- Be sure to differentiate reemergence of symptoms requiring reinstitution of treatment from withdrawal symptoms
- Benzodiazepine-dependent anxiety patients and insulin-dependent diabetics are not addicted to their medications. When benzodiazepine-dependent patients stop their medication, disease symptoms can reemerge, disease symptoms can worsen (rebound), and/or withdrawal symptoms can emerge

Pharmacokinetics

- Long half-life compared to other benzodiazepine anxiolytics (elimination half-life approximately 30–40 hours)
- Substrate for CYP450 3A4
- Food does not affect absorption

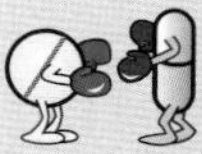

Drug Interactions

- Increased depressive effects when taken with other CNS depressants (see Warnings below)
- Inhibitors of CYP450 3A4 may affect the clearance of clonazepam, but dosage adjustment usually not necessary
- Flumazenil (used to reverse the effects of benzodiazepines) may precipitate seizures and should not be used in patients treated for seizure disorders with clonazepam
- Use of clonazepam with valproate may cause absence status

Other Warnings/ Precautions

- Boxed warning regarding the increased risk of CNS depressant effects when benzodiazepines and opioid medications are used together, including specifically the risk of slowed or difficulty breathing and death

- If alternatives to the combined use of benzodiazepines and opioids are not available, clinicians should limit the dosage and duration of each drug to the minimum possible while still achieving therapeutic efficacy
- Patients and their caregivers should be warned to seek medical attention if unusual dizziness, lightheadedness, sedation, slowed or difficulty breathing, or unresponsiveness occur
- Dosage changes should be made in collaboration with prescriber
- Use with caution in patients with pulmonary disease; rare reports of death after initiation of benzodiazepines in patients with severe pulmonary impairment
- History of drug or alcohol abuse often creates greater risk for dependency
- Clonazepam may induce grand mal seizures in patients with multiple seizure disorders
- Use only with extreme caution if patient has obstructive sleep apnea
- Some depressed patients may experience a worsening of suicidal ideation
- Some patients may exhibit abnormal thinking or behavioral changes similar to those caused by other CNS depressants (i.e., either depressant actions or disinhibiting actions)

Do Not Use

- If patient has angle-closure glaucoma
- If patient has severe liver disease
- If there is a proven allergy to clonazepam or any benzodiazepine

SPECIAL POPULATIONS

Renal Impairment

- Dose should be reduced

Hepatic Impairment

- Dose should be reduced

Cardiac Impairment

- Benzodiazepines have been used to treat anxiety associated with acute myocardial infarction

Elderly

- Should receive lower doses and be monitored

Children and Adolescents

- Seizures – up to 10 years or 30 kg – 0.01–0.03 mg/kg per day divided into 2–3 doses; maximum dose 0.05 mg/kg per day
- Safety and efficacy not established in panic disorder
- For anxiety, children and adolescents should generally receive lower doses and be more closely monitored
- Long-term effects of clonazepam in children/adolescents are unknown

Pregnancy

- Effective June 30, 2015, the US FDA requires changes to the content and format of pregnancy and lactation information in prescription drug labels, including the elimination of the pregnancy letter categories; the Pregnancy and Lactation Labeling Rule (PLLR or final rule) applies only to prescription drugs and will be phased in gradually for drugs approved on or after June 30, 2001
- Possible increased risk of birth defects when benzodiazepines taken during pregnancy
- Because of the potential risks, clonazepam is not generally recommended as treatment for anxiety during pregnancy, especially during the first trimester
- Drug should be tapered if discontinued
- Infants whose mothers received a benzodiazepine late in pregnancy may experience withdrawal effects
- Neonatal flaccidity has been reported in infants whose mothers took a benzodiazepine during pregnancy
- Seizures, even mild seizures, may cause harm to the embryo/fetus

Breast Feeding

- Some drug is found in mother's breast milk

* Recommended either to discontinue drug or bottle feed

- Effects on infant have been observed and include feeding difficulties, sedation, and weight loss

THE ART OF PSYCHOPHARMACOLOGY

Potential Advantages

- Rapid onset of action
- Less sedation than some other benzodiazepines
- Longer duration of action than some other benzodiazepines
- Availability of oral disintegrating wafer

Potential Disadvantages

- Development of tolerance may require dose increases, especially in seizure disorders
- Abuse especially risky in past or present substance abusers

Primary Target Symptoms

- Frequency and duration of seizures
- Spike and wave discharges in absence seizures (petit mal)
- Panic attacks
- Anxiety

Pearls

✻ One of the most popular benzodiazepines for anxiety, especially among psychiatrists
- Is a very useful adjunct to SSRIs and SNRIs in the treatment of numerous anxiety disorders
- Not effective for treating psychosis as a monotherapy, but can be used as an adjunct to antipsychotics
- Not effective for treating bipolar disorder as a monotherapy, but can be used as an adjunct to mood stabilizers and antipsychotics
- Generally used as second-line treatment for petit mal seizures if succinimides are ineffective
- Can be used as an adjunct or as monotherapy for seizure disorders
- Clonazepam is the only benzodiazepine that is used as a solo maintenance treatment for seizure disorders

✻ Easier to taper than some other benzodiazepines because of long half-life

✻ May have less abuse potential than some other benzodiazepines

✻ May cause less depression, euphoria, or dependence than some other benzodiazepines

✻ Clonazepam is often considered a "longer-acting alprazolam-like anxiolytic" with improved tolerability features in terms of less euphoria, abuse, dependence, and withdrawal problems, but this has not been proven
- When using to treat insomnia, remember that insomnia may be a symptom of some other primary disorder itself, and thus warrant evaluation for comorbid psychiatric and/or medical conditions
- Though not systematically studied, benzodiazepines have been used effectively to treat catatonia and are the initial recommended treatment

Suggested Reading

Davidson JR, Moroz G. Pivotal studies of clonazepam in panic disorder. Psychopharmacol Bull 1998;34:169–74.

DeVane CL, Ware MR, Lydiard RB. Pharmacokinetics, pharmacodynamics, and treatment issues of benzodiazepines: alprazolam, adinazolam, and clonazepam. Psychopharmacol Bull 1991;27:463–73.

Iqbal MM, Sobhan T, Ryals T. Effects of commonly used benzodiazepines on the fetus, the neonate, and the nursing infant. Psychiatr Serv 2002;53:39–49.

Panayiotopoulos CP. Treatment of typical absence seizures and related epileptic syndromes. Paediatr Drugs 2001;3:379–403.

THERAPEUTICS

Brands
- Duraclon (injection)
- Catapres
- Kapvay

see index for additional brand names

Generic? Yes (not for transdermal)

Class
- Neuroscience-based Nomenclature: norepinephrine receptor agonist (N-RA)
- Antihypertensive; centrally acting alpha 2 agonist hypotensive agent, nonstimulant for ADHD

Commonly Prescribed for
(bold for FDA approved)
- **Hypertension**
- **Attention deficit hyperactivity disorder (ADHD) (Kapvay)**
- Attention deficit hyperactivity disorder (ADHD)
- Tourette's syndrome
- Substance withdrawal, including opiates and alcohol
- Anxiety disorders, including posttraumatic stress disorder (PTSD) and social anxiety disorder
- Clozapine-induced hypersalivation
- Menopausal flushing
- Severe pain in cancer patients that is not adequately relieved by opioid analgesics alone (combination with opiates)

How the Drug Works
- For ADHD, theoretically has central actions on postsynaptic alpha 2 receptors in the prefrontal cortex
- For hypertension, stimulates alpha 2 adrenergic receptors in the brain stem, reducing sympathetic outflow from the CNS and decreasing peripheral resistance, renal vascular resistance, heart rate, and blood pressure
- An imidazoline, so also interacts at imidazoline receptors

How Long Until It Works
- For ADHD, can take a few weeks to see maximum therapeutic benefits
- Blood pressure may be lowered 30–60 minutes after first dose; greatest reduction seen after 2–4 hours
- May take several weeks to control blood pressure adequately

If It Works
- The goal of treatment of ADHD is reduction of symptoms of inattentiveness, motor hyperactivity, and/or impulsiveness that disrupt social, school, and/or occupational functioning
- Continue treatment until all symptoms are under control or improvement is stable and then continue treatment indefinitely as long as improvement persists
- Reevaluate the need for treatment periodically
- Treatment for ADHD begun in childhood may need to be continued into adolescence and adulthood if continued benefit is documented
- For hypertension, continue treatment indefinitely and check blood pressure regularly

If It Doesn't Work
- Consider adjusting dose or switching to another agent
- Consider behavioral therapy
- Consider the presence of noncompliance and counsel patient and parents
- Consider evaluation for another diagnosis or for a comorbid condition (e.g., bipolar disorder, substance abuse, medical illness, etc.)

Best Augmenting Combos for Partial Response or Treatment Resistance
- Best to attempt another monotherapy prior to augmenting for ADHD
- Possibly combination with stimulants (with caution as benefits of combination poorly documented and there are some reports of serious adverse events)
- Combinations for ADHD should be for the expert, while monitoring the patient closely, and when other treatment options have failed
- Chlorthalidone, thiazide-type diuretics, and furosemide for hypertension

Tests
- Blood pressure should be checked regularly during treatment

SIDE EFFECTS

How Drug Causes Side Effects

- Excessive actions on alpha 2 receptors and/or on imidazoline receptors

Notable Side Effects

✽ Dry mouth

✽ Dizziness, constipation, sedation

- Weakness, fatigue, impotence, loss of libido, insomnia, headache
- Major depression
- Dermatologic reactions (especially with transdermal clonidine)
- Hypotension, occasional syncope
- Tachycardia
- Nervousness, agitation
- Nausea, vomiting

Life-Threatening or Dangerous Side Effects

- Sinus bradycardia, atrioventricular block
- During withdrawal, hypertensive encephalopathy, cerebrovascular accidents, and death (rare)

Weight Gain

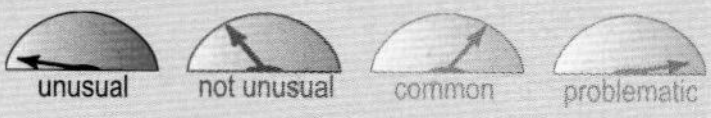

- Reported but not expected

Sedation

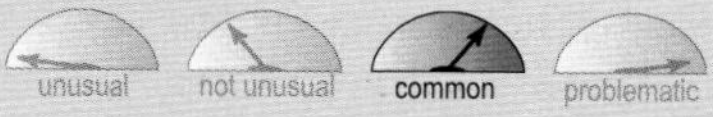

- Many experience and/or can be significant in amount
- Some patients may not tolerate it
- Can abate with time

What to Do About Side Effects

- Wait
- Take larger dose at bedtime to avoid daytime sedation
- Switch to another medication with better evidence of efficacy

✽ For withdrawal and discontinuation reactions, may need to reinstate clonidine and taper very slowly when stabilized

Best Augmenting Agents for Side Effects

- Dose reduction or switching to another agent may be more effective since most side effects cannot be improved with an augmenting agent

DOSING AND USE

Usual Dosage Range

- Extended-release for ADHD: 0.1–0.4 mg/day in divided doses
- Immediate-release for hypertension: 0.2–0.6 mg/day in divided doses
- Opioid withdrawal: 0.1 mg 3 times daily (can be higher in inpatient setting)

Dosage Forms

- Extended-release tablet 0.1 mg, 0.2 mg
- Immediate-release tablet 0.1 mg scored, 0.2 mg scored, 0.3 mg scored
- Topical (7 day administration) 0.1 mg/24 hours, 0.2 mg/24 hours, 0.3 mg/24 hours
- Injection 0.1 mg/mL, 0.5 mg/mL

How to Dose

- Oral (for ADHD): initial 0.1 mg at bedtime; can increase by 0.1 mg/day each week with dosing divided and larger dose at bedtime; maximum dose generally 0.4 mg/day in divided doses
- For opioid withdrawal: 0.1 mg 3 times daily; next dose should be withheld if blood pressure falls below 90/60 mm Hg; outpatients should not be given more than a 3-day supply, detoxification can usually be achieved in 4–6 days for short-acting opioids
- Oral (for hypertension): initial 0.1 mg in 2 divided doses, morning and night; can increase by 0.1 mg/day each week; maximum dose generally 2.4 mg/day
- Topical (for hypertension): apply once every 7 days in hairless area; change location with each application
- Injection (for hypertension): initial 30 mcg/hr; maximum 40 mcg/hr; 500 mg/mL must be diluted

Dosing Tips

- Extended-release tablet should not be chewed, crushed, or broken before swallowing, as this could alter controlled-release properties
- Do not substitute different clonidine products for each other on a mg-per-mg basis, because they have different pharmacokinetic profiles
- Adverse effects are dose-related and usually transient

- The last dose of the day should occur at bedtime so that blood pressure is controlled overnight
- If clonidine is terminated abruptly, rebound hypertension may occur within 2–4 days, so taper dose in decrements of no more than 0.1 mg every 3 to 7 days when discontinuing
- Using clonidine in combination with another antihypertensive agent may attenuate the development of tolerance to clonidine's antihypertensive effects
- The likelihood of severe discontinuation reactions with CNS and cardiovascular symptoms may be greater after administration of high doses of clonidine

✽ In patients who have developed localized contact sensitization to transdermal clonidine, continuing transdermal dosing on other skin areas or substituting with oral clonidine may be associated with the development of a generalized skin rash, urticaria, or angioedema

✽ If administered with a beta blocker, stop the beta blocker first for several days before the gradual discontinuation of clonidine in cases of planned discontinuation

Overdose

- Hypotension, hypertension, miosis, respiratory depression, seizures, bradycardia, hypothermia, coma, sedation, decreased reflexes, weakness, irritability, dysrhythmia

Long-Term Use

- Patients may develop tolerance to the antihypertensive effects

✽ Studies have not established the utility of clonidine for long-term CNS uses

✽ Be aware that forgetting to take clonidine or running out of medication can lead to abrupt discontinuation and associated withdrawal reactions and complications

Habit Forming

- Reports of some abuse by opiate addicts
- Reports of some abuse by non-opioid dependent patients

How to Stop

✽ Discontinuation reactions are common and sometimes severe

- Sudden discontinuation can result in nervousness, agitation, headache, and tremor, with rapid rise in blood pressure
- Rare instances of hypertensive encephalopathy, cerebrovascular accident, and death have been reported after clonidine withdrawal
- Taper over 2–4 days or longer to avoid rebound effects (nervousness, increased blood pressure)
- If administered with a beta blocker, stop the beta blocker first for several days before the gradual discontinuation of clonidine

Pharmacokinetics

- Half-life 12–16 hours
- Metabolized by the liver
- Excreted renally

Drug Interactions

- The likelihood of severe discontinuation reactions with CNS and cardiovascular symptoms may be greater when clonidine is combined with beta blocker treatment
- Increased depressive and sedative effects when taken with other CNS depressants
- TCAs may reduce the hypotensive effects of clonidine
- Corneal lesions in rats increased by use of clonidine with amitriptyline
- Use of clonidine with agents that affect sinus node function or AV nodal function (e.g., digitalis, calcium channel blockers, beta blockers) may result in bradycardia or AV block

Other Warnings/ Precautions

- There have been cases of hypertensive encephalopathy, cerebrovascular accidents, and death after abrupt discontinuation
- If used with a beta blocker, the beta blocker should be stopped several days before tapering clonidine
- In patients who have developed localized contact sensitization to transdermal clonidine, continuing transdermal dosing on other skin areas or substituting with oral clonidine may be associated with the development of a generalized skin rash, urticaria, or angioedema
- Injection is not recommended for use in managing obstetrical, postpartum or peri-operative pain

- Certain transdermal patches containing even small traces of aluminum or other metals in the adhesive backing can cause skin burns if worn during MRI, so warn patients taking the transdermal formulation about this possibility and advise them to disclose this information if they need an MRI

Do Not Use
- If there is a proven allergy to clonidine

SPECIAL POPULATIONS

Renal Impairment
- Use with caution and possibly reduce dose

Hepatic Impairment
- Use with caution

Cardiac Impairment
- Use with caution in patients with recent myocardial infarction, severe coronary insufficiency, cerebrovascular disease

Elderly
- Elderly patients may tolerate a lower initial dose better
- Elderly patients may be more sensitive to sedative effects

Children and Adolescents
- Safety and efficacy not established for children under age 6
- Children may be more sensitive to hypertensive effects of withdrawing treatment

* Because children commonly have gastrointestinal illnesses that lead to vomiting, they may be more likely to abruptly discontinue clonidine and therefore be more susceptible to hypertensive episodes resulting from abrupt inability to take medication

- Children may be more likely to experience CNS depression with overdose and may even exhibit signs of toxicity with 0.1 mg of clonidine
- Injection may be used in pediatric cancer patients with severe pain unresponsive to other medications

Pregnancy
- Effective June 30, 2015, the US FDA requires changes to the content and format of pregnancy and lactation information in prescription drug labels, including the elimination of the pregnancy letter categories; the Pregnancy and Lactation Labeling Rule (PLLR or final rule) applies only to prescription drugs and will be phased in gradually for drugs approved on or after June 30, 2001
- Controlled studies have not been conducted in pregnant women
- Some animal studies have shown adverse effects
- Use in women of childbearing potential requires weighing potential benefits to the mother against potential risks to the fetus

* For ADHD patients, clonidine should generally be discontinued before anticipated pregnancies

Breast Feeding
- Some drug is found in mother's breast milk
- No adverse effects have been reported in nursing infants
- If irritability or sedation develop in nursing infant, may need to discontinue drug or bottle feed

THE ART OF PSYCHOPHARMACOLOGY

Potential Advantages
- No known abuse potential; not a controlled substance

Potential Disadvantages
- Not well studied in adults with ADHD
- Withdrawal reactions
- Noncompliant patients
- Patients on concomitant CNS medications

Primary Target Symptoms
- Concentration
- Motor hyperactivity
- Oppositional and impulsive behavior
- High blood pressure

Pearls

✻ Clonidine extended-release is approved for ADHD in children ages 6–17

- As monotherapy or in combination with methylphenidate for ADHD with conduct disorder or oppositional defiant disorder, may improve aggression, oppositional, and conduct disorder symptoms
- Clonidine is sometimes used in combination with stimulants to reduce side effects and enhance therapeutic effects on motor hyperactivity
- Doses of 0.1 mg in 3 divided doses have been reported to reduce stimulant-induced insomnia as well as impulsivity

✻ Clonidine may also be effective for treatment of tic disorders, including Tourette's syndrome

- May suppress tics especially in severe Tourette's syndrome, and may be even better at reducing explosive violent behaviors in Tourette's syndrome
- Sedation is often unacceptable in various patients despite improvement in CNS symptoms and leads to discontinuation of treatment, especially for ADHD and Tourette's syndrome
- Considered an investigational treatment for most other CNS applications
- May block the autonomic symptoms in anxiety and panic disorders (e.g., palpitations, sweating) and improve subjective anxiety as well
- May be useful in decreasing the autonomic arousal of PTSD
- May be useful as an as-needed medication for stage fright or other predictable socially phobic situations
- May also be useful when added to SSRIs for reducing arousal and dissociative symptoms in PTSD
- May block autonomic symptoms of opioid withdrawal (e.g., palpitations, sweating) especially in inpatients, but muscle aches, irritability, and insomnia may not be well suppressed by clonidine
- Often prescribed with naltrexone to suppress symptoms of opioid withdrawal; this requires monitoring of the patient for 8 hours on the first day due to the potential severity of naltrexone-induced withdrawal and the potential blood pressure effects of clonidine
- May be useful in decreasing the hypertension, tachycardia, and tremulousness associated with alcohol withdrawal, but not the seizures or delirium tremens in complicated alcohol withdrawal
- Clonidine may improve social relationships, affectual responses, and sensory responses in autistic disorder
- Clonidine may reduce the incidence of menopausal flushing
- Growth hormone response to clonidine may be reduced during menses
- Clonidine stimulates growth hormone secretion (no chronic effects have been observed)
- Alcohol may reduce the effects of clonidine on growth hormone

✻ Guanfacine is a related centrally active alpha 2 agonist hypotensive agent that has been used for similar CNS applications but has not been as widely investigated or used as clonidine

✻ Guanfacine may be tolerated better than clonidine in some patients (e.g., sedation) or it may work better in some patients for CNS applications than clonidine, but no head-to-head trials

Suggested Reading

American Psychiatric Association. Practice guideline for the treatment of patients with substance use disorders, second edition. Am J Psychiatry 2007;164(4):1–86.

Burris JF. The USA experience with the clonidine transdermal therapeutic system. Clin Auton Res 1993;3:391–6.

Croxtall JD. Clonidine extended-release: in attention-deficit hyperactivity disorder. Paediatr Drugs 2011;13(5):329–36.

Gavras I, Manolis AJ, Gayras H. The alpha2-adrenergic receptors in hypertension and heart failure: experimental and clinical studies. J Hypertens 2001;19:2115–24.

Neil MJ. Clonidine: clinical pharmacology and therapeutic use in pain management. Curr Clin Pharmacol 2011;6(4):280–7.

CLORAZEPATE

THERAPEUTICS

Brands • Azene
• Tranxene

see index for additional brand names

Generic? Yes

Class

- Neuroscience-based Nomenclature: GABA positive allosteric modulator (GABA-PAM)
- Benzodiazepine (anxiolytic)

Commonly Prescribed for

(bold for FDA approved)

- **Anxiety disorder**
- **Symptoms of anxiety**
- **Acute alcohol withdrawal**
- Partial seizures (adjunct)
- Catatonia

How the Drug Works

- Binds to benzodiazepine receptors at the GABA-A ligand-gated chloride channel complex
- Enhances the inhibitory effects of GABA
- Boosts chloride conductance through GABA-regulated channels
- Inhibits neuronal activity presumably in amygdala-centered fear circuits to provide therapeutic benefits in anxiety disorders

How Long Until It Works

- Some immediate relief with first dosing is common; can take several weeks with daily dosing for maximal therapeutic benefit

If It Works

- For short-term symptoms of anxiety – after a few weeks, discontinue use or use on an "as-needed" basis
- For chronic anxiety disorders, the goal of treatment is complete remission of symptoms as well as prevention of future relapses
- For chronic anxiety disorders, treatment most often reduces or even eliminates symptoms, but not a cure since symptoms can recur after medicine stopped
- For long-term symptoms of anxiety, consider switching to an SSRI or SNRI for long-term maintenance
- If long-term maintenance with a benzodiazepine is necessary, continue treatment for 6 months after symptoms resolve, and then taper dose slowly
- If symptoms reemerge, consider treatment with an SSRI or SNRI, or consider restarting the benzodiazepine; sometimes benzodiazepines have to be used in combination with SSRIs or SNRIs for best results

If It Doesn't Work

- Consider switching to another agent or adding an appropriate augmenting agent
- Consider psychotherapy, especially cognitive behavioral psychotherapy
- Consider presence of concomitant substance abuse
- Consider presence of clorazepate abuse
- Consider another diagnosis, such as a comorbid medical condition

Best Augmenting Combos for Partial Response or Treatment Resistance

- Benzodiazepines are frequently used as augmenting agents for antipsychotics and mood stabilizers in the treatment of psychotic and bipolar disorders
- Benzodiazepines are frequently used as augmenting agents for SSRIs and SNRIs in the treatment of anxiety disorders
- Not generally rational to combine with other benzodiazepines
- Caution if using as an anxiolytic concomitantly with other sedative hypnotics for sleep

Tests

- In patients with seizure disorders, concomitant medical illness, and/or those with multiple concomitant long-term medications, periodic liver tests and blood counts may be prudent

SIDE EFFECTS

How Drug Causes Side Effects

- Same mechanism for side effects as for therapeutic effects – namely due to excessive actions at benzodiazepine receptors

- Long-term adaptations in benzodiazepine receptors may explain the development of dependence, tolerance, and withdrawal
- Side effects are generally immediate, but immediate side effects often disappear in time

Notable Side Effects

✻ Sedation, fatigue, depression
✻ Dizziness, ataxia, slurred speech, weakness
✻ Forgetfulness, confusion
✻ Nervousness
- Rare hallucinations, mania
- Rare hypotension
- Hypersalivation, dry mouth

Life-Threatening or Dangerous Side Effects

- Respiratory depression, especially when taken with CNS depressants in overdose
- Rare hepatic dysfunction, renal dysfunction, blood dyscrasias

Weight Gain

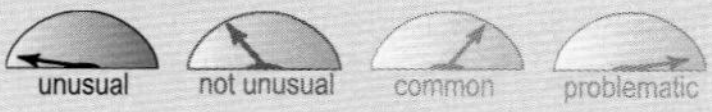

- Reported but not expected

Sedation

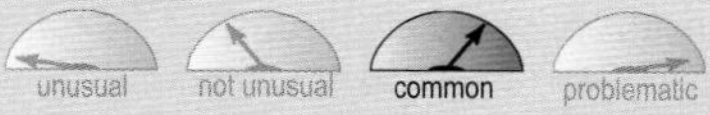

- Many experience and/or can be significant in amount
- Especially at initiation of treatment or when dose increases
- Tolerance often develops over time

What to Do About Side Effects

- Wait
- Wait
- Wait
- Lower the dose
- Take largest dose at bedtime to avoid sedative effects during the day
- Switch to another agent
- Administer flumazenil if side effects are severe or life-threatening

Best Augmenting Agents for Side Effects

- Many side effects cannot be improved with an augmenting agent

DOSING AND USE

Usual Dosage Range

- Anxiety: 15–60 mg/day in divided doses
- Alcohol withdrawal: 30–60 mg/day in divided doses

Dosage Forms

- Tablet 3.75 mg scored, 7.5 mg scored, 15 mg scored, 22.5 mg single dose, 11.25 mg single dose half strength

How to Dose

- Anxiety: initial 15 mg/day in divided doses; adjust dose as needed on subsequent days; single-dose tablet may be given once daily at bedtime after patient is stable; maximum generally 90 mg/day
- Alcohol withdrawal: initial 30 mg, then 30–60 mg in divided doses; second day 45–90 mg in divided doses; third day 22.5–45 mg in divided doses; fourth day 15–30 mg in divided doses; after fourth day decrease dose gradually and discontinue when patient is stable; maximum generally 90 mg/day
- Epilepsy: initial 7.5 mg 3 times/day; increase by 7.5 mg weekly; maximum generally 90 mg/day

Dosing Tips

- Use lowest possible effective dose for the shortest possible period of time (a benzodiazepine-sparing strategy)
- Assess need for continued treatment regularly
- Risk of dependence may increase with dose and duration of treatment
- For interdose symptoms of anxiety, can either increase dose or maintain same total daily dose but divide into more frequent doses
- Can also use an as-needed occasional "top up" dose for interdose anxiety
- Because anxiety disorders can require higher doses, the risk of dependence may be greater in these patients
- Frequency of dosing in practice is often greater than predicted from half-life, as duration of biological activity is often shorter than pharmacokinetic terminal half-life

Overdose
- Fatalities can occur; hypotension, tiredness, ataxia, confusion, coma

Long-Term Use
- Evidence of efficacy for up to 16 weeks
- Risk of dependence, particularly for periods longer than 12 weeks and especially in patients with past or current polysubstance abuse

Habit Forming
- Clorazepate is a Schedule IV drug
- Patients may develop dependence and/or tolerance with long-term use

How to Stop
- Patients with history of seizure may seize upon withdrawal, especially if withdrawal is abrupt
- Taper by 7.5 mg every 3 days to reduce chances of withdrawal effects
- For difficult to taper cases, consider reducing dose much more slowly after reaching 30 mg/day, perhaps by as little as 3.75 mg per week or less
- For other patients with severe problems discontinuing a benzodiazepine, dosing may need to be tapered over many months (i.e., reduce dose by 1% every 3 days by crushing tablet and suspending or dissolving in 100 mL of fruit juice and then disposing of 1 mL while drinking the rest; 3–7 days later, dispose of 2 mL, and so on). This is both a form of very slow biological tapering and a form of behavioral desensitization
- Be sure to differentiate reemergence of symptoms requiring reinstitution of treatment from withdrawal symptoms
- Benzodiazepine-dependent anxiety patients and insulin-dependent diabetics are not addicted to their medications. When benzodiazepine-dependent patients stop their medication, disease symptoms can reemerge, disease symptoms can worsen (rebound), and/or withdrawal symptoms can emerge

Pharmacokinetics
- Elimination half-life 40–50 hours

Drug Interactions
- Increased depressive effects when taken with other CNS depressants (see Warnings below)

Other Warnings/ Precautions
- Boxed warning regarding the increased risk of CNS depressant effects when benzodiazepines and opioid medications are used together, including specifically the risk of slowed or difficulty breathing and death
- If alternatives to the combined use of benzodiazepines and opioids are not available, clinicians should limit the dosage and duration of each drug to the minimum possible while still achieving therapeutic efficacy
- Patients and their caregivers should be warned to seek medical attention if unusual dizziness, lightheadedness, sedation, slowed or difficulty breathing, or unresponsiveness occur
- Dosage changes should be made in collaboration with prescriber
- Use with caution in patients with pulmonary disease; rare reports of death after initiation of benzodiazepines in patients with severe pulmonary impairment
- History of drug or alcohol abuse often creates greater risk for dependency
- Some depressed patients may experience a worsening of suicidal ideation
- Some patients may exhibit abnormal thinking or behavioral changes similar to those caused by other CNS depressants (i.e., either depressant actions or disinhibiting actions)

Do Not Use
- If patient has angle-closure glaucoma
- If there is a proven allergy to clorazepate or any benzodiazepine

SPECIAL POPULATIONS

Renal Impairment
- Initial 7.5–15 mg/day in divided doses or in 1 dose at bedtime

Hepatic Impairment
- Initial 7.5–15 mg/day in divided doses or in 1 dose at bedtime

Cardiac Impairment

- Benzodiazepines have been used to treat anxiety associated with acute myocardial infarction

Elderly

- Initial 7.5–15 mg/day in divided doses or in 1 dose at bedtime

Children and Adolescents

- Not recommended for use in children under age 9
- Recommended initial dose: 7.5 mg twice a day

Pregnancy

- Effective June 30, 2015, the US FDA requires changes to the content and format of pregnancy and lactation information in prescription drug labels, including the elimination of the pregnancy letter categories; the Pregnancy and Lactation Labeling Rule (PLLR or final rule) applies only to prescription drugs and will be phased in gradually for drugs approved on or after June 30, 2001
- Possible increased risk of birth defects when benzodiazepines taken during pregnancy
- Because of the potential risks, clorazepate is not generally recommended as treatment for anxiety during pregnancy, especially during the first trimester
- Drug should be tapered if discontinued
- Infants whose mothers received a benzodiazepine late in pregnancy may experience withdrawal effects
- Neonatal flaccidity has been reported in infants whose mothers took a benzodiazepine during pregnancy
- Seizures, even mild seizures, may cause harm to the embryo/fetus

Breast Feeding

- Some drug is found in mother's breast milk

✻ Recommended either to discontinue drug or bottle feed

- Effects of benzodiazepines on nursing infants have been reported and include feeding difficulties, sedation, and weight loss

THE ART OF PSYCHOPHARMACOLOGY

Potential Advantages

- Rapid onset of action

Potential Disadvantages

- Euphoria may lead to abuse
- Abuse especially risky in past or present substance abusers

Primary Target Symptoms

- Panic attacks
- Anxiety
- Incidence of seizures (adjunct)

Pearls

- Can be very useful as an adjunct to SSRIs and SNRIs in the treatment of numerous anxiety disorders
- Not effective for treating psychosis as a monotherapy, but can be used as an adjunct to antipsychotics
- Not effective for treating bipolar disorder as a monotherapy, but can be used as an adjunct to mood stabilizers and antipsychotics

✻ More commonly used than some other benzodiazepines for treating alcohol withdrawal

- May both cause depression and treat depression in different patients
- When using to treat insomnia, remember that insomnia may be a symptom of some other primary disorder itself, and thus warrant evaluation for comorbid psychiatric and/or medical conditions
- Though not systematically studied, benzodiazepines have been used effectively to treat catatonia and are the initial recommended treatment

Suggested Reading

Griffith JL, Murray GB. Clorazepate in the treatment of complex partial seizures with psychic symptomatology. J Nerv Ment Dis 1985;173:185–6.

Kiejna A, Kantorska-Janiec M, Malyszczak K. [The use of chlorazepate dipotassium (Tranxene) in the states of restlessness and agitation]. Psychiatr Pol 1997;31:753–60.

Mielke L, Breinbauer B, Schubert M, et al. [Comparison of the effectiveness of orally administered clorazepate dipotassium and nordiazepam on preoperative anxiety]. Anaesthesiol Reanim 1995;20:144–8.

Rickels K, Schweizer E, Csanalosi I, Case WG, Chung H. Long-term treatment of anxiety and risk of withdrawal. Prospective comparison of clorazepate and buspirone. Arch Gen Psychiatry 1988;45:444–50.

THERAPEUTICS

Brands
- Clozaril
- Leponex
- Versacloz (oral suspension)
- Fazaclo ODT (oral disintegrating tablet)

see index for additional brand names

Generic? Yes

Class
- Neuroscience-based Nomenclature: dopamine, serotonin, norepinephrine receptor antagonist (DSN-RAn)
- Atypical antipsychotic (serotonin-dopamine antagonist; second-generation antipsychotic; also a mood stabilizer)

Commonly Prescribed for
(bold for FDA approved)
- **Treatment-resistant schizophrenia**
- **Reduction in risk of recurrent suicidal behavior in patients with schizophrenia or schizoaffective disorder**
- Treatment-resistant bipolar disorder
- Violent aggressive patients with psychosis and other brain disorders not responsive to other treatments

How the Drug Works
- Blocks dopamine 2 receptors, reducing positive symptoms of psychosis and stabilizing affective symptoms
- Blocks serotonin 2A receptors, causing enhancement of dopamine release in certain brain regions and thus reducing motor side effects and possibly improving cognitive and affective symptoms
- Interactions at a myriad of other neurotransmitter receptors may contribute to clozapine's efficacy

✽ Specifically, interactions at 5HT2C and 5HT1A receptors may contribute to efficacy for cognitive and affective symptoms in some patients

- Mechanism of efficacy for psychotic patients who do not respond to conventional antipsychotics is unknown

How Long Until It Works
- Likelihood of response depends on achieving trough plasma levels of at least 350 ng/mL
- Median time to response after achieving therapeutic plasma levels (350 ng/mL) is approximately 3 weeks
- If there is no response after 3 weeks of therapeutic plasma levels, recheck plasma levels and continue titration

If It Works
- In strictly defined refractory schizophrenia, 50–60% of patients will respond to clozapine
- The response rate to other atypical antipsychotic in the refractory patient population ranges from 0–9%
- Can improve negative symptoms, as well as aggressive, cognitive, and affective symptoms in schizophrenia
- Most schizophrenic patients do not have a total remission of symptoms but rather a reduction of symptoms by about a third
- Many patients with bipolar disorder and other disorders with psychotic, aggressive, violent, impulsive, and other types of behavioral disturbances may respond to clozapine when other agents have failed
- Perhaps 5–15% of schizophrenic patients can experience an overall improvement of greater than 50–60%, especially when receiving stable treatment for more than a year

✽ Such patients are considered super-responders or "awakeners" since they may be well enough to be employed, live independently, and sustain long-term relationships; super-responders are anecdotally reported more often with clozapine than with some other antipsychotics

- Treatment may not only reduce mania but also prevent recurrences of mania in bipolar disorder

If It Doesn't Work
- Obtain clozapine plasma levels and continue titration
- Levels greater than 700 ng/mL are often not well tolerated
- No evidence to support dosing that results in plasma levels greater than 1,000 ng/mL
- Some patients may respond better if switched to a conventional antipsychotic

✽ Some patients may require augmentation with a conventional antipsychotic or with an atypical antipsychotic (especially risperidone or amisulpride), but these are the most refractory of all psychotic patients and such treatment can be expensive

✽ Consider augmentation with valproate or lamotrigine
- Consider noncompliance and switch to another antipsychotic with fewer side effects or to an antipsychotic that can be given by depot injection
- Consider initiating rehabilitation and psychotherapy such as cognitive remediation
- Consider presence of concomitant drug abuse

Best Augmenting Combos for Partial Response or Treatment Resistance

- Valproic acid (valproate, divalproex, divalproex ER)
- Lamotrigine
- Conventional antipsychotics
- Benzodiazepines
- Lithium

Tests

- Lower ANC threshold for starting clozapine:
  - General population: ≥1,500/μL
  - Benign ethnic neutropenia (BEN): ≥1,000/μL
- Testing for myocarditis:
  - Myocarditis is rare and only occurs in the first 6 weeks of treatment
  - Baseline: check troponin I/T, C-reactive protein (CRP)
  - Weekly troponin I/T and CRP for the first month
  - Fever is usually benign and self-limited; suspicion of myocarditis should only be raised based on elevated troponin and other features of myocarditis
  - Clozapine should be stopped if troponin ≥ 2x upper limits of normal or CRP >100 mg/L
- Cardiomyopathy is a late complication; consider annual ECG

Before starting an atypical antipsychotic

✽ Weigh all patients and track BMI during treatment
- Get baseline personal and family history of diabetes, obesity, dyslipidemia, hypertension, and cardiovascular disease

✽ Get waist circumference (at umbilicus), blood pressure, fasting plasma glucose, and fasting lipid profile
- Determine if the patient is
  - overweight (BMI 25.0–29.9)
  - obese (BMI ≥30)
  - has pre-diabetes (fasting plasma glucose 100–125 mg/dL)
  - has diabetes (fasting plasma glucose >126 mg/dL)
  - has hypertension (BP >140/90 mm Hg)
  - has dyslipidemia (increased total cholesterol, LDL cholesterol, and triglycerides; decreased HDL cholesterol)
- Treat or refer such patients for treatment, including nutrition and weight management, physical activity counseling, smoking cessation, and medical management

Monitoring after starting an atypical antipsychotic

✽ BMI monthly for 3 months, then quarterly

✽ Consider monitoring fasting triglycerides monthly for several months in patients at high risk for metabolic complications and when initiating or switching antipsychotics

✽ Blood pressure, fasting plasma glucose, fasting lipids within 3 months and then annually, but earlier and more frequently for patients with diabetes or who have gained >5% of initial weight
- Treat or refer for treatment and consider switching to another atypical antipsychotic for patients who become overweight, obese, pre-diabetic, diabetic, hypertensive, or dyslipidemic while receiving an atypical antipsychotic

✽ Even in patients without known diabetes, be vigilant for the rare but life-threatening onset of diabetic ketoacidosis, which always requires immediate treatment, by monitoring for the rapid onset of polyuria, polydipsia, weight loss, nausea, vomiting, dehydration, rapid respiration, weakness and clouding of sensorium, even coma
- Liver function testing, ECG, general physical exam, and assessment of baseline cardiac status before starting treatment
- Liver tests may be necessary during treatment in patients who develop nausea, vomiting, or anorexia

SIDE EFFECTS

How Drug Causes Side Effects

- By blocking alpha 1 adrenergic receptors, it can cause orthostatic hypotension, tachycardia, dizziness, and sedation
- By blocking muscarinic 1 receptors, it can cause sialorrhea, constipation, sometimes with paralytic ileus, and sedation
- By blocking histamine 1 receptors in the brain, it can cause sedation and possibly weight gain
- Mechanism of weight gain and increased risk of diabetes and dyslipidemia with atypical antipsychotics is unknown but insulin regulation may be impaired by blocking pancreatic M3 muscarinic receptors
- By blocking dopamine 2 receptors in the striatum, it can cause motor side effects (very rare)

Notable Side Effects

- Orthostasis
- Sialorrhea
- Constipation
- Sedation
- Tachycardia
- Weight gain
- Dyslipidemia and hyperglycemia
- Benign fever (~20%)
- Rare tardive dyskinesia (no reports have directly implicated clozapine in the development of tardive dyskinesia)

Life-Threatening or Dangerous Side Effects

- Severe neutropenia
- Myocarditis (only in first 6 weeks of treatment)
- Paralytic ileus
- Seizures (risk increases with dose)
- Hyperglycemia, in some cases extreme and associated with ketoacidosis or hyperosmolar coma or death, has been reported in patients taking atypical antipsychotics
- Pulmonary embolism (may include deep vein thrombosis or respiratory symptoms)
- Dilated cardiomyopathy
- Increased risk of death and cerebrovascular events in elderly patients with dementia-related psychosis
- Neuroleptic malignant syndrome (more likely when clozapine is used with another agent)

Weight Gain

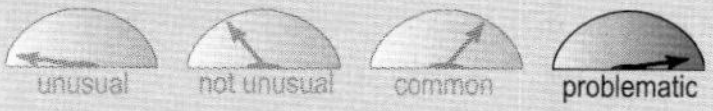

- Frequent and can be significant in amount
- May increase risk for aspiration events
- Should be managed aggressively
- More than for some other antipsychotics, but never say always as not a problem in everyone

Sedation

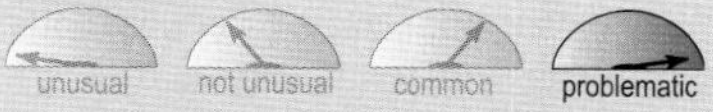

- Frequent and can be significant in amount
- Some patients may not tolerate it
- More than for some other antipsychotics, but never say always as not a problem in everyone
- Can wear off over time
- Can reemerge as dose increases and then wear off again over time

What To Do About Side Effects

- Slow titration to minimize orthostasis and sedation
  - Minimize use of other alpha 1 antagonists
  - If orthostasis remains a problem, Florines 0.1–0.3 mg qd for volume expansion (contraindicated in congestive heart failure)
  - Take at bedtime to help reduce daytime sedation
- Sialorrhea management
  - Atropine 1% drops, 1–3 drops sublingually at bedtime; can use up to 3 times per day if needed
  - Ipratropium bromide 0.06% spray, 1–3 sprays intra-orally at bedtime; can use up to 3 times per day if needed
  - Avoid use of systemic anticholinergic agents, which increase risk of ileus (benztropine, glycopyrrolate, etc.)
- Constipation management
  - Avoid psyllium as it may worsen symptoms
  - All patients should receive docusate 250 mg when starting clozapine
  - If needed, add Miralax 17 g
  - If docusate + Miralax are ineffective, add either bisacodyl or sennosides
  - If constipation still remains a problem, prescribe lubiprostone 8–24 mcg twice per day

- Weight gain and metabolic effects
  - Consider prophylactic metformin; start at 500 mg for 1 week, then increase dose
  - All patients should be referred for lifestyle management and exercise
- Tachycardia
  - Atenolol 12.5 mg qd, increase to keep resting HR <100 bpm
- Chest pain during the first 6 weeks
  - Obtain workup for myocarditis
- Fever
  - In the absence of elevated troponin and myocarditis symptoms, fever is usually self-limited and there is no need to stop clozapine
- Seizures
  - Valproate for myoclonic or generalized seizures
  - Avoid phenytoin and carbamazepine because of kinetic interactions

Best Augmenting Agents for Side Effects

- Many side effects cannot be improved with an augmenting agent

DOSING AND USE

Usual Dosage Range

- Depends on plasma levels; threshold for response is trough plasma level of 350 ng/mL

Dosage Forms

- Tablet 12.5 mg, 25 mg scored, 50 mg, 100 mg scored
- Orally disintegrating tablet 12.5 mg, 25 mg, 50 mg, 100 mg, 150 mg, 200 mg
- Oral suspension 50 mg/mL

How to Dose

- Initial 25 mg at night; increase by 25–50 mg/day every 48–72 hours as tolerated
- Obtain trough plasma level on 200 mg at bedtime
- Threshold for response is 350 ng/mL
- Levels greater than 700 ng/mL are often not well tolerated
- No evidence to support dosing that results in plasma levels greater than 1,000 ng/mL
- Doses greater than 500 mg per day may require a split dose
- See also The Art of Switching, after Pearls

Dosing Tips

- Because of the monitoring schedule, prescriptions are generally given 1 week at a time for the first 6 months, then every 2 weeks for months 6–12, and then monthly after 12 months
- Plasma half-life suggests twice daily administration, but in practice it may be given once a day at night
- Prior to initiating treatment with clozapine, a baseline ANC must be at least 1500/μL for the general population and at least 1000/μL for patients with documented benign ethnic neutropenia (BEN)

Recommended ANC Monitoring for the General Population		
ANC Level	**Recommendation**	**ANC Monitoring**
Normal range (at least 1,500 μL)	Initiate treatment If treatment is interrupted for <30 days, continue monitoring as before If treatment is interrupted for 30 days or more, monitor as if new patient	First 6 months: weekly Second 6 months: every 2 weeks After 1 year: every month
Mild neutropenia (1,000–1,499 μL)	Continue treatment	Confirm all initial reports of ANC <1,500/μL with a repeat ANC measurement within 24 hours Monitor 3 times/week until ANC ≥1,500/μL Once ANC ≥1,500/μL, return to patient's last "normal range" ANC monitoring interval
Moderate neutropenia (500–999 μL)	Interrupt treatment for suspected clozapine-induced neutropenia Recommend hematology consultation	Confirm all initial reports of ANC <1,500/μL with a repeat ANC measurement within 24 hours Monitor ANC daily until ≥1,000/μL THEN Monitor 3 times/week until ANC ≥1,500/μL Once ANC ≥1,500/μL, check ANC weekly for 4 weeks, then return to patient's last "normal range" ANC monitoring interval
Severe neutropenia (<500 μL)	Interrupt treatment for suspected clozapine-induced neutropenia Recommend hematology consultation Do not rechallenge unless prescriber determines benefits outweigh risks	Confirm all initial reports of ANC <1,500/μL with a repeat ANC measurement within 24 hours Monitor ANC daily until ≥1,000/μL THEN Monitor 3 times/week until ANC ≥1,500/μL If patient is rechallenged, resume treatment as a new patient under "normal range" monitoring once ANC ≥1,500/μL

Recommended ANC Monitoring for BEN Patients		
ANC Level	**Recommendation**	**ANC Monitoring**
Normal BEN range (established ANC Baseline ≥1,000 μL)	Obtain at least 2 baseline ANC levels before initiating treatment If treatment is interrupted for <30 days, continue monitoring as before If treatment is interrupted for 30 days or more, monitor as if new patient	First 6 months: weekly Second 6 months: every 2 weeks After 1 year: every month
BEN neutropenia (500–999 μL)	Continue treatment Recommend hematology consultation	Confirm all initial reports of ANC <1,500/μL with a repeat ANC measurement within 24 hours Monitor 3 times/week until ANC ≥1,000/μL or ≥patient's known baseline Once ANC ≥1,000/μL or above patient's known baseline, check ANC weekly for 4 weeks, then return to patient's last "normal BEN range" ANC monitoring interval
BEN severe neutropenia (<500 μL)	Interrupt treatment for suspected clozapine-induced neutropenia Recommend hematology consultation Do not rechallenge unless prescriber determines benefits outweigh risks	Confirm all initial reports of ANC <1,500/μL with a repeat ANC measurement within 24 hours Monitor ANC daily until ≥500/μL THEN Monitor 3 times/week until ANC ≥patient's baseline If patient is rechallenged, resume treatment as a new patient under "normal BEN range" monitoring once ANC ≥1,000/μL or at patient's known baseline

- If treatment is discontinued for more than 2 days, reinitiate with 12.5 mg once or twice daily; if that dose is tolerated, the dose may be increased to the previously therapeutic dose more quickly than recommended for initial treatment
- If abrupt discontinuation of clozapine is necessary, the patient must be covered for cholinergic rebound; those with higher clozapine plasma levels may need extremely high doses of anticholinergic medications to prevent delirium and other rebound symptoms
- Slow off-titration is preferred if possible to avoid cholinergic rebound and rebound psychosis

Overdose
- Sometimes lethal; changes in heart rhythm, excess salivation, respiratory depression, altered state of consciousness

Long-Term Use
- Treatment to reduce risk of suicidal behavior should be continued for at least 2 years
- Medication of choice for treatment-refractory schizophrenia

Habit Forming
- No

How to Stop
- See The Art of Switching section of individual agents for how to stop clozapine, generally over at least 4 weeks
- See Tables for guidance on stopping due to neutropenia

✻ Rapid discontinuation may lead to rebound psychosis and worsening of symptoms

Pharmacokinetics
- Half-life 5–16 hours
- Metabolized primarily by CYP450 1A2 and to a lesser extent by CYP450 2D6 and 3A4

Drug Interactions
- Use clozapine plasma levels to guide treatment due to propensity for drug interactions
- In presence of a strong CYP450 1A2 inhibitor (e.g., fluvoxamine, ciprofloxacin): use 1/3 the dose of clozapine
- In the presence of a strong CYP450 1A2 inducer (e.g., cigarette smoke), clozapine plasma levels are decreased
- May need to decrease clozapine dose by up to 50% during periods of extended smoking cessation (>1 week)
- Strong CYP450 2D6 inhibitors (e.g., bupropion, duloxetine, paroxetine, fluoxetine) can raise clozapine levels; dose adjustment may be necessary
- Strong CYP450 3A4 inhibitors (e.g., ketoconazole) can raise clozapine levels; dose adjustment may be necessary
- Clozapine may enhance effects of antihypertensive drugs

Other Warnings/ Precautions
- Use with caution in patients on other anticholinergic agents (benztropine, trihexyphenidyl, olanzapine, quetiapine, chlorpromazine, oxybutynin, and other antimuscarinics)
- Should not be used in conjunction with agents that are known to cause neutropenia
- Myocarditis is rare and only occurs in the first 6 weeks of treatment
- Cardiomyopathy is a late complication (consider annual ECG)
- Use with caution in patients with glaucoma
- Use with caution in patients with enlarged prostate

Do Not Use
- In patients with myeloproliferative disorder
- In patients with uncontrolled epilepsy
- In patients with paralytic ileus
- In patients with CNS depression
- If there is a proven allergy to clozapine

SPECIAL POPULATIONS

Renal Impairment
- Should be used with caution

Hepatic Impairment
- Should be used with caution

Cardiac Impairment
- Should be used with caution, particularly if patient is taking concomitant antihypertensive or alpha 1 antagonist

Elderly

- Some patients may tolerate lower doses better
- Although atypical antipsychotics are commonly used for behavioral disturbances in dementia, no agent has been approved for treatment of elderly patients with dementia-related psychosis
- Elderly patients with dementia-related psychosis treated with atypical antipsychotics are at an increased risk of death compared to placebo, and also have an increased risk of cerebrovascular events

Children and Adolescents

- Safety and efficacy have not been established
- Preliminary research has suggested efficacy in early-onset treatment-resistant schizophrenia
- Children and adolescents taking clozapine should be monitored more often than adults

Pregnancy

- Effective June 30, 2015, the US FDA requires changes to the content and format of pregnancy and lactation information in prescription drug labels, including the elimination of the pregnancy letter categories; the Pregnancy and Lactation Labeling Rule (PLLR or final rule) applies only to prescription drugs and will be phased in gradually for drugs approved on or after June 30, 2001
- Controlled studies have not been conducted in pregnant women
- There is a risk of abnormal muscle movements and withdrawal symptoms in newborns whose mothers took an antipsychotic during the third trimester; symptoms may include agitation, abnormally increased or decreased muscle tone, tremor, sleepiness, severe difficulty breathing, and difficulty feeding
- Animal studies have not shown adverse effects
- Psychotic symptoms may worsen during pregnancy and some form of treatment may be necessary
- Clozapine should be used only when the potential benefits outweigh potential risks to the fetus
- National Pregnancy Registry for Atypical Antipsychotics: 1-866-961-2388 or http://womensmentalhealth.org/clinical-and-research-programs/pregnancyregistry/

Breast Feeding

- Unknown if clozapine is secreted in human breast milk, but all psychotropics assumed to be secreted in breast milk
- ✻ Recommended either to discontinue drug or bottle feed
- Infants of women who choose to breast feed while on clozapine should be monitored for possible adverse effects

THE ART OF PSYCHOPHARMACOLOGY

Potential Advantages

- ✻ Treatment-resistant schizophrenia
- ✻ Violent, aggressive patients
- ✻ Patients with tardive dyskinesia
- ✻ Patients with suicidal behavior

Potential Disadvantages

- ✻ Patients with diabetes, obesity, and/or dyslipidemia
- Sialorrhea, sedation, and orthostatis may be intolerable for some

Primary Target Symptoms

- Positive symptoms of psychosis
- Negative symptoms of psychosis
- Cognitive symptoms
- Affective symptoms
- Suicidal behavior
- Violence and aggression

Pearls

- ✻ Clozapine is the gold standard treatment for refractory schizophrenia
- ✻ Clozapine is not used first line due to side effects and monitoring burden
- ✻ However, some studies have shown that clozapine was associated with the lowest risk of mortality among the antipsychotics, causing the study authors to question if its use should continue to be restricted to resistant cases

- May reduce violence and aggression in difficult cases, including forensic cases
- * Reduces suicide in schizophrenia
- May reduce substance abuse
- May improve tardive dyskinesia
- Little or no prolactin elevation, motor side effects, or tardive dyskinesia
- Clinical improvements often continue slowly over several years
- Cigarette smoke can decrease clozapine levels and patients may be at risk for relapse if they begin or increase smoking
- More weight gain than many other antipsychotics – does not mean every patient gains weight
- Patients can have much better responses to clozapine than to any other agent, but not always
- For treatment-resistant patients, especially those with impulsivity, aggression, violence, and self-harm, long-term polypharmacy with 2 atypical antipsychotics or with 1 atypical antipsychotic and 1 conventional antipsychotic may be useful or even necessary while closely monitoring
- In such cases, it may be beneficial to combine 1 depot antipsychotic with 1 oral antipsychotic
- To treat constipation and reduce risk of paralytic ileus and bowel obstruction, taper off other anticholinergic agents and start all patients routinely on docusate
- The US FDA has changed the requirements for monitoring, prescribing, dispensing, and receiving clozapine in order to address concerns related to neutropenia; in addition to updating the prescribing information for clozapine, the FDA has approved a new, shared risk evaluation and mitigation strategy (REMS)
- The Clozapine REMS program replaces the six existing clozapine registries, which are maintained by individual clozapine manufacturers. Prescribers, pharmacies, and patients will now be required to enroll in a single centralized program; patients already treated with clozapine will be automatically transferred. In order to prescribe and dispense clozapine, prescribers and pharmacies will be required to be certified in the Clozapine REMS Program. Visit the Clozapine REMS Program homepage for more information.

THE ART OF SWITCHING

Switching from Oral Antipsychotics to Clozapine

- With aripiprazole, amisulpride, and paliperidone ER, immediate stop is possible; begin clozapine at middle dose
- With risperidone, ziprasidone, iloperidone, and lurasidone, begin clozapine gradually, titrating over at least 2 weeks to allow patients to become tolerant to the sedating effect

* Benzodiazepine or anticholinergic medication can be administered during cross-titration to help alleviate side effects such as insomnia, agitation, and/or psychosis. However, use with caution in combination with clozapine as this can increase the risk of circulatory collapse.

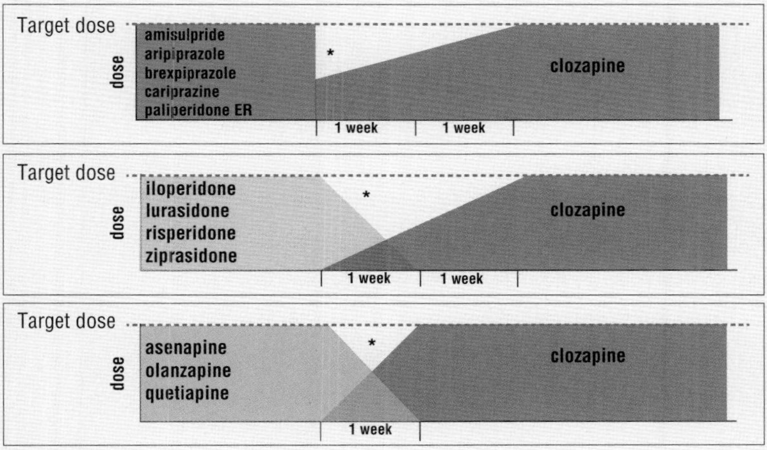

Suggested Reading

Bird AM, Smith TL, Walton AE. Current treatment strategies for clozapine-induced sialorrhea. Ann Pharmacother 2011;45(5):667–75.

Conley RR, Carpenter WT Jr, Tamminga CA. Time to clozapine response in a standardized trial. Am J Psychiatry 1997;154(9):1243–7.

Ronaldson KJ, Fitzgerald PD, McNeil JJ. Clozapine-induced myocarditis, a widely overlooked adverse reaction. Acta Psychiatr Scand 2015;132:231–40.

Rosenheck RA, Davis S, Covell N, et al. Does switching to a new antipsychotic improve outcomes? Data from the CATIE Trial. Schizophr Res 2009;170(1):22–9.

Schulte P. What is an adequate trial with clozapine?: therapeutic drug monitoring and time to response in treatment-refractory schizophrenia. Clin Pharmacokinet 2003;42:607–18.

Tiihonen J, Lonnqvist J, Wahlbeck K, et al. 11-year follow-up of mortality in patients with schizophrenia: a population-based cohort study (FIN11 study). Lancet 2009; 374(9690):620–7.

THERAPEUTICS

Brands • Tercian

see index for additional brand names

Generic? Not in the USA

Class

- Conventional antipsychotic (neuroleptic, phenothiazine, dopamine 2 antagonist, serotonin dopamine antagonist)

Commonly Prescribed for

(bold for FDA approved)

- Schizophrenia
- ✻ Anxiety associated with psychosis (short-term)
- Anxiety associated with nonpsychotic disorders, including mood disorders and personality disorders (short-term)
- Severe depression
- Bipolar disorder
- Other psychotic disorders
- Acute agitation/aggression (injection)
- Benzodiazepine withdrawal

How the Drug Works

- Blocks dopamine 2 receptors, reducing positive symptoms of psychosis
- ✻ Although classified as a conventional antipsychotic, cyamemazine is a potent serotonin 2A antagonist
- Affinity at a myriad of other neurotransmitter receptors may contribute to cyamemazine's efficacy
- ✻ Specifically, antagonist actions at 5HT2C receptors may contribute to notable anxiolytic effects in many patients
- 5HT2C antagonist actions may also contribute to antidepressant actions in severe depression and to improvement of cognitive and negative symptoms of schizophrenia in some patients

How Long Until It Works

- Psychotic symptoms can improve with high doses within 1 week, but it may take several weeks for full effect on behavior
- Anxiolytic actions can improve with low doses within 1 week, but it may take several days to weeks for full effect on behavior

If It Works

- High doses most often reduce positive symptoms in schizophrenia but do not eliminate them
- Low doses most often reduce anxiety symptoms in psychotic and nonpsychotic disorders
- Most schizophrenia patients do not have a total remission of symptoms but rather a reduction of symptoms by about a third
- Continue treatment in schizophrenia until reaching a plateau of improvement
- After reaching a satisfactory plateau, continue treatment for at least a year, after first episode of psychosis in schizophrenia
- For second and subsequent episodes of psychosis in schizophrenia, treatment may need to be indefinite
- For symptomatic treatment of anxiety in psychotic and nonpsychotic disorders, treatment may also need to be indefinite while monitoring the risks versus the benefits of long-term treatment
- Reduces symptoms of acute psychotic mania but not proven as a mood stabilizer or as an effective maintenance treatment in bipolar disorder
- After reducing acute psychotic symptoms in mania, consider switching to a mood stabilizer and/or an atypical antipsychotic for long-term mood stabilization and maintenance

If It Doesn't Work

- For treatment of psychotic symptoms, consider trying one of the first-line atypical antipsychotics (risperidone, olanzapine, quetiapine, ziprasidone, aripiprazole, paliperidone, amisulpiride)
- Consider trying another conventional antipsychotic
- If 2 or more antipsychotic monotherapies do not work, consider clozapine
- For treatment of anxiety symptoms, consider adding a benzodiazepine or switching to a benzodiazepine

Best Augmenting Combos for Partial Response or Treatment Resistance

- Generally, best to switch to another agent
- Augmentation of conventional antipsychotics has not been systematically studied

- Addition of a mood-stabilizing anticonvulsant such as valproate, carbamazepine, or lamotrigine may be helpful in both schizophrenia and bipolar mania
- Augmentation with lithium in bipolar mania may be helpful
- Addition of a benzodiazepine, especially for short-term agitation
- Addition of antidepressants for severe depression

Tests

✻ Since conventional antipsychotics are frequently associated with weight gain, before starting treatment, weigh all patients and determine if the patient is already overweight (BMI 25.0–29.9) or obese BMI ≥30)

- Before giving a drug that can cause weight gain to an overweight or obese patient, consider determining whether the patient already has pre-diabetes (fasting glucose 100–125 mg/dL), diabetes (fasting plasma glucose >125 mg/dL), or dyslipidemia (increased total cholesterol, LDL cholesterol and triglycerides; decreased HDL cholesterol), and treat or refer such patients for treatment, including nutrition and weight management, physical activity counseling, smoking cessation, and medical management

✻ Monitor weight and BMI during treatment

✻ Consider monitoring fasting triglycerides monthly for several months in patients at high risk for metabolic complications and when initiating or switching antipsychotics

✻ While giving a drug to a patient who has gained >5% of initial weight, consider evaluating for the presence of pre-diabetes, diabetes, or dyslipidemia, or consider switching to a different antipsychotic

- Should check blood pressure in the elderly before starting and for the first few weeks of treatment
- Monitoring elevated prolactin levels of dubious clinical benefit
- Patients with low white blood cell count (WBC) or history of drug-induced leucopenia/neutropenia should have complete blood count (CBC) monitored frequently during the first few months and cyamemazine should be discontinued at the first sign of decline of WBC in the absence of other causative factors

SIDE EFFECTS

How Drug Causes Side Effects

- By blocking dopamine 2 receptors in the striatum, it can cause motor side effects at antipsychotic (high) doses
- Much lower propensity to cause motor side effects at low doses used to treat anxiety
- By blocking dopamine 2 receptors in the pituitary, it can cause elevations in prolactin, but unlike other conventional antipsychotics, prolactin elevations at low doses of cyamemazine are uncommon or transient
- By blocking dopamine 2 receptors excessively in the mesocortical and mesolimbic dopamine pathways, especially at high doses, it can cause worsening of negative and cognitive symptoms (neuroleptic-induced deficit syndrome)
- Anticholinergic actions, especially at high doses, may cause sedation, blurred vision, constipation, dry mouth
- Antihistamine actions may contribute to anxiolytic actions at low doses and to sedation and weight gain at high doses
- By blocking alpha 1 adrenergic receptors, cyamemazine can cause dizziness, sedation, and hypotension especially at high doses
- Mechanism of weight gain and any possible increased incidence of diabetes and dyslipidemia with conventional antipsychotics is unknown

Notable Side Effects

✻ Neuroleptic-induced deficit syndrome (unusual at low doses)

- Akathisia
- Extrapyramidal symptoms, parkinsonism, tardive dyskinesia (unusual at low doses)
- Galactorrhea, amenorrhea (unusual at low doses)
- Hypotension, tachycardia (unusual at low doses)
- Dry mouth, constipation, vision disturbance, urinary retention
- Sedation
- Decreased sweating
- Weight gain (may be unusual at low doses)
- Sexual dysfunction
- Metabolic effects, glucose tolerance

Life-Threatening or Dangerous Side Effects

- Rare neuroleptic malignant syndrome
- Rare seizures
- Rare jaundice, agranulocytosis
- Increased risk of death and cerebrovascular events in elderly patients with dementia-related psychosis

Weight Gain

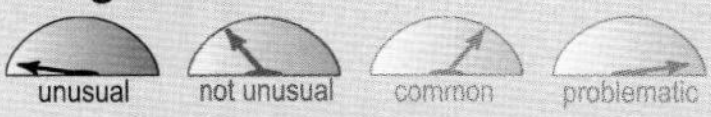

- Reported but not expected especially at low doses

Sedation

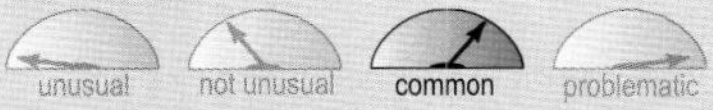

- Many experience and/or can be significant in amount, especially at high doses
- Sedation is usually dose-dependent and may not be experienced as sedation but as anxiolytic actions on anxiety and aggression at low doses where cyamemazine may function as an atypical antipsychotic (e.g., <300 mg/day; especially 25–100 mg/day)

What to Do About Side Effects

- Wait
- Wait
- Wait
- For motor symptoms, add an anticholinergic agent
- Reduce the dose
- For sedation, give at night
- Switch to an atypical antipsychotic
- Weight loss, exercise programs, and medical management for high BMIs, diabetes, dyslipidemia

Best Augmenting Agents for Side Effects

- Benztropine or trihexyphenidyl for motor side effects
- Benzodiazepines may be helpful for akathisia
- Many side effects cannot be improved with an augmenting agent

DOSING AND USE

Usual Dosage Range

- 50–300 mg at bedtime for treatment of psychosis
- 25–100 mg for anxiety; duration of treatment 4 weeks
- Children (ages 6 and older): 1–4 mg/kg per day
- Injection: 25–100 mg/day

Dosage Forms

- Tablet 25 mg, 100 mg
- Oral solution 40 mg/mL
- Injection 50 mg/5 mL

How to Dose

- Psychosis: usual maintenance dose 50–300 mg at bedtime; maximum dose 600 mg/day divided into 2 or 3 doses; after 2 weeks consider reducing to lowest effective dose
- Anxiety (adults): usual dose 25–100 mg/day; reduce dose if unacceptable sedation; maximum duration of treatment 4 weeks
- Anxiety (children): usual dose 1–4 mg/kg per day

Dosing Tips

- Has conventional antipsychotic properties at originally recommended high doses (300–600 mg/day)
- ✻ Binding studies, PET studies and clinical observations suggest that cyamemazine may be "atypical" with low motor side effects or prolactin elevations at low doses (below 300 mg/day)
- ✻ Clinical evidence suggests substantial anxiolytic benefits at 25–100 mg/day in many patients
- ✻ Clinical evidence suggests low EPS, little prolactin elevation yet demonstrable anxiolytic, anti-aggression and antidepressant actions at doses below 300 mg/day
- Robust antipsychotic actions on positive symptoms may require dosing above 300 mg/day
- Low doses up to 100 mg/day may be used to augment partial responders to other conventional or atypical antipsychotics, especially for anxiolytic actions
- Treatment should be suspended if absolute neutrophil count falls below 1,000/mm^3

Overdose
- Extrapyramidal symptoms, sedation, hypotension, coma, respiratory depression

Long-Term Use
- Some side effects may be irreversible (e.g., tardive dyskinesia)

Habit Forming
- No

How to Stop
- Slow down titration (over 6–8 weeks), especially when simultaneously beginning a new antipsychotic while switching (i.e., cross-titration)
- Rapid oral discontinuation of high doses of phenothiazines in psychotic patients may lead to rebound psychosis and worsening of symptoms
- If antiparkinsonian agents are being used, they should generally be continued for a few weeks after high-dose cyamemazine is discontinued

Pharmacokinetics
- Half-life 10 hours

Drug Interactions
- May decrease the effects of levodopa; contraindicated for use with dopamine agonists other than levodopa
- May increase the effects of antihypertensive drugs except for guanethidine, whose antihypertensive actions phenothiazines may antagonize
- May enhance QTc prolongation of other drugs capable of prolonging QTc interval
- Additive effects may occur if used with CNS depressants
- Anticholinergic effects may occur if used with atropine or related compounds
- Some patients taking a neuroleptic and lithium have developed an encephalopathic syndrome similar to neuroleptic malignant syndrome
- Epinephrine may lower blood pressure; diuretics and alcohol may increase risk of hypotension when administered with a phenothiazine

Other Warnings/ Precautions
- If signs of neuroleptic malignant syndrome develop, treatment should be immediately discontinued
- Use cautiously in patients with respiratory disorders
- Use cautiously in patients with alcohol withdrawal or convulsive disorders because phenothiazines can lower seizure threshold
- Do not use epinephrine in event of overdose as interaction with some pressor agents may lower blood pressure
- Avoid undue exposure to sunlight
- Avoid extreme heat exposure
- Use with caution in patients with respiratory disorders, glaucoma, or urinary retention
- Antiemetic effects of phenothiazines may mask signs of other disorders or overdose; suppression of cough reflex may cause asphyxia
- Observe for signs of ocular toxicity (corneal and lenticular deposits) as for other phenothiazines
- Use only with caution or at low doses, if at all, in Parkinson's disease or Lewy body dementia
- Because cyamemazine may dose-dependently prolong QTc interval, use with caution in patients who have bradycardia or who are taking drugs that can induce bradycardia (e.g., beta blockers, calcium channel blockers, clonidine, digitalis)
- Because cyamemazine may dose-dependently prolong QTc interval, use with caution in patients who have hyperkalemia and/or hypomagnesemia or who are taking drugs that can induce hypokalemia and/ or magnesemia (e.g., diuretics, stimulant laxatives, intravenous amphotericin B, glucocorticoids, tetracosaclides)
- Cyamemazine can increase the QTc interval, potentially causing torsades de pointes-type arrhythmia or sudden death

Do Not Use
- If there is a history of QTc prolongation or cardiac arrhythmia, recent acute myocardial infarction, uncompensated heart failure
- ✻ If QTc interval greater than 450 msec or if taking an agent capable of prolonging the QTc interval

- If patient is taking sultopride
- If patient is in a comatose state or has CNS depression
- If there is the presence of blood dyscrasias, bone marrow depression, or liver disease
- If there is subcortical brain damage
- If patient has sensitivity to or intolerance of gluten (tablets contain gluten)
- If patient has congenital galactosemy, does not adequately absorb glucose/galactose, or has lactase deficit (tablets contain lactose)
- If patient is intolerant of fructose, does not adequately absorb glucose/galactose, or has sugar-isomaltase deficit (oral solution only; oral solution contains saccharose)
- If there is a proven allergy to cyamemazine
- If there is a known sensitivity to any phenothiazine

SPECIAL POPULATIONS

Renal Impairment
- Use with caution

Hepatic Impairment
- Use with caution

Cardiac Impairment
- Cardiovacular toxicity can occur, especially orthostatic hypotension

Elderly
- Elderly patients may be more susceptible to adverse effects
- Lower doses should be used and patient should be monitored closely
- Generally, doses above 100 mg/day are not recommended
- Elderly patients with dementia-related psychosis treated with antipsychotics are at an increased risk of death compared to placebo, and also have an increased risk of cerebrovascular events

Children and Adolescents
- Sometimes used for severe behavioral disturbances in children ages 6 and older
- Oral solution is preferable to the other formulations

Pregnancy
- There is a risk of abnormal muscle movements and withdrawal symptoms in newborns whose mothers took an antipsychotic during the third trimester; symptoms may include agitation, abnormally increased or decreased muscle tone, tremor, sleepiness, severe difficulty breathing, and difficulty feeding
- Reports of extrapyramidal symptoms, jaundice, hyperreflexia, hyporeflexia in infants whose mothers took a phenothiazine during pregnancy
- Phenothiazines should only be used during pregnancy if clearly needed
- Psychotic symptoms may worsen during pregnancy and some form of treatment may be necessary
- Atypical antipsychotics may be preferable to phenothiazines or anticonvulsant mood stabilizers if treatment is required during pregnancy

Breast Feeding
- Unknown if cyamemazine is secreted in human breast milk, but all psychotropics assumed to be secreted in breast milk

✻ Recommended either to discontinue drug or bottle feed

THE ART OF PSYCHOPHARMACOLOGY

Potential Advantages
- For anxiety in patients with psychotic illnesses
- For anxiety in patients with nonpsychotic illnesses
- For severe depression

Potential Disadvantages
- Patients with tardive dyskinesia
- Children
- Elderly

Primary Target Symptoms
- Anxiety associated with psychosis
- Anxiety

- Aggression
- Agitation
- Positive symptoms of psychosis
- Severe depression

Pearls

- One of the most frequently prescribed antipsychotics in France, especially as a low-dose anxiolytic for psychotic patients
- * Appears to have unique anxiolytic actions at low doses without rebound anxiety following discontinuation
- * Low doses rarely associated with motor side effects or with prolactin elevation
- * Recently discovered to be a serotonin dopamine antagonist with more potent binding of 5HT2A and 5HT2C receptors than D2 receptors (binding studies and PET scans)
- Low doses appear to saturate 5HT2A receptors in frontal cortex while not saturating D2 receptors in the striatum, accounting for apparent atypical antipsychotic and anxiolytic properties at low doses
- May be useful second-line therapy in facilitating benzodiazepine withdrawal for those patients in whom substitution with another benzodiazepine is not effective or is not appropriate

Suggested Reading

Lemoine P, Kermadi I, Garcia-Acosta S, Garay RP, Dib M. Double-blind, comparative study of cyamemazine vs. bromazepam in the benzodiazepine withdrawal syndrome. Prog Neuropsychopharmacol Biol Psychiatry 2006;30(1):131–7.

Hameg A, Bayle F, Nuss P, Dupuis P, et al. Affinity of cyamemazine, an anxiolytic antipsychotic drug, for human recombinant dopamine vs. serotonin receptor subtypes. Biochem Pharmacol 2003;65(3):435–40.

Hode Y, Reimold M, Demazieres A, et al. A positron emission tomography (PET) study of cerebral dopamine D2 and serotonine 5-HT2A receptor occupancy in patients treated with cyamemazine (Tercian). Psychopharmacology (Berl) 2005;180(2):377–84.

THERAPEUTICS

Brands • Norpramin
see index for additional brand names

Generic? Yes

Class
- Neuroscience-based Nomenclature: norepinephrine reuptake inhibitor (N-RI)
- Tricyclic antidepressant (TCA)
- Predominantly a norepinephrine/noradrenaline reuptake inhibitor

Commonly Prescribed for
(bold for FDA approved)
- **Depression**
- Anxiety
- Insomnia
- Neuropathic pain/chronic pain
- Treatment-resistant depression

How the Drug Works
- Boosts neurotransmitter norepinephrine/noradrenaline
- Blocks norepinephrine reuptake pump (norepinephrine transporter), presumably increasing noradrenergic neurotransmission
- Since dopamine is inactivated by norepinephrine reuptake in frontal cortex, which largely lacks dopamine transporters, desipramine can thus increase dopamine neurotransmission in this part of the brain
- A more potent inhibitor of norepinephrine reuptake pump than serotonin reuptake pump (serotonin transporter)
- At high doses may also boost neurotransmitter serotonin and presumably increase serotonergic neurotransmission

How Long Until It Works
- May have immediate effects in treating insomnia or anxiety
- Onset of therapeutic actions usually not immediate, but often delayed 2–4 weeks
- If it is not working within 6–8 weeks for depression, it may require a dosage increase or it may not work at all
- May continue to work for many years to prevent relapse of symptoms

If It Works
- The goal of treatment of depression is complete remission of current symptoms as well as prevention of future relapses
- The goal of treatment of chronic neuropathic pain is to reduce symptoms as much as possible, especially in combination with other treatments
- Treatment of depression most often reduces or even eliminates symptoms, but not a cure since symptoms can recur after medicine stopped
- Treatment of chronic neuropathic pain may reduce symptoms, but rarely eliminates them completely, and is not a cure since symptoms can recur after medicine is stopped
- Continue treatment of depression until all symptoms are gone (remission)
- Once symptoms of depression are gone, continue treating for 1 year for the first episode of depression
- For second and subsequent episodes of depression, treatment may need to be indefinite
- Use in anxiety disorders and chronic pain may also need to be indefinite, but long-term treatment is not well studied in these conditions

If It Doesn't Work
- Many depressed patients have only a partial response where some symptoms are improved but others persist (especially insomnia, fatigue, and problems concentrating)
- Other depressed patients may be nonresponders, sometimes called treatment-resistant or treatment-refractory
- Consider increasing dose, switching to another agent, or adding an appropriate augmenting agent
- Consider psychotherapy
- Consider evaluation for another diagnosis or for a comorbid condition (e.g., medical illness, substance abuse, etc.)
- Some patients may experience apparent lack of consistent efficacy due to activation of latent or underlying bipolar disorder, and require antidepressant discontinuation and a switch to a mood stabilizer

Best Augmenting Combos for Partial Response or Treatment Resistance

- Lithium, buspirone, thyroid hormone (for depression)
- Gabapentin, tiagabine, other anticonvulsants, even opiates if done by experts while monitoring carefully in difficult cases (for chronic pain)

Tests

- Baseline ECG is recommended for patients over age 50
- ✻ Monitoring of plasma drug levels is available
- ✻ Since tricyclic and tetracyclic antidepressants are frequently associated with weight gain, before starting treatment, weigh all patients and determine if the patient is already overweight (BMI 25.0–29.9) or obese (BMI ≥30)
- Before giving a drug that can cause weight gain to an overweight or obese patient, consider determining whether the patient already has pre-diabetes (fasting plasma glucose 100–125 mg/dL), diabetes (fasting plasma glucose >126 mg/dL), or dyslipidemia (increased total cholesterol, LDL cholesterol, and triglycerides; decreased HDL cholesterol), and treat or refer such patients for treatment, including nutrition and weight management, physical activity counseling, smoking cessation, and medical management
- ✻ Monitor weight and BMI during treatment
- ✻ While giving a drug to a patient who has gained >5% of initial weight, consider evaluating for the presence of pre-diabetes, diabetes, or dyslipidemia, or consider switching to a different antidepressant
- EKGs may be useful for selected patients (e.g., those with personal or family history of QTc prolongation; cardiac arrhythmia; recent myocardial infarction; uncompensated heart failure; or taking agents that prolong QTc interval such as pimozide, thioridazine, selected antiarrhythmics, moxifloxacin, sparfloxacin, etc.)
- Patients at risk for electrolyte disturbances (e.g., patients on diuretic therapy) should have baseline and periodic serum potassium and magnesium measurements

SIDE EFFECTS

How Drug Causes Side Effects

- ✻ Anticholinergic activity for desipramine may be somewhat less than for some other TCAs, yet can still explain the presence, if lower incidence, of sedative effects, dry mouth, constipation, and blurred vision
- Sedative effects and weight gain may be due to antihistamine properties
- Blockade of alpha adrenergic 1 receptors may explain dizziness, sedation, and hypotension
- Cardiac arrhythmias and seizures, especially in overdose, may be caused by blockade of ion channels

Notable Side Effects

- Blurred vision, constipation, urinary retention, increased appetite, dry mouth, nausea, diarrhea, heartburn, unusual taste in mouth, weight gain
- Fatigue, weakness, dizziness, sedation, headache, anxiety, nervousness, restlessness
- Sexual dysfunction, sweating

Life-Threatening or Dangerous Side Effects

- Paralytic ileus, hyperthermia (TCAs + anticholinergic agents)
- Lowered seizure threshold and rare seizures
- Orthostatic hypotension, sudden death, arrhythmias, tachycardia
- QTc prolongation
- Hepatic failure, extrapyramidal symptoms
- Increased intraocular pressure
- Blood dyscrasias
- Rare induction of mania
- Rare activation of suicidal ideation and behavior (suicidality) (short-term studies did not show an increase in the risk of suicidality with antidepressants compared to placebo beyond age 24)

Weight Gain

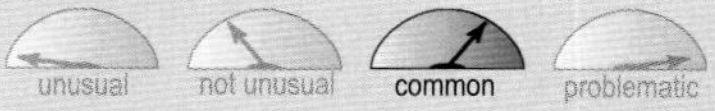

- Many experience and/or can be significant in amount
- Can increase appetite and carbohydrate craving

Sedation

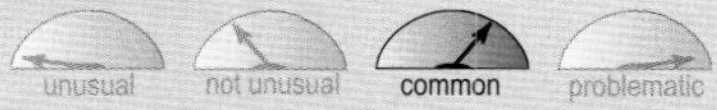

- Many experience and/or can be significant in amount
- Tolerance to sedative effects may develop with long-term use

What to Do About Side Effects

- Wait
- Wait
- Wait
- Lower the dose
- Switch to an SSRI or newer antidepressant

Best Augmenting Agents for Side Effects

- Many side effects cannot be improved with an augmenting agent

DOSING AND USE

Usual Dosage Range

- 100–200 mg/day (for depression)
- 50–150 mg/day (for chronic pain)

Dosage Forms

- Tablets 10 mg, 25 mg, 50 mg, 75 mg, 100 mg, 150 mg

How to Dose

- Initial 25 mg/day at bedtime; increase by 25 mg every 3–7 days
- 75 mg/day once daily or in divided doses; gradually increase dose to achieve desired therapeutic effect; maximum dose 300 mg/day

Dosing Tips

- If given in a single dose, should generally be administered at bedtime because of its sedative properties
- If given in split doses, largest dose should generally be given at bedtime because of its sedative properties
- If patients experience nightmares, split dose and do not give large dose at bedtime
- Patients treated for chronic pain may only require lower doses (e.g., 50–75 mg/day)
- Risk of seizure increases with dose

✻ Monitoring plasma levels of desipramine is recommended in patients who do not respond to the usual dose or whose treatment is regarded as urgent

- If intolerable anxiety, insomnia, agitation, akathisia, or activation occur either upon dosing initiation or discontinuation, consider the possibility of activated bipolar disorder, and switch to a mood stabilizer or an atypical antipsychotic

Overdose

- Death may occur, and may be more likely than with other TCAs; convulsions, cardiac dysrhythmias, severe hypotension, CNS depression, coma, changes in EKG

Long-Term Use

- Safe

Habit Forming

- No

How to Stop

- Taper to avoid withdrawal effects
- Even with gradual dose reduction some withdrawal symptoms may appear within the first 2 weeks
- Many patients tolerate 50% dose reduction for 3 days, then another 50% reduction for 3 days, then discontinuation
- If withdrawal symptoms emerge during discontinuation, raise dose to stop symptoms and then restart withdrawal much more slowly

Pharmacokinetics

- Substrate for CYP450 2D6 and 1A2
- Is the active metabolite of imipramine, formed by demethylation via CYP450 1A2
- Half-life approximately 24 hours
- Food does not affect absorption

Drug Interactions

- Tramadol increases the risk of seizures in patients taking TCAs
- Use of TCAs with anticholinergic drugs may result in paralytic ileus or hyperthermia
- Fluoxetine, paroxetine, bupropion, duloxetine, and other CYP450 2D6 inhibitors may increase TCA concentrations
- Cimetidine may increase plasma concentrations of TCAs and cause anticholinergic symptoms
- Phenothiazines or haloperidol may raise TCA blood concentrations

- May alter effects of antihypertensive drugs; may inhibit hypotensive effects of clonidine
- Use of TCAs with sympathomimetic agents may increase sympathetic activity
- Methylphenidate may inhibit metabolism of TCAs
- Activation and agitation, especially following switching or adding antidepressants, may represent the induction of a bipolar state, especially a mixed dysphoric bipolar II condition sometimes associated with suicidal ideation, and require the addition of lithium, a mood stabilizer or an atypical antipsychotic, and/or discontinuation of desipramine

Other Warnings/ Precautions

- Add or initiate other antidepressants with caution for up to 2 weeks after discontinuing desipramine
- Generally, do not use with MAOIs, including 14 days after MAOIs are stopped; do not start an MAOI for at least 5 half-lives (5 to 7 days for most drugs) after discontinuing desipramine, but see Pearls
- Use with caution in patients with history of seizures, urinary retention, angle-closure glaucoma, hyperthyroidism
- Use caution when prescibing in patients with a family history of sudden death, cardiac dysrhythmias, and cardiac conduction disturbances
- Some patients may have seizures before cardiac dysrhythmias and death
- TCAs can increase QTc interval, especially at toxic doses, which can be attained not only by overdose but also by combining with drugs that inhibit TCA metabolism via CYP450 2D6, potentially causing torsade de pointes-type arrhythmia or sudden death
- Because TCAs can prolong QTc interval, use with caution in patients who have bradycardia or who are taking drugs that can induce bradycardia (e.g., beta blockers, calcium channel blockers, clonidine, digitalis)
- Because TCAs can prolong QTc interval, use with caution in patients who have hypokalemia and/or hypomagnesemia or who are taking drugs that can induce hypokalemia and/or magnesemia (e.g., diuretics, stimulant laxatives, intravenous amphotericin B, glucocorticoids, tetracosactide)
- When treating children, carefully weigh the risks and benefits of pharmacological treatment against the risks and benefits of nontreatment with antidepressants and make sure to document this in the patient's chart
- Distribute the brochures provided by the FDA and the drug companies
- Warn patients and their caregivers about the possibility of activating side effects and advise them to report such symptoms immediately
- Monitor patients for activation of suicidal ideation, especially children and adolescents

Do Not Use

- If patient is recovering from myocardial infarction
- If patient is taking agents capable of significantly prolonging QTc interval (e.g., pimozide, thioridazine, selected antiarrhythmics, moxifloxacin, sparfloxacin)
- If there is a history of QTc prolongation or cardiac arrhythmia, recent acute myocardial infarction, uncompensated heart failure
- If patient is taking drugs that inhibit TCA metabolism, including CYP450 2D6 inhibitors, except by an expert
- If there is reduced CYP450 2D6 function, such as patients who are poor 2D6 metabolizers, except by an expert and at low doses
- If there is a proven allergy to desipramine, imipramine, or lofepramine

SPECIAL POPULATIONS

Renal Impairment

- Use with caution; may need to lower dose
- May need to monitor plasma levels

Hepatic Impairment

- Use with caution; may need to lower dose
- May need to monitor plasma levels

Cardiac Impairment

- Baseline ECG is recommended
- TCAs have been reported to cause arrhythmias, prolongation of conduction

time, orthostatic hypotension, sinus tachycardia, and heart failure, especially in the diseased heart
- Myocardial infarction and stroke have been reported with TCAs
- TCAs produce QTc prolongation, which may be enhanced by the existence of bradycardia, hypokalemia, congenital or acquired long QTc interval, which should be evaluated prior to administering desipramine
- Use with caution if treating concomitantly with a medication likely to produce prolonged bradycardia, hypokalemia, slowing of intracardiac conduction, or prolongation of the QTc interval
- Avoid TCAs in patients with a known history of QTc prolongation, recent acute myocardial infarction, and uncompensated heart failure
- TCAs may cause a sustained increase in heart rate in patients with ischemic heart disease and may worsen (decrease) heart rate variability, an independent risk of mortality in cardiac populations
- Since SSRIs may improve (increase) heart rate variability in patients following a myocardial infarct and may improve survival as well as mood in patients with acute angina or following a myocardial infarction, these are more appropriate agents for cardiac population than tricyclic/tetracyclic antidepressants

✻ Risk/benefit ratio may not justify use of TCAs in cardiac impairment

Elderly

- Baseline ECG is recommended for patients over age 50
- May be more sensitive to anticholinergic, cardiovascular, hypotensive, and sedative effects
- Initial dose 25–50 mg/day, raise to 100 mg/day; maximum 150 mg/day
- May be useful to monitor plasma levels in elderly patients
- Reduction in the risk of suicidality with antidepressants compared to placebo in adults age 65 and older

Children and Adolescents

- Carefully weigh the risks and benefits of pharmacological treatment against the risks and benefits of nontreatment with antidepressants and make sure to document this in the patient's chart
- Monitor patients face-to-face regularly, particularly during the first several weeks of treatment
- Use with caution, observing for activation of known or unknown bipolar disorder and/or suicidal ideation, and inform parents or guardians of this risk so they can help observe child or adolescent patients
- Not recommended for use in children under age 12
- Several studies show lack of efficacy of TCAs for depression
- May be used to treat enuresis or hyperactive/impulsive behaviors
- May reduce tic symptoms
- Some cases of sudden death have occurred in children taking TCAs
- Adolescents: initial dose 25–50 mg/day, increase to 100 mg/day; maximum dose 150 mg/day
- May be useful to monitor plasma levels in children and adolescents

Pregnancy

- Effective June 30, 2015, the US FDA requires changes to the content and format of pregnancy and lactation information in prescription drug labels, including the elimination of the pregnancy letter categories; the Pregnancy and Lactation Labeling Rule (PLLR or final rule) applies only to prescription drugs and will be phased in gradually for drugs approved on or after June 30, 2001
- Controlled studies have not been conducted in pregnant women
- Crosses the placenta
- Adverse effects have been reported in infants whose mothers took a TCA (lethargy, withdrawal symptoms, fetal malformations)
- Must weigh the risk of treatment (first trimester fetal development, third trimester newborn delivery) to the child against the risk of no treatment (recurrence of depression, maternal health, infant bonding) to the mother and child
- For many patients this may mean continuing treatment during pregnancy

Breast Feeding

- Some drug is found in mother's breast milk
- ✻ Recommended either to discontinue drug or bottle feed
- Immediate postpartum period is a high-risk time for depression, especially in women who have had prior depressive episodes, so drug may need to be reinstituted late in the third trimester or shortly after childbirth to prevent a recurrence during the postpartum period
- Must weigh benefits of breast feeding with risks and benefits of antidepressant treatment versus nontreatment to both the infant and the mother
- For many patients this may mean continuing treatment during breast feeding

THE ART OF PSYCHOPHARMACOLOGY

Potential Advantages

- Patients with insomnia
- Severe or treatment-resistant depression
- Patients for whom therapeutic drug monitoring is desirable

Potential Disadvantages

- Pediatric and geriatric patients
- Patients concerned with weight gain
- Cardiac patients

Primary Target Symptoms

- Depressed mood
- Chronic pain

Pearls

- TCAs are often a first-line treatment option for chronic pain
- TCAs are no longer generally considered a first-line option for depression because of their side effect profile
- TCAs continue to be useful for severe or treatment-resistant depression
- Noradrenergic reuptake inhibitors such as desipramine can be used as a second-line treatment for smoking cessation, cocaine dependence, and attention deficit disorder
- TCAs may aggravate psychotic symptoms
- Alcohol should be avoided because of additive CNS effects
- Underweight patients may be more susceptible to adverse cardiovascular effects
- Children, patients with inadequate hydration, and patients with cardiac disease may be more susceptible to TCA-induced cardiotoxicity than healthy adults
- For the expert only: although generally prohibited, a heroic but potentially dangerous treatment for severely treatment-resistant patients is to give a tricyclic/tetracyclic antidepressant other than clomipramine simultaneously with an MAOI for patients who fail to respond to numerous other antidepressants
- If this option is elected, start the MAOI with the tricyclic/tetracyclic antidepressant simultaneously at low doses after appropriate drug washout, then alternately increase doses of these agents every few days to a week as tolerated
- Although very strict dietary and concomitant drug restrictions must be observed to prevent hypertensive crises and serotonin syndrome, the most common side effects of MAOI/tricyclic or tetracyclic combinations may be weight gain and orthostatic hypotension
- Patients on TCAs should be aware that they may experience symptoms such as photosensitivity or blue-green urine
- SSRIs may be more effective than TCAs in women, and TCAs may be more effective than SSRIs in men
- Not recommended for first-line use in children with ADHD because of the availability of safer treatments with better documented efficacy and because of desipramine's potential for sudden death in children
- ✻ Desipramine is one of the few TCAs where monitoring of plasma drug levels has been well studied
- ✻ Fewer anticholinergic side effects than some other TCAs
- Since tricyclic/tetracyclic antidepressants are substrates for CYP450 2D6, and 7% of the population (especially Caucasians) may have a genetic variant leading to reduced activity of 2D6, such patients may not safely tolerate normal doses of tricyclic/tetracyclic antidepressants and may require dose reduction

- Phenotypic testing may be necessary to detect this genetic variant prior to dosing with a tricyclic/tetracyclic antidepressant, especially in vulnerable populations such as children, elderly, cardiac populations, and those on concomitant medications
- Patients who seem to have extraordinarily severe side effects at normal or low doses may have this phenotypic CYP450 2D6 variant and require low doses or switching to another antidepressant not metabolized by 2D6

Suggested Reading

Anderson IM. Meta-analytical studies on new antidepressants. Br Med Bull 2001;57:161–78.

Anderson IM. Selective serotonin reuptake inhibitors versus tricyclic antidepressants: a meta-analysis of efficacy and tolerability. J Aff Disorders 2000;58:19–36.

Janowsky DS, Byerley B. Desipramine: an overview. J Clin Psychiatry 1984;45:3–9.

Levin FR, Lehman AF. Meta-analysis of desipramine as an adjunct in the treatment of cocaine addiction. J Clin Psychopharmacol 1991;11:374–8.

THERAPEUTICS

Brands • Pristiq

see index for additional brand names

Generic? No

Class

- Neuroscience-based Nomenclature: serotonin norepinephrine reuptake inhibitor (SN-RI)
- SNRI (dual serotonin and norepinephrine reuptake inhibitor); often classified as an antidepressant, but it is not just an antidepressant

Commonly Prescribed for

(bold for FDA approved)

- **Major depressive disorder**
- Vasomotor symptoms
- Fibromyalgia
- Generalized anxiety disorder (GAD)
- Social anxiety disorder (social phobia)
- Panic disorder
- Posttraumatic stress disorder (PTSD)
- Premenstrual dysphoric disorder (PMDD)

How the Drug Works

- Boosts neurotransmitters serotonin, norepinephrine/noradrenaline, and dopamine
- Blocks serotonin reuptake pump (serotonin transporter), presumably increasing serotonergic neurotransmission
- Blocks norepinephrine reuptake pump (norepinephrine transporter), presumably increasing noradrenergic neurotransmission
- Desensitizes both serotonin 1A receptors and beta adrenergic receptors
- Since dopamine is inactivated by norepinephrine reuptake in frontal cortex, which largely lacks dopamine transporters, desvenlafaxine can increase dopamine neurotransmission in this part of the brain

How Long Until It Works

- Onset of therapeutic actions usually not immediate, but often delayed 2–4 weeks
- If it is not working within 6 or 8 weeks for depression, it may require a dosage increase or it may not work at all
- May continue to work for many years to prevent relapse of depressive symptoms
- Vasomotor symptoms in perimenopausal women with or without depression may improve within 1 week

If It Works

- The goal of treatment is complete remission of current symptoms as well as prevention of future relapses
- Treatment most often reduces or even eliminates symptoms, but not a cure since symptoms can recur after medicine stopped
- Continue treatment until all symptoms are gone (remission) or significantly reduced
- Once symptoms are gone, continue treating for 1 year for the first episode of depression
- For second and subsequent episodes of depression, treatment may need to be indefinite

If It Doesn't Work

- Many patients have only a partial response where some symptoms are improved but others persist (especially insomnia, fatigue, and problems concentrating)
- Other patients may be nonresponders, sometimes called treatment-resistant or treatment-refractory
- Some patients who have an initial response may relapse even though they continue treatment, sometimes called "poop-out"
- Consider increasing dose, switching to another agent, or adding an appropriate augmenting agent
- Consider psychotherapy
- Consider evaluation for another diagnosis or for a comorbid condition (e.g., medical illness, substance abuse, etc.)
- Some patients may experience apparent lack of consistent efficacy due to activation of latent or underlying bipolar disorder, and require antidepressant discontinuation and switch to a mood stabilizer

Best Augmenting Combos for Partial Response or Treatment Resistance

- Mirtazapine ("California rocket fuel"; a potentially powerful dual serotonin and norepinephrine combination, but observe for activation of bipolar disorder and suicidal ideation)
- Bupropion, reboxetine, nortriptyline, desipramine, maprotiline, atomoxetine (all potentially powerful enhancers of noradrenergic action, but observe for activation of bipolar disorder and suicidal ideation)

- Modafinil, especially for fatigue, sleepiness, and lack of concentration
- Mood stabilizers or atypical antipsychotics for bipolar depression, psychotic depression, or treatment-resistant depression
- Benzodiazepines
- If all else fails for anxiety disorders, consider gabapentin or tiagabine
- Hypnotics or trazodone for insomnia
- Classically, lithium, buspirone, or thyroid hormone

Tests

- Check blood pressure before initiating treatment and regularly during treatment

SIDE EFFECTS

How Drug Causes Side Effects

- Theoretically due to increases in serotonin and norepinephrine concentrations at receptors in parts of the brain and body other than those that cause therapeutic actions (e.g., unwanted actions of serotonin in sleep centers causing insomnia, unwanted actions of norepinephrine on acetylcholine release causing constipation and dry mouth, etc.)
- Most side effects are immediate but often go away with time

Notable Side Effects

- Most side effects increase with higher doses, at least transiently
- Insomnia, sedation, anxiety, dizziness
- Nausea, vomiting, constipation, decreased appetite
- Sexual dysfunction (abnormal ejaculation/orgasm, impotence)
- Sweating
- SIADH (syndrome of inappropriate antidiuretic hormone secretion)
- Hyponatremia
- Increase in blood pressure

Life-Threatening or Dangerous Side Effects

- Rare seizures
- Rare induction of hypomania
- Rare activation of suicidal ideation and behavior (suicidality) (short-term studies did not show an increase in the risk of suicidality with antidepressants compared to placebo beyond age 24)

Weight Gain

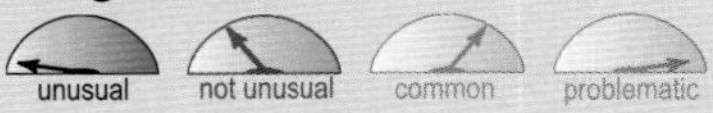

- Reported but not expected

Sedation

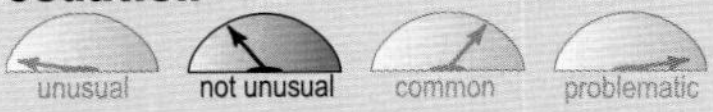

- Occurs in significant minority
- May also be activating in some patients

What to Do About Side Effects

- Wait
- Wait
- Wait
- Lower the dose
- In a few weeks, switch or add other drugs

Best Augmenting Agents for Side Effects

- Often best to try another antidepressant monotherapy prior to resorting to augmentation strategies to treat side effects
- Trazodone or a hypnotic for insomnia
- Bupropion, sildenafil, vardenafil, or tadalafil for sexual dysfunction
- Benzodiazepines for jitteriness and anxiety, especially at initiation of treatment and especially for anxious patients
- Mirtazapine for insomnia, agitation, and gastrointestinal side effects
- Many side effects are dose-dependent (i.e., they increase as dose increases, or they reemerge until tolerance redevelops)
- Many side effects are time-dependent (i.e., they start immediately upon dosing and upon each dose increase, but go away with time)
- Activation and agitation may represent the induction of a bipolar state, especially a mixed dysphoric bipolar II condition sometimes associated with suicidal ideation, and require the addition of lithium, a mood stabilizer or an atypical antipsychotic, and/or discontinuation of desvenlafaxine

DOSING AND USE

Usual Dosage Range

- Depression: 50 mg once daily

Dosage Forms

- Tablet (extended-release) 50 mg, 100 mg

How to Dose

- Initial dose 50 mg once daily; maximum recommended dose generally 100 mg once daily; doses up to 400 mg once daily have been shown to be effective but higher doses are associated with increased side effects

Dosing Tips

- Desvenlafaxine is the active metabolite O-desmethylvenlafaxine (ODV) of venlafaxine, and is formed as the result of CYP450 2D6
- More potent at the serotonin transporter (SERT) than at the norepinephrine transporter (NET), but has greater inhibition of NET relative to SERT compared to venlafaxine
- Nonresponders at lower doses may try higher doses to be assured of the benefits of dual SNRI action
- For vasomotor symptoms, current data suggest that a dose of 100 mg/day is effective
- Do not break or chew tablets, as this will alter controlled-release properties
- For some patients with severe problems discontinuing desvenlafaxine, it may be useful to add an SSRI with a long half-life, especially fluoxetine, prior to taper of desvenlafaxine. While maintaining fluoxetine dosing, first slowly taper desvenlafaxine and then taper fluoxetine
- Be sure to differentiate between reemergence of symptoms requiring reinstitution of treatment and withdrawal symptoms
- May dose up to 400 mg/day in patients who do not respond to lower doses, if tolerated

Overdose

- No fatalities have been reported as monotherapy; headache, vomiting, agitation, dizziness, nausea, constipation, diarrhea, dry mouth, paresthesia, tachycardia
- Desvenlafaxine is the active metabolite of venlafaxine; fatal toxicity index data from the UK suggest a higher rate of deaths from overdose with venlafaxine than with SSRIs; it is unknown whether this is related to differences in patients who receive venlafaxine or to potential cardiovascular toxicity of venlafaxine

Long-Term Use

- See doctor regularly to monitor blood pressure

Habit Forming

- No

How to Stop

- Taper to avoid withdrawal effects (dizziness, nausea, diarrhea, sweating, anxiety, irritability)
- Recommended taper schedule is to give a fully daily dose (50 mg) less frequently
- If withdrawal symptoms emerge during discontinuation, raise dose to stop symptoms and then restart withdrawal much more slowly

Pharmacokinetics

- Active metabolite of venlafaxine
- Half-life 9–13 hours
- Minimally metabolized by CYP450 3A4
- Food does not affect absorption

Drug Interactions

- Tramadol increases the risk of seizures in patients taking an antidepressant
- Can cause a fatal "serotonin syndrome" when combined with MAOIs, so do not use with MAOIs or for at least 14 days after MAOIs are stopped
- Do not start an MAOI for at least 5 half-lives (5 to 7 days for most drugs) after discontinuing desvenlafaxine
- Can rarely cause weakness, hyperreflexia, and incoordination when combined with sumatriptan or possibly other triptans, requiring careful monitoring of patient
- Possible increased risk of bleeding, especially when combined with anticoagulants (e.g., warfarin, NSAIDs)
- NSAIDs may impair effectiveness of SSRIs
- Potent inhibitors of CYP450 3A4 may increase plasma levels of desvenlafaxine, but the clinical significance of this is unknown

- Few known adverse drug interactions
- False-positive urine immunoassay screening tests for phencyclidine (PCP) and amphetamine have been reported in patients taking desvenlafaxine, due to a lack of specificity of the screening tests. False-positive test results may be expected for several days following discontinuation of desvenlafaxine

Other Warnings/ Precautions

- Use with caution in patients with history of seizure
- Use with caution in patients with heart disease
- Use with caution in patients with bipolar disorder unless treated with concomitant mood-stabilizing agent
- When treating children, carefully weigh the risks and benefits of pharmacological treatment against the risks and benefits of nontreatment with antidepressants and make sure to document this in the patient's chart
- Distribute the brochures provided by the FDA and the drug companies
- Warn patients and their caregivers about the possibility of activating side effects and advise them to report such symptoms immediately
- Monitor patients for activation of suicidal ideation, especially children and adolescents

Do Not Use

- If patient has uncontrolled angle-closure glaucoma
- If patient is taking an MAOI
- If there is a proven allergy to desvenlafaxine or venlafaxine

SPECIAL POPULATIONS

Renal Impairment

- For moderate impairment, recommended dose is 50 mg/day
- For severe impairment, recommended dose is 50 mg every other day
- Patients on dialysis should not receive subsequent dose until dialysis is completed

Hepatic Impairment

- Doses greater than 100 mg/day not recommended

Cardiac Impairment

- Drug should be used with caution
- Hypertension should be controlled prior to initiation of desvenlafaxine and should be monitored regularly during treatment
- Desvenlafaxine has a dose-dependent effect on increasing blood pressure
- Desvenlafaxine is the active metabolite of venlafaxine, which is contraindicated in patients with heart disease in the UK
- Venlafaxine can block cardiac ion channels in vitro and worsens (i.e., reduces) heart rate variability in depression, perhaps due to norepinephrine reuptake inhibition

Elderly

- Some patients may tolerate lower doses better
- Risk of SIADH with SSRIs is higher in the elderly
- Reduction in the risk of suicidality with antidepressants compared to placebo in adults age 65 and older

Children and Adolescents

- Carefully weigh the risks and benefits of pharmacological treatment against the risks and benefits of nontreatment with antidepressants and make sure to document this in the patient's chart
- Monitor patients face-to-face regularly, particularly during the first several weeks of treatment
- Use with caution, observing for activation of known or unknown bipolar disorder and/ or suicidal ideation, and inform parents or guardians of this risk so they can help observe child or adolescent patients

Pregnancy

- Effective June 30, 2015, the US FDA requires changes to the content and format of pregnancy and lactation information in prescription drug labels, including the elimination of the pregnancy letter categories; the Pregnancy and Lactation

Labeling Rule (PLLR or final rule) applies only to prescription drugs and will be phased in gradually for drugs approved on or after June 30, 2001
- Controlled studies have not been conducted in pregnant women
- Not generally recommended for use during pregnancy, especially during first trimester
- Nonetheless, continuous treatment during pregnancy may be necessary and has not been proven to be harmful to the fetus
- Must weigh the risk of treatment (first trimester fetal development, third trimester newborn delivery) to the child against the risk of no treatment (recurrence of depression, maternal health, infant bonding) to the mother and child
- For many patients this may mean continuing treatment during pregnancy
- Exposure to SSRIs late in pregnancy may be associated with increased risk of gestational hypertension and preeclampsia
- Neonates exposed to SSRIs or SNRIs late in the third trimester have developed complications requiring prolonged hospitalization, respiratory support, and tube feeding; reported symptoms are consistent with either a direct toxic effect of SSRIs and SNRIs or, possibly, a drug discontinuation syndrome, and include respiratory distress, cyanosis, apnea, seizures, temperature instability, feeding difficulty, vomiting, hypoglycemia, hypotonia, hypertonia, hyperreflexia, tremor, jitteriness, irritability, and constant crying

Breast Feeding

- Some drug is found in mother's breast milk
- Trace amounts may be present in nursing children whose mothers are on desvenlafaxine
- If child becomes irritable or sedated, breast feeding or drug may need to be discontinued
- Immediate postpartum period is a high-risk time for depression, especially in women who have had prior depressive episodes, so drug may need to be reinstituted late in the third trimester or shortly after childbirth to prevent a recurrence during the postpartum period
- Must weigh benefits of breast feeding with risks and benefits of antidepressant treatment versus nontreatment to both the infant and the mother
- For many patients, this may mean continuing treatment during breast feeding

THE ART OF PSYCHOPHARMACOLOGY

Potential Advantages

- Patients with retarded depression
- Patients with atypical depression
- Patients with depression may have higher remission rates on SNRIs than on SSRIs
- Depressed patients with somatic symptoms, fatigue, and pain
- Depressed patients with vasomotor symptoms
- Patients who do not respond or remit on treatment with SSRIs

Potential Disadvantages

- Patients sensitive to nausea
- Patients with borderline or uncontrolled hypertension
- Patients with cardiac disease

Primary Target Symptoms

- Depressed mood
- Energy, motivation, and interest
- Sleep disturbance
- Physical symptoms
- Pain

Pearls

- Because desvenlafaxine is only minimally metabolized by CYP450 3A4 and is not metabolized at all by CYP450 2D6, as venlafaxine is, it should have more consistent plasma levels than venlafaxine
- In addition, although desvenlafaxine, like venlafaxine, is more potent at the serotonin transporter (SERT) than the norepinephrine transporter (NET), it has relatively greater actions on NET versus SERT than venlafaxine does at comparable doses
- The greater potency for NET may make it a preferable agent for conditions theoretically associated with targeting norepinephrine actions, such as vasomotor symptoms and fibromyalgia

- May be particularly helpful for hot flushes in perimenopausal women
- May be effective in patients who fail to respond to SSRIs
- May be used in combination with other antidepressants for treatment-refractory cases
- May be effective in a broad array of anxiety disorders and possibly adult ADHD, although it has not been studied in these conditions
- May be associated with higher depression remission rates than SSRIs
- Because of recent studies from the UK that suggest a higher rate of deaths from overdose with venlafaxine than with SSRIs, and because of its potential to affect heart function, venlafaxine can only be prescribed in the UK by specialist doctors and is contraindicated there in patients with heart disease
- Overdose data are from fatal toxicity index studies, which do not take into account patient characteristics or whether drug use was first- or second-line
- Venlafaxine's toxicity in overdose is less than that for TCAs

Suggested Reading

Deecher DC, Beyer CE, Johnston G, et al. Desvenlafaxine succinate: a new serotonin and norepinephrine reuptake inhibitor. J Pharmacol Exp Ther 2006;318(2):657–65.

Lieberman DZ, Montgomery SA, Tourian KA, et al. A pooled analysis of two placebo-controlled trials of desvenlafaxine in major depressive disorder. Int Clin Psychopharmacol 2008;23(4):188–97.

Speroff L, Gass M, Constantine G. Efficacy and tolerability of desvenlafaxine succinate treatment for menopausal vasomotor symptoms: a randomized controlled trial. Obstet Gynecol 2008;111(1):77–87.

DEXTROMETHORPHAN

THERAPEUTICS

Brands • Nuedexta (in combination with quinidine)

see index for additional brand names

Generic? No

Class

- Noncompetitive NMDA receptor antagonist and sigma 1 agonist

Commonly Prescribed for

(bold for FDA approved)

- **Pseudobulbar affect (PBA)**
- Diabetic peripheral neuropathic pain
- Unstable mood and affect in PTSD and mild traumatic brain injury
- Third-line for treatment-resistant depression

How the Drug Works

- Dextromethorphan reduces glutamate neurotransmission through blocking NMDA receptors and by acting as an agonist at sigma 1 receptors
- Dextromethorphan also has affinity for the serotonin transporter and may therefore modulate serotonin levels
- Quinidine increases availability of dextromethorphan by inhibiting its metabolism via CYP450 2D6

How Long Until It Works

- In clinical trials the rate of pseudobulbar affect episodes was significantly decreased beginning at day 15

If It Works

- Reduces the frequency and severity of episodes of uncontrollable laughing and/or crying

If It Doesn't Work

- Consider switching to a TCA or an SSRI

Best Augmenting Combos for Partial Response or Treatment Resistance

- Often best to attempt another monotherapy prior to resorting to augmentation strategies

Tests

- None for healthy individuals

SIDE EFFECTS

How Drug Causes Side Effects

- Presumably mechanism related, including central actions at sigma and NMDA receptors causing dissociative symptoms, euphoria, or sedation

Notable Side Effects

- Dizziness, asthenia
- Diarrhea, vomiting
- Cough, peripheral edema
- Urinary tract infection
- Euphoria

Life-Threatening or Dangerous Side Effects

- Immune-mediated thrombocytopenia
- Hepatotoxicity
- Dose-dependent QT prolongation

Weight Gain

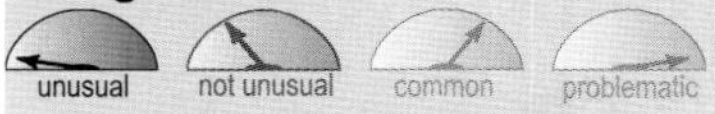

- Reported but not expected

Sedation

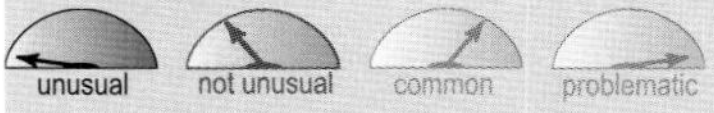

- Reported but not expected

What to Do About Side Effects

- Wait
- Wait
- Wait
- In a few weeks, switch to another agent or add other drugs

Best Augmenting Agents for Side Effects

- Often best to try another agent prior to resorting to augmentation strategies to treat side effects
- Many side effects are dose-dependent (i.e., they increase as dose increases, or they reemerge until tolerance redevelops)
- Many side effects are time-dependent (i.e., they start immediately upon dosing and upon each dose increase, but go away with time)

DOSING AND USE

Usual Dosage Range
- 20 mg/10 mg twice per day

Dosage Forms
- Capsule 20 mg/10 mg (dextromethorphan/quinidine)

How to Dose
- Initial 20 mg/10 mg once per day; after 7 days increase to 20 mg/10 mg twice per day

Dosing Tips
- Some patients may tolerate and respond to doses higher than the approved doses, but few controlled studies of high doses

Overdose
- Nausea, dizziness, headache, ventricular arrhythmias, hypotension, coma, respiratory depression, seizures, tachycardia, hyperexcitability, toxic psychosis

Long-Term Use
- Not evaluated

Habit Forming
- No

How to Stop
- Taper not necessary

Pharmacokinetics
- Elimination half-life of dextromethorphan is approximately 13 hours
- Elimination half-life of quinidine is approximately 7 hours
- Dextromethorphan is metabolized by CYP450 2D6, while quinidine inhibits CYP450 2D6
- Quinidine is metabolized by CYP450 3A4

Drug Interactions
- Via CYP450 2D6 inhibition, dextromethorphan/quinidine could increase plasma concentrations of drugs metabolized by CYP450 2D6 (e.g., desipramine), potentially requiring dose reduction of the substrate
- Can cause a fatal "serotonin syndrome" when combined with MAOIs, so do not use with MAOIs or for at least 14 days after MAOIs are stopped
- Do not start an MAOI for at least 5 half-lives (5 to 7 days for most drugs) after discontinuing dextromethorphan/quinidine
- Via P-glycoprotein inhibition, quinidine could increase plasma concentrations of P-glycoprotein substrates such as digoxin, potentially requiring dose reduction of the substrate
- Can theoretically cause serotonin syndrome when combined with serotonin reuptake inhibitors, but not well studied

Other Warnings/ Precautions
- Quinidine can cause immune-mediated thrombocytopenia that can be severe or fatal; dextromethorphan/quinidine should be discontinued immediately if thrombocytopenia occurs unless it is clearly not drug-related, and should not be restarted in sensitized patients
- Quinidine has been associated with a lupus-like syndrome involving polyarthritis
- ECG should be monitored if patient must take an agent that prolongs QT interval or that inhibits CYP450 3A4
- Anticholinergic effects of quinidine may lead to worsening in myasthenia gravis and other sensitive conditions

Do Not Use
- If patient is taking an MAOI
- If patient is taking another medication containing quinidine, quinine, or mefloquine
- If patient has a history of quinidine, quinine, or mefloquine-induced thrombocytopenia, hepatitis, or other hypersensitivity reaction
- If patient has prolonged QT interval, congenital long QT syndrome, history suggestive of torsades de pointes, or heart failure
- If patient has complete atrioventricular block (AV) without implanted pacemaker, or patients at high risk of complete AV block
- If patient is taking a drug that prolongs QT interval and is metabolized by CYP450 2D6 (e.g., thioridazine, pimozide)
- If there is a proven allergy to dextromethorphan or quinidine

SPECIAL POPULATIONS

Renal Impairment
- Dose adjustment not necessary in patients with mild to moderate impairment

Hepatic Impairment
- Dose adjustment not necessary in patients with mild to moderate impairment

Cardiac Impairment
- Contraindicated in patients with prolonged QT interval, congenital long QT syndrome, history suggestive of torsades de pointes, and heart failure
- Monitor ECG in patients with left ventricular hypertrophy or left ventricular dysfunction

Elderly
- Some patients may tolerate lower doses better

Children and Adolescents
- Safety and efficacy have not been established
- Use with caution, observing for activation of known or unknown bipolar disorder and/or suicidal ideation, and strongly consider informing parents or guardian of this risk so they can help observe child or adolescent patients

Pregnancy
- Effective June 30, 2015, the US FDA requires changes to the content and format of pregnancy and lactation information in prescription drug labels, including the elimination of the pregnancy letter categories; the Pregnancy and Lactation Labeling Rule (PLLR or final rule) applies only to prescription drugs and will be phased in gradually for drugs approved on or after June 30, 2001
- Controlled studies have not been conducted in pregnant women
- Some animal studies have shown adverse effects

Breast Feeding
- Unknown if dextromethorphan/quinidine is secreted in human breast milk, but all psychotropics assumed to be secreted in breast milk
- If child becomes irritable or sedated, breast feeding or drug may need to be discontinued
- Must weigh benefits of breast feeding with risks and benefits of antidepressant treatment versus nontreatment to both the infant and the mother

THE ART OF PSYCHOPHARMACOLOGY

Potential Advantages
- No other approved agent for PBA

Potential Disadvantages
- CYP450 2D6 poor metabolizers may require dose reduction
- In patients with past substance abuse, especially of dextromethorphan, ketamine, or PCP

Primary Target Symptoms
- Uncontrollable crying
- Uncontrollable laughter

Pearls
- Quinidine is intended to increase the actions of dextromethorphan by inhibiting its metabolism by CYP450 2D6; therefore, poor metabolizers of CYP450 2D6 may not benefit as much from this treatment while still experiencing adverse effects associated with quinidine
- Affective instability in Alzheimer disease may be treatable with this agent, including agitation, allowing antipsychotics to be avoided in this population
- Some men express emotional lability as laughter and anger rather than laughter and crying
- Affective instability in PTSD and in mild traumatic brain injury may be improved by dextromethorphan/quinidine
- Similar binding properties to ketamine suggest possible efficacy in both treatment-resistant depression and chronic pain

Suggested Reading

Brooks BR, Thisted RA, Appel SH, et al. Treatment of pseudobulbar affect in ALS with dextromethorphan/quinidine: a randomized trial. Neurology 2004;63(8):1364–70.

Garnock-Jones KP. Dextromethorphan/quinidine in pseudobulbar affect. CNS Drugs 2011;25(5):435–45.

The Medical Letter Inc. Dextromethorphan/quinidine (neudexta) for pseudobulbar affect. Med Lett Drugs Ther 2011;53(1366):46–7.

Pioro EP, Brooks BR, Cummings J, et al. Dextromethorphan plus ultra low-dose quinidine reduces pseudobulbar affect. Ann Neurol 2010;68(5):693–702.

THERAPEUTICS

Brands • Valium
• Diastat

see index for additional brand names

Generic? Yes (not Diastat)

Class
- Neuroscience-based Nomenclature: GABA positive allosteric modulator (GABA-PAM)
- Benzodiazepine (anxiolytic, muscle relaxant, anticonvulsant)

Commonly Prescribed for
(bold for FDA approved)
- **Anxiety disorder**
- **Symptoms of anxiety (short-term)**
- **Acute agitation, tremor, impending or acute delirium tremens and hallucinosis in acute alcohol withdrawal**
- **Skeletal muscle spasm due to reflex spasm to local pathology**
- **Spasticity caused by upper motor neuron disorder**
- **Athetosis**
- **Stiffman syndrome**
- **Convulsive disorder (adjunctive)**
- **Anxiety during endoscopic procedures (adjunctive) (injection only)**
- **Preoperative anxiety (injection only)**
- **Anxiety relief prior to cardioversion (intravenous)**
- **Initial treatment of status epilepticus (injection only)**
- Insomnia
- Catatonia

How the Drug Works
- Binds to benzodiazepine receptors at the GABA-A ligand-gated chloride channel complex
- Enhances the inhibitory effects of GABA
- Boosts chloride conductance through GABA-regulated channels
- Inhibits neuronal activity presumably in amygdala-centered fear circuits to provide therapeutic benefits in anxiety disorders
- Inhibiting actions in cerebral cortex may provide therapeutic benefits in seizure disorders
- Inhibitory actions in spinal cord may provide therapeutic benefits for muscle spasms

How Long Until It Works
- Some immediate relief with first dosing is common; can take several weeks with daily dosing for maximal therapeutic benefit

If It Works
- For short-term symptoms of anxiety or muscle spasms – after a few weeks, discontinue use or use on an "as-needed" basis
- Chronic muscle spasms may require chronic diazepam treatment
- For chronic anxiety disorders, the goal of treatment is complete remission of symptoms as well as prevention of future relapses
- For chronic anxiety disorders, treatment most often reduces or even eliminates symptoms, but not a cure since symptoms can recur after medicine stopped
- For long-term symptoms of anxiety, consider switching to an SSRI or SNRI for long-term maintenance
- If long-term maintenance with a benzodiazepine is necessary, continue treatment for 6 months after symptoms resolve, and then taper dose slowly
- If symptoms reemerge, consider treatment with an SSRI or SNRI, or consider restarting the benzodiazepine; sometimes benzodiazepines have to be used in combination with SSRIs or SNRIs for best results

If It Doesn't Work
- Consider switching to another agent or adding an appropriate augmenting agent
- Consider psychotherapy, especially cognitive behavioral psychotherapy
- Consider presence of concomitant substance abuse
- Consider presence of diazepam abuse
- Consider another diagnosis, such as a comorbid medical condition

Best Augmenting Combos for Partial Response or Treatment Resistance
- Benzodiazepines are frequently used as augmenting agents for antipsychotics and mood stabilizers in the treatment of psychotic and bipolar disorders
- Benzodiazepines are frequently used as augmenting agents for SSRIs and SNRIs in the treatment of anxiety disorders

- Not generally rational to combine with other benzodiazepines
- Caution if using as an anxiolytic concomitantly with other sedative hypnotics for sleep

Tests

- In patients with seizure disorders, concomitant medical illness, and/or those with multiple concomitant long-term medications, periodic liver tests and blood counts may be prudent

SIDE EFFECTS

How Drug Causes Side Effects

- Same mechanism for side effects as for therapeutic effects – namely due to excessive actions at benzodiazepine receptors
- Long-term adaptations in benzodiazepine receptors may explain the development of dependence, tolerance, and withdrawal
- Side effects are generally immediate, but immediate side effects often disappear in time

Notable Side Effects

✻ Sedation, fatigue, depression
✻ Dizziness, ataxia, slurred speech, weakness
✻ Forgetfulness, confusion
✻ Hyperexcitability, nervousness
✻ Pain at injection site
- Rare hallucinations, mania
- Rare hypotension
- Hypersalivation, dry mouth

Life-Threatening or Dangerous Side Effects

- Respiratory depression, especially when taken with CNS depressants in overdose
- Rare hepatic dysfunction, renal dysfunction, blood dyscrasias

Weight Gain

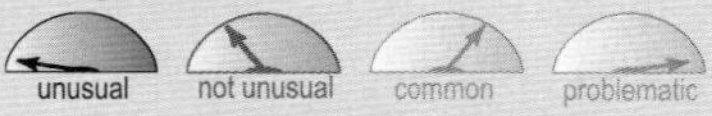

- Reported but not expected

Sedation

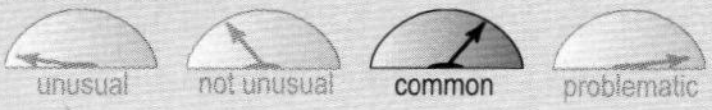

- Many experience and/or can be significant in amount
- Especially at initiation of treatment or when dose increases
- Tolerance often develops over time

What to Do About Side Effects

- Wait
- Wait
- Wait
- Lower the dose
- Take largest dose at bedtime to avoid sedative effects during the day
- Switch to another agent
- Administer flumazenil if side effects are severe or life-threatening

Best Augmenting Agents for Side Effects

- Many side effects cannot be improved with an augmenting agent

DOSING AND USE

Usual Dosage Range

- Oral: 4–40 mg/day in divided doses
- Intravenous (adults): 5 mg/minute
- Intravenous (children): 0.25 mg/kg every 3 minutes

Dosage Forms

- Tablet 2 mg scored, 5 mg scored, 10 mg scored
- Liquid 5 mg/5 mL, concentrate 5 mg/mL
- Injection vial 5 mg/mL; 10 mL, boxes of 1; 2 mL boxes of 10
- Rectal gel 5 mg/mL; 2.5 mg, 5 mg, 10 mg, 15 mg, 20 mg

How to Dose

- Oral (anxiety, muscle spasm, seizure): 2–10 mg, 2–4 times/day
- Oral (alcohol withdrawal): initial 10 mg, 3–4 times/day for 1 day; reduce to 5 mg, 3–4 times/day; continue treatment as needed
- Liquid formulation should be mixed with water or fruit juice, applesauce, or pudding
- Because of risk of respiratory depression, rectal diazepam treatment should not be given more than once in 5 days or more than twice during a treatment course, especially for alcohol withdrawal or status epilepticus

Dosing Tips

* ✻ Only benzodiazepine with a formulation specifically for rectal administration
* ✻ One of the few benzodiazepines available in an oral liquid formulation
* ✻ One of the few benzodiazepines available in an injectable formulation
* Diazepam injection is intended for acute use; patients who require long-term treatment should be switched to the oral formulation
* Use lowest possible effective dose for the shortest possible period of time (a benzodiazepine-sparing strategy)
* Assess need for continued treatment regularly
* Risk of dependence may increase with dose and duration of treatment
* For interdose symptoms of anxiety, can either increase dose or maintain same total daily dose but divide into more frequent doses
* Can also use an as-needed occasional "top up" dose for interdose anxiety
* Because some anxiety disorder patients and muscle spasm patients can require doses higher than 40 mg/day or more, the risk of dependence may be greater in these patients
* Frequency of dosing in practice is often greater than predicted from half-life, as duration of biological activity is often shorter than pharmacokinetic terminal half-life

Overdose

* Fatalities can occur; hypotension, tiredness, ataxia, confusion, coma

Long-Term Use

* Evidence of efficacy up to 16 weeks
* Risk of dependence, particularly for treatment periods longer than 12 weeks and especially in patients with past or current polysubstance abuse
* Not recommended for long-term treatment of seizure disorders

Habit Forming

* Diazepam is a Schedule IV drug
* Patients may develop dependence and/or tolerance with long-term use

How to Stop

* Patients with history of seizure may seize upon withdrawal, especially if withdrawal is abrupt
* Taper by 2 mg every 3 days to reduce chances of withdrawal effects
* For difficult to taper cases, consider reducing dose much more slowly after reaching 20 mg/day, perhaps by as little as 0.5–1 mg every week or less
* For other patients with severe problems discontinuing a benzodiazepine, dosing may need to be tapered over many months (i.e., reduce dose by 1% every 3 days by crushing tablet and suspending or dissolving in 100 mL of fruit juice and then disposing of 1 mL while drinking the rest; 3–7 days later, dispose of 2 mL, and so on). This is both a form of very slow biological tapering and a form of behavioral desensitization
* Be sure to differentiate reemergence of symptoms requiring reinstitution of treatment from withdrawal symptoms
* Benzodiazepine-dependent anxiety patients and insulin-dependent diabetics are not addicted to their medications. When benzodiazepine-dependent patients stop their medication, disease symptoms can reemerge, disease symptoms can worsen (rebound), and/or withdrawal symptoms can emerge

Pharmacokinetics

* Elimination half-life 20–50 hours
* Substrate for CYP450 2C19 and 3A4
* Food does not affect absorption

Drug Interactions

* Increased depressive effects when taken with other CNS depressants (see Warnings below)
* Cimetidine may reduce the clearance and raise the levels of diazepam
* Flumazenil (used to reverse the effects of benzodiazepines) may precipitate seizures and should not be used in patients treated for seizure disorders with diazepam

Other Warnings/ Precautions

* Boxed warning regarding the increased risk of CNS depressant effects when benzodiazepines and opioid medications are

used together, including specifically the risk of slowed or difficulty breathing and death
- If alternatives to the combined use of benzodiazepines and opioids are not available, clinicians should limit the dosage and duration of each drug to the minimum possible while still achieving therapeutic efficacy
- Patients and their caregivers should be warned to seek medical attention if unusual dizziness, lightheadedness, sedation, slowed or difficulty breathing, or unresponsiveness occur
- Dosage changes should be made in collaboration with prescriber
- Use with caution in patients with pulmonary disease; rare reports of death after initiation of benzodiazepines in patients with severe pulmonary impairment
- History of drug or alcohol abuse often creates greater risk for dependency
- Some depressed patients may experience a worsening of suicidal ideation
- Some patients may exhibit abnormal thinking or behavioral changes similar to those caused by other CNS depressants (i.e., either depressant actions or disinhibiting actions)

Do Not Use
- If angle-closure glaucoma
- If there is a proven allergy to diazepam or any benzodiazepine

SPECIAL POPULATIONS

Renal Impairment
- Initial 2–2.5 mg, 1–2 times/day; increase gradually as needed

Hepatic Impairment
- Initial 2–2.5 mg, 1–2 times/day; increase gradually as needed

Cardiac Impairment
- Benzodiazepines have been used to treat anxiety associated with acute myocardial infarction
- Diazepam may be used as an adjunct during cardiovascular emergencies

Elderly
- Initial 2–2.5 mg, 1–2 times/day; increase gradually as needed

Children and Adolescents
- 6 months and up: initial 1–2.5 mg, 3–4 times/day; increase gradually as needed
- Parenteral: 30 days or older
- Rectal: 2 years or older
- Long-term effects of diazepam in children/adolescents are unknown
- Should generally receive lower doses and be more closely monitored

Pregnancy
- Effective June 30, 2015, the US FDA requires changes to the content and format of pregnancy and lactation information in prescription drug labels, including the elimination of the pregnancy letter categories; the Pregnancy and Lactation Labeling Rule (PLLR or final rule) applies only to prescription drugs and will be phased in gradually for drugs approved on or after June 30, 2001
- Possible increased risk of birth defects when benzodiazepines taken during pregnancy
- Because of the potential risks, diazepam is not generally recommended as treatment for anxiety during pregnancy, especially during the first trimester
- Drug should be tapered if discontinued
- Infants whose mothers received a benzodiazepine late in pregnancy may experience withdrawal effects
- Neonatal flaccidity has been reported in infants whose mothers took a benzodiazepine during pregnancy
- Seizures, even mild seizures, may cause harm to the embryo/fetus

Breast Feeding
- Unknown if diazepam is secreted in human breast milk, but all psychotropics assumed to be secreted in breast milk

✻ Recommended either to discontinue drug or bottle feed
- Effects of benzodiazepines on nursing infants have been reported and include feeding difficulties, sedation, and weight loss

THE ART OF PSYCHOPHARMACOLOGY

Potential Advantages
- Rapid onset of action
- Availability of oral liquid, rectal, and injectable dosage formulations

Potential Disadvantages
- Euphoria may lead to abuse
- Abuse especially risky in past or present substance abusers
- Can be sedating at doses necessary to treat moderately severe anxiety disorders

Primary Target Symptoms
- Panic attacks
- Anxiety
- Incidence of seizures (adjunct)
- Muscle spasms

Pearls
- Can be a useful adjunct to SSRIs and SNRIs in the treatment of numerous anxiety disorders, but not used as frequently as other benzodiazepines for this purpose
- Not effective for treating psychosis as a monotherapy, but can be used as an adjunct to antipsychotics
- Not effective for treating bipolar disorder as a monotherapy, but can be used as an adjunct to mood stabilizers and antipsychotics

* ✻ Diazepam is often the first choice benzodiazepine to treat status epilepticus, and is administered either intravenously or rectally
- Because diazepam suppresses stage 4 sleep, it may prevent night terrors in adults
- May both cause depression and treat depression in different patients
- Was once one of the most commonly prescribed drugs in the world and the most commonly prescribed benzodiazepine

* ✻ Remains a popular benzodiazepine for treating muscle spasms
- A commonly used benzodiazepine to treat sleep disorders

* ✻ Remains a popular benzodiazepine to treat acute alcohol withdrawal
- Not especially useful as an oral anticonvulsant

* ✻ Multiple dosage formulations (oral tablet, oral liquid, rectal gel, injectable) allow more flexibility of administration compared to most other benzodiazepines
- When using to treat insomnia, remember that insomnia may be a symptom of some other primary disorder itself, and thus warrant evaluation for comorbid psychiatric and/or medical conditions
- Though not systematically studied, benzodiazepines have been used effectively to treat catatonia and are the initial recommended treatment

Suggested Reading

Ashton H. Guidelines for the rational use of benzodiazepines. When and what to use. Drugs 1994;48:25–40.

De Negri M, Baglietto MG. Treatment of status epilepticus in children. Paediatr Drugs 2001;3:411–20.

Mandelli M, Tognoni G, Garattini S. Clinical pharmacokinetics of diazepam. Clin Pharmacokinet 1978;3:72–91.

Rey E, Treluver JM, Pons G. Pharmacokinetic optimization of benzodiazepine therapy for acute seizures. Focus on delivery routes. Clin Pharmacokinet 1999;36:409–24.

DIPHENHYDRAMINE

THERAPEUTICS

Brands • Benadryl, Sominex
see index for additional brand names

Generic? Yes

Class
• Antihistamine; anticholinergic agent

Commonly Prescribed for
(bold for FDA approved)
- **Allergy symptoms**
- **Motion sickness**
- **Occasional sleeplessness**
- **Antiparkinsonism**
- Extrapyramidal disorders

How the Drug Works (for extrapyramidal disorders)
- Diminishes the excess acetylcholine activity caused by removal of dopamine inhibition when dopamine receptors are blocked
- Also has potent histamine 1 antagonist properties

How Long Until It Works (for extrapyramidal disorders)
- For extrapyramidal disorders and parkinsonism, onset of action can be within minutes or hours

If It Works (for extrapyramidal disorders)
- Reduces motor side effects
- Does not lessen the ability of antipsychotics to cause tardive dyskinesia

If It Doesn't Work (for extrapyramidal disorders)
- Consider switching to trihexyphenidyl, benztropine, or a benzodiazepine
- Disorders that develop after prolonged antipsychotic use may not respond to treatment
- Consider discontinuing the agent that precipitated the EPS

Best Augmenting Combos for Partial Response or Treatment Resistance
- If ineffective, switch to another agent rather than augment
- Diphenhydramine itself is an augmenting agent to antipsychotics

Tests
- None for healthy individuals

SIDE EFFECTS

How Drug Causes Side Effects
- Blocking histamine 1 receptors can cause sedation
- Preventing the action of acetylcholine on muscarinic receptors can cause anticholinergic effects such as dry mouth, blurred vision, constipation

Notable Side Effects
- Sedation, dizziness
- Constipation, nausea
- Dry mouth, blurred vision

Life-Threatening or Dangerous Side Effects
- Rare convulsions (at high doses)
- Urinary retention
- Tachycardia, cardiac arrhythmias
- Confusion
- Paralytic ileus/bowel obstruction

Weight Gain
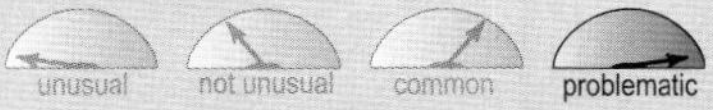

- Frequent and can be significant in amount

Sedation
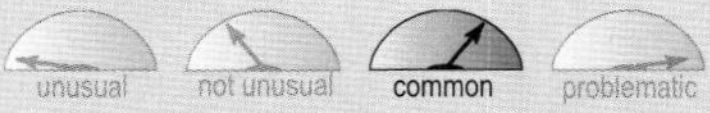

- Many experience and/or can be significant in amount

What to Do About Side Effects
- For confusion or hallucinations, discontinue use
- For sedation, lower the dose and/or take the entire dose at night
- For dry mouth, chew gum or drink water
- For urinary retention, obtain a urological evaluation; may need to discontinue use

Best Augmenting Agents for Side Effects
- Many side effects cannot be improved with an augmenting agent

DOSING AND USE

Usual Dosage Range
- Oral: 50 mg/day
- Injection: 10–50 mg

Dosage Forms
- Injection 50 mg/mL
- Capsule 50 mg
- Elixir 12.5 mg/5 mL
- Also available in formulations in combination with other medications

How to Dose
- Injection: 10–50 mg intravenously at a rate not exceeding 25 mg/min or deep intramuscularly; can dose at 100 mg if required; maximum daily dose 400 mg

Dosing Tips
- If drug-induced EPS occur soon after initiation of a neuroleptic drug, they are likely to be transient; thus, attempt to withdraw diphenhydramine after 1–2 weeks to determine if still needed
- The injection should be used for parkinsonism only if oral therapy is impossible or contraindicated

Overdose
- CNS depression, CNS stimulation (more likely in pediatric patients), dry mouth, dilated pupils, flushing, gastrointestinal symptoms

Long-Term Use
- Safe
- Effectiveness may decrease over time, even after a few doses, but side effects such as cognitive impairment and sedation may persist

Habit Forming
- No

How to Stop
- Tapering generally not necessary

Pharmacokinetics
- Plasma half-life approximately 8 hours; may be longer in children and in the elderly

Drug Interactions
- May potentiate the effects of other CNS depressants
- If anticholinergic agents are used with diphenhydramine, the anticholinergic effects may be enhanced

Other Warnings/ Precautions
- Use with caution in patients with a history of bronchial asthma, lower respiratory disease, increased intraocular pressure, hyperthyroidism, cardiovascular disease, or hypertension
- May have additive effects if taken with anticholinergic agents

Do Not Use
- If patient is breast feeding
- In neonates or premature infants
- In patients with glaucoma, particularly angle-closure glaucoma
- In patients with pyloric or duodenal obstruction, stenosing peptic ulcers, prostate hypertrophy, or bladder neck obstructions
- If patient is taking an MAOI
- If there is a proven allergy to diphenhydramine

SPECIAL POPULATIONS

Renal Impairment
- No dose adjustment necessary

Hepatic Impairment
- No dose adjustment necessary

Cardiac Impairment
- Not systematically evaluated in patients with cardiac impairment

Elderly
- Some patients may tolerate lower doses better
- Diphenhydramine injection is preferred for parkinsonism in the elderly who are unable to tolerate more potent agents

Children and Adolescents

- Not recommended for children under age 12
- Injection: 5 mg/kg/24 hours or 150 mg/m^2/24 hours; maximum daily dose 300 mg; divide into 4 doses; can be given intravenously at a rate not exceeding 25 mg/min, or deep intramuscularly
- Contraindicated in neonates and premature infants

Pregnancy

- Effective June 30, 2015, the US FDA requires changes to the content and format of pregnancy and lactation information in prescription drug labels, including the elimination of the pregnancy letter categories; the Pregnancy and Lactation Labeling Rule (PLLR or final rule) applies only to prescription drugs and will be phased in gradually for drugs approved on or after June 30, 2001
- Controlled studies have not been conducted in pregnant women
- Animal studies have not shown adverse effects

Breast Feeding

- Contraindicated

THE ART OF PSYCHOPHARMACOLOGY

Potential Advantages

- Mild cases of parkinsonism

Potential Disadvantages

- Can be too sedating for some patients
- Can cause confusion in elderly patients and in patients with dementia

Primary Target Symptoms

- Extrapyramidal disorders

Pearls

- Can be useful for occasional insomnia
- Patients with cognitive impairment may do poorly
- Can cause cognitive side effects with chronic use, so periodic trials of discontinuation may be useful to justify continuous use, especially in institutional settings when used as an adjunct to antipsychotics
- Can be abused in institutional or correctional settings

Suggested Reading

Gonzalez F. Diphenhydramine may be useful as a palliative treatment for patients dying with Parkinson's disease and tremors: a case report and discussion. Am J Hosp Palliat Care 2010;26(6):474–5.

DISULFIRAM

THERAPEUTICS

Brands • Antabuse
see index for additional brand names

Generic? Yes

Class
- Alcohol dependence treatment

Commonly Prescribed for
(bold for FDA approved)
- **Maintenance of alcohol abstinence**

How the Drug Works
- Irreversibly inhibits aldehyde dehydrogenase, the enzyme involved in second-stage metabolism of alcohol
- Alcohol is metabolized to acetaldehyde, which in turn is metabolized by aldehyde dehydrogenase; thus, disulfiram blocks this second-stage metabolism
- If alcohol is consumed by a patient taking disulfiram, toxic levels of acetaldehyde build up, causing unpleasant side effects
- This aversive experience ideally leads to negative conditioning, in which patients abstain from alcohol in order to avoid the unpleasant effects

How Long Until It Works
- Disulfiram's effects are immediate; patients should not take disulfiram until at least 12 hours after drinking

If It Works
- Increases abstinence from alcohol

If It Doesn't Work
- Patients who drink alcohol while taking disulfiram can experience side effects, including alcohol toxicity
- Evaluate for and address contributing factors
- Consider switching to another agent

Best Augmenting Combos for Partial Response or Treatment Resistance
- Augmentation with behavioral, educational, and/or supportive therapy in groups or as an individual is probably key to successful treatment

Tests
- Baseline and follow-up liver function tests

SIDE EFFECTS

How Drug Causes Side Effects
- When alcohol is consumed by a patient taking disulfiram, levels of acetaldehyde build up, causing side effects of alcohol toxicity
- One of disulfiram's metabolites is carbon disulfide, which may be excreted through the lungs; this could account for the side effect of metallic taste

Notable Side Effects
- Metallic taste, dermatitis, sedation
- Flushing, headache, tachycardia, nausea, vomiting (if alcohol is consumed)

Life-Threatening or Dangerous Side Effects
- Hepatotoxicity
- Myocardial infarction, congestive heart failure, respiratory depression, other signs of alcohol toxicity (if alcohol is consumed)

Weight Gain
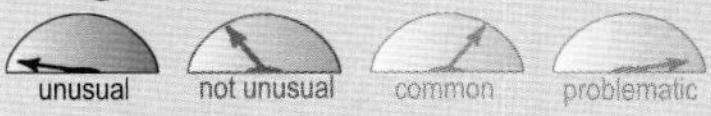

- Reported but not expected

Sedation
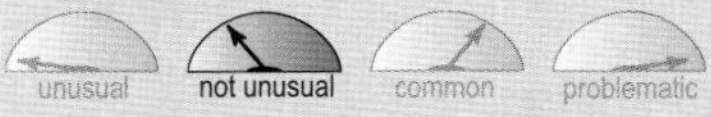

- Occurs in significant minority

What to Do About Side Effects
- Wait
- Reduce dose
- Take at night to reduce sedation

Best Augmenting Agents for Side Effects
- Dose reduction or switching to another agent may be more effective since most side effects cannot be improved with an augmenting agent

DOSING AND USE

Usual Dosage Range
- 250–500 mg/day; 1-year duration

Dosage Forms
- Tablet 250 mg, 500 mg scored

How to Dose
- The patient should not take disulfiram until at least 12 hours after drinking
- Initial 250–500 mg/day for 1–2 weeks
- Usually dosed in the morning but can be dosed at night if sedation is a problem
- Maintenance dose usually 250 mg/day; maximum dose 500 mg/day

Dosing Tips
- The patient must be fully informed of the disulfiram-alcohol reaction
- The patient should be advised not to consume any food or beverages containing alcohol or to use any alcohol-containing preparations (e.g., cough syrup)
- The patient should be warned that reactions may occur up to 2 weeks after disulfiram is stopped
- The patient should carry an emergency card stating that he or she is taking disulfiram

Overdose
- Unknown

Long-Term Use
- Maintenance treatment should be continued until the patient is recovered

Habit Forming
- No

How to Stop
- Taper not necessary
- A disulfiram-alcohol reaction may occur for up to 2 weeks after disulfiram is stopped

Pharmacokinetics
- Half-life of parent drug is 60–120 hours
- Half-life of metabolites is 13.9 hours (diethyldithiocarbamate) and 8.9 hours (carbon disulfide)

Drug Interactions
- Disulfiram may increase blood levels of phenytoin; baseline and follow-up levels of phenytoin should be taken
- Disulfiram may prolong prothrombin time, requiring dose adjustment of oral anticoagulants
- Use with isoniazid may lead to unsteady gait or change in mental status

Other Warnings/ Precautions
- Disulfiram should not be given to a patient in a state of alcohol intoxication or without the patient's full knowledge
- Not recommended for patients older than age 60 or for those with severe pulmonary disease, chronic renal failure, diabetes, peripheral neuropathy, seizures, cirrhosis, or portal hypertension
- Use with extreme caution in patients with hypothyroidism, epilepsy, cerebral damage
- Patients taking disulfiram should not be exposed to ethylene dibromide or its vapors, as this has resulted in a higher incidence of tumors in rats

Do Not Use
- If the patient is in a state of alcohol intoxication
- Without the patient's full knowledge
- For at least 12 hours after the patient last drank
- If patient is taking metronidazole, amprenavir, ritonavir, or sertraline
- If patient has psychosis
- If patient has cardiovascular disease
- If there is a proven allergy to disulfiram
- If there is a proven allergy to thiuram derivatives

SPECIAL POPULATIONS

Renal Impairment
- Not recommended for patients with chronic renal failure

Hepatic Impairment
- Not recommended

Cardiac Impairment
- Contraindicated

Elderly
- Not generally recommended for patients older than age 60
- Some patients may tolerate lower doses better

Children and Adolescents
- Safety and efficacy have not been established

Pregnancy
- Effective June 30, 2015, the US FDA requires changes to the content and format of pregnancy and lactation information in prescription drug labels, including the elimination of the pregnancy letter categories; the Pregnancy and Lactation Labeling Rule (PLLR or final rule) applies only to prescription drugs and will be phased in gradually for drugs approved on or after June 30, 2001
- Controlled studies have not been conducted in pregnant women
- Some animal studies have shown adverse effects
- Pregnant women needing to stop drinking may consider behavioral therapy before pharmacotherapy
- Not generally recommended for use during pregnancy, especially during first trimester

Breast Feeding
- Unknown if disulfiram is secreted in human breast milk, but all psychotropics assumed to be secreted in breast milk

* Recommended either to discontinue drug or bottle feed

THE ART OF PSYCHOPHARMACOLOGY

Potential Advantages
- Individuals who are motivated to abstain from alcohol

Potential Disadvantages
- Adherence rates can be low

Primary Target Symptoms
- Alcohol dependence

Pearls
- Some evidence of efficacy in comorbid alcohol use disorder and PTSD
- Preliminary evidence of efficacy for use in cocaine dependence, both alone and comorbid with alcohol use disorder

Suggested Reading

Barth KS, Malcolm RJ. Disulfiram: an old therapeutic with new applications. CNS Neurol Disord Drug Targets 2010;9(1):5–12.

Jorgensen CH, Pedersen B, Tonnesen H. The efficacy of disulfiram for the treatment of alcohol use disorder. Alcohol Clin Exp Res 2011;35(10):1749–58.

Pani PP, Troqu E, Vacca R, et al. Disulfiram for the treatment of cocaine dependence. Cochrane Database Syst Rev 2010;20(1):CD007024.

THERAPEUTICS

Brands
- Aricept
- Memac

see index for additional brand names

Generic? Yes

Class
- Neuroscience-based Nomenclature: acetylcholine enzyme inhibitor (ACh-EI)
- Cholinesterase inhibitor (selective acetylcholinesterase inhibitor); cognitive enhancer

Commonly Prescribed for
(bold for FDA approved)
- **Alzheimer disease (mild, moderate, and severe)**
- Memory disorders in other conditions
- Mild cognitive impairment

How the Drug Works
- * Reversibly but noncompetitively inhibits centrally active acetylcholinesterase (AChE), making more acetylcholine available
- Increased availability of acetylcholine compensates in part for degenerating cholinergic neurons in neocortex that regulate memory
- Does not inhibit butyrylcholinesterase
- May release growth factors or interfere with amyloid deposition

How Long Until It Works
- May take up to 6 weeks before any improvement in baseline memory or behavior is evident
- May take months before any stabilization in degenerative course is evident

If It Works
- May improve symptoms and slow progression of disease, but does not reverse the degenerative process

If It Doesn't Work
- Consider adjusting dose, switching to a different cholinesterase inhibitor or adding an appropriate augmenting agent
- Reconsider diagnosis and rule out other conditions such as depression or a dementia other than Alzheimer disease

Best Augmenting Combos for Partial Response or Treatment Resistance
- * Atypical antipsychotics to reduce behavioral disturbances
- * Antidepressants if concomitant depression, apathy, or lack of interest
- * Memantine for moderate to severe Alzheimer disease
- Divalproex, carbamazepine, or oxcarbazepine for behavioral disturbances
- Not rational to combine with another cholinesterase inhibitor

Tests
- None for healthy individuals

SIDE EFFECTS

How Drug Causes Side Effects
- Peripheral inhibition of acetylcholinesterase can cause gastrointestinal side effects
- Central inhibition of acetylcholinesterase may contribute to nausea, vomiting, weight loss, and sleep disturbances

Notable Side Effects
- * Nausea, diarrhea, vomiting, appetite loss, increased gastric acid secretion, weight loss
- Insomnia, dizziness
- Muscle cramps, fatigue, depression, abnormal dreams

Life-Threatening or Dangerous Side Effects
- Rare seizures
- Rare syncope

Weight Gain
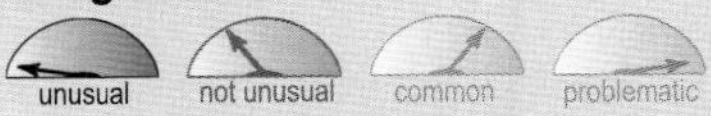

- Reported but not expected
- Some patients may experience weight loss

Sedation
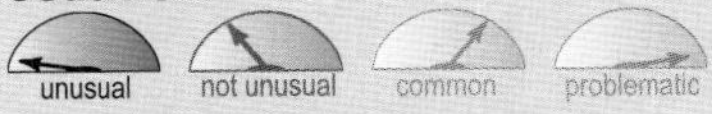

- Reported but not expected

What to Do About Side Effects
- Wait
- Wait

- Wait
- Take in daytime to reduce insomnia
- Use slower dose titration
- Consider lowering dose, switching to a different agent or adding an appropriate augmenting agent

Best Augmenting Agents for Side Effects

- Hypnotics or trazodone may improve insomnia
- Many side effects cannot be improved with an augmenting agent

DOSING AND USE

Usual Dosage Range

- 5–10 mg at night

Dosage Forms

- Tablet 5 mg, 10 mg, 23 mg
- Orally disintegrating tablet 5 mg, 10 mg

How to Dose

- Initial 5 mg/day; may increase to 10 mg/day after 4–6 weeks

Dosing Tips

- Side effects occur more frequently at higher doses than at lower doses
- Slower titration (e.g., 6 weeks to 10 mg/day) may reduce the risk of side effects
- Food does not affect the absorption of donepezil
- Probably best to utilize highest tolerated dose within the usual dosage range
- Some off-label uses for cognitive disturbances other than Alzheimer disease have anecdotally utilized doses higher than 10 mg/day

✽ When switching to another cholinesterase inhibitor, probably best to cross-titrate from one to the other to prevent precipitous decline in function if the patient washes out of one drug entirely

Overdose

- Can be lethal; nausea, vomiting, excess salivation, sweating, hypotension, bradycardia, collapse, convulsions, muscle weakness (weakness of respiratory muscles can lead to death)

Long-Term Use

- Drug may lose effectiveness in slowing degenerative course of Alzheimer disease after 6 months
- Can be effective in some patients for several years

Habit Forming

- No

How to Stop

- Taper to avoid withdrawal effects
- Discontinuation may lead to notable deterioration in memory and behavior, which may not be restored when drug is restarted or another cholinesterase inhibitor is initiated

Pharmacokinetics

- Metabolized by CYP450 2D6 and CYP450 3A4
- Elimination half-life approximately 70 hours

Drug Interactions

- Donepezil may increase the effects of anesthetics and should be discontinued prior to surgery
- Inhibitors of CYP450 2D6 and CYP450 3A4 may inhibit donepezil metabolism and increase its plasma levels
- Inducers of CYP450 2D6 and CYP450 3A4 may increase clearance of donepezil and decrease its plasma levels
- Donepezil may interact with anticholinergic agents and the combination may decrease the efficacy of both
- May have synergistic effect if administered with cholinomimetics (e.g., bethanechol)
- Bradycardia may occur if combined with beta blockers
- Theoretically, could reduce the efficacy of levodopa in Parkinson's disease
- Not rational to combine with another cholinesterase inhibitor

Other Warnings/ Precautions

- May exacerbate asthma or other pulmonary disease
- Increased gastric acid secretion may increase the risk of ulcers
- Bradycardia or heart block may occur in patients with or without cardiac impairment

Do Not Use
- If there is a proven allergy to donepezil

SPECIAL POPULATIONS

Renal Impairment
- Few data available but dose adjustment is most likely unnecessary

Hepatic Impairment
- Few data available; may need to lower dose

Cardiac Impairment
- Should be used with caution
- Syncopal episodes have been reported with the use of donepezil

Elderly
- Some patients may tolerate lower doses better
- Use of cholinesterase inhibitors may be associated with increased rates of syncope, bradycardia, pacemaker insertion, and hip fracture in older adults with dementia

Children and Adolescents
- Safety and efficacy have not been established
- Preliminary reports of efficacy as an adjunct in attention deficit hyperactivity disorder (ADHD) (ages 8–17)

Pregnancy
- Effective June 30, 2015, the US FDA requires changes to the content and format of pregnancy and lactation information in prescription drug labels, including the elimination of the pregnancy letter categories; the Pregnancy and Lactation Labeling Rule (PLLR or final rule) applies only to prescription drugs and will be phased in gradually for drugs approved on or after June 30, 2001
- Controlled studies have not been conducted in pregnant women

✽ Not recommended for use in pregnant women or women of childbearing potential

Breast Feeding
- Unknown if donepezil is secreted in human breast milk, but all psychotropics assumed to be secreted in breast milk

✽ Recommended either to discontinue drug or bottle feed

- Donepezil is not recommended for use in nursing women

THE ART OF PSYCHOPHARMACOLOGY

Potential Advantages
- Once a day dosing
- May be used in vascular dementia
- May work in some patients who do not respond to other cholinesterase inhibitors
- May work in some patients who do not tolerate other cholinesterase inhibitors

Potential Disadvantages
- Patients with insomnia

Primary Target Symptoms
- Memory loss in Alzheimer disease
- Behavioral symptoms in Alzheimer disease
- Memory loss in other dementias

Pearls
- A fixed-dose combination of memantine extended-release and donepezil has been approved for the treatment of moderate to severe Alzheimer's dementia in patients stabilized on memantine and donepezil
- Dramatic reversal of symptoms of Alzheimer disease is not generally seen with cholinesterase inhibitors
- Can lead to therapeutic nihilism among prescribers and lack of an appropriate trial of a cholinesterase inhibitor

✽ Perhaps only 50% of Alzheimer patients are diagnosed, and only 50% of those diagnosed are treated, and only 50% of those treated are given a cholinesterase inhibitor, and then only for 200 days in a disease that lasts 7–10 years

- Must evaluate lack of efficacy and loss of efficacy over months, not weeks

✽ Treats behavioral and psychological symptoms of Alzheimer dementia as well as cognitive symptoms (i.e., especially

apathy, disinhibition, delusions, anxiety, cooperation, pacing)
- Patients who complain themselves of memory problems may have depression, whereas patients whose spouses or children complain of the patient's memory problems may have Alzheimer disease
- Treat the patient but ask the caregiver about efficacy
- What you see may depend upon how early you treat
- The first symptoms of Alzheimer disease are generally mood changes; thus, Alzheimer disease may initially be diagnosed as depression
- Women may experience cognitive symptoms in perimenopause as a result of hormonal changes that are not a sign of dementia or Alzheimer disease
- Aggressively treat concomitant symptoms with augmentation (e.g., atypical antipsychotics for agitation, antidepressants for depression)
- If treatment with antidepressants fails to improve apathy and depressed mood in the elderly, it is possible that this represents early Alzheimer disease and a cholinesterase inhibitor like donepezil may be helpful
- What to expect from a cholinesterase inhibitor:
  - Patients do not generally improve dramatically although this can be observed in a significant minority of patients
  - Onset of behavioral problems and nursing home placement can be delayed
  - Functional outcomes, including activities of daily living, can be preserved
  - Caregiver burden and stress can be reduced
- Delay in progression in Alzheimer disease is not evidence of disease-modifying actions of cholinesterase inhibition
- Cholinesterase inhibitors like donepezil depend upon the presence of intact targets for acetylcholine for maximum effectiveness and thus may be most effective in the early stages of Alzheimer disease
- The most prominent side effects of donepezil are gastrointestinal effects, which are usually mild and transient

✻ May cause more sleep disturbances than some other cholinesterase inhibitors
- For patients with intolerable side effects, generally allow a washout period with resolution of side effects prior to switching to another cholinesterase inhibitor
- Weight loss can be a problem in Alzheimer patients with debilitation and muscle wasting
- Women over 85, particularly with low body weights, may experience more adverse effects
- Use with caution in underweight or frail patients
- Cognitive improvement may be linked to substantial (>65%) inhibition of acetylcholinesterase
- Donepezil has greater action on CNS acetylcholinesterase than on peripheral acetylcholinesterase
- Some Alzheimer patients who fail to respond to donepezil may respond to another cholinesterase inhibitor
- Some Alzheimer patients who fail to respond to another cholinesterase inhibitor may respond when switched to donepezil
- To prevent potential clinical deterioration, generally switch from long-term treatment with one cholinesterase inhibitor to another without a washout period

✻ Donepezil may slow the progression of mild cognitive impairment to Alzheimer disease

✻ May be useful for dementia with Lewy bodies (DLB, constituted by early loss of attentiveness and visual perception with possible hallucinations, Parkinson-like movement problems, fluctuating cognition such as daytime drowsiness and lethargy, staring into space for long periods, episodes of disorganized speech)
- May decrease delusions, apathy, agitation, and hallucinations in dementia with Lewy bodies

✻ May be useful for vascular dementia (e.g., acute onset with slow stepwise progression that has plateaus, often with gait abnormalities, focal signs, imbalance, and urinary incontinence)
- May be helpful for dementia in Down's syndrome
- Suggestions of utility in some cases of treatment-resistant bipolar disorder
- Theoretically, may be useful for ADHD, but not yet proven
- Theoretically, could be useful in any memory condition characterized by cholinergic deficiency (e.g., some cases of brain injury, cancer chemotherapy-induced cognitive changes, etc.)

Suggested Reading

Bentue-Ferrer D, Tribut O, Polard E, Allain H. Clinically significant drug interactions with cholinesterase inhibitors: a guide for neurologists. CNS Drugs 2003;17:947–63.

Birks JS, Harvey R. Donepezil for dementia due to Alzheimer's disease. Cochrane Database Syst Rev 2003;(1):CD001190.

Bonner LT, Peskind ER. Pharmacologic treatments of dementia. Med Clin North Am 2002;86:657–74.

Jones RW. Have cholinergic therapies reached their clinical boundary in Alzheimer's disease? Int J Geriatr Psychiatry 2003;18(Suppl 1): S7–13.

Seltzer B. Donepezil: an update. Expert Opin Pharmacother 2007;8(7):1011–23.

DOTHIEPIN

THERAPEUTICS

Brands • Prothiaden

see index for additional brand names

Generic? In UK

Class

- Neuroscience-based Nomenclature: serotonin, norepinephrine multi-modal (SN-MM)
- Tricyclic antidepressant (TCA)
- Serotonin and norepinephrine/noradrenaline reuptake inhibitor

Commonly Prescribed for

(bold for FDA approved)

- Major depressive disorder
- Anxiety
- Insomnia
- Neuropathic pain/chronic pain
- Treatment-resistant depression

How the Drug Works

- Boosts neurotransmitters serotonin and norepinephrine/noradrenaline
- Blocks serotonin reuptake pump (serotonin transporter), presumably increasing serotonergic neurotransmission
- Blocks norepinephrine reuptake pump (norepinephrine transporter), presumably increasing noradrenergic neurotransmission
- Presumably desensitizes both serotonin 1A receptors and beta adrenergic receptors
- Since dopamine is inactivated by norepinephrine reuptake in frontal cortex, which largely lacks dopamine transporters, dothiepin can increase dopamine neurotransmission in this part of the brain

How Long Until It Works

- May have immediate effects in treating insomnia or anxiety
- Onset of therapeutic actions usually not immediate, but often delayed 2–4 weeks
- If it is not working within 6–8 weeks for depression, it may require a dosage increase or it may not work at all
- May continue to work for many years to prevent relapse of symptoms

If It Works

- The goal of treatment of depression is complete remission of current symptoms as well as prevention of future relapses
- The goal of treatment of chronic neuropathic pain is to reduce symptoms as much as possible, especially in combination with other treatments
- Treatment of depression most often reduces or even eliminates symptoms, but not a cure since symptoms can recur after medicine stopped
- Treatment of chronic neuropathic pain may reduce symptoms, but rarely eliminates them completely, and is not a cure since symptoms can recur after medicine is stopped
- Continue treatment of depression until all symptoms are gone (remission)
- Once symptoms of depression are gone, continue treating for 1 year for the first episode of depression
- For second and subsequent episodes of depression, treatment may need to be indefinite
- Use in anxiety disorders and chronic pain may also need to be indefinite, but long-term treatment is not well studied in these conditions

If It Doesn't Work

- Many depressed patients have only a partial response where some symptoms are improved but others persist (especially insomnia, fatigue, and problems concentrating)
- Other depressed patients may be nonresponders, sometimes called treatment-resistant or treatment-refractory
- Consider increasing dose, switching to another agent or adding an appropriate augmenting agent
- Consider psychotherapy
- Consider evaluation for another diagnosis or for a comorbid condition (e.g., medical illness, substance abuse, etc.)
- Some patients may experience apparent lack of consistent efficacy due to activation of latent or underlying bipolar disorder, and require antidepressant discontinuation and a switch to a mood stabilizer

Best Augmenting Combos for Partial Response or Treatment Resistance

- Lithium, buspirone, thyroid hormone (for depression)
- Gabapentin, tiagabine, other anticonvulsants, even opiates if done by experts while monitoring carefully in difficult cases (for chronic pain)

Tests

- Baseline ECG is recommended for patients over age 50

✻ Since tricyclic and tetracyclic antidepressants are frequently associated with weight gain, before starting treatment, weigh all patients and determine if the patient is already overweight (BMI 25.0–29.9) or obese (BMI ≥30)

- Before giving a drug that can cause weight gain to an overweight or obese patient, consider determining whether the patient already has pre-diabetes (fasting plasma glucose 100–125 mg/dL), diabetes (fasting plasma glucose >126 mg/dL), or dyslipidemia (increased total cholesterol, LDL cholesterol, and triglycerides; decreased HDL cholesterol), and treat or refer such patients for treatment including nutrition and weight management, physical activity counseling, smoking cessation, and medical management

✻ Monitor weight and BMI during treatment

✻ While giving a drug to a patient who has gained >5% of initial weight, consider evaluating for the presence of pre-diabetes, diabetes, or dyslipidemia, or consider switching to a different antidepressant

- EKGs may be useful for selected patients (e.g., those with personal or family history of QTc prolongation; cardiac arrhythmia; recent myocardial infarction; uncompensated heart failure; or taking agents that prolong QTc interval such as pimozide, thioridazine, selected antiarrhythmics, moxifloxacin, sparfloxacin, etc.)
- Patients at risk for electrolyte disturbances (e.g., patients on diuretic therapy) should have baseline and periodic serum potassium and magnesium measurements

SIDE EFFECTS

How Drug Causes Side Effects

- Anticholinergic activity may explain sedative effects, dry mouth, constipation, and blurred vision
- Sedative effects and weight gain may be due to antihistamine properties
- Blockade of alpha adrenergic 1 receptors may explain dizziness, sedation, and hypotension
- Cardiac arrhythmias and seizures, especially in overdose, may be caused by blockade of ion channels

Notable Side Effects

- Blurred vision, constipation, urinary retention, increased appetite, dry mouth, nausea, diarrhea, heartburn, unusual taste in mouth, weight gain
- Fatigue, weakness, dizziness, sedation, headache, anxiety, nervousness, restlessness
- Sexual dysfunction, sweating

Life-Threatening or Dangerous Side Effects

- Paralytic ileus, hyperthermia (TCAs + anticholinergic agents)
- Lowered seizure threshold and rare seizures
- Orthostatic hypotension, sudden death, arrhythmias, tachycardia
- QTc prolongation
- Hepatic failure, extrapyramidal symptoms
- Increased intraocular pressure
- Rare induction of mania
- Rare activation of suicidal ideation and behavior (suicidality) (short-term studies did not show an increase in the risk of suicidality with antidepressants compared to placebo beyond age 24)

Weight Gain

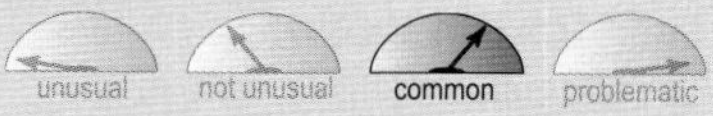

- Many experience and/or can be significant in amount
- Can increase appetite and carbohydrate craving

Sedation

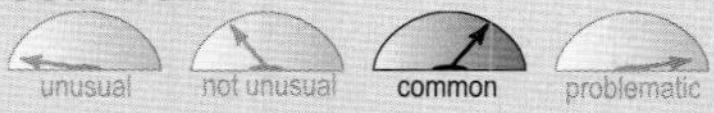

- Many experience and/or can be significant in amount
- Tolerance to sedative effect may develop with long-term use

What to Do About Side Effects

- Wait
- Wait
- Wait
- Lower the dose
- Switch to an SSRI or newer antidepressant

Best Augmenting Agents for Side Effects

- Many side effects cannot be improved with an augmenting agent

DOSING AND USE

Usual Dosage Range

- 75–150 mg/day

Dosage Forms

- Capsule 25 mg
- Tablet 75 mg

How to Dose

- 75 mg/day once daily or in divided doses; gradually increase dose to achieve desired therapeutic effect; maximum dose 300 mg/day

Dosing Tips

- If given in a single dose, should generally be administered at bedtime because of its sedative properties
- If given in split doses, largest dose should generally be given at bedtime because of its sedative properties
- If patients experience nightmares, split dose and do not give large dose at bedtime
- Patients treated for chronic pain may only require lower doses
- Risk of seizure increases with dose
- If intolerable anxiety, insomnia, agitation, akathisia, or activation occur either upon dosing initiation or discontinuation, consider the possibility of activated bipolar disorder, and switch to a mood stabilizer or an atypical antipsychotic

Overdose

- Death may occur; convulsions, cardiac dysrhythmias, severe hypotension, CNS depression, coma, changes in EKG

Long-Term Use

- Safe

Habit Forming

- No

How to Stop

- Taper to avoid withdrawal effects
- Even with gradual dose reduction some withdrawal symptoms may appear within the first 2 weeks
- Many patients tolerate 50% dose reduction for 3 days, then another 50% reduction for 3 days, then discontinuation
- If withdrawal symptoms emerge during discontinuation, raise dose to stop symptoms and then restart withdrawal much more slowly

Pharmacokinetics

- Substrate for CYP450 2D6
- Half-life approximately 14–40 hours

Drug Interactions

- Tramadol increases the risk of seizures in patients taking TCAs
- Use of TCAs with anticholinergic drugs may result in paralytic ileus or hyperthermia
- Fluoxetine, paroxetine, bupropion, duloxetine, and other CYP450 2D6 inhibitors may increase TCA concentrations
- Cimetidine may increase plasma concentrations of TCAs and cause anticholinergic symptoms
- Phenothiazines or haloperidol may raise TCA blood concentrations
- May alter effects of antihypertensive drugs; may inhibit hypotensive effects of clonidine
- Use of TCAs with sympathomimetic agents may increase sympathetic activity
- Methylphenidate may inhibit metabolism of TCAs
- Activation and agitation, especially following switching or adding antidepressants, may represent the

induction of a bipolar state, especially a mixed dysphoric bipolar II condition sometimes associated with suicidal ideation, and require the addition of lithium, a mood stabilizer or an atypical antipsychotic, and/or discontinuation of dothiepin

Other Warnings/ Precautions

- Add or initiate other antidepressants with caution for up to 2 weeks after discontinuing dothiepin
- Generally, do not use with MAOIs, including 14 days after MAOIs are stopped; do not start an MAOI for at least 5 half-lives (5 to 7 days for most drugs) after discontinuing dothiepin, but see Pearls
- Use with caution in patients with history of seizures, urinary retention, angle-closure glaucoma, hyperthyroidism, and in patients recovering from myocardial infarction
- TCAs can increase QTc interval, especially at toxic doses, which can be attained not only by overdose but also by combining with drugs that inhibit TCA metabolism via CYP450 2D6, potentially causing torsade de pointes-type arrhythmia or sudden death
- Because TCAs can prolong QTc interval, use with caution in patients who have bradycardia or who are taking drugs that can induce bradycardia (e.g., beta blockers, calcium channel blockers, clonidine, digitalis)
- Because TCAs can prolong QTc interval, use with caution in patients who have hypokalemia and/or hypomagnesemia or who are taking drugs that can induce hypokalemia and/or magnesemia (e.g., diuretics, stimulant laxatives, intravenous amphotericin B, glucocorticoids, tetracosactide)
- When treating children, carefully weigh the risks and benefits of pharmacological treatment against the risks and benefits of nontreatment with antidepressants and make sure to document this in the patient's chart
- Distribute the brochures provided by the FDA and the drug companies
- Warn patients and their caregivers about the possibility of activating side effects and advise them to report such symptoms immediately
- Monitor patients for activation of suicidal ideation, especially children and adolescents

Do Not Use

- If patient is recovering from myocardial infarction
- If patient is taking agents capable of significantly prolonging QTc interval (e.g., pimozide, thioridazine, selected antiarrhythmics, moxifloxacin, sparfloxacin)
- If there is a history of QTc prolongation or cardiac arrhythmia, recent acute myocardial infarction, uncompensated heart failure
- If patient is taking drugs that inhibit TCA metabolism, including CYP450 2D6 inhibitors, except by an expert
- If there is reduced CYP450 2D6 function, such as patients who are poor 2D6 metabolizers, except by an expert and at low doses
- If there is a proven allergy to dothiepin

SPECIAL POPULATIONS

Renal Impairment

- Use with caution

Hepatic Impairment

- Use with caution

Cardiac Impairment

- Baseline ECG is recommended
- TCAs have been reported to cause arrhythmias, prolongation of conduction time, orthostatic hypotension, sinus tachycardia, and heart failure, especially in the diseased heart
- Myocardial infarction and stroke have been reported with TCAs
- TCAs produce QTc prolongation, which may be enhanced by the existence of bradycardia, hypokalemia, congenital or acquired long QTc interval, which should be evaluated prior to administering dothiepin
- Use with caution if treating concomitantly with a medication likely to produce prolonged bradycardia, hypokalemia, slowing of intracardiac conduction, or prolongation of the QTc interval

- Avoid TCAs in patients with a known history of QTc prolongation, recent acute myocardial infarction, and uncompensated heart failure
- TCAs may cause a sustained increase in heart rate in patients with ischemic heart disease and may worsen (decrease) heart rate variability, an independent risk of mortality in cardiac populations
- Since SSRIs may improve (increase) heart rate variability in patients following a myocardial infarct and may improve survival as well as mood in patients with acute angina or following a myocardial infarction, these are more appropriate agents for cardiac population than tricyclic/tetracyclic antidepressants

✻ Risk/benefit ratio may not justify use of TCAs in cardiac impairment

Elderly

- Baseline ECG is recommended for patients over age 50
- May be more sensitive to anticholinergic, cardiovascular, hypotensive, and sedative effects
- Reduction in the risk of suicidality with antidepressants compared to placebo in adults age 65 and older

Children and Adolescents

- Carefully weigh the risks and benefits of pharmacological treatment against the risks and benefits of nontreatment with antidepressants and make sure to document this in the patient's chart
- Monitor patients face-to-face regularly, particularly during the first several weeks of treatment
- Use with caution, observing for activation of known or unknown bipolar disorder and/or suicidal ideation, and inform parents or guardians of this risk so they can help observe child or adolescent patients
- Not recommended for use in children under age 18
- Several studies show lack of efficacy of TCAs for depression
- May be used to treat enuresis or hyperactive/impulsive behaviors
- Some cases of sudden death have occurred in children taking TCAs

Pregnancy

- Controlled studies have not been conducted in pregnant women
- Crosses the placenta
- Adverse effects have been reported in infants whose mothers took a TCA (lethargy, withdrawal symptoms, fetal malformations)
- Not generally recommended for use during pregnancy, especially during first trimester
- Must weigh the risk of treatment (first trimester fetal development, third trimester newborn delivery) to the child against the risk of no treatment (recurrence of depression, maternal health, infant bonding) to the mother and child
- For many patients this may mean continuing treatment during pregnancy

Breast Feeding

- Some drug is found in mother's breast milk

✻ Recommended either to discontinue drug or bottle feed

- Immediate postpartum period is a high-risk time for depression, especially in women who have had prior depressive episodes, so drug may need to be reinstituted late in the third trimester or shortly after childbirth to prevent a recurrence during the postpartum period
- Must weigh benefits of breast feeding with risks and benefits of antidepressant treatment versus nontreatment to both the infant and the mother
- For many patients this may mean continuing treatment during breast feeding

THE ART OF PSYCHOPHARMACOLOGY

Potential Advantages

- Patients with insomnia
- Severe or treatment-resistant depression
- Anxious depression

Potential Disadvantages

- Pediatric and geriatric patients
- Patients concerned with weight gain
- Cardiac patients

Primary Target Symptoms

- Depressed mood
- Chronic pain

Pearls

- ✽ Close structural similarity to amitriptyline
- TCAs are often a first-line treatment option for chronic pain
- TCAs are no longer generally considered a first-line option for depression because of their side effect profile
- TCAs continue to be useful for severe or treatment-resistant depression
- TCAs may aggravate psychotic symptoms
- Alcohol should be avoided because of additive CNS effects
- Underweight patients may be more susceptible to adverse cardiovascular effects
- Children, patients with inadequate hydration, and patients with cardiac disease may be more susceptible to TCA-induced cardiotoxicity than healthy adults
- For the expert only: a heroic treatment (but potentially dangerous) for severely treatment-resistant patients is to give simultaneously with MAOIs for patients who fail to respond to numerous other antidepressants, but generally recommend a different TCA than dothiepin for this use
- If this option is elected, start the MAOI with the tricyclic/tetracyclic antidepressant simultaneously at low doses after appropriate drug washout, then alternately increase doses of these agents every few days to a week as tolerated
- Although very strict dietary and concomitant drug restrictions must be observed to prevent hypertensive crises and serotonin syndrome, the most common side effects of MAOI and tricyclic/tetracyclic antidepressant combinations may be weight gain and orthostatic hypotension
- Patients on TCAs should be aware that they may experience symptoms such as photosensitivity or blue-green urine
- SSRIs may be more effective than TCAs in women, and TCAs may be more effective than SSRIs in men
- Since tricyclic/tetracyclic antidepressants are substrates for CYP450 2D6, and 7% of the population (especially Caucasians) may have a genetic variant leading to reduced activity of 2D6, such patients may not safely tolerate normal doses of tricyclic/tetracyclic antidepressants and may require dose reduction
- Phenotypic testing may be necessary to detect this genetic variant prior to dosing with a tricyclic/tetracyclic antidepressant, especially in vulnerable populations such as children, elderly, cardiac populations, and those on concomitant medications
- Patients who seem to have extraordinarily severe side effects at normal or low doses may have this phenotypic CYP450 2D6 variant and require low doses or switching to another antidepressant not metabolized by 2D6

Suggested Reading

Anderson IM. Meta-analytical studies on new antidepressants. Br Med Bull 2001; 57:161–78.

Anderson IM. Selective serotonin reuptake inhibitors versus tricyclic antidepressants: a meta-analysis of efficacy and tolerability. J Aff Disorders 2000;58:19–36.

Donovan S, Dearden L, Richardson L. The tolerability of dothiepin: a review of clinical studies between 1963 and 1990 in over 13,000 depressed patients. Prog Neuropsychopharmacol Biol Psychiatry 1994; 18:1143–62.

Lancaster SG, Gonzalez JP. Dothiepin. A review of its pharmacodynamic and pharmacokinetic properties, and therapeutic efficacy in depressive illness. Drugs 1989;38:123–47.

THERAPEUTICS

Brands • Sinequan, Silenor
see index for additional brand names

Generic? Yes

Class

- Neuroscience-based Nomenclature: serotonin, norepinephrine multi-modal (SN-MM)
- Tricyclic antidepressant (TCA)
- Serotonin and norepinephrine/noradrenaline reuptake inhibitor
- Antihistamine

Commonly Prescribed for

(bold for FDA approved)

- **Psychoneurotic patient with depression and/or anxiety**
- **Depression and/or anxiety associated with alcoholism**
- **Depression and/or anxiety associated with organic disease**
- **Psychotic depressive disorders with associated anxiety**
- **Involutional depression**
- **Manic-depressive disorder**
- **Insomnia (difficulty with sleep maintenance) (Silenor only)**

✻ Pruritus/itching (topical)
- Dermatitis, atopic (topical)
- Lichen simplex chronicus (topical)
- Anxiety
- Neuropathic pain/chronic pain
- Treatment-resistant depression

How the Drug Works

At antidepressant doses:

- Boosts neurotransmitters serotonin and norepinephrine/noradrenaline
- Blocks serotonin reuptake pump (serotonin transporter), presumably increasing serotonergic neurotransmission
- Blocks norepinephrine reuptake pump (norepinephrine transporter), presumably increasing noradrenergic neurotransmission
- Presumably desensitizes both serotonin 1A receptors and beta adrenergic receptors
- Since dopamine is inactivated by norepinephrine reuptake in frontal cortex, which largely lacks dopamine transporters, doxepin can thus increase dopamine neurotransmission in this part of the brain
- May be effective in treating skin conditions because of its strong antihistamine properties

At hypnotic doses (3–6 mg/day):

- Selectively and potently blocks histamine 1 receptors, presumably decreasing wakefulness and thus promoting sleep

How Long Until It Works

- May have immediate effects in treating insomnia or anxiety
- Onset of therapeutic actions in depression is usually not immediate, but often delayed 2–4 weeks
- If it is not working within 6–8 weeks for depression, it may require a dosage increase or it may not work at all
- May continue to work for many years to prevent relapse of depressive symptoms
- May also work long-term for insomnia (studied for up to 12 weeks)

If It Works

- The goal of treatment of depression is complete remission of current symptoms as well as prevention of future relapses
- The goal of treatment of insomnia is to improve quality of sleep, including effects on total wake time and number of nighttime awakenings.
- The goal of treatment of chronic neuropathic pain is to reduce symptoms as much as possible, especially in combination with other treatments
- Treatment of depression most often reduces or even eliminates symptoms, but not a cure since symptoms can recur after medicine stopped
- Treatment of chronic neuropathic pain may reduce symptoms, but rarely eliminates them completely, and is not a cure since symptoms can recur after medicine is stopped
- Continue treatment of depression until all symptoms are gone (remission)
- Once symptoms of depression are gone, continue treating for 1 year for the first episode of depression
- For second and subsequent episodes of depression, treatment may need to be indefinite

- Use in anxiety disorders, chronic pain, and skin conditions may also need to be indefinite, but long-term treatment is not well studied in these conditions

If It Doesn't Work

- Many depressed patients have only a partial response where some symptoms are improved but others persist (especially insomnia, fatigue, and problems concentrating)
- Other depressed patients may be nonresponders, sometimes called treatment-resistant or treatment-refractory
- Consider increasing dose, switching to another agent or adding an appropriate augmenting agent
- Consider psychotherapy
- Consider evaluation for another diagnosis or for a comorbid condition (e.g., medical illness, substance abuse, etc.)
- Some patients may experience apparent lack of consistent efficacy due to activation of latent or underlying bipolar disorder, and require antidepressant discontinuation and a switch to a mood stabilizer
- If insomnia does not improve after 7–10 days, it may be a manifestation of a primary psychiatric or physical illness such as obstructive sleep apnea or restless leg syndrome, which requires independent evaluation

Best Augmenting Combos for Partial Response or Treatment Resistance

- Lithium, buspirone, thyroid hormone (for depression)
- Trazodone, GABA-ergic sedative hypnotics (for insomnia)
- Gabapentin, tiagabine, other anticonvulsants, even opiates if done by experts while monitoring carefully in difficult cases (for chronic pain)

Tests

- Baseline ECG is recommended for patients over age 50 (not for Silenor)

✽ Since tricyclic and tetracyclic antidepressants are frequently associated with weight gain, before starting treatment, weigh all patients and determine if the patient is already overweight (BMI 25.0–29.9) or obese (BMI ≥30)

- Before giving a drug that can cause weight gain to an overweight or obese patient, consider determining whether the patient already has pre-diabetes (fasting plasma glucose 100–125 mg/dL), diabetes (fasting plasma glucose >126 mg/dL), or dyslipidemia (increased total cholesterol, LDL cholesterol, and triglycerides; decreased HDL cholesterol), and treat or refer such patients for treatment including nutrition and weight management, physical activity counseling, smoking cessation, and medical management

✽ Monitor weight and BMI during treatment

✽ While giving a drug to a patient who has gained >5% of initial weight, consider evaluating for the presence of pre-diabetes, diabetes, or dyslipidemia, or consider switching to a different antidepressant

- EKGs may be useful for selected patients (e.g., those with personal or family history of QTc prolongation; cardiac arrhythmia; recent myocardial infarction; uncompensated heart failure; or taking agents that prolong QTc interval such as pimozide, thioridazine, selected antiarrhythmics, moxifloxacin, sparfloxacin, etc.)
- Patients at risk for electrolyte disturbances (e.g., patients on diuretic therapy) should have baseline and periodic serum potassium and magnesium measurements

SIDE EFFECTS

How Drug Causes Side Effects

- At antidepressant doses, anticholinergic activity may explain sedative effects, dry mouth, constipation, and blurred vision
- Sedative effects and weight gain may be due to antihistamine properties
- At antidepressant doses, blockade of alpha adrenergic 1 receptors may explain dizziness, sedation, and hypotension
- Cardiac arrhythmias and seizures, especially in overdose, may be caused by blockade of ion channels

Notable Side Effects

Antidepressant Doses

- Blurred vision, constipation, urinary retention, increased appetite, dry mouth, nausea, diarrhea, heartburn, unusual taste in mouth, weight gain

- Fatigue, weakness, dizziness, sedation, headache, anxiety, nervousness, restlessness
- Sexual dysfunction, sweating
- Topical: burning, stinging, itching, or swelling at application site

Hypnotic Doses
- Few side effects at low doses (3–6 mg/day), the most common being somnolence/sedation

Life-Threatening or Dangerous Side Effects
- Paralytic ileus, hyperthermia (TCAs + anticholinergic agents)
- Lowered seizure threshold and rare seizures
- Orthostatic hypotension, sudden death, arrhythmias, tachycardia
- QTc prolongation
- Hepatic failure, extrapyramidal symptoms
- Increased intraocular pressure, increased psychotic symptoms
- Rare induction of mania
- Rare activation of suicidal ideation and behavior (suicidality) (short-term studies did not show an increase in the risk of suicidality with antidepressants compared to placebo beyond age 24)

Weight Gain
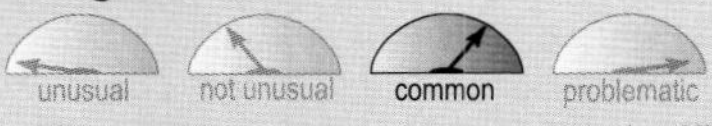

- Many experience and/or can be significant in amount (antidepressant doses)
- Can increase appetite and carbohydrate craving
- Weight gain is unusual at hypnotic doses

Sedation
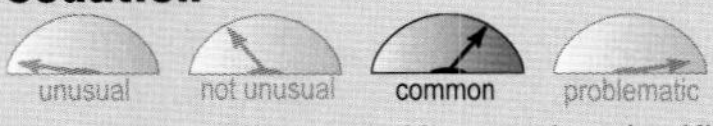

- Many experience and/or can be significant in amount
- Tolerance to sedative effect may develop with long-term use
- Sedation is not unusual at hypnotic doses

What to Do About Side Effects
- Wait
- Wait
- Wait
- Lower the dose
- Switch to an SSRI or newer antidepressant
- Switch to another hypnotic

Best Augmenting Agents for Side Effects
- Many side effects cannot be improved with an augmenting agent

DOSING AND USE

Usual Dosage Range
- 75–150 mg/day for depression
- 3–6 mg at bedtime for insomnia

Dosage Forms
- Capsule 10 mg, 25 mg, 50 mg, 75 mg, 100 mg, 150 mg
- Solution 10 mg/mL
- Topical 5%
- Tablet 3 mg, 6 mg

How to Dose
- Initial 25 mg/day at bedtime; increase by 25 mg every 3–7 days
- 75 mg/day; increase gradually until desired efficacy is achieved; can be dosed once a day at bedtime or in divided doses; maximum dose 300 mg/day
- Topical: apply thin film 4 times a day (or every 3–4 hours while awake)
- Insomnia: 6 mg once daily, 30 minutes before bedtime; should not be taken within 3 hours of a meal; maximum dose 6 mg/day

Dosing Tips
- If given in a single antidepressant dose, should generally be administered at bedtime because of its sedative properties
- If given in split antidepressant doses, largest dose should generally be given at bedtime because of its sedative properties
- If patients experience nightmares, split antidepressant dose and do not give large dose at bedtime
- Patients treated for chronic pain may only require lower doses
- Patients treated for insomnia may benefit from doses of 3–6 mg at bedtime
- Liquid formulation should be diluted with water or juice, excluding grape juice
- 150-mg capsule available only for maintenance use, not initial therapy

✽ Topical administration is absorbed systematically and can cause the

same systematic side effects as oral administration
- If intolerable anxiety, insomnia, agitation, akathisia, or activation occur either upon dosing initiation or discontinuation, consider the possibility of activated bipolar disorder, and switch to a mood stabilizer or an atypical antipsychotic

Overdose
- Death may occur; convulsions, cardiac dysrhythmias, severe hypotension, CNS depression, coma, changes in EKG

Long-Term Use
- Safe

Habit Forming
- No

How to Stop
- At antidepressant doses, taper to avoid withdrawal effects
- Even with gradual dose reduction some withdrawal symptoms may appear within the first 2 weeks
- Many patients tolerate 50% dose reduction for 3 days, then another 50% reduction for 3 days, then discontinuation
- If withdrawal symptoms emerge during discontinuation, raise dose to stop symptoms and then restart withdrawal much more slowly
- Taper not necessary for low doses (3–6 mg/day); withdrawal effects generally not observed

Pharmacokinetics
- Substrate for CYP450 2D6
- Half-life approximately 8–24 hours

Drug Interactions
- Tramadol increases the risk of seizures in patients taking TCAs
- Use of TCAs with anticholinergic drugs may result in paralytic ileus or hyperthermia
- Fluoxetine, paroxetine, bupropion, duloxetine, and other CYP450 2D6 inhibitors may increase TCA concentrations
- Cimetidine may increase plasma concentrations of TCAs and cause anticholinergic symptoms
- Phenothiazines or haloperidol may raise TCA blood concentrations
- May alter effects of antihypertensive drugs; may inhibit hypotensive effects of clonidine
- Use with sympathomimetic agents may increase sympathetic activity
- Methylphenidate may inhibit metabolism of TCAs
- Most drug interactions may be less likely at low doses (1–6 mg/day) due to the lack of effects on receptors other than the histamine 1 receptors
- Activation and agitation, especially following switching or adding antidepressants, may represent the induction of a bipolar state, especially a mixed dysphoric bipolar II condition sometimes associated with suicidal ideation, and require the addition of lithium, a mood stabilizer or an atypical antipsychotic, and/or discontinuation of doxepin

Other Warnings/ Precautions
- Add or initiate other antidepressants with caution for up to 2 weeks after discontinuing doxepin
- Generally, do not use with MAOIs, including 14 days after MAOIs are stopped; do not start an MAOI for at least 5 half-lives (5 to 7 days for most drugs) after discontinuing doxepin, but see Pearls
- Use with caution in patients with history of seizures, urinary retention, angle-closure glaucoma, hyperthyroidism
- TCAs can increase QTc interval, especially at toxic doses, which can be attained not only by overdose but also by combining with drugs that inhibit TCA metabolism via CYP450 2D6, potentially causing torsade de pointes-type arrhythmia or sudden death
- Because TCAs can prolong QTc interval, use with caution in patients who have bradycardia or who are taking drugs that can induce bradycardia (e.g., beta blockers, calcium channel blockers, clonidine, digitalis)
- Because TCAs can prolong QTc interval, use with caution in patients who have hypokalemia and/or hypomagnesemia or who are taking drugs that can induce hypokalemia and/or magnesemia (e.g.,

diuretics, stimulant laxatives, intravenous amphotericin B, glucocorticoids, tetracosactide)
- When treating children, carefully weigh the risks and benefits of pharmacological treatment against the risks and benefits of nontreatment with antidepressants and make sure to document this in the patient's chart
- Distribute the brochures provided by the FDA and the drug companies
- Warn patients and their caregivers about the possibility of activating side effects and advise them to report such symptoms immediately
- Monitor patients for activation of suicidal ideation, especially children and adolescents

Do Not Use

- If patient is recovering from myocardial infarction
- If patient is taking agents capable of significantly prolonging QTc interval (e.g., pimozide, thioridazine, selected antiarrhythmics, moxifloxacin, sparfloxacin)
- If there is a history of QTc prolongation or cardiac arrhythmia, recent acute myocardial infarction, uncompensated heart failure
- If patient is taking drugs that inhibit TCA metabolism, including CYP450 2D6 inhibitors, except by an expert
- If there is reduced CYP450 2D6 function, such as patients who are poor 2D6 metabolizers, except by an expert and at low doses
- If patient has angle-closure glaucoma or severe urinary retention
- If there is a proven allergy to doxepin

SPECIAL POPULATIONS

Renal Impairment

- Use with caution

Hepatic Impairment

- Use with caution – may need lower than usual adult dose

Cardiac Impairment

- Baseline ECG is recommended (not for Silenor)
- TCAs have been reported to cause arrhythmias, prolongation of conduction time, orthostatic hypotension, sinus tachycardia, and heart failure, especially in the diseased heart
- Myocardial infarction and stroke have been reported with TCAs
- TCAs produce QTc prolongation, which may be enhanced by the existence of bradycardia, hypokalemia, congenital or acquired long QTc interval, which should be evaluated prior to administering doxepin
- Use with caution if treating concomitantly with a medication likely to produce prolonged bradycardia, hypokalemia, slowing of intracardiac conduction, or prolongation of the QTc interval
- Avoid TCAs in patients with a known history of QTc prolongation, recent acute myocardial infarction, and uncompensated heart failure
- TCAs may cause a sustained increase in heart rate in patients with ischemic heart disease and may worsen (decrease) heart rate variability, an independent risk of mortality in cardiac populations
- Since SSRIs may improve (increase) heart rate variability in patients following a myocardial infarct and may improve survival as well as mood in patients with acute angina or following a myocardial infarction, these are more appropriate agents for cardiac population than tricyclic/tetracyclic antidepressants

✽ Risk/benefit ratio may not justify use of TCAs in cardiac impairment

Elderly

- Baseline ECG is recommended for patients over age 50 (not for Silenor)
- May be more sensitive to anticholinergic, cardiovascular, hypotensive, and sedative effects
- Low-dose doxepin (3–6 mg/day) has been studied and found effective for insomnia in elderly patients; recommended dose is 3 mg/day
- Reduction in the risk of suicidality with antidepressants compared to placebo in adults age 65 and older

Children and Adolescents

- Carefully weigh the risks and benefits of pharmacological treatment against

the risks and benefits of nontreatment with antidepressants and make sure to document this in the patient's chart
- Monitor patients face-to-face regularly, particularly during the first several weeks of treatment
- Use with caution, observing for activation of known or unknown bipolar disorder and/or suicidal ideation, and inform parents or guardians of this risk so they can help observe child or adolescent patients
- Not recommended for use in children under age 12
- Several studies show lack of efficacy of TCAs for depression
- May be used to treat enuresis or hyperactive/impulsive behaviors
- Some cases of sudden death have occurred in children taking TCAs
- Initial dose 25–50 mg/day; maximum 100 mg/day

Pregnancy

- Effective June 30, 2015, the US FDA requires changes to the content and format of pregnancy and lactation information in prescription drug labels, including the elimination of the pregnancy letter categories; the Pregnancy and Lactation Labeling Rule (PLLR or final rule) applies only to prescription drugs and will be phased in gradually for drugs approved on or after June 30, 2001
- Controlled studies have not been conducted in pregnant women
- Crosses the placenta
- Adverse effects have been reported in infants whose mothers took a TCA (lethargy, withdrawal symptoms, fetal malformations)
- Not generally recommended for use during pregnancy, especially during first trimester
- Must weigh the risk of treatment (first trimester fetal development, third trimester newborn delivery) to the child against the risk of no treatment (recurrence of depression, maternal health, infant bonding) to the mother and child
- For many patients this may mean continuing treatment during pregnancy for depression

Breast Feeding

- Some drug is found in mother's breast milk
- Significant drug levels have been detected in some nursing infants

✻ Recommended either to discontinue drug or bottle feed

- Immediate postpartum period is a high-risk time for depression, especially in women who have had prior depressive episodes, so drug may need to be reinstituted late in the third trimester or shortly after childbirth to prevent a recurrence during the postpartum period
- Must weigh benefits of breast feeding with risks and benefits of antidepressant treatment versus nontreatment to both the infant and the mother
- For many patients this may mean continuing treatment during breast feeding

THE ART OF PSYCHOPHARMACOLOGY

Potential Advantages

- Patients with insomnia
- Severe or treatment-resistant depression
- Patients with neurodermatitis and itching

Potential Disadvantages

- Pediatric and geriatric patients
- Patients concerned with weight gain
- Cardiac patients

Primary Target Symptoms

- Depressed mood
- Anxiety
- Disturbed sleep, energy
- Somatic symptoms
- Itching skin

Pearls

✻ Only TCA available in topical formulation

✻ Topical administration may reduce symptoms in patients with various neurodermatitis syndromes, especially itching

- Although low doses are specifically approved for sleep maintenance in insomnia they may also work for sleep onset in insomnia
- At low doses, one of the few hypnotics that is not a controlled substance, because it

has no risk of dependence, withdrawal, or abuse
- At low doses, there is no tolerance to hypnotic actions seen
- At low doses, there is little or no weight gain
- At low doses doxepin is selective for the histamine 1 receptor and thus can improve sleep without causing side effects associated with other neurotransmitter systems
- In particular, low-dose doxepin does not appear to cause anticholinergic symptoms, memory impairment, or weight gain, nor is there evidence of tolerance, rebound insomnia, or withdrawal effects
- TCAs are often a first-line treatment option for chronic pain
- TCAs are no longer generally considered a first-line option for depression because of their side effect profile
- TCAs continue to be useful for severe or treatment-resistant depression
- TCAs may aggravate psychotic symptoms
- Alcohol should be avoided because of additive CNS effects
- Underweight patients may be more susceptible to adverse cardiovascular effects
- Children, patients with inadequate hydration, and patients with cardiac disease may be more susceptible to TCA-induced cardiotoxicity than healthy adults
- For the expert only: although generally prohibited, a heroic but potentially dangerous treatment for severely treatment-resistant patients is to give a tricyclic/tetracyclic antidepressant other than clomipramine simultaneously with an MAOI for patients who fail to respond to numerous other antidepressants
- If this option is elected, start the MAOI with the tricyclic/tetracyclic antidepressant simultaneously at low doses after appropriate drug washout, then alternately increase doses of these agents every few days to a week as tolerated
- Although very strict dietary and concomitant drug restrictions must be observed to prevent hypertensive crises and serotonin syndrome, the most common side effects of MAOI/tricyclic or tetracyclic combinations may be weight gain and orthostatic hypotension
- Patients on TCAs should be aware that they may experience symptoms such as photosensitivity or blue-green urine
- SSRIs may be more effective than TCAs in women, and TCAs may be more effective than SSRIs in men
- Since tricyclic/tetracyclic antidepressants are substrates for CYP450 2D6, and 7% of the population (especially Caucasians) may have a genetic variant leading to reduced activity of 2D6, such patients may not safely tolerate normal doses of tricyclic/tetracyclic antidepressants and may require dose reduction
- Phenotypic testing may be necessary to detect this genetic variant prior to dosing with a tricyclic/tetracyclic antidepressant, especially in vulnerable populations such as children, elderly, cardiac populations, and those on concomitant medications
- Patients who seem to have extraordinarily severe side effects at normal or low doses may have this phenotypic CYP450 2D6 variant and require low doses or switching to another antidepressant not metabolized by 2D6

Suggested Reading

Anderson IM. Meta-analytical studies on new antidepressants. Br Med Bull 2001;57:161–78.

Anderson IM. Selective serotonin reuptake inhibitors versus tricyclic antidepressants: a meta-analysis of efficacy and tolerability. J Aff Disorders 2000;58:19–36.

Godfrey RG. A guide to the understanding and use of tricyclic antidepressants in the overall management of fibromyalgia and other chronic pain syndromes. Arch Intern Med 1996;156:1047–52.

Roth T, Rogowski R, Hull S, et al. Efficacy and safety of doxepin 1 mg, 3 mg, and 6 mg in adults with primary insomnia. Sleep 2007;30(11):1555–61.

Singh H, Becker PM. Novel therapeutic usage of low-dose doxepin hydrochloride. Expert Opin Investig Drugs 2007;16(8):1295–305.

Stahl SM. Selective histamine 1 antagonism: novel hypnotic and pharmacologic actions challenge classical notions of antihistamines. CNS Spectrums 2008;13(12):855–65.

THERAPEUTICS

Brands • Cymbalta
see index for additional brand names

Generic? Yes

Class
- Neuroscience-based Nomenclature: serotonin norepinephrine reuptake inhibitor (SN-RI)
- SNRI (dual serotonin and norepinephrine reuptake inhibitor); may be classified as an antidepressant, but it is not just an antidepressant

Commonly Prescribed for
(bold for FDA approved)
- **Major depressive disorder**
- **Diabetic peripheral neuropathic pain (DPNP)**
- **Fibromyalgia**
- **Generalized anxiety disorder, acute and maintenance**
- **Chronic musculoskeletal pain**
- Stress urinary incontinence
- Neuropathic pain/chronic pain
- Other anxiety disorders

How the Drug Works
- Boosts neurotransmitters serotonin, norepinephrine/noradrenaline, and dopamine
- Blocks serotonin reuptake pump (serotonin transporter), presumably increasing serotonergic neurotransmission
- Blocks norepinephrine reuptake pump (norepinephrine transporter), presumably increasing noradrenergic neurotransmission
- Presumably desensitizes both serotonin 1A receptors and beta adrenergic receptors
- Since dopamine is inactivated by norepinephrine reuptake in frontal cortex, which largely lacks dopamine transporters, duloxetine can increase dopamine neurotransmission in this part of the brain
- Weakly blocks dopamine reuptake pump (dopamine transporter), and may increase dopamine neurotransmission

How Long Until It Works
- Onset of therapeutic actions usually not immediate, but often delayed 2–4 weeks for depression
- If it is not working within 6–8 weeks for depression, it may require a dosage increase or it may not work at all
- Can reduce neuropathic pain within a week, but onset can take longer
- May continue to work for many years to prevent relapse of depressive symptoms or prevent worsening of painful symptoms
- Vasomotor symptoms in perimenopausal women with or without depression may improve within 1 week

If It Works
- The goal of treatment of depression and anxiety disorders is complete remission of current symptoms as well as prevention of future relapses
- The goal of treatment of diabetic peripheral neuropathic pain and fibromyalgia and chronic neuropathic pain is to reduce symptoms as much as possible, especially in combination with other treatments
- Treatment of depression most often reduces or even eliminates symptoms, but is not a cure since symptoms can recur after medicine stopped
- Treatment of diabetic peripheral neuropathic pain, fibromyalgia, and chronic neuropathic pain may reduce symptoms, but rarely eliminates them completely, and is not a cure since symptoms can recur after medicine is stopped
- Continue treatment of depression and anxiety disorders until all symptoms are gone (remission)
- Once symptoms of depression are gone, continue treating for 1 year for the first episode of depression
- For second and subsequent episodes of depression, treatment may need to be indefinite
- Use in anxiety disorders may also need to be indefinite
- Use in diabetic peripheral neuropathic pain, fibromyalgia, and chronic neuropathic pain may also need to be indefinite, but long-term treatment is not well studied in these conditions

If It Doesn't Work
- Many patients have only a partial response where some symptoms are improved but others persist (especially insomnia, fatigue, and problems concentrating)

- Other patients may be nonresponders, sometimes called treatment-resistant or treatment-refractory
- Some depressed patients who have an initial response may relapse even though they continue treatment, sometimes called "poop-out"
- Consider increasing dose, switching to another agent or adding an appropriate augmenting agent
- Consider psychotherapy for depression or biofeedback or hypnosis for pain
- Consider evaluation for another diagnosis or for a comorbid condition (e.g., medical illness, substance abuse, etc.)
- Consider the presence of noncompliance and counsel the patient
- Some patients may experience apparent lack of consistent efficacy due to activation of latent or underlying bipolar disorder, and require antidepressant discontinuation and a switch to a mood stabilizer

Best Augmenting Combos for Partial Response or Treatment Resistance

✽ Augmentation experience is limited compared to other antidepressants and treatments for neuropathic pain

✽ Adding other agents to duloxetine for treating depression could follow the same practice for augmenting SSRIs or other SNRIs if done by experts while monitoring carefully in difficult cases

- Although no controlled studies and little clinical experience, adding other agents for treating diabetic peripheral neuropathic pain and fibromyalgia and neuropathic pain could theoretically include gabapentin, pregabalin, and tiagabine, if done by experts while monitoring carefully in difficult cases
- Mirtazapine ("California rocket fuel" for depression; a potentially powerful dual serotonin and norepinephrine combination, but observe for activation of bipolar disorder and suicidal ideation)
- Bupropion, reboxetine, nortriptyline, desipramine, maprotiline, atomoxetine (all potentially powerful enhancers of noradrenergic action for depression, but observe for activation of bipolar disorder and suicidal ideation)
- Modafinil, especially for fatigue, sleepiness, and lack of concentration
- Mood stabilizers or atypical antipsychotics for bipolar depression, psychotic depression, or treatment-resistant depression
- Benzodiazepines
- If all else fails for anxiety disorders, consider gabapentin, pregabalin, or tiagabine
- Hypnotics or trazodone for insomnia
- Classically, lithium, buspirone, or thyroid hormone for depression

Tests

- Check blood pressure before initiating treatment and regularly during treatment

SIDE EFFECTS

How Drug Causes Side Effects

- Theoretically due to increases in serotonin and norepinephrine concentrations at receptors in parts of the brain and body other than those that cause therapeutic actions (e.g., unwanted actions of serotonin in sleep centers causing insomnia, unwanted actions of norepinephrine on acetylcholine release causing decreased appetite, increased blood pressure, urinary retention, etc.)
- Most side effects are immediate but often go away with time

Notable Side Effects

- Nausea, diarrhea, decreased appetite, dry mouth, constipation (dose-dependent)
- Insomnia, sedation, dizziness
- Sexual dysfunction (men: abnormal ejaculation/orgasm, impotence, decreased libido; women: abnormal orgasm)
- Sweating
- Increase in blood pressure (up to 2 mm Hg)
- Urinary retention

Life-Threatening or Dangerous Side Effects

- Rare seizures
- Rare induction of hypomania
- Rare activation of suicidal ideation, suicide attempts, and completed suicide
- Short-term studies did not show an increase in the risk of suicidality with antidepressants compared to placebo beyond age 24

Weight Gain

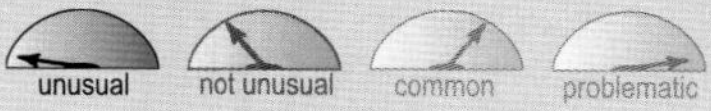

- Reported but not expected

Sedation

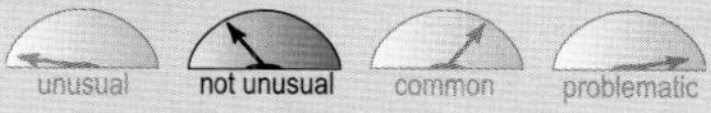

- Occurs in significant minority
- May also be activating in some patients

What to Do About Side Effects

- Wait
- Wait
- Wait
- Lower the dose
- In a few weeks, switch or add other drugs

Best Augmenting Agents for Side Effects

- For urinary hesitancy, give an alpha 1 blocker such as tamsulosin
- Often best to try another antidepressant monotherapy prior to resorting to augmentation strategies to treat side effects
- Trazodone or a hypnotic for insomnia
- Bupropion, sildenafil, vardenafil, or tadalafil for sexual dysfunction
- Benzodiazepines for jitteriness and anxiety, especially at initiation of treatment and especially for anxious patients
- Mirtazapine for insomnia, agitation, and gastrointestinal side effects
- Many side effects are dose-dependent (i.e., they increase as dose increases, or they reemerge until tolerance redevelops)
- Many side effects are time-dependent (i.e., they start immediately upon dosing and upon each dose increase, but go away with time)
- Activation and agitation may represent the induction of a bipolar state, especially a mixed dysphoric bipolar II condition sometimes associated with suicidal ideation, and require the addition of lithium, a mood stabilizer or an atypical antipsychotic, and/or discontinuation of duloxetine

DOSING AND USE

Usual Dosage Range

- 40–60 mg/day in 1–2 doses for depression
- 60 mg once daily for diabetic peripheral neuropathic pain and fibromyalgia
- 60 mg once daily for generalized anxiety disorder
- 40 mg twice daily for stress urinary incontinence

Dosage Forms

- Capsule 20 mg, 30 mg, 60 mg

How to Dose

- For depression, initial 40 mg/day in 2 doses; can increase to 60 mg/day in 1–2 doses if necessary; maximum dose generally 120 mg/day
- For neuropathic pain and fibromyalgia initial 30 mg once daily; increase to 60 mg once daily after 1 week; maximum dose generally 60 mg/day
- For generalized anxiety, initial 60 mg once daily; maximum dose generally 120 mg/day

Dosing Tips

- Studies have not demonstrated increased efficacy beyond 60 mg/day
- ✻ Some patients may require up to or more than 120 mg/day, but clinical experience is quite limited with high dosing
- In relapse prevention studies in depression, a significant percentage of patients who relapsed on 60 mg/day responded and remitted when the dose was increased to 120 mg/day
- In neuropathic pain and fibromyalgia doses above 60 mg/day have been associated with increased side effects without an increase in efficacy
- Some studies suggest that both serotonin and norepinephrine reuptake blockade are present at 40–60 mg/day
- Do not chew or crush and do not sprinkle on food or mix with food, but rather always swallow whole to avoid affecting enteric coating
- Some patients may require dosing above 120 mg/day in 2 divided doses, but this should be done with caution and by experts

Overdose
- Rare fatalities have been reported; serotonin syndrome, sedation, vomiting, seizures, coma, change in blood pressure

Long-Term Use
- Blood pressure should be monitored regularly

Habit Forming
- No

How to Stop
- Taper to avoid withdrawal effects (dizziness, nausea, vomiting, headache, paresthesias, irritability)
- Many patients tolerate 50% dose reduction for 3 days, then another 50% reduction for 3 days, then discontinuation

✻ If withdrawal symptoms emerge during discontinuation, raise dose to stop symptoms and then restart withdrawal much more slowly

Pharmacokinetics
- Elimination half-life approximately 12 hours
- Metabolized mainly by CYP450 2D6 and CYP450 1A2
- Inhibitor of CYP450 2D6 (probably clinically significant) and CYP450 1A2 (probably not clinically significant)
- Absorption may be delayed by up to 3 hours and clearance may be increased by one-third after an evening dose as compared to a morning dose
- Food does not affect absorption

Drug Interactions
- Can increase TCA levels; use with caution with TCAs or when switching from a TCA to duloxetine
- Can cause a fatal "serotonin syndrome" when combined with MAOIs, so do not use with MAOIs or for at least 14 days after MAOIs are stopped
- Possible increased risk of bleeding, especially when combined with anticoagulants (e.g., warfarin, NSAIDs)
- Do not start an MAOI for at least 5 half-lives (5 to 7 days for most drugs) after discontinuing duloxetine
- Inhibitors of CYP450 1A2, such as fluvoxamine, increase plasma levels of duloxetine and may require a dosage reduction of duloxetine
- Cigarette smoking induces CYP450 1A2 and may reduce plasma levels of duloxetine, but dosage modifications are not recommended for smokers

✻ Inhibitors of CYP450 2D6, such as paroxetine, fluoxetine, and quinidine, may increase plasma levels of duloxetine and require a dosage reduction of duloxetine

- Via CYP450 1A2 inhibition, duloxetine could theoretically reduce clearance of theophylline and clozapine; however, studies of coadministration with theophylline did not demonstrate significant effects of duloxetine on theophylline pharmacokinetics
- Via CYP450 2D6 inhibition, duloxetine could theoretically interfere with the analgesic actions of codeine, and increase the plasma levels of some beta blockers and of atomoxetine
- Via CYP450 2D6 inhibition, duloxetine could theoretically increase concentrations of thioridazine and cause dangerous cardiac arrhythmias

Other Warnings/ Precautions
- Use with caution in patients with history of seizures
- Use with caution in patients with bipolar disorder unless treated with concomitant mood-stabilizing agent
- Rare reports of hepatotoxicity; although causality has not been established, duloxetine should be discontinued in patients who develop jaundice or other evidence of significant liver dysfunction
- When treating children, carefully weigh the risks and benefits of pharmacological treatment against the risks and benefits of nontreatment with antidepressants and make sure to document this in the patient's chart
- Distribute the brochures provided by the FDA and the drug companies
- Warn patients and their caregivers about the possibility of activating side effects and advise them to report such symptoms immediately
- Monitor patients for activation of suicidal ideation, especially children and adolescents

- Duloxetine may increase blood pressure, so blood pressure should be monitored during treatment

Do Not Use
- If patient has uncontrolled angle-closure glaucoma
- If patient has substantial alcohol use
- If patient is taking an MAOI
- If patient is taking thioridazine
- If there is a proven allergy to duloxetine

SPECIAL POPULATIONS

Renal Impairment
- Dose adjustment generally not necessary for mild to moderate impairment
- Not recommended for use in patients with end-stage renal disease (requiring dialysis) or severe renal impairment

Hepatic Impairment
- Not to be administered to patients with any hepatic insufficiency
- Not recommended for use in patients with substantial alcohol use
- Increased risk of elevation of serum transaminase levels

Cardiac Impairment
- Drug should be used with caution
- Duloxetine may raise blood pressure

Elderly
- Some patients may tolerate lower doses better
- Reduction in the risk of suicidality with antidepressants compared to placebo in adults age 65 and older

Children and Adolescents
- Carefully weigh the risks and benefits of pharmacological treatment against the risks and benefits of nontreatment with antidepressants and make sure to document this in the patient's chart
- Monitor patients face-to-face regularly, particularly during the first several weeks of treatment
- Use with caution, observing for activation of known or unknown bipolar disorder and/or suicidal ideation, and inform parents or guardians of this risk so they can help observe child or adolescent patients
- Not studied, but can be used by experts

Pregnancy
- Effective June 30, 2015, the US FDA requires changes to the content and format of pregnancy and lactation information in prescription drug labels, including the elimination of the pregnancy letter categories; the Pregnancy and Lactation Labeling Rule (PLLR or final rule) applies only to prescription drugs and will be phased in gradually for drugs approved on or after June 30, 2001
- Controlled studies have not been conducted in pregnant women
- Not generally recommended for use during pregnancy, especially during first trimester
- Nonetheless, continuous treatment during pregnancy may be necessary and has not been proven to be harmful to the fetus
- Must weigh the risk of treatment (first trimester fetal development, third trimester newborn delivery) to the child against the risk of no treatment (recurrence of depression, maternal health, infant bonding) to the mother and child
- For many patients this may mean continuing treatment during pregnancy
- Neonates exposed to SSRIs or SNRIs late in the third trimester have developed complications requiring prolonged hospitalization, respiratory support, and tube feeding; reported symptoms are consistent with either a direct toxic effect of SSRIs and SNRIs or, possibly, a drug discontinuation syndrome, and include respiratory distress, cyanosis, apnea, seizures, temperature instability, feeding difficulty, vomiting, hypoglycemia, hypotonia, hypertonia, hyperreflexia, tremor, jitteriness, irritability, and constant crying

Breast Feeding
- Some drug is found in mother's breast milk
- If child becomes irritable or sedated, breast feeding or drug may need to be discontinued
- Immediate postpartum period is a high-risk time for depression, especially in women who have had prior depressive episodes,

so drug may need to be reinstituted late in the third trimester or shortly after childbirth to prevent a recurrence during the postpartum period
- Must weigh benefits of breast feeding with risks and benefits of antidepressant treatment versus nontreatment to both the infant and the mother
- For many patients, this may mean continuing treatment during breast feeding

THE ART OF PSYCHOPHARMACOLOGY

Potential Advantages

- Patients with physical symptoms of depression
- Patients with retarded depression
- Patients with atypical depression
- Patients with comorbid anxiety
- Patients with depression may have higher remission rates on SNRIs than on SSRIs
- Depressed patients with somatic symptoms, fatigue, and pain
- Patients who do not respond or do not remit on treatment with SSRIs

Potential Disadvantages

- Patients with urologic disorders, prostate disorders (e.g., older men)
- Patients sensitive to nausea

Primary Target Symptoms

- Depressed mood
- Energy, motivation, and interest
- Sleep disturbance
- Anxiety
- Physical symptoms
- Pain

Pearls

✻ Duloxetine has well-documented efficacy for the painful physical symptoms of depression
- Duloxetine has only somewhat greater potency for serotonin reuptake blockade than for norepinephrine reuptake blockade, but this is of unclear clinical significance as a differentiator from other SNRIs
- No head-to-head studies, but may have less hypertension than venlafaxine XR
- Powerful pro-noradrenergic actions may occur at doses greater than 60 mg/day
- Not well studied in ADHD, but may be effective

✻ Approved in many countries for stress urinary incontinence
- Patients may have higher remission rate for depression on SNRIs than on SSRIs
- Add or switch to or from pro-noradrenergic agents (e.g., atomoxetine, reboxetine, other SNRIs, mirtazapine, maprotiline, nortriptyline, desipramine, bupropion) with caution
- Add or switch to or from CYP450 2D6 substrates with caution (e.g., atomoxetine, maprotiline, nortriptyline, desipramine)
- Mechanism of action as SNRI suggests it may be effective in some patients who fail to respond to SSRIs

Suggested Reading

Arnold LM, Pritchett YL, D'Souza DN, et al. Duloxetine for the treatment of fibromyalgia in women: pooled results from two randomized, placebo-controlled trials. J Womens Health (Larchmt) 2007;16(8):1145–56.

Bymaster FP, Dreshfield-Ahmad LJ, Threlkeld PG, et al. Comparative affinity of duloxetine and venlafaxine for serotonin and norepinephrine transporters in vitro and in vivo, human serotonin receptor subtypes, and other neuronal receptors. Neuropsychopharmacology 2001;25(6):871–80.

Hartford J, Kornstein S, Liebowitz M, et al. Duloxetine as an SNRI treatment for generalized anxiety disorder: results from placebo and active-controlled trial. Int Clin Psychopharmacol 2007;22(3):167–74.

Muller N, Schennach R, Riedel M, Moller HJ. Duloxetine in the treatment of major psychiatric and neuropathic disorders. Expert Rev Neurother 2008;8(4):527–36.

Zinner NR. Duloxetine: a serotonin-noradrenaline re-uptake inhibitor for the treatment of stress urinary incontinence. Expert Opin Investig Drugs 2003;12(9):1559–66.

THERAPEUTICS

Brands • Lexapro

see index for additional brand names

Generic? Yes

Class

- Neuroscience-based Nomenclature: serotonin reuptake inhibitor (S-RI)
- SSRI (selective serotonin reuptake inhibitor); often classified as an antidepressant, but it is not just an antidepressant

Commonly Prescribed for

(bold for FDA approved)

- **Major depressive disorder (ages 12 and older)**
- **Generalized anxiety disorder (GAD)**
- Panic disorder
- Obsessive-compulsive disorder (OCD)
- Posttraumatic stress disorder (PTSD)
- Social anxiety disorder (social phobia)
- Premenstrual dysphoric disorder (PMDD)

How the Drug Works

- Boosts neurotransmitter serotonin
- Blocks serotonin reuptake pump (serotonin transporter)
- Desensitizes serotonin receptors, especially serotonin 1A autoreceptors
- Presumably increases serotonergic neurotransmission

How Long Until It Works

- Onset of therapeutic actions usually not immediate, but often delayed 2–4 weeks
- If it is not working within 6–8 weeks, it may require a dosage increase or it may not work at all
- May continue to work for many years to prevent relapse of symptoms

If It Works

- The goal of treatment is complete remission of current symptoms as well as prevention of future relapses
- Treatment most often reduces or even eliminates symptoms, but not a cure since symptoms can recur after medicine stopped
- Continue treatment until all symptoms are gone (remission) or significantly reduced (e.g., OCD, PTSD)
- Once symptoms gone, continue treating for 1 year for the first episode of depression
- For second and subsequent episodes of depression, treatment may need to be indefinite
- Use in anxiety disorders may also need to be indefinite

If It Doesn't Work

- Many patients have only a partial response where some symptoms are improved but others persist (especially insomnia, fatigue, and problems concentrating in depression)
- Other patients may be nonresponders, sometimes called treatment-resistant or treatment-refractory
- Some patients who have an initial response may relapse even though they continue treatment, sometimes called "poop-out"
- Consider increasing dose, switching to another agent or adding an appropriate augmenting agent
- Consider psychotherapy
- Consider evaluation for another diagnosis or for a comorbid condition (e.g., medical illness, substance abuse, etc.)
- Some patients may experience apparent lack of consistent efficacy due to activation of latent or underlying bipolar disorder, and require antidepressant discontinuation and a switch to a mood stabilizer

Best Augmenting Combos for Partial Response or Treatment Resistance

- Trazodone, especially for insomnia
- Bupropion, mirtazapine, reboxetine, or atomoxetine (use combinations of antidepressants with caution as this may activate bipolar disorder and suicidal ideation)
- Modafinil, especially for fatigue, sleepiness, and lack of concentration
- Mood stabilizers or atypical antipsychotics for bipolar depression, psychotic depression, treatment-resistant depression, or treatment-resistant anxiety disorders
- Benzodiazepines
- If all else fails for anxiety disorders, consider gabapentin or tiagabine
- Hypnotics for insomnia
- Classically, lithium, buspirone, or thyroid hormone

Tests
- None for healthy individuals

SIDE EFFECTS

How Drug Causes Side Effects
- Theoretically due to increases in serotonin concentrations at serotonin receptors in parts of the brain and body other than those that cause therapeutic actions (e.g., unwanted actions of serotonin in sleep centers causing insomnia, unwanted actions of serotonin in the gut causing diarrhea, etc.)
- Increasing serotonin can cause diminished dopamine release and might contribute to emotional flattening, cognitive slowing, and apathy in some patients
- Most side effects are immediate but often go away with time, in contrast to most therapeutic effects which are delayed and are enhanced over time

✻ As escitalopram has no known important secondary pharmacologic properties, its side effects are presumably all mediated by its serotonin reuptake blockade

Notable Side Effects
- Sexual dysfunction (men: delayed ejaculation, erectile dysfunction; men and women: decreased sexual desire, anorgasmia)
- Gastrointestinal (decreased appetite, nausea, diarrhea, constipation, dry mouth)
- Mostly central nervous system (insomnia but also sedation, agitation, tremors, headache, dizziness)
- Note: patients with diagnosed or undiagnosed bipolar or psychotic disorders may be more vulnerable to CNS-activating actions of SSRIs
- Autonomic (sweating)
- Bruising and rare bleeding
- Rare hyponatremia (mostly in elderly patients and generally reversible on discontinuation of escitalopram
- SIADH (syndrome of inappropriate antidiuretic hormone secretion)

Life-Threatening or Dangerous Side Effects
- Rare seizures
- Rare induction of mania
- Rare activation of suicidal ideation and behavior (suicidality) (short-term studies did not show an increase in the risk of suicidality with antidepressants compared to placebo beyond age 24)

Weight Gain
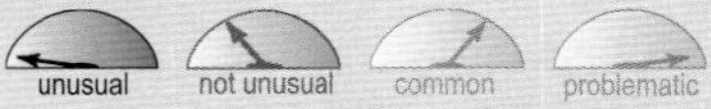

- Reported but not expected

Sedation
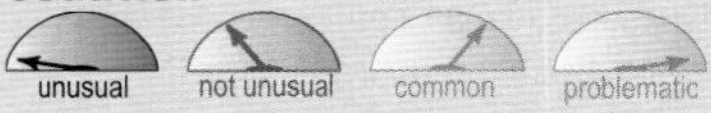

- Reported but not expected

What to Do About Side Effects
- Wait
- Wait
- Wait
- In a few weeks, switch to another agent or add other drugs

Best Augmenting Agents for Side Effects
- Often best to try another SSRI or another antidepressant monotherapy prior to resorting to augmentation strategies to treat side effects
- Trazodone or a hypnotic for insomnia
- Bupropion, sildenafil, vardenafil, or tadalafil for sexual dysfunction
- Bupropion for emotional flattening, cognitive slowing, or apathy
- Mirtazapine for insomnia, agitation, and gastrointestinal side effects
- Benzodiazepines for jitteriness and anxiety, especially at initiation of treatment and especially for anxious patients
- Many side effects are dose-dependent (i.e., they increase as dose increases, or they reemerge until tolerance redevelops)
- Many side effects are time-dependent (i.e., they start immediately upon dosing and upon each dose increase, but go away with time)
- Activation and agitation may represent the induction of a bipolar state, especially a mixed dysphoric bipolar II condition sometimes associated with suicidal ideation, and require the addition of lithium, a mood stabilizer or an atypical antipsychotic, and/or discontinuation of escitalopram

DOSING AND USE

Usual Dosage Range
- 10–20 mg/day

Dosage Forms
- Tablets 5 mg, 10 mg (scored), 20 mg (scored)
- Capsule 5 mg, 10 mg, 20 mg
- Oral solution 5 mg/5 mL

How to Dose
- Initial 10 mg/day; increase to 20 mg/day if necessary; single dose administration, morning or evening

Dosing Tips
- Given once daily, any time of day tolerated
- ✽ 10 mg of escitalopram may be comparable in efficacy to 40 mg of citalopram with fewer side effects
- Thus, give an adequate trial of 10 mg prior to giving 20 mg
- Some patients require dosing with 30 or 40 mg
- If intolerable anxiety, insomnia, agitation, akathisia, or activation occur either upon dosing initiation or discontinuation, consider the possibility of activated bipolar disorder and switch to a mood stabilizer or an atypical antipsychotic

Overdose
- Few reports of escitalopram overdose, but probably similar to citalopram overdose
- Rare fatalities have been reported in citalopram overdose, both in combination with other drugs and alone
- Symptoms associated with citalopram overdose include vomiting, sedation, heart rhythm disturbances, dizziness, sweating, nausea, tremor, and rarely amnesia, confusion, coma, convulsions

Long-Term Use
- Safe

Habit Forming
- No

How to Stop
- Taper not usually necessary
- However, tapering to avoid potential withdrawal reactions generally prudent
- Many patients tolerate 50% dose reduction for 3 days, then another 50% reduction for 3 days, then discontinuation
- If withdrawal symptoms emerge during discontinuation, raise dose to stop symptoms and then restart withdrawal much more slowly

Pharmacokinetics
- Mean terminal half-life 27–32 hours
- Steady-state plasma concentrations achieved within 1 week
- No significant actions on CYP450 enzymes

Drug Interactions
- Tramadol increases the risk of seizures in patients taking an antidepressant
- Can cause a fatal "serotonin syndrome" when combined with MAOIs, so do not use with MAOIs or for at least 14 days after MAOIs are stopped
- Do not start an MAOI for at least 5 half-lives (5 to 7 days for most drugs) after discontinuing escitalopram
- Could theoretically cause weakness, hyperreflexia, and incoordination when combined with sumatriptan or possibly other triptans, requiring careful monitoring of patient
- Possible increased risk of bleeding, especially when combined with anticoagulants (e.g., warfarin, NSAIDs)
- NSAIDs may impair effectiveness of SSRIs
- Few known adverse drug interactions

Other Warnings/ Precautions
- Use with caution in patients with history of seizures
- Use with caution in patients with bipolar disorder unless treated with concomitant mood-stabilizing agent
- When treating children, carefully weigh the risks and benefits of pharmacological treatment against the risks and benefits of nontreatment with antidepressants and make sure to document this in the patient's chart
- Distribute the brochures provided by the FDA and the drug companies

- Warn patients and their caregivers about the possibility of activating side effects and advise them to report such symptoms immediately
- Monitor patients for activation of suicidal ideation, especially children and adolescents

Do Not Use

- If patient is taking an MAOI
- If patient is taking pimozide
- If there is a proven allergy to escitalopram or citalopram

SPECIAL POPULATIONS

Renal Impairment

- No dose adjustment for mild to moderate impairment
- Use cautiously in patients with severe impairment

Hepatic Impairment

- Recommended dose 10 mg/day

Cardiac Impairment

- Not systematically evaluated in patients with cardiac impairment
- Preliminary data suggest that citalopram is safe in patients with cardiac impairment, suggesting that escitalopram is also safe
- Treating depression with SSRIs in patients with acute angina or following myocardial infarction may reduce cardiac events and improve survival as well as mood

Elderly

- Recommended dose 10 mg/day
- Risk of SIADH with SSRIs is higher in the elderly
- Reduction in the risk of suicidality with antidepressants compared to placebo in adults age 65 and older

Children and Adolescents

- Approved for depression in adolescents ages 12–17
- Carefully weigh the risks and benefits of pharmacological treatment against the risks and benefits of nontreatment with antidepressants and make sure to document this in the patient's chart
- Monitor patients face-to-face regularly, particularly during the first several weeks of treatment
- Use with caution, observing for activation of known or unknown bipolar disorder and/or suicidal ideation, and inform parents or guardians of this risk so they can help observe child or adolescent patients

Pregnancy

- Effective June 30, 2015, the US FDA requires changes to the content and format of pregnancy and lactation information in prescription drug labels, including the elimination of the pregnancy letter categories; the Pregnancy and Lactation Labeling Rule (PLLR or final rule) applies only to prescription drugs and will be phased in gradually for drugs approved on or after June 30, 2001
- Controlled studies have not been conducted in pregnant women
- Not generally recommended for use during pregnancy, especially during first trimester
- Nonetheless, continuous treatment during pregnancy may be necessary and has not been proven to be harmful to the fetus
- At delivery there may be more bleeding in the mother and transient irritability or sedation in the newborn
- Must weigh the risk of treatment (first trimester fetal development, third trimester newborn delivery) to the child against the risk of no treatment (recurrence of depression, maternal health, infant bonding) to the mother and child
- For many patients, this may mean continuing treatment during pregnancy
- Exposure to SSRIs early in pregnancy may be associated with increased risk of septal heart defects (absolute risk is small)
- SSRI use beyond the 20th week of pregnancy may be associated with increased risk of pulmonary hypertension in newborns, although this is not proven
- Exposure to SSRIs late in pregnancy may be associated with increased risk of gestational hypertension and preeclampsia
- Neonates exposed to SSRIs or SNRIs late in the third trimester have developed complications requiring prolonged hospitalization, respiratory support,

and tube feeding; reported symptoms are consistent with either a direct toxic effect of SSRIs and SNRIs or, possibly, a drug discontinuation syndrome, and include respiratory distress, cyanosis, apnea, seizures, temperature instability, feeding difficulty, vomiting, hypoglycemia, hypotonia, hypertonia, hyperreflexia, tremor, jitteriness, irritability, and constant crying

Breast Feeding

- Some drug is found in mother's breast milk
- Trace amounts may be present in nursing children whose mothers are on escitalopram
- If child becomes irritable or sedated, breast feeding or drug may need to be discontinued
- Immediate postpartum period is a high-risk time for depression, especially in women who have had prior depressive episodes, so drug may need to be reinstituted late in the third trimester or shortly after childbirth to prevent a recurrence during the postpartum period
- Must weigh benefits of breast feeding with risks and benefits of antidepressant treatment versus nontreatment to both the infant and the mother
- For many patients, this may mean continuing treatment during breast feeding

THE ART OF PSYCHOPHARMACOLOGY

Potential Advantages

- Patients taking concomitant medications (few drug interactions and fewer even than with citalopram)
- Patients requiring faster onset of action

Potential Disadvantages

- More expensive than citalopram in markets where citalopram is generic

Primary Target Symptoms

- Depressed mood
- Anxiety
- Panic attacks, avoidant behavior, re-experiencing, hyperarousal
- Sleep disturbance, both insomnia and hypersomnia

Pearls

- ✻ May be among the best-tolerated antidepressants
- May have less sexual dysfunction than some other SSRIs
- May be better tolerated than citalopram
- Can cause cognitive and affective "flattening"
- ✻ R-citalopram may interfere with the binding of S-citalopram at the serotonin transporter
- ✻ For this reason, S-citalopram may be more than twice as potent as R,S-citalopram (i.e., citalopram)
- Thus, 10 mg starting dose of S-citalopram may have the therapeutic efficacy of 40 mg of R,S-citalopram
- Thus, escitalopram may have faster onset and better efficacy with reduced side effects compared to R,S-citalopram
- Some data may actually suggest remission rates comparable to SNRIs, but this is not proven
- ✻ Escitalopram is commonly used with augmenting agents, as it is the SSRI with the least interaction at either CYP450 2D6 or 3A4, therefore causing fewer pharmacokinetically mediated drug interactions with augmenting agents than other SSRIs
- SSRIs may be less effective in women over 50, especially if they are not taking estrogen
- SSRIs may be useful for hot flushes in perimenopausal women
- Some postmenopausal women's depression will respond better to escitalopram plus estrogen augmentation than to escitalopram alone
- Nonresponse to escitalopram in elderly may require consideration of mild cognitive impairment or Alzheimer disease

Suggested Reading

Baldwin DS, Reines EH, Guiton C, Weiller E. Escitalopram therapy for major depression and anxiety disorders. Ann Pharmacother 2007;41(10):1583–92.

Bareggi SR, Mundo E, Dell–Osso B, Altamura AC. The use of escitalopram beyond major depression: pharmacological aspects, efficacy and tolerability in anxiety disorders. Expert Opin Drug Metab Toxicol 2007;3(5):741–53.

Burke WJ. Escitalopram. Expert Opin Investig Drugs 2002;11(10):1477–86.

ESTAZOLAM

THERAPEUTICS

Brands • ProSom

see index for additional brand names

Generic? Yes

Class

- Neuroscience-based Nomenclature: GABA positive allosteric modulator (GABA-PAM)
- Benzodiazepine (hypnotic)

Commonly Prescribed for

(bold for FDA approved)

- **Insomnia characterized by difficulty in falling asleep, frequent nocturnal awakenings, and/or early morning awakenings**
- Catatonia

How the Drug Works

- Binds to benzodiazepine receptors at the GABA-A ligand-gated chloride channel complex
- Enhances the inhibitory effects of GABA
- Boosts chloride conductance through GABA-regulated channels
- Inhibitory actions in sleep centers may provide sedative hypnotic effects

How Long Until It Works

- Generally takes effect in less than an hour

If It Works

- Improves quality of sleep
- Effects on total wake-time and number of nighttime awakenings may be decreased over time

If It Doesn't Work

- If insomnia does not improve after 7–10 days, it may be a manifestation of a primary psychiatric or physical illness such as obstructive sleep apnea or restless leg syndrome, which requires independent evaluation
- Increase the dose
- Improve sleep hygiene
- Switch to another agent

Best Augmenting Combos for Partial Response or Treatment Resistance

- Generally, best to switch to another agent
- Trazodone
- Agents with antihistamine actions (e.g., diphenhydramine, TCAs)

Tests

- In patients with seizure disorders, concomitant medical illness, and/or those with multiple concomitant long-term medications, periodic liver tests and blood counts may be prudent

SIDE EFFECTS

How Drug Causes Side Effects

- Same mechanism for side effects as for therapeutic effects – namely due to excessive actions at benzodiazepine receptors
- Actions at benzodiazepine receptors that carry over to next day can cause daytime sedation, amnesia, and ataxia
- Long-term adaptations in benzodiazepine receptors may explain the development of dependence, tolerance, and withdrawal

Notable Side Effects

- ✻ Sedation, fatigue, depression
- ✻ Dizziness, ataxia, slurred speech, weakness
- ✻ Forgetfulness, confusion
- ✻ Hyperexcitability, nervousness
- Rare hallucinations, mania
- Rare hypotension
- Hypersalivation, dry mouth
- Rebound insomnia when withdrawing from long-term treatment

Life-Threatening or Dangerous Side Effects

- Respiratory depression, especially when taken with CNS depressants in overdose
- Rare hepatic dysfunction, renal dysfunction, blood dyscrasias

Weight Gain

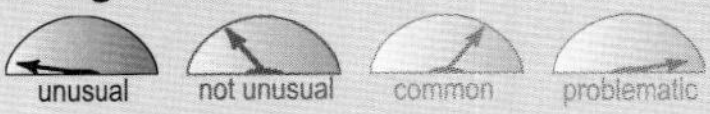

- Reported but not expected

Sedation

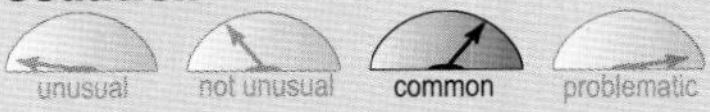

- Many experience and/or can be significant in amount

What to Do About Side Effects

- Wait
- To avoid problems with memory, take estazolam only if planning to have a full night's sleep
- Lower the dose
- Switch to a shorter-acting sedative hypnotic
- Switch to a non-benzodiazepine hypnotic
- Administer flumazenil if side effects are severe or life-threatening

Best Augmenting Agents for Side Effects

- Many side effects cannot be improved with an augmenting agent

DOSING AND USE

Usual Dosage Range

- 1–2 mg/day at bedtime

Dosage Forms

- Tablet 1 mg scored, 2 mg scored

How to Dose

- Initial 1 mg/day at bedtime; increase to 2 mg/day at bedtime if ineffective

Dosing Tips

- Use lowest possible effective dose and assess need for continued treatment regularly
- Estazolam should generally not be prescribed in quantities greater than a 1-month supply
- Patients with lower body weights may require lower doses
- Risk of dependence may increase with dose and duration of treatment

Overdose

- No death reported in monotherapy; sedation, slurred speech, poor coordination, confusion, coma, respiratory depression

Long-Term Use

- Not generally intended for long-term use
- Evidence of efficacy up to 12 weeks

Habit Forming

- Estazolam is a Schedule IV drug
- Some patients may develop dependence and/or tolerance; risk may be greater with higher doses
- History of drug addiction may increase risk of dependence

How to Stop

- If taken for more than a few weeks, taper to reduce chances of withdrawal effects
- Patients with seizure history may seize upon sudden withdrawal
- Rebound insomnia may occur the first 1–2 nights after stopping
- For patients with severe problems discontinuing a benzodiazepine, dosing may need to be tapered over many months (i.e., reduce dose by 1% every 3 days by crushing tablet and suspending or dissolving in 100 mL of fruit juice and then disposing of 1 mL while drinking the rest; 3–7 days later, dispose of 2 mL, and so on). This is both a form of very slow biological tapering and a form of behavioral desensitization

Pharmacokinetics

- Half-life 10–24 hours
- Inactive metabolites

Drug Interactions

- Increased clearance and thus decreased estazolam levels in smokers
- Increased depressive effects when taken with other CNS depressants (see Warnings below)

Other Warnings/ Precautions

- Boxed warning regarding the increased risk of CNS depressant effects when benzodiazepines and opioid medications are used together, including specifically the risk of slowed or difficulty breathing and death
- If alternatives to the combined use of benzodiazepines and opioids are not available, clinicians should limit the dosage and duration of each drug to the minimum possible while still achieving therapeutic efficacy
- Patients and their caregivers should be warned to seek medical attention if unusual dizziness, lightheadedness, sedation, slowed or difficulty breathing, or unresponsiveness occur

- Insomnia may be a symptom of a primary disorder, rather than a primary disorder itself
- Some patients may exhibit abnormal thinking or behavioral changes similar to those caused by other CNS depressants (i.e., either depressant actions or disinhibiting actions)
- Some depressed patients may experience a worsening of suicidal ideation
- Use only with extreme caution in patients with impaired respiratory function or obstructive sleep apnea
- Estazolam should be administered only at bedtime

Do Not Use

- If patient is pregnant
- If patient has angle-closure glaucoma
- If there is a proven allergy to estazolam or any benzodiazepine

SPECIAL POPULATIONS

Renal Impairment

- Drug should be used with caution

Hepatic Impairment

- Drug should be used with caution

Cardiac Impairment

- Benzodiazepines have been used to treat insomnia associated with acute myocardial infarction

Elderly

- No dose adjustment in healthy patients
- Debilitated patients: recommended initial dose of 0.5 mg/day

Children and Adolescents

- Safety and efficacy have not been established
- Long-term effects of estazolam in children/adolescents are unknown
- Should generally receive lower doses and be more closely monitored

Pregnancy

- Contraindicated for use in pregnancy
- Effective June 30, 2015, the US FDA requires changes to the content and format of pregnancy and lactation information in prescription drug labels, including the elimination of the pregnancy letter categories; the Pregnancy and Lactation Labeling Rule (PLLR or final rule) applies only to prescription drugs and will be phased in gradually for drugs approved on or after June 30, 2001
- Infants whose mothers received a benzodiazepine late in pregnancy may experience withdrawal effects
- Neonatal flaccidity has been reported in infants whose mothers took a benzodiazepine during pregnancy

Breast Feeding

- Unknown if estazolam is secreted in human breast milk, but all psychotropics assumed to be secreted in breast milk
- ✻ Recommended either to discontinue drug or bottle feed
- Effects on infant have been observed and include feeding difficulties, sedation, and weight loss

THE ART OF PSYCHOPHARMACOLOGY

Potential Advantages

- Transient insomnia

Potential Disadvantages

- Smokers (may need higher dose)

Primary Target Symptoms

- Time to sleep onset
- Total sleep time
- Nighttime awakenings

Pearls

- If tolerance develops, it may result in increased anxiety during the day and/or increased wakefulness during the latter part of the night
- Best short-term use is for less than 10 consecutive days, and for less than half of the nights in a month
- Drug holidays may restore drug effectiveness if tolerance develops
- Though not systematically studied, benzodiazepines have been used effectively to treat catatonia and are the initial recommended treatment

Suggested Reading

Pierce MW, Shu VS. Efficacy of estazolam. The United States clinical experience. Am J Med 1990;88:S6–11.

Pierce MW, Shu VS, Groves LJ. Safety of estazolam. The United States clinical experience. Am J Med 1990;88:S12–17.

Vogel GW, Morris D. The effects of estazolam on sleep, performance, and memory: a long-term sleep laboratory study of elderly insomniacs. J Clin Pharmacol 1992;32:647–51.

THERAPEUTICS

Brands • Lunesta

see index for additional brand names

Generic? Yes

Class

- Neuroscience-based Nomenclature: GABA positive allosteric modulator (GABA-PAM)
- Non-benzodiazepine hypnotic; alpha 1 isoform selective agonist of GABA-A/ benzodiazepine receptors

Commonly Prescribed for

(bold for FDA approved)

- **Insomnia**
- Primary insomnia
- Chronic insomnia
- Transient insomnia
- Insomnia secondary to psychiatric or medical conditions
- Residual insomnia following treatment with antidepressants

How the Drug Works

- May bind selectively to a subtype of the benzodiazepine receptor, the alpha 1 isoform
- May enhance GABA inhibitory actions that provide sedative hypnotic effects more selectively than other actions of GABA
- Boosts chloride conductance through GABA-regulated channels
- Inhibitory actions in sleep centers may provide sedative hypnotic effects

How Long Until It Works

- Generally takes effect in less than an hour

If It Works

- Improves quality of sleep
- Effects on total wake-time and number of nighttime awakenings may be decreased over time

If It Doesn't Work

- If insomnia does not improve after 7–10 days, it may be a manifestation of a primary psychiatric or physical illness such as obstructive sleep apnea or restless leg syndrome, which requires independent evaluation
- Increase the dose
- Improve sleep hygiene
- Switch to another agent

Best Augmenting Combos for Partial Response or Treatment Resistance

- Generally, best to switch to another agent
- Trazodone
- Agents with antihistamine actions (e.g., diphenhydramine, TCAs)

Tests

- None for healthy individuals

SIDE EFFECTS

How Drug Causes Side Effects

- Actions at benzodiazepine receptors that carry over to the next day can cause daytime sedation, amnesia, and ataxia
- * Chronic studies of eszopiclone suggest lack of notable tolerance or dependence developing over time

Notable Side Effects

- * Unpleasant taste
- Sedation
- Dizziness
- Dose-dependent amnesia
- Nervousness
- Dry mouth, headache

Life-Threatening or Dangerous Side Effects

- Respiratory depression, especially when taken with other CNS depressants in overdose
- Rare angioedema

Weight Gain

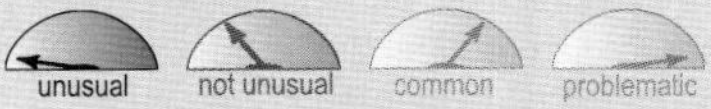

(unusual)

- Reported but not expected

Sedation

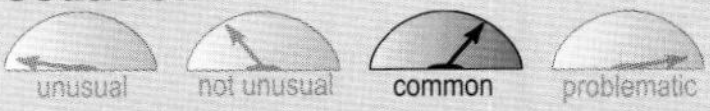

(common)

- Many experience and/or can be significant in amount
- Next day carryover sedation following nighttime dosing uncommon

What to Do About Side Effects

- Wait

- To avoid problems with memory, take eszopiclone only if planning to have a full night's sleep
- Lower the dose
- Switch to a shorter-acting sedative hypnotic
- Administer flumazenil if side effects are severe or life-threatening

Best Augmenting Agents for Side Effects

- Many side effects cannot be improved with an augmenting agent

DOSING AND USE

Usual Dosage Range

- 2–3 mg at bedtime

Dosage Forms

- Tablet 1 mg, 2 mg, 3 mg

How to Dose

- No titration, take dose at bedtime

Dosing Tips

- Not restricted to short-term use
- No notable development of tolerance or dependence seen in studies up to 6 months
- Recent study adding eszopiclone to patients with major depression and only a partial response to fluoxetine showed improvement not only in residual insomnia, but in other residual symptoms of depression as well
- Most studies were done with 3-mg dose or less at night, but some patients with insomnia associated with psychiatric disorders may require higher dosing
- However, doses higher than 3 mg may be associated with carryover effects, hallucinations, or other CNS adverse effects
- To avoid problems with memory or carryover sedation, only take eszopiclone if planning to have a full night's sleep
- Most notable side effect may be unpleasant taste
- Other side effects can include sedation, dizziness, dose-dependent amnesia, nervousness, dry mouth, and headache

Overdose

- Few reports of eszopiclone overdose, but probably similar to zopiclone overdose
- Rare fatalities have been reported in zopiclone overdose
- Symptoms associated with zopiclone overdose include clumsiness, mood changes, sedation, weakness, breathing trouble, unconsciousness

Long-Term Use

- No development of tolerance was seen in studies up to 6 months

Habit Forming

- Eszopiclone is a Schedule IV drug
- Some patients could develop dependence and/or tolerance with drugs of this class; risk may be theoretically greater with higher doses
- History of drug addiction may theoretically increase risk of dependence

How to Stop

- Rebound insomnia may occur the first night after stopping
- If taken for more than a few weeks, taper to reduce chances of withdrawal effects

Pharmacokinetics

- Metabolized by CYP450 3A4 and 2E1
- Terminal elimination half-life approximately 6 hours
- Heavy high-fat meal slows absorption, which could reduce effect on sleep latency

Drug Interactions

- Increased depressive effects when taken with other CNS depressants
- Inhibitors of CYP450 3A4, such as nefazodone and fluvoxamine, could increase plasma levels of eszopiclone
- Inducers of CYP450 3A4, such as rifampicin, could decrease plasma levels of eszopiclone

Other Warnings/ Precautions

- Insomnia may be a symptom of a primary disorder, rather than a primary disorder itself

- Some patients may exhibit abnormal thinking or behavioral changes similar to those caused by other CNS depressants (i.e., either depressant actions or disinhibiting actions)
- Some depressed patients may experience a worsening of suicidal ideation
- Use only with caution in patients with impaired respiratory function or obstructive sleep apnea
- Eszopiclone should only be administered at bedtime

Do Not Use

- If there is a proven allergy to eszopiclone or zopiclone
- Rare angioedema has occurred with sedative hypnotic use and could potentially cause fatal airway obstruction if it involves the throat, glottis, or larynx; thus if angioedema occurs treatment should be discontinued
- Sleep driving and other complex behaviors, such as eating and preparing food and making phone calls, have been reported in patients taking sedative hypnotics

SPECIAL POPULATIONS

Renal Impairment

- Dose adjustment not generally necessary

Hepatic Impairment

- Dose adjustment not generally recommended for mild-to-moderate hepatic impairment
- For severe impairment, recommended initial dose 1 mg at bedtime; maximum dose 2 mg at bedtime

Cardiac Impairment

- Dosage adjustment may not be necessary

Elderly

- May be more susceptible to adverse effects
- Initial dose 1 mg at bedtime; maximum dose generally 2 mg at bedtime

Children and Adolescents

- Safety and efficacy have not been established
- Long-term effects of eszopiclone in children/adolescents are unknown
- Should generally receive lower doses and be more closely monitored

Pregnancy

- Effective June 30, 2015, the US FDA requires changes to the content and format of pregnancy and lactation information in prescription drug labels, including the elimination of the pregnancy letter categories; the Pregnancy and Lactation Labeling Rule (PLLR or final rule) applies only to prescription drugs and will be phased in gradually for drugs approved on or after June 30, 2001
- Controlled studies have not been conducted in pregnant women
- Infants whose mothers took sedative hypnotics during pregnancy may experience some withdrawal symptoms
- Neonatal flaccidity has been reported in infants whose mothers took sedative hypnotics during pregnancy

Breast Feeding

- Unknown if eszopiclone is secreted in human breast milk, but all psychotropics assumed to be secreted in breast milk
- ✻ Recommended either to discontinue drug or bottle feed

THE ART OF PSYCHOPHARMACOLOGY

Potential Advantages

- Primary insomnia
- Chronic insomnia
- Those who require long-term treatment
- Those with depression whose insomnia does not resolve with antidepressant treatment

Potential Disadvantages

- More expensive than some other sedative hypnotics

Primary Target Symptoms

- Time to sleep onset
- Nighttime awakenings
- Total sleep time

Pearls

* May be preferred over benzodiazepines because of its rapid onset of action, short duration of effect, and safety profile
- Eszopiclone is the best documented agent to be safe for long-term use, with little or no suggestion of tolerance, dependence, or abuse
- May even be safe to consider in patients with a past history of substance abuse who require treatment with a hypnotic
- May be preferred over benzodiazepine hypnotics, which all cause tolerance, dependence, and abuse as a class
- Not a benzodiazepine itself but binds to the benzodiazepine receptor
- May be a preferred agent in primary insomnia
- Targeting insomnia may prevent the onset of depression and maintain remission after recovery from depression
- Rebound insomnia does not appear to be common

Suggested Reading

Eszopiclone: esopiclone, estorra, S-zopiclone, zopiclone–Sepracor. Drugs R D 2005;6(2):111–15.

Krystal AD, Walsh JK, Laska E, et al. Sustained efficacy of eszopiclone over 6 months of nightly treatment: results of a randomized, double-blind, placebo-controlled study in adults with chronic insomnia. Sleep 2003;26(7):793–9.

Zammit GK, McNabb LJ, Caron J, Amato DA, Roth T. Efficacy and safety of eszopiclone across 6-weeks of treatment for primary insomnia. Curr Med Res Opin 2004;20(12):1979–91.

FLIBANSERIN

THERAPEUTICS

Brands • Addyi

see index for additional brand names

Generic? No

Class

- Serotonin 1A agonist and serotonin 2A antagonist

Commonly Prescribed for

(bold for FDA approved)

- **Acquired, generalized hypoactive sexual desire disorder (HSDD) in premenopausal women**

How the Drug Works

- Sexual dysfunction is theoretically linked to an imbalance in central excitatory and inhibitory sexual signals
- HSDD hypothetically results from excessive inhibitory signals, inadequate excitatory signals, or a combination of the two
- Flibanserin hypothetically counteracts this imbalance in HSDD through its ability to both reduce inhibitory signals and enhance excitatory signals
- Specifically, flibanserin increases the release of dopamine and norepinephrine, which are excitatory sexual signals, and reduces the release of serotonin, an inhibitory sexual signal

How Long Until It Works

- In clinical trials, improvement was seen at 4 weeks

If It Works

- Increases number of satisfying sexual events and ratings on sexual desire scores
- Reduces distress related to sexual dysfunction

If It Doesn't Work

- If there is no improvement after 8 weeks, discontinue use

Best Augmenting Combos for Partial Response or Treatment Resistance

- None known
- Theoretically, bupropion augmentation could be considered, but no published trials

Tests

- None for healthy individuals

SIDE EFFECTS

How Drug Causes Side Effects

- Most common side effects (e.g., notable side effects below) likely caused by 5HT1A agonism and/or 5HT2A antagonism
- Hypotension, dizziness, and syncope of flibanserin as a monotherapy is theoretically related to its 5HT1A agonist actions
- Weak alpha 1 antagonist actions may also contribute to hypotension and dizziness of flibanserin, especially when given in combination with alcohol, which is contraindicated

Notable Side Effects

- Somnolence
- Nausea
- Fatigue
- Insomnia
- Dry mouth

Life-Threatening or Dangerous Side Effects

- Dizziness, syncope, especially when combined with alcohol

Weight Gain

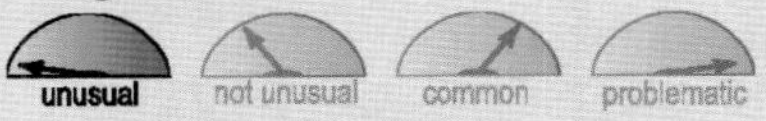

- Reported but not expected

Sedation

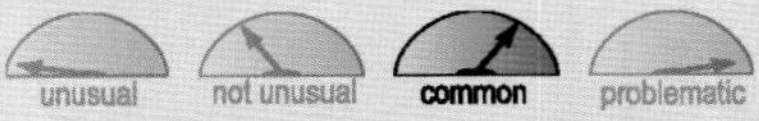

- Many experience and/or can be significant in amount

What to Do About Side Effects

- Wait
- Wait
- Wait
- Review any concomitant medications and consider reducing the dose or

discontinuing agents that may be interacting with flibanserin
- Switch to another treatment option

Best Augmenting Agents for Side Effects
- Many side effects cannot be improved with an augmenting agent

DOSING AND USE

Usual Dosage Range
- 100 mg once daily at bedtime

Dosage Forms
- Tablet 100 mg

How to Dose
- Flibanserin is dosed at bedtime to reduce the risk of hypotension, syncope, and somnolence

Overdose
- Limited experience

Long-Term Use
- Not studied
- However, flibanserin is recommended for long-term use with close monitoring

Habit Forming
- No

How to Stop
- Taper not necessary but may be better tolerated in some patients

Pharmacokinetics
- Metabolized primarily by CYP450 3A4 and to a lesser extent by CYP450 2C19
- Mean terminal half-life approximately 11 hours

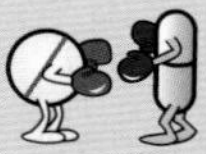

Drug Interactions
- The risk of hypotension, syncope, and CNS depression with flibanserin is increased in the presence of alcohol; therefore, the concomitant use of alcohol and flibanserin is contraindicated
- The risk of hypotension, syncope, and CNS depression with flibanserin is increased in the presence of moderate or strong CYP450 3A4 inhibitors; therefore, the concomitant use of moderate/strong CYP450 3A4 inhibitors and flibanserin is contraindicated
- If the patient requires a moderate or strong CYP450 3A4 inhibitor, flibanserin should be discontinued at least 2 days prior to starting the CYP450 3A4 inhibitor
- If the patient is taking a moderate or strong CYP450 3A4 inhibitor, it should be discontinued 2 weeks prior to starting flibanserin
- Concomitant use of flibanserin and weak CYP450 3A4 inhibitors may increase flibanserin exposure, potentially increasing risk of adverse effects
- Concomitant use of flibanserin and CNS depressants may increase the risk of adverse effects such as somnolence
- Concomitant use of flibanserin and CYP450 3A4 inducers may decrease exposure to flibanserin and is not recommended
- Concomitant use of flibanserin and CYP450 2C19 inhibitors may increase flibanserin exposure, potentially increasing risk of adverse effects
- Use of flibanserin in patients who are poor CYP450 2C19 metabolizers may increase flibanserin exposure, potentially increasing risk of adverse effects
- Concomitant use of flibanserin and P-glycoprotein substrates (e.g., digoxin) may increase concentrations of the P-glycoprotein substrate; monitoring is required for P-glycoprotein substrates that have narrow therapeutic index (e.g., digoxin)

Other Warnings/ Precautions
- Flibanserin can cause severe hypotension and loss of consciousness, with increased risk in the presence of alcohol or CYP450 3A4 inhibitors; for that reason, flibanserin is available only through a risk evaluation and mitigation strategy (REMS), which includes elements to assure safe use (ETASU)

Do Not Use
- In the presence of alcohol
- With moderate/strong CYP450 3A4 inhibitors
- In patients with hepatic impairment
- If there is a proven allergy to flibanserin

SPECIAL POPULATIONS

Renal Impairment
- Exposure may be increased

Hepatic Impairment
- Contraindicated; flibanserin exposure increases 4.5-fold in patients with hepatic impairment

Cardiac Impairment
- Use in patients with cardiac impairment has not been studied

Elderly
- Some elderly patients may theoretically tolerate lower doses better but this has not been formally studied

Children and Adolescents
- Safety and efficacy have not been established

Pregnancy
- Effective June 30, 2015, the US FDA requires changes to the content and format of pregnancy and lactation information in prescription drug labels, including the elimination of the pregnancy letter categories; the Pregnancy and Lactation Labeling Rule (PLLR or final rule) applies only to prescription drugs and will be phased in gradually for drugs approved on or after June 30, 2001
- Controlled studies have not been conducted in pregnant women
- In animal studies, fetal toxicity occurred only in the presence of significant maternal toxicity including reductions in weight gain and sedation
- In animal studies, decreased fetal weight, structural anomalies, and increases in fetal loss occurred with flibanserin at exposures greater than 15 times those achieved with recommended human doses

Breast Feeding
- Unknown if flibanserin is secreted in human breast milk, but all psychotropics assumed to be secreted in breast milk
- Breastfeeding is not recommended during treatment with flibanserin

THE ART OF PSYCHOPHARMACOLOGY

Potential Advantages
- Only agent approved for the treatment of HSDD

Potential Disadvantages
- Patients who drink alcohol
- Patients who take concomitant medications that may interact with flibanserin's pharmacokinetic and pharmacodynamic properties

Primary Target Symptoms
- Reduced sexual desire

Pearls
- Flibanserin is the first treatment to be approved for sexual dysfunction in females
- Flibanserin is not approved for treatment in postmenopausal women and is not indicated to enhance sexual performance
- May act on reward circuits in the CNS to enhance motivation and interest
- If not effective for HSDD, consider avoiding any concomitant use of agents that either enhance serotonin activity (such as SSRIs or SNRIs) or diminish dopamine activity (such as antipsychotics)
- Theoretically, may wish to avoid concomitant use with agents that have potent alpha 1 antagonist actions that may enhance the possibility of hypotension

Suggested Reading

Deeks ED. Flibanserin: first global approval. Drugs 2015;75(15):1855–22.

Dhanuka I, Simon JA. Flibanserin for the treatment of hypoactive sexual desire disorder in premenopausal women. Expert Opin Pharmacother 2015;16(16):2523–9.

Stahl SM. Mechanism of action of flibanserin, a multifunctional serotonin agonist and antagonist (MSAA), in hypoactive sexual desire disorder. CNS Spectr 2015;20(1):1–6.

Stahl SM, Sommer B, Allers KA. Multifunctional pharmacology of flibanserin: Possible mechanism of therapeutic action in Hypoactive Sexual Desire Disorder. J Sex Med. 2011;8:15–27.

FLUMAZENIL

THERAPEUTICS

Brands • Romazicon
• Anexate
• Lanexat

see index for additional brand names

Generic? Yes

Class

• Benzodiazepine receptor antagonist

Commonly Prescribed for

(bold for FDA approved)

• **Reversal of sedative effects of benzodiazepines after general anesthesia has been induced and/or maintained with benzodiazepines**
• **Reversal of sedative effects of benzodiazepines after sedation has been produced with benzodiazepines for diagnostic and therapeutic procedures**
• **Management of benzodiazepine overdose**
• **Reversal of conscious sedation induced with benzodiazepines (pediatric patients)**

How the Drug Works

• Blocks benzodiazepine receptors at GABA-A ligand-gated chloride channel complex, preventing benzodiazepines from binding there

How Long Until It Works

• Onset of action 1–2 minutes; peak effect 6–10 minutes

If It Works

✻ Reverses sedation and psychomotor retardation rapidly, but may not restore memory completely
✻ Patients treated for benzodiazepine overdose may experience CNS excitation
✻ Patients who receive flumazenil to reverse benzodiazepine effects should be monitored for up to 2 hours for resedation, respiratory depression, or other lingering benzodiazepine effects
• Flumazenil has not been shown to treat hypoventilation due to benzodiazepine treatment

If It Doesn't Work

• Sedation is most likely not due to a benzodiazepine, and treatment with flumazenil should be discontinued and other causes of sedation investigated

Best Augmenting Combos for Partial Response or Treatment Resistance

• None – flumazenil is basically used as a monotherapy antidote to reverse the actions of benzodiazepines

Tests

• None for healthy individuals

SIDE EFFECTS

How Drug Causes Side Effects

• Blocks benzodiazepine receptors at GABA-A ligand-gated chloride channel complex, preventing benzodiazepines from binding there

Notable Side Effects

• May precipitate benzodiazepine withdrawal in patients dependent upon or tolerant to benzodiazepines
• Dizziness, injection site pain, sweating, headache, blurred vision

Life-Threatening or Dangerous Side Effects

• Seizures
• Death (majority occurred in patients with severe underlying disease or who overdosed with non-benzodiazepines)
• Cardiac dysrhythmia

Weight Gain

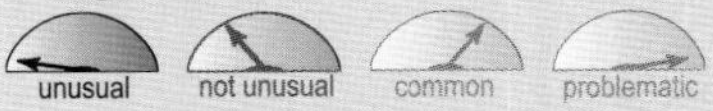

• Reported but not expected

Sedation

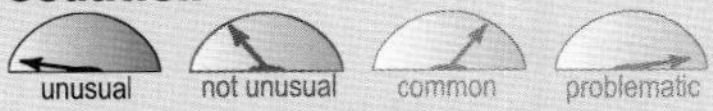

• Reported but not expected
• Patients may experience resedation if the effects of flumazenil wear off before the effects of the benzodiazepine

What to Do About Side Effects
- Monitor patient
- Restrict ambulation because of dizziness, blurred vision, and possibility of resedation

Best Augmenting Agents for Side Effects
- None – augmenting agents are not appropriate to treat side effects associated with flumazenil use

DOSING AND USE

Usual Dosage Range
- 0.4–1 mg generally causes complete antagonism of therapeutic doses of benzodiazepines
- 1–3 mg generally reverses benzodiazepine overdose

Dosage Forms
- Intravenous 0.1 mg/mL – 5 mL multiple-use vial, 10 mL multiple-use vial

How to Dose
- Conscious sedation, general anesthesia: 0.2 mg (2 mL) over 15 seconds; can administer 0.2 mg again after 45 seconds; can administer 0.2 mg each additional 60 seconds; maximum 1 mg
- Benzodiazepine overdose: 0.2 mg over 30 seconds; can administer 0.3 mg over next 30 seconds; can administer 0.5 mg over 30 seconds after 1 minute; maximum 5 mg

Dosing Tips
- May need to administer follow-up doses to reverse actions of benzodiazepines that have a longer half-life than flumazenil (i.e., longer than 1 hour)

Overdose
- Anxiety, agitation, increased muscle tone, hyperesthesia, convulsions

Long-Term Use
- Not a long-term treatment

Habit Forming
- No

How to Stop
- N/A

Pharmacokinetics
- Terminal half-life 41–79 minutes

Drug Interactions
- Food increases its clearance

Other Warnings/ Precautions
- Flumazenil may induce seizures, particularly in patients tolerant to or dependent on benzodiazepines, or who have overdosed on cyclic antidepressants, received recent/repeated doses of parenteral benzodiazepines, or have jerking or convulsion during overdose
- Patients dependent on benzodiazepines or receiving benzodiazepines to suppress seizures in cyclic antidepressant overdose should receive the minimally effective dose of flumazenil
- Use with caution in patients with head injury
- Greater risk of resedation if administered to a patient who took a long-acting benzodiazepine or a large dose of a short-acting benzodiazepine
- Flumazenil may induce panic attacks in patients with panic disorder
- Use with caution in cases of mixed overdose because toxic effects of other drugs used in overdose (e.g., convulsions) may appear when the effects of the benzodiazepine are reversed

Do Not Use
- Should not be used until after effects of neuromuscular blockers have been reversed
- If benzodiazepine was prescribed to control a life-threatening condition (e.g., status epilepticus, intracranial pressure)
- If there is a high risk of seizure
- If patient exhibits signs of serious cyclic antidepressant overdose
- If there is a proven allergy to flumazenil or benzodiazepines

SPECIAL POPULATIONS

Renal Impairment
- Dosage adjustment may not be necessary

Hepatic Impairment
- Prolongation of half-life
- Moderate: clearance reduced by half
- Severe: clearance reduced by three-quarters

Cardiac Impairment
- Dosage adjustment may not be necessary

Elderly
- Dosage adjustment may not be necessary

Children and Adolescents
- More variability of pharmacokinetics than in adults
- Safety and efficacy established for reversal of conscious sedation for children over age 1
- Initial 0.01 mg/kg (up to 0.2 mg) over 15 seconds; same dosing pattern as adults; maximum 0.05 mg/kg or 1 mg
- Safety and efficacy for reversal of benzodiazepine overdose, general anesthesia induction or resuscitation of a newborn have not been established, but anecdotal data suggest similar safety and efficacy as for conscious sedation

Pregnancy
- Effective June 30, 2015, the US FDA requires changes to the content and format of pregnancy and lactation information in prescription drug labels, including the elimination of the pregnancy letter categories; the Pregnancy and Lactation Labeling Rule (PLLR or final rule) applies only to prescription drugs and will be phased in gradually for drugs approved on or after June 30, 2001
- Controlled studies have not been conducted in pregnant women
- Not recommended to treat the effects of benzodiazepines during labor and delivery because the effects on the infant have not been studied

Breast Feeding
- Unknown if flumazenil is secreted in human breast milk, but all psychotropics assumed to be secreted in breast milk
- If treatment with flumazenil is necessary, it should be administered with caution

THE ART OF PSYCHOPHARMACOLOGY

Potential Advantages
- To reverse a low dose of a short-acting benzodiazepine

Potential Disadvantages
- May be too short-acting

Primary Target Symptoms
- Effects of benzodiazepines
- Sedative effects
- Recall and psychomotor impairments
- Ventilatory depression

Pearls
- Can precipitate benzodiazepine withdrawal seizures

✻ Can wear off before the benzodiazepine it is reversing

✻ Can precipitate anxiety or panic in conscious patients with anxiety disorders

Suggested Reading

Malizia AL, Nutt DJ. The effects of flumazenil in neuropsychiatric disorders. Clin Neuropharmacol 1995;18:215–32.

McCloy RF. Reversal of conscious sedation by flumazenil: current status and future prospects. Acta Anaesthesiol Scand Suppl 1995;108:35–42.

Weinbroum AA, Flaishon R, Sorkine P, Szold O, Rudick V. A risk-benefit assessment of flumazenil in the management of benzodiazepine overdose. Drug Saf 1997;17:181–96.

Whitwam JG. Flumazenil and midazolam in anaesthesia. Acta Anaesthesiol Scand Suppl 1995;108:15–22.

Whitwam JG, Amrein R. Pharmacology of flumazenil. Acta Anaesthesiol Scand Suppl 1995;108:3–14.

FLUNITRAZEPAM

THERAPEUTICS

Brands • Rohypnol

see index for additional brand names

Generic? No

Class

- Neuroscience-based Nomenclature: GABA positive allosteric modulator (GABA-PAM)
- Benzodiazepine (hypnotic)

Commonly Prescribed for

(bold for FDA approved)

- Short-term treatment of insomnia (severe, disabling)
- Catatonia

How the Drug Works

- Binds to benzodiazepine receptors at the GABA-A ligand-gated chloride channel complex
- Enhances the inhibitory effects of GABA
- Boosts chloride conductance through GABA-regulated channels
- Inhibitory actions in sleep centers may provide sedative hypnotic effects

How Long Until It Works

- Generally takes effect in less than an hour

If It Works

- Improves quality of sleep
- Effects on total wake-time and number of nighttime awakenings may be decreased over time

If It Doesn't Work

- If insomnia does not improve after 7–10 days, it may be a manifestation of a primary psychiatric or physical illness such as obstructive sleep apnea or restless leg syndrome, which requires independent evaluation
- Increase the dose
- Improve sleep hygiene
- Switch to another agent

Best Augmenting Combos for Partial Response or Treatment Resistance

- Generally, best to switch to another agent
- Trazodone
- Agents with antihistamine actions (e.g., diphenhydramine, TCAs)

Tests

- In patients with seizure disorders, concomitant medical illness, and/or those with multiple concomitant long-term medications, periodic liver tests and blood counts may be prudent

SIDE EFFECTS

How Drug Causes Side Effects

- Same mechanism for side effects as for therapeutic effects – namely due to excessive actions at benzodiazepine receptors
- Actions at benzodiazepine receptors that carry over to next day can cause daytime sedation, amnesia, and ataxia
- Long-term adaptations in benzodiazepine receptors may explain the development of dependence, tolerance, and withdrawal

Notable Side Effects

- * Sedation, fatigue, depression
- * Dizziness, ataxia, slurred speech, weakness
- * Forgetfulness, confusion
- * Hyperexcitability, nervousness
- Rare hallucinations, mania
- Rare hypotension
- Hypersalivation, dry mouth
- Rebound insomnia when withdrawing from long-term treatment

Life-Threatening or Dangerous Side Effects

- Respiratory depression, especially when taken with CNS depressants in overdose
- Rare hepatic dysfunction, renal dysfunction, blood dyscrasias

Weight Gain

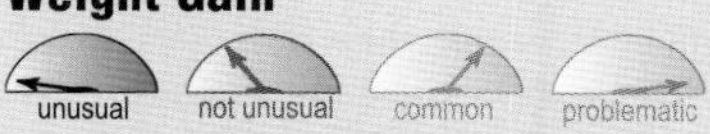

- Reported but not expected

Sedation

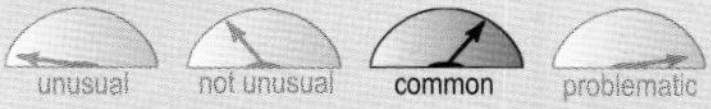

- Many experience and/or can be significant in amount

What to Do About Side Effects
- Wait
- To avoid problems with memory, only take flunitrazepam if planning to have a full night's sleep
- Lower the dose
- Switch to a shorter-acting sedative hypnotic
- Switch to a non-benzodiazepine hypnotic
- Administer flumazenil if side effects are severe or life-threatening

Best Augmenting Agents for Side Effects
- Many side effects cannot be improved with an augmenting agent

DOSING AND USE

Usual Dosage Range
- 0.5–1 mg/day at bedtime

Dosage Forms
- Tablet 0.5 mg, 1 mg, 2 mg, 4 mg

How to Dose
- Initial 0.5–1 mg/day at bedtime; maximum generally 2 mg/day at bedtime

Dosing Tips
- Use lowest possible effective dose and assess need for continued treatment regularly
- Flunitrazepam should generally not be prescribed in quantities greater than a 1-month supply
- Patients with lower body weights may require lower doses
- Risk of dependence may increase with dose and duration of treatment
- Use doses over 1 mg only in exceptional circumstances
- Patients who request or who require doses over 1 mg may be more likely to have present or past substance abuse
- Flunitrazepam is 10 times more potent than diazepam

Overdose
- Sedation, slurred speech, poor coordination, confusion, coma, respiratory depression

Long-Term Use
- Not generally intended for long-term use
- Use is not recommended to exceed 4 weeks

Habit Forming
- Some patients may develop dependence and/or tolerance; risk may be greater with higher doses
- History of drug addiction may increase risk of dependence
- Currently classified as Schedule III by the World Health Organization
- Currently classified as a Schedule IV drug in the USA, but not legally available in the USA

How to Stop
- If taken for more than a few weeks, taper to reduce chances of withdrawal effects
- Patients with seizure history may seize upon sudden withdrawal
- Rebound insomnia may occur the first 1–2 nights after stopping
- For patients with severe problems discontinuing a benzodiazepine, dosing may need to be tapered over many months (i.e., reduce dose by 1% every 3 days by crushing tablet and suspending or dissolving in 100 mL of fruit juice and then disposing of 1 mL while drinking the rest; 3–7 days later, dispose of 2 mL, and so on). This is both a form of very slow biological tapering and a form of behavioral desensitization

Pharmacokinetics
- Elimination half-life 16–35 hours
- Half-life of active metabolite 23–33 hours

Drug Interactions
- Increased depressive effects when taken with other CNS depressants (see Warnings below)
- Cisapride may hasten the absorption of flunitrazepam and thus cause a temporary increase in the sedative effects of flunitrazepam

Other Warnings/ Precautions
- Boxed warning regarding the increased risk of CNS depressant effects when benzodiazepines and opioid medications

are used together, including specifically the risk of slowed or difficulty breathing and death
- If alternatives to the combined use of benzodiazepines and opioids are not available, clinicians should limit the dosage and duration of each drug to the minimum possible while still achieving therapeutic efficacy
- Patients and their caregivers should be warned to seek medical attention if unusual dizziness, lightheadedness, sedation, slowed or difficulty breathing, or unresponsiveness occur
- Insomnia may be a symptom of a primary disorder, rather than a primary disorder itself
- Some patients may exhibit abnormal thinking or behavioral changes similar to those caused by other CNS depressants (i.e., either depressant actions or disinhibiting actions)
- Some depressed patients may experience a worsening of suicidal ideation
- Use only with extreme caution in patients with impaired respiratory function or obstructive sleep apnea
- Flunitrazepam should be administered only at bedtime

Do Not Use
- If patient is pregnant
- If patient has severe chronic hypercapnia, myasthenia gravis, severe respiratory insufficiency, sleep apnea, or severe hepatic insufficiency
- In children
- If patient has angle-closure glaucoma
- If there is a proven allergy to flunitrazepam or any benzodiazepine

SPECIAL POPULATIONS

Renal Impairment
- Drug should be used with caution

Hepatic Impairment
- Dose should be lowered
- Should not be used in patients with severe hepatic insufficiency, as it may precipitate encephalopathy

Cardiac Impairment
- Benzodiazepines have been used to treat insomnia associated with acute myocardial infarction

Elderly
- Initial starting dose 0.5 mg at bedtime; maximum generally 1 mg/day at bedtime
- Paradoxical reactions with restlessness and agitation are more likely to occur in the elderly

Children and Adolescents
- Safety and efficacy have not been established
- Not recommended for use in children or adolescents
- Paradoxical reactions with restlessness and agitation are more likely to occur in children

Pregnancy
- Positive evidence of risk to human fetus; contraindicated for use in pregnancy
- Infants whose mothers received a benzodiazepine late in pregnancy may experience withdrawal effects
- Neonatal flaccidity has been reported in infants whose mothers took a benzodiazepine during pregnancy

Breast Feeding
- Unknown if flunitrazepam is secreted in human breast milk, but all psychotropics assumed to be secreted in breast milk
- * Recommended either to discontinue drug or bottle feed
- Effects on infant have been observed and include feeding difficulties, sedation, and weight loss

THE ART OF PSYCHOPHARMACOLOGY

Potential Advantages
- For severe, disabling insomnia unresponsive to other sedative hypnotics

Potential Disadvantages
- For those who need treatment for longer than a few weeks
- For those with current or past substance abuse

Primary Target Symptoms
- Time to sleep onset
- Total sleep time
- Nighttime awakenings

Pearls

* Psychiatric symptoms and "paradoxical" reactions may be quite severe with flunitrazepam and may be more frequent than with other benzodiazepines
* "Paradoxical" reactions include symptoms such as restlessness, agitation, irritability, aggressiveness, delusions, rage, nightmares, hallucinations, psychosis, inappropriate behavior, and other adverse behavioral effects
* Although legally available in Europe, Mexico, South America, and many other countries, it is not legally available in the USA
* Although currently classified as a Schedule IV drug, the USA drug enforcement agency is considering reclassifying it as Schedule I
* Has earned a reputation as a "date rape drug" in which sexual predators have allegedly slipped flunitrazepam into women's drinks to induce sexual relations
* Flunitrazepam, especially in combination with alcohol, is claimed to reduce the woman's judgment, inhibitions, or physical ability to resist sexual advances, as well as to reduce or eliminate her recall of the events
* Until 1999 was colorless, but a colorimetric compound is now added that turns the drug blue when added to a liquid, making it obvious that a drink was tampered with
* Illicit use since 1999 has fallen in part due to this additive
* Illicit use has also fallen in the USA due to the Drug-Induced Rape Prevention and Punishment act of 1996, making it punishable to commit a violent crime using a controlled substance such as flunitrazepam
* Street names for flunitrazepam, based in part upon its trade name of Rohypnol, manufacturer Roche, and the presence of RO-2 on the surface of the tablets, include "roofies," "ruffies," "roapies," "la roacha," "roach-2," "Mexican valium," "rope," "roache vitamins," and others
* If tolerance develops, it may result in increased anxiety during the day and/or increased wakefulness during the latter part of the night
* Best short-term use is for less than 10 consecutive days, and for less than half of the nights in a month
* Drug holidays may restore drug effectiveness if tolerance develops
* Though not systematically studied, benzodiazepines have been used effectively to treat catatonia and are the initial recommended treatment

Suggested Reading

Simmons MM, Cupp MJ. Use and abuse of flunitrazepam. Ann Pharmacother 1998;32(1):117–19.

Woods JH, Winger G. Abuse liability of flunitrazepam. J Clin Psychopharmacol 1997;17(3 Suppl 2):S1–57.

THERAPEUTICS

Brands
- Prozac
- Prozac weekly
- Sarafem

see index for additional brand names

Generic? Yes

Class
- Neuroscience-based Nomenclature: serotonin reuptake inhibitor (S-RI)
- SSRI (selective serotonin reuptake inhibitor); often classified as an antidepressant, but it is not just an antidepressant

Commonly Prescribed for
(bold for FDA approved)
- **Major depressive disorder (ages 8 and older)**
- **Obsessive-compulsive disorder (OCD) (ages 7 and older)**
- **Premenstrual dysphoric disorder (PMDD)**
- **Bulimia nervosa**
- **Panic disorder**
- **Bipolar depression [in combination with olanzapine (Symbyax)]**
- **Treatment-resistant depression [in combination with olanzapine (Symbyax)]**
- Social anxiety disorder (social phobia)
- Posttraumatic stress disorder (PTSD)

How the Drug Works
- Boosts neurotransmitter serotonin
- Blocks serotonin reuptake pump (serotonin transporter)
- Desensitizes serotonin receptors, especially serotonin 1A receptors
- Presumably increases serotonergic neurotransmission

✻ Fluoxetine also has antagonist properties at 5HT2C receptors, which could increase norepinephrine and dopamine neurotransmission

How Long Until It Works
✻ Some patients may experience increased energy or activation early after initiation of treatment
- Onset of therapeutic actions usually not immediate, but often delayed 2–4 weeks
- If it is not working within 6–8 weeks, it may require a dosage increase or it may not work at all
- May continue to work for many years to prevent relapse of symptoms

If It Works
- The goal of treatment is complete remission of current symptoms as well as prevention of future relapses
- Treatment most often reduces or even eliminates symptoms, but not a cure since symptoms can recur after medicine stopped
- Continue treatment until all symptoms are gone (remission) or significantly reduced (e.g., OCD, PTSD)
- Once symptoms are gone, continue treating for 1 year for the first episode of depression
- For second and subsequent episodes of depression, treatment may need to be indefinite
- For anxiety disorders and bulimia, treatment may also need to be indefinite

If It Doesn't Work
- Many patients have only a partial response where some symptoms are improved but others persist (especially insomnia, fatigue, and problems concentrating in depression)
- Other patients may be nonresponders, sometimes called treatment-resistant or treatment-refractory
- Some patients who have an initial response may relapse even though they continue treatment, sometimes called "poop-out"
- Consider increasing dose, switching to another agent or adding an appropriate augmenting agent
- Consider psychotherapy
- Consider evaluation for another diagnosis or for a comorbid condition (e.g., medical illness, substance abuse, etc.)
- Some patients may experience apparent lack of consistent efficacy due to activation of latent or underlying bipolar disorder, and require antidepressant discontinuation and a switch to a mood stabilizer

Best Augmenting Combos for Partial Response or Treatment Resistance
- Trazodone, especially for insomnia

- Bupropion, mirtazapine, reboxetine, or atomoxetine (add with caution and at lower doses since fluoxetine could theoretically raise atomoxetine levels); use combinations of antidepressants with caution as this may activate bipolar disorder and suicidal ideation
- Modafinil, especially for fatigue, sleepiness, and lack of concentration
- Mood stabilizers or atypical antipsychotics for bipolar depression, psychotic depression, treatment-resistant depression, or treatment-resistant anxiety disorders

✻ Fluoxetine has been specifically studied in combination with olanzapine (olanzapine-fluoxetine combination) with excellent results for bipolar depression, treatment-resistant unipolar depression, and psychotic depression

- Benzodiazepines
- If all else fails for anxiety disorders, consider gabapentin or tiagabine
- Hypnotics for insomnia
- Classically, lithium, buspirone, or thyroid hormone

Tests
- None for healthy individuals

SIDE EFFECTS

How Drug Causes Side Effects
- Theoretically due to increases in serotonin concentrations at serotonin receptors in parts of the brain and body other than those that cause therapeutic actions (e.g., unwanted actions of serotonin in sleep centers causing insomnia, unwanted actions of serotonin in the gut causing diarrhea, etc.)
- Increasing serotonin can cause diminished dopamine release and might contribute to emotional flattening, cognitive slowing, and apathy in some patients
- Most side effects are immediate but often go away with time, in contrast to most therapeutic effects which are delayed and are enhanced over time

✻ Fluoxetine's unique 5HT2C antagonist properties could contribute to agitation, anxiety, and undesirable activation, especially early in dosing

Notable Side Effects
- Sexual dysfunction (men: delayed ejaculation, erectile dysfunction; men and women: decreased sexual desire, anorgasmia)
- Gastrointestinal (decreased appetite, nausea, diarrhea, constipation, dry mouth)
- Mostly CNS (insomnia but also sedation, agitation, tremors, headache, dizziness)
- Note: patients with diagnosed or undiagnosed bipolar or psychotic disorders may be more vulnerable to CNS-activating actions of SSRIs
- Autonomic (sweating)
- Bruising and rare bleeding
- SIADH (syndrome of inappropriate antidiuretic hormone secretion)

Life-Threatening or Dangerous Side Effects
- Rare seizures
- Rare induction of mania
- Rare activation of suicidal ideation and behavior (suicidality) (short-term studies did not show an increase in the risk of suicidality with antidepressants compared to placebo beyond age 24)

Weight Gain
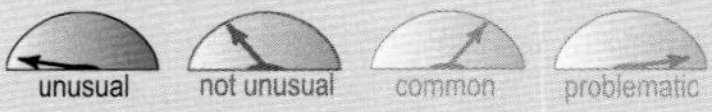

- Reported but not expected
- Possible weight loss, especially short-term

Sedation
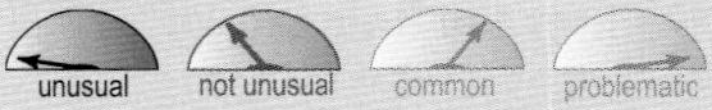

- Reported but not expected

What to Do About Side Effects
- Wait
- Wait
- Wait
- If fluoxetine is activating, take in the morning to help reduce insomnia
- Reduce dose to 10 mg, and either stay at this dose if tolerated and effective, or consider increasing again to 20 mg or more if tolerated but not effective at 10 mg
- In a few weeks, switch or add other drugs

Best Augmenting Agents for Side Effects
- Often best to try another SSRI or another antidepressant monotherapy prior to

resorting to augmentation strategies to treat side effects
- Trazodone or a hypnotic for insomnia
- Bupropion, sildenafil, vardenafil, or tadalafil for sexual dysfunction
- Bupropion for emotional flattening, cognitive slowing, or apathy
- Mirtazapine for insomnia, agitation, and gastrointestinal side effects
- Benzodiazepines for jitteriness and anxiety, especially at initiation of treatment and especially for anxious patients
- Many side effects are dose-dependent (i.e., they increase as dose increases, or they reemerge until tolerance redevelops)
- Many side effects are time-dependent (i.e., they start immediately upon dosing and upon each dose increase, but go away with time)
- Activation and agitation may represent the induction of a bipolar state, especially a mixed dysphoric bipolar II condition sometimes associated with suicidal ideation, and require the addition of lithium, a mood stabilizer or an atypical antipsychotic, and/or discontinuation of fluoxetine

DOSING AND USE

Usual Dosage Range
- 20–80 mg for depression and anxiety disorders
- 60–80 mg for bulimia

Dosage Forms
- Capsules 10 mg, 20 mg, 40 mg, 60 mg
- Tablet 10 mg
- Liquid 20 mg/5 mL–120 mL bottles
- Weekly capsule 90 mg

How to Dose
- Depression and OCD: initial dose 20 mg/day in morning, usually wait a few weeks to assess drug effects before increasing dose; maximum dose generally 80 mg/day
- Bulimia: initial dose 60 mg/day in morning; some patients may need to begin at lower dose and titrate over several days

Dosing Tips
- The long half-lives of fluoxetine and its active metabolites mean that dose changes will not be fully reflected in plasma for several weeks, lengthening titration to final dose and extending withdrawal from treatment
- Give once daily, often in the mornings, but at any time of day tolerated
- Often available in capsules, not tablets, so unable to break capsules in half
- Occasional patients are dosed above 80 mg
- Liquid formulation easiest for doses below 10 mg when used for cases that are very intolerant to fluoxetine or for very slow up and down titration needs
- ✽ For some patients, weekly dosing with the weekly formulation may enhance compliance
- The more anxious and agitated the patient, the lower the starting dose, the slower the titration, and the more likely the need for a concomitant agent such as trazodone or a benzodiazepine
- If intolerable anxiety, insomnia, agitation, akathisia, or activation occur either upon dosing initiation or discontinuation, consider the possibility of activated bipolar disorder and switch to a mood stabilizer or an atypical antipsychotic

Overdose
- Rarely lethal in monotherapy overdose; respiratory depression especially with alcohol, ataxia, sedation, possible seizures

Long-Term Use
- Safe

Habit Forming
- No

How to Stop
- Taper rarely necessary since fluoxetine tapers itself after immediate discontinuation, due to the long half-life of fluoxetine and its active metabolites

Pharmacokinetics
- Active metabolite (norfluoxetine) has 2 week half-life
- Parent drug has 2–3 day half-life
- Inhibits CYP450 2D6
- Inhibits CYP450 3A4

Drug Interactions
- Tramadol increases the risk of seizures in patients taking an antidepressant

- Can increase TCA levels; use with caution with TCAs or when switching from a TCA to fluoxetine
- Can cause a fatal "serotonin syndrome" when combined with MAOIs, so do not use with MAOIs or for at least 14 days after MAOIs are stopped
- Do not start an MAOI for at least 5 weeks after discontinuing fluoxetine
- May displace highly protein bound drugs (e.g., warfarin)
- Can rarely cause weakness, hyperreflexia, and incoordination when combined with sumatriptan, or possibly with other triptans, requiring careful monitoring of patient
- Possible increased risk of bleeding, especially when combined with anticoagulants (e.g.,warfarin, NSAIDs)
- NSAIDs may impair effectiveness of SSRIs
- Via CYP450 2D6 inhibition, could theoretically interfere with the analgesic actions of codeine, and increase the plasma levels of some beta blockers and of atomoxetine
- Via CYP450 2D6 inhibition, fluoxetine could theoretically increase concentrations of thioridazine and cause dangerous cardiac arrhythmias
- May reduce the clearance of diazepam or trazodone, thus increasing their levels
- Via CYP450 3A4 inhibition, may increase the levels of alprazolam, buspirone, and triazolam
- Via CYP450 3A4 inhibition, fluoxetine could theoretically increase concentrations of certain cholesterol lowering HMG CoA reductase inhibitors, especially simvastatin, atorvastatin, and lovastatin, but not pravastatin or fluvastatin, which would increase the risk of rhabdomyolysis; thus, coadministration of fluoxetine with certain HMG CoA reductase inhibitors should proceed with caution
- Via CYP450 3A4 inhibition, fluoxetine could theoretically increase the concentrations of pimozide, and cause QTc prolongation and dangerous cardiac arrhythmias

Other Warnings/ Precautions

- ✻ Add or initiate other antidepressants with caution for up to 5 weeks after discontinuing fluoxetine
- Use with caution in patients with history of seizure
- Use with caution in patients with bipolar disorder unless treated with concomitant mood-stabilizing agent
- When treating children, carefully weigh the risks and benefits of pharmacological treatment against the risks and benefits of nontreatment with antidepressants and make sure to document this in the patient's chart
- Distribute the brochures provided by the FDA and the drug companies
- Warn patients and their caregivers about the possibility of activating side effects and advise them to report such symptoms immediately
- Monitor patients for activation of suicidal ideation, especially children and adolescents

Do Not Use

- If patient is taking an MAOI
- If patient is taking thioridazine
- If patient is taking pimozide
- If patient is taking tamoxifen
- If there is a proven allergy to fluoxetine

SPECIAL POPULATIONS

Renal Impairment

- No dose adjustment
- Not removed by hemodialysis

Hepatic Impairment

- Lower dose or give less frequently, perhaps by half

Cardiac Impairment

- Preliminary research suggests that fluoxetine is safe in these patients
- Treating depression with SSRIs in patients with acute angina or following myocardial infarction may reduce cardiac events and improve survival as well as mood

Elderly

- Some patients may tolerate lower doses better
- Risk of SIADH with SSRIs is higher in the elderly
- Reduction in the risk of suicidality with antidepressants compared to placebo in adults age 65 and older

Children and Adolescents

- Carefully weigh the risks and benefits of pharmacological treatment against the risks and benefits of nontreatment with antidepressants and make sure to document this in the patient's chart
- Monitor patients face-to-face regularly, particularly during the first several weeks of treatment
- Use with caution, observing for activation of known or unknown bipolar disorder and/or suicidal ideation, and inform parents or guardians of this risk so they can help observe child or adolescent patients
- Approved for OCD and depression
- Adolescents often receive adult dose, but doses slightly lower for children
- Children taking fluoxetine may have slower growth; long-term effects are unknown

Pregnancy

- Effective June 30, 2015, the US FDA requires changes to the content and format of pregnancy and lactation information in prescription drug labels, including the elimination of the pregnancy letter categories; the Pregnancy and Lactation Labeling Rule (PLLR or final rule) applies only to prescription drugs and will be phased in gradually for drugs approved on or after June 30, 2001
- Controlled studies have not been conducted in pregnant women
- Not generally recommended for use during pregnancy, especially during first trimester
- Nonetheless, continuous treatment during pregnancy may be necessary and has not been proven to be harmful to the fetus
- Current patient registries of children whose mothers took fluoxetine during pregnancy do not show adverse consequences
- At delivery there may be more bleeding in the mother and transient irritability or sedation in the newborn
- Must weigh the risk of treatment (first trimester fetal development, third trimester newborn delivery) to the child against the risk of no treatment (recurrence of depression, maternal health, infant bonding) to the mother and child
- For many patients this may mean continuing treatment during pregnancy
- Exposure to SSRIs early in pregnancy may be associated with increased risk of septal heart defects (absolute risk is small)
- SSRI use beyond the 20th week of pregnancy may be associated with increased risk of pulmonary hypertension in newborns, although this is not proven
- Exposure to SSRIs late in pregnancy may be associated with increased risk of gestational hypertension and preeclampsia
- Neonates exposed to SSRIs or SNRIs late in the third trimester have developed complications requiring prolonged hospitalization, respiratory support, and tube feeding; reported symptoms are consistent with either a direct toxic effect of SSRIs and SNRIs or, possibly, a drug discontinuation syndrome, and include respiratory distress, cyanosis, apnea, seizures, temperature instability, feeding difficulty, vomiting, hypoglycemia, hypotonia, hypertonia, hyperreflexia, tremor, jitteriness, irritability, and constant crying

Breast Feeding

- Some drug is found in mother's breast milk
- Trace amounts may be present in nursing children whose mothers are on fluoxetine
- If child becomes irritable or sedated, breast feeding or drug may need to be discontinued
- Immediate postpartum period is a high-risk time for depression, especially in women who have had prior depressive episodes, so drug may need to be reinstituted late in the third trimester or shortly after childbirth to prevent a recurrence during the postpartum period
- Must weigh benefits of breast feeding with risks and benefits of antidepressant treatment versus nontreatment to both the infant and the mother
- For many patients this may mean continuing treatment during breast feeding

THE ART OF PSYCHOPHARMACOLOGY

Potential Advantages

- Patients with atypical depression (hypersomnia, increased appetite)
- Patients with fatigue and low energy
- Patients with comorbid eating and affective disorders
- Generic is less expensive than brand name where available
- Patients for whom weekly administration is desired
- Children with OCD or depression

Potential Disadvantages

- Patients with anorexia
- Initiating treatment in anxious, agitated patients
- Initiating treatment in severe insomnia

Primary Target Symptoms

- Depressed mood
- Energy, motivation, and interest
- Anxiety (eventually, but can actually increase anxiety, especially short-term)
- Sleep disturbance, both insomnia and hypersomnia (eventually, but may actually cause insomnia, especially short-term)

Pearls

* May be a first-line choice for atypical depression (e.g., hypersomnia, hyperphagia, low energy, mood reactivity)
- Consider avoiding in agitated insomniacs
- Can cause cognitive and affective "flattening"
- Not as well tolerated as some other SSRIs for panic disorder and other anxiety disorders, especially when dosing is initiated, unless given with co-therapies such as benzodiazepines or trazodone
- Long half-life; even longer lasting active metabolite
* Actions at 5HT2C receptors may explain its activating properties
* Actions at 5HT2C receptors may explain in part fluoxetine's efficacy in combination with olanzapine for bipolar depression and treatment-resistant depression, since both agents have this property
- For sexual dysfunction, can augment with bupropion, sildenafil, vardenafil, or tadalafil, or switch to a non-SSRI such as bupropion or mirtazapine
- Mood disorders can be associated with eating disorders (especially in adolescent females) and be treated successfully with fluoxetine
- SSRIs may be less effective in women over 50, especially if they are not taking estrogen
- SSRIs may be useful for hot flushes in perimenopausal women
- Some postmenopausal women's depression will respond better to fluoxetine plus estrogen augmentation than to fluoxetine alone
- Nonresponse to fluoxetine in elderly may require consideration of mild cognitive impairment or Alzheimer disease
- SSRIs may not cause as many patients to attain remission of depression as some other classes of antidepressants (e.g., SNRIs)
- A single pill containing both fluoxetine and olanzapine is available for combination treatment of bipolar depression, psychotic depression, and treatment-resistant unipolar depression

Suggested Reading

Anderson IM. Selective serotonin reuptake inhibitors versus tricyclic antidepressants: a meta-analysis of efficacy and tolerability. J Affect Disord 2000;58:19–36.

Beasley CM Jr, Ball SG, Nilsson ME, et al. Fluoxetine and adult suicidality revisited: an updated meta-analysis using expanded data sources from placebo-controlled trials. J Clin Psychopharmacol 2007;27(6):682–6.

March JS, Silva S, Petrycki S, et al. The treatment for adolescents with depression study (TADS): long-term effectiveness and safety outcomes. Arch Gen Psychiatry 2007;64(10):1132–43.

Wagstaff AJ, Goa KL. Once-weekly fluoxetine. Drugs 2001;61:2221–8.

THERAPEUTICS

Brands • Depixol
see index for additional brand names

Generic? No

Class

- Neuroscience-based Nomenclature: dopamine receptor antagonist (D-RAn)
- Conventional antipsychotic (neuroleptic, thioxanthene, dopamine 2 antagonist)

Commonly Prescribed for

(bold for FDA approved)

- Schizophrenia
- Depression (low dose)
- Other psychotic disorders
- Bipolar disorder

How the Drug Works

- Blocks dopamine 2 receptors, reducing positive symptoms of psychosis

How Long Until It Works

- With injection, psychotic symptoms can improve within a few days, but it may take 1–2 weeks for notable improvement
- With oral formulation, psychotic symptoms can improve within 1 week, but it may take several weeks for full effect on behavior

If It Works

- Most often reduces positive symptoms in schizophrenia but does not eliminate them
- Most schizophrenic patients do not have a total remission of symptoms but rather a reduction of symptoms by about a third
- Continue treatment in schizophrenia until reaching a plateau of improvement
- After reaching a satisfactory plateau, continue treatment for at least a year after first episode of psychosis in schizophrenia
- For second and subsequent episodes of psychosis in schizophrenia, treatment may need to be indefinite
- Reduces symptoms of acute psychotic mania but not proven as a mood stabilizer or as an effective maintenance treatment in bipolar disorder
- After reducing acute psychotic symptoms in mania, switch to a mood stabilizer and/or an atypical antipsychotic for mood stabilization and maintenance

If It Doesn't Work

- Consider trying one of the first-line atypical antipsychotics (risperidone, olanzapine, quetiapine, ziprasidone, aripiprazole, paliperidone, amisulpride)
- Consider trying another conventional antipsychotic
- If 2 or more antipsychotic monotherapies do not work, consider clozapine

Best Augmenting Combos for Partial Response or Treatment Resistance

- Augmentation of conventional antipsychotics has not been systematically studied
- Addition of a mood-stabilizing anticonvulsant such as valproate, carbamazepine, or lamotrigine may be helpful in both schizophrenia and bipolar mania
- Augmentation with lithium in bipolar mania may be helpful
- Addition of a benzodiazepine, especially short-term for agitation

Tests

✻ Since conventional antipsychotics are frequently associated with weight gain, before starting treatment, weigh all patients and determine if the patient is already overweight (BMI 25.0–29.9) or obese (BMI ≥30)

- Before giving a drug that can cause weight gain to an overweight or obese patient, consider determining whether the patient already has pre-diabetes (fasting plasma glucose 100–125 mg/dL), diabetes (fasting plasma glucose >126 mg/dL), or dyslipidemia (increased total cholesterol, LDL cholesterol, and triglycerides; decreased HDL cholesterol), and treat or refer such patients for treatment, including nutrition and weight management, physical activity counseling, smoking cessation, and medical management

✻ Monitor weight and BMI during treatment

✻ Consider monitoring fasting triglycerides monthly for several months in patients at high risk for metabolic complications and when initiating or switching antipsychotics

✻ While giving a drug to a patient who has gained >5% of initial weight, consider evaluating for the presence of pre-diabetes,

diabetes, or dyslipidemia, or consider switching to a different antipsychotic
- Monitoring elevated prolactin levels of dubious clinical benefit
- Patients with low white blood cell count (WBC) or history of drug-induced leucopenia/neutropenia should have complete blood count (CBC) monitored frequently during the first few months and flupenthixol should be discontinued at the first sign of decline of WBC in the absence of other causative factors

SIDE EFFECTS

How Drug Causes Side Effects
- By blocking dopamine 2 receptors in the striatum, it can cause motor side effects
- By blocking dopamine 2 receptors in the pituitary, it can cause elevations in prolactin
- By blocking dopamine 2 receptors excessively in the mesocortical and mesolimbic dopamine pathways, especially at high doses, it can cause worsening of negative and cognitive symptoms (neuroleptic-induced deficit syndrome)
- Anticholinergic actions may cause sedation, blurred vision, constipation, dry mouth
- Antihistaminic actions may cause sedation, weight gain
- By blocking alpha 1 adrenergic receptors, it can cause dizziness, sedation, and hypotension
- Mechanism of weight gain and any possible increased incidence of diabetes or dyslipidemia with conventional antipsychotics is unknown

Notable Side Effects
✻ Neuroleptic-induced deficit syndrome
✻ Extrapyramidal symptoms (more common at start of treatment), parkinsonism
✻ Insomnia, restlessness, agitation, sedation
✻ Tardive dyskinesia (risk increases with duration of treatment and with dose)
✻ Galactorrhea, amenorrhea
- Tachycardia
- Weight gain
- Hypomania
- Rare eosinophilia

Life-Threatening or Dangerous Side Effects
- Rare neuroleptic malignant syndrome
- Rare seizures
- Rare jaundice, leucopenia
- Increased risk of death and cerebrovascular events in elderly patients with dementia-related psychosis

Weight Gain
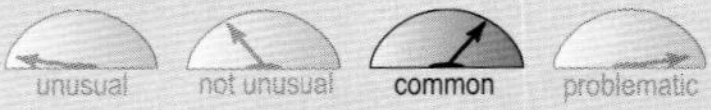

- Many experience and/or can be significant in amount

Sedation
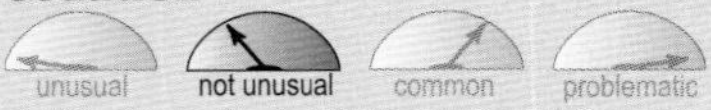

- Occurs in significant minority

What to Do About Side Effects
- Wait
- Wait
- Wait
- For motor symptoms, add an anticholinergic agent
- Reduce the dose
- For sedation, give at night
- Switch to an atypical antipsychotic
- Weight loss, exercise programs, and medical management for high BMIs, diabetes, dyslipidemia

Best Augmenting Agents for Side Effects
- Benztropine or trihexyphenidyl for motor side effects
- Sometimes amantadine can be helpful for motor side effects
- Benzodiazepines may be helpful for akathisia
- Many side effects cannot be improved with an augmenting agent

DOSING AND USE

Usual Dosage Range
- Oral 3–6 mg/day in divided doses
- Intramuscular 40–120 mg every 1–4 weeks

Dosage Forms
- Tablet 0.5 mg, 3 mg
- Injection 20 mg/mL, 100 mg/mL

How to Dose

- Oral: initial 1 mg 3 times a day; increase by 1 mg every 2–3 days; maximum generally 18 mg/day
- Intramuscular: initial dose 20 mg for patients who have not been exposed to long-acting depot antipsychotics, 40 mg for patients who have previously demonstrated tolerance to long-acting depot antipsychotics; after 4–10 days can give additional 20 mg dose; maximum 200 mg every 1–4 weeks

Dosing Tips

- The peak of action for the decanoate is usually 7–10 days, and doses generally have to be administered every 2–3 weeks
- May have more activating effects at low doses, which can sometimes be useful as a second-line, short-term treatment of depression
- Some evidence that flupenthixol may improve anxiety and depression at low doses
- Treatment should be suspended if absolute neutrophil count falls below 1,000/mm^3

Overdose

- Agitation, confusion, sedation, extrapyramidal symptoms, respiratory collapse, circulatory collapse

Long-Term Use

- Safe

Habit Forming

- No

How to Stop

- Slow down-titration of oral formulation (over 6–8 weeks), especially when simultaneously beginning a new antipsychotic while switching (i.e., cross-titration)
- Rapid oral discontinuation may lead to rebound psychosis and worsening of symptoms
- If antiparkinson agents are being used, they should be continued for a few weeks after flupenthixol is discontinued

Pharmacokinetics

- Oral: maximum plasma concentrations within 3-8 hours
- Intramuscular: rate-limiting half-life approximately 8 days with single dose, approximately 17 days with multiple doses

Drug Interactions

- May decrease the effects of levodopa, dopamine agonists
- May increase the effects of antihypertensive drugs except for guanethidine, whose antihypertensive actions flupenthixol may antagonize
- CNS effects may be increased if used with other CNS depressants
- Combined use with epinephrine may lower blood pressure
- Ritonavir may increase plasma levels of flupenthixol
- May increase carbamazepine plasma levels
- Some patients taking a neuroleptic and lithium have developed an encephalopathic syndrome similar to neuroleptic malignant syndrome

Other Warnings/ Precautions

- If signs of neuroleptic malignant syndrome develop, treatment should be immediately discontinued
- Use cautiously in patients with alcohol withdrawal or convulsive disorders because of possible lowering of seizure threshold
- In epileptic patients, dose 10–20 mg every 15 days for intramuscular formulation
- Use with caution if at all in patients with Parkinson's disease, severe arteriosclerosis, or Lewy body dementia
- Possible antiemetic effect of flupenthixol may mask signs of other disorders or overdose; suppression of cough reflex may cause asphyxia
- Avoid extreme heat exposure
- Do not use epinephrine in event of overdose as interaction with some pressor agents may lower blood pressure

Do Not Use

- If patient is taking a large concomitant dose of a sedative hypnotic
- If patient has CNS depression
- If patient is comatose or if there is brain damage
- If there is blood dyscrasia
- If patient has pheochromocytoma

- If patient has liver damage
- If patient has a severe cardiovascular disorder
- If patient has renal insufficiency
- If patient has cerebrovascular insufficiency
- If there is a proven allergy to flupenthixol

SPECIAL POPULATIONS

Renal Impairment
- Oral: recommended to take half or less of usual adult dose
- Intramuscular: recommended dose schedule generally 10–20 mg every 15 days

Hepatic Impairment
- Use with caution
- Oral: recommended to take half or less of usual adult dose

Cardiac Impairment
- Use with caution
- Oral: recommended to take half or less of usual adult dose

Elderly
- Intramuscular: recommended initial dose generally 5 mg; recommended dose schedule generally 10–20 mg every 15 days
- Oral: recommended to take half or less of usual adult dose
- Although conventional antipsychotics are commonly used for behavioral disturbances in dementia, no agent has been approved for treatment of elderly patients with dementia-related psychosis
- Elderly patients with dementia-related psychosis treated with antipsychotics are at increased risk of death compared to placebo, and also have an increased risk of cerebrovascular events

Children and Adolescents
- Not recommended for use in children

Pregnancy
- Not recommended for use during pregnancy
- There is a risk of abnormal muscle movements and withdrawal symptoms in newborns whose mothers took an antipsychotic during the third trimester; symptoms may include agitation, abnormally increased or decreased muscle tone, tremor, sleepiness, severe difficulty breathing, and difficulty feeding
- Reports of extrapyramidal symptoms, jaundice, hyperreflexia, hyporeflexia in infants whose mothers took a conventional antipsychotic during pregnancy
- Psychotic symptoms may worsen during pregnancy and some form of treatment may be necessary
- Atypical antipsychotics may be preferable to conventional antipsychotics or anticonvulsant mood stabilizers if treatment is required during pregnancy

Breast Feeding
- Some drug is found in mother's breast milk
- ✻ Recommended either to discontinue drug or bottle feed

THE ART OF PSYCHOPHARMACOLOGY

Potential Advantages
- Noncompliant patients

Potential Disadvantages
- Children
- Elderly
- Patients with tardive dyskinesia

Primary Target Symptoms
- Positive symptoms of psychosis
- Negative symptoms of psychosis
- Aggressive symptoms

Pearls
- Less sedation and orthostatic hypotension but more extrapyramidal symptoms than some other conventional antipsychotics
- Patients have very similar antipsychotic responses to any conventional antipsychotic, which is different from atypical antipsychotics where antipsychotic responses of individual patients can occasionally vary greatly from one atypical antipsychotic to another

- Patients with inadequate responses to atypical antipsychotics may benefit from a trial of augmentation with a conventional antipsychotic such as flupenthixol or from switching to a conventional antipsychotic such as flupenthixol
- However, long-term polypharmacy with a combination of a conventional antipsychotic such as flupenthixol with an atypical antipsychotic may combine their side effects without clearly augmenting the efficacy of either
- For treatment-resistant patients, especially those with impulsivity, aggression, violence, and self-harm, long-term polypharmacy with 2 atypical antipsychotics or with 1 atypical antipsychotic and 1 conventional antipsychotic may be useful or even necessary while closely monitoring
- In such cases, it may be beneficial to combine 1 depot antipsychotic with 1 oral antipsychotic
- Although a frequent practice by some prescribers, adding 2 conventional antipsychotics together has little rationale and may reduce tolerability without clearly enhancing efficacy

Suggested Reading

Gerlach J. Depot neuroleptics in relapse prevention: advantages and disadvantages. Int Clin Psychopharmacol 1995;(9 Suppl 5):S17–20.

Quraishi S, David A. Depot flupenthixol decanoate for schizophrenia or other similar psychotic disorders. Cochrane Database Syst Rev 2000;(2):CD001470.

Soyka M, De Vry J. Flupenthixol as a potential pharmacotreatment of alcohol and cocaine abuse/dependence. Eur Neuropsychopharmacol 2000;10(5):325–32.

THERAPEUTICS

Brands • Prolixin

see index for additional brand names

Generic? Yes

Class

- Conventional antipsychotic (neuroleptic, phenothiazine, dopamine 2 antagonist)

Commonly Prescribed for

(bold for FDA approved)

- **Psychotic disorders**
- Bipolar disorder

How the Drug Works

- Blocks dopamine 2 receptors, reducing positive symptoms of psychosis

How Long Until It Works

- Psychotic symptoms can improve within 1 week, but it may take several weeks for full effect on behavior

If It Works

- Most often reduces positive symptoms in schizophrenia but does not eliminate them
- Most schizophrenic patients do not have a total remission of symptoms but rather a reduction of symptoms by about a third
- Continue treatment in schizophrenia until reaching a plateau of improvement
- After reaching a satisfactory plateau, continue treatment for at least a year after first episode of psychosis in schizophrenia
- For second and subsequent episodes of psychosis in schizophrenia, treatment may need to be indefinite
- Reduces symptoms of acute psychotic mania but not proven as a mood stabilizer or as an effective maintenance treatment in bipolar disorder
- After reducing acute psychotic symptoms in mania, switch to a mood stabilizer and/or an atypical antipsychotic for mood stabilization and maintenance

If It Doesn't Work

- Consider trying one of the first-line atypical antipsychotics (risperidone, olanzapine, quetiapine, ziprasidone, aripiprazole, paliperidone, amisulpride, asenapine, iloperidone, lurasidone)
- Consider trying another conventional antipsychotic
- If 2 or more antipsychotic monotherapies do not work, consider clozapine

Best Augmenting Combos for Partial Response or Treatment Resistance

- Augmentation of conventional antipsychotics has not been systematically studied
- Addition of a mood-stabilizing anticonvulsant such as valproate, carbamazepine, or lamotrigine may be helpful in both schizophrenia and bipolar mania
- Augmentation with lithium in bipolar mania may be helpful
- Addition of a benzodiazepine, especially short-term for agitation

Tests

- ❋ Since conventional antipsychotics are frequently associated with weight gain, before starting treatment, weigh all patients and determine if the patient is already overweight (BMI 25.0–29.9) or obese (BMI ≥30)
- Before giving a drug that can cause weight gain to an overweight or obese patient, consider determining whether the patient already has pre-diabetes (fasting plasma glucose 100–125 mg/dL), diabetes (fasting plasma glucose >126 mg/dL), or dyslipidemia (increased total cholesterol, LDL cholesterol, and triglycerides; decreased HDL cholesterol), and treat or refer such patients for treatment, including nutrition and weight management, physical activity counseling, smoking cessation, and medical management
- ❋ Monitor weight and BMI during treatment
- ❋ Consider monitoring fasting triglycerides monthly for several months in patients at high risk for metabolic complications and when initiating or switching anitpsychotics
- ❋ While giving a drug to a patient who has gained >5% of initial weight, consider evaluating for the presence of pre-diabetes, diabetes, or dyslipidemia, or consider switching to a different antipsychotic
- Should check blood pressure in the elderly before starting and for the first few weeks of treatment

- Monitoring elevated prolactin levels of dubious clinical benefit
- Phenothiazines may cause false-positive phenylketonuria results
- Patients with low white blood cell count (WBC) or history of drug-induced leucopenia/neutropenia should have complete blood count (CBC) monitored frequently during the first few months and fluphenazine should be discontinued at the first sign of decline of WBC in the absence of other causative factors

SIDE EFFECTS

How Drug Causes Side Effects

- By blocking dopamine 2 receptors in the striatum, it can cause motor side effects
- By blocking dopamine 2 receptors in the pituitary, it can cause elevations in prolactin
- By blocking dopamine 2 receptors excessively in the mesocortical and mesolimbic dopamine pathways, especially at high doses, it can cause worsening of negative and cognitive symptoms (neuroleptic-induced deficit syndrome)
- Anticholinergic actions may cause sedation, blurred vision, constipation, dry mouth
- Antihistaminic actions may cause sedation, weight gain
- By blocking alpha 1 adrenergic receptors, it can cause dizziness, sedation, and hypotension
- Mechanism of weight gain and any possible increased incidence of diabetes or dyslipidemia with conventional antipsychotics is unknown

Notable Side Effects

✽ Neuroleptic-induced deficit syndrome
✽ Akathisia
✽ Priapism
✽ Extrapyramidal symptoms, parkinsonism, tardive dyskinesia, tardive dystonia
✽ Galactorrhea, amenorrhea

- Dizziness, sedation
- Dry mouth, constipation, urinary retention, blurred vision
- Decreased sweating, depression
- Sexual dysfunction
- Hypotension, tachycardia, syncope
- Weight gain

Life-Threatening or Dangerous Side Effects

- Rare neuroleptic malignant syndrome
- Rare jaundice, agranulocytosis
- Rare seizures
- Increased risk of death and cerebrovascular events in elderly patients with dementia-related psychosis

Weight Gain

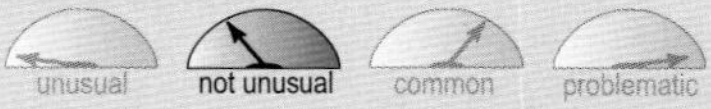

- Occurs in significant minority

Sedation

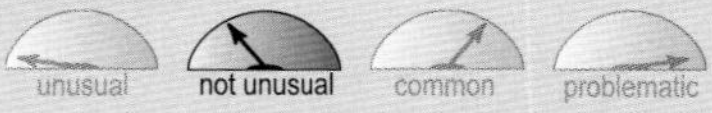

- Occurs in significant minority

What to Do About Side Effects

- Wait
- Wait
- Wait
- For motor symptoms, add an anticholinergic agent
- Reduce the dose
- For sedation, take at night
- Switch to an atypical antipsychotic
- Weight loss, exercise programs, and medical management for high BMIs, diabetes, dyslipidemia

Best Augmenting Agents for Side Effects

- Benztropine or trihexyphenidyl for motor side effects
- Sometimes amantadine can be helpful for motor side effects
- Benzodiazepines may be helpful for akathisia
- Many side effects cannot be improved with an augmenting agent

DOSING AND USE

Usual Dosage Range

- Oral: 1–20 mg/day maintenance
- Intramuscular: generally 1/3 to 1/2 the oral dose
- Decanoate for intramuscular or subcutaneous administration: 12.5–100 mg/2 weeks maintenance (see Fluphenazine Decanoate section after Pearls for dosing and use)

Dosage Forms
- Tablet 1 mg, 2.5 mg scored, 5 mg scored, 10 mg scored
- Decanoate for long-acting intramuscular or subcutaneous administration 25 mg/mL
- Injection for acute intramuscular administration 2.5 mg/mL
- Elixir 2.5 mg/5 mL
- Concentrate 5 mg/mL

How to Dose
- Oral: initial 0.5–10 mg/day in divided doses; maximum 40 mg/day
- Intramuscular (short-acting): initial 1.25 mg; 2.5–10 mg/day can be given in divided doses every 6–8 hours; maximum dose generally 10 mg/day

Dosing Tips – Oral
- Patients receiving atypical antipsychotics may occasionally require a "top up" of a conventional antipsychotic to control aggression or violent behavior
- Fluphenazine tablets 2.5 mg, 5 mg, and 10 mg contain tartrazine, which can cause allergic reactions, especially in patients sensitive to aspirin
- Oral solution should not be mixed with drinks containing caffeine, tannic acid (tea), or pectinates (apple juice)
- Treatment should be suspended if absolute neutrophil count falls below 1,000/mm^3

Overdose
- Extrapyramidal symptoms, coma, hypotension, sedation, seizures, respiratory depression

Long-Term Use
- Some side effects may be irreversible (e.g., tardive dyskinesia)

Habit Forming
- No

How to Stop
- Slow down-titration of oral formulation (over 6 to 8 weeks), especially when simultaneously beginning a new antipsychotic while switching (i.e., cross-titration)
- Rapid oral discontinuation may lead to rebound psychosis and worsening of symptoms
- If antiparkinson agents are being used, they should be continued for a few weeks after fluphenazine is discontinued

Pharmacokinetics
- Mean half-life of oral formulation approximately 15 hours
- Mean half-life of intramuscular formulation approximately 6.8–9.6 days

Drug Interactions
- May decrease the effects of levodopa, dopamine agonists
- May increase the effects of antihypertensive drugs except for guanethidine, whose antihypertensive actions fluphenazine may antagonize
- Additive effects may occur if used with CNS depressants
- Additive anticholinergic effects may occur if used with atropine or related compounds
- Alcohol and diuretics may increase the risk of hypotension
- Some patients taking a neuroleptic and lithium have developed an encephalopathic syndrome similar to neuroleptic malignant syndrome
- Combined use with epinephrine may lower blood pressure

Other Warnings/ Precautions
- If signs of neuroleptic malignant syndrome develop, treatment should be immediately discontinued
- Use cautiously in patients with alcohol withdrawal or convulsive disorders because of possible lowering of seizure threshold
- Avoid undue exposure to sunlight
- Use cautiously in patients with respiratory disorders
- Avoid extreme heat exposure
- Antiemetic effect can mask signs of other disorders or overdose
- Do not use epinephrine in event of overdose as interaction with some pressor agents may lower blood pressure
- Use only with caution if at all in Parkinson's disease or Lewy body dementia

Do Not Use
- If patient is in a comatose state or has CNS depression
- If patient is taking cabergoline, pergolide, or metrizamide
- If there is a proven allergy to fluphenazine
- If there is a known sensitivity to any phenothiazine

SPECIAL POPULATIONS

Renal Impairment
- Use with caution; titration should be slower

Hepatic Impairment
- Use with caution; titration should be slower

Cardiac Impairment
- Cardiovascular toxicity can occur, especially orthostatic hypotension

Elderly
- Titration should be slower; lower initial dose (1–2.5 mg/day)
- Elderly patients may be more susceptible to adverse effects
- Although conventional antipsychotics are commonly used for behavioral disturbances in dementia, no agent has been approved for treatment of elderly patients with dementia-related psychosis
- Elderly patients with dementia-related psychosis treated with antipsychotics are at an increased risk of death compared to placebo, and also have an increased risk of cerebrovascular events

Children and Adolescents
- Safety and efficacy not established
- Decanoate and enanthate injectable formulations are contraindicated in children under age 12
- Generally consider second-line after atypical antipsychotics

Pregnancy
- Effective June 30, 2015, the US FDA requires changes to the content and format of pregnancy and lactation information in prescription drug labels, including the elimination of the pregnancy letter categories; the Pregnancy and Lactation Labeling Rule (PLLR or final rule) applies only to prescription drugs and will be phased in gradually for drugs approved on or after June 30, 2001
- There is a risk of abnormal muscle movements and withdrawal symptoms in newborns whose mothers took an antipsychotic during the third trimester; symptoms may include agitation, abnormally increased or decreased muscle tone, tremor, sleepiness, severe difficulty breathing, and difficulty feeding
- Reports of extrapyramidal symptoms, jaundice, hyperreflexia, hyporeflexia in infants whose mothers took a phenothiazine during pregnancy
- Fluphenazine should only be used during pregnancy if clearly indicated
- Psychotic symptoms may worsen during pregnancy and some form of treatment may be necessary
- Atypical antipsychotics may be preferable to conventional antipsychotics or anticonvulsant mood stabilizers if treatment is required during pregnancy

Breast Feeding
- Some drug is found in mother's breast milk
- Effects on infant have been observed (dystonia, tardive dyskinesia, sedation)
- ✻ Recommended either to discontinue drug or bottle feed

THE ART OF PSYCHOPHARMACOLOGY

Potential Advantages
- Intramuscular formulation for (emergency use
- Relatively rapid onset of LAI (but see fluphenazine decanoate after Pearls section)

Potential Disadvantages
- Patients with tardive dyskinesia
- Children
- Elderly

Primary Target Symptoms
- Positive symptoms of psychosis
- Motor and autonomic hyperactivity
- Violent or aggressive behavior

Pearls
- Fluphenazine is a high-potency phenothiazine
- Less risk of sedation and orthostatic hypotension but greater risk of extrapyramidal symptoms than with low potency phenothiazines

- Not shown to be effective for behavioral problems in mental retardation
- Patients have very similar antipsychotic responses to any conventional antipsychotic, which is different from atypical antipsychotics where antipsychotic responses of individual patients can occasionally vary greatly from one atypical antipsychotic to another
- Patients with inadequate responses to atypical antipsychotics may benefit from a trial of augmentation with a conventional antipsychotic such as fluphenazine or from switching to a conventional antipsychotic such as fluphenazine
- However, long-term polypharmacy with a combination of a conventional antipsychotic such as fluphenazine with an atypical antipsychotic may combine their side effects without clearly augmenting the efficacy of either
- For treatment-resistant patients, especially those with impulsivity, aggression, violence, and self-harm, long-term polypharmacy with 2 atypical antipsychotics or with 1 atypical antipsychotic and 1 conventional antipsychotic may be useful or even necessary while closely monitoring
- In such cases, it may be beneficial to combine 1 depot antipsychotic with 1 oral antipsychotic
- Although a frequent practice by some prescribers, adding 2 conventional antipsychotics together has little rationale and may reduce tolerability without clearly enhancing efficacy

Fluphenazine Decanoate

Vehicle	Sesame Oil
Tmax	0.3–1.5 days
T1/2 with multiple dosing	14 days
Able to be loaded	Yes
Time to reach steady state	4–6 weeks with loading
Dosing schedule (maintenance)	2 weeks
Injection site	Intramuscular or subcutaneous
Needle gauge	21
Dosage forms	25 mg
Injection volume	25 mg/mL

Usual Dosage Range

- 12.5–100 mg/2 weeks maintenance

How to Dose

- Conversion from oral: can either supplement with oral formulation at half-dose for at least 2 weeks OR use weekly loading injections of 1.6 times the oral daily dose (mg/day) for 4–6 weeks

Dosing Tips

- With LAIs, the absorption rate constant is slower than the elimination rate constant, thus resulting in "flip-flop" kinetics—i.e., time to steady-state is a function of absorption rate, while concentration at steady-state is a function of elimination rate
- In general, 5 half-lives of any medication are needed to achieve 97% of steady-state levels
- The long half-lives of depot antipsychotics mean that one must either adequately load the dose (if possible) or provide oral supplementation
- The failure to adequately load the dose leads either to prolonged cross-titration from oral antipsychotic or to sub-therapeutic antipsychotic plasma levels for weeks or months in patients who are not receiving (or adhering to) oral supplementation
- Because plasma antipsychotic levels increase gradually over time, dose requirements may ultimately decrease from initial; obtaining periodic plasma levels can be beneficial to prevent unnecessary plasma level creep
- The time to get a blood level for patients receiving LAI is the morning of the day they will receive their next injection
- Advantages: Early peak (see following graph) may be beneficial in the management of acute patients
- Disadvantages: Early peak also carries risk of EPS or akathisia in first 48 hours; 2-week injection schedule; higher incidence of local site reactions (due to sesame oil vehicle)
- Response threshold is 0.81 ng/mL; plasma levels greater than 2–3 ng/mL are generally not well tolerated

SWITCHING FROM ORAL ANTIPSYCHOTICS TO FLUPHENAZINE DECANOATE

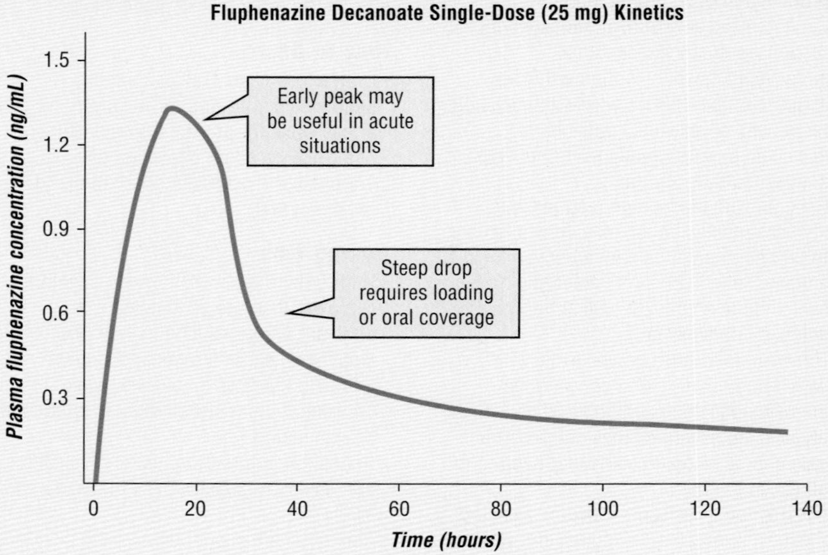

- Discontinuation of oral antipsychotic can begin immediately if adequate loading is pursued; otherwise, supplement with oral formulation at half-dose for at least 2 weeks
- How to discontinue oral formulations
  - Down-titration is not required for: amisulpride, aripiprazole, brexpiprazole, cariprazine, paliperidone ER
  - 1-week down-titration is required for: iloperidone, lurasidone, risperidone, ziprasidone
  - 3–4-week down-titration is required for: asenapine, olanzapine, quetiapine
  - 4+-week down-titration is required for: clozapine
  - For patients taking benzodiazepine or anticholinergic medication, this can be continued during cross-titration to help alleviate side effects such as insomnia, agitation, and/or psychosis. Once the patient is stable on LAI, these can be tapered one at a time as appropriate.

Suggested Reading

Adams CE, Eisenbruch M. Depot fluphenazine for schizophrenia. Cochrane Database Syst Rev 2000;(2):CD000307.

David A, Adams CE, Eisenbruch M, Quraishi S, Rathbone J. Depot fluphenazine decanoate and enanthate for schizophrenia. Cochrane Database Syst Rev 2005;25(1):CD000307.

Ereshefsky L, Saklad SR, Jann MW. Future of depot neuroleptic therapy: pharmacokinetic and pharmacodynamic approaches. J Clin Psychiatry 1984;45(suppl):50–9.

King DJ. Drug treatment of the negative symptoms of schizophrenia. Eur Neuropsychopharmacol 1998;8(1):33–42.

Matar HE, Almerie MQ. Oral fluphenazine versus placebo for schizophrenia. Cochrane Database Syst Rev 2007;24(1):CD006352.

Milton GV, Jann MW. Emergency treatment of psychotic symptoms. Pharmacokinetic considerations for antipsychotic drugs. Clin Pharmacokinet 1995;28(6):494–504.

FLURAZEPAM

THERAPEUTICS

Brands • Dalmane

see index for additional brand names

Generic? Yes

Class

- Neuroscience-based Nomenclature: GABA positive allosteric modulator (GABA-PAM)
- Benzodiazepine (hypnotic)

Commonly Prescribed for

(bold for FDA approved)

- **Insomnia characterized by difficulty in falling asleep, frequent nocturnal awakenings, and/or early morning awakening**
- **Recurring insomnia or poor sleeping habits**
- **Acute or chronic medical situations requiring restful sleep**
- Catatonia

How the Drug Works

- Binds to benzodiazepine receptors at the GABA-A ligand-gated chloride channel complex
- Enhances the inhibitory effects of GABA
- Boosts chloride conductance through GABA-regulated channels
- Inhibitory actions in sleep centers may provide sedative hypnotic effects

How Long Until It Works

- Generally takes effect in less than an hour

If It Works

- Improves quality of sleep
- Effects on total wake-time and number of nighttime awakenings may be decreased over time

If It Doesn't Work

- If insomnia does not improve after 7–10 days, it may be a manifestation of a primary psychiatric or physical illness such as obstructive sleep apnea or restless leg syndrome, which requires independent evaluation
- Increase the dose
- Improve sleep hygiene
- Switch to another agent

Best Augmenting Combos for Partial Response or Treatment Resistance

- Generally, best to switch to another agent
- Trazodone
- Agents with antihistamine actions (e.g., diphenhydramine, TCAs)

Tests

- In patients with seizure disorders, concomitant medical illness, and/or those with multiple concomitant long-term medications, periodic liver tests and blood counts may be prudent

SIDE EFFECTS

How Drug Causes Side Effects

- Same mechanism for side effects as for therapeutic effects – namely due to excessive actions at benzodiazepine receptors
- Actions at benzodiazepine receptors that carry over to the next day can cause daytime sedation, amnesia, and ataxia
- Long-term adaptations in benzodiazepine receptors may explain the development of dependence, tolerance, and withdrawal

Notable Side Effects

- ❋ Sedation, fatigue, depression
- ❋ Dizziness, ataxia, slurred speech, weakness
- ❋ Forgetfulness, confusion
- ❋ Hyperexcitability, nervousness
- Rare hallucinations, mania
- Rare hypotension
- Hypersalivation, dry mouth
- Rebound insomnia when withdrawing from long-term treatment

Life-Threatening or Dangerous Side Effects

- Respiratory depression, especially when taken with CNS depressants in overdose
- Rare hepatic dysfunction, renal dysfunction, blood dyscrasias

Weight Gain

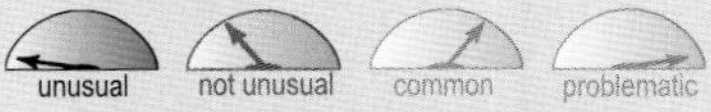

- Reported but not expected

Sedation

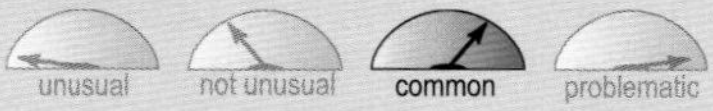

- Many experience and/or can be significant in amount

What to Do About Side Effects

- Wait
- To avoid problems with memory, only take flurazepam if planning to have a full night's sleep
- Lower the dose
- Switch to a shorter-acting sedative hypnotic
- Switch to a non-benzodiazepine hypnotic
- Administer flumazenil if side effects are severe or life-threatening

Best Augmenting Agents for Side Effects

- Many side effects cannot be improved with an augmenting agent

DOSING AND USE

Usual Dosage Range

- 15–30 mg/day at bedtime for 7–10 days

Dosage Forms

- Capsule 15 mg, 30 mg

How to Dose

- 15 mg/day at bedtime; may increase to 30 mg/day at bedtime if ineffective

Dosing Tips

* Because flurazepam tends to accumulate over time, perhaps not the best hypnotic for chronic nightly use
- Use lowest possible effective dose and assess need for continued treatment regularly
- Flurazepam should generally not be prescribed in quantities greater than a 1-month supply
- Patients with lower body weights may require lower doses
- Risk of dependence may increase with dose and duration of treatment

Overdose

- No death reported in monotherapy; sedation, slurred speech, poor coordination, confusion, coma, respiratory depression

Long-Term Use

- Not generally intended for long-term use
* Because of its relatively longer half-life, flurazepam may cause some daytime sedation and/or impaired motor/cognitive function, and may do so progressively over time

Habit Forming

- Flurazepam is a Schedule IV drug
- Some patients may develop dependence and/or tolerance; risk may be greater with higher doses
- History of drug addiction may increase risk of dependence

How to Stop

- If taken for more than a few weeks, taper to reduce chances of withdrawal effects
- Patients with seizure history may seize upon sudden withdrawal
- Rebound insomnia may occur the first 1–2 nights after stopping
- For patients with severe problems discontinuing a benzodiazepine, dosing may need to be tapered over many months (i.e., reduce dose by 1% every 3 days by crushing tablet and suspending or dissolving in 100 mL of fruit juice and then disposing of 1 mL while drinking the rest; 3–7 days later, dispose of 2 mL, and so on). This is both a form of very slow biological tapering and a form of behavioral desensitization

Pharmacokinetics

- Elimination half-life approximately 24–100 hours
- Active metabolites

Drug Interactions

- Cimetidine may decrease flurazepam clearance and thus raise flurazepam levels
- Flurazepam and kava combined use may affect clearance of either drug
- Increased depressive effects when taken with other CNS depressants (see Warnings below)

Other Warnings/ Precautions

- Boxed warning regarding the increased risk of CNS depressant effects when benzodiazepines and opioid medications are used together, including specifically the risk of slowed or difficulty breathing and death
- If alternatives to the combined use of benzodiazepines and opioids are not available, clinicians should limit the dosage and duration of each drug to the minimum possible while still achieving therapeutic efficacy
- Patients and their caregivers should be warned to seek medical attention if unusual dizziness, lightheadedness, sedation, slowed or difficulty breathing, or unresponsiveness occur
- Insomnia may be a symptom of a primary disorder, rather than a primary disorder itself
- Some patients may exhibit abnormal thinking or behavioral changes similar to those caused by other CNS depressants (i.e., either depressant actions or disinhibiting actions)
- Some depressed patients may experience a worsening of suicidal ideation
- Use only with extreme caution in patients with impaired respiratory function or obstructive sleep apnea
- Flurazepam should be administered only at bedtime

Do Not Use

- If patient is pregnant
- If patient has angle-closure glaucoma
- If there is a proven allergy to flurazepam or any benzodiazepine

SPECIAL POPULATIONS

Renal Impairment

- Recommended dose: 15 mg/day

Hepatic Impairment

- Recommended dose: 15 mg/day

Cardiac Impairment

- Benzodiazepines have been used to treat insomnia associated with acute myocardial infarction

Elderly

- Recommended dose: 15 mg/day

Children and Adolescents

- Safety and efficacy have not been established
- Long-term effects of flurazepam in children/adolescents are unknown
- Should generally receive lower doses and be more closely monitored

Pregnancy

- Contraindicated for use in pregnancy
- Effective June 30, 2015, the US FDA requires changes to the content and format of pregnancy and lactation information in prescription drug labels, including the elimination of the pregnancy letter categories; the Pregnancy and Lactation Labeling Rule (PLLR or final rule) applies only to prescription drugs and will be phased in gradually for drugs approved on or after June 30, 2001
- Infants whose mothers received a benzodiazepine late in pregnancy may experience withdrawal effects
- Neonatal flaccidity has been reported in infants whose mothers took a benzodiazepine during pregnancy

Breast Feeding

- Unknown if flurazepam is secreted in human breast milk, but all psychotropics assumed to be secreted in breast milk

✻ Recommended either to discontinue drug or bottle feed

- Effects on infant have been observed and include feeding difficulties, sedation, and weight loss

THE ART OF PSYCHOPHARMACOLOGY

Potential Advantages

- Transient insomnia

Potential Disadvantages

- Chronic nightly insomnia

Primary Target Symptoms

- Time to sleep onset
- Total sleep time
- Nighttime awakenings

Pearls

✻ Flurazepam has a longer half-life than some other sedative hypnotics, so it may be less likely to cause rebound insomnia on discontinuation
- Flurazepam may not be as effective on the first night as it is on subsequent nights
- Was once one of the most widely used hypnotics

✻ Long-term accumulation of flurazepam and its active metabolites may cause insidious onset of confusion or falls, especially in the elderly
- Though not systematically studied, benzodiazepines have been used effectively to treat catatonia and are the initial recommended treatment

Suggested Reading

Greenblatt DJ. Pharmacology of benzodiazepine hypnotics. J Clin Psychiatry 1992;53(Suppl):S7–13.

Hilbert JM, Battista D. Quazepam and flurazepam: differential pharmacokinetic and pharmacodynamic characteristics. J Clin Psychiatry 1991;52(Suppl):S21–6.

Johnson LC, Chernik DA, Sateia MJ. Sleep, performance, and plasma levels in chronic insomniacs during 14-day use of flurazepam and midazolam: an introduction. J Clin Psychopharmacol 1990;10(4 Suppl):S5–9.

Roth T, Roehrs TA. A review of the safety profiles of benzodiazepine hypnotics. J Clin Psychiatry 1991;52(Suppl):S38–41.

THERAPEUTICS

Brands • Luvox
• Luvox CR

see index for additional brand names

Generic? Yes (not for fluvoxamine CR)

Class

- Neuroscience-based Nomenclature: serotonin reuptake inhibitor (S-RI)
- SSRI (selective serotonin reuptake inhibitor); often classified as an antidepressant, but it is not just an antidepressant

Commonly Prescribed for

(bold for FDA approved)

- **Obsessive-compulsive disorder (OCD) (fluvoxamine and fluvoxamine CR)**
- **Social anxiety disorder (fluvoxamine CR)**
- Depression
- Panic disorder
- Generalized anxiety disorder (GAD)
- Posttraumatic stress disorder (PTSD)

How the Drug Works

- Boosts neurotransmitter serotonin
- Blocks serotonin reuptake pump (serotonin transporter)
- Desensitizes serotonin receptors, especially serotonin 1A receptors
- Presumably increases serotonergic neurotransmission
- ✱ Fluvoxamine also binds at sigma 1 receptors

How Long Until It Works

- ✱ Some patients may experience relief of insomnia or anxiety early after initiation of treatment
- Onset of therapeutic actions usually not immediate, but often delayed 2–4 weeks
- If it is not working within 6–8 weeks, it may require a dosage increase or it may not work at all
- May continue to work for many years to prevent relapse of symptoms

If It Works

- The goal of treatment is complete remission of current symptoms as well as prevention of future relapses
- Treatment most often reduces or even eliminates symptoms, but not a cure since symptoms can recur after medicine stopped
- Continue treatment until all symptoms are gone (remission) or significantly reduced (e.g., OCD)
- Once symptoms gone, continue treating for 1 year for the first episode of depression
- For second and subsequent episodes of depression, treatment may need to be indefinite
- Use in anxiety disorders may also need to be indefinite

If It Doesn't Work

- Many patients have only a partial response where some symptoms are improved but others persist (especially insomnia, fatigue, and problems concentrating in depression)
- Other patients may be nonresponders, sometimes called treatment-resistant or treatment-refractory
- Some patients who have an initial response may relapse even though they continue treatment, sometimes called "poop-out"
- Consider increasing dose, switching to another agent or adding an appropriate augmenting agent
- Consider psychotherapy
- Consider evaluation for another diagnosis or for a comorbid condition (e.g., medical illness, substance abuse, etc.)
- Some patients may experience apparent lack of consistent efficacy due to activation of latent or underlying bipolar disorder, and require antidepressant discontinuation and a switch to a mood stabilizer

Best Augmenting Combos for Partial Response or Treatment Resistance

- For the expert, consider cautious addition of clomipramine for treatment-resistant OCD
- Trazodone, especially for insomnia
- Bupropion, mirtazapine, reboxetine, or atomoxetine (use combinations of antidepressants with caution as this may activate bipolar disorder and suicidal ideation)
- Modafinil, especially for fatigue, sleepiness, and lack of concentration
- Mood stabilizers or atypical antipsychotics for bipolar depression, psychotic depression, treatment-resistant depression, or treatment-resistant anxiety disorders

- Benzodiazepines
- If all else fails for anxiety disorders, consider gabapentin or tiagabine
- Hypnotics for insomnia
- Classically, lithium, buspirone, or thyroid hormone
- In Europe and Japan, augmentation is more commonly administered for the treatment of depression and anxiety disorders, especially with benzodiazepines and lithium
- In the USA, augmentation is more commonly administered for the treatment of OCD, especially with atypical antipsychotics, buspirone, or even clomipramine; clomipramine should be added with caution and at low doses as fluvoxamine can alter clomipramine metabolism and raise its levels

Tests
- None for healthy individuals

SIDE EFFECTS

How Drug Causes Side Effects
- Theoretically due to increases in serotonin concentrations at serotonin receptors in parts of the brain and body other than those that cause therapeutic actions (e.g., unwanted actions of serotonin in sleep centers causing insomnia, unwanted actions of serotonin in the gut causing diarrhea, etc.)
- Increasing serotonin can cause diminished dopamine release and might contribute to emotional flattening, cognitive slowing, and apathy in some patients
- Most side effects are immediate but often go away with time, in contrast to most therapeutic effects which are delayed and are enhanced over time

✻ Fluvoxamine's sigma 1 agonist properties may contribute to sedation and fatigue in some patients

Notable Side Effects
- Sexual dysfunction (men: delayed ejaculation, erectile dysfunction; men and women: decreased sexual desire, anorgasmia)
- Gastrointestinal (decreased appetite, nausea, diarrhea, constipation, dry mouth)
- Mostly CNS (insomnia but also sedation, agitation, tremors, headache, dizziness)
- Note: patients with diagnosed or undiagnosed bipolar or psychotic disorders may be more vulnerable to CNS-activating actions of SSRIs
- Autonomic (sweating)
- Bruising and rare bleeding
- Rare hyponatremia

Life-Threatening or Dangerous Side Effects
- Rare seizures
- Rare induction of mania
- Rare activation of suicidal ideation and behavior (suicidality) (short-term studies did not show an increase in the risk of suicidality with antidepressants compared to placebo beyond age 24)

Weight Gain

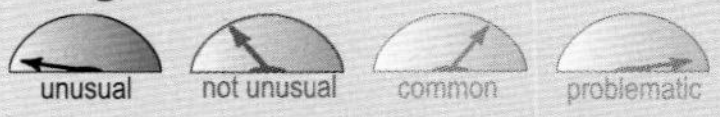

- Reported but not expected
- Patients may actually experience weight loss

Sedation

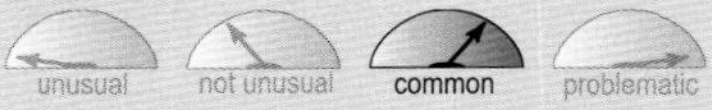

- Many experience and/or can be significant in amount

What to Do About Side Effects
- Wait
- Wait
- Wait
- If fluvoxamine is sedating, take at night to reduce drowsiness
- Reduce dose
- In a few weeks, switch or add other drugs

Best Augmenting Agents for Side Effects
- Often best to try another SSRI or another antidepressant monotherapy prior to resorting to augmentation strategies to treat side effects
- Trazodone or a hypnotic for insomnia
- Bupropion, sildenafil, vardenafil, or tadalafil for sexual dysfunction
- Bupropion for emotional flattening, cognitive slowing, or apathy

- Mirtazapine for insomnia, agitation, and gastrointestinal side effects
- Benzodiazepines for jitteriness and anxiety, especially at initiation of treatment and especially for anxious patients
- Many side effects are dose-dependent (i.e., they increase as dose increases, or they reemerge until tolerance redevelops)
- Many side effects are time-dependent (i.e., they start immediately upon dosing and upon each dose increase, but go away with time)
- Activation and agitation may represent the induction of a bipolar state, especially a mixed dysphoric bipolar II condition sometimes associated with suicidal ideation, and require the addition of lithium, a mood stabilizer or an atypical antipsychotic, and/or discontinuation of fluvoxamine

DOSING AND USE

Usual Dosage Range

- 100–300 mg/day for OCD
- 100–200 mg/day for depression
- 100–300 mg/day for social anxiety disorder

Dosage Forms

- Tablets 25 mg, 50 mg scored, 100 mg scored
- Controlled-release capsules 100 mg, 150 mg

How to Dose

- For immediate-release, initial 50 mg/day; increase by 50 mg/day in 4–7 days; usually wait a few weeks to assess drug effects before increasing dose further, but can increase by 50 mg/day every 4–7 days until desired efficacy is reached; maximum 300 mg/day
- For immediate-release, doses below 100 mg/day usually given as a single dose at bedtime; doses above 100 mg/day can be divided into two doses to enhance tolerability, with the larger dose administered at night, but can also be given as a single dose at bedtime
- For controlled-release, initial 100 mg/day; increase by 50 mg/day each week until desired efficacy is reached; maximum generally 300 mg/day

Dosing Tips

- 50-mg and 100-mg tablets are scored, so to save costs, give 25 mg as half of 50 mg tablet, and give 50 mg as half of 100 mg tablet
- To improve tolerability of immediate-release formulation, dosing can either be given once a day, usually all at night, or split either symmetrically or asymmetrically, usually with more of the dose given at night
- Some patients take more than 300 mg/day
- Controlled-release capsules should not be chewed or crushed
- If intolerable anxiety, insomnia, agitation, akathisia, or activation occur either upon dosing initiation or discontinuation, consider the possibility of activated bipolar disorder and switch to a mood stabilizer or an atypical antipsychotic

Overdose

- Rare fatalities have been reported, both in combination with other drugs and alone; sedation, dizziness, vomiting, diarrhea, irregular heartbeat, seizures, coma, breathing difficulty

Long-Term Use

- Safe

Habit Forming

- No

How to Stop

- Taper to avoid withdrawal effects (dizziness, nausea, stomach cramps, sweating, tingling, dysesthesias)
- Many patients tolerate 50% dose reduction for 3 days, then another 50% reduction for 3 days, then discontinuation
- If withdrawal symptoms emerge during discontinuation, raise dose to stop symptoms and then restart withdrawal much more slowly

Pharmacokinetics

- Parent drug has 9–28 hour half-life
- Inhibits CYP450 3A4
- Inhibits CYP450 1A2
- Inhibits CYP450 2C9/2C19

Drug Interactions

- Tramadol increases the risk of seizures in patients taking an antidepressant
- Can increase tricyclic antidepressant levels; use with caution with TCAs
- Can cause a fatal "serotonin syndrome" when combined with MAOIs, so do not use with MAOIs or for at least 14 days after MAOIs are stopped
- Do not start an MAOI for at least 5 half-lives (5 to 7 days for most drugs) after discontinuing fluvoxamine
- May displace highly protein-bound drugs (e.g., warfarin)
- Can rarely cause weakness, hyperreflexia, and incoordination when combined with sumatriptan or possibly with other triptans, requiring careful monitoring of patient
- Possible increased risk of bleeding, especially when combined with anticoagulants (e.g., warfarin, NSAIDs)
- NSAIDs may impair effectiveness of SSRIs
- Via CYP450 1A2 inhibition, fluvoxamine may reduce clearance of theophylline and clozapine, thus raising their levels and requiring their dosing to be lowered
- Fluvoxamine administered with either caffeine or theophylline can thus cause jitteriness, excessive stimulation, or rarely seizures, so concomitant use should proceed cautiously
- Metabolism of fluvoxamine may be enhanced in smokers and thus its levels lowered, requiring higher dosing
- Via CYP450 3A4 inhibition, fluvoxamine may reduce clearance of carbamazepine and benzodiazepines such as alprazolam and triazolam, and thus require dosage reduction
- Via CYP450 3A4 inhibition, fluvoxamine could theoretically increase concentrations of certain cholesterol lowering HMG CoA reductase inhibitors, especially simvastatin, atorvastatin, and lovastatin, but not pravastatin or fluvastatin, which would increase the risk of rhabdomyolysis; thus, coadministration of fluvoxamine with certain HMG CoA reductase inhibitors should proceed with caution
- Via CYP450 3A4 inhibition, fluvoxamine could theoretically increase the concentrations of pimozide, and cause QTc prolongation and dangerous cardiac arrhythmias

Other Warnings/ Precautions

- Add or initiate other antidepressants with caution for up to 2 weeks after discontinuing fluvoxamine
- Use with caution in patients with history of seizure
- Use with caution in patients with bipolar disorder unless treated with concomitant mood-stabilizing agent
- May cause photosensitivity
- When treating children, carefully weigh the risks and benefits of pharmacological treatment against the risks and benefits of nontreatment with antidepressants and make sure to document this in the patient's chart
- Distribute the brochures provided by the FDA and the drug companies
- Warn patients and their caregivers about the possibility of activating side effects and advise them to report such symptoms immediately
- Monitor patients for activation of suicidal ideation, especially children and adolescents

Do Not Use

- If patient is taking an MAOI
- If patient is taking thioridazine, pimozide, tizanidine, alosetron, or ramelteon
- If there is a proven allergy to fluvoxamine

SPECIAL POPULATIONS

Renal Impairment

- Consider lower initial dose

Hepatic Impairment

- Lower dose or give less frequently, perhaps by half; use slower titration

Cardiac Impairment

- Preliminary research suggests that fluvoxamine is safe in these patients
- Treating depression with SSRIs in patients with acute angina or following myocardial infarction may reduce cardiac events and improve survival as well as mood

Elderly
- May require lower initial dose and slower titration
- Reduction in the risk of suicidality with antidepressants compared to placebo in adults age 65 and older

Children and Adolescents
- Immediate-release approved for ages 8–17 for OCD
- 8–17: initial 25 mg/day at bedtime; increase by 25 mg/day every 4–7 days; maximum 200 mg/day; doses above 50 mg/day should be divided into 2 doses with the larger dose administered at bedtime
- Preliminary evidence suggests efficacy for other anxiety disorders and depression in children and adolescents
- Carefully weigh the risks and benefits of pharmacological treatment against the risks and benefits of nontreatment with antidepressants and make sure to document this in the patient's chart
- Monitor patients face-to-face regularly, particularly during the first several weeks of treatment
- Use with caution, observing for activation of known or unknown bipolar disorder and/or suicidal ideation, and inform parents or guardians of this risk so they can help observe child or adolescent patients

Pregnancy
- Effective June 30, 2015, the US FDA requires changes to the content and format of pregnancy and lactation information in prescription drug labels, including the elimination of the pregnancy letter categories; the Pregnancy and Lactation Labeling Rule (PLLR or final rule) applies only to prescription drugs and will be phased in gradually for drugs approved on or after June 30, 2001
- Controlled studies have not been conducted in pregnant women
- Not generally recommended for use during pregnancy, especially during first trimester
- Nonetheless, continuous treatment during pregnancy may be necessary and has not been proven to be harmful to the fetus
- At delivery there may be more bleeding in the mother and transient irritability or sedation in the newborn
- Must weigh the risk of treatment (first trimester fetal development, third trimester newborn delivery) to the child against the risk of no treatment (recurrence of depression, maternal health, infant bonding) to the mother and child
- For many patients this may mean continuing treatment during pregnancy
- Exposure to SSRIs early in pregnancy may be associated with increased risk of septal heart defects (absolute risk is small)
- SSRI use beyond the 20th week of pregnancy may be associated with increased risk of pulmonary hypertension in newborns, although this is not proven
- Exposure to SSRIs late in pregnancy may be associated with increased risk of gestational hypertension and preeclampsia
- Neonates exposed to SSRIs or SNRIs late in the third trimester have developed complications requiring prolonged hospitalization, respiratory support, and tube feeding; reported symptoms are consistent with either a direct toxic effect of SSRIs and SNRIs or, possibly, a drug discontinuation syndrome, and include respiratory distress, cyanosis, apnea, seizures, temperature instability, feeding difficulty, vomiting, hypoglycemia, hypotonia, hypertonia, hyperreflexia, tremor, jitteriness, irritability, and constant crying

Breast Feeding
- Some drug is found in mother's breast milk
- Trace amounts may be present in nursing children whose mothers are on fluvoxamine
- If child becomes irritable or sedated, breast feeding or drug may need to be discontinued
- Immediate postpartum period is a high-risk time for depression, especially in women who have had prior depressive episodes, so drug may need to be reinstituted late in the third trimester or shortly after childbirth to prevent a recurrence during the postpartum period
- Must weigh benefits of breast feeding with risks and benefits of antidepressant treatment versus nontreatment to both the infant and the mother
- For many patients this may mean continuing treatment during breast feeding

THE ART OF PSYCHOPHARMACOLOGY

Potential Advantages

- Patients with mixed anxiety/depression
- Generic is less expensive than brand name where available

Potential Disadvantages

- Patients with irritable bowel or multiple gastrointestinal complaints
- Can require dose titration and twice daily dosing

Primary Target Symptoms

- Depressed mood
- Anxiety

Pearls

* ✻ Often a preferred treatment of anxious depression as well as major depressive disorder comorbid with anxiety disorders
- Some withdrawal effects, especially gastrointestinal effects
- May have lower incidence of sexual dysfunction than other SSRIs
- Preliminary research suggests that fluvoxamine is efficacious in obsessive-compulsive symptoms in schizophrenia when combined with antipsychotics
- Not FDA approved for depression, but used widely for depression in many countries
- CR formulation may be better tolerated than immediate-release formulation, particularly with less sedation
- SSRIs may be less effective in women over 50, especially if they are not taking estrogen
- SSRIs may be useful for hot flushes in perimenopausal women
* ✻ Actions at sigma 1 receptors may explain in part fluvoxamine's sometimes rapid onset effects in anxiety disorders and insomnia
* ✻ Actions at sigma 1 receptors may explain potential advantages of fluvoxamine for psychotic depression and delusional depression
* ✻ For treatment-resistant OCD, consider cautious combination of fluvoxamine and clomipramine by an expert
- Normally, clomipramine (CMI), a potent serotonin reuptake blocker, at steady state is metabolized extensively to its active metabolite desmethyl-clomipramine (de-CMI), a potent noradrenergic reuptake blocker
- Thus, at steady state, plasma drug activity is generally more noradrenergic (with higher de-CMI levels) than serotonergic (with lower parent CMI levels)
- Addition of a CYP450 1A2 inhibitor, fluvoxamine, blocks this conversion and results in higher CMI levels than de-CMI levels
- Thus, addition of the SSRI fluvoxamine to CMI in treatment-resistant OCD can powerfully enhance serotonergic activity, not only due to the inherent serotonergic activity of fluvoxamine, but also due to a favorable pharmacokinetic interaction inhibiting CYP450 1A2 and thus converting CMI's metabolism to a more powerful serotonergic portfolio of parent drug

Suggested Reading

Cheer SM, Figgitt DP. Spotlight on fluvoxamine in anxiety disorders in children and adolescents. CNS Drugs 2002;16:139–44.

Edwards JG, Anderson I. Systematic review and guide to selection of selective serotonin reuptake inhibitors. Drugs 1999;57:507–33.

Figgitt DP, McClellan KJ. Fluvoxamine. An updated review of its use in the management of adults with anxiety disorders. Drugs 2000;60:925–54.

Omori M, Watanabe N, Nakagawa A, et al. Fluvoxamine versus other anti-depressive agents for depression. Cochrane Database Syst Rev 2010;17(3):CD006114.

Pigott TA, Seay SM. A review of the efficacy of selective serotonin reuptake inhibitors in obsessive-compulsive disorder. J Clin Psychiatry 1999;60:101–6.

THERAPEUTICS

Brands • Neurontin
• Horizant

see index for additional brand names

Generic? Yes (not for extended release)

Class

- Neuroscience-based Nomenclature: glutamate, voltage-gated calcium channel blocker (Glu-CB)
- Anticonvulsant, antineuralgic for chronic pain, alpha 2 delta ligand at voltage-sensitive calcium channels

Commonly Prescribed for

(bold for FDA approved)

- **Partial seizures with or without secondary generalization (adjunctive)**
- **Postherpetic neuralgia**
- **Restless leg syndrome (extended release)**
- Neuropathic pain/chronic pain
- Anxiety (adjunctive)
- Bipolar disorder (adjunctive)

How the Drug Works

- Is a leucine analogue and is transported both into the blood from the gut and also across the blood-brain barrier into the brain from the blood by the system L transport system
- ✻ Binds to the alpha 2 delta subunit of voltage-sensitive calcium channels
- This closes N and P/Q presynaptic calcium channels, diminishing excessive neuronal activity and neurotransmitter release
- Although structurally related to gamma-aminobutyric acid (GABA), no known direct actions on GABA or its receptors

How Long Until It Works

- Should reduce seizures by 2 weeks
- Should also reduce pain in postherapeutic neuralgia by 2 weeks; some patients respond earlier
- May reduce pain in other neuropathic pain syndromes within a few weeks
- If it is not reducing pain within 6–8 weeks, it may require a dosage increase or it may not work at all
- May reduce anxiety in a variety of disorders within a few weeks
- Not yet clear if it has mood-stabilizing effects in bipolar disorder or antineuralgic actions in chronic neuropathic pain, but some patients may respond and if so, would be expected to show clinical effects starting by 2 weeks although it may take several weeks to months to optimize

If It Works

- The goal of treatment is complete remission of symptoms (e.g., seizures)
- The goal of treatment of chronic neuropathic pain is to reduce symptoms as much as possible, especially in combination with other treatments
- Treatment of chronic neuropathic pain most often reduces but does not eliminate symptoms and is not a cure since symptoms usually recur after medicine stopped
- Continue treatment until all symptoms are gone or until improvement is stable and then continue treating indefinitely as long as improvement persists

If It Doesn't Work (for neuropathic pain or bipolar disorder)

- ✻ May only be effective in a subset of bipolar patients, in some patients who fail to respond to other mood stabilizers, or it may not work at all
- Many patients have only a partial response where some symptoms are improved but others persist or continue to wax and wane without stabilization of pain or mood
- Other patients may be nonresponders, sometimes called treatment-resistant or treatment-refractory
- Consider increasing dose, switching to another agent or adding an appropriate augmenting agent
- Consider biofeedback or hypnosis for pain
- Consider the presence of noncompliance and counsel patient
- Switch to another agent with fewer side effects
- Consider evaluation for another diagnosis or for a comorbid condition (e.g., medical illness, substance abuse, etc.)

Best Augmenting Combos for Partial Response or Treatment Resistance

- ✻ Gabapentin is itself an augmenting agent to numerous other anticonvulsants in treating epilepsy; and to lithium, atypical

antipsychotics and other anticonvulsants in the treatment of bipolar disorder
- For postherpetic neuralgia, gabapentin can decrease concomitant opiate use

✻ For neuropathic pain, gabapentin can augment TCAs and SNRIs as well as tiagabine, other anticonvulsants and even opiates if done by experts while carefully monitoring in difficult cases
- For anxiety, gabapentin is a second-line treatment to augment SSRIs, SNRIs, or benzodiazepines

Tests
- None for healthy individuals
- False positive readings with the Ames N-Multistix SG® dipstick test for urinary protein have been reported when gabapentin was administered with other anticonvulsants

SIDE EFFECTS

How Drug Causes Side Effects
- CNS side effects may be due to excessive blockade of voltage-sensitive calcium channels

Notable Side Effects
✻ Sedation (dose-dependent), dizziness

✻ Ataxia (dose-dependent), fatigue, nystagmus, tremor
- Peripheral edema
- Blurred vision
- Vomiting, dyspepsia, diarrhea, dry mouth, constipation, weight gain
- Additional effects in children under age 12: hostility, emotional lability, hyperkinesia, thought disorder, weight gain

Life-Threatening or Dangerous Side Effects
- Anaphylaxis and angioedema
- Sudden unexplained deaths have occurred in epilepsy (unknown if related to gabapentin use)
- Rare activation of suicidal ideation and behavior (suicidality)

Weight Gain
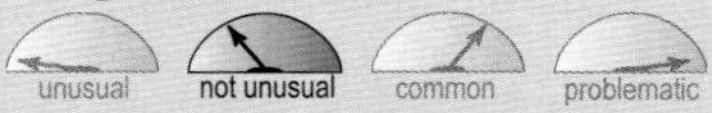

- Occurs in significant minority

Sedation
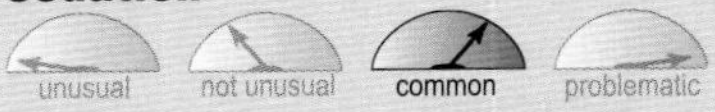

- Many experience and/or can be significant in amount
- Dose-related; can be problematic at high doses
- Can wear off with time, but may not wear off at high doses

What to Do About Side Effects
- Wait
- Wait
- Wait
- Take more of the dose at night to reduce daytime sedation
- Lower the dose
- Switch to another agent

Best Augmenting Agents for Side Effects
- Many side effects cannot be improved with an augmenting agent

DOSING AND USE

Usual Dosage Range
- 900–1,800 mg/day in 3 divided doses (immediate-release)

Dosage Forms
- Capsule 100 mg, 300 mg, 400 mg, 800 mg
- Tablet 100 mg, 300 mg, 400 mg, 600 mg, 800 mg
- Tablet extended-release 300 mg, 600 mg
- Liquid 250 mg/5 mL – 470 mL bottle

How to Dose
- Postherpetic neuralgia (immediate-release): 300 mg on day 1; on day 2 increase to 600 mg in 2 doses; on day 3 increase to 900 mg in 3 doses; maximum dose generally 1,800 mg/day in 3 doses
- Postherpetic neuralgia (extended-release): 600 mg in the morning on day 1; on day 4 increase to 600 mg twice daily
- Restless leg syndrome (extended-release): 600 mg once daily at about 5 pm
- Seizures (ages 12 and older): initial 900 mg/day in 3 doses; recommended dose generally 1,800 mg/day in 3 doses; maximum dose generally 3,600 mg/day;

time between any 2 doses should usually not exceed 12 hours
- Seizures (under age 13): see Children and Adolescents

Dosing Tips
- Gabapentin should not be taken until 2 hours after administration of an antacid
- If gabapentin is added to a second anticonvulsant, the titration period should be at least a week to improve tolerance to sedation
- Some patients need to take immediate-release gabapentin only twice daily in order to experience adequate symptomatic relief for pain or anxiety
- At the high end of the dosing range, tolerability may be enhanced by splitting immediate-release dose into more than 3 divided doses
- Half-tablets not used within several days of breaking the scored tablet should be discarded
- Do not break or chew extended-release tablets, as this could alter controlled-release properties
- Extended-release tablets should be taken with food
- For intolerable sedation, can give most of the dose at night and less during the day
- To improve slow-wave sleep, may need to take gabapentin only at bedtime

Overdose
- No fatalities; slurred speech, sedation, double vision, diarrhea

Long-Term Use
- Safe

Habit Forming
- No

How to Stop
- Taper over a minimum of 1 week
- Epilepsy patients may seize upon withdrawal, especially if withdrawal is abrupt

* Rapid discontinuation may increase the risk of relapse in bipolar disorder

- Discontinuation symptoms uncommon

Pharmacokinetics
- Gabapentin is not metabolized but excreted intact renally
- Not protein bound
- Elimination half-life approximately 5–7 hours

Drug Interactions
- Antacids may reduce the bioavailability of gabapentin, so gabapentin should be administered approximately 2 hours before antacid medication
- Naproxen may increase absorption of gabapentin
- Morphine and hydrocodone may increase plasma AUC (area under the curve) values of gabapentin and thus gabapentin plasma levels over time

Other Warnings/ Precautions
- Depressive effects may be increased by other CNS depressants (alcohol, MAOIs, other anticonvulsants, etc.)
- Dizziness and sedation could increase the chances of accidental injury (falls) in the elderly
- Pancreatic acinar adenocarcinomas have developed in male rats that were given gabapentin, but clinical significance is unknown
- Development of new tumors or worsening of tumors has occurred in humans taking gabapentin; it is unknown whether gabapentin affected the development or worsening of tumors
- Warn patients and their caregivers about the possibility of activation of suicidal ideation and advise them to report such side effects immediately

Do Not Use
- If there is a proven allergy to gabapentin or pregabalin

SPECIAL POPULATIONS

Renal Impairment

- Gabapentin is renally excreted, so the dose may need to be lowered

Immediate-Release	
Creatinine Clearance (mL/min)	**Dosing**
30–59	400–1,400 mg/day in 2 doses
16–29	200–700 mg/day in 1 dose
<16	100–300 mg/day in 1 dose
<16 on hemodialysis	May need supplemental doses following dialysis

Extended-Release for Restless Leg Syndrome	
Creatinine Clearance (mL/min)	**Dosing**
30–59	Initial 300 mg/day; increase to 600 mg/day if needed
15–29	300 mg/day
<15	300 mg every other day
<15 on hemodialysis	Not recommended

Extended-Release for Postherpetic Neuralgia	
Creatinine Clearance (mL/min)	**Dosing**
30–59	Initial 300 mg in the morning; on day 4 increase to 300 mg twice daily; increase to 600 mg twice daily if needed
15–29	Initial 300 mg in the morning on days 1 and 3; on day 4 increase to 300 mg in the morning; increase to 300 mg twice daily if needed
<15	300 mg every other day in the morning; increase to 300 mg/day in the morning if needed
<15 on hemodialysis	300 mg following dialysis; increase to 600 mg following dialysis if needed

- Can be removed by hemodialysis; patients receiving hemodialysis may require supplemental doses of gabapentin
- Use in renal impairment has not been studied in children under age 12

Hepatic Impairment

- No available data but not metabolized by the liver and clinical experience suggests normal dosing

Cardiac Impairment

- No specific recommendations

Elderly

- Some patients may tolerate lower doses better
- Elderly patients may be more susceptible to adverse effects, including peripheral edema and ataxia

Children and Adolescents

- Approved for use starting at age 3 as adjunct treatment for partial seizures
- Ages 5–12: initial 10–15 mg/kg per day in 3 doses; titrate over 3 days to 25–35 mg/kg per day given in 3 doses; maximum dose generally 50 mg/kg per day; time between any 2 doses should usually not exceed 12 hours
- Ages 3–4: initial 10–15 mg/kg per day in 3 doses; titrate over 3 days to 40 mg/kg per day; maximum dose generally 50 mg/kg per day; time between any 2 doses should usually not exceed 12 hours

Pregnancy

- Effective June 30, 2015, the US FDA requires changes to the content and format of pregnancy and lactation information in prescription drug labels, including the elimination of the pregnancy letter categories; the Pregnancy and Lactation Labeling Rule (PLLR or final rule) applies only to prescription drugs and will be phased in gradually for drugs approved on or after June 30, 2001
- Controlled studies have not been conducted in pregnant women
- Use in women of childbearing potential requires weighing potential benefits to the mother against the risks to the fetus
- Antiepileptic Drug Pregnancy Registry: (888) 233-2334
- Taper drug if discontinuing
- Seizures, even mild seizures, may cause harm to the embryo/fetus

* Lack of convincing efficacy for treatment of bipolar disorder or psychosis suggests risk/benefit ratio is in favor of discontinuing gabapentin during pregnancy for these indications
* For bipolar patients, gabapentin should generally be discontinued before anticipated pregnancies
* For bipolar patients, given the risk of relapse in the postpartum period, mood-stabilizer treatment, especially with agents with better evidence of efficacy than gabapentin, should generally be restarted immediately after delivery if patient is unmedicated during pregnancy
* Atypical antipsychotics may be preferable to gabapentin if treatment of bipolar disorder is required during pregnancy
- Bipolar symptoms may recur or worsen during pregnancy and some form of treatment may be necessary

Breast Feeding

- Some drug is found in mother's breast milk
* Recommended either to discontinue drug or bottle feed
- If drug is continued while breast feeding, infant should be monitored for possible adverse effects
- If infant becomes irritable or sedated, breast feeding or drug may need to be discontinued
* Bipolar disorder may recur during the postpartum period, particularly if there is a history of prior postpartum episodes of either depression or psychosis
* Relapse rates may be lower in women who receive prophylactic treatment for postpartum episodes of bipolar disorder
- Atypical antipsychotics and anticonvulsants such as valproate may be safer and more effective than gabapentin during the postpartum period when treating a nursing mother with bipolar disorder

THE ART OF PSYCHOPHARMACOLOGY

Potential Advantages

- Chronic neuropathic pain
- Has relatively mild side effect profile
- Has few pharmacokinetic drug interactions
- Treatment-resistant bipolar disorder

Potential Disadvantages

- Usually requires 3 times a day dosing
- Poor documentation of efficacy for many off-label uses, especially bipolar disorder

Primary Target Symptoms

- Seizures
- Pain
- Anxiety

Pearls

- Gabapentin is generally well-tolerated, with only mild adverse effects
- Well studied in epilepsy and postherpetic neuralgia
* Most use is off label
* Off-label use for first-line treatment of neuropathic pain may be justified
* Off-label use for second-line treatment of anxiety may be justified
* Off-label use as an adjunct for bipolar disorder may not be justified
* Misperceptions about gabapentin's efficacy in bipolar disorder have led to its use in more patients than other agents with proven efficacy, such as lamotrigine
* Off-label use as an adjunct for schizophrenia may not be justified
- May be useful for some patients in alcohol withdrawal
* One of the few agents that enhances slow-wave delta sleep, which may be helpful in chronic neuropathic pain syndromes
* May be a useful adjunct for fibromyalgia
- Drug absorption and clinical efficacy may not necessarily be proportionately increased at high doses, and thus response to high doses may not be consistent

Suggested Reading

MacDonald KJ, Young LT. Newer antiepileptic drugs in bipolar disorder. CNS Drugs 2002;16:549–62.

Marson AG, Kadir ZA, Hutton JL, Chadwick DW. Gabapentin for drug-resistant partial epilepsy. Cochrane Database Syst Rev 2000;(2):CD001415.

Moore RA, Wiffen PJ, Derry S, McQuay HJ. Gabapentin for chronic neuropathic pain and fibromyalgia in adults. Cochrane Database Syst Rev 2011;16(3):CD007938.

Stahl SM. Anticonvulsants and the relief of chronic pain: pregabalin and gabapentin as alpha(2)delta ligands at voltage-gated calcium channels. J Clin Psychiatry 2004;65:596–7.

Stahl SM. Anticonvulsants as anxiolytics, part 2: Pregabalin and gabapentin as alpha(2)delta ligands at voltage-gated calcium channels. J Clin Psychiatry 2004;65:460–1.

THERAPEUTICS

Brands
- Razadyne
- Razadyne ER

see index for additional brand names

Generic? Yes

Class
- Neuroscience-based Nomenclature: acetylcholine multi-modal; enzyme inhibitor; receptor PAM (ACh-MM)
- Cholinesterase inhibitor (acetylcholinesterase inhibitor); also an allosteric nicotinic cholinergic modulator; cognitive enhancer

Commonly Prescribed for
(bold for FDA approved)
- **Alzheimer disease (mild to moderate)**
- Memory disturbances in other dementias
- Memory disturbances in other conditions
- Mild cognitive impairment

How the Drug Works
* Reversibly and competitively inhibits centrally active acetylcholinesterase (AChE), making more acetylcholine available
- Increased availability of acetylcholine compensates in part for degenerating cholinergic neurons in neocortex that regulate memory
* Modulates nicotinic receptors, which enhances actions of acetylcholine
- Nicotinic modulation may also enhance the actions of other neurotransmitters by increasing the release of dopamine, norepinephrine, serotonin, GABA, and glutamate
- Does not inhibit butyrylcholinesterase
- May release growth factors or interfere with amyloid deposition

How Long Until It Works
- May take up to 6 weeks before any improvement in baseline memory or behavior is evident
- May take months before any stabilization in degenerative course is evident

If It Works
- May improve symptoms and slow progression of disease, but does not reverse the degenerative process

If It Doesn't Work
- Consider adjusting dose, switching to a different cholinesterase inhibitor or adding an appropriate augmenting agent
- Reconsider diagnosis and rule out other conditions such as depression or a dementia other than Alzheimer disease

Best Augmenting Combos for Partial Response or Treatment Resistance
* Atypical antipsychotics to reduce behavioral disturbances
* Antidepressants if concomitant depression, apathy, or lack of interest
* Memantine for moderate to severe Alzheimer disease
- Divalproex, carbamazepine, or oxcarbazepine for behavioral disturbances
- Not rational to combine with another cholinesterase inhibitor

Tests
- None for healthy individuals

SIDE EFFECTS

How Drug Causes Side Effects
- Peripheral inhibition of acetylcholinesterase can cause gastrointestinal side effects
- Central inhibition of acetylcholinesterase may contribute to nausea, vomiting, weight loss, and sleep disturbances

Notable Side Effects
* Nausea, diarrhea, vomiting, appetite loss, increased gastric acid secretion, weight loss
- Headache, dizziness
- Fatigue, depression

Life-Threatening or Dangerous Side Effects
- Rare seizures
- Rare syncope

Weight Gain
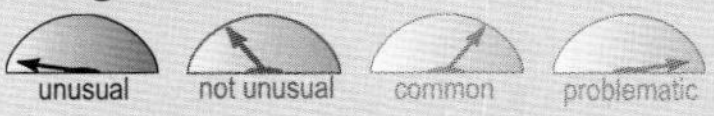

- Reported but not expected
- Some patients may experience weight loss

Sedation

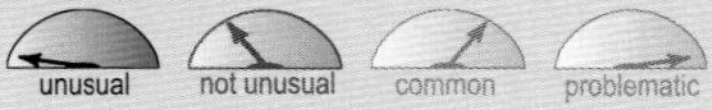

- Reported but not expected

What to Do About Side Effects

- Wait
- Wait
- Wait
- Use slower dose titration
- Consider lowering dose, switching to a different agent or adding an appropriate augmenting agent

Best Augmenting Agents for Side Effects

- Many side effects cannot be improved with an augmenting agent

DOSING AND USE

Usual Dosage Range

- 16–24 mg/day

Dosage Forms

- Tablet 4 mg, 8 mg, 12 mg
- Extended-release capsule 8 mg, 16 mg, 24 mg
- Liquid 4 mg/mL – 100 mL bottle

How to Dose

- Immediate-release: initial 4 mg twice daily; after 4 weeks may increase dose to 8 mg twice daily; after 4 more weeks may increase to 12 mg twice daily
- Extended-release: same titration schedule as immediate-release but dosed once a day in the morning, preferably with food

Dosing Tips

- Gastrointestinal side effects may be reduced if drug is administered with food
- Gastrointestinal side effects may also be reduced if dose is titrated slowly
- Probably best to utilize highest tolerated dose within the usual dosing range

* When switching to another cholinesterase inhibitor, probably best to cross-titrate from one to the other to prevent precipitous decline in function if the patient washes out of one drug entirely

Overdose

- Can be lethal; nausea, vomiting, excess salivation, sweating, hypotension, bradycardia, collapse, convulsions, muscle weakness (weakness of respiratory muscles can lead to death)

Long-Term Use

- Drug may lose effectiveness in slowing degenerative course of Alzheimer disease after 6 months
- Can be effective in some patients for several years

Habit Forming

- No

How to Stop

- Taper not necessary
- Discontinuation may lead to notable deterioration in memory and behavior, which may not be restored when drug is restarted or another cholinesterase inhibitor is initiated

Pharmacokinetics

- Terminal elimination half-life approximately 7 hours
- Metabolized by CYP450 2D6 and 3A4

Drug Interactions

- Galantamine may increase the effects of anesthetics and should be discontinued prior to surgery
- Inhibitors of CYP450 2D6 and CYP450 3A4 may inhibit galantamine metabolism and raise galantamine plasma levels
- Galantamine may interact with anticholinergic agents and the combination may decrease the efficacy of both
- Cimetidine may increase bioavailability of galantamine
- May have synergistic effect if administered with cholinomimetics (e.g., bethanechol)
- Bradycardia may occur if combined with beta blockers
- Theoretically, could reduce the efficacy of levodopa in Parkinson's disease
- Not rational to combine with another cholinesterase inhibitor

Other Warnings/ Precautions

- May exacerbate asthma or other pulmonary disease
- Increased gastric acid secretion may increase the risk of ulcers
- Bradycardia or heart block may occur in patients with or without cardiac impairment

Do Not Use

- If there is a proven allergy to galantamine

SPECIAL POPULATIONS

Renal Impairment

- Should be used with caution
- Not recommended for use in patients with severe renal impairment

Hepatic Impairment

- Should be used with caution
- Reduction of clearance may increase with the degree of hepatic impairment
- Not recommended for use in patients with severe hepatic impairment

Cardiac Impairment

- Should be used with caution
- Syncopal episodes have been reported with the use of galantamine

Elderly

- Clearance is reduced in elderly patients
- Use of cholinesterase inhibitors may be associated with increased rates of syncope, bradycardia, pacemaker insertion, and hip fracture in older adults with dementia

Children and Adolescents

- Safety and efficacy have not been established

Pregnancy

- Effective June 30, 2015, the US FDA requires changes to the content and format of pregnancy and lactation information in prescription drug labels, including the elimination of the pregnancy letter categories; the Pregnancy and Lactation Labeling Rule (PLLR or final rule) applies only to prescription drugs and will be phased in gradually for drugs approved on or after June 30, 2001
- Controlled studies have not been conducted in pregnant women
- Animal studies do not show adverse effects
- ✻ Not recommended for use in pregnant women or in women of childbearing potential

Breast Feeding

- Unknown if galantamine is secreted in human breast milk, but all psychotropics assumed to be secreted in breast milk
- ✻ Recommended either to discontinue drug or bottle feed
- Galantamine is not recommended for use in nursing women

THE ART OF PSYCHOPHARMACOLOGY

Potential Advantages

- Alzheimer disease with cerebrovascular disease
- Theoretically, nicotinic modulation may provide added therapeutic benefits for memory and behavior in some Alzheimer patients
- Theoretically, nicotinic modulation may also provide efficacy for cognitive disorders other than Alzheimer disease

Potential Disadvantages

- Patients who have difficulty taking a medication twice daily

Primary Target Symptoms

- Memory loss in Alzheimer disease
- Behavioral symptoms in Alzheimer disease
- Memory loss in other dementias

Pearls

- Dramatic reversal of symptoms of Alzheimer disease is not generally seen with cholinesterase inhibitors
- Can lead to therapeutic nihilism among prescribers and lack of an appropriate trial of a cholinesterase inhibitor
- ✻ Perhaps only 50% of Alzheimer patients are diagnosed, and only 50% of those diagnosed are treated, and only 50% of

those treated are given a cholinesterase inhibitor, and then only for 200 days in a disease that lasts 7–10 years
- Must evaluate lack of efficacy and loss of efficacy over months, not weeks
- ✻ Treats behavioral and psychological symptoms of Alzheimer dementia as well as cognitive symptoms (i.e., especially apathy, disinhibition, delusions, anxiety, cooperation, pacing)
- Patients who complain themselves of memory problems may have depression, whereas patients whose spouses or children complain of the patient's memory problems may have Alzheimer disease
- Treat the patient but ask the caregiver about efficacy
- What you see may depend upon how early you treat
- The first symptoms of Alzheimer disease are generally mood changes; thus, Alzheimer disease may initially be diagnosed as depression
- Women may experience cognitive symptoms in perimenopause as a result of hormonal changes that are not a sign of dementia or Alzheimer disease
- Aggressively treat concomitant symptoms with augmentation (e.g., atypical antipsychotics for agitation, antidepressants for depression)
- If treatment with antidepressants fails to improve apathy and depressed mood in the elderly, it is possible that this represents early Alzheimer disease and a cholinesterase inhibitor like galantamine may be helpful
- What to expect from a cholinesterase inhibitor:
  - Patients do not generally improve dramatically although this can be observed in a significant minority of patients
  - Onset of behavioral problems and nursing home placement can be delayed
  - Functional outcomes, including activities of daily living, can be preserved
  - Caregiver burden and stress can be reduced
- Delay in progression in Alzheimer disease is not evidence of disease-modifying actions of cholinesterase inhibition
- Cholinesterase inhibitors like galantamine depend upon the presence of intact targets for acetylcholine for maximum effectiveness and thus may be most effective in the early stages of Alzheimer disease
- The most prominent side effects of galantamine are gastrointestinal effects, which are usually mild and transient
- For patients with intolerable side effects, generally allow a washout period with resolution of side effects prior to switching to another cholinesterase inhibitor
- Weight loss can be a problem in Alzheimer patients with debilitation and muscle wasting
- Women over 85, particularly with low body weights, may experience more adverse effects
- Use with caution in underweight or frail patients
- Cognitive improvement may be linked to substantial (>65%) inhibition of acetylcholinesterase
- ✻ Galantamine is a natural product present in daffodils and snowdrops
- New extended-release formulation allows for once daily dosing
- ✻ Novel dual action uniquely combines acetylcholinesterase inhibition with allosteric nicotine modulation
- ✻ Novel dual action should theoretically enhance cholinergic actions but incremental clinical benefits have been difficult to demonstrate
- ✻ Actions at nicotinic receptors enhance not only the release of acetylcholine but also that of other neurotransmitters, which may boost attention and improve behaviors caused by deficiencies in those neurotransmitters in Alzheimer disease
- Some Alzheimer patients who fail to respond to another cholinesterase inhibitor may respond when switched to galantamine
- Some Alzheimer patients who fail to respond to galantamine may respond to another cholinesterase inhibitor
- To prevent potential clinical deterioration, generally switch from long-term treatment with one cholinesterase inhibitor to another without a washout period
- ✻ Galantamine may slow the progression of mild cognitive impairment to Alzheimer disease

✻ May be useful for dementia with Lewy bodies (DLB, constituted by early loss of attentiveness and visual perception with possible hallucinations, Parkinson-like movement problems, fluctuating cognition such as daytime drowsiness and lethargy, staring into space for long periods, episodes of disorganized speech)
- May decrease delusions, apathy, agitation, and hallucinations in dementia with Lewy bodies

✻ May be useful for vascular dementia (e.g., acute onset with slow stepwise progression that has plateaus, often with gait abnormalities, focal signs, imbalance, and urinary incontinence)
- May be helpful for dementia in Down's syndrome
- Suggestions of utility in some cases of treatment-resistant bipolar disorder
- Theoretically, may be useful for ADHD, but not yet proven
- Theoretically, could be useful in any memory condition characterized by cholinergic deficiency (e.g., some cases of brain injury, cancer chemotherapy-induced cognitive changes, etc.)

Suggested Reading

Bentue-Ferrer D, Tribut O, Polard E, Allain H. Clinically significant drug interactions with cholinesterase inhibitors: a guide for neurologists. CNS Drugs 2003;17:947–63.

Bonner LT, Peskind ER. Pharmacologic treatments of dementia. Med Clin North Am 2002;86:657–74.

Coyle J, Kershaw P. Galantamine, a cholinesterase inhibitor that allosterically modulates nicotinic receptors: effects on the course of Alzheimer's disease. Biol Psychiatry 2001;49:289–99.

Jones RW. Have cholinergic therapies reached their clinical boundary in Alzheimer's disease? Int J Geriatr Psychiatry 2003;18(Suppl 1): S7–13.

Olin J, Schneider L. Galantamine for Alzheimer's disease. Cochrane Database Syst Rev 2002;(3):CD001747.

Stahl SM. Cholinesterase inhibitors for Alzheimer's disease. Hosp Pract (Off Ed) 1998;33:131–6.

Stahl SM. The new cholinesterase inhibitors for Alzheimer's disease, part 1. J Clin Psychiatry 2000;61:710–11.

Stahl SM. The new cholinesterase inhibitors for Alzheimer's disease, part 2. J Clin Psychiatry 2000;61:813–14.

THERAPEUTICS

Brands • Intuniv
• Tenex

see index for additional brand names

Generic? Yes (not for guanfacine ER)

Class

- Neuroscience-based Nomenclature: norepinephrine receptor agonist (N-RA)
- Centrally acting alpha 2A agonist; antihypertensive; nonstimulant for ADHD

Commonly Prescribed for

(bold for FDA approved)

- **Hypertension**
- **Attention deficit hyperactivity disorder (ADHD) in children ages 6–17 (Intuniv, adjunct and monotherapy)**
- Oppositional defiant disorder
- Conduct disorder
- Pervasive developmental disorders
- Motor tics
- Tourette's syndrome

How the Drug Works

- For ADHD, theoretically has central actions on postsynaptic alpha 2A receptors in the prefrontal cortex
- Guanfacine is 15–20 times more selective for alpha 2A receptors than for alpha 2B or alpha 2C receptors
- The prefrontal cortex is thought to be responsible for modulation of working memory, attention, impulse, control, and planning
- For hypertension, stimulates alpha 2A adrenergic receptors in the brain stem, reducing sympathetic outflow from the CNS and decreasing peripheral resistance, renal vascular resistance, heart rate, and blood pressure

How Long Until It Works

- For ADHD, can take a few weeks to see maximum therapeutic benefits
- Blood pressure may be lowered 30–60 minutes after first dose; greatest reduction seen after 2–4 hours
- May take several weeks to control blood pressure adequately

If It Works

- The goal of treatment of ADHD is reduction of symptoms of inattentiveness, motor hyperactivity, and/or impulsiveness that disrupt social, school, and/or occupational functioning
- Continue treatment until all symptoms are under control or improvement is stable and then continue treatment indefinitely as long as improvement persists
- Some studies of up to 2 years
- Reevaluate the need for treatment periodically
- Treatment for ADHD begun in childhood may need to be continued into adolescence and adulthood if continued benefit is documented

If It Doesn't Work

- Consider adjusting dose or switching to another agent
- Consider behavioral therapy
- Consider the presence of noncompliance and counsel patient and parents
- Consider evaluation for another diagnosis or for a comorbid condition (e.g., bipolar disorder, substance abuse, medical illness, etc.)

Best Augmenting Combos for Partial Response or Treatment Resistance

- Best to attempt another monotherapy prior to augmenting for ADHD
- Possibly combination with stimulants (with caution)
- Combinations for ADHD should be for the expert, while monitoring the patient closely, and when other treatment options have failed
- Chlorthalidone, thyazide-type diuretics, and furosemide for hypertension

Tests

- Blood pressure should be checked regularly during treatment

SIDE EFFECTS

How Drug Causes Side Effects

- Excessive actions on alpha 2A receptors, nonselective actions on alpha 2B and alpha 2C receptors

Notable Side Effects

- Sedation, dizziness
- Dry mouth, constipation, abdominal pain

- Fatigue, weakness
- Hypotension

Life-Threatening or Dangerous Side Effects

- Sinus bradycardia, hypotension (dose-related)

Weight Gain

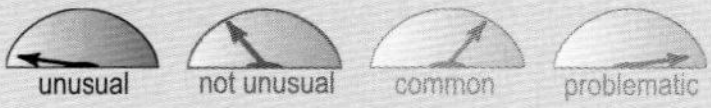

- Reported but not expected

Sedation

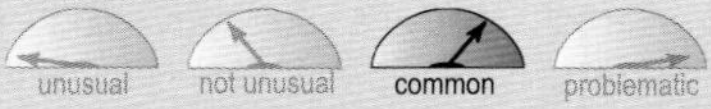

- Many experience and/or can be significant in amount
- Some patients may not tolerate it
- Can abate with time
- May be less sedation with extended-release formulation

What to Do About Side Effects

- Wait
- Adjust dose
- If side effects persist, discontinue use

Best Augmenting Agents for Side Effects

- Dose reduction or switching to another agent may be more effective since most side effects cannot be improved with an augmenting agent

DOSING AND USE

Usual Dosage Range

- Immediate-release: 1–2 mg/day
- Extended-release: 1–4 mg/day

Dosage Forms

- Immediate-release tablet 1 mg, 2 mg, 3 mg
- Extended-release: 1 mg, 2 mg, 3 mg, 4 mg

How to Dose

- Immediate-release: initial 1 mg/day at bedtime; after 3–4 weeks can increase to 2 mg/day
- Extended-release: initial 1 mg/day; can increase by 1 mg/week; maximum dose 4 mg/day

Dosing Tips

- Adverse effects are dose-related and usually transient
- Doses greater than 2 mg/day are associated with increased side effects
- If guanfacine is terminated abruptly, rebound hypertension may occur within 2–4 days
- For hypertension, dose can be raised to 2 mg/day if 1 mg/day is ineffective, but 2 mg may have no more efficacy than 1 mg
- For extended-release formulation, do not administer with high-fat meals because this increases exposure
- Extended-release tablets should not be crushed, chewed, or broken
- Extended-release and immediate-release tablets have different pharmacokinetic properties, so do not substitute on a mg-per-mg basis
- Consider dosing extended-release on a mg/kg basis (0.05 mg/kg to 0.12 mg/kg)

Overdose

- Drowsiness, lethargy, bradycardia, hypotension

Long-Term Use

- Shown to be safe and effective for treatment of hypertension
- Studies of up to 2 years in ADHD

Habit Forming

- No

How to Stop

- Taper to avoid rebound effects (nervousness, increased blood pressure)

Pharmacokinetics

- Pharmacokinetic properties differ for immediate- and extended-release fomulations
- Metabolized by CYP450 3A4

Drug Interactions

- CYP450 3A inhibitors such as nefazodone, fluoxetine, fluvoxamine, and ketoconazole, may decrease clearance of guanfacine and raise guanfacine levels significantly
- CYP450 3A inducers may increase clearance of guanfacine and lower guanfacine levels significantly

- Do not administer extended-release with high-fat meals, because this increases exposure
- Combined use with valproate may increase plasma concentrations of valproate
- Increased depressive effects when taken with other CNS depressants
- Phenobarbital and phenytoin may reduce plasma concentrations of guanfacine

Other Warnings/ Precautions

- Excessive heat (e.g., saunas) may exacerbate some of the side effects, such as dizziness and drowsiness
- Use with caution in patients with severe coronary insufficiency, recent myocardial infarction, cerebrovascular disease, or chronic renal or hepatic failure

Do Not Use

- If there is a proven allergy to guanfacine

SPECIAL POPULATIONS

Renal Impairment

- Patients should receive lower doses

Hepatic Impairment

- Use with caution

Cardiac Impairment

- Use with caution in patients with recent myocardial infarction, severe coronary insufficiency, cerebrovascular disease
- Use with caution in patients at risk for hypotension, bradycardia, heart block, or syncope

Elderly

- Elimination half-life may be longer in elderly patients
- Elderly patients may be more sensitive to sedative effects

Children and Adolescents

- Safety and efficacy not established in children under age 6
- Some reports of mania and aggressive behavior in ADHD patients taking guanfacine

Pregnancy

- Effective June 30, 2015, the US FDA requires changes to the content and format of pregnancy and lactation information in prescription drug labels, including the elimination of the pregnancy letter categories; the Pregnancy and Lactation Labeling Rule (PLLR or final rule) applies only to prescription drugs and will be phased in gradually for drugs approved on or after June 30, 2001
- Controlled studies have not been conducted in pregnant women
- Animal studies do not show adverse effects
- Use in women of childbearing potential requires weighing potential benefits to the mother against potential risks to the fetus

Breast Feeding

- Unknown if guanfacine is secreted in human breast milk, but all psychotropics assumed to be secreted in breast milk
- Recommended either to discontinue drug or bottle feed

THE ART OF PSYCHOPHARMACOLOGY

Potential Advantages

- No known abuse potential; not a controlled substance
- Not a stimulant
- For oppositional behavior associated with ADHD
- Less sedation than clonidine

Potential Disadvantages

- Not well studied in adults with ADHD

Primary Target Symptoms

- Concentration
- Motor hyperactivity
- Oppositional and impulsive behavior
- High blood pressure

Pearls

- Guanfacine has been shown to be effective in both children and adults, and guanfacine extended-release is approved for ADHD in children ages 6–17

- Guanfacine can also be used to treat tic disorders, including Tourette's syndrome
- Although both guanfacine and clonidine are alpha 2 adrenergic agonists, guanfacine is relatively selective for alpha 2A receptors, whereas clonidine binds not only alpha 2A, 2B, and 2C receptors but also imidazoline receptors, causing more sedation, hypotension, and side effects than guanfacine
- May be used as monotherapy or in combination with stimulants for the treatment of oppositional behavior in children with or without ADHD

Suggested Reading

Arnsten AF, Scahill L, Findling RL. alpha2-Adrenergic receptor agonists for the treatment of attention-deficit/hyperactivity disorder: emerging concepts from new data. J Child Adolesc Psychopharmacol 2007;17(4):393–406.

Biederman J, Melmed RD, Patel A, et al. Long-term, open-label extension study of guanfacine extended-release in children and adolescents with ADHD. CNS Spectr 2008;13(12):1047–55.

Posey DJ, McDougal CJ. Guanfacine and guanfacine extended-release: treatment for ADHD and related disorders. CNS Drug Rev 2007;13(4):465–74.

Sallee FR, Lyne A, Wigal T, McGough J. Long-term safety and efficacy of guanfacine extended-release in children and adolescents with attention-deficit/hyperactivity disorder. J Child Adolesc Psychopharmacol 2009;19(3):215–26.

Sallee FR, McGough J, Wigal T, et al. Guanfacine extended-release in children and adolescents with attention-deficit/hyperactivity disorder: a placebo-controlled trial. J Am Acad Child Adolesc Psychiatry 2009;48(2):155–65.

Spencer TJ, Greenbaum M, Ginsberg LD, Murphy WR. Safety and effectiveness of coadministration of guanfacine extended-release and psychostimulants in children and adolescents with attention-deficit/hyperactivity disorder. J Child Adolesc Psychopharmacol 2009;19(5):501–10.

THERAPEUTICS

Brands • Haldol

see index for additional brand names

Generic? Yes

Class

- Neuroscience-based Nomenclature: dopamine receptor antagonist (D-RAn)
- Conventional antipsychotic (neuroleptic, butyrophenone, dopamine 2 antagonist)

Commonly Prescribed for

(bold for FDA approved)

- **Manifestations of psychotic disorders (oral, immediate-release injection)**
- **Tics and vocal utterances in Tourette's syndrome (oral, immediate-release injection)**
- **Second-line treatment of severe behavior problems in children of combative, explosive hyperexcitability (oral, immediate-release injection)**
- **Second-line short-term treatment of hyperactive children (oral, immediate-release injection)**
- **Treatment of schizophrenic patients who require prolonged parenteral antipsychotic therapy (depot intramuscular decanoate)**
- Bipolar disorder
- Behavioral disturbances in dementias
- Delirium (with lorazepam)

How the Drug Works

- Blocks dopamine 2 receptors, reducing positive symptoms of psychosis and possibly combative, explosive, and hyperactive behaviors
- Blocks dopamine 2 receptors in the nigrostriatal pathway, improving tics and other symptoms in Tourette's syndrome

How Long Until It Works

- Psychotic symptoms can improve within 1 week, but it may take several weeks for full effect on behavior

If It Works

- Most often reduces positive symptoms in schizophrenia but does not eliminate them
- Most schizophrenic patients do not have a total remission of symptoms but rather a reduction of symptoms by about a third
- Continue treatment in schizophrenia until reaching a plateau of improvement
- After reaching a satisfactory plateau, continue treatment for at least a year after first episode of psychosis in schizophrenia
- For second and subsequent episodes of psychosis in schizophrenia, treatment may need to be indefinite
- Reduces symptoms of acute psychotic mania but not proven as a mood stabilizer or as an effective maintenance treatment in bipolar disorder
- After reducing acute psychotic symptoms in mania, switch to a mood stabilizer and/or an atypical antipsychotic for mood stabilization and maintenance

If It Doesn't Work

- Consider trying one of the first-line atypical antipsychotics (risperidone, olanzapine, quetiapine, ziprasidone, aripiprazole, paliperidone, asenapine, iloperidone, lurasidone, amisulpride)
- Consider trying another conventional antipsychotic
- If 2 or more antipsychotic monotherapies do not work, consider clozapine

Best Augmenting Combos for Partial Response or Treatment Resistance

- Augmentation of conventional antipsychotics has not been systematically studied
- Addition of a mood-stabilizing anticonvulsant such as valproate, carbamazepine, or lamotrigine may be helpful in both schizophrenia and bipolar mania
- Augmentation with lithium in bipolar mania may be helpful
- Addition of a benzodiazepine, especially short-term for agitation

Tests

- ✻ Since conventional antipsychotics are frequently associated with weight gain, before starting treatment, weigh all patients and determine if the patient is already overweight (BMI 25.0–29.9) or obese (BMI ≥30)
- Before giving a drug that can cause weight gain to an overweight or obese patient, consider determining whether the patient already has pre-diabetes (fasting plasma glucose 100–125 mg/dL), diabetes

(fasting plasma glucose >126 mg/dL), or dyslipidemia (increased total cholesterol, LDL cholesterol, and triglycerides; decreased HDL cholesterol), and treat or refer such patients for treatment, including nutrition and weight management, physical activity counseling, smoking cessation, and medical management

✱ Monitor weight and BMI during treatment
✱ Consider monitoring fasting triglycerides monthly for several months in patients at high risk for metabolic complications and when initiating or switching antipsychotics
✱ While giving a drug to a patient who has gained >5% of initial weight, consider evaluating for the presence of pre-diabetes, diabetes, or dyslipidemia, or consider switching to a different antipsychotic
- Should check blood pressure in the elderly before starting and for the first few weeks of treatment
- Monitoring elevated prolactin levels of dubious clinical benefit
- Patients with low white blood cell count (WBC) or history of drug-induced leucopenia/neutropenia should have complete blood count (CBC) monitored frequently during the first few months and haloperidol should be discontinued at the first sign of decline of WBC in the absence of other causative factors

SIDE EFFECTS

How Drug Causes Side Effects
- By blocking dopamine 2 receptors in the striatum, it can cause motor side effects
- By blocking dopamine 2 receptors in the pituitary, it can cause elevations in prolactin
- By blocking dopamine 2 receptors excessively in the mesocortical and mesolimbic dopamine pathways, especially at high doses, it can cause worsening of negative and cognitive symptoms (neuroleptic-induced deficit syndrome)
- By blocking alpha 1 adrenergic receptors, it can cause dizziness, sedation, and hypotension
- Mechanism of weight gain and any possible increased incidence of diabetes or dyslipidemia with conventional antipsychotics is unknown

Notable Side Effects
✱ Neuroleptic-induced deficit syndrome
✱ Akathisia
✱ Extrapyramidal symptoms, parkinsonism, tardive dyskinesia, tardive dystonia
✱ Galactorrhea, amenorrhea
- Dizziness, sedation
- Dry mouth, constipation, urinary retention, blurred vision
- Decreased sweating
- Hypotension, tachycardia, hypertension
- Weight gain

Life-Threatening or Dangerous Side Effects
- Rare neuroleptic malignant syndrome
- Rare seizures
- Rare jaundice, agranulocytosis, leukopenia
- Increased risk of death and cerebrovascular events in elderly patients with dementia-related psychosis

Weight Gain
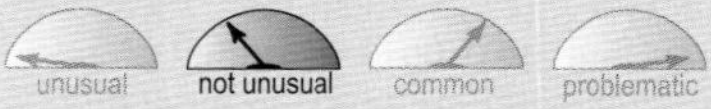

- Occurs in significant minority

Sedation
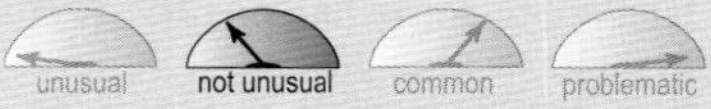

- Sedation is usually transient

What to Do About Side Effects
- Wait
- Wait
- Wait
- For motor symptoms, add an anticholinergic agent
- Reduce the dose
- For sedation, give at night
- Switch to an atypical antipsychotic
- Weight loss, exercise programs, and medical management for high BMIs, diabetes, dyslipidemia

Best Augmenting Agents for Side Effects
- Benztropine or trihexyphenidyl for motor side effects
- Sometimes amantadine can be helpful for motor side effects
- Benzodiazepines may be helpful for akathisia
- Many side effects cannot be improved with an augmenting agent

DOSING AND USE

Usual Dosage Range

- 1–40 mg/day orally
- Immediate-release injection 2–5 mg each dose
- Decanoate injection 10–20 times the previous daily dose of oral antipsychotic (see Haloperidol Decanoate section after Pearls for dosing and use)

Dosage Forms

- Tablet 0.5 mg scored, 1 mg scored, 2 mg scored, 5 mg scored, 10 mg scored, 20 mg scored
- Concentrate 2 mg/mL
- Solution 1 mg/mL
- Injection 5 mg/mL (immediate-release)
- Decanoate injection 50 mg /mL, 100 mg/mL

How to Dose

- Oral: initial 1–15 mg/day; can give once daily or in divided doses at the beginning of treatment during rapid dose escalation; increase as needed; can be dosed up to 100 mg/day; safety not established for doses over 100 mg/day
- Immediate-release injection: initial dose 2–5 mg; subsequent doses may be given as often as every hour; patient should be switched to oral administration as soon as possible

Dosing Tips – Oral

- Haloperidol is frequently dosed too high
- Some studies suggest that patients who respond well to low doses of haloperidol (e.g., approximately 2 mg/day) may have efficacy similar to atypical antipsychotics for both positive and negative symptoms of schizophrenia
- Higher doses may actually induce or worsen negative symptoms of schizophrenia
- Low doses, however, may not have beneficial actions for treatment-resistant cases or violence
- One of the only antipsychotics with a depot formulation lasting for up to a month
- Treatment should be suspended if absolute neutrophil count falls below $1,000/mm^3$

Overdose

- Fatalities have been reported; extrapyramidal symptoms, hypotension, sedation, respiratory depression, shock-like state

Long-Term Use

- Often used for long-term maintenance
- Some side effects may be irreversible (e.g., tardive dyskinesia)

Habit Forming

- No

How to Stop

- Slow down-titration of oral formulation (over 6–8 weeks), especially when simultaneously beginning a new antipsychotic while switching (i.e., cross-titration)
- Rapid oral discontinuation may lead to rebound psychosis and worsening of symptoms
- If antiparkinson agents are being used, they should be continued for a few weeks after haloperidol is discontinued

Pharmacokinetics

- Decanoate half-life approximately 3 weeks
- Oral half-life approximately 12–38 hours

Drug Interactions

- May decrease the effects of levodopa, dopamine agonists
- May increase the effects of antihypertensive drugs except for guanethidine, whose antihypertensive actions haloperidol may antagonize
- Additive effects may occur if used with CNS depressants; dose of other agent should be reduced
- Some pressor agents (e.g., epinephrine) may interact with haloperidol to lower blood pressure
- Haloperidol and anticholinergic agents together may increase intraocular pressure
- Reduces effects of anticoagulants
- Plasma levels of haloperidol may be lowered by rifampin
- Some patients taking haloperidol and lithium have developed an encephalopathic syndrome similar to neuroleptic malignant syndrome

- May enhance effects of antihypertensive drugs

Other Warnings/ Precautions

- If signs of neuroleptic malignant syndrome develop, treatment should be immediately discontinued
- Use with caution in patients with respiratory disorders
- Avoid extreme heat exposure
- If haloperidol is used to treat mania, patients may experience a rapid switch to depression
- Patients with thyrotoxicosis may experience neurotoxicity
- Use only with caution if at all in Parkison's disease or Lewy body dementia
- Higher doses and IV administration may be associated with increased risk of QT prolongation and torsades de pointes; use particular caution if patient has a QT-prolonging condition, underlying cardiac abnormalities, hypothyroidism, familial long-QT syndrome, or is taking a drug known to prolong QT interval

Do Not Use

- If patient is in comatose state or has CNS depression
- If patient has Parkinson's disease
- If there is a proven allergy to haloperidol

SPECIAL POPULATIONS

Renal Impairment

- Use with caution

Hepatic Impairment

- Use with caution

Cardiac Impairment

- Use with caution because of risk of orthostatic hypertension
- Possible increased risk of QT prolongation or torsades de pointes at higher doses or with IV administration

Elderly

- Lower doses should be used and patient should be monitored closely
- Elderly patients may be more susceptible to respiratory side effects and hypotension
- Although conventional antipsychotics are commonly used for behavioral disturbances in dementia, no agent has been approved for treatment of elderly patients with dementia-related psychosis
- Elderly patients with dementia-related psychosis treated with antipsychotics are at an increased risk of death compared to placebo, and also have an increased risk of cerebrovascular events

Children and Adolescents

- Safety and efficacy have not been established; not intended for use under age 3
- Oral: initial 0.5 mg/day; target dose 0.05–0.15 mg/kg per day for psychotic disorders; 0.05–0.075 mg/kg per day for nonpsychotic disorders
- Generally consider second-line after atypical antipsychotics

Pregnancy

- Effective June 30, 2015, the US FDA requires changes to the content and format of pregnancy and lactation information in prescription drug labels, including the elimination of the pregnancy letter categories; the Pregnancy and Lactation Labeling Rule (PLLR or final rule) applies only to prescription drugs and will be phased in gradually for drugs approved on or after June 30, 2001
- Controlled studies have not been conducted in pregnant women
- There is a risk of abnormal muscle movements and withdrawal symptoms in newborns whose mothers took an antipsychotic during the third trimester; symptoms may include agitation, abnormally increased or decreased muscle tone, tremor, sleepiness, severe difficulty breathing, and difficulty feeding
- Reports of extrapyramidal symptoms, jaundice, hyperreflexia, hyporeflexia in infants whose mothers took a conventional antipsychotic during pregnancy
- Reports of limb deformity in infants whose mothers took haloperidol during pregnancy
- Haloperidol should generally not be used during the first trimester

- Haloperidol should only be used during pregnancy if clearly needed
- Psychotic symptoms may worsen during pregnancy and some form of treatment may be necessary
- Atypical antipsychotics may be preferable to conventional antipsychotics or anticonvulsant mood stabilizers if treatment is required during pregnancy

Breast Feeding

- Some drug is found in mother's breast milk
- ✽ Recommended either to discontinue drug or bottle feed

THE ART OF PSYCHOPHARMACOLOGY

Potential Advantages

- Intramuscular formulation for emergency use
- 4-week depot formulation for noncompliance
- Low-dose responders may have comparable positive and negative symptom efficacy to atypical antipsychotics
- Low-cost, effective treatment

Potential Disadvantages

- Patients with tardive dyskinesia or who wish to avoid tardive dyskinesia and extrapyramidal symptoms
- Vulnerable populations such as children or elderly
- Patients with notable cognitive or mood symptoms

Primary Target Symptoms

- Positive symptoms of psychosis
- Violent or aggressive behavior

Pearls

- Prior to the introduction of atypical antipsychotics, haloperidol was one of the most preferred antipsychotics
- Haloperidol may still be a useful antipsychotic, especially at low doses for those patients who require management with a conventional antipsychotic or who cannot afford an atypical antipsychotic
- Low doses may not induce negative symptoms, but high doses may
- Not clearly effective for improving cognitive or affective symptoms of schizophrenia
- May be effective for bipolar maintenance, but there may be more tardive dyskinesia when affective disorders are treated with a conventional antipsychotic long-term
- Less sedating than many other conventional antipsychotics, especially "low potency" phenothiazines
- Haloperidol is often used to treat delirium, generally in combination with lorazepam, with the haloperidol dose 2 times the lorazepam dose
- Haloperidol's long-acting intramuscular formulation lasts up to 4 weeks, whereas some other long-acting intramuscular antipsychotics may last only up to 2 weeks
- Decanoate administration is intended for patients with chronic schizophrenia who have been stabilized on oral antipsychotic medication
- Patients have very similar antipsychotic responses to any conventional antipsychotic, which is different from atypical antipsychotics where antipsychotic responses of individual patients can occasionally vary greatly from one atypical antipsychotic to another
- Patients receiving atypical antipsychotics may occasionally require a "top up" of a conventional antipsychotic such as haloperidol to control aggression or violent behavior
- Patients with inadequate responses to atypical antipsychotics may benefit from a trial of augmentation with a conventional antipsychotic such as haloperidol or from switching to a conventional antipsychotic such as haloperidol
- However, long-term polypharmacy with a combination of a conventional antipsychotic such as haloperidol with an atypical antipsychotic may combine their side effects without clearly augmenting the efficacy of either
- For treatment-resistant patients, especially those with impulsivity, aggression, violence, and self-harm, long-term polypharmacy with 2 atypical antipsychotics or with 1 atypical antipsychotic and 1 conventional antipsychotic may be useful or even necessary while closely monitoring
- In such cases, it may be beneficial to combine 1 depot antipsychotic with 1 oral antipsychotic

HALOPERIDOL DECANOATE

Haloperidol Decanoate Properties	
Vehicle	Sesame oil
Tmax	3–9 days
T1/2 with multiple dosing	21 days
Time to reach steady state	4 weeks with loading
Able to be loaded	Yes
Dosing schedule (maintenance)	4 weeks
Injection site	Intramuscular
Needle gauge	21
Dosage forms	50 mg, 100 mg
Injection volume	50 or 100 mg/mL; not to exceed 3 mL

Usual Dosage Range

- 10–20 times the previous oral dose

How to Dose

- Conversion from oral: loading with 20 times the oral daily dose (mg/day) for the first month, divided into 2 biweekly injections; weekly loading is an alternate option; may require oral coverage for the first week

Dosing Tips

- With LAIs, the absorption rate constant is slower than the elimination rate constant, thus resulting in "flip-flop" kinetics—i.e., time to steady-state is a function of absorption rate, while concentration at steady-state is a function of elimination rate
- The rate-limiting step for plasma drug levels for LAIs is not drug metabolism, but rather slow absorption from the injection site
- In general, 5 half-lives of any medication are needed to achieve 97% of steady-state levels
- The long half-lives of depot antipsychotics mean that one must either adequately load the dose (if possible) or provide oral supplementation
- The failure to adequately load the dose leads either to prolonged cross-titration from oral antipsychotic or to sub-therapeutic antipsychotic plasma levels for weeks or months in patients who are not receiving (or adhering to) oral supplementation
- Because plasma antipsychotic levels increase gradually over time, dose requirements may ultimately decrease from initial; obtaining periodic plasma levels can be beneficial to prevent unnecessary plasma level creep
- The time to get a blood level for patients receiving LAI is the morning of the day they will receive their next injection
- Advantages: reliable conversion formula from oral dosing, established loading regimens
- Disadvantages: higher incidence of local site reactions (due to sesame oil vehicle); even with loading, may require oral coverage for at least a week
- Response threshold is generally 3–5 ng/mL; plasma levels greater than 20 ng/mL are generally not well tolerated
- Single injection volumes greater than 300 (3 mL) are not tolerated, so patients who require higher doses typically receive the monthly dose as split injections every 2 weeks
- A loading strategy advocated by some is to give 300 mg LAI every 1–2 weeks for 2 doses and then measure plasma drug concentrations just prior to a third loading dose to see if a third dose is necessary

SWITCHING FROM ORAL ANTIPSYCHOTICS TO HALOPERIDOL DECANOATE

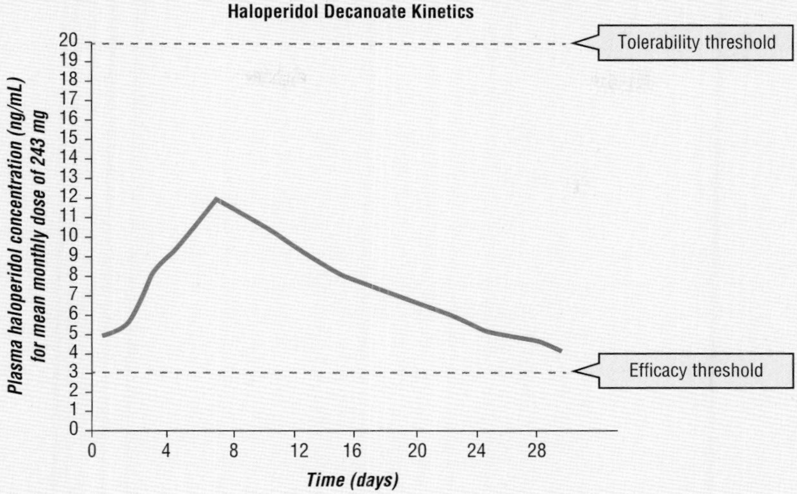

- Discontinuation of oral antipsychotic can begin immediately if adequate loading is pursued; however, oral coverage may still be necessary for the first week
- How to discontinue oral formulations
  - Down-titration is not required for: amisulpride, aripiprazole, brexpiprazole, cariprazine, paliperidone ER
  - 1-week down-titration is required for: iloperidone, lurasidone, risperidone, ziprasidone
  - 3–4-week down-titration is required for: asenapine, olanzapine, quetiapine
  - 4+-week down-titration is required for: clozapine
  - For patients taking benzodiazepine or anticholinergic medication, this can be continued during cross-titration to help alleviate side effects such as insomnia, agitation, and/or psychosis. Once the patient is stable on LAI, these can be tapered one at a time as appropriate.

Suggested Reading

Cipriani A, Rendell JM, Geddes JR. Haloperidol alone or in combination for acute mania. Cochrane Database Syst Rev 2006;19(3):CD004362.

Huf G, Alexander J, Allen MH, Raveendran NS. Haloperidol plus promethazine for psychosis-induced aggression. Cochrane Database Syst Rev 2009;8(3):CD005146.

Joy CB, Adams CE, Lawrie SM. Haloperidol versus placebo for schizophrenia. Cochrane Database Syst Rev 2006;18(4):CD003082.

Leucht C, Kitzmantel M, Chua L, Kane J, Leucht S. Haloperidol versus chlorpromazine for schizophrenia. Cochrane Database Syst Rev 2008;23(1):CD004278.

HYDROXYZINE

THERAPEUTICS

Brands
- Atarax
- Marax
- Vistaril

see index for additional brand names

Generic? Yes

Class
- Neuroscience-based Nomenclature: histamine receptor antagonist (H-RAn)
- Antihistamine (anxiolytic, hypnotic, antiemetic)

Commonly Prescribed for
(bold for FDA approved)
- **Anxiety and tension associated with psychoneurosis**
- **Adjunct in organic disease states in which anxiety is manifested**
- **Pruritus due to allergic conditions**
- **Histamine-mediated pruritus**
- **Premedication sedation**
- **Sedation following general anesthesia**
- **Acute disturbance/hysteria (injection)**
- **Anxiety withdrawal symptoms in alcoholics or patients with delirium tremens (injection)**
- **Adjunct in pre/postoperative and pre/postpartum patients to allay anxiety, control emesis, and reduce narcotic dose (injection)**
- **Nausea and vomiting (injection)**
- Insomnia

How the Drug Works
- Blocks histamine 1 receptors

How Long Until It Works
- 15–20 minutes (oral administration)
- Some immediate relief with first dosing is common; can take several weeks with daily dosing for maximal therapeutic benefit in chronic conditions

If It Works
- For short-term symptoms of anxiety – after a few weeks, discontinue use or use on an "as-needed" basis
- For chronic anxiety disorders, the goal of treatment is complete remission of symptoms as well as prevention of future relapses
- For chronic anxiety disorders, treatment most often reduces or even eliminates symptoms, but not a cure since symptoms can recur after medicine stopped
- For long-term symptoms of anxiety, consider switching to an SSRI or SNRI for long-term maintenance
- If long-term maintenance is necessary, continue treatment for 6 months after symptoms resolve, and then taper dose slowly
- If symptoms reemerge, consider treatment with an SSRI or SNRI, or consider restarting hydroxyzine

If It Doesn't Work
- Consider switching to another agent or adding an appropriate augmenting agent

Best Augmenting Combos for Partial Response or Treatment Resistance
- Hydroxyzine can be used as an adjunct to SSRIs or SNRIs in treating anxiety disorders

Tests
- None for healthy individuals
- Hydroxyzine may cause falsely elevated urinary concentrations of 17-hydroxycorticosteroids in certain lab tests (e.g., Porter-Silber reaction, Glenn-Nelson method)

SIDE EFFECTS

How Drug Causes Side Effects
- Blocking histamine 1 receptors can cause sedation

Notable Side Effects
- Dry mouth, sedation, tremor

Life-Threatening or Dangerous Side Effects
- Rare convulsions (generally at high doses)
- Rare cardiac arrest, death (intramuscular formulation combined with CNS depressants)
- Bronchodilation
- Respiratory depression

Weight Gain

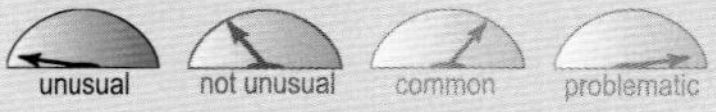

- Reported but not expected

Sedation

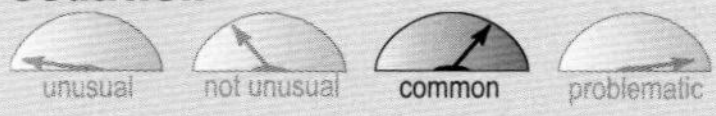

- Many experience and/or can be significant in amount
- Sedation is usually transient

What to Do About Side Effects

- Wait
- Wait
- Wait
- Switch to another agent

Best Augmenting Agents for Side Effects

- Many side effects cannot be improved with an augmenting agent

DOSING AND USE

Usual Dosage Range

- Anxiety: 50–100 mg 4 times a day
- Sedative: 50–100 mg oral, 25–100 mg intramuscular injection
- Pruritus: 75 mg/day divided into 3–4 doses

Dosage Forms

- Tablet 10 mg, 25 mg, 50 mg, 100 mg
- Capsule 25 mg, 50 mg, 100 mg
- Oral liquid 10 mg/5 mL, 25 mg/5 mL
- Intramuscular 25 mg/mL, 50 mg/mL, 100 mg/2 mL

How to Dose

- Oral dosing does not require titration
- Emergency intramuscular injection: initial 50–100 mg, repeat every 4–6 hours as needed
- Hydroxyzine intramuscular injection should not be given in the lower or mid-third of the arm and should only be given in the deltoid area if it is well-developed
- In adults, hydroxyzine intramuscular injections may be given in the upper outer quadrant of the buttock or in the mid-lateral thigh

Dosing Tips

- Hydroxyzine may be administered intramuscularly initially, but should be changed to oral administration as soon as possible
- Tolerance usually develops to sedation, allowing higher dosing over time

Overdose

- Sedation, hypotension, possible QTc prolongation

Long-Term Use

- Evidence of efficacy for up to 16 weeks

Habit Forming

- No

How to Stop

- Taper generally not necessary

Pharmacokinetics

- Rapidly absorbed from gastrointestinal tract
- Mean elimination half-life approximately 20 hours

Drug Interactions

- If hydroxyzine is taken in conjunction with another CNS depressant, the dose of the CNS depressant should be reduced by half
- If hydroxyzine is used pre- or post-operatively, the dose of narcotic can be reduced
- If anticholinergic agents are used with hydroxyzine, the anticholinergic effects may be enhanced
- Hydroxyzine may reverse the vasopressor effect of epinephrine; patients requiring a vasopressor agent should use norepinephrine or metaraminol instead

Other Warnings/ Precautions

- Hydroxyzine should not be administered subcutaneously, intra-arterially, or intravenously

Do Not Use

- If patient is in early stages of pregnancy
- If there is a proven allergy to hydroxyzine

SPECIAL POPULATIONS

Renal Impairment

- Dosage adjustment may not be necessary

Hepatic Impairment

- Dosage adjustment may not be necessary

Cardiac Impairment

- Hydroxyzine may be used to treat anxiety associated with cardiac impairment

Elderly

- Some patients may tolerate lower doses better
- Elderly patients may be more sensitive to sedative and anticholinergic effects
- Should be avoided in elderly patients with dementia

Children and Adolescents

- Anxiety, pruritus (6 and older): 50–100 mg/day in divided doses
- Anxiety, pruritus (under 6): 50 mg/day in divided doses
- Sedative: 0.6 mg/kg oral, 0.5 mg/lb intramuscular injection
- Small children should not receive hydroxyzine by intramuscular injection in the periphery of the upper quadrant of the buttock unless absolutely necessary because of risk of damage to the sciatic nerve
- Hyperactive children should be monitored for paradoxical effects

Pregnancy

- ❋ Hydroxyzine is contraindicated in early pregnancy
- Effective June 30, 2015, the US FDA requires changes to the content and format of pregnancy and lactation information in prescription drug labels, including the elimination of the pregnancy letter categories; the Pregnancy and Lactation Labeling Rule (PLLR or final rule) applies only to prescription drugs and will be phased in gradually for drugs approved on or after June 30, 2001
- Hydroxyzine intramuscular injection can be used prepartum, reducing narcotic requirements by up to 50%

Breast Feeding

- Unknown if hydroxyzine is secreted in human breast milk, but all psychotropics assumed to be secreted in breast milk
- ❋ Recommended either to discontinue drug or bottle feed

THE ART OF PSYCHOPHARMACOLOGY

Potential Advantages

- Has multiple formulations, including oral capsules, tablets, and liquid, as well as injectable
- No abuse liability, dependence, or withdrawal

Potential Disadvantages

- Patients with severe anxiety disorders
- Elderly patients
- Dementia patients

Primary Target Symptoms

- Anxiety
- Skeletal muscle tension
- Itching
- Nausea, vomiting

Pearls

- ❋ A preferred anxiolytic for patients with dermatitis or skin symptoms such as pruritis
- Anxiolytic actions may be proportional to sedating actions
- Hydroxyzine tablets are made with 1,1,1-trichloroethane, which destroys ozone
- Hydroxyzine by intramuscular injection may be used to treat agitation during alcohol withdrawal
- Hydroxyzine may not be as effective as benzodiazepines or newer agents in the management of anxiety

Suggested Reading

Diehn F, Tefferi A. Pruritus in polycythaemia vera: prevalence, laboratory correlates and management. Br J Haematol 2001;115:619–21.

Ferreri M, Hantouche EG. Recent clinical trials of hydroxyzine in generalized anxiety disorder. Acta Psychiatr Scand Suppl 1998;393:102–8.

Guaiana G, Barbui C, Cipriani A. Hydroxyzine for generalised anxiety disorder. Cochrane Database Syst Rev 2010;8(12):CD006815.

Paton DM, Webster DR. Clinical pharmacokinetics of H1-receptor antagonists (the antihistamines). Clin Pharmacokinet 1985;10:477–97.

THERAPEUTICS

Brands • FANAPT
see index for additional brand names

Generic? No

Class

- Neuroscience-based Nomenclature: dopamine and serotonin receptor antagonist (DS-RAn)
- Atypical antipsychotic (serotonin-dopamine antagonist; second-generation antipsychotic; also a mood stabilizer)

Commonly Prescribed for

(bold for FDA approved)

- **Schizophrenia**
- **Schizophrenia maintenance**
- Acute mania/mixed mania
- Other psychotic disorders
- Bipolar maintenance
- Bipolar depression
- Treatment-resistant depression
- Behavioral disturbances in dementia
- Behavioral disturbances in children and adolescents
- Disorders associated with problems with impulse control

How the Drug Works

- Blocks dopamine 2 receptors, reducing positive symptoms of psychosis and stabilizing affective symptoms
- Blocks serotonin 2A receptors, causing enhancement of dopamine release in certain brain regions and thus reducing motor side effects and possibly improving cognitive and affective symptoms
- Blockade of central alpha 1 adrenergic receptors may contribute to low potential for EPS

How Long Until It Works

- Psychotic symptoms can improve within 1 week, but it may take several weeks for full effect on behavior as well as on cognition
- Slow titration may delay antipsychotic effects during the first 1 to 2 weeks compared to some other antipsychotic drugs that do not require similar titration
- Classically recommended to wait at least 4–6 weeks to determine efficacy of drug, but in practice some patients may require up to 16–20 weeks to show a good response, especially on cognitive symptoms

If It Works

- Most often reduces positive symptoms but does not eliminate them
- Can improve negative symptoms, as well as aggressive, cognitive, and affective symptoms in schizophrenia
- Most schizophrenia patients do not have a total remission of symptoms but rather a reduction of symptoms by about a third
- Perhaps 5–15% of schizophrenia patients can experience an overall improvement of greater than 50–60%, especially when receiving stable treatment for more than a year
- Such patients are considered super-responders or "awakeners" since they may be well enough to be employed, live independently, and sustain long-term relationships
- Continue treatment until reaching a plateau of improvement
- After reaching a satisfactory plateau, continue treatment for at least a year after first episode of psychosis
- For second and subsequent episodes of psychosis, treatment may need to be indefinite
- Even for first episodes of psychosis, it may be preferable to continue treatment

If It Doesn't Work

- Try one of the other atypical antipsychotics (risperidone, olanzapine, quetiapine, ziprasidone, aripiprazole, paliperidone, asenapine, lurasidone, amisulpride)
- If 2 or more antipsychotic monotherapies do not work, consider clozapine
- Some patients may require treatment with a conventional antipsychotic
- If no first-line atypical antipsychotic is effective, consider higher doses or augmentation with valproate or lamotrigine
- Consider noncompliance and switch to another antipsychotic with fewer side effects or to an antipsychotic that can be given by depot injection (a depot formulation of iloperidone is in clinical testing)

- Consider initiating rehabilitation and psychotherapy such as cognitive remediation
- Consider presence of concomitant drug abuse

Best Augmenting Combos for Partial Response or Treatment Resistance

- Valproic acid (valproate, divalproex, divalproex ER)
- Other mood-stabilizing anticonvulsants (carbamazepine, oxcarbazepine, lamotrigine)
- Lithium
- Benzodiazepines

Tests

Before starting an atypical antipsychotic

✽ Weigh all patients and track BMI during treatment
- Get baseline personal and family history of diabetes, obesity, dyslipidemia, hypertension, and cardiovascular disease

✽ Get waist circumference (at umbilicus), blood pressure, fasting plasma glucose, and fasting lipid profile
- Determine if the patient is
  - overweight (BMI 25.0–29.9)
  - obese (BMI ≥30)
  - has pre-diabetes (fasting plasma glucose 100–125 mg/dL)
  - has diabetes (fasting plasma glucose >126 mg/dL)
  - has hypertension (BP >140/90 mm Hg)
  - has dyslipidemia (increased total cholesterol, LDL cholesterol, and triglycerides; decreased HDL cholesterol)
- Treat or refer such patients for treatment, including nutrition and weight management, physical activity counseling, smoking cessation, and medical management

Monitoring after starting an atypical antipsychotic

✽ BMI monthly for 3 months, then quarterly

✽ Consider monitoring fasting triglycerides monthly for several months in patients at high risk for metabolic complications and when initiating or switching antipsychotics

✽ Blood pressure, fasting plasma glucose, fasting lipids within 3 months and then annually, but earlier and more frequently for patients with diabetes or who have gained >5% of initial weight
- Treat or refer for treatment and consider switching to another atypical antipsychotic for patients who become overweight, obese, pre-diabetic, diabetic, hypertensive, or dyslipidemic while receiving an atypical antipsychotic

✽ Even in patients without known diabetes, be vigilant for the rare but life-threatening onset of diabetic ketoacidosis, which always requires immediate treatment, by monitoring for the rapid onset of polyuria, polydipsia, weight loss, nausea, vomiting, dehydration, rapid respiration, weakness, and clouding of sensorium, even coma
- Patients with low white blood cell count (WBC) or history of drug-induced leucopenia/neutropenia should have complete blood count (CBC) monitored frequently during the first few months and iloperidone should be discontinued at the first sign of decline in WBC in the absence of other causative factors
- Patients at risk for electrolyte disturbances (e.g., patients on diuretic therapy) should have baseline and periodic serum potassium and magnesium measurements

SIDE EFFECTS

How Drug Causes Side Effects

- By blocking alpha 1 adrenergic receptors, it can cause dizziness, sedation, and hypotension
- By blocking dopamine 2 receptors in the striatum, it can cause motor side effects
- By blocking dopamine 2 receptors in the pituitary, it can cause elevations in prolactin
- Mechanism of weight gain and increased incidence of diabetes and dyslipidemia with atypical antipsychotics is unknown

Notable Side Effects

✽ Orthostatic hypotension
- Sedation, dose-dependent dizziness, fatigue
- Dry mouth, nasal congestion
- Dose-dependent weight gain

✽ May increase risk for diabetes and dyslipidemia
- Dose-dependent tachycardia
- Rare tardive dyskinesia (much reduced risk compared to conventional antipsychotics)

Life-Threatening or Dangerous Side Effects

- Hyperglycemia, in some cases extreme and associated with ketoacidosis or hyperosmolar coma or death, has been reported in patients taking atypical antipsychotics
- Increased risk of death and cerebrovascular events in elderly patients with dementia-related psychosis
- Rare neuroleptic malignant syndrome (much reduced risk compared to conventional antipsychotics)
- Rare seizures

Weight Gain

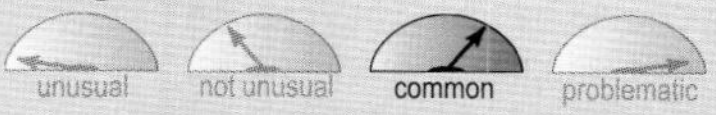

- Many experience and/or can be significant in amount
- May be less than for some antipsychotics, more than for others

Sedation

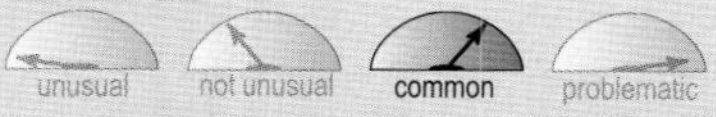

- Many experience and/or can be significant in amount

What to Do About Side Effects

- Wait
- Wait
- Wait
- Anticholinergics may reduce motor side effects when present
- Weight loss, exercise programs, and medical management for high BMIs, diabetes, dyslipidemia
- Switch to another atypical antipsychotic

Best Augmenting Agents for Side Effects

- Benztropine or trihexyphenidyl for motor side effects
- Many side effects cannot be improved with an augmenting agent

DOSING AND USE

Usual Dosage Range

- 12–24 mg/day in 2 divided doses

Dosage Forms

- Tablet 1 mg, 2 mg, 4 mg, 6 mg, 8 mg, 10 mg, 12 mg

How to Dose

- Initial 2 mg in 2 divided doses on day 1; 4 mg in 2 divided doses on day 2; 8 mg in 2 divided doses on day 3; 12 mg in 2 divided doses on day 4; 16 mg in 2 divided doses on day 5; 20 mg in 2 divided doses on day 6; 24 mg in 2 divided doses on day 7
- Maximum dose studied is 32 mg/day

Dosing Tips

- May titrate even slower in patients who develop side effects, especially orthostasis, or when adding or switching from another drug with alpha 1 antagonist properties
- Patients most vulnerable to side effects during titration would be those sensitive to orthostasis (e.g., the young, the elderly, those with cardiovascular problems, those taking concomitant vasoactive drugs)
- Slow dosing could lead to delayed onset of antipsychotic effects
- Once daily use seems theoretically possible because the half-life of iloperidone is 18–33 hours
- Some patients may respond to doses greater than 24 mg/day if tolerated
- Treatment should be suspended if absolute neutrophil count falls below 1,000/mm^3
- If treatment is discontinued for more than 3 days, it may need to be restarted following the initial titration schedule in order to maximize tolerability
- Iloperidone should be discontinued in patients with persistent QTc measurements of more than 500 msec

Overdose

- Sedation, tachycardia, hypotension

Long-Term Use

- Not studied, but long-term maintenance treatment is often necessary for schizophrenia

Habit Forming

- No

How to Stop
- Down-titration, especially when simultaneously beginning a new antipsychotic while switching (i.e., cross-titration)
- Rapid discontinuation could theoretically lead to rebound psychosis and worsening of symptoms

Pharmacokinetics
- Half-life 18–33 hours
- Metabolized by CYP450 2D6 and 3A4
- Food does not affect absorption

Drug Interactions
- May increase effects of antihypertensive agents
- May antagonize levodopa, dopamine agonists
- May enhance QTc prolongation of other drugs capable of prolonging QTc interval
- Inhibitors of CYP450 2D6 (e.g., paroxetine, fluoxetine, duloxetine, quinidine) may increase plasma levels of iloperidone and require a dosage reduction by one-half of iloperidone
- Inhibitors of CYP450 3A4 (e.g., nefazodone, fluvoxamine, fluoxetine, ketoconazole) may increase plasma levels of iloperidone and require a dosage reduction by one-half of iloperidone

Other Warnings/ Precautions
- Use with caution in patients with conditions that predispose to hypotension (dehydration, overheating)
- Dysphagia has been associated with antipsychotic use, and iloperidone should be used cautiously in patients at risk for aspiration pneumonia
- Iloperidone prolongs QTc interval more than some other antipsychotics, an effect that is augmented by concomitant use of drugs that inhibit iloperidone metabolism
- Priapism has been reported with iloperidone

Do Not Use
- If patient is taking agents capable of significantly prolonging QTc interval (e.g., pimozide, thioridazine, selected antiarrhythmics, moxifloxacin, sparfloxacin)
- If there is a history of QTc prolongation or cardiac arrhythmia, recent acute myocardial infarction, uncompensated heart failure
- If there is a proven allergy to iloperidone

SPECIAL POPULATIONS

Renal Impairment
- Dose adjustment not generally necessary

Hepatic Impairment
- Not recommended for patients with hepatic impairment

Cardiac Impairment
- Drug should be used with caution because of risk of orthostatic hypotension
- Not recommended for patients with significant cardiovascular illness

Elderly
- Some patients may tolerate lower doses better
- Although atypical antipsychotics are commonly used for behavioral disturbances in dementia, no agent has been approved for treatment of elderly patients with dementia-related psychosis
- Elderly patients with dementia-related psychosis treated with atypical antipsychotics are at an increased risk of death compared to placebo, and also have an increased risk of cerebrovascular events

Children and Adolescents
- Safety and efficacy have not been established
- Children and adolescents using iloperidone may need to be monitored more often than adults

Pregnancy
- Effective June 30, 2015, the US FDA requires changes to the content and format of pregnancy and lactation information in prescription drug labels, including the elimination of the pregnancy letter categories; the Pregnancy and Lactation Labeling Rule (PLLR or final rule) applies only to prescription drugs and will be

phased in gradually for drugs approved on or after June 30, 2001
- Controlled studies have not been conducted in pregnant women
- There is a risk of abnormal muscle movements and withdrawal symptoms in newborns whose mothers took an antipsychotic during the third trimester; symptoms may include agitation, abnormally increased or decreased muscle tone, tremor, sleepiness, severe difficulty breathing, and difficulty feeding
- Psychotic symptoms may worsen during pregnancy and some form of treatment may be necessary
- Iloperidone may be preferable to anticonvulsant mood stabilizers if treatment is required during pregnancy
- National Pregnancy Registry for Atypical Antipsychotics: 1-866-961-2388 or http://womensmentalhealth.org/clinical-and-research-programs/pregnancyregistry/

Breast Feeding

- Unknown if iloperidone is secreted in human breast milk, but all psychotropics assumed to be secreted in breast milk
- ✻ Recommended either to discontinue drug or bottle feed
- Infants of women who choose to breast feed while on iloperidone should be monitored for possible adverse effects

THE ART OF PSYCHOPHARMACOLOGY

Potential Advantages

- Some cases of psychosis and bipolar disorder refractory to treatment with other antipsychotics
- Patients wishing to avoid EPS

Potential Disadvantages

- Patients requiring rapid onset of antipsychotic action without dosage titration
- Patients noncompliant with twice daily dosing
- Cognitive symptoms
- Unstable mood (both depression and mania)
- Aggressive symptoms

Primary Target Symptoms

- Positive symptoms of psychosis
- Negative symptoms of psychosis

Pearls

- Not approved for mania, but all atypical antipsychotics approved for acute treatment of schizophrenia have proven effective in the acute treatment of mania as well
- Seems to have placebo-level EPS, including little or no akathisia
- Potent alpha 1 blocking properties suggest potential utility in PTSD (e.g., nightmares, as for prazosin)
- Binding properties suggest theoretical efficacy in depression, but studies and clinical experience are required to confirm this
- QTc warning similar to that for ziprasidone, where this has not materialized into a significant clinical problem
- A 4-week depot preparation is in clinical testing
- Early studies indicate iloperidone's efficacy may be linked to pharmacogenomic markers such as ciliary neurotrophic factor (CNTF), and others
- Patients with inadequate responses to atypical antipsychotics may benefit from determination of plasma drug levels and, if low, a dosage increase even beyond the usual prescribing limits
- For treatment-resistant patients, especially those with impulsivity, aggression, violence, and self-harm, long-term polypharmacy with 2 atypical antipsychotics or with 1 atypical antipsychotic and 1 conventional antipsychotic may be useful or even necessary while closely monitoring
- In such cases, it may be beneficial to combine 1 depot antipsychotic with 1 oral antipsychotic

THE ART OF SWITCHING

Switching from Oral Antipsychotics to Iloperidone

- With aripiprazole, amisulpride, and paliperidone ER, immediate stop is possible
- Clinical experience has shown that quetiapine, olanzapine, and asenapine should be tapered off slowly over a period of 3–4 weeks, to allow patients to readapt to the withdrawal of blocking cholinergic, histaminergic, and alpha-1 receptors
- Clozapine should always be tapered off slowly, over a period of 4 weeks or more

* Benzodiazepine or anticholinergic medication can be administered during cross-titration to help alleviate side effects such as insomnia, agitation, and/or psychosis

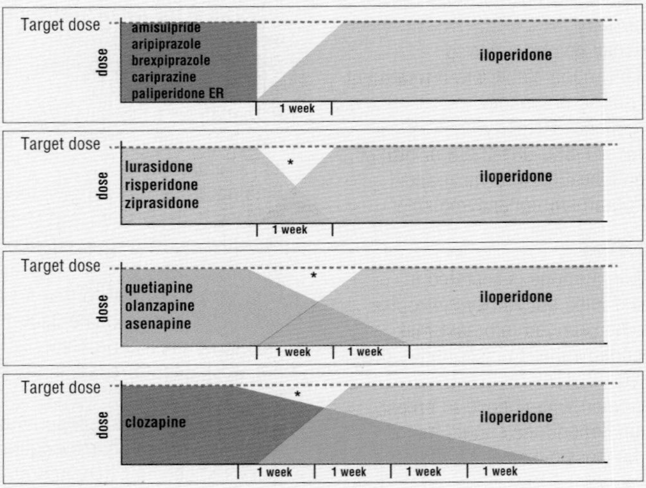

Suggested Reading

Albers LJ, Musenga A, Raggi MA. Iloperidone: a new benzisoxazole atypical antipsychotic drug. Is it novel enough to impact the crowded atypical antipsychotic market? Expert Opin Investig Drugs 2008;17:61–75.

Citrome L. Iloperidone for schizophrenia: a review of the efficacy and safety profile for this newly commercialized second-generation antipsychotics. Int J Clin Pract 2009;63: 1237–48.

Kane JM, Lauriello J, Laska E, Di Marino M, Wolfgang CD. Long-term efficacy and safety of iloperidone: results from 3 clinical trials for the treatment of schizophrenia. J Clin Psychopharmacol 2008;28(2 Suppl 1):S29–35.

Tarazi F, Stahl SM. Iloperidone, asenapine and lurasidone: a primer on their current status. Exp Opin Pharmacother 2012;13(13):1911–22.

Volpi S, Potkin SG, Malhotra AK, Licamele L, Lavedan C. Applicability of a genetic signature for enhanced iloperidone efficacy in the treatment of schizophrenia. J Clin Psychiatry 2009;70:801–9.

IMIPRAMINE

THERAPEUTICS

Brands • Tofranil

see index for additional brand names

Generic? Yes

Class

- Neuroscience-based Nomenclature: serotonin norepinephrine reuptake inhibitor (SN-RI)
- Tricyclic antidepressant (TCA)
- Serotonin and norepinephrine/noradrenaline reuptake inhibitor

Commonly Prescribed for

(bold for FDA approved)

- **Depression**
- * Enuresis
- Anxiety
- Insomnia
- Neuropathic pain/chronic pain
- Treatment-resistant depression
- Cataplexy syndrome

How the Drug Works

- Boosts neurotransmitters serotonin and norepinephrine/noradrenaline
- Blocks serotonin reuptake pump (serotonin transporter), presumably increasing serotonergic neurotransmission
- Blocks norepinephrine reuptake pump (norepinephrine transporter), presumably increasing noradrenergic neurotransmission
- Presumably desensitizes both serotonin 1A receptors and beta adrenergic receptors
- Since dopamine is inactivated by norepinephrine reuptake in frontal cortex, which largely lacks dopamine transporters, imipramine can increase dopamine neurotransmission in this part of the brain
- May be effective in treating enuresis because of its anticholinergic properties

How Long Until It Works

- May have immediate effects in treating insomnia or anxiety
- Onset of therapeutic actions usually not immediate, but often delayed 2–4 weeks
- If it is not working within 6–8 weeks for depression, it may require a dosage increase or it may not work at all
- May continue to work for many years to prevent relapse of symptoms

If It Works

- The goal of treatment of depression is complete remission of current symptoms as well as prevention of future relapses
- The goal of treatment of chronic neuropathic pain is to reduce symptoms as much as possible, especially in combination with other treatments
- Treatment of depression most often reduces or even eliminates symptoms, but not a cure since symptoms can recur after medicine stopped
- Treatment of chronic neuropathic pain may reduce symptoms, but rarely eliminates them completely, and is not a cure since symptoms can recur after medicine is stopped
- Continue treatment of depression until all symptoms are gone (remission)
- Once symptoms of depression are gone, continue treating for 1 year for the first episode of depression
- For second and subsequent episodes of depression, treatment may need to be indefinite
- Use in anxiety disorders and chronic pain may also need to be indefinite, but long-term treatment is not well studied in these conditions

If It Doesn't Work

- Many depressed patients have only a partial response where some symptoms are improved but others persist (especially insomnia, fatigue, and problems concentrating)
- Other depressed patients may be nonresponders, sometimes called treatment-resistant or treatment-refractory
- Consider increasing dose, switching to another agent or adding an appropriate augmenting agent
- Consider psychotherapy
- Consider evaluation for another diagnosis or for a comorbid condition (e.g., medical illness, substance abuse, etc.)
- Some patients may experience apparent lack of consistent efficacy due to activation of latent or underlying bipolar disorder, and require antidepressant discontinuation and a switch to a mood stabilizer

Best Augmenting Combos for Partial Response or Treatment Resistance

- Lithium, buspirone, thyroid hormone (for depression)
- Gabapentin, tiagabine, other anticonvulsants, even opiates if done by experts while monitoring carefully in difficult cases (for chronic pain)

Tests

- Baseline EKG is recommended for patients over age 50
- ✻ Since tricyclic and tetracyclic antidepressants are frequently associated with weight gain, before starting treatment, weigh all patients and determine if the patient is already overweight (BMI 25.0–29.9) or obese (BMI ≥30)
- Before giving a drug that can cause weight gain to an overweight or obese patient, consider determining whether the patient already has pre-diabetes (fasting plasma glucose 100–125 mg/dL), diabetes (fasting plasma glucose >126 mg/dL), or dyslipidemia (increased total cholesterol, LDL cholesterol, and triglycerides; decreased HDL cholesterol), and treat or refer such patients for treatment, including nutrition and weight management, physical activity counseling, smoking cessation, and medical management
- ✻ Monitor weight and BMI during treatment
- ✻ While giving a drug to a patient who has gained >5% of initial weight, consider evaluating for the presence of pre-diabetes, diabetes, or dyslipidemia, or consider switching to a different antidepressant
- EKGs may be useful for selected patients (e.g., those with personal or family history of QTc prolongation; cardiac arrhythmia; recent myocardial infarction; uncompensated heart failure; or taking agents that prolong QTc interval such as pimozide, thioridazine, selected antiarrhythmics, moxifloxacin, sparfloxacin, etc.)
- Patients at risk for electrolyte disturbances (e.g., patients on diuretic therapy) should have baseline and periodic serum potassium and magnesium measurements

SIDE EFFECTS

How Drug Causes Side Effects

- Anticholinergic activity may explain sedative effects, dry mouth, constipation, and blurred vision
- Sedative effects and weight gain may be due to antihistamine properties
- Blockade of alpha adrenergic 1 receptors may explain dizziness, sedation, and hypotension
- Cardiac arrhythmias and seizures, especially in overdose, may be caused by blockade of ion channels

Notable Side Effects

- Blurred vision, constipation, urinary retention, increased appetite, dry mouth, nausea, diarrhea, heartburn, unusual taste in mouth, weight gain
- Fatigue, weakness, dizziness, sedation, headache, anxiety, nervousness, restlessness
- Sexual dysfunction, sweating

Life-Threatening or Dangerous Side Effects

- Paralytic ileus, hyperthermia (TCAs + anticholinergic agents)
- Lowered seizure threshold and rare seizures
- Orthostatic hypotension, sudden death, arrhythmias, tachycardia
- QTc prolongation
- Hepatic failure, extrapyramidal symptoms
- Increased intraocular pressure, increased psychotic symptoms
- Rare induction of mania
- Rare activation of suicidal ideation and behavior (suicidality) (short-term studies did not show an increase in the risk of suicidality with antidepressants compared to placebo beyond age 24)

Weight Gain

unusual | not unusual | **common** | problematic

- Many experience and/or can be significant in amount
- Can increase appetite and carbohydrate craving

Sedation

unusual | not unusual | **common** | problematic

- Many experience and/or can be significant in amount
- Tolerance to sedative effects may develop with long-term use

What to Do About Side Effects
- Wait
- Wait
- Wait
- Lower the dose
- Switch to an SSRI or newer antidepressant

Best Augmenting Agents for Side Effects
- Many side effects cannot be improved with an augmenting agent

DOSING AND USE

Usual Dosage Range
- 50–150 mg/day

Dosage Forms
- Capsule 75 mg, 100 mg, 125 mg, 150 mg
- Tablet 10 mg, 25 mg, 50 mg

How to Dose
- Initial 25 mg/day at bedtime; increase by 25 mg every 3–7 days
- 75–100 mg/day once daily or in divided doses; gradually increase daily dose to achieve desired therapeutic effects; dose at bedtime for daytime sedation and in morning for insomnia; maximum dose 300 mg/day

Dosing Tips
- If given in a single dose, should generally be administered at bedtime because of its sedative properties
- If given in split doses, largest dose should generally be given at bedtime because of its sedative properties
- If patients experience nightmares, split dose and do not give large dose at bedtime
- Patients treated for chronic pain may only require lower doses
- Tofranil-PM(r) (imipramine pamoate) 100- and 125-mg capsules contain the dye tartrazine (FD&C yellow No. 5), which may cause allergic reactions in some patients; this reaction is more likely in patients with sensitivity to aspirin
- If intolerable anxiety, insomnia, agitation, akathisia, or activation occur either upon dosing initiation or discontinuation, consider the possibility of activated bipolar disorder, and switch to a mood stabilizer or an atypical antipsychotic

Overdose
- Death may occur; convulsions, cardiac dysrhythmias, severe hypotension, CNS depression, coma, changes in EKG

Long-Term Use
- Safe

Habit Forming
- No

How to Stop
- Taper to avoid withdrawal effects
- Even with gradual dose reduction some withdrawal symptoms may appear within the first 2 weeks
- Many patients tolerate 50% dose reduction for 3 days, then another 50% reduction for 3 days, then discontinuation
- If withdrawal symptoms emerge during discontinuation, raise dose to stop symptoms and then restart withdrawal much more slowly

Pharmacokinetics
- Substrate for CYP450 2D6 and 1A2
- Metabolized to an active metabolite, desipramine, a predominantly norepinephrine reuptake inhibitor, by demethylation via CYP450 1A2
- Food does not affect absorption

Drug Interactions
- Tramadol increases the risk of seizures in patients taking TCAs
- Use of TCAs with anticholinergic drugs may result in paralytic ileus or hyperthermia
- Fluoxetine, paroxetine, bupropion, duloxetine, and other CYP450 2D6 inhibitors may increase TCA concentrations
- Fluvoxamine, a CYP450 1A2 inhibitor, can decrease the conversion of imipramine to desmethylimipramine (desipramine) and increase imipramine plasma concentrations
- Cimetidine may increase plasma concentrations of TCAs and cause anticholinergic symptoms

- Phenothiazines or haloperidol may raise TCA blood concentrations
- May alter effects of antihypertensive drugs; may inhibit hypotensive effects of clonidine
- Use with sympathomimetic agents may increase sympathetic activity
- Methylphenidate may inhibit metabolism of TCAs
- Activation and agitation, especially following switching or adding antidepressants, may represent the induction of a bipolar state, especially a mixed dysphoric bipolar II condition sometimes associated with suicidal ideation, and require the addition of lithium, a mood stabilizer or an atypical antipsychotic, and/or discontinuation of imipramine

Other Warnings/ Precautions

- Add or initiate other antidepressants with caution for up to 2 weeks after discontinuing imipramine
- Generally, do not use with MAO inhibitors, including 14 days after MAOIs are stopped; do not start an MAOI for at least 5 half-lives (5 to 7 days for most drugs) after discontinuing imipramine, but see Pearls
- Use with caution in patients with history of seizure, urinary retention, angle-closure glaucoma, hyperthyroidism
- TCAs can increase QTc interval, especially at toxic doses, which can be attained not only by overdose but also by combining with drugs that inhibit its metabolism via CYP450 2D6, potentially causing torsade de pointes-type arrhythmia or sudden death
- Because TCAs can prolong QTc interval, use with caution in patients who have bradycardia or who are taking drugs that can induce bradycardia (e.g., beta blockers, calcium channel blockers, clonidine, digitalis)
- Because TCAs can prolong QTc interval, use with caution in patients who have hypokalemia and/or hypomagnesemia or who are taking drugs that can induce hypokalemia and/or magnesemia (e.g., diuretics, stimulant laxatives, intravenous amphotericin B, glucocorticoids, tetracosactide)
- When treating children, carefully weigh the risks and benefits of pharmacological treatment against the risks and benefits of nontreatment with antidepressants and make sure to document this in the patient's chart
- Distribute the brochures provided by the FDA and the drug companies
- Warn patients and their caregivers about the possibility of activating side effects and advise them to report such symptoms immediately
- Monitor patients for activation of suicidal ideation, especially children and adolescents

Do Not Use

- If patient is recovering from myocardial infarction
- If patient is taking agents capable of significantly prolonging QTc interval (e.g., pimozide, thioridazine, selected antiarrhythmics, moxifloxacin, sparfloxacin)
- If there is a history of QTc prolongation or cardiac arrhythmia, recent acute myocardial infarction, uncompensated heart failure
- If patient is taking drugs that inhibit TCA metabolism, including CYP450 2D6 inhibitors, except by an expert
- If there is reduced CYP450 2D6 function, such as patients who are poor 2D6 metabolizers, except by an expert and at low doses
- If there is a proven allergy to imipramine, desipramine, or lofepramine

SPECIAL POPULATIONS

Renal Impairment

- Cautious use; may need lower dose

Hepatic Impairment

- Cautious use; may need lower dose

Cardiac Impairment

- Baseline EKG is recommended
- TCAs have been reported to cause arrhythmias, prolongation of conduction time, orthostatic hypotension, sinus tachycardia, and heart failure, especially in the diseased heart
- Myocardial infarction and stroke have been reported with TCAs
- TCAs produce QTc prolongation, which may be enhanced by the existence of bradycardia, hypokalemia, congenital or acquired long QTc interval, which should be evaluated prior to administering imipramine

- Use with caution if treating concomitantly with a medication likely to produce prolonged bradycardia, hypokalemia, slowing of intracardiac conduction, or prolongation of the QTc interval
- Avoid TCAs in patients with a known history of QTc prolongation, recent acute myocardial infarction, and uncompensated heart failure
- TCAs may cause a sustained increase in heart rate in patients with ischemic heart disease and may worsen (decrease) heart rate variability, an independent risk of mortality in cardiac populations
- Since SSRIs may improve (increase) heart rate variability in patients following a myocardial infarct and may improve survival as well as mood in patients with acute angina or following a myocardial infarction, these are more appropriate agents for cardiac population than tricyclic/tetracyclic antidepressants

✻ Risk/benefit ratio may not justify use of TCAs in cardiac impairment

Elderly

- Baseline EKG is recommended for patients over age 50
- May be more sensitive to anticholinergic, cardiovascular, hypotensive, and sedative effects
- Initial 30–40 mg/day; maximum dose 100 mg/day
- Reduction in the risk of suicidality with antidepressants compared to placebo in adults age 65 and older

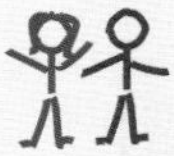

Children and Adolescents

- Carefully weigh the risks and benefits of pharmacological treatment against the risks and benefits of nontreatment with antidepressants and make sure to document this in the patient's chart
- Monitor patients face-to-face regularly, particularly during the first several weeks of treatment
- Use with caution, observing for activation of known or unknown bipolar disorder and/or suicidal ideation, and inform parents or guardians of this risk so they can help observe child or adolescent patients
- Used age 6 and older for enuresis; age 12 and older for other disorders
- Several studies show lack of efficacy of TCAs for depression
- May be used to treat hyperactive/impulsive behaviors
- Some cases of sudden death have occurred in children taking TCAs
- Adolescents: initial 30–40 mg/day; maximum 100 mg/day
- Children: initial 1.5 mg/kg per day; maximum 5 mg/kg per day
- Functional enuresis: 50 mg/day (age 6–12) or 75 mg/day (over 12)

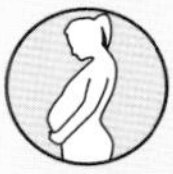

Pregnancy

- Effective June 30, 2015, the US FDA requires changes to the content and format of pregnancy and lactation information in prescription drug labels, including the elimination of the pregnancy letter categories; the Pregnancy and Lactation Labeling Rule (PLLR or final rule) applies only to prescription drugs and will be phased in gradually for drugs approved on or after June 30, 2001
- Controlled studies have not been conducted in pregnant women
- Crosses the placenta
- Should be used only if potential benefits outweigh potential risks
- Adverse effects have been reported in infants whose mothers took a TCA (lethargy, withdrawal symptoms, fetal malformations)
- Evaluate for treatment with an antidepressant with a better risk/benefit ratio

Breast Feeding

- Some drug is found in mother's breast milk

✻ Recommended either to discontinue drug or bottle feed

- Immediate postpartum period is a high-risk time for depression, especially in women who have had prior depressive episodes, so drug may need to be reinstituted late in the third trimester or shortly after childbirth to prevent a recurrence during the postpartum period
- Must weigh benefits of breast feeding with risks and benefits of antidepressant treatment versus nontreatment to both the infant and the mother
- For many patients this may mean continuing treatment during breast feeding

THE ART OF PSYCHOPHARMACOLOGY

Potential Advantages
- Patients with insomnia
- Severe or treatment-resistant depression
- Patients with enuresis

Potential Disadvantages
- Pediatric and geriatric patients
- Patients concerned with weight gain
- Cardiac patients

Primary Target Symptoms
- Depressed mood
- Chronic pain

Pearls
- Was once one of the most widely prescribed agents for depression
- ✻ Probably the most preferred TCA for treating enuresis in children
- ✻ Preference of some prescribers for imipramine over other TCAs for the treatment of enuresis is based more upon art and anecdote and empiric clinical experience than comparative clinical trials with other TCAs
- TCAs are no longer generally considered a first-line treatment option for depression because of their side effect profile
- TCAs may aggravate psychotic symptoms
- Alcohol should be avoided because of additive CNS effects
- Underweight patients may be more susceptible to adverse cardiovascular effects
- Children, patients with inadequate hydration, and patients with cardiac disease may be more susceptible to TCA-induced cardiotoxicity than healthy adults
- For the expert only: although generally prohibited, a heroic but potentially dangerous treatment for severely treatment-resistant patients is to give a tricyclic/tetracyclic antidepressant other than clomipramine simultaneously with an MAOI for patients who fail to respond to numerous other antidepressants
- If this option is elected, start the MAOI with the tricyclic/tetracyclic antidepressant simultaneously at low doses after appropriate drug washout, then alternately increase doses of these agents every few days to a week as tolerated
- Although very strict dietary and concomitant drug restrictions must be observed to prevent hypertensive crises and serotonin syndrome, the most common side effects of MAOI/tricyclic or tetracyclic combinations may be weight gain and orthostatic hypotension
- Patients on TCAs should be aware that they may experience symptoms such as photosensitivity or blue-green urine
- SSRIs may be more effective than TCAs in women, and TCAs may be more effective than SSRIs in men
- Since tricyclic/tetracyclic antidepressants are substrates for CYP450 2D6, and 7% of the population (especially Caucasians) may have a genetic variant leading to reduced activity of 2D6, such patients may not safely tolerate normal doses of tricyclic/tetracyclic antidepressants and may require dose reduction
- Phenotypic testing may be necessary to detect this genetic variant prior to dosing with a tricyclic/tetracyclic antidepressant, especially in vulnerable populations such as children, elderly, cardiac populations, and those on concomitant medications
- Patients who seem to have extraordinarily severe side effects at normal or low doses may have this phenotypic CYP450 2D6 variant and require low doses or switching to another antidepressant not metabolized by 2D6

Suggested Reading

Anderson IM. Meta-analytical studies on new antidepressants. Br Med Bull 2001;57:161–78.

Anderson IM. Selective serotonin reuptake inhibitors versus tricyclic antidepressants: a meta-analysis of efficacy and tolerability. J Aff Disorders 2000;58:19–36.

Preskorn SH. Comparison of the tolerability of bupropion, fluoxetine, imipramine, nefazodone, paroxetine, sertraline, and venlafaxine. J Clin Psychiatry 1995;56(Suppl 6):S12–21.

Workman EA, Short DD. Atypical antidepressants versus imipramine in the treatment of major depression: a meta-analysis. J Clin Psychiatry 1993;54:5–12.

THERAPEUTICS

Brands • Marplan

see index for additional brand names

Generic? Not in USA

Class

- Neuroscience-based Nomenclature: serotonin, norepinephrine, dopamine enzyme inhibitor (SN-EI)
- Monoamine oxidase inhibitor (MAOI)

Commonly Prescribed for

(bold for FDA approved)

- **Depression**
- Treatment-resistant depression
- Treatment-resistant panic disorder
- Treatment-resistant social anxiety disorder

How the Drug Works

- Irreversibly blocks monoamine oxidase (MAO) from breaking down norepinephrine, serotonin, and dopamine
- This presumably boosts noradrenergic, serotonergic, and dopaminergic neurotransmission

How Long Until It Works

- Onset of therapeutic actions usually not immediate, but often delayed 2–4 weeks
- If it is not working within 6–8 weeks, it may require a dosage increase or it may not work at all
- May continue to work for many years to prevent relapse of symptoms

If It Works

- The goal of treatment is complete remission of current symptoms as well as prevention of future relapses
- Treatment most often reduces or even eliminates symptoms, but not a cure since symptoms can recur after medicine stopped
- Continue treatment until all symptoms are gone (remission)
- Once symptoms are gone, continue treating for 1 year for the first episode of depression
- For second and subsequent episodes of depression, treatment may need to be indefinite
- Use in anxiety disorders may also need to be indefinite

If It Doesn't Work

- Many patients have only a partial response where some symptoms are improved but others persist (especially insomnia, fatigue, and problems concentrating)
- Other patients may be nonresponders, sometimes called treatment-resistant or treatment-refractory
- Some patients who have an initial response may relapse even though they continue treatment, sometimes called "poop-out"
- Consider increasing dose, switching to another agent, or adding an appropriate augmenting agent
- Consider psychotherapy
- Consider evaluation for another diagnosis or for a comorbid condition (e.g., medical illness, substance abuse, etc.)
- Some patients may experience apparent lack of consistent efficacy due to activation of latent or underlying bipolar disorder, and require antidepressant discontinuation and a switch to a mood stabilizer

Best Augmenting Combos for Partial Response or Treatment Resistance

✻ Augmentation of MAOIs has not been systematically studied, and this is something for the expert, to be done with caution and with careful monitoring

✻ A stimulant such as d-amphetamine or methylphenidate (with caution; may activate bipolar disorder and suicidal ideation; may elevate blood pressure)

- Lithium
- Mood-stabilizing anticonvulsants
- Atypical antipsychotics (with special caution for those agents with monoamine reuptake blocking properties, such as ziprasidone and zotepine)

Tests

- Patients should be monitored for changes in blood pressure
- Patients receiving high doses or long-term treatment should have hepatic function evaluated periodically

✻ Since MAOIs are frequently associated with weight gain, before starting treatment, weigh all patients and determine if the patient is already overweight (BMI 25.0–29.9) or obese (BMI ≥30)

- Before giving a drug that can cause weight gain to an overweight or obese patient, consider determining whether the patient already has pre-diabetes (fasting plasma glucose 100–125 mg/dL), diabetes (fasting plasma glucose >126 mg/dL), or dyslipidemia (increased total cholesterol, LDL cholesterol, and triglycerides; decreased HDL cholesterol), and treat or refer such patients for treatment, including nutrition and weight management, physical activity counseling, smoking cessation, and medical management

✻ Monitor weight and BMI during treatment

✻ While giving a drug to a patient who has gained >5% of initial weight, consider evaluating for the presence of pre-diabetes, diabetes, or dyslipidemia, or consider switching to a different antidepressant

SIDE EFFECTS

How Drug Causes Side Effects

- Theoretically due to increases in monoamines in parts of the brain and body and at receptors other than those that cause therapeutic actions (e.g., unwanted actions of serotonin in sleep centers causing insomnia, unwanted actions of norepinephrine on vascular smooth muscle causing hypertension, etc.)
- Side effects are generally immediate, but immediate side effects often disappear in time

Notable Side Effects

- Dizziness, sedation, headache, sleep disturbances, fatigue, weakness, tremor, movement problems, blurred vision, increased sweating
- Constipation, dry mouth, nausea, change in appetite, weight gain
- Sexual dysfunction
- Orthostatic hypotension (dose-related); syncope may develop at high doses

Life-Threatening or Dangerous Side Effects

- Hypertensive crisis (especially when MAOIs are used with certain tyramine-containing foods or prohibited drugs)
- Induction of mania
- Rare activation of suicidal ideation and behavior (suicidality) (short-term studies did not show an increase in the risk of suicidality with antidepressants compared to placebo beyond age 24)
- Seizures
- Hepatotoxicity

Weight Gain

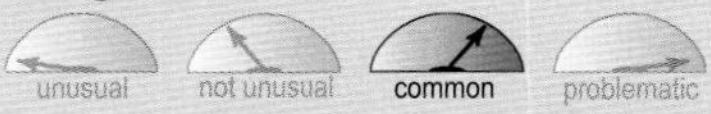

- Many experience and/or can be significant in amount

Sedation

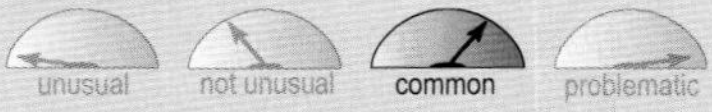

- Many experience and/or can be significant in amount
- Can also cause activation

What to Do About Side Effects

- Wait
- Wait
- Wait
- Lower the dose
- Take at night if daytime sedation
- Switch after appropriate washout to an SSRI or newer antidepressant

Best Augmenting Agents for Side Effects

- Trazodone (with caution) for insomnia
- Benzodiazepines for insomnia

✻ Single oral or sublingual dose of a calcium channel blocker (e.g., nifedipine) for urgent treatment of hypertension due to drug interaction or dietary tyramine

- Many side effects cannot be improved with an augmenting agent

DOSING AND USE

Usual Dosage Range

- 40–60 mg/day

Dosage Forms
- Tablet 10 mg

How to Dose
- Initial 10 mg twice a day; increase by 10 mg/day every 2–4 days; dosed 2–4 times/day; maximum dose 60 mg/day

Dosing Tips
- Orthostatic hypotension, especially at high doses, may require splitting into 3 or 4 daily doses
- Patients receiving high doses may need to be evaluated periodically for effects on the liver
- Little evidence to support efficacy of isocarboxazid at doses below 30 mg/day

Overdose
- Dizziness, sedation, ataxia, headache, insomnia, restlessness, anxiety, irritability; cardiovascular effects, confusion, respiratory depression, or coma may also occur

Long-Term Use
- May require periodic evaluation of hepatic function
- MAOIs may lose some efficacy long-term

Habit Forming
- Some patients have developed dependence to MAOIs

How to Stop
- Generally no need to taper, as drug wears off slowly over 2–3 weeks

Pharmacokinetics
- Clinical duration of action may be up to 14 days due to irreversible enzyme inhibition

Drug Interactions
- Tramadol may increase the risk of seizures in patients taking an MAOI
- Can cause a fatal "serotonin syndrome" when combined with drugs that block serotonin reuptake, so do not use with a serotonin reuptake inhibitor or for 5 half-lives after stopping the serotonin reuptake inhibitor (see Table 1 after Pearls)
- Hypertensive crisis with headache, intracranial bleeding, and death may result from combining MAOIs with sympathomimetic drugs (e.g., amphetamines, methylphenidate, cocaine, dopamine, epinephrine, norepinephrine, and related compounds methyldopa, levodopa, *L*-tryptophan, *L*-tyrosine, and phenylalanine)
- Do not combine with another MAOI, alcohol, or guanethidine
- Adverse drug reactions can results from combining MAOIs with tricyclic/tetracyclic antidepressants and related compounds, including carbamazepine, cyclobenzaprine, and mirtazapine, and should be avoided except by experts to treat difficult cases (see Pearls)
- MAOIs in combination with spinal anesthesia may cause combined hypotensive effects
- Combination of MAOIs and CNS depressants may enhance sedation and hypotension

Other Warnings/ Precautions
- Use requires low tyramine diet (see Table 2 after Pearls)
- Patient and prescriber must be vigilant to potential interactions with any drug, including antihypertensives and over-the-counter cough/cold preparations
- Over-the-counter medications to avoid include cough and cold preparations, including those containing dextromethorphan, nasal decongestants (tablets, drops, or spray), hay-fever medications, sinus medications, asthma inhalant medications, anti-appetite medications, weight reducing preparations, "pep" pills (see Table 3 after Pearls)
- Use cautiously in patients receiving reserpine, anesthetics, disulfiram, metrizamide, anticholinergic agents
- Isocarboxazid is not recommended for use in patients who cannot be monitored closely
- When treating children, carefully weigh the risks and benefits of pharmacological treatment against the risks and benefits of nontreatment with antidepressants and make sure to document this in the patient's chart

- Distribute the brochures provided by the FDA and the drug companies
- Warn patients and their caregivers about the possibility of activating side effects and advise them to report such symptoms immediately
- Monitor patients for activation of suicidal ideation, especially children and adolescents

Do Not Use

- If patient is taking meperidine (pethidine)
- If patient is taking a sympathomimetic agent or taking guanethidine
- If patient is taking another MAOI
- If patient is taking any agent that can inhibit serotonin reuptake (e.g., SSRIs, sibutramine, tramadol, milnacipran, duloxetine, venlafaxine, clomipramine, etc.)
- If patient is taking diuretics, dextromethorphan
- If patient has pheochromocytoma
- If patient has cardiovascular or cerebrovascular disease
- If patient has frequent or severe headaches
- If patient is undergoing elective surgery and requires general anesthesia
- If patient has a history of liver disease or abnormal liver function tests
- If patient is taking a prohibited drug
- If patient is not compliant with a low tyramine diet
- If there is a proven allergy to isocarboxazid

SPECIAL POPULATIONS

Renal Impairment

- Use with caution – drug may accumulate in plasma
- May require lower than usual adult dose

Hepatic Impairment

- Not for use in hepatic impairment

Cardiac Impairment

- Contraindicated in patients with congestive heart failure or hypertension
- Any other cardiac impairment may require lower than usual adult dose
- Patients with angina pectoris or coronary artery disease should limit their exertion

Elderly

- Initial dose lower than usual adult dose
- Elderly patients may have greater sensitivity to adverse effects
- Reduction in the risk of suicidality with antidepressants compared to placebo in adults age 65 and older

Children and Adolescents

- Not recommended for use in children under age 16
- Carefully weigh the risks and benefits of pharmacological treatment against the risks and benefits of nontreatment with antidepressants and make sure to document this in the patient's chart
- Distribute the brochures provided by the FDA and the drug companies
- Warn patients and their caregivers about the possibility of activating side effects and advise them to report such symptoms immediately
- Use with caution, observing for activation of known or unknown bipolar disorder and/or suicidal ideation, and inform parents or guardians of this risk so they can help observe child or adolescent patients

Pregnancy

- Effective June 30, 2015, the US FDA requires changes to the content and format of pregnancy and lactation information in prescription drug labels, including the elimination of the pregnancy letter categories; the Pregnancy and Lactation Labeling Rule (PLLR or final rule) applies only to prescription drugs and will be phased in gradually for drugs approved on or after June 30, 2001
- Controlled studies have not been conducted in pregnant women
- Not generally recommended for use during pregnancy, especially during first trimester
- Should evaluate patient for treatment with an antidepressant with a better risk/benefit ratio

Breast Feeding

- Some drug is found in mother's breast milk
- Immediate postpartum period is a high-risk time for depression, especially in women who have had prior depressive episodes, so drug may need to be reinstituted late

in the third trimester or shortly after childbirth to prevent a recurrence during the postpartum period
- Should evaluate patient for treatment with an antidepressant with a better risk/benefit ratio

THE ART OF PSYCHOPHARMACOLOGY

Potential Advantages
- Atypical depression
- Severe depression
- Treatment-resistant depression or anxiety disorders

Potential Disadvantages
- Requires compliance to dietary restrictions, concomitant drug restrictions
- Patients with cardiac problems or hypertension
- Multiple daily doses

Primary Target Symptoms
- Depressed mood
- Somatic symptoms
- Sleep and eating disturbances
- Psychomotor retardation
- Morbid preoccupation

Pearls
- MAOIs are generally reserved for second-line use after SSRIs, SNRIs, and combinations of newer antidepressants have failed
- Despite little utilization, some patients respond to isocarboxazid who do not respond to other antidepressants including other MAOIs
- Patient should be advised not to take any prescription or over-the-counter drugs without consulting their doctor because of possible drug interactions with the MAOI
- Headache is often the first symptom of hypertensive crisis
- The rigid dietary restrictions may reduce compliance (see Table 2 after Pearls)
- Mood disorders can be associated with eating disorders (especially in adolescent females), and isocarboxazid can be used to treat both depression and bulimia
- MAOIs are a viable second-line treatment option in depression, but are not frequently used

✻ Myths about the danger of dietary tyramine can be exaggerated, but prohibitions against concomitant drugs often not followed closely enough
- Orthostatic hypotension, insomnia, and sexual dysfunction are often the most troublesome common side effects

✻ MAOIs should be for the expert, especially if combining with agents of potential risk (e.g., stimulants, trazodone, TCAs)

✻ MAOIs should not be neglected as therapeutic agents for the treatment-resistant
- Although generally prohibited, a heroic but potentially dangerous treatment for severely treatment-resistant patients is for an expert to give a tricyclic/tetracyclic antidepressant other than clomipramine simultaneously with an MAOI for patients who fail to respond to numerous other antidepressants
- Use of MAOIs with clomipramine is always prohibited because of the risk of serotonin syndrome and death
- Amoxapine may be the preferred trycyclic/tetracyclic antidepressant to combine with an MAOI in heroic cases due to its theoretically protective 5HT2A antagonist properties
- If this option is elected, start the MAOI with the tricyclic/tetracyclic antidepressant simultaneously at low doses after appropriate drug washout, then alternately increase doses of these agents every few days to a week as tolerated
- Although very strict dietary and concomitant drug restrictions must be observed to prevent hypertensive crises and serotonin syndrome, the most common side effects of MAOI and tricyclic/tetracyclic combinations may be weight gain and orthostatic hypotension

Table 1. Drugs contraindicated due to risk of serotonin syndrome/toxicity

Do Not Use:			
Antidepressants	**Drugs of Abuse**	**Opioids**	**Other**
SSRIs	MDMA (ecstasy)	Meperidine	Non-subcutaneous sumatriptan
SNRIs	Cocaine	Tramadol	Chlorpheniramine
Clomipramine	Methamphetamine	Methadone	Brompheniramine
St. John's wort	High-dose or injected amphetamine	Fentanyl	Dextromethorphan
			Procarbazine?

Table 2. Dietary guidelines for patients taking MAOIs

Foods to avoid*	Foods allowed
Dried, aged, smoked, fermented, spoiled, or improperly stored meat, poultry, and fish	Fresh or processed meat, poultry, and fish; properly stored pickled or smoked fish
Broad bean pods	All other vegetables
Aged cheeses	Processed cheese slices, cottage cheese, ricotta cheese, yogurt, cream cheese
Tap and unpasteurized beer	Canned or bottled beer and alcohol
Marmite	Brewer's and baker's yeast
Sauerkraut, kimchee	
Soy products/tofu	Peanuts
Banana peel	Bananas, avocados, raspberries
Tyramine-containing nutritional supplement	

*Not necessary for 6-mg transdermal or low-dose oral selegiline

Table 3. Drugs that boost norepinephrine: should only be used with caution with MAOIs

Use With Caution:			
Decongestants	**Stimulants**	**Antidepressants with norepinephrine reuptake inhibition**	**Other**
Phenylephrine	Amphetamines	Most tricyclics	Phentermine
Pseudoephedrine	Methylphenidate	NRIs	Local anesthetics containing vasoconstrictors
	Cocaine	NDRIs	
	Methamphetamine		
	Modafinil		Tapentadol
	Armodafinil		

Suggested Reading

Kennedy SH. Continuation and maintenance treatments in major depression: the neglected role of monoamine oxidase inhibitors. J Psychiatry Neurosci 1997;22:127–31.

Larsen JK, Rafaelsen OJ. Long-term treatment of depression with isocarboxazide. Acta Psychiatr Scand 1980;62(5):456–63.

Lippman SB, Nash K. Monoamine oxidase inhibitor update. Potential adverse food and drug interactions. Drug Saf 1990;5:195–204.

THERAPEUTICS

Brands • Ketalar

see index for additional brand names

Generic? Yes

Class

- *N*-methyl-D-aspartate (NMDA) receptor antagonist

Commonly Prescribed for

(bold for FDA approved)

- **Induction and maintenance of general anesthesia**
- Pain/neuropathic pain
- Sedation
- Treatment-resistant depression (experimental)

How the Drug Works

- Ketamine is a noncompetitive open channel inhibitor of the NMDA receptor; specifically, it binds to the phencyclidine site of the NMDA receptor
- This leads to downstream glutamate release and consequent stimulation of other glutamate receptors, including AMPA receptors
- Theoretically, ketamine may have antidepressant effects at low (subanesthetic) doses because activation of AMPA receptors leads to activation of signal transduction cascades that cause the expression of synaptic proteins and an increase in the density of dendritic spines
- Low (subanesthetic) doses also produce analgesia and modulate central sensitization, hyperalgesia, and opioid tolerance

How Long Until It Works

- For treatment-resistant depression, antidepressant effects can occur within hours
- For neuropathic pain, effects can occur within hours but may take weeks for full effect

If It Works

- For treatment-resistant depression, can immediately alleviate depressed mood and suicidal ideation, but antidepressant effects last only a few days
- For neuropathic pain, can continue to use as long as it is beneficial

If It Doesn't Work

- Try a traditional antidepressant or electroconvulsive therapy (ECT) for treatment-resistant depression
- Try traditional analgesics and treatments for neuropathic pain

Best Augmenting Combos for Partial Response or Treatment Resistance

- For neuropathic pain, may use cautiously with opioids
- For treatment-resistant depression, combinations have not been systematically studied

Tests

- None for healthy individuals

SIDE EFFECTS

How Drug Causes Side Effects

- Direct effect on NMDA receptors

Notable Side Effects

- When used as an anesthesia induction/maintenance agent (generally at doses >2 mg/kg IV), it may produce emergent psychosis, including auditory and visual hallucinations, restlessness, disorientation, vivid dreams, and irrational behavior. Spontaneous involuntary movements, nystagmus, hypertonus, and vocalizations are also common. These adverse effects are uncommon with very low-dose therapy.
- CSF pressure increased, erythema (transient), morbilliform rash (transient), anorexia, pain/erythema at the injection site, exanthema at the injection site, skeletal muscle tone enhanced, intraocular pressure increased, bronchial secretions increased, potential for dependence with prolonged use, emergence reactions (includes confusion, dreamlike state, excitement, irrational behavior, vivid imagery)
- Psychotomimetic phenomena (euphoria, dysphasia, blunted affect, psychomotor retardation, vivid dreams, nightmares,

impaired attention, memory and judgment, illusions, hallucinations, altered body image), delirium, dizziness, diplopia, blurred vision, nystagmus, altered hearing, hypertension, tachycardia, hypersalivation, nausea and vomiting, erythema and pain at injection site
- Urinary tract toxicity
- When used at higher doses in anesthesia, tonic-clonic movements are very common (>10%); however, these have not been reported after oral use or with the lower parenteral doses used for analgesia

Life-Threatening or Dangerous Side Effects

- Syncope or cardiac arrhythmias
- Hypertension/hypotension
- Anaphylaxis
- CNS depression
- Respiratory depression/apnea
- Airway obstruction/laryngospasm

Weight Gain

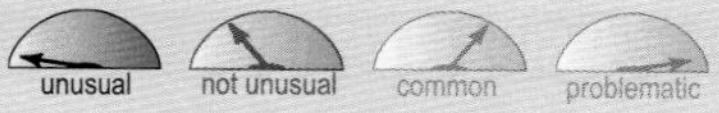

- Reported but not expected

Sedation

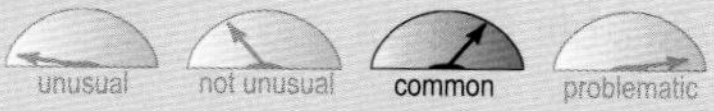

- Many experience and/or can be significant in amount

What to Do About Side Effects

- Pretreatment with a benzodiazepine reduces incidence of psychosis by >50%
- For CNS side effects, discontinuation of nonessential centrally acting medications may help

Best Augmenting Agents for Side Effects

- Many side effects cannot be improved with an augmenting agent

DOSING AND USE

Usual Dosage Range

- Oral: 10–50 mg
- IV infusion: 1–10 μg/kg per minute

Dosage Forms

- Oral solution: 50 mg/mL
- Injection: 50 mg/mL

How to Dose

- For pain (oral): initial 10 mg; titrate up as appropriate
- For pain (IM): 2–4 mg/kg
- For pain (IV): 0.2–0.075 mg/kg

For pain (continuous IV infusion): 2–7 μg/kg per minute

Dosing Tips

- Slow titration can reduce side effects
- Food does not affect absorption
- For oral use: to prepare 100 mL of 50 mg/5 mL ketamine oral solution
  - 2 x 10 mL vials of generic ketamine 50 mg/mL for injection (cheapest concentration)
  - 80 mL purified water
  - Store in a refrigerator with an expiry date of 1 week from manufacture
  - Patients can add their own flavoring, e.g., fruit cordial, just before use to disguise the bitter taste
- For sublingual use:
  - Place under the tongue and ask patient not to swallow for 2 minutes
  - Use a high concentration to minimize dose volume; retaining >2 mL is difficult
  - Start with 10 mg
- Incompatibility
  - Ketamine forms precipitates with barbiturates and diazepam (manufacturer's data on file); do not mix
  - Mixing lorazepam with ketamine is also not recommended; compatibility data are lacking, and there is a risk of adsorption of lorazepam to the tubing

Overdose

- Restlessness, psychosis, hallucinations, stupor

Long-Term Use

- Safe

Habit Forming

- No

How to Stop

- Taper not necessary

Pharmacokinetics
- Plasma half-life: alpha: 10–15 minutes; beta: 2.5 hours; 1–3 hours IM; 2.5–3 hours orally; 12 hours norketamine
- Metabolized by CYP450 2B6, 2C9, and 3A4

Drug Interactions
- Use with caution with other drugs that are NMDA antagonists (amantadine, memantine, dextromethorphan)
- Ketamine may increase the effects of other sedatives, including benzodiazepines, barbiturates, opioids, anesthetics, and alcohol
- CYP3A4 inhibitors (e.g., clarithromycin, ketoconazole) can increase plasma concentrations of ketamine and reduce those of norketamine, but the clinical relevance of this is unclear
- Plasma concentrations of ketamine are increased by diazepam
- Barbiturates and hydroxyzine may increase the effects of ketamine; avoid combination

Other Warnings/ Precautions
- Use with caution in patients with current or past history of psychiatric disorder; epilepsy, glaucoma, hypertension, heart failure, ischemic heart disease, and a history of cerebrovascular accidents

Do Not Use
- If patient has a condition in which an increase in blood pressure would be hazardous
- If patient has schizophrenia or another psychotic disorder
- If patient has a condition in which an increase in intraocular pressure would be hazardous
- If there is a proven allergy to ketamine

SPECIAL POPULATIONS

Renal Impairment
- Reduce dose for moderate impairment
- Should not be used in severe impairment

Hepatic Impairment
- Dose reduction not necessary

Cardiac Impairment
- Use with caution

Elderly
- Some patients may tolerate lower doses better

Children and Adolescents
- Safety and efficacy have not been established

Pregnancy
- Effective June 30, 2015, the US FDA requires changes to the content and format of pregnancy and lactation information in prescription drug labels, including the elimination of the pregnancy letter categories; the Pregnancy and Lactation Labeling Rule (PLLR or final rule) applies only to prescription drugs and will be phased in gradually for drugs approved on or after June 30, 2001
- Controlled studies have not been conducted in pregnant women
- Use only if potential benefits outweigh the potential risks to the fetus

Breast Feeding
- Unknown if ketamine is secreted in human breast milk, but all psychotropics assumed to be secreted in breast milk

* Recommended either to discontinue drug or bottle feed

THE ART OF PSYCHOPHARMACOLOGY

Potential Advantages
- For pain, may be especially useful when used in conjunction with opioids
- Severely treatment-resistant depression, suicidal ideation

Potential Disadvantages
- May produce dysphoria, nightmares, excitement (uncommon with very low-dose therapy)
- Antidepressant effects are short-lived

Primary Target Symptoms
- Pain
- Treatment-resistant depression

Pearls

- Actions in treatment-resistant depression are transient, lasting only a few days following infusion
- The use of ketamine can cause urinary tract symptoms (e.g., frequency, urgency, urge incontinence, dysuria, and hematuria); the causal agent has not been determined, but direct irritation by ketamine and/or its metabolites is a possibility. (Investigations have revealed interstitial cystitis, detrusor overactivity, decreased bladder capacity; symptoms generally settle several weeks after stopping ketamine.)
- May be used in combination with anticholinergic agents to decrease hypersalivation
- Do not mix with barbiturates or diazepam (precipitation may occur)
- Bronchodilation is beneficial in asthmatic or chronic obstructive pulmonary disease (COPD) patients. Laryngeal reflexes may remain intact or may be obtunded.
- The direct myocardial depressant action of ketamine can be seen in stressed, catecholamine-deficient patients
- Ketamine releases endogenous catecholamines (epinephrine, norepinephrine), which maintain blood pressure and heart rate, and increase myocardial oxygen demand
- Ketamine increases cerebral metabolism and cerebral blood flow while producing a noncompetitive block of the neuronal postsynaptic NMDA receptor
- Lowers seizure threshold
- Recent laboratory/clinical studies support the use of low-dose ketamine to improve postoperative analgesia/outcome
- May be especially beneficial for refractory neuropathic pain/complex regional pain syndrome
- May be especially beneficial when used in conjunction with opioids
- (S)-ketamine is available in a preservative-free solution in Europe; however, it currently is not approved by the FDA. S(+)-ketamine may be more potent and have fewer side effects when used intravenously than the racemate. Although not rigorously tested and not available in the USA; some European investigators have utilized the preservation-free solution for intrathecal/epidural use – this is not recommended

Suggested Reading

Cohen SP, Liao W, Gupta A, Plunkett A. Ketamine in pain management. Adv Psychosom Med 2011;30:139–61.

Duman RS, Voleti B. Signaling pathways underlying the pathophysiology and treatment of depression: novel mechanisms for rapid-acting agents. Trends Neurosci 2012;35(1):47–56.

Schwartzman RJ, Alexander GM, Grothusen JR. The use of ketamine in complex regional pain syndrome: possible mechanisms. Expert Rev Neurother 2011;11(5):719–34.

Stahl SM. Mechanism of action of ketamine. CNS Spectrums 2013;18(4):171–4.

Zarate CA Jr, Singh JB, Carlson PH, et al. A randomized trial of an N-methyl-D-aspartate antagonist in treatment-resistant major depression. Arch Gen Psychiatry 2006;63(8):856–64.

THERAPEUTICS

Brands
- Lamictal
- Labileno
- Lamictin

see index for additional brand names

Generic? Yes

Class
- Neuroscience-based Nomenclature: glutamate, voltage-gated sodium channel blocker (Glu-CB)
- Anticonvulsant, mood stabilizer, voltage-sensitive sodium channel antagonist

Commonly Prescribed for
(bold for FDA approved)
- **Maintenance treatment of bipolar I disorder**
- **Partial seizures (adjunctive; adults and children ages 2 and older)**
- **Generalized seizures of Lennox-Gastaut syndrome (adjunctive; adults and children ages 2 and older)**
- **Primary generalized tonic-clonic seizures (adjunctive; adults and children ages 2 and older)**
- **Conversion to monotherapy in adults (16 and older) with partial seizures who are receiving treatment with carbamazepine, phenytoin, phenobarbital, primidone, or valproate**
- Bipolar depression
- Bipolar mania (adjunctive and second-line)
- Psychosis, schizophrenia (adjunctive)
- Neuropathic pain/chronic pain
- Major depressive disorder (adjunctive)
- Other seizure types and as initial monotherapy for epilepsy

How the Drug Works
- ✻ Acts as a use-dependent blocker of voltage-sensitive sodium channels
- ✻ Interacts with the open channel conformation of voltage-sensitive sodium channels
- ✻ Interacts at a specific site of the alpha pore-forming subunit of voltage-sensitive sodium channels
- Inhibits release of glutamate and asparate

How Long Until It Works
- May take several weeks to improve bipolar depression
- May take several weeks to months to optimize an effect on mood stabilization
- Can reduce seizures by 2 weeks, but may take several weeks to months to reduce seizures

If It Works
- The goal of treatment is complete remission of symptoms (e.g., seizures, depression, pain)
- Continue treatment until all symptoms are gone or until improvement is stable and then continue treating indefinitely as long as improvement persists
- Continue treatment indefinitely to avoid recurrence of mania, depression, and/or seizures
- Treatment of chronic neuropathic pain may reduce but does not eliminate pain symptoms and is not a cure since pain usually recurs after medicine stopped

If It Doesn't Work (for bipolar disorder)
- ✻ Many patients have only a partial response where some symptoms are improved but others persist or continue to wax and wane without stabilization of mood
- Other patients may be nonresponders, sometimes called treatment-resistant or treatment-refractory
- Consider increasing dose, switching to another agent, or adding an appropriate augmenting agent
- Consider adding psychotherapy
- Consider biofeedback or hypnosis for pain
- Consider the presence of noncompliance and counsel patient
- Switch to another mood stabilizer with fewer side effects
- Consider evaluation for another diagnosis or for a comorbid condition (e.g., medical illness, substance abuse, etc.)

Best Augmenting Combos for Partial Response or Treatment Resistance (for bipolar disorder)
- Lithium
- Atypical antipsychotics (especially risperidone, olanzapine, quetiapine, ziprasidone, and aripiprazole)
- ✻ Valproate (with caution and at half dose of lamotrigine in the presence of valproate,

because valproate can double lamotrigine levels)

✱ Antidepressants (with caution because antidepressants can destabilize mood in some patients, including induction of rapid cycling or suicidal ideation; in particular consider bupropion; also SSRIs, SNRIs, others; generally avoid TCAs, MAOIs)

Tests

- None required
- The value of monitoring plasma concentrations of lamotrigine has not been established
- Because lamotrigine binds to melanin-containing tissues, opthalmological checks may be considered

SIDE EFFECTS

How Drug Causes Side Effects

- CNS side effects theoretically due to excessive actions at voltage-sensitive sodium channels
- Rash hypothetically an allergic reaction

Notable Side Effects

✱ Benign rash (approximately 10%)

- Dose dependent: blurred or double vision, dizziness, ataxia
- Sedation, headache, tremor, insomnia, poor coordination, fatigue
- Nausea (dose-dependent), vomiting, dyspepsia, rhinitis
- Additional effects in pediatric patients with epilepsy: infection, pharyngitis, asthenia

Life-Threatening or Dangerous Side Effects

✱ Rare serious rash (risk may be greater in pediatric patients but still rare)

- Rare multi-organ failure associated with Stevens-Johnson syndrome, toxic epidermal necrolysis, or drug hypersensitivity syndrome
- Rare blood dyscrasias
- Rare aseptic meningitis
- Rare sudden unexplained deaths have occurred in epilepsy (unknown if related to lamotrigine use)
- Withdrawal seizures upon abrupt withdrawal
- Rare activation of suicidal ideation and behavior (suicidality)

Weight Gain

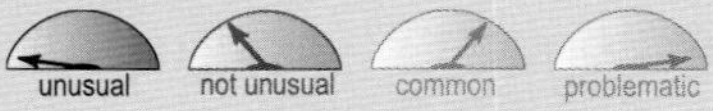

- Reported but not expected

Sedation

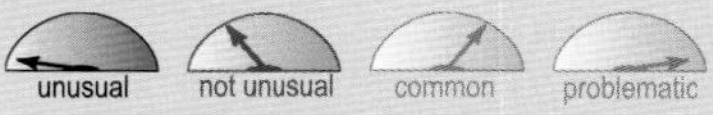

- Reported but not expected
- Dose-related
- Can wear off with time

What to Do About Side Effects

- Wait
- Take at night to reduce daytime sedation
- Divide dosing to twice daily

✱ If patient develops signs of a rash with benign characteristics (i.e., a rash that peaks within days, settles in 10–14 days, is spotty, nonconfluent, nontender, has no systemic features, and laboratory tests are normal):

- Reduce lamotrigine dose or stop dosage increase
- Warn patient to stop drug and contact physician if rash worsens or new symptoms emerge
- Prescribe antihistamine and/or topical corticosteroid for pruritis
- Monitor patient closely

✱ If patient develops signs of a rash with serious characteristics (i.e., a rash that is confluent and widespread, or purpuric or tender; with any prominent involvement of neck or upper trunk; any involvement of eyes, lips, mouth, etc.; any associated fever, malaise, pharyngitis, anorexia, or lymphadenopathy; abnormal laboratory tests for complete blood count, liver function, urea, creatinine):

- Stop lamotrigine (and valproate if administered)
- Monitor and investigate organ involvement (hepatic, renal, hematologic)
- Patient may require hospitalization
- Monitor patient very closely

Best Augmenting Agents for Side Effects

- Antihistamines and/or topical corticosteroid for rash, pruritis
- Many side effects cannot be improved with an augmenting agent

DOSING AND USE

Usual Dosage Range

- Monotherapy for bipolar disorder: 100–200 mg/day
- Adjunctive treatment for bipolar disorder: 100 mg/day in combination with valproate; 400 mg/day in combination with enzyme-inducing antiepileptic drugs such as carbamazepine, phenobarbital, phenytoin, and primidone
- Monotherapy for seizures in patients over age 12: 300–500 mg/day in 2 doses
- Adjunctive treatment for seizures in patients over age 12: 100–400 mg/day for regimens containing valproate; 100–200 mg/day for valproate alone; 300–500 mg/day in 2 doses for regimens not containing valproate
- Patients ages 2–12 with epilepsy are dosed based on body weight and concomitant medications

Dosage Forms

- Tablet 25 mg, 50 mg, 100 mg, 150 mg, 200 mg, 250 mg
- Chewable tablet 2 mg, 5 mg, 25 mg, 100 mg
- Orally disintegrating tablet 25 mg, 50 mg, 100 mg, 200 mg
- Extended-release tablet 25 mg, 50 mg, 100 mg, 200 mg, 250 mg, 300 mg

How to Dose

✻ Bipolar disorder (monotherapy, see chart): for the first 2 weeks administer 25 mg/day; at week 3 increase to 50 mg/day; at week 5 increase to 100 mg/day; at week 6 increase to 200 mg/day; maximum dose generally 200 mg/day

✻ Bipolar disorder (adjunct to valproate): for the first 2 weeks administer 25 mg every other day; at week 3 increase to 25 mg/day; at week 5 increase to 50 mg/day; at week 6 increase to 100 mg/day; maximum dose generally 100 mg/day

- Bipolar disorder (adjunct to enzyme-inducing antiepileptic drugs): for the first 2 weeks administer 50 mg/day; at week 3 increase to 100 mg/day in divided doses; starting at week 5 increase by 100 mg/day each week; maximum dose generally 400 mg/day in divided doses
- When lamotrigine is added to epilepsy treatment that includes valproate (ages 12 and older): for the first 2 weeks administer 25 mg every other day; at week 3 increase to 25 mg/day; every 1–2 weeks can increase by 25–50 mg/day; usual maintenance dose 100–400 mg/day in 1–2 doses or 100–200 mg/day if lamotrigine is added to valproate alone
- When lamotrigine is added to epilepsy treatment that includes carbamazepine, phenytoin, phenobarbital, or primidone (without valproate) (ages 12 and older): for the first 2 weeks administer 50 mg/day; at week 3 increase to 100 mg/day in 2 doses; every 1–2 weeks can increase by 100 mg/day; usual maintenance dose 300–500 mg/day in 2 doses

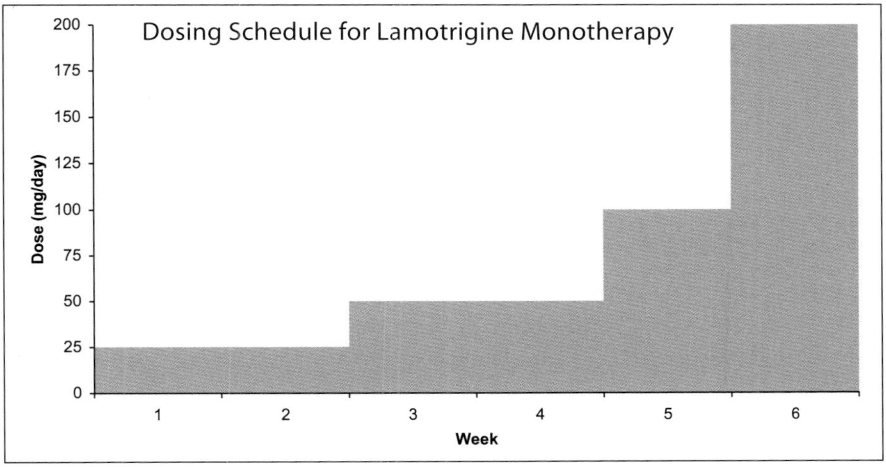

- When converting from a single enzyme-inducing antiepileptic drug to lamotrigine monotherapy for epilepsy: titrate as described above to 500 mg/day in 2 doses while maintaining dose of previous medication; decrease first drug in 20% decrements each week over the next 4 weeks
- When converting from valproate to lamotrigine monotherapy for epilepsy: titrate as described above to 200 mg/day while maintaining dose of valproate, then gradually increase lamotrigine up to 500 mg/day while gradually discontinuing valproate
- Seizures (under age 12): see Children and Adolescents

Dosing Tips

✽ Very slow dose titration may reduce the incidence of skin rash
- Therefore, dose should not be titrated faster than recommended because of possible risk of increased side effects, including rash
- If patient stops taking lamotrigine for 5 days or more it may be necessary to restart the drug with the initial dose titration, as rashes have been reported on reexposure
- Advise patient to avoid new medications, foods, or products during the first 3 months of lamotrigine treatment in order to decrease the risk of unrelated rash; patient should also not start lamotrigine within 2 weeks of a viral infection, rash, or vaccination

✽ If lamotrigine is added to patients taking valproate, remember that valproate inhibits lamotrigine metabolism and therefore titration rate and ultimate dose of lamotrigine should be reduced by 50% to reduce the risk of rash

✽ Thus, if concomitant valproate is discontinued after lamotrigine dose is stabilized, then the lamotrigine dose should be cautiously doubled over at least 2 weeks in equal increments each week following discontinuation of valproate
- Also, if concomitant enzyme-inducing antiepileptic drugs such as carbamazepine, phenobarbital, phenytoin, and primidone are discontinued after lamotrigine dose is stabilized, then the lamotrigine dose should be maintained for 1 week following discontinuation of the other drug and then reduced by half over 2 weeks in equal decrements each week
- Since oral contraceptives and pregnancy can decrease lamotrigine levels, adjustments to the maintenance dose of lamotrigine are recommended in women taking, starting, or stopping oral contraceptives, becoming pregnant, or after delivery
- Chewable dispersible tablets should only be administered as whole tablets; dose should be rounded down to the nearest whole tablet
- Chewable dispersible tablets can be dispersed by adding the tablet to liquid (enough to cover the drug); after approximately 1 minute the solution should be stirred and then consumed immediately in its entirety
- Orally disintegrating tablet should be placed onto the tongue and moved around in the mouth; the tablet will disintegrate rapidly and can be swallowed with or without food or water
- Do not break or chew extended-release tablets, as this could alter controlled-release properties

Overdose

- Some fatalities have occurred; ataxia, nystagmus, seizures, coma, intraventricular conduction delay

Long-Term Use

- Safe

Habit Forming

- No

How to Stop

- Taper over at least 2 weeks

✽ Rapid discontinuation can increase the risk of relapse in bipolar disorder
- Patients with epilepsy may seize upon withdrawal, especially if withdrawal is abrupt
- Discontinuation symptoms uncommon

Pharmacokinetics

- Elimination half-life in healthy volunteers approximately 33 hours after a single dose of lamotrigine
- Elimination half-life in patients receiving concomitant valproate treatment

approximately 59 hours after a single dose of lamotrigine
- Elimination half-life in patients receiving concomitant enzyme-inducing antiepileptic drugs (such as carbamazepine, phenobarbital, phenytoin, and primidone) approximately 14 hours after a single dose of lamotrigine
- Metabolized in the liver through glucorunidation but not through the CYP450 enzyme system
- Inactive metabolite
- Renally excreted
- Lamotrigine inhibits dihydrofolate reductase and may therefore reduce folate concentrations
- Rapidly and completely absorbed; bioavailability not affected by food

Drug Interactions

✱ Valproate increases plasma concentrations and half-life of lamotrigine, requiring lower doses of lamotrigine (half or less)

✱ Use of lamotrigine with valproate may be associated with an increased incidence of rash

- Enzyme-inducing antiepileptic drugs (e.g., carbamazepine, phenobarbital, phenytoin, primidone) may increase the clearance of lamotrigine and lower its plasma levels
- Oral contraceptives may decrease plasma levels of lamotrigine
- No likely pharmacokinetic interactions of lamotrigine with lithium, oxcarbazepine, atypical antipsychotics, or antidepressants
- False-positive urine immunoassay screening tests for phencyclidine (PCP) have been reported in patients taking lamotrigine due to a lack of specificity of the screening tests

Other Warnings/ Precautions

✱ Life-threatening rashes have developed in association with lamotrigine use; lamotrigine should generally be discontinued at the first sign of serious rash

✱ Risk of rash may be increased with higher doses, faster dose escalation, concomitant use of valproate, or in children under age 12

- Patient should be instructed to report any symptoms of hypersensitivity immediately (fever; flu-like symptoms; rash; blisters on skin or in eyes, mouth, ears, nose, or genital areas; swelling of eyelids, conjunctivitis, lymphadenopathy)
- Aseptic meningitis has been reported rarely in association with lamotrigine use
- Patients should be advised to report any symptoms of aseptic meningitis immediately; these include headache, chills, fever, vomiting and nausea, a stiff neck, and sensitivity to light
- Depressive effects may be increased by other CNS depressants (alcohol, MAOIs, other anticonvulsants, etc.)
- A small number of people may experience a worsening of seizures
- May cause photosensitivity
- Lamotrigine binds to tissue that contains melanin, so for long-term treatment ophthalmological checks may be considered
- Warn patients and their caregivers about the possibility of activation of suicidal ideation and advise them to report such side effects immediately

Do Not Use

- If there is a proven allergy to lamotrigine

SPECIAL POPULATIONS

Renal Impairment

- Lamotrigine is renally excreted, so the maintenance dose may need to be lowered
- Can be removed by hemodialysis; patients receiving hemodialysis may require supplemental doses of lamotrigine

Hepatic Impairment

- Dose adjustment not necessary in mild impairment
- Initial, escalation, and maintenance doses should be reduced by 25% in patients with moderate and severe liver impairment without ascites and 50% in patients with severe liver impairment with ascites

Cardiac Impairment

- Clinical experience is limited
- Drug should be used with caution

Elderly

- Some patients may tolerate lower doses better
- Elderly patients may be more susceptible to adverse effects

Children and Adolescents

- Ages 2 and older: approved as add-on for Lennox-Gastaut syndrome
- Ages 2 and older: approved as add-on for partial seizures
- No other use of lamotrigine is approved for patients under 16 years of age
- ✱ Risk of rash is increased in pediatric patients, especially in children under 12 and in children taking valproate
- When lamotrigine is added to treatment that includes valproate (ages 2–12): for the first 2 weeks administer 0.15 mg/kg per day in 1–2 doses rounded down to the nearest whole tablet; at week 3 increase to 0.3 mg/kg per day in 1–2 doses rounded down to the nearest whole tablet; every 1–2 weeks can increase by 0.3 mg/kg per day rounded down to the nearest whole tablet; usual maintenance dose 1–5 mg/kg per day in 1–2 doses (maximum generally 200 mg/day) or 1–3 mg/kg per day in 1–2 doses if lamotrigine is added to valproate alone
- When lamotrigine is added to treatment with carbamazepine, phenytoin, phenobarbital, or primidone (without valproate) (ages 2–12): for the first 2 weeks administer 0.6 mg/kg per day in 2 doses rounded down to the nearest whole tablet; at week 3 increase to 1.2 mg/kg per day in 2 doses rounded down to the nearest whole tablet; every 1–2 weeks can increase by 1.2 mg/kg per day rounded down to the nearest whole tablet; usual maintenance dose 5–15 mg/kg per day in 2 doses (maximum dose generally 400 mg per day)
- Clearance of lamotrigine may be influenced by weight, such that patients weighing less than 30 kg may require an increase of up to 50% for maintenance doses

Pregnancy

- Effective June 30, 2015, the US FDA requires changes to the content and format of pregnancy and lactation information in prescription drug labels, including the elimination of the pregnancy letter categories; the Pregnancy and Lactation Labeling Rule (PLLR or final rule) applies only to prescription drugs and will be phased in gradually for drugs approved on or after June 30, 2001
- Controlled studies have not been conducted in pregnant women
- Use in women of childbearing potential requires weighing potential benefits to the mother against the risks to the fetus
- Pregnancy registry data show increased risk of isolated cleft palate or cleft lip deformity with first trimester exposure
- ✱ If treatment with lamotrigine is continued, plasma concentrations of lamotrigine may be reduced during pregnancy, possibly requiring increased doses with dose reduction following delivery
- Pregnancy exposure registry for lamotrigine: (800) 336–2176
- Taper drug if discontinuing
- Seizures, even mild seizures, may cause harm to the embryo/fetus
- Recurrent bipolar illness during pregnancy can be quite disruptive
- ✱ For bipolar patients, lamotrigine should generally be discontinued before anticipated pregnancies
- ✱ For bipolar patients in whom treatment is discontinued, given the risk of relapse in the postpartum period, lamotrigine should generally be restarted immediately after delivery
- ✱ Atypical antipsychotics may be preferable to lithium or anticonvulsants such as lamotrigine if treatment of bipolar disorder is required during pregnancy, but lamotrigine may be preferable to other anticonvulsants such as valproate if anticonvulsant treatment is required during pregnancy
- Bipolar symptoms may recur or worsen during pregnancy and some form of treatment may be necessary

Breast Feeding

- Some drug is found in mother's breast milk
- ✱ Generally recommended either to discontinue drug or bottle feed
- If drug is continued while breast feeding, infant should be monitored for possible adverse effects

- If infant shows signs of irritability or sedation, drug may need to be discontinued

✽ Bipolar disorder may recur during the postpartum period, particularly if there is a history of prior postpartum episodes of either depression or psychosis

✽ Relapse rates may be lower in women who receive prophylactic treatment for postpartum episodes of bipolar disorder

- Atypical antipsychotics and anticonvulsants such as valproate may be preferable to lithium or lamotrigine during the postpartum period when breast feeding

THE ART OF PSYCHOPHARMACOLOGY

Potential Advantages

- Depressive stages of bipolar disorder (bipolar depression)
- To prevent recurrences of both depression and mania in bipolar disorder

Potential Disadvantages

- May not be as effective in the manic stage of bipolar disorder

Primary Target Symptoms

- Incidence of seizures
- Unstable mood, especially depression, in bipolar disorder
- Pain

Pearls

✽ Lamotrigine is a first-line treatment option that may be best for patients with bipolar depression

✽ Seems to be more effective in treating depressive episodes than manic episodes in bipolar disorder (treats from below better than it treats from above)

✽ Seems to be effective in preventing both manic relapses as well as depressive relapses (stabilizes both from above and from below) although it may be even better for preventing depressive relapses than for preventing manic relapses

✽ Despite convincing evidence of efficacy in bipolar disorder, is often used less frequently than anticonvulsants without convincing evidence of efficacy in bipolar disorder (e.g., gabapentin or topiramate)

✽ Low levels of use may be based upon exaggerated fears of skin rashes or lack of knowledge about how to manage skin rashes if they occur

✽ May actually be one of the best tolerated mood stabilizers with little weight gain or sedation

- Actual risk of serious skin rash may be comparable to agents erroneously considered "safer" including carbamazepine, phenytoin, phenobarbital, and zonisamide
- Rashes are common even in placebo-treated patients in clinical trials of bipolar patients (5–10%) due to non-drug related causes including eczema, irritant, and allergic contact dermatitis, such as poison ivy and insect bite reactions

✽ To manage rashes in bipolar patients receiving lamotrigine, realize that rashes that occur within the first 5 days or after 8–12 weeks of treatment are rarely drug-related, and learn the clinical distinctions between a benign rash and a serious rash (see What to Do About Side Effects section)

- Rash, including serious rash, appears riskiest in younger children, in those who are receiving concomitant valproate, and/or in those receiving rapid lamotrigine titration and/or high dosing
- Risk of serious rash is less than 1% and has been declining since slower titration, lower dosing, adjustments to use of concomitant valproate administration, and limitations on use in children under 12 have been implemented
- Incidence of serious rash is very low (approaching zero) in recent studies of bipolar patients
- Benign rashes related to lamotrigine may affect up to 10% of patients and resolve rapidly with drug discontinuation

✽ Given the limited treatment options for bipolar depression, patients with benign rashes can even be rechallenged with lamotrigine 5–12 mg/day with very slow titration after risk/benefit analysis if they are informed, reliable, closely monitored, and warned to stop lamotrigine and contact their physician if signs of hypersensitivity occur

- Only a third of bipolar patients experience adequate relief with a monotherapy, so most patients need multiple medications for best control
- Lamotrigine is useful in combination with atypical antipsychotics and/or lithium for acute mania
- Usefulness for bipolar disorder in combination with anticonvulsants other than valproate is not well demonstrated; such combinations can be expensive and are possibly ineffective or even irrational
- May be useful as an adjunct to atypical antipsychotics for rapid onset of action in schizophrenia
- May be useful as an adjunct to antidepressants in major depressive disorder
- Early studies suggest possible utility for patients with neuropathic pain such as diabetic peripheral neuropathy, HIV-associated neuropathy, and other pain conditions including migraine

Suggested Reading

Calabrese JR, Bowden CL, Sachs GS, et al. A double-blind placebo-controlled study of lamotrigine monotherapy in outpatients with bipolar I depression. J Clin Psych 1999;60:79–88.

Calabrese JR, Sullivan JR, Bowden CL, et al. Rash in multicenter trials of lamotrigine in mood disorders: clinical relevance and management. J Clin Psychiatry 2002;63:1012–19.

Culy CR, Goa KL. Lamotrigine. A review of its use in childhood epilepsy. Paediatr Drugs 2000;2:299–330.

Cunningham M, Tennis P, and the International Lamotrigine Pregnancy Registry Scientific Advisory Committee. Lamotrigine and the risk of malformations in pregnancy. Neurology 2005;64:955–60.

Goodwin GM, Bowden CL, Calabrese JR, et al. A pooled analysis of 2 placebo-controlled 18-month trials of lamotrigine and lithium maintenance treatment in bipolar I disorder. J Clin Psychiatry 2004;65:432–41.

Green B. Lamotrigine in mood disorders. Curr Med Res Opin 2003;19:272–7.

THERAPEUTICS

Brands • Keppra
• Keppra XR

see index for additional brand names

Generic? Yes

Class

- Anticonvulsant, synaptic vesicle protein SV2A modulator

Commonly Prescribed for

(bold for FDA approved)

- **Adjunct therapy for partial seizures in patients with epilepsy (≥16 years of age for extended-release, ≥4 years of age for immediate-release)**
- **Adjunct therapy for myoclonic seizures in juvenile myoclonic epilepsy (ages 12 and older)**
- **Adjunct therapy for primary generalized tonic-clonic seizures in idiopathic generalized epilepsy (ages 6 and older)**
- Neuropathic pain/chronic pain
- Mania

How the Drug Works

- ✻ Binds to synaptic vesicle protein SV2A, which is involved in synaptic vesicle exocytosis
- Opposes the activity of negative modulators of GABA- and glycine-gated currents and partially inhibits N-type calcium currents in neuronal cells

How Long Until It Works

- Should reduce seizures by 2 weeks
- Not yet clear if it has mood-stabilizing effects in bipolar disorder or antineuralgic actions in chronic neuropathic pain, but some patients may respond and if so, would be expected to show clinical effects starting by 2 weeks although it may take several weeks to months to optimize clinical effects

If It Works

- The goal of treatment is complete remission of symptoms (e.g., seizures, mania, pain)
- The goal of treatment of chronic neuropathic pain is to reduce symptoms as much as possible, especially in combination with other treatments
- Treatment of chronic neuropathic pain most often reduces but does not eliminate symptoms and is not a cure since symptoms usually recur after medicine stopped
- Continue treatment until all symptoms are gone or until mood is stable and then continue treating indefinitely as long as improvement persists
- Continue treatment indefinitely to avoid recurrence of seizures, mania, and pain

If It Doesn't Work (for bipolar disorder or neuropathic pain)

- ✻ May be effective only in a subset of bipolar patients, in some patients who fail to respond to other mood stabilizers, or it may not work at all
- Many patients have only a partial response where some symptoms are improved but others persist or continue to wax and wane without stabilization of pain or mood
- Other patients may be nonresponders, sometimes called treatment-resistant or treatment-refractory
- Consider increasing dose or switching to another agent with better demonstrated efficacy in bipolar disorder or neuropathic pain

Best Augmenting Combos for Partial Response or Treatment Resistance

- Levetiracetam is itself a second-line augmenting agent to numerous other anticonvulsants, lithium, and atypical antipsychotics for bipolar disorder and to gabapentin, tiagabine, other anticonvulsants, SNRIs, and TCAs for neuropathic pain

Tests

- None for healthy individuals

SIDE EFFECTS

How Drug Causes Side Effects

- CNS side effects may be due to excessive actions on SV2A synaptic vesicle proteins or to actions on various voltage-sensitive ion channels

Notable Side Effects

- ✻ Sedation, dizziness, ataxia, asthenia

- Hematologic abnormalities (decrease in red blood cell count and hemoglobin)

Life-Threatening or Dangerous Side Effects

- Rare severe dermatologic reactions [Stevens-Johnson syndrome (SJS), toxic epidermal necrolysis (TEN)]
- Activation of suicidal ideation and acts (rare)
- Changes in behavior (aggression, agitation, anxiety, hostility)
- Rare activation of suicidal ideation and behavior (suicidality)

Weight Gain

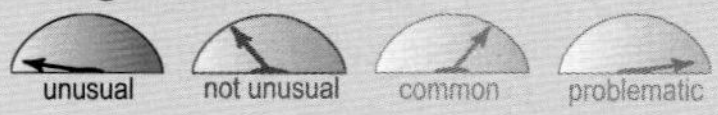

- Reported but not expected

Sedation

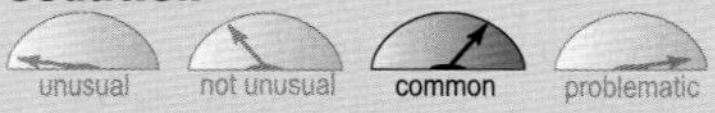

- Many experience and/or can be significant in amount

What to Do About Side Effects

- Wait
- Wait
- Wait
- Take more of the dose at night to reduce daytime sedation
- Lower the dose
- Switch to another agent

Best Augmenting Agents for Side Effects

- Many side effects cannot be improved with an augmenting agent

DOSING AND USE

Usual Dosage Range

- 1,000–3,000 mg/day in 2 doses

Dosage Forms

- Tablet 250 mg, 500 mg, 750 mg
- Extended-release tablet 500 mg, 750 mg
- Oral solution 100 mg/mL

How to Dose

- Initial 1,000 mg/day in 1 (extended-release) or 2 (immediate-release) doses; after 2 weeks can increase by 1,000 mg/day every 2 weeks; maximum dose generally 3,000 mg/day

Dosing Tips

- For intolerable sedation, can give most of the dose at night and less during the day
- Some patients may tolerate and respond to doses greater than 3,000 mg/day

Overdose

- No fatalities; sedation, agitation, aggression, respiratory depression, coma

Long-Term Use

- Safe

Habit Forming

- No

How to Stop

- Taper
- Epilepsy patients may seize upon withdrawal, especially if withdrawal is abrupt
- * Rapid discontinuation can increase the risk of relapse in bipolar disorder
- Discontinuation symptoms uncommon

Pharmacokinetics

- Elimination half-life approximately 6–8 hours
- Inactive metabolites
- Not metabolized by CYP450 enzymes
- Does not inhibit/induce CYP450 enzymes
- Renally excreted

Drug Interactions

- Because levetiracetam is not metabolized by CYP450 enzymes and does not inhibit or induce CYP450 enzymes, it is unlikely to have significant pharmacokinetic drug interactions

Other Warnings/ Precautions

- Depressive effects may be increased by other CNS depressants (alcohol, MAOIs, other anticonvulsants, etc.)
- Warn patients and their caregivers about the possibility of activation of suicidal ideation and advise them to report such side effects immediately

- Monitor patients for behavioral symptoms (aggression, agitation, anger, anxiety, apathy, depression, hostility, irritability) as well as for possible psychotic symptoms or suicidality

Do Not Use

- If there is a proven allergy to levetiracetam

SPECIAL POPULATIONS

Renal Impairment

- Recommended dose for patients with mild impairment may be between 500 mg and 1,500 mg twice a day
- Recommended dose for patients with moderate impairment may be between 250 mg and 750 mg twice a day
- Recommended dose for patients with severe impairment may be between 250 mg and 500 mg twice a day
- Patients on dialysis may require doses between 500 mg and 1,000 mg once a day, with a supplemental dose of 250–500 mg following dialysis

Hepatic Impairment

- Dose adjustment usually not necessary

Cardiac Impairment

- No specific recommendations

Elderly

- Some patients may tolerate lower doses better
- Elderly patients may be more susceptible to adverse effects

Children and Adolescents

- Safety and efficacy not established under age 16
- Children may require higher doses than adults; dosing should be adjusted according to weight

Pregnancy

- Effective June 30, 2015, the US FDA requires changes to the content and format of pregnancy and lactation information in prescription drug labels, including the elimination of the pregnancy letter categories; the Pregnancy and Lactation Labeling Rule (PLLR or final rule) applies only to prescription drugs and will be phased in gradually for drugs approved on or after June 30, 2001
- Controlled studies have not been conducted in pregnant women
- Use in women of childbearing potential requires weighing potential benefits to the mother against the risks to the fetus
- Antiepileptic Drug Pregnancy Registry: (888) 233–2334
- Taper drug if discontinuing
- Seizures, even mild seizures, may cause harm to the embryo/fetus
- Lack of convincing efficacy for treatment of bipolar disorder or chronic neuropathic pain suggests risk/benefit ratio is in favor of discontinuing levetiracetam during pregnancy for these indications

✽ For bipolar patients, given the risk of relapse in the postpartum period, mood-stabilizer treatment, especially with agents with better evidence of efficacy than levetiracetam, should generally be restarted immediately after delivery if patient is unmedicated during pregnancy

✽ For bipolar patients, levetiracetam should generally be discontinued before anticipated pregnancies

✽ Atypical antipsychotics may be preferable to levetiracetam if treatment of bipolar disorder is required during pregnancy

- Bipolar symptoms may recur or worsen during pregnancy and some form of treatment may be necessary

Breast Feeding

- Some drug is found in mother's breast milk

✽ Recommended either to discontinue drug or bottle feed

- If drug is continued while breast feeding, infant should be monitored for possible adverse effects
- If infant becomes irritable or sedated, breast feeding or drug may need to be discontinued

✽ Bipolar disorder may recur during the postpartum period, particularly if there is a history of prior postpartum episodes of either depression or psychosis

* Relapse rates may be lower in women who receive prophylactic treatment for postpartum episodes of bipolar disorder
- Atypical antipsychotics and anticonvulsants such as valproate may be safer than levetiracetam during the postpartum period when breast feeding

THE ART OF PSYCHOPHARMACOLOGY

Potential Advantages

- Patients on concomitant drugs (lack of drug interactions)
- Treatment-refractory bipolar disorder
- Treatment-refractory neuropathic pain

Potential Disadvantages

- Patients noncompliant with twice daily dosing
- Efficacy for bipolar disorder or neuropathic pain not well documented

Primary Target Symptoms

- Seizures
- Pain
- Mania

Pearls

- Well studied in epilepsy
* Off-label use second-line and as an augmenting agent may be justified for bipolar disorder and neuropathic pain unresponsive to other treatments
* Unique mechanism of action suggests utility where other anticonvulsants fail to work
* Unique mechanism of action as modulator of synaptic vesicle release suggests theoretical utility for clinical conditions that are hypothetically linked to excessively activated neuronal circuits, such as anxiety disorders and neuropathic pain as well as epilepsy

Suggested Reading

Ben-Menachem E. Levetiracetam: treatment in epilepsy. Expert Opin Pharmacother 2003;4(11):2079–88.

French J. Use of levetiracetam in special populations. Epilepsia 2001;42(Suppl 4):S40–3.

Leppik IE. Three new drugs for epilepsy: levetiracetam, oxcarbazepine, and zonisamide. J Child Neurol 2002;17(Suppl 1):S53–7.

Lynch BA, Lambeng N, Nocka K, et al. The synaptic vesicle protein SV2A is the binding site for the antiepileptic drug levetiracetam. Proc Natl Acad Sci USA 2004;101:9861–6.

Pinto A, Sander JW. Levetiracetam: a new therapeutic option for refractory epilepsy. Int J Clin Pract 2003;57(7):616–21.

THERAPEUTICS

Brands • Fetzima

see index for additional brand names

Generic? No

Class

- Neuroscience-based Nomenclature: serotonin, norepinephrine reuptake inhibitor (SN-RI)
- SNRI (dual serotonin and norepinephrine reuptake inhibitor); antidepressant

Commonly Prescribed for

(bold for FDA approved)

- **Major depressive disorder**
- Fibromyalgia
- Neuropathic pain/chronic pain

How the Drug Works

- Boosts neurotransmitters serotonin, norepinephrine/noradrenaline, and dopamine
- Blocks norepinephrine reuptake pump (norepinephrine transporter), presumably increasing noradrenergic neurotransmission
- Blocks serotonin reuptake pump (serotonin transporter), presumably increasing serotonergic neurotransmission
- Presumably desensitizes both serotonin 1A receptors and beta adrenergic receptors
- Since dopamine is inactivated by norepinephrine reuptake in frontal cortex, which largely lacks dopamine transporters, levomilnacipran can increase dopamine neurotransmission in this part of the brain

How Long Until It Works

- Onset of therapeutic actions is usually not immediate, but often delayed 2–4 weeks
- If it is not working within 6 or 8 weeks, it may require a dosage increase (off label), or it may not work at all
- May continue to work for many years to prevent relapse of symptoms

If It Works

- The goal of treatment of depression is complete remission of current symptoms as well as prevention of future relapses
- Treatment of depression most often reduces or even eliminates symptoms, but not a cure since symptoms can recur after medicine stopped
- Continue treatment of depression until all symptoms are gone (remission) or significantly reduced
- Once symptoms gone, continue treating for 1 year for the first episode of depression
- For second and subsequent episodes of depression, treatment may need to be indefinite

If It Doesn't Work

- Many depressed patients only have a partial response where some symptoms are improved but others persist (especially insomnia, fatigue, and problems concentrating)
- Other depressed patients may be nonresponders, sometimes called treatment-resistant or treatment-refractory
- Some depressed patients who have an initial response may relapse even though they continue treatment, sometimes called "poop-out"
- Consider increasing dose, switching to another agent, or adding an appropriate augmenting agent
- Consider psychotherapy
- Consider evaluation for another diagnosis or for a comorbid condition (e.g., medical illness, substance abuse, etc.)
- Some patients may experience apparent lack of consistent efficacy due to activation of latent or underlying bipolar disorder, and require antidepressant discontinuation and switch to a mood stabilizer

Best Augmenting Combos for Partial Response or Treatment Resistance

- Augmentation experience is limited compared to other antidepressants
- Benzodiazepines can reduce insomnia and anxiety
- Bupropion, mirtazapine, reboxetine, or atomoxetine (use combinations of antidepressants with caution as this may activate bipolar disorder and suicidal ideation)
- Modafinil, especially for fatigue, sleepiness, and lack of concentration
- Mood stabilizers or atypical antipsychotics for bipolar depression, psychotic depression, or treatment-resistant depression
- Hypnotics or trazodone for insomnia

- Classically, lithium, buspirone, or thyroid hormone

Tests

- Check heart rate and blood pressure before initiating treatment and regularly during treatment

SIDE EFFECTS

How Drug Causes Side Effects

- Theoretically due to increases in serotonin and norepinephrine concentrations at receptors in parts of the brain and body other than those that cause therapeutic actions (e.g., unwanted actions of serotonin in sleep centers causing insomnia, unwanted actions of norepinephrine on acetylcholine release causing urinary retention or constipation)
- Most side effects are immediate but often go away with time, in contrast to most therapeutic effects, which are delayed and are enhanced over time

Notable Side Effects

- Nausea, vomiting, constipation
- Hyperhidrosis
- Tachycardia, heart rate increase, palpitations
- Erectile dysfunction
- Urinary hesitancy or retention

Life-Threatening or Dangerous Side Effects

- Rare seizures
- Rare induction of mania and activation of suicidal ideation

Weight Gain

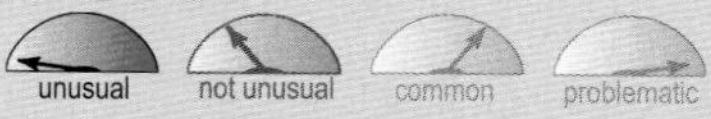

- Reported but not expected

Sedation

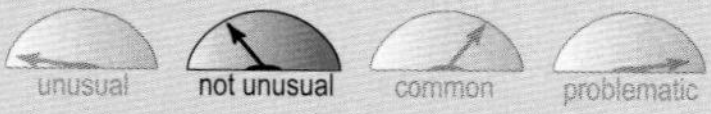

- Occurs in significant minority

What to Do About Side Effects

- Wait
- Wait
- Wait
- Lower the dose
- In a few weeks, switch to another agent or add other drugs

Best Augmenting Agents for Side Effects

- ✻ For urinary hesitancy, give an alpha 1 blocker such as tamsulosin or naftopidil
- Often best to try another antidepressant monotherapy prior to resorting to augmentation strategies to treat side effects
- Trazodone or a hypnotic for insomnia
- Bupropion, sildenafil, vardenafil, or tadalafil for sexual dysfunction
- Benzodiazepines for anxiety, agitation
- Mirtazapine for insomnia, agitation, and gastrointestinal side effects
- Many side effects are time-dependent (i.e., they start immediately upon dosing and upon each dose increase, but go away with time)
- Activation and agitation may represent the induction of a bipolar state, especially a mixed dysphoric bipolar II condition sometimes associated with suicidal ideation, and require the addition of lithium, a mood stabilizer, or an atypical antipsychotic, and/or discontinuation of levomilnacipran

DOSING AND USE

Usual Dosage Range

- 40–120 mg once daily

Dosage Forms

- Extended-release capsule 20 mg, 40 mg, 80 mg, 120 mg

How to Dose

- Initial dose 20 mg once daily for 2 days, then increase to 40 mg once daily; can increase by 40 mg/day every 2 or more days; maximum recommended dose 120 mg once daily

Dosing Tips

- Can be taken with or without food
- Do not break or chew levomilnacipran capsules, as this will alter controlled-release properties

- If intolerable anxiety, insomnia, agitation, akathisia, or activation occur either upon dosing initiation or discontinuation, consider the possibility of activating a bipolar disorder and switch to a mood stabilizer or an atypical antipsychotic

Overdose
- No fatalities have been reported; experience is limited

Long-Term Use
- Has not been evaluated in controlled studies, but long-term treatment of major depressive disorder is generally necessary

Habit Forming
- No

How to Stop
- Taper is prudent, but usually not necessary

Pharmacokinetics
- Metabolized by CYP450 3A4; renally excreted
- Terminal elimination half-life approximately 12 hours

Drug Interactions
- Tramadol increases the risk of seizures in patients taking an antidepressant
- Can cause a fatal "serotonin syndrome" when combined with MAOIs, so do not use with MAOIs or for at least 14 days after MAOIs are stopped
- Do not start an MAOI for at least 5 half-lives (5 to 7 days for most drugs) after discontinuing levomilnacipran
- Strong CYP450 3A4 inhibitors, such as ketoconazole, can increase plasma levels of levomilnacipran; do not exceed 80 mg once daily of levomilnacipran if used with a strong CYP450 3A4 inhibitor
- Alcohol may interact with the extended-release properties of levomilnacipran, causing a pronounced accelerated drug release ("drug dumping"); thus, taking levomilnacipran with alcohol is not recommended
- Possible increased risk of bleeding, especially when combined with anticoagulants (e.g., warfarin, NSAIDs)
- Switching from or addition of other norepinephrine reuptake inhibitors should be done with caution, as the additive pro-noradrenergic effects may enhance therapeutic actions in depression, but also enhance noradrenergically mediated side effects

Other Warnings/ Precautions
- Use with caution in patients with history of seizures
- Use with caution in patients with bipolar disorder unless treated with concomitant mood-stabilizing agent
- Use with caution in patients with controlled angle-closure glaucoma
- Not approved in children, so when treating children off label, carefully weigh the risks and benefits of pharmacological treatment against the risks and benefits of non-treatment with antidepressants and make sure to document this in the patient's chart
- Distribute the brochures provided by the FDA and the drug companies
- Warn patients and their caregivers about the possibility of activating side effects and advise them to report such symptoms immediately
- Monitor patients for activation of suicidal ideation, especially children and adolescents

Do Not Use
- If patient has uncontrolled angle-closure glaucoma
- If patient is taking an MAOI
- If there is a proven allergy to levomilnacipran or milnacipran

SPECIAL POPULATIONS

Renal Impairment
- Maximum dose 80 mg once daily for moderate impairment
- Maximum dose 40 mg once daily for severe impairment

Hepatic Impairment
- Dose adjustment not necessary

Cardiac Impairment
- Not systematically evaluated in patients with cardiac impairment
- Drug should be used with caution

Elderly
- Some patients may tolerate lower doses better
- Reduction in risk of suicidality with antidepressants compared to placebo in adults age 65 and older

Children and Adolescents
- Safety and efficacy have not been established
- Carefully weigh the risks and benefits of pharmacological treatment against the risks and benefits of nontreatment with antidepressants and make sure to document this in the patient's chart
- Monitor patients face-to-face regularly, particularly during the first several weeks of treatment
- Use with caution, observing for activation of known or unknown bipolar disorder and/or suicidal ideation, and strongly consider informing parents or guardian of this risk so they can help observe child or adolescent patients

Pregnancy
- Effective June 30, 2015, the US FDA requires changes to the content and format of pregnancy and lactation information in prescription drug labels, including the elimination of the pregnancy letter categories; the Pregnancy and Lactation Labeling Rule (PLLR or final rule) applies only to prescription drugs and will be phased in gradually for drugs approved on or after June 30, 2001
- Controlled studies have not been conducted in pregnant women
- Not generally recommended for use during pregnancy, especially during first trimester
- Nonetheless, continuous treatment during pregnancy may be necessary and has not been proven to be harmful to the fetus
- At delivery there may be more bleeding in the mother and transient irritability or sedation in the newborn
- Must weigh the risk of treatment (first trimester fetal development, third trimester newborn delivery) to the child against the risk of no treatment (recurrence of depression, maternal health, infant bonding) to the mother and child
- For many patients, this may mean continuing treatment during pregnancy
- Exposure to serotonin reuptake inhibitors early in pregnancy may be associated with increased risk of septal heart defects (absolute risk is small)
- Use of serotonin reuptake inhibitors beyond the 20th week of pregnancy may be associated with increased risk of pulmonary hypertension in newborns, although this is not proven
- Exposure to serotonin reuptake inhibitors late in pregnancy may be associated with increased risk of gestational hypertension and preeclampsia
- Neonates exposed to SSRIs or SNRIs late in the third trimester have developed complications requiring prolonged hospitalization, respiratory support, and tube feeding; reported symptoms are consistent with either a direct toxic effect of SSRIs and SNRIs or, possibly, a drug discontinuation syndrome, and include respiratory distress, cyanosis, apnea, seizures, temperature instability, feeding difficulty, vomiting, hypoglycemia, hypotonia, hypertonia, hyperreflexia, tremor, jitteriness, irritability, and constant crying

Breast Feeding
- Unknown if levomilnacipran is secreted in human breast milk, but all psychotropics assumed to be secreted in breast milk
- If child becomes irritable or sedated, breast feeding or drug may need to be discontinued
- Immediate postpartum period is a high-risk time for depression, especially in women who have had prior depressive episodes, so drug may need to be reinstituted late in the third trimester or shortly after childbirth to prevent a recurrence during the postpartum period
- Must weigh benefits of breast feeding with risks and benefits of antidepressant treatment versus nontreatment to both the infant and the mother
- For many patients, this may mean continuing treatment during breast feeding

THE ART OF PSYCHOPHARMACOLOGY

Potential Advantages
- Patients with depression may have higher remission rates on SNRIs than on SSRIs
- Depressed patients with somatic symptoms, fatigue, and pain

Potential Disadvantages
- Cost
- Patients with urologic disorders, prostate disorders
- Patients with borderline or uncontrolled hypertension
- Patients with agitation and anxiety (short-term)

Primary Target Symptoms
- Depressed mood
- Physical symptoms

Pearls
✻ Has greater potency for norepinephrine reuptake blockade than for serotonin reuptake blockade, but this is of unclear clinical significance as a differentiating feature from other SNRIs, although it might contribute to theoretical effects in fibromyalgia and chronic pain

✻ Potent noradrenergic actions may account for possibly higher incidence of sweating and urinary hesitancy than some other SNRIs
- Urinary hesitancy more common in men than women and in older men than in younger men
- Alpha 1 antagonists such as tamsulosin or naftopidil can reverse urinary hesitancy or retention
- Alpha 1 antagonists given prophylactically may prevent urinary hesitancy or retention in patients at higher risk, such as elderly men with borderline urine flow
- Nonresponse to levomilnacipran in elderly may require consideration of mild cognitive impairment or Alzheimer disease

Suggested Reading

Auclair AL, Martel JC, Assié MB, et al. Levomilnacipran (F2695), a norepinephrine-preferring SNRI: profile in vitro and in models of depression and anxiety. Neuropharmacology 2013;70:338–47.

Citrome L. Levomilnacipran for major depressive disorder: a systematic review of the efficacy and safety profile for this newly approved antidepressant – what is the number needed to treat, number needed to harm and likelihood to be helped or harmed? Int J Clin Pract 2013;67:1089–104.

Mago R, Forero G, Greenberg WM, Gommoll C, Chen C. Safety and tolerability of levomilnacipran ER in major depressive disorder: results from an open-label, 48-week extension study. Clin Drug Investig 2013;33:761–71.

THERAPEUTICS

Brands • Vyvanse
see index for additional brand names

Generic? No

Class
- Neuroscience-based Nomenclature: dopamine and norepinephrine reuptake inhibitor and releaser (DN-RIRe)
- Stimulant

Commonly Prescribed for
(bold for FDA approved)
- **Attention deficit hyperactivity disorder (ADHD) (ages 6 and older)**
- **Binge eating disorder**
- Narcolepsy
- Treatment-resistant depression

How the Drug Works
* Lisdexamfetamine is a prodrug of dextroamphetamine and is thus not active until after it has been absorbed by the intestinal tract and converted to dextroamphetamine (active component) and l-lysine
* Once converted to dextroamphetamine, it increases norepinephrine and especially dopamine actions by blocking their reuptake and facilitating their release
- Enhancement of dopamine and norepinephrine in certain brain regions (e.g., dorsolateral prefrontal cortex) may improve attention, concentration, executive dysfunction, and wakefulness
- Enhancement of dopamine actions in other brain regions (e.g., basal ganglia) may improve hyperactivity
- Enhancement of dopamine and norepinephrine in yet other brain regions (e.g., medial prefrontal cortex, hypothalamus) may improve depression, fatigue, and sleepiness

How Long Until It Works
- Some immediate effects can be seen with first dosing
- Can take several weeks to attain maximum therapeutic benefit

If It Works (for ADHD)
- The goal of treatment of ADHD is reduction of symptoms of inattentiveness, motor hyperactivity, and/or impulsiveness that disrupt social, school, and/or occupational functioning
- Continue treatment until all symptoms are under control or improvement is stable and then continue treatment indefinitely as long as improvement persists
- Reevaluate the need for treatment periodically
- Treatment for ADHD begun in childhood may need to be continued into adolescence and adulthood if continued benefit is documented

If It Doesn't Work (for ADHD)
- Consider adjusting dose or switching to another formulation of d-amphetamine or to another agent
- Consider behavioral therapy
- Consider the presence of noncompliance and counsel patients and parents
- Consider evaluation for another diagnosis or for a comorbid condition (e.g., bipolar disorder, substance abuse, medical illness, etc.)
* Some ADHD patients and some depressed patients may experience lack of consistent efficacy due to activation of latent or underlying bipolar disorder, and require either augmenting with a mood stabilizer or switching to a mood stabilizer

Best Augmenting Combos for Partial Response or Treatment Resistance
* Best to attempt other monotherapies prior to augmenting
- For the expert, can combine with modafinil or atomoxetine for ADHD
- For the expert, can occasionally combine with atypical antipsychotics in highly treatment-resistant cases of bipolar disorder or ADHD
- For the expert, can combine with antidepressants to boost antidepressant efficacy in highly treatment-resistant cases of depression while carefully monitoring patient

Tests
- Before treatment, assess for presence of cardiac disease (history, family history, physical exam)

- Blood pressure should be monitored regularly
- In children, monitor weight and height

SIDE EFFECTS

How Drug Causes Side Effects
- Increases in norepinephrine especially peripherally can cause autonomic side effects, including tremor, tachycardia, hypertension, and cardiac arrhythmias
- Increases in norepinephrine and dopamine centrally can cause CNS side effects such as insomnia, agitation, psychosis, and substance abuse

Notable Side Effects
✽ Insomnia, headache, exacerbation of tics, nervousness, irritability, overstimulation, tremor, dizziness

✽ Anorexia, nausea, dry mouth, constipation, diarrhea, weight loss

- Can temporarily slow normal growth in children (controversial)
- Sexual dysfunction long-term (impotence, libido changes), but can also improve sexual dysfunction short-term

Life-Threatening or Dangerous Side Effects
- Psychotic episodes
- Seizures
- Palpitations, tachycardia, hypertension
- Rare activation of hypomania, mania, or suicidal ideation (controversial)
- Cardiovascular adverse effects, sudden death in patients with preexisting cardiac structural abnormalities

Weight Gain
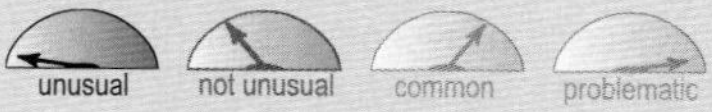

- Reported but not expected
- Some patients may experience weight loss

Sedation
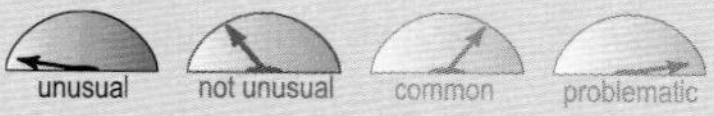

- Reported but not expected
- Activation much more common than sedation

What to Do About Side Effects
- Wait
- Adjust dose
- Switch to another long-acting stimulant
- Switch to another agent
- For insomnia, avoid dosing in afternoon/evening

Best Augmenting Agents for Side Effects
- Beta blockers for peripheral autonomic side effects
- Dose reduction or switching to another agent may be more effective since most side effects cannot be improved with an augmenting agent

DOSING AND USE

Usual Dosage Range
- ADHD: 30–70 mg/day
- Binge eating disorder: 50–70 mg/day

Dosage Forms
- Capsule 10 mg, 20 mg, 30 mg, 40 mg, 50 mg, 60 mg, 70 mg

How to Dose
- Initial 30 mg/day in the morning; can increase by 10–20 mg each week; maximum dose generally 70 mg/day
- Binge eating disorder: initial 30 mg/day in the morning; can increase by 20 mg each week; maximum dose generally 70 mg/day

Dosing Tips
- 10–12 hour duration of clinical action
- Capsules can either be taken whole or they can be opened and the contents dissolved in water
- When taken in water, the entire solution should be consumed immediately
- Dose of a single capsule should not be divided
- Once daily dosing can be an important practical element in stimulant utilization, eliminating the hassle and pragmatic difficulties of lunchtime dosing at school, including storage problems, potential diversion, and the need for a medical professional to supervise dosing away from home

- Avoid dosing after the morning because of the risk of insomnia

✻ May be possible to dose only during the school week for some ADHD patients

✻ May be able to give drug holidays for patients with ADHD over the summer in order to reassess therapeutic utility and effects on growth suppression as well as to assess any other side effects and the need to reinstitute stimulant treatment for the next school term

- Can be taken with or without food

Overdose

- Rarely fatal; panic, hyperreflexia, rhabdomyolysis, rapid respiration, confusion, coma, hallucination, convulsion, arrhythmia, change in blood pressure, circulatory collapse

Long-Term Use

- Can be used long-term for ADHD when ongoing monitoring documents continued efficacy
- Dependence and/or abuse may develop
- Tolerance to therapeutic effects may develop in some patients
- Long-term stimulant use may be associated with growth suppression in children (controversial)
- Periodic monitoring of weight, blood pressure, CBC, platelet counts, and liver function may be prudent

Habit Forming

- Schedule II drug
- Patients may develop tolerance, psychological dependence
- Theoretically less abuse potential than other stimulants when taken as directed because it is inactive until it reaches the gut and thus has delayed time to onset as well as long duration of action

How to Stop

- Taper to avoid withdrawal effects
- Withdrawal following chronic therapeutic use may unmask symptoms of the underlying disorder and may require follow-up and reinstitution of treatment
- Careful supervision is required during withdrawal from abuse use since severe depression may occur

Pharmacokinetics

- 1 hour to maximum concentration of lisdexamfetamine, 3.5 hours to maximum concentration of dextroamphetamine
- Duration of clinical action 10–12 hours

Drug Interactions

- May affect blood pressure and should be used cautiously with agents used to control blood pressure
- Gastrointestinal acidifying agents (guanethidine, reserpine, glutamic acid, ascorbic acid, fruit juices, etc.) and urinary acidifying agents (ammonium chloride, sodium phosphate, etc.) lower amphetamine plasma levels, so such agents can be useful to administer after an overdose but may also lower therapeutic efficacy of amphetamines
- Gastrointestinal alkalinizing agents (sodium bicarbonate, etc.) and urinary alkalinizing agents (acetazolamide, some thiazides) increase amphetamine plasma levels and potentiate amphetamine's actions
- Desipramine and protryptiline can cause striking and sustained increases in brain concentrations of d-amphetamine and may also add to d-amphetamine's cardiovascular effects
- Theoretically, other agents with norepinephrine reuptake blocking properties, such as venlafaxine, duloxetine, atomoxetine, milnacipran, and reboxetine, could also add to amphetamine's CNS and cardiovascular effects
- Amphetamines may counteract the sedative effects of antihistamines
- Haloperidol, chlorpromazine, and lithium may inhibit stimulatory effects of amphetamine
- Theoretically, atypical antipsychotics should also inhibit stimulatory effects of amphetamines
- Theoretically, amphetamines could inhibit the antipsychotic actions of antipsychotics
- Theoretically, amphetamines could inhibit the mood-stabilizing actions of atypical antipsychotics in some patients
- Combinations of amphetamines with mood stabilizers (lithium, anticonvulsants, atypical antipsychotics) is generally something for experts only, when

monitoring patients closely and when other options fail
- Absorption of phenobarbital, phenytoin, and ethosuximide is delayed by amphetamines
- Amphetamines inhibit adrenergic blockers and enhance adrenergic effects of norepinephrine
- Amphetamines may antagonize hypotensive effects of Veratrum alkaloids and other antihypertensives
- Amphetamines increase the analgesic effects of meperidine
- Amphetamines contribute to excessive CNS stimulation if used with large doses of propoxyphene
- Amphetamines can raise plasma corticosteroid levels
- MAOIs slow absorption of amphetamines and thus potentiate their actions, which can cause headache, hypertension, and rarely hypertensive crisis and malignant hyperthermia, sometimes with fatal results
- Use with MAOIs, including within 14 days of MAOI use, is not advised, but this can sometimes be considered by experts who monitor depressed patients closely when other treatment options for depression fail

Other Warnings/ Precautions
- Use with caution in patients with any degree of hypertension, hyperthyroidism, or history of drug abuse
- Children who are not growing or gaining weight should stop treatment, at least temporarily
- May worsen motor and phonic tics
- May worsen symptoms of thought disorder and behavior disturbance in psychotic patients
- Stimulants have a high potential for abuse and must be used with caution in anyone with a current or past history of substance abuse or alcoholism or in emotionally unstable patients
- Administration of stimulants for prolonged periods of time should be avoided whenever possible or done only with close monitoring, as it may lead to marked tolerance and drug dependence, including psychological dependence with varying degrees of abnormal behavior
- Particular attention should be paid to the possibility of subjects obtaining stimulants for nontherapeutic use or distribution to others and the drugs should in general be prescribed sparingly with documentation of appropriate use
- Usual dosing has been associated with sudden death in children with structural cardiac abnormalities
- Not an appropriate first-line treatment for depression or for normal fatigue
- May lower the seizure threshold
- Emergence or worsening of activation and agitation may represent the induction of a bipolar state, especially a mixed dysphoric bipolar II condition sometimes associated with suicidal ideation, and require the addition of a mood stabilizer and/or discontinuation of lisdexamfetamine

Do Not Use
- If patient has extreme anxiety or agitation
- If patient has motor tics or Tourette's syndrome or if there is a family history of Tourette's, unless administered by an expert in cases when the potential benefits for ADHD outweigh the risks of worsening tics
- Should generally not be administered with an MAOI, including within 14 days of MAOI use, except in heroic circumstances and by an expert
- If patient has arteriosclerosis, cardiovascular disease, or severe hypertension
- If patient has glaucoma
- If patient has structural cardiac abnormalities
- If patient has hyperthyroidism
- If there is a proven allergy to any sympathomimetic agent

SPECIAL POPULATIONS

Renal Impairment
- Severe impairment: maximum dose 50 mg/day
- End-stage renal disease: maximum dose 30 mg/day

Hepatic Impairment
- Use with caution

Cardiac Impairment

- Use with caution, particularly in patients with recent myocardial infarction or other conditions that could be negatively affected by increased blood pressure
- Do not use in patients with structural cardiac abnormalities, cardiac myopathy, serious heart arrhythmia, or coronary artery disease

Elderly

- Some patients may tolerate lower doses better

Children and Adolescents

- Safety and efficacy not established in children under age 6
- Use in young children should be reserved for the expert
- d-amphetamine may worsen symptoms of behavioral disturbance and thought disorder in psychotic children
- d-amphetamine has acute effects on growth hormone; long-term effects are unknown but weight and height should be monitored during long-term treatment
- Sudden death in children and adolescents with serious heart problems has been reported
- American Heart Association recommends EKG prior to initiating stimulant treatment in children, although not all experts agree

Pregnancy

- Effective June 30, 2015, the US FDA requires changes to the content and format of pregnancy and lactation information in prescription drug labels, including the elimination of the pregnancy letter categories; the Pregnancy and Lactation Labeling Rule (PLLR or final rule) applies only to prescription drugs and will be phased in gradually for drugs approved on or after June 30, 2001
- Controlled studies have not been conducted in pregnant women
- There is a greater risk of premature birth and low birth weight in infants whose mothers take d-amphetamine during pregnancy
- Infants whose mothers take d-amphetamine during pregnancy may experience withdrawal symptoms
- In animal studies, d-amphetamine caused delayed skeletal ossification and decreased post-weaning weight gain in rats; no major malformations occurred in rat or rabbit studies
- Use in women of childbearing potential requires weighing potential benefits to the mother against potential risks to the fetus
- For ADHD patients, lisdexamfetamine should generally be discontinued before anticipated pregnancies

Breast Feeding

- Some drug is found in mother's breast milk
- * Recommended either to discontinue drug or bottle feed
- If infant shows signs of irritability, drug may need to be discontinued

THE ART OF PSYCHOPHARMACOLOGY

Potential Advantages

- Only approved treatment for binge eating disorder
- Although restricted as a Schedule II controlled substance like other stimulants, as a prodrug lisdexamfetamine may have less propensity for abuse, intoxication, or dependence than other stimulants
- May be particularly useful in adult patients without prior diagnosis and treatment of ADHD as a child to prevent abuse and diversion since lisdexamfetamine may be less abusable than other stimulants

Potential Disadvantages

- Patients with current or past substance abuse
- Patients with current or past bipolar disorder or psychosis

Primary Target Symptoms

- Concentration, attention span
- Motor hyperactivity
- Impulsiveness
- Binge eating
- Physical and mental fatigue
- Daytime sleepiness
- Depression

Pearls

- First medication approved for the treatment of binge eating disorder
- Theoretically, efficacy in binge eating disorder is due to controlled-release of a stimulant enhancing tonic over phasic dopamine neuronal firing
- Theoretically, binge eating in binge eating disorder could be due to a shift from reward-related eating to habit, and from impulsivity to compulsivity due to a shift of control of dopamine from dorsal to ventral striatum, which can be reversed by lisdexamfetamine
- May be useful for treatment of depressive symptoms in medically ill elderly patients
- May be useful for treatment of post-stroke depression
- A classical augmentation strategy for treatment-refractory depression
- Specifically, may be useful for treatment of cognitive dysfunction and fatigue as residual symptoms of major depressive disorder unresponsive to multiple prior treatments
- May also be useful for the treatment of cognitive impairment, depressive symptoms, and severe fatigue in patients with HIV infection and in cancer patients
- Can be used to potentiate opioid analgesia and reduce sedation, particularly in end-of-life management
- Some patients respond to or tolerate lisdexamfetamine better than methylphenidate or amphetamine and vice versa

✻ Despite warnings, can be a useful adjunct to MAOIs for heroic treatment of highly refractory mood disorders when monitored with vigilance

✻ Can reverse sexual dysfunction caused by psychiatric illness and by some drugs such as SSRIs, including decreased libido, erectile dysfunction, delayed ejaculation, and anorgasmia

- Atypical antipsychotics may be useful in treating stimulant or psychotic consequences of overdose
- Half-life and duration of clinical action tend to be shorter in younger children
- Drug abuse may actually be lower in ADHD adolescents treated with stimulants than in ADHD adolescents who are not treated

Suggested Reading

Biederman J, Boellner SW, Childress A, et al. Lisdexamfetamine dimesylate and mixed amphetamine salts extended-release in children with ADHD: a double-blind, placebo-controlled, crossover analog classroom study. Biol Psychiatry 2007;62(9):970–6.

Biederman J, Krishnan S, Zhang Y, McGough JJ, Findling RL. Efficacy and tolerability of lisdexamfetamine dimesylate (NRP-104) in children with attention-deficit/hyperactivity disorder: a phase III, multicenter, randomized, double-blind, forced dose, parallel-group study. Clin Ther 2007;29(3):450–63.

THERAPEUTICS

Brands
- Eskalith
- Eskalith CR
- Lithobid slow-release tablets
- Lithostat tablets
- Lithium carbonate tablets
- Lithium citrate syrup

see index for additional brand names

Generic? Yes

Class
- Neuroscience-based Nomenclature: lithium enzyme interactions (Li-Eint)
- Mood stabilizer

Commonly Prescribed for
(bold for FDA approved)
- **Manic episodes of manic-depressive illness**
- **Maintenance treatment for manic-depressive patients with a history of mania**
- Bipolar depression
- Major depressive disorder (adjunctive)
- Vascular headache
- Neutropenia

How the Drug Works
- Unknown and complex
- Alters sodium transport across cell membranes in nerve and muscle cells
- Alters metabolism of neurotransmitters including catecholamines and serotonin

✻ May alter intracellular signaling through actions on second messenger systems
- Specifically, inhibits inositol monophosphatase, possibly affecting neurotransmission via phosphatidyl inositol second messenger system
- Also reduces protein kinase C activity, possibly affecting genomic expression associated with neurotransmission
- Increases cytoprotective proteins, activates signaling cascade utilized by endogenous growth factors, and increases gray matter content, possibly by activating neurogenesis and enhancing trophic actions that maintain synapses

How Long Until It Works
- 1–3 weeks

If It Works
- The goal of treatment is complete remission of symptoms (i.e., mania and/or depression)
- Continue treatment until all symptoms are gone or until improvement is stable and then continue treating indefinitely as long as improvement persists
- Continue treatment indefinitely to avoid recurrence of mania or depression

If It Doesn't Work

✻ Many patients have only a partial response where some symptoms are improved but others persist or continue to wax and wane without stabilization of mood
- Other patients may be nonresponders, sometimes called treatment-resistant or treatment-refractory
- Consider checking plasma drug level, increasing dose, switching to another agent or adding an appropriate augmenting agent
- Consider adding psychotherapy
- Consider the presence of noncompliance and counsel patient
- Switch to another mood stabilizer with fewer side effects
- Consider evaluation for another diagnosis or for a comorbid condition (e.g., medical illness, substance abuse, etc.)

Best Augmenting Combos for Partial Response or Treatment Resistance
- Valproate
- Atypical antipsychotics (especially risperidone, olanzapine, quetiapine, ziprasidone, and aripiprazole)
- Lamotrigine

✻ Antidepressants (with caution because antidepressants can destabilize mood in some patients, including induction of rapid cycling or suicidal ideation; in particular consider bupropion; also SSRIs, SNRIs, others; generally avoid TCAs, MAOIs)

Tests

✻ Before initiating treatment, kidney function tests (including creatinine and urine specific gravity) and thyroid function tests; electrocardiogram for patients over 50
- Repeat kidney function tests 1–2 times/year

* Frequent tests to monitor trough lithium plasma levels (about 12 hours after last dose; should generally be between 1.0 and 1.5 mEq/L for acute treatment, 0.6 and 1.2 mEq/L for chronic treatment)
* Initial monitoring: every 1–2 weeks until desired serum concentration is achieved, then every 2–3 months for the first 6 months
* Stable monitoring: every 6–12 months
* One-off monitoring after dose change, other medication change, illness change (not before 1 week)
* Since lithium is frequently associated with weight gain, before starting treatment, weigh all patients and determine if the patient is already overweight (BMI 25.0–29.9) or obese (BMI ≥30)
- Before giving a drug that can cause weight gain to an overweight or obese patient, consider determining whether the patient already has pre-diabetes (fasting plasma glucose 100–125 mg/dL), diabetes (fasting plasma glucose >126 mg/dL), or dyslipidemia (increased total cholesterol, LDL cholesterol, and triglycerides; decreased HDL cholesterol), and treat or refer such patients for treatment, including nutrition and weight management, physical activity counseling, smoking cessation, and medical management
* Monitor weight and BMI during treatment
* While giving a drug to a patient who has gained >5% of initial weight, consider evaluating for the presence of pre-diabetes, diabetes, or dyslipidemia, or consider switching to a different agent

SIDE EFFECTS

How Drug Causes Side Effects
- Unknown and complex
- CNS side effects theoretically due to excessive actions at the same or similar sites that mediate its therapeutic actions
- Some renal side effects theoretically due to lithium's actions on ion transport

Notable Side Effects
* Ataxia, dysarthria, delirium, tremor, memory problems
* Polyuria, polydipsia (nephrogenic diabetes insipidus)
* Diarrhea, nausea
* Weight gain
- Euthyroid goiter or hypothyroid goiter, possibly with increased TSH and reduced thyroxine levels
- Acne, rash, alopecia
- Leukocytosis
- Side effects are typically dose-related

Life-Threatening or Dangerous Side Effects
- Lithium toxicity
- Renal impairment (interstitial nephritis)
- Nephrogenic diabetes insipidus
- Arrhythmia, cardiovascular changes, sick sinus syndrome, bradycardia, hypotension
- T wave flattening and inversion
- Rare pseudotumor cerebri
- Rare seizures

Weight Gain

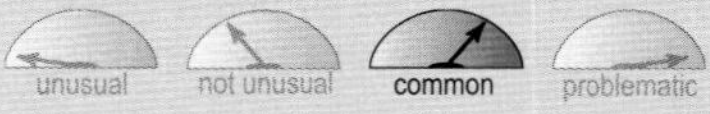

- Many experience and/or can be significant in amount
- Can become a health problem in some
- May be associated with increased appetite

Sedation

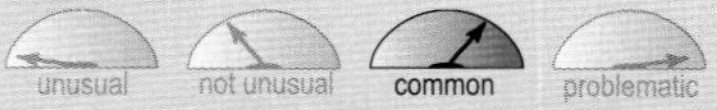

- Many experience and/or can be significant in amount
- May wear off with time

What to Do About Side Effects
- Wait
- Wait
- Wait
- Lower the dose
* Take entire dose at night as long as efficacy persists all day long with this administration
* Change to a different lithium preparation (e.g., controlled-release)
* Reduce dosing from 3 times/day to 2 times/day
- If signs of lithium toxicity occur, discontinue immediately
- For stomach upset, take with food
- For tremor, avoid caffeine
- Switch to another agent

Best Augmenting Agents for Side Effects

* ✻ Propranolol 20–30 mg 2–3 times/day may reduce tremor
* For the expert, cautious addition of a diuretic (e.g., chlorothiazide 50 mg/day) while reducing lithium dose by 50% and monitoring plasma lithium levels may reduce polydipsia and polyuria that does not go away with time alone
* Many side effects cannot be improved with an augmenting agent

DOSING AND USE

Usual Dosage Range

* Mania: recommended 1.0–1.5 mEq/L
* Depression: recommended 0.6–1.0 mEq/L
* Maintenance: recommended 0.7–1.0 mEq/L
* Liquid: 10 mL three times/day (acute mania); 5 mL 3–4 times/day (long-term)

Dosage Forms

* Tablet 300 mg (slow-release), 450 mg (controlled-release)
* Capsule 150 mg, 300 mg, 600 mg
* Liquid 8 mEq/5 mL

How to Dose

* Start 300 mg 2–3 times/day and adjust dosage upward as indicated by plasma lithium levels

Dosing Tips

* ✻ Sustained-release formulation may reduce gastric irritation, lower peak lithium plasma levels, and diminish peak dose side effects (i.e., side effects occurring 1–2 hours after each dose of standard lithium carbonate may be improved by sustained-release formulation)
* Lithium sulfate and other dosage strengths for lithium are available in Europe
* Check therapeutic blood levels as "trough" levels about 12 hours after the last dose
* After stabilization, some patients may do best with a once daily dose at night
* Responses in acute mania may take 7–14 days even with adequate plasma lithium levels
* ✻ Some patients apparently respond to doses as low as 300 mg twice a day, even with plasma lithium levels below 0.5 mEq/L
* Use the lowest dose of lithium associated with adequate therapeutic response
* Lower doses and lower plasma lithium levels (<0.6 mEq/L) are often adequate and advisable in the elderly
* ✻ Rapid discontinuation increases the risk of relapse and possibly suicide, so lithium may need to be tapered slowly over 3 months if it is to be discontinued after long-term maintenance

Overdose

* Fatalities have occurred; tremor, dysarthria, delirium, coma, seizures, autonomic instability

Long-Term Use

* Indicated for long-term prevention of relapse
* May cause reduced kidney function
* Requires regular therapeutic monitoring of lithium levels as well as of kidney function and thyroid function

Habit Forming

* No

How to Stop

* Taper gradually over 3 months to avoid relapse
* Rapid discontinuation increases the risk of relapse, and possibly suicide
* Discontinuation symptoms uncommon

Pharmacokinetics

* Half life 18–30 hours
* Lower absorption on empty stomach

Drug Interactions

* ✻ Non-steroidal anti-inflammatory agents, including ibuprofen and selective COX-2 inhibitors (cyclooxygenase 2), can <u>increase</u> plasma lithium concentrations; add with caution to patients stabilized on lithium
* ✻ Diuretics, especially thiazides, can <u>increase</u> plasma lithium concentrations; add with caution to patients stabilized on lithium
* Angiotensin-converting enzyme inhibitors can <u>increase</u> plasma lithium concentrations; add with caution to patients stabilized on lithium
* Metronidazole can lead to lithium toxicity through decreased renal clearance

- Acetazolamide, alkalizing agents, xanthine preparations, and urea may lower lithium plasma concentrations
- Methyldopa, carbamazepine, and phenytoin may interact with lithium to increase its toxicity
- Use lithium cautiously with calcium channel blockers, which may also increase lithium toxicity
- Use of lithium with an SSRI may raise risk of dizziness, confusion, diarrhea, agitation, tremor
- Some patients taking haloperidol and lithium have developed an encephalopathic syndrome similar to neuroleptic malignant syndrome
- Lithium may prolong effects of neuromuscular blocking agents
- No likely pharmacokinetic interactions of lithium with mood-stabilizing anticonvulsants or atypical antipsychotics

Other Warnings/ Precautions

❋ Toxic levels are near therapeutic levels; signs of toxicity include tremor, ataxia, diarrhea, vomiting, sedation
- Monitor for dehydration; lower dose if patient exhibits signs of infection, excessive sweating, diarrhea
- Closely monitor patients with thyroid disorders
- Lithium may cause unmasking of Brugada syndrome; consultation with a cardiologist is recommended if patients develop unexplained syncope or palpitations after starting lithium

Do Not Use

- If patient has severe kidney disease
- If patient has severe cardiovascular disease
- If patient has Brugada syndrome
- If patient has severe dehydration
- If patient has sodium depletion
- If there is a proven allergy to lithium

SPECIAL POPULATIONS

Renal Impairment

- Not recommended for use in patients with severe impairment
- Some experts recommend no dosing modification for glomerular filtration rate (GFR)>50 mL/min

Hepatic Impairment

- No special indications

Cardiac Impairment

- Not recommended for use in patients with severe impairment
- Lithium can cause reversible T-wave changes, sinus bradycardia, sick sinus syndrome, or heart block

Elderly

- Likely that elderly patients will require lower doses to achieve therapeutic serum levels
- Elderly patients may be more sensitive to adverse effects

❋ Neurotoxicity, including delirium and other mental status changes, may occur even at therapeutic doses in elderly and organically compromised patients
- Lower doses and lower plasma lithium levels (<0.6 mEg/L) are often adequate and advisable in the elderly

Children and Adolescents

- Safety and efficacy not established in children under age 12
- Use only with caution
- Younger children tend to have more frequent and severe side effects
- Children should be monitored more frequently

Pregnancy

- Effective June 30, 2015, the US FDA requires changes to the content and format of pregnancy and lactation information in prescription drug labels, including the elimination of the pregnancy letter categories; the Pregnancy and Lactation Labeling Rule (PLLR or final rule) applies only to prescription drugs and will be phased in gradually for drugs approved on or after June 30, 2001

❋ Evidence of increased risk of major birth defects (perhaps 2–3 times the general population), but probably lower than with some other mood stabilizers (e.g., valproate)
- Evidence of increase in cardiac anomalies (especially Ebstein's anomaly) in infants

whose mothers took lithium during pregnancy
- No long-term neurobehavioral effects of late-term neonatal lithium exposure have been observed
- If lithium is continued, monitor serum lithium levels every 4 weeks, then every week beginning at 36 weeks
- Dehydration due to morning sickness may cause rapid increases in lithium levels
- Lithium administration during delivery may be associated with hypotonia in the infant; most recommend withholding lithium for 24–48 hours before delivery
- Monitoring during delivery should include fluid balance
- After delivery, monitor for 48 hours for "floppy baby syndrome"
- Use in women of childbearing potential requires weighing potential benefits to the mother against the risks to the fetus
- Recurrent bipolar illness during pregnancy can be quite disruptive
- Taper drug if discontinuing
- Given the risk of bipolar relapse in the postpartum period, lithium should generally be restarted immediately after delivery
- This may mean no breast feeding, since lithium can be found in breast milk, possibly at full therapeutic levels

* Atypical antipsychotics may be preferable to lithium or anticonvulsants if treatment of bipolar disorder is required during pregnancy

- Bipolar symptoms may recur or worsen during pregnancy and some form of treatment may be necessary

Breast Feeding

- Some drug is found in mother's breast milk, possibly at full therapeutic levels since lithium is soluble in breast milk

* Recommended either to discontinue drug or bottle feed
* Bipolar disorder may recur during the postpartum period, particularly if there is a history of prior postpartum episodes of either depression or psychosis
* Relapse rates may be lower in women who receive prophylactic treatment for postpartum episodes of bipolar disorder

- Atypical antipsychotics and anticonvulsants such as valproate may be safer than lithium during the postpartum period when breast feeding

THE ART OF PSYCHOPHARMACOLOGY

Potential Advantages

- Euphoric mania
- Treatment-resistant depression
- Reduces suicide risk
- Works well in combination with atypical antipsychotics and/or mood-stabilizing anticonvulsants such as valproate

Potential Disadvantages

- Dysphoric mania
- Mixed mania, rapid-cycling mania
- Depressed phase of bipolar disorder
- Patients unable to tolerate weight gain, sedation, gastrointestinal effects, renal effects, and other side effects
- Requires blood monitoring

Primary Target Symptoms

- Unstable mood
- Mania

Pearls

* Lithium was the original mood stabilizer and is still a first-line treatment option but may be underutilized since it is an older agent and is less promoted for use in bipolar disorder than newer agents
* May be best for euphoric mania; patients with rapid-cycling and mixed state types of bipolar disorder generally do less well on lithium
* Seems to be more effective in treating manic episodes than depressive episodes in bipolar disorder (treats from above better than it treats from below)
* May also be more effective in preventing manic relapses than in preventing depressive episodes (stabilizes from above better than it stabilizes from below)
* May decrease suicide and suicide attempts not only in bipolar I disorder but also in bipolar II disorder and in unipolar depression
* Due to its narrow therapeutic index, lithium's toxic side effects occur at doses close to its therapeutic effects

- Close therapeutic monitoring of plasma drug levels is required during lithium treatment; lithium is the first psychiatric drug that required blood level monitoring
- Probably less effective than atypical antipsychotics for severe, excited,

disturbed, hyperactive, or psychotic patients with mania
- Due to delayed onset of action, lithium monotherapy may not be the first choice in acute mania, but rather may be used as an adjunct to atypical antipsychotics, benzodiazepines, and/or valproate loading
- After acute symptoms of mania are controlled, some patients can be maintained on lithium monotherapy
- However, only a third of bipolar patients experience adequate relief with a monotherapy, so most patients need multiple medications for best control
- Lithium is not a convincing augmentation agent to atypical antipsychotics for the treatment of schizophrenia
- Lithium is one of the most useful adjunctive agents to augment antidepressants for treatment-resistant unipolar depression
- Lithium may be useful for a number of patients with episodic, recurrent symptoms with or without affective illness, including episodic rage, anger or violence, and self-destructive behavior; such symptoms may be associated with psychotic or nonpsychotic illnesses, personality disorders, organic disorders, or mental retardation
- Lithium is better tolerated during acute manic phases than when manic symptoms have abated
- Adverse effects generally increase in incidence and severity as lithium serum levels increase
- Although not recommended for use in patients with severe renal or cardiovascular disease, dehydration, or sodium depletion, lithium can be administered cautiously in a hospital setting to such patients, with lithium serum levels determined daily
- Lithium-induced weight gain may be more common in women than in men

Suggested Reading

Baldessarini RJ, Tondo L, Davis P, et al. Decreased risk of suicides and attempts during long-term lithium treatment: a meta-analytic review. Bipolar Disord 2006;8(5 Pt 2):625–39.

Goodwin FK. Rationale for using lithium in combination with other mood stabilizers in the management of bipolar disorder. J Clin Psychiatry 2003;64(Suppl 5):S18–24.

Goodwin GM, Bowden CL, Calabrese JR, et al. A pooled analysis of 2 placebo-controlled 18-month trials of lamotrigine and lithium maintenance treatment in bipolar I disorder. J Clin Psychiatry 2004;65:432–41.

Malhi GS, Tanious M. Optimal frequency of lithium administration in the treatment of bipolar disorder: clinical and dosing considerations. CNS Drugs 2011;25(4):289–98.

Tueth MJ, Murphy TK, Evans DL. Special considerations: use of lithium in children, adolescents, and elderly populations. J Clin Psychiatry 1998;59(Suppl 6):S66–73.

THERAPEUTICS

Brands
- Deprimyl
- Gamanil

see index for additional brand names

Generic? Yes

Class
- Neuroscience-based Nomenclature: serotonin, norepinephrine reuptake inhibitor (SN-RI)
- Tricyclic antidepressant (TCA)
- Predominantly a norepinephrine/ noradrenaline reuptake inhibitor

Commonly Prescribed for
(bold for FDA approved)
- Major depressive disorder
- Anxiety
- Insomnia
- Neuropathic pain/chronic pain
- Treatment-resistant depression

How the Drug Works
- Boosts neurotransmitter norepinephrine/ noradrenaline
- Blocks norepinephrine reuptake pump (norepinephrine transporter), presumably increasing noradrenergic neurotransmission
- Since dopamine is inactivated by norepinephrine reuptake in frontal cortex, which largely lacks dopamine transporters, lofepramine can increase dopamine neurotransmission in this part of the brain
- A more potent inhibitor of norepinephrine reuptake pump than serotonin reuptake pump (serotonin transporter)
- At high doses may also boost neurotransmitter serotonin and presumably increase serotonergic neurotransmission

How Long Until It Works
- May have immediate effects in treating insomnia or anxiety
- Onset of therapeutic actions usually not immediate, but often delayed 2–4 weeks
- If it is not working within 6–8 weeks for depression, it may require a dosage increase or it may not work at all
- May continue to work for many years to prevent relapse of symptoms

If It Works
- The goal of treatment of depression is complete remission of current symptoms as well as prevention of future relapses
- The goal of treatment of chronic neuropathic pain is to reduce symptoms as much as possible, especially in combination with other treatments
- Treatment of depression most often reduces or even eliminates symptoms, but not a cure since symptoms can recur after medicine stopped
- Treatment of chronic neuropathic pain may reduce symptoms, but rarely eliminates them completely, and is not a cure since symptoms can recur after medicine is stopped
- Continue treatment of depression until all symptoms are gone (remission)
- Once symptoms of depression are gone, continue treating for 1 year for the first episode of depression
- For second and subsequent episodes of depression, treatment may need to be indefinite
- Use in anxiety disorders and chronic pain may also need to be indefinite, but long-term treatment is not well studied in these conditions

If It Doesn't Work
- Many depressed patients have only a partial response where some symptoms are improved but others persist (especially insomnia, fatigue, and problems concentrating)
- Other depressed patients may be nonresponders, sometimes called treatment-resistant or treatment-refractory
- Consider increasing dose, switching to another agent or adding an appropriate augmenting agent
- Consider psychotherapy
- Consider evaluation for another diagnosis or for a comorbid condition (e.g., medical illness, substance abuse, etc.)
- Some patients may experience apparent lack of consistent efficacy due to activation of latent or underlying bipolar disorder, and require antidepressant discontinuation and a switch to a mood stabilizer

Best Augmenting Combos for Partial Response or Treatment Resistance

- Lithium, buspirone, thyroid hormone (for depression)
- Gabapentin, tiagabine, other anticonvulsants, even opiates if done by experts while monitoring carefully in difficult cases (for chronic pain)

Tests

- Baseline ECG is recommended for patients over age 50

❋ Since tricyclic and tetracyclic antidepressants are frequently associated with weight gain, before starting treatment, weigh all patients and determine if the patient is already overweight (BMI 25.0–29.9) or obese (BMI ≥30)

- Before giving a drug that can cause weight gain to an overweight or obese patient, consider determining whether the patient already has pre-diabetes (fasting plasma glucose 100–125 mg/dL), diabetes (fasting plasma glucose >126 mg/dL), or dyslipidemia (increased total cholesterol, LDL cholesterol, and triglycerides; decreased HDL cholesterol), and treat or refer such patients for treatment, including nutrition and weight management, physical activity counseling, smoking cessation, and medical management

❋ Monitor weight and BMI during treatment

❋ While giving a drug to a patient who has gained >5% of initial weight, consider evaluating for the presence of pre-diabetes, diabetes, or dyslipidemia, or consider switching to a different antidepressant

- EKGs may be useful for selected patients (e.g., those with personal or family history of QTc prolongation; cardiac arrhythmia; recent myocardial infarction; uncompensated heart failure; or taking agents that prolong QTc interval such as pimozide, thioridazine, selected antiarrhythmics, moxifloxacin, sparfloxacin, etc.)
- Patients at risk for electrolyte disturbances (e.g., patients on diuretic therapy) should have baseline and periodic serum potassium and magnesium measurements

SIDE EFFECTS

How Drug Causes Side Effects

- Anticholinergic activity may explain sedative effects, dry mouth, constipation, and blurred vision
- Sedative effects and weight gain may be due to antihistamine properties
- Blockade of alpha adrenergic 1 receptors may explain dizziness, sedation, and hypotension
- Cardiac arrhythmias and seizures, especially in overdose, may be caused by blockade of ion channels

Notable Side Effects

- Blurred vision, constipation, urinary retention, increased appetite, dry mouth, nausea, diarrhea, heartburn, unusual taste in mouth, weight gain
- Fatigue, weakness, dizziness, sedation, headache, anxiety, nervousness, restlessness
- Sexual dysfunction, sweating

Life-Threatening or Dangerous Side Effects

- Paralytic ileus, hyperthermia (TCAs + anticholinergic agents)
- Lowered seizure threshold and rare seizures
- Orthostatic hypotension, sudden death, arrhythmias, tachycardia
- QTc prolongation
- Hepatic failure, extrapyramidal symptoms
- Increased intraocular pressure
- Rare induction of mania
- Rare activation of suicidal ideation and behavior (suicidality) (short-term studies did not show an increase in the risk of suicidality with antidepressants compared to placebo beyond age 24)

Weight Gain

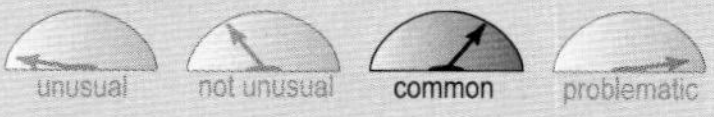

- Many experience and/or can be significant in amount
- Can increase appetite and carbohydrate craving

Sedation

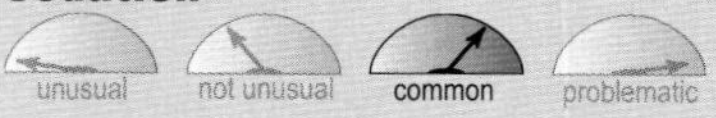

- Many experience and/or can be significant in amount
- Tolerance to sedative effect may develop with long-term use

What to Do About Side Effects

- Wait
- Wait
- Wait
- Lower the dose
- Switch to an SSRI or newer antidepressant

Best Augmenting Agents for Side Effects

- Many side effects cannot be improved with an augmenting agent

DOSING AND USE

Usual Dosage Range

- 140–210 mg/day

Dosage Forms

- Tablet 70 mg multiscored
- Liquid 70 mg/5mL

How to Dose

- Initial 70 mg/day once daily or in divided doses; gradually increase daily dose to achieve desired therapeutic effects; dose at bedtime for daytime sedation and in morning for insomnia; maximum dose 280 mg/day for inpatients, 210 mg/day for outpatients

Dosing Tips

- If given in a single dose, should generally be administered at bedtime because of its sedative properties
- If given in split doses, largest dose should generally be given at bedtime because of its sedative properties
- If patients experience nightmares, split dose and do not give large dose at bedtime
- Unusual dose compared to most TCAs
- Patients treated for chronic pain may only require lower doses
- If intolerable anxiety, insomnia, agitation, akathisia, or activation occur either upon dosing initiation or discontinuation, consider the possibility of activated bipolar disorder, and switch to a mood stabilizer or an atypical antipsychotic

Overdose

- Death may occur; convulsions, cardiac dysrhythmias, severe hypotension, CNS depression, coma, changes in EKG

Long-Term Use

- Safe

Habit Forming

- No

How to Stop

- Taper to avoid withdrawal effects
- Even with gradual dose reduction some withdrawal symptoms may appear within the first 2 weeks
- Many patients tolerate 50% dose reduction for 3 days, then another 50% reduction for 3 days, then discontinuation
- If withdrawal symptoms emerge during discontinuation, raise dose to stop symptoms and then restart withdrawal much more slowly

Pharmacokinetics

- Substrate for CYP450 2D6
- Half-life of parent compound approximately 1.5–6 hours

* Major metabolite is the antidepressant desipramine, with a half-life of approximately 24 hours

Drug Interactions

- Tramadol increases the risk of seizures in patients taking TCAs
- Use of TCAs with anticholinergic drugs may result in paralytic ileus or hyperthermia
- Fluoxetine, paroxetine, bupropion, duloxetine, and other CYP450 2D6 inhibitors may increase TCA concentrations
- Cimetidine may increase plasma concentrations of TCAs and cause anticholinergic symptoms
- Phenothiazines or haloperidol may raise TCA blood concentrations
- May alter effects of antihypertensive drugs; may inhibit hypotensive effects of clonidine
- Use with sympathomimetic agents may increase sympathetic activity

- Methylphenidate may inhibit metabolism of TCAs
- Activation and agitation, especially following switching or adding antidepressants, may represent the induction of a bipolar state, especially a mixed dysphoric bipolar II condition sometimes associated with suicidal ideation, and require the addition of lithium, a mood stabilizer or an atypical antipsychotic, and/or discontinuation of lofepramine

Other Warnings/ Precautions

- Add or initiate other antidepressants with caution for up to 2 weeks after discontinuing lofepramine
- Generally, do not use with MAOIs, including 14 days after MAOIs are stopped; do not start an MAOI for at least 5 half-lives (5 to 7 days for most drugs) after discontinuing lofepramine, but see Pearls
- Use with caution in patients with history of seizure, urinary retention, angle-closure glaucoma, hyperthyroidism
- TCAs can increase QTc interval, especially at toxic doses, which can be attained not only by overdose but also by combining with drugs that inhibit its metabolism via CYP450 2D6, potentially causing torsade de pointes-type arrhythmia or sudden death
- Because TCAs can prolong QTc interval, use with caution in patients who have bradycardia or who are taking drugs that can induce bradycardia (e.g., beta blockers, calcium channel blockers, clonidine, digitalis)
- Because TCAs can prolong QTc interval, use with caution in patients who have hypokalemia and/or hypomagnesemia or who are taking drugs that can induce hypokalemia and/or magnesemia (e.g., diuretics, stimulant laxatives, intravenous amphotericin B, glucocorticoids, tetracosactide)
- When treating children, carefully weigh the risks and benefits of pharmacological treatment against the risks and benefits of nontreatment with antidepressants and make sure to document this in the patient's chart
- Distribute the brochures provided by the FDA and the drug companies
- Warn patients and their caregivers about the possibility of activating side effects and advise them to report such symptoms immediately
- Monitor patients for activation of suicidal ideation, especially children and adolescents

Do Not Use

- If patient is recovering from myocardial infarction
- If patient is taking agents capable of significantly prolonging QTc interval (e.g., pimozide, thioridazine, selected antiarrhythmics, moxifloxacin, sparfloxacin)
- If there is a history of QTc prolongation or cardiac arrhythmia, recent acute myocardial infarction, uncompensated heart failure
- If patient is taking drugs that inhibit TCA metabolism, including CYP450 2D6 inhibitors, except by an expert
- If there is reduced CYP450 2D6 function, such as patients who are poor 2D6 metabolizers, except by an expert and at low doses
- If there is a proven allergy to lofepramine, desipramine, or imipramine

SPECIAL POPULATIONS

Renal Impairment

- Use with caution

Hepatic Impairment

- Use with caution

Cardiac Impairment

- Baseline ECG is recommended
- TCAs have been reported to cause arrhythmias, prolongation of conduction time, orthostatic hypotension, sinus tachycardia, and heart failure, especially in the diseased heart
- Myocardial infarction and stroke have been reported with TCAs
- TCAs produce QTc prolongation, which may be enhanced by the existence of bradycardia, hypokalemia, congenital or acquired long QTc interval, which should be evaluated prior to administering lofepramine

- Use with caution if treating concomitantly with a medication likely to produce prolonged bradycardia, hypokalemia, slowing of intracardiac conduction, or prolongation of the QTc interval
- Avoid TCAs in patients with a known history of QTc prolongation, recent acute myocardial infarction, and uncompensated heart failure
- TCAs may cause a sustained increase in heart rate in patients with ischemic heart disease and may worsen (decrease) heart rate variability, an independent risk of mortality in cardiac populations
- Since SSRIs may improve (increase) heart rate variability in patients following a myocardial infarct and may improve survival as well as mood in patients with acute angina or following a myocardial infarction, these are more appropriate agents for cardiac population than tricyclic/tetracyclic antidepressants

✻ Risk/benefit ratio may not justify use of TCAs in cardiac impairment

Elderly

- Baseline ECG is recommended for patients over age 50
- May be more sensitive to anticholinergic, cardiovascular, hypotensive, and sedative effects
- Reduction in the risk of suicidality with antidepressants compared to placebo in adults age 65 and older

Children and Adolescents

- Carefully weigh the risks and benefits of pharmacological treatment against the risks and benefits of nontreatment with antidepressants and make sure to document this in the patient's chart
- Monitor patients face-to-face regularly, particularly during the first several weeks of treatment
- Use with caution, observing for activation of known or unknown bipolar disorder and/or suicidal ideation, and inform parents or guardians of this risk so they can help observe child or adolescent patients
- Not recommended for use under age 18
- Several studies show lack of efficacy of TCAs for depression
- May be used to treat enuresis or hyperactive/impulsive behaviors
- Some cases of sudden death have occurred in children taking TCAs

Pregnancy

- Effective June 30, 2015, the US FDA requires changes to the content and format of pregnancy and lactation information in prescription drug labels, including the elimination of the pregnancy letter categories; the Pregnancy and Lactation Labeling Rule (PLLR or final rule) applies only to prescription drugs and will be phased in gradually for drugs approved on or after June 30, 2001
- Crosses the placenta
- Adverse effects have been reported in infants whose mothers took a TCA (lethargy, withdrawal symptoms, fetal malformations)
- Not generally recommended for use during pregnancy, especially during first trimester
- Must weigh the risk of treatment (first trimester fetal development, third trimester newborn delivery) to the child against the risk of no treatment (recurrence of depression, maternal health, infant bonding) to the mother and child
- For many patients this may mean continuing treatment during pregnancy

Breast Feeding

- Some drug is found in mother's breast milk

✻ Recommended either to discontinue drug or bottle feed

- Immediate postpartum period is a high-risk time for depression, especially in women who have had prior depressive episodes, so drug may need to be reinstituted late in the third trimester or shortly after childbirth to prevent a recurrence during the postpartum period
- Must weigh benefits of breast feeding with risks and benefits of antidepressant treatment versus nontreatment to both the infant and the mother
- For many patients this may mean continuing treatment during breast feeding

THE ART OF PSYCHOPHARMACOLOGY

Potential Advantages

- Patients with insomnia
- Severe or treatment-resistant depression
- Anxious depression

Potential Disadvantages
- Pediatric and geriatric patients
- Patients concerned with weight gain
- Cardiac patients

Primary Target Symptoms
- Depressed mood

Pearls
- TCAs are often a first-line treatment option for chronic pain
- TCAs are no longer generally considered a first-line option for depression because of their side effect profile
- TCAs continue to be useful for severe or treatment-resistant depression
- Noradrenergic reuptake inhibitors such as lofepramine can be used as a second-line treatment for smoking cessation, cocaine dependence, and attention deficit disorder
- * Lofepramine is a short-acting prodrug of the TCA desipramine
- * Fewer anticholinergic side effects, particularly sedation, than some other tricyclics
- Once a popular TCA in the UK but not widely marketed throughout the world
- TCAs may aggravate psychotic symptoms
- Alcohol should be avoided because of additive CNS effects
- Underweight patients may be more susceptible to adverse cardiovascular effects
- Children, patients with inadequate hydration, and patients with cardiac disease may be more susceptible to TCA-induced cardiotoxicity than healthy adults
- For the expert only: although generally prohibited, a heroic treatment (but potentially dangerous) for severely treatment-resistant patients is to give a tricyclic/tetracyclic antidepressant other than clomipramine simultaneously with an MAOI for patients who fail to respond to numerous other antidepressants
- If this option is elected, start the MAOI with the tricyclic/tetracyclic antidepressant simultaneously at low doses after appropriate drug washout, then alternately increase doses of these agents every few days to a week as tolerated
- Although very strict dietary and concomitant drug restrictions must be observed to prevent hypertensive crises and serotonin syndrome, the most common side effects of MAOI/tricyclic or tetracyclic combinations may be weight gain and orthostatic hypotension
- Patients on TCAs should be aware that they may experience symptoms such as photosensitivity or blue-green urine
- SSRIs may be more effective than TCAs in women, and TCAs may be more effective than SSRIs in men
- Since tricyclic/tetracyclic antidepressants are substrates for CYP450 2D6, and 7% of the population (especially Caucasians) may have a genetic variant leading to reduced activity of 2D6, such patients may not safely tolerate normal doses of tricyclic/tetracyclic antidepressants and may require dose reduction
- Phenotypic testing may be necessary to detect this genetic variant prior to dosing with a tricyclic/tetracyclic antidepressant, especially in vulnerable populations such as children, elderly, cardiac populations, and those on concomitant medications
- Patients who seem to have extraordinarily severe side effects at normal or low doses may have this phenotypic CYP450 2D6 variant and require low doses or switching to another antidepressant not metabolized by 2D6

Suggested Reading

Anderson IM. Meta-analytical studies on new antidepressants. Br Med Bull 2001;57:161–78.

Anderson IM. Selective serotonin reuptake inhibitors versus tricyclic antidepressants: a meta-analysis of efficacy and tolerability. J Aff Disorders 2000;58:19–36.

Kerihuel JC, Dreyfus JF. Meta-analyses of the efficacy and tolerability of the tricyclic antidepressant lofepramine. J Int Med Res 1991;19:183–201.

Lancaster SG, Gonzales JP. Lofepramine. A review of its pharmacodynamic and pharmacokinetic properties, and therapeutic efficacy in depressive illness. Drugs 1989;37:123–40.

THERAPEUTICS

Brands • Meilax

see index for additional brand names

Generic? No

Class

- Benzodiazepine (anxiolytic)

Commonly Prescribed for

(bold for FDA approved)

- Anxiety, tension, depression, or sleep disorder in patients with neurosis
- Anxiety, tension, depression, or sleep disorder in patients with psychosomatic disease
- Catatonia

How the Drug Works

- Binds to benzodiazepine receptors at the GABA-A ligand-gated chloride channel complex
- Enhances the inhibitory effects of GABA
- Boosts chloride conductance through GABA-regulated channels
- Inhibits neuronal activity presumably in amygdala-centered fear circuits to provide therapeutic benefits in anxiety disorders

How Long Until It Works

- Some immediate relief with first dosing is common; can take several weeks with daily dosing for maximal therapeutic benefit

If It Works

- For short-term symptoms of anxiety – after a few weeks, discontinue use or use on an "as-needed" basis
- For chronic anxiety disorders, the goal of treatment is complete remission of symptoms as well as prevention of future relapses
- For chronic anxiety disorders, treatment most often reduces or even eliminates symptoms, but not a cure since symptoms can recur after medicine stopped
- For long-term symptoms of anxiety, consider switching to an SSRI or SNRI for long-term maintenance
- If long-term maintenance with a benzodiazepine is necessary, continue treatment for 6 months after symptoms resolve, and then taper dose slowly
- If symptoms reemerge, consider treatment with an SSRI or SNRI, or consider restarting the benzodiazepine; sometimes benzodiazepines have to be used in combination with SSRIs or SNRIs for best results

If It Doesn't Work

- Consider switching to another agent or adding an appropriate augmenting agent
- Consider psychotherapy, especially cognitive behavioral psychotherapy
- Consider presence of concomitant substance abuse
- Consider presence of loflazepate abuse
- Consider another diagnosis, such as a comorbid medical condition

Best Augmenting Combos for Partial Response or Treatment Resistance

- Benzodiazepines are frequently used as augmenting agents for antipsychotics and mood stabilizers in the treatment of psychotic and bipolar disorders
- Benzodiazepines are frequently used as augmenting agents for SSRIs and SNRIs in the treatment of anxiety disorders
- Not generally rational to combine with other benzodiazepines
- Caution if using as an anxiolytic concomitantly with other sedative hypnotics for sleep

Tests

- In patients with seizure disorders, concomitant medical illness, and/or those with multiple concomitant long-term medications, periodic liver tests and blood counts may be prudent

SIDE EFFECTS

How Drug Causes Side Effects

- Same mechanism for side effects as for therapeutic effects – namely due to excessive actions at benzodiazepine receptors
- Long-term adaptations in benzodiazepine receptors may explain the development of dependence, tolerance, and withdrawal

- Side effects are generally immediate, but immediate side effects often disappear in time

Notable Side Effects

✱ Sedation, fatigue, depression
✱ Dizziness, ataxia, slurred speech, weakness
✱ Forgetfulness, confusion
✱ Hyperexcitability, nervousness
- Rare hallucinations, mania
- Rare hypotension
- Hypersalivation, dry mouth

Life-Threatening or Dangerous Side Effects

- Respiratory depression, especially when taken with CNS depressants in overdose
- Rare hepatic dysfunction, renal dysfunction, blood dyscrasias

Weight Gain

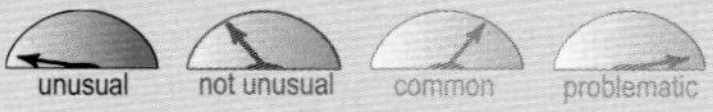

- Reported but not expected

Sedation

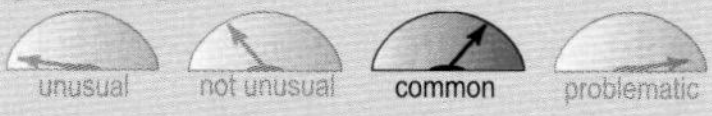

- Occurs in significant minority
- Especially at initiation of treatment or when dose increases
- Tolerance often develops over time

What to Do About Side Effects

- Wait
- Wait
- Wait
- Lower the dose
- Take largest dose at bedtime to avoid sedative effects during the day
- Switch to another agent
- Administer flumazenil if side effects are severe or life-threatening

Best Augmenting Agents for Side Effects

- Many side effects cannot be improved with an augmenting agent

DOSING AND USE

Usual Dosage Range

- 1 mg once or twice a day

Dosage Forms

- Tablet 1 mg, 2 mg

How to Dose

- Start at 1 mg, increase to 1 mg twice/day or 2 mg once a day in a few days if necessary

Dosing Tips

✱ Because of its long half-life, patients who require chronic treatment may need dose reduction after a few weeks due to drug accumulation
✱ Because of its long half-life, once daily dosing is the most frequent dosing generally necessary
✱ Because of its long half-life, some patients may have sustained benefits even if dosing is intermittently skipped on some days
- Use lowest possible effective dose for the shortest possible period of time (a benzodiazepine-sparing strategy)
- Assess need for continued treatment regularly
- Risk of dependence may increase with dose and duration of treatment
- For interdose symptoms of anxiety, can either increase dose or maintain same total daily dose but divide into more frequent doses
- Can also use an as-needed occasional “top up” dose for interdose anxiety
- Because panic disorder can require doses higher than 2 mg/day, the risk of dependence may be greater in these patients
- Some severely ill patients may require more than 2 mg/day
- Frequency of dosing in practice is often greater than predicted from half-life, as duration of biological activity is often shorter than pharmacokinetic terminal half-life, which is why once daily dosing is usually the favored option despite the long half-life

Overdose

- Sedation, confusion, poor coordination, diminished reflexes, coma

Long-Term Use

- Risk of dependence, particularly for treatment periods longer than 12 weeks and especially in patients with past or current polysubstance abuse

Habit Forming

- Patients may develop dependence and/or tolerance with long-term use

How to Stop

- Patients with history of seizures may seize upon withdrawal, especially if withdrawal is abrupt
- Taper by 0.5 mg every 3–7 days to reduce chances of withdrawal effects
- For difficult to taper cases, consider reducing dose much more slowly after reaching 3 mg/day, perhaps by as little as 0.25 mg every 7–10 days or slower
- For other patients with severe problems discontinuing a benzodiazepine, dosing may need to be tapered over many months (i.e., reduce dose by 1% every 3 days by crushing tablet and suspending or dissolving in 100 mL of fruit juice and then disposing of 1 mL while drinking the rest; 3–7 days later, dispose of 2 mL, and so on). This is both a form of very slow biological tapering and a form of behavioral desensitization
- Be sure to differentiate reemergence of symptoms requiring reinstitution of treatment from withdrawal symptoms
- Benzodiazepine-dependent anxiety patients and insulin-dependent diabetics are not addicted to their medications. When benzodiazepine-dependent patients stop their medication, disease symptoms can reemerge, disease symptoms can worsen (rebound), and/or withdrawal symptoms can emerge

Pharmacokinetics

- Elimination half-life approximately 122 hours (ultra-long half-life)

Drug Interactions

- Increased depressive effects when taken with other CNS depressants (see Warnings below)
- Cimetidine raises loflazepate plasma levels
- Rapid dose reduction or discontinuation of loflazepate during concomitant use with tetracyclic antidepressants such as maprotiline may result in convulsive seizures, possibly due to the loss of anticonvulsant actions that suppress the proconvulsant actions of tetracyclic antidepressants

Other Warnings/ Precautions

- Boxed warning regarding the increased risk of CNS depressant effects when benzodiazepines and opioid medications are used together, including specifically the risk of slowed or difficulty breathing and death
- If alternatives to the combined use of benzodiazepines and opioids are not available, clinicians should limit the dosage and duration of each drug to the minimum possible while still achieving therapeutic efficacy
- Patients and their caregivers should be warned to seek medical attention if unusual dizziness, lightheadedness, sedation, slowed or difficulty breathing, or unresponsiveness occur
- Dosage changes should be made in collaboration with prescriber
- Use with caution in patients with pulmonary disease; rare reports of death after initiation of benzodiazepines in patients with severe pulmonary impairment
- History of drug or alcohol abuse often creates greater risk for dependency
- Hypomania and mania have occurred in depressed patients taking loflazepate
- Use only with extreme caution if patient has obstructive sleep apnea
- Some depressed patients may experience a worsening of suicidal ideation
- Some patients may exhibit abnormal thinking or behavioral changes similar to those caused by other CNS depressants (i.e., either depressant actions or disinhibiting actions)

Do Not Use

- If patient has angle-closure glaucoma
- If patient has myasthenia gravis
- If there is a proven allergy to loflazepate or any benzodiazepine

SPECIAL POPULATIONS

Renal Impairment
- Drug should be used with caution

Hepatic Impairment
- Drug should be used with caution

Cardiac Impairment
- Benzodiazepines have been used to treat anxiety associated with acute myocardial infarction

Elderly
- Drug should be used with caution
- Should begin with lower starting dose

Children and Adolescents
- Safety and efficacy have not been established
- Benzodiazepines are often used in children and adolescents, especially short-term and at the lower end of the dosing scale
- Long-term effects of loflazepate in children/adolescents are unknown
- Should generally receive lower doses and be more closely monitored

Pregnancy
- Possible increased risk of birth defects when benzodiazepines taken during pregnancy
- Because of the potential risks, loflazepate is not generally recommended as treatment for anxiety during pregnancy, especially during the first trimester
- Drug should be tapered if discontinued
- Infants whose mothers received a benzodiazepine late in pregnancy may experience withdrawal effects
- Neonatal flaccidity has been reported in infants whose mothers took a benzodiazepine during pregnancy
- Seizures, even mild seizures, may cause harm to the embryo/fetus

Breast Feeding
- Some drug is found in mother's breast milk

✽ Recommended either to discontinue drug or bottle feed
- Effects on infant have been observed and include feeding difficulties, sedation, and weight loss

THE ART OF PSYCHOPHARMACOLOGY

Potential Advantages
- Patients who have interdose anxiety on shorter-acting benzodiazepines
- Patients who wish to take drug only once daily
- Patients who occasionally forget to take their dose

Potential Disadvantages
- Drug may accumulate in long-term users and require dosage reduction

Primary Target Symptoms
- Anxiety
- Tension

Pearls
✽ Is the only "ultra-long half-life" benzodiazepine with a half-life much longer than 24 hours

✽ Less interdose anxiety than other benzodiazepines

✽ Long half-life could theoretically reduce abuse and withdrawal symptoms
- Is a very useful adjunct to SSRIs and SNRIs in the treatment of numerous anxiety disorders
- Not effective for treating psychosis as a monotherapy, but can be used as an adjunct to antipsychotics
- Not effective for treating bipolar disorder as a monotherapy, but can be used as an adjunct to mood stabilizers and antipsychotics
- May both cause depression and treat depression in different patients
- Risk of seizure is greatest during the first 3 days after discontinuation of loflazepate, especially in those with prior seizures, head injuries or withdrawal from drugs of abuse
- Clinical duration of action may be shorter than plasma half-life, leading to dosing more frequently than 2–3 times daily in some patients
- When using to treat insomnia, remember that insomnia may be a symptom of some other primary disorder itself, and thus warrant evaluation for comorbid psychiatric and/or medical conditions
- Though not systematically studied, benzodiazepines have been used effectively to treat catatonia and are the initial recommended treatment

Suggested Reading

Ba BB, Iliadis A, Cano JP. Pharmacokinetic modeling of ethyl loflazepate (Victan) and its main active metabolites. Ann Biomed Eng 1989;17(6):633–46.

Chambon JP, Perio A, Demarne H, et al. Ethyl loflazepate: a prodrug from the benzodiazepine series designed to dissociate anxiolytic and sedative activities. Arzneimittelforschung 1985;35(10):1573–7.

Murasaki M, Mori A, Noguchi T, et al. Comparison of therapeutic efficacy of neuroses between CM6912 (ethyl loflazepate) and diazepam in a double-blind trial. Prog Neuropsychopharmacol Biol Psychiatry 1989;13(1–2):145–54.

THERAPEUTICS

Brands • Ativan

see index for additional brand names

Generic? Yes

Class

- Neuroscience-based Nomenclature: GABA positive allosteric modulator (GABA-PAM)
- Benzodiazepine (anxiolytic, anticonvulsant)

Commonly Prescribed for

(bold for FDA approved)

- **Anxiety disorder (oral)**
- **Anxiety associated with depressive symptoms (oral)**
- **Initial treatment of status epilepticus (injection)**
- **Preanesthetic (injection)**
- Insomnia
- Muscle spasm
- Alcohol withdrawal psychosis
- Headache
- Panic disorder
- Acute mania (adjunctive)
- Acute psychosis (adjunctive)
- Delirium (with haloperidol)
- Catatonia

How the Drug Works

- Binds to benzodiazepine receptors at the GABA-A ligand-gated chloride channel complex
- Enhances the inhibitory effects of GABA
- Boosts chloride conductance through GABA-regulated channels
- Inhibits neuronal activity presumably in amygdala-centered fear circuits to provide therapeutic benefits in anxiety disorders
- Inhibitory actions in cerebral cortex may provide therapeutic benefits in seizure disorders

How Long Until It Works

- Some immediate relief with first dosing is common; can take several weeks for maximal therapeutic benefit with daily dosing

If It Works

- For short-term symptoms of anxiety – after a few weeks, discontinue use or use on an "as-needed" basis
- For chronic anxiety disorders, the goal of treatment is complete remission of symptoms as well as prevention of future relapses
- For chronic anxiety disorders, treatment most often reduces or even eliminates symptoms, but not a cure since symptoms can recur after medicine stopped
- For long-term symptoms of anxiety, consider switching to an SSRI or SNRI for long-term maintenance
- If long-term maintenance with a benzodiazepine is necessary, continue treatment for 6 months after symptoms resolve, and then taper dose slowly
- If symptoms reemerge, consider treatment with an SSRI or SNRI, or consider restarting the benzodiazepine; sometimes benzodiazepines have to be used in combination with SSRIs or SNRIs for best results

If It Doesn't Work

- Consider switching to another agent or adding an appropriate augmenting agent
- Consider psychotherapy, especially cognitive behavioral psychotherapy
- Consider presence of concomitant substance abuse
- Consider presence of lorazepam abuse
- Consider another diagnosis such as a comorbid medical condition

Best Augmenting Combos for Partial Response or Treatment Resistance

- Benzodiazepines are frequently used as augmenting agents for antipsychotics and mood stabilizers in the treatment of psychotic and bipolar disorders
- Benzodiazepines are frequently used as augmenting agents for SSRIs and SNRIs in the treatment of anxiety disorders
- Not generally rational to combine with other benzodiazepines
- Caution if using as an anxiolytic concomitantly with other sedative hypnotics for sleep

Tests

- In patients with seizure disorders, concomitant medical illness, and/or those with multiple concomitant long-term medications, periodic liver tests and blood counts may be prudent

SIDE EFFECTS

How Drug Causes Side Effects
- Same mechanism for side effects as for therapeutic effects – namely due to excessive actions at benzodiazepine receptors
- Long-term adaptations in benzodiazepine receptors may explain the development of dependence, tolerance, and withdrawal
- Side effects are generally immediate, but immediate side effects often disappear in time

Notable Side Effects
✽ Sedation, fatigue, depression
✽ Dizziness, ataxia, slurred speech, weakness
✽ Forgetfulness, confusion
✽ Hyperexcitability, nervousness
✽ Pain at injection site
- Rare hallucinations, mania
- Rare hypotension
- Hypersalivation, dry mouth

Life-Threatening or Dangerous Side Effects
- Respiratory depression, especially when taken with CNS depressants in overdose
- Rare hepatic dysfunction, renal dysfunction, blood dyscrasias

Weight Gain
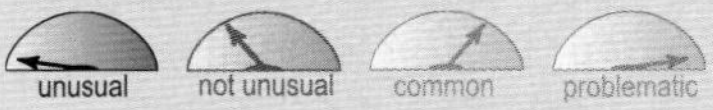

- Reported but not expected

Sedation
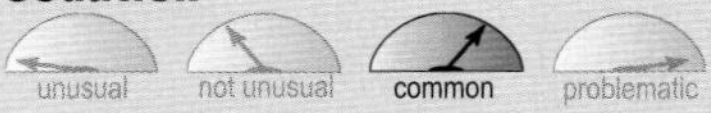

- Many experience and/or can be significant in amount
- Especially at initiation of treatment or when dose increases
- Tolerance often develops over time

What to Do About Side Effects
- Wait
- Wait
- Wait
- Lower the dose
- Take largest dose at bedtime to avoid sedative effects during the day
- Switch to another agent
- Administer flumazenil if side effects are severe or life-threatening

Best Augmenting Agents for Side Effects
- Many side effects cannot be improved with an augmenting agent

DOSING AND USE

Usual Dosage Range
- Oral: 2–6 mg/day in divided doses, largest dose at bedtime
- Injection: 4 mg administered slowly
- Catatonia: 1–2 mg per dose

Dosage Forms
- Tablet 0.5 mg, 1 mg, 2 mg
- Liquid 0.5 mg/5mL, 2 mg/mL
- Injection 1 mg/0.5mL, 2 mg/mL, 4 mg/mL

How to Dose
- Oral: initial 2–3 mg/day in 2–3 doses; increase as needed, starting with evening dose; maximum generally 10 mg/day
- Injection: initial 4 mg administered slowly; after 10–15 minutes may administer again
- Take liquid formulation with water, soda, applesauce, or pudding
- Catatonia: initial 1–2 mg; can repeat in 3 hours and then again in another 3 hours if necessary

Dosing Tips
✽ One of the few benzodiazepines available in an oral liquid formulation
✽ One of the few benzodiazepines available in an injectable formulation
- Lorazepam injection is intended for acute use; patients who require long-term treatment should be switched to the oral formulation
- Use lowest possible effective dose for the shortest possible period of time (a benzodiazepine-sparing strategy)
- Assess need for continued treatment regularly
- Risk of dependence may increase with dose and duration of treatment
- For interdose symptoms of anxiety, can either increase dose or maintain same total daily dose but divide into more frequent doses

- Can also use an as-needed occasional "top up" dose for interdose anxiety
- Because panic disorder can require doses higher than 6 mg/day, the risk of dependence may be greater in these patients
- Some severely ill patients may require 10 mg/day or more
- Frequency of dosing in practice is often greater than predicted from half-life, as duration of biological activity is often shorter than pharmacokinetic terminal half-life

Overdose

- Fatalities can occur; hypotension, tiredness, ataxia, confusion, coma

Long-Term Use

- Evidence of efficacy up to 16 weeks
- Risk of dependence, particularly for treatment periods longer than 12 weeks and especially in patients with past or current polysubstance abuse

Habit Forming

- Lorazepam is a Schedule IV drug
- Patients may develop dependence and/or tolerance with long-term use

How to Stop

- Patients with history of seizure may seize upon withdrawal, especially if withdrawal is abrupt
- Taper by 0.5 mg every 3 days to reduce chances of withdrawal effects
- For difficult to taper cases, consider reducing dose much more slowly once reaching 3 mg/day, perhaps by as little as 0.25 mg per week or less
- For other patients with severe problems discontinuing a benzodiazepine, dosing may need to be tapered over many months (i.e., reduce dose by 1% every 3 days by crushing tablet and suspending or dissolving in 100 mL of fruit juice and then disposing of 1 mL while drinking the rest; 3–7 days later, dispose of 2 mL, and so on). This is both a form of very slow biological tapering and a form of behavioral desensitization
- Be sure to differentiate reemergence of symptoms requiring reinstitution of treatment from withdrawal symptoms
- Benzodiazepine-dependent anxiety patients and insulin-dependent diabetics are not addicted to their medications. When benzodiazepine-dependent patients stop their medication, disease symptoms can reemerge, disease symptoms can worsen (rebound), and/or withdrawal symptoms can emerge

Pharmacokinetics

- Elimination half-life 10–20 hours
- No active metabolites
- Food does not affect absorption

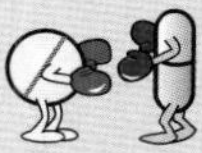

Drug Interactions

- Increased depressive effects when taken with other CNS depressants (see Warnings below)
- Valproate and probenecid may reduce clearance and raise plasma concentrations of lorazepam
- Oral contraceptives may increase clearance and lower plasma concentrations of lorazepam
- Flumazenil (used to reverse the effects of benzodiazepines) may precipitate seizures and should not be used in patients treated for seizure disorders with lorazepam

Other Warnings/ Precautions

- Boxed warning regarding the increased risk of CNS depressant effects when benzodiazepines and opioid medications are used together, including specifically the risk of slowed or difficulty breathing and death
- If alternatives to the combined use of benzodiazepines and opioids are not available, clinicians should limit the dosage and duration of each drug to the minimum possible while still achieving therapeutic efficacy
- Patients and their caregivers should be warned to seek medical attention if unusual dizziness, lightheadedness, sedation, slowed or difficulty breathing, or unresponsiveness occur
- Dosage changes should be made in collaboration with prescriber
- Use with caution in patients with pulmonary disease; rare reports of death after initiation of benzodiazepines in patients with severe pulmonary impairment

- History of drug or alcohol abuse often creates greater risk for dependency
- Use oral formulation only with extreme caution if patient has obstructive sleep apnea; injection is contraindicated in patients with sleep apnea
- Some depressed patients may experience a worsening of suicidal ideation
- Some patients may exhibit abnormal thinking or behavioral changes similar to those caused by other CNS depressants (i.e., either depressant actions or disinhibiting actions)

Do Not Use

- If patient has angle-closure glaucoma
- If patient has sleep apnea (injection)
- Must not be given intra-arterially because it may cause arteriospasm and result in gangrene
- If there is a proven allergy to lorazepam or any benzodiazepine

SPECIAL POPULATIONS

Renal Impairment

- 1–2 mg/day in 2–3 doses

Hepatic Impairment

- 1–2 mg/day in 2–3 doses
- Because of its short half-life and inactive metabolites, lorazepam may be a preferred benzodiazepine in some patients with liver disease

Cardiac Impairment

- Benzodiazepines have been used to treat anxiety associated with acute myocardial infarction
- Rare reports of QTc prolongation in patients with underlying arrhythmia
- Lorazepam may be used as an adjunct to control drug-induced cardiovascular emergencies

Elderly

- 1–2 mg/day in 2–3 doses
- May be more sensitive to sedative or respiratory effects

Children and Adolescents

- Oral: safety and efficacy not established in children under age 12
- Injection: safety and efficacy not established in children under age 18
- Long-term effects of lorazepam in children/adolescents are unknown
- Should generally receive lower doses and be more closely monitored

Pregnancy

- Effective June 30, 2015, the US FDA requires changes to the content and format of pregnancy and lactation information in prescription drug labels, including the elimination of the pregnancy letter categories; the Pregnancy and Lactation Labeling Rule (PLLR or final rule) applies only to prescription drugs and will be phased in gradually for drugs approved on or after June 30, 2001
- Possible increased risk of birth defects when benzodiazepines taken during pregnancy
- Because of the potential risks, lorazepam is not generally recommended as treatment for anxiety during pregnancy, especially during the first trimester
- Drug should be tapered if discontinued
- Infants whose mothers received a benzodiazepine late in pregnancy may experience withdrawal effects
- Neonatal flaccidity has been reported in infants whose mothers took a benzodiazepine during pregnancy
- Seizures, even mild seizures, may cause harm to the embryo/fetus

Breast Feeding

- Some drug is found in mother's breast milk

✱ Recommended either to discontinue drug or bottle feed

- Effects on infant have been observed and include feeding difficulties, sedation, and weight loss

THE ART OF PSYCHOPHARMACOLOGY

Potential Advantages

- Rapid onset of action
- Availability of oral liquid as well as injectable dosage formulations

Potential Disadvantages

- Euphoria may lead to abuse
- Abuse especially risky in past or present substance abusers
- Possibly more sedation than some other benzodiazepines commonly used to treat anxiety

Primary Target Symptoms

- Panic attacks
- Anxiety
- Muscle spasms
- Incidence of seizures (adjunct)

Pearls

* One of the most popular and useful benzodiazepines for treatment of agitation associated with psychosis, bipolar disorder, and other disorders, especially in the inpatient setting; this is due in part to useful sedative properties and flexibility of administration with oral tablets, oral liquid, or injectable formulations, which is often useful in treating uncooperative patients
- Is a very useful adjunct to SSRIs and SNRIs in the treatment of numerous anxiety disorders
- Though not systematically studied, benzodiazepines, and lorazepam in particular, have been used effectively to treat catatonia and are the initial recommended treatment
- Not effective for treating psychosis as a monotherapy, but can be used as an adjunct to antipsychotics
- Not effective for treating bipolar disorder as a monotherapy, but can be used as an adjunct to mood stabilizers and antipsychotics
- Because of its short half-life and inactive metabolites, lorazepam may be preferred over some benzodiazepines for patients with liver disease

* Lorazepam may be preferred over other benzodiazepines for the treatment of delirium
- When treating delirium, lorazepam is often combined with haloperidol, with the haloperidol dose 2 times the lorazepam dose

* Lorazepam is often used to induce pre-operative anterograde amnesia to assist in anesthesiology
- May both cause depression and treat depression in different patients
- Clinical duration of action may be shorter than plasma half-life, leading to dosing more frequently than 2–3 times daily in some patients
- When using to treat insomnia, remember that insomnia may be a symptom of some other primary disorder itself, and thus warrant evaluation for comorbid psychiatric and/or medical conditions

Suggested Reading

Bonnet MH, Arand DL. The use of lorazepam TID for chronic insomnia. Int Clin Psychopharmacol 1999;14:81–9.

Greenblatt DJ. Clinical pharmacokinetics of oxazepam and lorazepam. Clin Pharmacokinet 1981;6:89–105.

Starreveld E, Starreveld AA. Status epilepticus. Current concepts and management. Can Fam Physician 2000;46:1817–23.

Wagner BK, O'Hara DA, Hammond JS. Drugs for amnesia in the ICU. Am J Crit Care 1997;6:192–201.

LORCASERIN

THERAPEUTICS

Brands • Belviq, Belviq XR
see index for additional brand names

Generic? No

Class
- Serotonin 2C agonist; weight management medication

Commonly Prescribed for
(bold for FDA approved)
- **Chronic weight management (adjunct to reduced-calorie diet and increased physical activity) in adults with an initial BMI of at least 30 kg/m^2 (obese) or at least 27 kg/m^2 (overweight) in the presence of at least 1 weight-related comorbid condition**

How the Drug Works
- Selectively activates serotonin 2C receptors on anorexigenic pro-opiomelanocortin neurons in the hypothalamus

How Long Until It Works
- Significant weight loss (at least 5%) is generally achieved by week 12

If It Works
- Patients may achieve 5–10% reduction from baseline in body weight

If It Doesn't Work
- Discontinue if 5% weight loss is not achieved by week 12

Best Augmenting Combos for Partial Response or Treatment Resistance
- Lorcaserin itself should be administered in conjunction with reduced-calorie diet and increased physical activity
- Often best to try another strategy prior to resorting to augmentation

Tests
- Consider periodic monitoring of complete blood count during treatment with lorcaserin
- Measurement of blood glucose levels prior to starting lorcaserin and during lorcaserin treatment is recommended in patients with type 2 diabetes

SIDE EFFECTS

How Drug Causes Side Effects
- Serotonin 2C agonist actions in parts of the brain and body other than those that cause therapeutic actions
- Agonist actions at serotonin 2C receptors could theoretically diminish norepinephrine and dopamine neurotransmission in some brain areas

Notable Side Effects
- Nausea, constipation, dry mouth
- Fatigue, headache, dizziness
- Prolactin elevation

Life-Threatening or Dangerous Side Effects
- Hypoglycemia
- Rare priapism
- Rare serotonin syndrome
- Theoretical activation of suicidal ideation
- Theoretical risk of pulmonary hypertension

Weight Gain
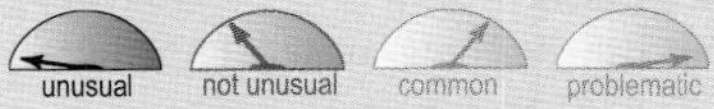

- Reported but not expected

Sedation
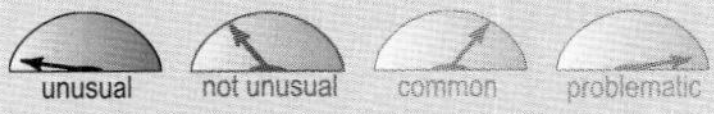

- Reported but not expected

What to Do About Side Effects
- Wait
- Wait
- Wait
- In a few weeks, switch to another agent

Best Augmenting Agents for Side Effects
- Often best to try another treatment prior to resorting to augmentation strategies to treat side effects

DOSING AND USE

Usual Dosage Range
- 20 mg/day

Dosage Forms
- Extended-release tablet 20 mg
- Tablet 10 mg

How to Dose
- 20 mg/day, in 1 dose (extended-release) or 2 doses (immediate-release)

Dosing Tips
- Can be taken with or without food
- No dose titration necessary

Overdose
- No overdoses have been reported
- Headache, nausea, dizziness, abdominal discomfort, euphoria, hallucination

Long-Term Use
- Has been evaluated in controlled studies up to 2 years

Habit Forming
- No
- Lorcaserin is a Schedule IV drug

How to Stop
- Taper not necessary

Pharmacokinetics
- Plasma half-life approximately 11 hours
- Inhibits CYP450 2D6

Drug Interactions
- Use extreme caution if administering lorcaserin with an agent that affects the serotonergic neurotransmitter system due to the potential risk of serotonin toxicity
- Via CYP450 2D6 inhibition, lorcaserin could increase plasma concentrations of drugs metabolized by CYP450 2D6 (e.g., desipramine), potentially requiring dose reduction of the substrate

Other Warnings/ Precautions
- Lorcaserin has not been studied in combination with insulin; weight loss may increase the risk of hypoglycemia in patients with type 2 diabetes mellitus treated with insulin and/or insulin secretagogues, and medication adjustments may be necessary

Do Not Use
- If patient is pregnant
- If patient is taking an agent that is a serotonin 2B agonist and known to increase the risk for cardiac valvulopathy (e.g., cabergoline)
- If there is a proven allergy to lorcaserin

SPECIAL POPULATIONS

Renal Impairment
- No dose adjustment necessary in patients with mild impairment
- Use with caution in patients with moderate impairment
- Not recommended in patients with severe impairment or end-stage renal disease

Hepatic Impairment
- No dose adjustment necessary in patients with mild to moderate impairment
- Use with caution in patients with severe impairment

Cardiac Impairment
- Not systematically evaluated in patients with cardiac impairment
- Use with caution in patients with congestive heart failure, bradycardia, or a history of heart block greater than first degree

Elderly
- Some patients may tolerate lower doses better

Children and Adolescents
- Safety and efficacy have not been established
- Not recommended for use in children or adolescents

Pregnancy
- Contraindicated in pregnancy

Breast Feeding

- Unknown if lorcaserin is secreted in human breast milk, but all psychotropics assumed to be secreted in breast milk
- Recommended to discontinue drug or bottle feed

THE ART OF PSYCHOPHARMACOLOGY

Potential Advantages

- For some patients who have failed to respond to or tolerate other treatments for obesity
- For patients who do not wish to take an agent with higher controlled substance designation
- For patients who do not wish to take a stimulant or who have past stimulant abuse

Potential Disadvantages

- Patients taking serotonergic agents concomitantly
- Women who are pregnant or who wish to become pregnant

Primary Target Symptoms

- Excess weight

Pearls

- In clinical studies patients who did not lose at least 5% of baseline body weight by week 12 were unlikely to achieve at least 5% weight loss at week 52
- Pooled analysis shows that the risk of FDA-defined valvulopathy with lorcaserin is generally low and not statistically significantly different from placebo; thus, the FDA has concluded that lorcaserin is unlikely to elevate the risk of valvulopathy
- Unknown whether lorcaserin can be used safely or effectively with atypical antipsychotic agents that may cause weight gain, some of which have serotonin 2C antagonist properties
- Could theoretically be effective in binge eating disorder

Suggested Reading

Chan EW, He Y, Chui CS, et al. Efficacy and safety of lorcaserin in obese adults: a meta-analysis of 1-year randomized controlled trials (RCTs) and narrative review on short-term RCTs. Obes Rev 2013;14:383–92.

Colman E, Golden J, Roberts M, et al. The FDA's assessment of two drugs for chronic weight management. N Engl J Med 2012;367(17):1577–9.

Holes-Lewis KA, Malcolm R, O'Neil PM. Pharmacotherapy of obesity: clinical treatments and considerations. Am J Med Sci 2013;345(4):284–8.

Hoy SM. Lorcaserin: a review of its use in chronic weight management. Drugs 2013;73(5):463–73.

THERAPEUTICS

Brands • Loxitane
• Adasuve (Staccato loxapine, inhaled loxapine)
see index for additional brand names

Generic? Yes

Class

- Neuroscience-based Nomenclature: dopamine and serotonin receptor antagonist (DS-RAn)
- Conventional antipsychotic (neuroleptic, dopamine 2 antagonist, serotonin dopamine antagonist)

Commonly Prescribed for

(bold for FDA approved)

- **Schizophrenia**
- **Acute treatment of agitation associated with schizophrenia or bipolar disorder**
- Other psychotic disorders
- Bipolar disorder

How the Drug Works

- Blocks dopamine 2 receptors, reducing positive symptoms of psychosis
- ✻ Although classified as a conventional antipsychotic, loxapine is a potent serotonin 2A antagonist
- Serotonin 2A antagonist properties might be relevant at low doses, but generally are overwhelmed by high dosing

How Long Until It Works

- Psychotic symptoms can improve within 1 week, but it may take several weeks for full effect on behavior

If It Works

- Most often reduces positive symptoms in schizophrenia but does not eliminate them
- Most schizophrenic patients do not have a total remission of symptoms but rather a reduction of symptoms by about a third
- Continue treatment in schizophrenia until reaching a plateau of improvement
- After reaching a satisfactory plateau, continue treatment for at least a year after first episode of psychosis in schizophrenia
- For second and subsequent episodes of psychosis in schizophrenia, treatment may need to be indefinite
- Reduces symptoms of acute psychotic mania but not proven as a mood stabilizer or as an effective maintenance treatment in bipolar disorder
- After reducing acute psychotic symptoms in mania, switch to a mood stabilizer and/or an atypical antipsychotic for mood stabilization and maintenance

If It Doesn't Work

- Consider trying one of the first-line atypical antipsychotics (risperidone, olanzapine, quetiapine, ziprasidone, aripiprazole, paliperidone, asenapine, iloperidone, lurasidone, amisulpride)
- Consider trying another conventional antipsychotic
- If 2 or more antipsychotic monotherapies do not work, consider clozapine

Best Augmenting Combos for Partial Response or Treatment Resistance

- Augmentation of conventional antipsychotics has not been systematically studied
- Addition of a mood stabilizing anticonvulsant such as valproate, carbamazepine, or lamotrigine may be helpful in both schizophrenia and bipolar mania
- Augmentation with lithium in bipolar mania may be helpful
- Addition of a benzodiazepine, especially short-term for agitation

Tests

- ✻ Since conventional antipsychotics are frequently associated with weight gain, before starting treatment, weigh all patients and determine if the patient is already overweight (BMI 25.0–29.9) or obese (BMI ≥30)
- Before giving a drug that can cause weight gain to an overweight or obese patient, consider determining whether the patient already has pre-diabetes (fasting plasma glucose 100–125 mg/dL), diabetes (fasting plasma glucose >126 mg/dL), or dyslipidemia (increased total cholesterol, LDL cholesterol, and triglycerides; decreased HDL cholesterol), and treat or refer such patients for treatment, including nutrition and weight management, physical activity counseling, smoking cessation, and medical management
- ✻ Monitor weight and BMI during treatment

✱ Consider monitoring fasting triglycerides monthly for several months in patients at high risk for metabolic complications and when initiating or switching antipsychotics

✱ While giving a drug to a patient who has gained >5% of initial weight, consider evaluating for the presence of pre-diabetes, diabetes, or dyslipidemia, or consider switching to a different antipsychotic

- Should check blood pressure in the elderly before starting and for the first few weeks of treatment
- Monitoring elevated prolactin levels of dubious clinical benefit
- Patients with low white blood cell count (WBC) or history of drug-induced leucopenia/neutropenia should have complete blood count (CBC) monitored frequently during the first few months and loxapine should be discontinued at the first sign of decline of WBC in the absence of other causative factors

SIDE EFFECTS

How Drug Causes Side Effects

- By blocking dopamine 2 receptors in the striatum, it can cause motor side effects
- By blocking dopamine 2 receptors in the pituitary, it can cause elevations in prolactin
- By blocking dopamine 2 receptors excessively in the mesocortical and mesolimbic dopamine pathways, especially at high doses, it can cause worsening of negative and cognitive symptoms (neuroleptic-induced deficit syndrome)
- Anticholinergic actions may cause sedation, blurred vision, constipation, dry mouth
- Antihistaminic actions may cause sedation, weight gain
- By blocking alpha 1 adrenergic receptors, it can cause dizziness, sedation, and hypotension
- Mechanism of weight gain and any possible increased incidence of diabetes or dyslipidemia with conventional antipsychotics is unknown

Notable Side Effects

✱ Neuroleptic-induced deficit syndrome

✱ Akathisia

✱ Extrapyramidal symptoms, parkinsonism, tardive dyskinesia

✱ Galactorrhea, amenorrhea

- Sedation
- Dry mouth, constipation, vision disturbance, urninary retention
- Hypotension, tachycardia

Life-Threatening or Dangerous Side Effects

- Rare neuroleptic malignant syndrome
- Rare agranulocytosis
- Rare hepatocellular injury
- Rare seizures
- Increased risk of death and cerebrovascular events in elderly patients with dementia-related psychosis
- Bronchospasm, with the potential to lead to respiratory distress and respiratory arrest (inhalant)

Weight Gain

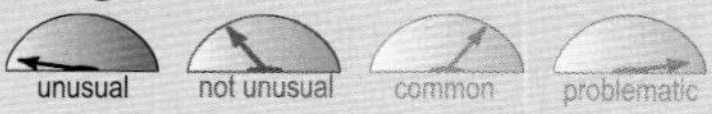

- Reported but not expected

Sedation

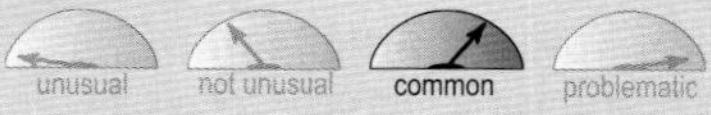

- Many experience and/or can be significant in amount
- Sedation is usually transient
- Sedation is usually dose-dependent and may not be experienced at low doses where loxapine may function as an atypical antipsychotic (e.g., <50 mg/day; especially 5–25 mg/day)

What to Do About Side Effects

- Wait
- Wait
- Wait
- For motor symptoms, add an anticholinergic agent
- Reduce the dose
- For sedation, give at night
- Switch to an atypical antipsychotic
- Weight loss, exercise programs, and medical management for high BMIs, diabetes, dyslipidemia

Best Augmenting Agents for Side Effects

- Benztropine or trihexyphenidyl for motor side effects

- Sometimes amantadine can be helpful for motor side effects
- Benzodiazepines may be helpful for akathisia
- Many side effects cannot be improved with an augmenting agent

DOSING AND USE

Usual Dosage Range

- 60–100 mg/day in divided doses

Dosage Forms

- Capsule 6.8 mg loxapine succinate equivalent to 5 mg loxapine, 13.6 mg loxapine succinate equivalent to 10 mg loxapine, 34.0 mg loxapine succinate equivalent to 25 mg loxapine, 68.1 mg loxapine succinate equivalent to 50 mg loxapine
- Oral liquid 25 mg/mL
- Injection 50 mg/mL
- Inhalant 10 mg unit in a single-use inhaler

How to Dose

- Initial 20 mg/day in 2 doses; titrate over 7–10 days to 60–100 mg/day in 2–4 doses; maximum generally 250 mg/day
- Take liquid formulation in orange or grapefruit juice
- Inhalation powder: 10 mg by oral inhalation using an inhaler; only 1 dose per 24 hours; must be administered by a health-care professional in a setting with immediate onsite access to equipment and personnel trained to manage acute bronchospasm, including advanced airway management

Dosing Tips

- Has conventional antipsychotic properties at originally recommended doses (i.e., starting at 10 mg twice a day, maintenance 60–100 mg/day, maximum 250 mg/day given in 2 divided doses)

✻ Binding studies, PET studies, and anecdotal clinical observations suggest that loxapine may be atypical at lower doses (perhaps 5–30 mg/day) but further studies needed

- Anecdotal evidence that many patients can be maintained at 20–60 mg/day as monotherapy
- To augment partial responders to an atypical antipsychotic, consider doses of loxapine as low as 5–60 mg/day, but use full doses if necessary
- No formal studies, but some patients may do well on once daily dosing, especially at night, rather than twice daily dosing
- Available as 5-mg and 10-mg capsules for low-dose use and as 25-mg and 50-mg capsules for routine use
- Available as a liquid dosage formulation
- Available for acute inhalation administration
- Prior to administering inhalation powder, screen all patients for a history of pulmonary disease, and examine patients (including chest auscultation) for respiratory abnormalities (e.g., wheezing)
- After administering inhalation powder, monitor patients for signs and symptoms of bronchospasm at least every 15 minutes for at least an hour
- Available for acute intramuscular administration (50 mg/mL)
- Intramuscular loxapine may have faster onset of action and superior efficacy for agitated/excited and aggressive behavior in some patients than intramuscular haloperidol
- In the acute situation, give 25–50 mg intramuscularly (0.5–1.0 mL of 50 mg/mL solution) with onset of action within 60 minutes
- When initiating therapy with an atypical antipsychotic in an acute situation, consider short-term intramuscular loxapine to "lead in" to orally administered atypical; e.g., initiate oral dosing of an atypical antipsychotic with 25–50 mg loxapine 2–3 times a day intramuscularly to achieve antipsychotic effects without extrapyramidal symptoms and sedation
- When using loxapine to "top-up" previously stabilized patients now decompensating, may use loxapine as single 25–50 mg doses as needed intramuscularly or as oral liquid or tablets
- Patients receiving atypical antipsychotics may occasionally require a "top up" of a conventional antipsychotic to control aggression or violent behavior
- Treatment should be suspended if absolute neutrophil count falls below 1,000/mm^3

Overdose
- Deaths have occurred; extrapyramidal symptoms, CNS depression, cardiovascular effects, hypotension, seizures, respiratory depression, renal failure, coma

Long-Term Use
- Some side effects may be irreversible (e.g., tardive dyskinesia)

Habit Forming
- No

How to Stop
- Slow down-titration of oral formulation (at least 4 weeks when possible), especially when simultaneously beginning a new antipsychotic while switching (i.e., cross-titration)
- Rapid oral discontinuation may lead to rebound psychosis and worsening of symptoms
- If antiparkinson agents are being used, they should be continued for a few weeks after loxapine is discontinued

Pharmacokinetics
- Half-life approximately 4 hours for oral formulation
- Half-life approximately 12 hours for intramuscular formulation
- Multiple active metabolites with longer half-lives than parent drug

✻ *N*-desmethyl loxapine is amoxapine, an antidepressant
- 8-hydroxyloxapine and 7-hydroxyloxapine are also serotonin-dopamine antagonists
- 8-hydroxyamoxapine and 7-hydroxyamoxapine are also serotonin-dopamine antagonists

Drug Interactions
- Respiratory depression may occur when loxapine is combined with lorazepam
- Additive effects may occur if used with CNS depressants
- May decrease the effects of levodopa, dopamine agonists
- Some patients taking a neuroleptic and lithium have developed an encephalopathic syndrome similar to neuroleptic malignant syndrome
- Combined use with epinephrine may lower blood pressure
- May increase the effects of antihypertensive drugs except for guanethidine, whose antihypertensive actions loxapine may antagonize

Other Warnings/ Precautions
- If signs of neuroleptic malignant syndrome develop, treatment should be immediately discontinued
- Use cautiously in patients with alcohol withdrawal or convulsive disorders because of possible lowering of seizure threshold
- Antiemetic effect can mask signs of other disorders or overdose
- Do not use epinephrine in event of overdose, as interaction with some pressor agents may lower blood pressure
- Use cautiously in patients with glaucoma, urinary retention
- Observe for signs of ocular toxicity (pigmentary retinopathy, lenticular pigmentation)
- Avoid extreme heat exposure
- Use only with caution if at all in Parkinson's disease or Lewy body dementia

Do Not Use
- If patient is in a comatose state or has CNS depression
- If patient has asthma or history of asthma, COPD, other lung disease associated with bronchospasm, acute respiratory signs/ symptoms, current use of medications to treat airways, history of bronchospasm following treatment with loxapine inhalation powder (inhalant only)
- If there is a proven allergy to loxapine
- If there is a known sensitivity to any dibenzoxazepine

SPECIAL POPULATIONS

Renal Impairment
- Use with caution

Hepatic Impairment
- Use with caution

Cardiac Impairment
- Use with caution

Elderly

- Some patients may tolerate lower doses better
- Although conventional antipsychotics are commonly used for behavioral disturbances in dementia, no agent has been approved for treatment of elderly patients with dementia-related psychosis
- Elderly patients with dementia-related psychosis treated with antipsychotics are at an increased risk of death compared to placebo, and also have an increased risk of cerebrovascular events

Children and Adolescents

- Safety and efficacy not established
- Generally, consider second-line after atypical antipsychotics

Pregnancy

- Effective June 30, 2015, the US FDA requires changes to the content and format of pregnancy and lactation information in prescription drug labels, including the elimination of the pregnancy letter categories; the Pregnancy and Lactation Labeling Rule (PLLR or final rule) applies only to prescription drugs and will be phased in gradually for drugs approved on or after June 30, 2001
- Controlled studies have not been conducted in pregnant women
- There is a risk of abnormal muscle movements and withdrawal symptoms in newborns whose mothers took an antipsychotic during the third trimester; symptoms may include agitation, abnormally increased or decreased muscle tone, tremor, sleepiness, severe difficulty breathing, and difficulty feeding
- Renal papillary abnormalities have been seen in rats during pregnancy
- Psychotic symptoms may worsen during pregnancy and some form of treatment may be necessary
- Atypical antipsychotics may be preferable to conventional antipsychotics or anticonvulsant mood stabilizers if treatment is required during pregnancy

Breast Feeding

- Unknown if loxapine is secreted in human breast milk, but all psychotropics assumed to be secreted in breast milk
- ✽ Recommended either to discontinue drug or bottle feed

THE ART OF PSYCHOPHARMACOLOGY

Potential Advantages

- Intramuscular formulation for emergency use

Potential Disadvantages

- Patients with tardive dyskinesia

Primary Target Symptoms

- Positive symptoms of psychosis
- Motor and autonomic hyperactivity
- Violent or aggressive behavior

Pearls

- ✽ Recently discovered to be a serotonin dopamine antagonist (binding studies and PET scans)
- ✽ Active metabolites are also serotonin dopamine antagonists with longer half-lives than parent drug, thus possibly allowing once daily treatment
- ✽ One active metabolite is an antidepressant (amoxapine, also known as *N*-desmethyl-loxapine)
- Theoretically, loxapine should have antidepressant actions, especially at high doses, but no controlled studies
- Theoretically, loxapine may have advantages for short-term use in some patients with psychotic depression
- Developed as a conventional antipsychotic; i.e., reduces positive symptoms, but causes extrapyramidal symptoms and prolactin elevations
- Lower extrapyramidal symptoms than haloperidol in some studies, but not fixed-dose studies and no low-dose studies
- ✽ Causes less weight gain than other antipsychotics, both atypical and conventional, and may even be associated with weight loss
- No formal studies of negative symptoms, but some studies show superiority to

conventional antipsychotics for emotional withdrawal and social competence

- Best use may be as low-cost augmentation agent to atypical antipsychotics
- ✻ Enhances efficacy in clozapine partial responders when given concomitantly with clozapine
- For previously stabilized patients with "breakthrough" agitation or incipient decompensation, "top-up" the atypical antipsychotic with as-needed intramuscular or oral single doses of loxapine
- An inhalation powder for acute agitation is available only through a restricted program under a Risk Evaluation and Mitigation Strategy (REMS) called the ADASUVE REMS
- Due to the risk of bronchospasm, loxapine inhalation powder should be administered only in an enrolled health-care facility that has immediate onsite access to equipment and personnel trained to manage acute bronchospasm, including advanced airway management (intubation and mechanical ventilation)
- Patients have very similar antipsychotic responses to any conventional antipsychotic, which is different from atypical antipsychotics where antipsychotic responses of individual patients can occasionally vary greatly from one atypical antipsychotic to another
- Patients with inadequate responses to atypical antipsychotics may benefit from determination of plasma levels and, if low, a dosage increase even beyond the usual prescribing limits
- Patients with inadequate responses to atypical antipsychotics may also benefit from a trial of augmentation with a conventional antipsychotic such as loxapine or from switching to a conventional antipsychotic such as loxapine
- However, long-term polypharmacy with a combination of a conventional antipsychotic such as loxapine with an atypical antipsychotic may combine their side effects without clearly augmenting the efficacy of either
- For treatment-resistant patients, especially those with impulsivity, aggression, violence, and self-harm, long-term polypharmacy with 2 atypical antipsychotics or with 1 atypical antipsychotic and 1 conventional antipsychotic may be useful or even necessary while closely monitoring. In such cases, it may be beneficial to combine 1 depot antipsychotic with 1 oral antipsychotic
- Although a frequent practice by some prescribers, adding 2 conventional antipsychotics together has little rationale and may reduce tolerability without clearly enhancing efficacy

Suggested Reading

Chakrabarti A, Bagnall A, Chue P, et al. Loxapine for schizophrenia. Cochrane Database Syst Rev 2007;17(4):CD001943.

Fenton M, Murphy B, Wood J, et al. Loxapine for schizophrenia. Cochrane Database Syst Rev 2000;(2): CD001943.

Heel RC, Brogden RN, Speight TM, Avery GS. Loxapine: a review of its pharmacological properties and therapeutic efficacy as an antipsychotic agent. Drugs 1978;15(3): 198–217.

Zisook S, Click MA Jr. Evaluations of loxapine succinate in the ambulatory treatment of acute schizophrenic episodes. Int Pharmacopsychiatry 1980;15(6):365–78.

THERAPEUTICS

Brands • LATUDA

see index for additional brand names

Generic? No

Class

- Neuroscience-based Nomenclature: dopamine, serotonin receptor antagonist (DS-RAn)
- Atypical antipsychotic (serotonin-dopamine antagonist; second generation antipsychotic; also a potential mood stabilizer)

Commonly Prescribed for

(bold for FDA approved)

- **Schizophrenia (ages 13 and older)**
- **Bipolar depression**
- Acute mania/mixed mania
- Other psychotic disorders
- Bipolar maintenance
- Treatment-resistant depression
- Behavioral disturbances in dementia
- Behavioral disturbances in children and adolescents
- Disorders associated with problems with impulse control

How the Drug Works

- Blocks dopamine 2 receptors, reducing positive symptoms of psychosis and stabilizing affective symptoms
- Blocks serotonin 2A receptors, causing enhancement of dopamine release in certain brain regions and thus reducing motor side effects and possibly improving cognition and affective symptoms
- Potently blocks serotonin 7 receptors, which may be beneficial for mood, sleep, cognitive impairment, and negative symptoms in schizophrenia, and also in bipolar disorder and major depressive disorder
- Partial agonist at 5HT1A receptors, and antagonist actions at serotonin 7 and alpha 2A and alpha 2C receptors, which may be beneficial for mood, anxiety and cognition in a number of disorders
- Lacks potent actions at dopamine D1, muscarinic M1, and histamine H1 receptors, theoretically suggesting less propensity for inducing cognitive impairment, weight gain, or sedation compared to other agents with these properties

How Long Until It Works

- Psychotic symptoms can improve within 1 week, but it may take several weeks for full effect on behavior as well as on cognition
- Classically recommended to wait at least 4–6 weeks to determine efficacy of drug, but in practice some patients may require up to 16–20 weeks to show a good response, especially on cognitive impairment and functional outcome

If It Works

- Most often reduces positive symptoms but does not eliminate them
- Can improve negative symptoms, as well as aggressive, cognitive, and affective symptoms in schizophrenia
- Most schizophrenia patients do not have a total remission of symptoms but rather a reduction of symptoms by about a third
- Perhaps 5–15% of schizophrenia patients can experience an overall improvement of greater than 50–60%, especially when receiving stable treatment for more than a year
- Such patients are considered super-responders or "awakeners" since they may be well enough to be employed, live independently, and sustain long-term relationships
- Continue treatment until reaching a plateau of improvement
- After reaching a satisfactory plateau, continue treatment for at least a year after first episode of psychosis
- For second and subsequent episodes of psychosis, treatment may need to be indefinite
- Even for first episodes of psychosis, it may be preferable to continue treatment

If It Doesn't Work

- Try one of the other atypical antipsychotics (risperidone, olanzapine, quetiapine, ziprasidone, aripiprazole, paliperidone, asenapine, iloperidone, amisulpride)
- If 2 or more antipsychotic monotherapies do not work, consider clozapine
- Some patients may require treatment with a conventional antipsychotic

- If no first-line atypical antipsychotic is effective, consider higher doses or augmentation with valproate or lamotrigine
- Consider noncompliance and switch to another antipsychotic with fewer side effects or to an antipsychotic that can be given by depot injection
- Consider initiating rehabilitation and psychotherapy
- Consider presence of concomitant drug abuse

Best Augmenting Combos for Partial Response or Treatment Resistance

- Valproic acid (valproate, divalproex, divalproex ER)
- Mood-stabilizing anticonvulsants (see drug interactions)
- Lithium
- Benzodiazepines

Tests

Before starting any atypical antipsychotic

✽ Weigh all patients and track BMI during treatment
- Get baseline personal and family history of diabetes, obesity, dyslipidemia, hypertension, and cardiovascular disease

✽ Get waist circumference (at umbilicus), blood pressure, fasting plasma glucose, and fasting lipid profile
- Determine if the patient is
  - overweight (BMI 25.0–29.9)
  - obese (BMI ≥30)
  - has pre-diabetes (fasting plasma glucose 100–125 mg/dL)
  - has diabetes (fasting plasma glucose ≥126 mg/dL)
  - has hypertension (BP >140/90 mm Hg)
  - has dyslipidemia (increased total cholesterol, LDL cholesterol, and triglycerides; decreased HDL cholesterol)
- Treat or refer such patients for treatment, including nutrition and weight management, physical activity counseling, smoking cessation, and medical management

Monitoring after starting any atypical antipsychotic

✽ BMI monthly for 3 months, then quarterly

✽ Consider monitoring fasting triglycerides monthly for several months in patients at high risk for metabolic complications and when initiating or switching antipsychotics

✽ Blood pressure, fasting plasma glucose, fasting lipids within 3 months and then annually, but earlier and more frequently for patients with diabetes or who have gained >5% of initial weight
- Treat or refer for treatment and consider switching to another atypical antipsychotic for patients who become overweight, obese, pre-diabetic, diabetic, hypertensive, or dyslipidemic while receiving an atypical antipsychotic

✽ Even in patients without known diabetes, be vigilant for the rare but life-threatening onset of diabetic ketoacidosis, which always requires immediate treatment, by monitoring for the rapid onset of polyuria, polydipsia, weight loss, nausea, vomiting, dehydration, rapid respiration, weakness, and clouding of sensorium, even coma
- Patients with low white blood cell count (WBC) or history of drug-induced leucopenia/neutropenia should have complete blood count (CBC) monitored frequently during the first few months and lurasidone should be discontinued at the first sign of decline in WBC in the absence of other causative factors (class warning)

SIDE EFFECTS

How Drug Causes Side Effects (Class effects)

- By blocking dopamine 2 receptors in the striatum, it can cause motor side effects
- By blocking dopamine 2 receptors in the pituitary, it can cause elevations in prolactin
- Mechanism of weight gain and increased incidence of diabetes and dyslipidemia with atypical antipsychotics is unknown

Notable Side Effects

- Dose-dependent sedation
- Akathisia
- Nausea
- Dose-dependent hyperprolactinemia
- May increase risk for diabetes and dyslipidemia
- Rare tardive dyskinesia (much reduced risk compared to conventional antipsychotics)

Life-Threatening or Dangerous Side Effects

- Tachycardia, first-degree AV block
- Hyperglycemia, in some cases extreme and associated with ketoacidosis or hyperosmolar coma or death, has been reported in patients taking atypical antipsychotics (class warning)
- Increased risk of death and cerebrovascular events in elderly patients with dementia-related psychosis (class warning)
- Rare neuroleptic malignant syndrome (much reduced risk compared to conventional antipsychotics) (class warning)
- Rare seizures (class warning)

Weight Gain

Short Term

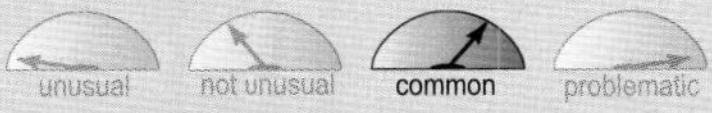

- Many experience about one- to two-pound weight gain greater than placebo in short term 6-week trials

Long Term

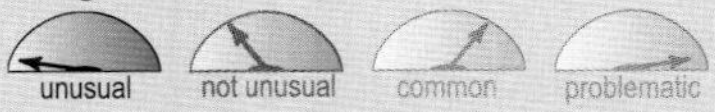

- Patients in long-term 52-week trials actually lost 1.5 pounds on average
- Clinical experience, however, is still limited
- Appears to be less weight gain than observed with some antipsychotics
- Many patients lost weight in long-term trials when switching from olanzapine to lurasidone

Sedation

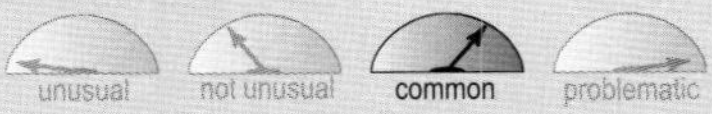

- May be higher in short-term trials than in long-term use

What to Do About Side Effects

- Wait
- Wait
- Wait
- Anticholinergics may reduce motor side effects when present
- Dose reduction may reduce akathisia when present
- Consider changing to nighttime dosing (with evening meal)
- Weight loss, exercise programs, and medical management for high BMIs, diabetes, dyslipidemia
- Switch to another atypical antipsychotic

Best Augmenting Agents for Side Effects

- Benztropine or trihexyphenidyl for motor side effects
- Beta blockers or benzodiazepines may reduce akathisia when present
- Many side effects cannot be improved with an augmenting agent

DOSING AND USE

Usual Dosage Range

- 40–80 mg/day for schizophrenia
- Some patients with schizophrenia may benefit from doses up to 160 mg/day
- 20–60 mg/day for bipolar depression
- Some patients with bipolar depression may benefit from doses up to 120 mg/day

Dosage Forms

- Tablet 20 mg, 40 mg, 60 mg, 80 mg, 120 mg

How to Dose

- Initial 40–80 mg once daily with food for schizophrenia
- Dose titration to initial dose of 40 mg/day is not required for schizophrenia
- Consider dose increases from 40 mg/day up to 160 mg/day as necessary and as tolerated for schizophrenia
- Initial 20 mg once daily with food for bipolar depression
- Can titrate to 120 mg/day in bipolar depression if necessary and tolerated

Dosing Tips

- Lurasidone should be taken with food (i.e., at least a small meal of a minimum of 350 calories)
- Lurasidone absorption can be decreased by up to 50% on an empty stomach and more consistent efficacy will be seen if dosing is done regularly with food
- Once daily dosing
- Giving lurasidone at bedtime can greatly reduce daytime sedation, akathisia, and EPS

- Starting dose for schizophrenia is 40 mg/day, which may be an adequate dose for some patients, especially first-episode and early-onset psychosis cases
- 40–80 mg per day was suggested by controlled clinical trials as adequate for many patients with schizophrenia
- Some patients with schizophrenia benefit from higher dosing, with controlled clinical trials up to 160 mg/day
- Higher doses than 160 mg/day may benefit more difficult patients with schizophrenia with treatment nonresponsiveness to other agents
- Higher dosing, however, may cause more side effects
- Dosing for bipolar depression or major depressive episodes with mixed features is generally lower than for schizophrenia, with a 20 mg starting dose; 20 mg/day may be an adequate dose for some patients
- Doses between 20 and 60 mg/day are generally as efficacious as doses between 60 and 120 mg/day for bipolar depression or major depressive episodes with mixed features
- Some patients with bipolar depression or major depressive episodes with mixed features may require higher doses

Overdose
- Limited data

Long-Term Use
- Not extensively studied past 52 weeks, but long-term maintenance treatment is often necessary for schizophrenia
- Should periodically reevaluate long-term usefulness in individual patients, but treatment may need to continue for many years in patients with schizophrenia

Habit Forming
- No

How to Stop
- Down-titration, especially when simultaneously beginning a new antipsychotic while switching (i.e., cross-titration)
- Rapid discontinuation could theoretically lead to rebound psychosis and worsening of symptoms

Pharmacokinetics
- Half-life 18–31 hours (shorter half-life better documented at the 40 mg dose)
- Metabolized by CYP450 3A4
- Cmax and bioavailability are reduced if taken without food

Drug Interactions
- Inhibitors of CYP450 3A4 (e.g., nefazodone, fluvoxamine, fluoxetine, ketoconazole) may increase plasma levels of lurasidone
- Coadministration of lurasidone with a strong CYP450 3A4 inhibitor (e.g., ketoconazole) or with a strong CYP450 3A4 inducer (e.g., rifampin) is contraindicated
- Coadministration of lurasidone with moderate CYP450 3A4 inhibitors can be considered; recommended starting dose is 20 mg/day; recommended maximum dose is 80 mg/day
- Moderate inducers of CYP450 3A4 may decrease plasma levels of lurasidone
- May increase effects of antihypertensive agents
- May antagonize levodopa, dopamine agonists

Other Warnings/ Precautions
- Use with caution in patients with conditions that predispose to hypotension (dehydration, overheating)
- Dysphagia has been associated with antipsychotic use, and lurasidone should be used cautiously in patients at risk for aspiration pneumonia

Do Not Use
- If patient is taking a strong CYP 3A4 inhibitor (e.g., ketoconazole) or inducer (e.g., rifampin)
- In patients with a history of angioedema
- If there is a proven allergy to lurasidone

SPECIAL POPULATIONS

Renal Impairment
- Moderate and severe impairment: initial 20 mg/day; maximum dose 80 mg/day

Hepatic Impairment

- Moderate impairment: initial 20 mg/day; maximum dose 80 mg/day
- Severe impairment: initial 20 mg/day; maximum dose 40 mg/day

Cardiac Impairment

- Should be used with caution because of theoretical risk of orthostatic hypotension, although low potency at alpha 1 receptors suggests this risk may be less than for some other antipsychotics
- Lurasidone does not have a warning for QTc prolongation

Elderly

- In general, no dose adjustment is necessary for elderly patients
- However, some elderly patients may tolerate lower doses better
- Although atypical antipsychotics are commonly used for behavioral disturbances in dementia, no agent has been approved for treatment of elderly patients with dementia-related psychosis
- Elderly patients with dementia-related psychosis treated with atypical antipsychotics are at an increased risk of death compared to placebo, and also have an increased risk of cerebrovascular events

Children and Adolescents

- Safety and efficacy have not been established
- Children and adolescents using lurasidone may need to be monitored more often than adults

Pregnancy

- Effective June 30, 2015, the US FDA requires changes to the content and format of pregnancy and lactation information in prescription drug labels, including the elimination of the pregnancy letter categories; the Pregnancy and Lactation Labeling Rule (PLLR or final rule) applies only to prescription drugs and will be phased in gradually for drugs approved on or after June 30, 2001
- Controlled studies have not been conducted in pregnant women
- Animal studies do not show adverse effects
- There is a risk of abnormal muscle movements and withdrawal symptoms in newborns whose mothers took an antipsychotic during the third trimester; symptoms may include agitation, abnormally increased or decreased muscle tone, tremor, sleepiness, severe difficulty breathing, and difficulty feeding
- Psychotic symptoms may worsen during pregnancy and some form of treatment may be necessary
- Lurasidone may be preferable to anticonvulsant mood stabilizers if treatment is required during pregnancy
- National Pregnancy Registry for Atypical Antipsychotics: 1-866-961-2388 or http://womensmentalhealth.org/clinical-and-research-programs/pregnancyregistry/

Breast Feeding

- Unknown if lurasidone is secreted in human breast milk, but all psychotropics assumed to be secreted in breast milk

✽ Recommended either to discontinue drug or bottle feed unless the potential benefit to the mother justifies the potential risk to the child

- Infants of women who choose to breast feed while on lurasidone should be monitored for possible adverse effects

THE ART OF PSYCHOPHARMACOLOGY

Potential Advantages

- Patients requiring rapid onset of antipsychotic action without dosage titration
- Patients who wish to take an antipsychotic once a day
- Patients experiencing weight gain from other antipsychotics or who wish to avoid weight gain

Potential Disadvantages

- Patients who cannot take a medication consistently with food

Primary Target Symptoms

- Positive symptoms of psychosis
- Negative symptoms of psychosis
- Cognitive symptoms
- Unstable mood (both depression and mania)
- Aggressive symptoms

Pearls

- Clinical trials suggest that lurasidone is well tolerated with a favorable balance of efficacy and safety
- One of the few "metabolically friendly" antipsychotics
  - Neutral for weight gain (1–2 pounds weight gain in short-term studies, with 1–2 pounds weight loss in long-term studies)
  - Neutral for lipids (triglycerides and cholesterol)
  - Neutral for glucose
- Only atypical antipsychotic documented not to cause QTc prolongation, and one of the few atypical antipsychotics without a QTc warning
- Seems to have low-level EPS, especially when dosed at bedtime
- Somnolence and akathisia are the most common side effects in short-term clinical trials of schizophrenia that dosed lurasidone in the daytime, but these adverse effects were reduced in a controlled study of lurasidone administered at night with food
- Nausea and occasional vomiting occurred in bipolar depression studies especially at higher doses
- Nausea and vomiting generally rapidly abates within a few days or can be avoided by slow dose titration and giving lower doses
- Prolactin elevations low and generally transient
- Agitation experienced by some patients
- Receptor binding profile suggests favorable potential as an antidepressant
  - 5HT7 antagonism is antidepressant in animal models and has pro-cognitive actions in animal models
  - 5HT7 antagonism and 5HT1A partial agonism enhance serotonin levels in animals treated with SSRIs/SNRIs, suggesting use for lurasidone as an augmenting agent to SSRIs/SNRIs in depression
  - 5HT7 antagonism plus the absence of D1, H1, and M1 antagonism suggest potential for cognitive improvement
  - Lack of D1 antagonist, anticholinergic, and antihistamine properties may explain relative lack of cognitive side effects in most patients
- One of the best studied agents for depression with mixed features, showing efficacy in a large randomized controlled trial
- Not approved for mania, but almost all atypical antipsychotics approved for acute treatment of schizophrenia have proven effective in the acute treatment of mania as well
- Patients with inadequate responses to atypical antipsychotics may benefit from determination of plasma drug levels and, if low, a dosage increase even beyond the usual prescribing limits
- Patients with inadequate responses to atypical antipsychotics may also benefit from a trial of augmentation with a conventional antipsychotic or switching to a conventional antipsychotic
- However, long-term polypharmacy with a combination of a conventional antipsychotic with an atypical antipsychotic may combine their side effects without clearly augmenting the efficacy of either
- For treatment-resistant patients, especially those with impulsivity, aggression, violence, and self-harm, long-term polypharmacy with 2 atypical antipsychotics or with 1 atypical antipsychotic and 1 conventional antipsychotic may be useful or even necessary while closely monitoring
- In such cases, it may be beneficial to combine 1 depot antipsychotic with 1 oral antipsychotic

THE ART OF SWITCHING

Switching from Oral Antipsychotics to Lurasidone

- With aripiprazole, amisulpride, and paliperidone ER, immediate stop is possible; begin lurasidone at an intermediate dose
- Clinical experience has shown that quetiapine, olanzapine, and asenapine should be tapered off slowly over a period of 3–4 weeks, to allow patients to readapt to the withdrawal of blocking cholinergic, histaminergic, and alpha-1 receptors
- Clozapine should always be tapered off slowly, over a period of 4 weeks or more

* Benzodiazepine or anticholinergic medication can be administered during cross-titration to help alleviate side effects such as insomnia, agitation, and/or psychosis

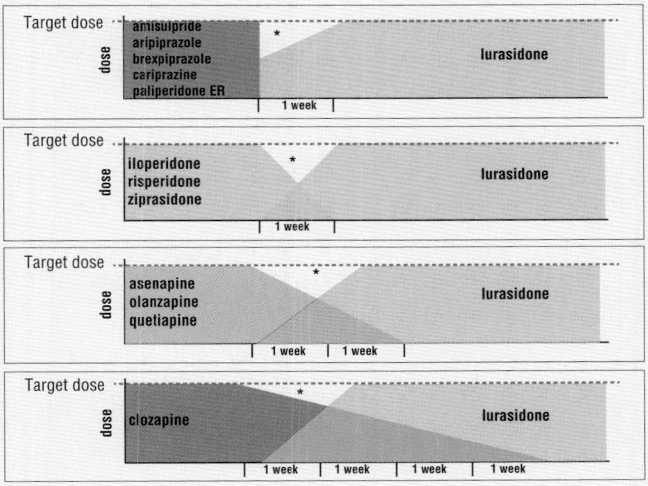

Suggested Reading

Ishibashi T, Horisawa T, Tokuda K, et al. Pharmacological profile of lurasidone, a novel antipsychotic agent with potent 5-hydroxytryptamine 7 (5-HT7) and 5-HT1A receptor activity. J Pharmacol Exp Ther 2010;334(1):171–81.

Meyer JM, Loebel AD, Schweizer E. Lurasidone: A new drug in development for schizophrenia. Expert Opin Investig Drugs 2009;18(11):1715–26.

Nakamura M, Ogasa M, Guarino J, et al. Lurasidone in the treatment of acute schizophrenia: A double-blind, placebo-controlled trial. J Clin Psychiatry 2009;70(6):829–36.

Stahl SM. The serotonin 7 receptor as a novel therapeutic target. J Clin Psychiatry 2010,71: 1414–15.

Tarazi F, Stahl SM. Iloperidone, asenapine and lurasidone: a primer on their current status. Exp Opin Pharmacother 2013;13(13):1911–22.

MAPROTILINE

THERAPEUTICS

Brands • Ludiomil

see index for additional brand names

Generic? Yes

Class

- Neuroscience-based Nomenclature: norepinephrine reuptake inhibitor (N-RI)
- Tricyclic antidepressant (TCA), sometimes classified as a tetracyclic antidepressant (tetra)
- Predominantly a norepinephrine/ noradrenaline reuptake inhibitor

Commonly Prescribed for

(bold for FDA approved)

- **Depression**
- Anxiety
- Insomnia
- Neuropathic pain/chronic pain
- Treatment-resistant depression

How the Drug Works

- Boosts neurotransmitter norepinephrine/ noradrenaline
- Blocks norepinephrine reuptake pump (norepinephrine transporter), presumably increasing noradrenergic neurotransmission
- Since dopamine is inactivated by norepinephrine reuptake in frontal cortex, which largely lacks dopamine transporters, maprotiline can thus increase dopamine neurotransmission in this part of the brain
- A more potent inhibitor of norepinephrine reuptake pump than serotonin reuptake pump (serotonin transporter)
- At high doses may also boost neurotransmitter serotonin and presumably increase serotonergic neurotransmission

How Long Until It Works

- Onset of therapeutic actions usually not immediate, but often delayed 2–4 weeks
- If it is not working within 6–8 weeks for depression, it may require a dosage increase or it may not work at all
- May continue to work for many years to prevent relapse of symptoms

If It Works

- The goal of treatment of depression is complete remission of current symptoms as well as prevention of future relapses
- The goal of treatment of chronic neuropathic pain is to reduce symptoms as much as possible, especially in combination with other treatments
- Treatment of depression most often reduces or even eliminates symptoms, but not a cure since symptoms can recur after medicine is stopped
- Treatment of chronic neuropathic pain may reduce symptoms, but rarely eliminates them completely, and is not a cure since symptoms can recur after medicine is stopped
- Continue treatment of depression until all symptoms are gone (remission)
- Once symptoms of depression are gone, continue treating for 1 year for the first episode of depression
- For second and subsequent episodes of depression, treatment may need to be indefinite
- Use in anxiety disorders and chronic pain may also need to be indefinite, but long-term treatment is not well studied in these conditions

If It Doesn't Work

- Many depressed patients have only a partial response where some symptoms are improved but others persist (especially insomnia, fatigue, and problems concentrating)
- Other depressed patients may be nonresponders, sometimes called treatment-resistant or treatment-refractory
- Consider increasing dose, switching to another agent or adding an appropriate augmenting agent
- Consider psychotherapy
- Consider evaluation for another diagnosis or for a comorbid condition (e.g., medical illness, substance abuse, etc.)
- Some patients may experience apparent lack of consistent efficacy due to activation of latent or underlying bipolar disorder, and require antidepressant discontinuation and a switch to a mood stabilizer

Best Augmenting Combos for Partial Response or Treatment Resistance

- Lithium, buspirone, thyroid hormone (for depression)
- Gabapentin, tiagabine, other anticonvulsants, even opiates if done by experts while monitoring carefully in difficult cases (for chronic pain)

Tests

- Baseline ECG is recommended for patients over age 50
- * Since tricyclic and tetracyclic antidepressants are frequently associated with weight gain, before starting treatment, weigh all patients and determine if the patient is already overweight (BMI 25.0–29.9) or obese (BMI ≥30)
- Before giving a drug that can cause weight gain to an overweight or obese patient, consider determining whether the patient already has pre-diabetes (fasting plasma glucose 100–125 mg/dL), diabetes (fasting plasma glucose >126 mg/dL), or dyslipidemia (increased total cholesterol, LDL cholesterol, and triglycerides; decreased HDL cholesterol), and treat or refer such patients for treatment, including nutrition and weight management, physical activity counseling, smoking cessation, and medical management
- * Monitor weight and BMI during treatment
- * While giving a drug to a patient who has gained >5% of initial weight, consider evaluating for the presence of pre-diabetes, diabetes, or dyslipidemia, or consider switching to a different antidepressant
- EKGs may be useful for selected patients (e.g., those with personal or family history of QTc prolongation; cardiac arrhythmia; recent myocardial infarction; uncompensated heart failure; or taking agents that prolong QTc interval such as pimozide, thioridazine, selected antiarrhythmics, moxifloxacin, sparfloxacin, etc.)
- Patients at risk for electrolyte disturbances (e.g., patients on diuretic therapy) should have baseline and periodic serum potassium and magnesium measurements

SIDE EFFECTS

How Drug Causes Side Effects

- Anticholinergic activity may explain sedative effects, dry mouth, constipation, and blurred vision
- Sedative effects and weight gain may be due to antihistamine properties
- Blockade of alpha adrenergic 1 receptors may explain dizziness, sedation, and hypotension
- Cardiac arrhythmias and seizures, especially in overdose, may be caused by blockade of ion channels

Notable Side Effects

- Blurred vision, constipation, urinary retention, increased appetite, dry mouth, nausea, diarrhea, heartburn, unusual taste in mouth, weight gain
- Fatigue, weakness, dizziness, sedation, headache, anxiety, nervousness, restlessness
- Sexual dysfunction (impotence, change in libido)
- Sweating, rash, itching

Life-Threatening or Dangerous Side Effects

- Paralytic ileus, hyperthermia (TCAs/ tetracylics + anticholinergic agents)
- Lowered seizure threshold and rare seizures
- Orthostatic hypotension, sudden death, arrhythmias, tachycardia
- QTc prolongation
- Hepatic failure, extrapyramidal symptoms
- Increased intraocular pressure
- Rare induction of mania
- Rare activation of suicidal ideation and behavior (suicidality) (short-term studies did not show an increase in the risk of suicidality with antidepressants compared to placebo beyond age 24)

Weight Gain

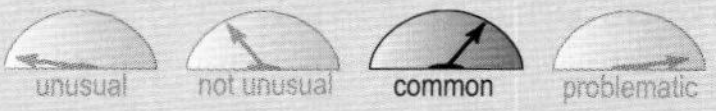

- Many experience and/or can be significant in amount
- Can increase appetite and carbohydrate craving

Sedation

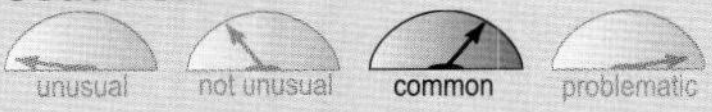

- Many experience and/or can be significant in amount
- Tolerance to sedative effect may develop with long-term use

What to Do About Side Effects

- Wait
- Wait
- Wait
- Lower the dose
- Switch to an SSRI or newer antidepressant

Best Augmenting Agents for Side Effects

- Many side effects cannot be improved with an augmenting agent

DOSING AND USE

Usual Dosage Range

- 75–150 mg/day (for depression)
- 50–150 mg/day (for chronic pain)

Dosage Forms

- Tablet 25 mg, 50 mg, 75 mg

How to Dose

- Initial 25 mg/day at bedtime; increase by 25 mg every 3–7 days
- 75 mg/day; after 2 weeks increase dose gradually by 25 mg/day; maximum dose generally 225 mg/day

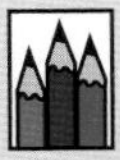

Dosing Tips

- If given in a single dose, should generally be administered at bedtime because of its sedative properties
- If given in split doses, largest dose should generally be given at bedtime because of its sedative properties
- If patients experience nightmares, split dose and do not give large dose at bedtime
- Patients treated for chronic pain may only require lower doses

✻ Risk of seizures increases with dose, especially with maprotiline above 200 mg/day

- If intolerable anxiety, insomnia, agitation, akathisia, or activation occur either upon dosing initiation or discontinuation, consider the possibility of activated bipolar disorder, and switch to a mood stabilizer or an atypical antipsychotic

Overdose

- Death may occur; convulsions, cardiac dysrhythmias, severe hypotension, CNS depression, coma, changes in EKG

Long-Term Use

- Safe

Habit Forming

- No

How to Stop

- Taper to avoid withdrawal effects
- Even with gradual dose reduction some withdrawal symptoms may appear within the first 2 weeks
- Many patients tolerate 50% dose reduction for 3 days, then another 50% reduction for 3 days, then discontinuation
- If withdrawal symptoms emerge during discontinuation, raise dose to stop symptoms and then restart withdrawal much more slowly

Pharmacokinetics

- Substrate for CYP450 2D6
- Mean half-life approximately 51 hours
- Peak plasma concentration 8–24 hours

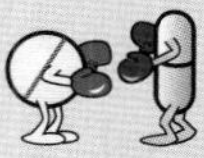

Drug Interactions

- Tramadol increases the risk of seizures in patients taking TCAs
- Use of TCAs/tetracyclics with anticholinergic drugs may result in paralytic ileus or hyperthermia
- Fluoxetine, paroxetine, bupropion, duloxetine, and other CYP450 2D6 inhibitors may increase TCA/tetracyclic concentrations
- Cimetidine may increase plasma concentrations of TCAs/tetracyclics and cause anticholinergic symptoms
- Phenothiazines or haloperidol may raise TCA/tetracyclic blood concentrations
- May alter effects of antihypertensive drugs; may inhibit hypotensive effects of clonidine
- Use with sympathomimetic agents may increase sympathetic activity

- Methylphenidate may inhibit metabolism of TCAs/tetracyclics
- Activation and agitation, especially following switching or adding antidepressants, may represent the induction of a bipolar state, especially a mixed dysphoric bipolar II condition sometimes associated with suicidal ideation, and require the addition of lithium, a mood stabilizer or an atypical antipsychotic, and/or discontinuation of maprotiline

Other Warnings/ Precautions

- Add or initiate other antidepressants with caution for up to 2 weeks after discontinuing maprotiline
- Generally, do not use with MAOIs, including 14 days after MAOIs are stopped; do not start an MAOI for at least 5 half-lives (5 to 7 days for most drugs) after discontinuing maprotiline, but see Pearls
- Use with caution in patients with history of seizures, urinary retention, angle-closure glaucoma, hyperthyroidism
- TCAs/tetracyclics can increase QTc interval, especially at toxic doses, which can be attained not only by overdose but also by combining with drugs that inhibit TCA/ tetracyclic metabolism via CYP450 2D6, potentially causing torsade de pointes-type arrhythmia or sudden death
- Because TCAs/tetracyclics can prolong QTc interval, use with caution in patients who have bradycardia or who are taking drugs that can induce bradycardia (e.g., beta blockers, calcium channel blockers, clonidine, digitalis)
- Because TCAs/tetracyclics can prolong QTc interval, use with caution in patients who have hypokalemia and/or hypomagnesemia or who are taking drugs that can induce hypokalemia and/or magnesemia (e.g., diuretics, stimulant laxatives, intravenous amphotericin B, glucocorticoids, tetracosactide)
- When treating children, carefully weigh the risks and benefits of pharmacological treatment against the risks and benefits of nontreatment with antidepressants and make sure to document this in the patient's chart
- Distribute the brochures provided by the FDA and the drug companies
- Warn patients and their caregivers about the possibility of activating side effects and advise them to report such symptoms immediately
- Monitor patients for activation of suicidal ideation, especially children and adolescents

Do Not Use

- If patient is recovering from myocardial infarction
- If patient is taking agents capable of significantly prolonging QTc interval (e.g., pimozide, thioridazine, selected antiarrhythmics, moxifloxacin, sparfloxacin)
- If there is a history of QTc prolongation or cardiac arrhythmia, recent acute myocardial infarction, uncompensated heart failure
- If patient is taking drugs that inhibit TCA/ tetracyclic metabolism, including CYP450 2D6 inhibitors, except by an expert
- If there is reduced CYP450 2D6 function, such as patients who are poor 2D6 metabolizers, except by an expert and at low doses
- If there is a proven allergy to maprotiline

SPECIAL POPULATIONS

Renal Impairment

- Use with caution

Hepatic Impairment

- Use with caution

Cardiac Impairment

- Baseline ECG is recommended
- TCAs/tetracyclics have been reported to cause arrhythmias, prolongation of conduction time, orthostatic hypotension, sinus tachycardia, and heart failure, especially in the diseased heart
- Myocardial infarction and stroke have been reported with TCAs/tetracyclics
- TCAs/tetracyclics produce QTc prolongation, which may be enhanced by the existence of bradycardia, hypokalemia, congenital or acquired long QTc interval, which should be evaluated prior to administering maprotiline
- Use with caution if treating concomitantly with a medication likely to produce

prolonged bradycardia, hypokalemia, slowing of intracardiac conduction, or prolongation of the QTc interval
- Avoid TCAs/tetracyclics in patients with a known history of QTc prolongation, recent acute myocardial infarction, and uncompensated heart failure
- TCAs/tetracyclics may cause a sustained increase in heart rate in patients with ischemic heart disease and may worsen (decrease) heart rate variability, an independent risk of mortality in cardiac populations
- Since SSRIs may improve (increase) heart rate variability in patients following a myocardial infarct and may improve survival as well as mood in patients with acute angina or following a myocardial infarction, these are more appropriate agents for cardiac population than tricyclic/tetracyclic antidepressants

✻ Risk/benefit ratio may not justify use of TCAs/tetracyclics in cardiac impairment

Elderly

- Baseline ECG is recommended for patients over age 50
- May be more sensitive to anticholinergic, cardiovascular, hypotensive, and sedative effects
- Usual dose generally 50–75 mg/day
- Reduction in the risk of suicidality with antidepressants compared to placebo in adults age 65 and older

Children and Adolescents

- Carefully weigh the risks and benefits of pharmacological treatment against the risks and benefits of nontreatment with antidepressants and make sure to document this in the patient's chart
- Monitor patients face-to-face regularly, particularly during the first several weeks of treatment
- Use with caution, observing for activation of known or unknown bipolar disorder and/or suicidal ideation, and inform parents or guardians of this risk so they can help observe child or adolescent patients
- Not recommended for use under age 18
- Several studies show lack of efficacy of TCAs/tetracyclics for depression
- May be used to treat enuresis or hyperactive/impulsive behaviors
- Some cases of sudden death have occurred in children taking TCAs/tetracyclics
- Maximum dose for children and adolescents is 75 mg/day

Pregnancy

- Effective June 30, 2015, the US FDA requires changes to the content and format of pregnancy and lactation information in prescription drug labels, including the elimination of the pregnancy letter categories; the Pregnancy and Lactation Labeling Rule (PLLR or final rule) applies only to prescription drugs and will be phased in gradually for drugs approved on or after June 30, 2001
- Controlled studies have not been conducted in pregnant women
- Animal studies do not show adverse effects
- Adverse effects have been reported in infants whose mothers took a TCA/tetracyclic (lethargy, withdrawal symptoms, fetal malformations)
- Must weigh the risk of treatment (first trimester fetal development, third trimester newborn delivery) to the child against the risk of no treatment (recurrence of depression, maternal health, infant bonding) to the mother and child
- For many patients this may mean continuing treatment during pregnancy

Breast Feeding

- Some drug is found in mother's breast milk

✻ Recommended either to discontinue drug or bottle feed

- Immediate postpartum period is a high-risk time for depression, especially in women who have had prior depressive episodes, so drug may need to be reinstituted late in the third trimester or shortly after childbirth to prevent a recurrence during the postpartum period
- Must weigh benefits of breast feeding with risks and benefits of antidepressant treatment versus nontreatment to both the infant and the mother
- For many patients this may mean continuing treatment during breast feeding

THE ART OF PSYCHOPHARMACOLOGY

Potential Advantages
- Patients with insomnia
- Severe or treatment-resistant depression

Potential Disadvantages
- Pediatric and geriatric patients
- Patients concerned with weight gain
- Cardiac patients
- Patients with seizure disorders

Primary Target Symptoms
- Depressed mood
- Chronic pain

Pearls
- Tricyclic/tetracyclic antidepressants are often a first-line treatment option for chronic pain
- Tricyclic/tetracyclic antidepressants are no longer generally considered a first-line treatment option for depression because of their side effect profile
- Tricyclic/tetracyclic antidepressants continue to be useful for severe or treatment-resistant depression

✻ May have somewhat increased risk of seizures compared to some other TCAs, especially at higher doses
- TCAs/tetracyclics may aggravate psychotic symptoms
- Alcohol should be avoided because of additive CNS effects
- Underweight patients may be more susceptible to adverse cardiovascular effects
- Children, patients with inadequate hydration, and patients with cardiac disease may be more susceptible to TCA/tetracyclic-induced cardiotoxicity than healthy adults
- For the expert only: a heroic treatment (but potentially dangerous) for severely treatment-resistant patients is to give simultaneously with MAOIs for patients who fail to respond to numerous other antidepressants
- If this option is elected, start the MAOI with the tricyclic/tetracyclic antidepressant simultaneously at low doses after appropriate drug washout, then alternately increase doses of these agents every few days to a week as tolerated
- Although very strict dietary and concomitant drug restrictions must be observed to prevent hypertensive crises and serotonin syndrome, the most common side effects of MAOI/tricyclic or tetracyclic combinations may be weight gain and orthostatic hypotension
- Patients on tricyclics/tetracyclics should be aware that they may experience symptoms such as photosensitivity or blue-green urine
- SSRIs may be more effective than TCAs/tetracyclics in women, and TCAs/tetracyclics may be more effective than SSRIs in men

✻ May have a more rapid onset of action than some other TCAs/tetracyclics
- Since tricyclic/tetracyclic antidepressants are substrates for CYP450 2D6, and 7% of the population (especially Caucasians) may have a genetic variant leading to reduced activity of 2D6, such patients may not safely tolerate normal doses of tricyclic/tetracyclic antidepressants and may require dose reduction
- Phenotypic testing may be necessary to detect this genetic variant prior to dosing with a tricyclic/tetracyclic antidepressant, especially in vulnerable populations such as children, elderly, cardiac populations, and those on concomitant medications
- Patients who seem to have extraordinarily severe side effects at normal or low doses may have this phenotypic CYP450 2D6 variant and require low doses or switching to another antidepressant not metabolized by 2D6

Suggested Reading

Anderson IM. Meta-analytical studies on new antidepressants. Br Med Bull 2001;57:161–78.

Anderson IM. Selective serotonin reuptake inhibitors versus tricyclic antidepressants: a meta-analysis of efficacy and tolerability. J Aff Disorders 2000;58:19–36.

Kane JM, Lieberman J. The efficacy of amoxapine, maprotiline, and trazodone in comparison to imipramine and amitriptyline: a review of the literature. Psychopharmacol Bull 1984;20:240–9.

MEMANTINE

THERAPEUTICS

Brands • Namenda
• Namenda XR

see index for additional brand names

Generic? Yes

Class

- Neuroscience-based Nomenclature: Glutamate receptor antagonist (Glu-RAn)
- NMDA receptor antagonist; *N*-methyl-d-aspartate (NMDA) subtype of glutamate receptor antagonist; cognitive enhancer

Commonly Prescribed for

(bold for FDA approved)

- **Alzheimer disease (moderate to severe)**
- Alzheimer disease (mild to moderate)
- Memory disorders in other conditions
- Mild cognitive impairment
- Chronic pain

How the Drug Works

* Is a low to moderate affinity noncompetitive (open-channel) NMDA receptor antagonist, which binds preferentially to the NMDA receptor-operated cation channels
- Presumably interferes with the postulated persistent activation of NMDA receptors by excessive glutamate release in Alzheimer disease

How Long Until It Works

- Memory improvement is not expected and it may take months before any stabilization in degenerative course is evident

If It Works

- May slow progression of disease, but does not reverse the degenerative process

If It Doesn't Work

- Consider adjusting dose, switching to a cholinesterase inhibitor or adding a cholinesterase inhibitor
- Reconsider diagnosis and rule out other conditions such as depression or a dementia other than Alzheimer disease

Best Augmenting Combos for Partial Response or Treatment Resistance

* Atypical antipsychotics to reduce behavioral disturbances
* Antidepressants if concomitant depression, apathy, or lack of interest
* May be combined with cholinesterase inhibitors
- Divalproex, carbamazepine, or oxcarbazepine for behavioral disturbances

Tests

- None for healthy individuals

SIDE EFFECTS

How Drug Causes Side Effects

- Presumably due to excessive actions at NMDA receptors

Notable Side Effects

- Dizziness, headache
- Constipation

Life-Threatening or Dangerous Side Effects

- Seizures (rare)

Weight Gain

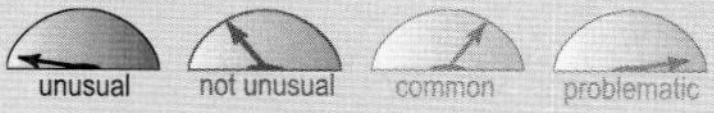

- Reported but not expected

Sedation

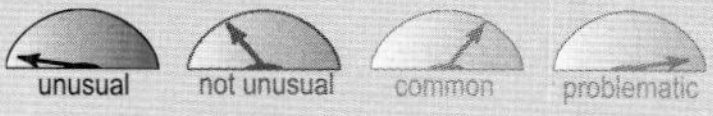

- Reported but not expected
- Fatigue may occur

What to Do About Side Effects

- Wait
- Wait
- Wait
- Consider lowering dose or switching to a different agent

Best Augmenting Agents for Side Effects

- Many side effects cannot be improved with an augmenting agent

DOSING AND USE

Usual Dosage Range

- 10 mg twice daily
- 28 mg once daily (extended-release)

Dosage Forms
- Tablet 5 mg, 10 mg
- Oral solution 2 mg/mL
- Extended-release capsule 7 mg, 14 mg, 21 mg, 28 mg

How to Dose
- Initial 5 mg/day; can increase by 5 mg each week; doses over 5 mg should be divided; maximum dose 10 mg twice daily
- Extended-release: initial 7 mg once daily; can increase by 7 mg each week; maximum dose 28 mg once daily

Dosing Tips
✻ Despite very long half-life, is generally dosed twice daily, although some data suggest once daily is safe and tolerable
- Both the patient and the patient's caregiver should be instructed on how to dose memantine since patients themselves have moderate to severe dementia and may require assistance

✻ Memantine is unlikely to affect pharmacokinetics of acetylcholinesterase inhibitors
- Absorption not affected by food

Overdose
- No fatalities have been reported; restlessness, psychosis, visual hallucinations, sedation, stupor, loss of consciousness

Long-Term Use
- Drug may lose effectiveness in slowing degenerative course of Alzheimer disease after 6 months

Habit Forming
- No

How to Stop
- No known withdrawal symptoms
- Theoretically, discontinuation could lead to notable deterioration in memory and behavior which may not be restored when drug is restarted or a cholinesterase inhibitor is initiated

Pharmacokinetics
- Little metabolism; mostly excreted unchanged in the urine
- Terminal elimination half-life approximately 60–80 hours
- Minimal inhibition of CYP450 enzymes

Drug Interactions
- No interactions with drugs metabolized by CYP450 enzymes
- Drugs that raise the urine pH (e.g., carbonic anhydrase inhibitors, sodium bicarbonate) may reduce elimination of memantine and raise plasma levels of memantine

✻ No interactions with cholinesterase inhibitors

Other Warnings/ Precautions
✻ Use cautiously if coadministering with other NMDA antagonists such as amantadine, ketamine, and dextromethorphan

Do Not Use
- If there is a proven allergy to memantine

SPECIAL POPULATIONS

Renal Impairment
- No dose adjustment in mild or moderate impairment
- Reduce dose in severe impairment

Hepatic Impairment
- Not likely to require dosage adjustment

Cardiac Impairment
- Not likely to require dosage adjustment

Elderly
- Pharmacokinetics similar to younger adults

Children and Adolescents
- Memantine use has not been studied in children or adolescents

Pregnancy

- Effective June 30, 2015, the US FDA requires changes to the content and format of pregnancy and lactation information in prescription drug labels, including the elimination of the pregnancy letter categories; the Pregnancy and Lactation Labeling Rule (PLLR or final rule) applies only to prescription drugs and will be phased in gradually for drugs approved on or after June 30, 2001
- Controlled studies have not been conducted in pregnant women
- Animal studies do not show adverse effects
- ✻ Not recommended for use in pregnant women or women of childbearing potential

Breast Feeding

- Unknown if memantine is secreted in human breast milk, but all psychotropics assumed to be secreted in breast milk
- ✻ Recommended either to discontinue drug or bottle feed
- Memantine is not recommended for use in nursing women

THE ART OF PSYCHOPHARMACOLOGY

Potential Advantages

- In patients with more advanced Alzheimer disease

Potential Disadvantages

- Unproven to be effective in mild to moderate Alzheimer disease
- Patients who have difficulty taking a medication twice daily

Primary Target Symptoms

- Memory loss in Alzheimer disease
- Behavioral symptoms in Alzheimer disease
- Memory loss in other dementias

Pearls

- ✻ Memantine's actions are somewhat like the natural inhibition of NMDA receptors by magnesium, and thus memantine is a sort of "artificial magnesium"
- Theoretically, NMDA antagonism of memantine is strong enough to block chronic low-level overexcitation of glutamate receptors associated with Alzheimer disease, but not strong enough to interfere with periodic high level utilization of glutamate for plasticity, learning, and memory
- Structurally related to the antiparkinsonian and anti-influenza agent amantadine, which is also a weak NMDA antagonist
- ✻ Memantine is well tolerated with a low incidence of adverse effects
- Antagonist actions at 5HT3 receptors have unknown clinical consequences but may contribute to low incidence of gastrointestinal side effects
- A fixed-dose combination of memantine extended-release and donepezil has been approved for the treatment of moderate to severe Alzheimer's dementia in patients stabilized on memantine and donepezil
- Treat the patient but ask the caregiver about efficacy
- Delay in progression of Alzheimer disease is not evidence of disease-modifying actions of NMDA antagonism
- May or may not be effective in vascular dementia
- Under investigation for dementia associated with HIV/AIDS
- May or may not be effective in chronic neuropathic pain
- ✻ Theoretically, could be useful for any condition characterized by moderate overactivation of NMDA glutamate receptors (possibly neurodegenerative conditions or even bipolar disorder, anxiety disorders, or chronic neuropathic pain), but this is not proven

Suggested Reading

Areosa SA, Sherriff F. Memantine for dementia. Cochrane Database Syst Rev 2003;(3):CD003154.

Doggrell S. Is memantine a breakthrough in the treatment of moderate-to-severe Alzheimer's disease? Expert Opin Pharmacother 2003;4:1857–60.

Mobius HJ. Memantine: update on the current evidence. Int J Geriatr Psychiatry 2003;18(Suppl 1):S47–54.

Sani G, Serra G, Kotzalidis GD, et al. The role of memantine in the treatment of psychiatric disorders other than the dementias: a review of current preclinical and clinical evidence. CNS Drugs 2012;26(8):663–90.

Tariot PN, Federoff HJ. Current treatment for Alzheimer disease and future prospects. Alzheimer Dis Assoc Disord 2003;17(Suppl 4): S105–13.

THERAPEUTICS

Brands
- Serentil
- *Lidanil*

see index for additional brand names

Generic? Yes

Class
- Conventional antipsychotic (neuroleptic, phenothiazine, dopamine 2 antagonist)

Commonly Prescribed for
(bold for FDA approved)
- **Management of schizophrenic patients who fail to respond adequately to treatment with other antipsychotic drugs**

How the Drug Works
- Blocks dopamine 2 receptors, reducing positive symptoms of psychosis

How Long Until It Works
- Psychotic symptoms can improve within 1 week, but it may take several weeks for full effect on behavior

If It Works
- Is a second-line treatment option
- ✻ Should evaluate for switching to an antipsychotic with a better risk/benefit ratio

If It Doesn't Work
- Consider trying one of the first-line atypical antipsychotics (risperidone, olanzapine, quetiapine, ziprasidone, aripiprazole, paliperidone, asenapine, iloperidone, lurasidone, amisulpride)
- Consider trying another conventional antipsychotic
- If 2 or more antipsychotic monotherapies do not work, consider clozapine

Best Augmenting Combos for Partial Response or Treatment Resistance
- Augmentation of mesoridazine has not been systematically studied and can be dangerous, especially with drugs that can prolong QTc interval

Tests
- ✻ Baseline EKG and serum potassium levels should be determined
- ✻ Periodic evaluation of EKG and serum potassium levels
- Serum magnesium levels may also need to be monitored
- ✻ Since conventional antipsychotics are frequently associated with weight gain, before starting treatment, weigh all patients and determine if the patient is already overweight (BMI 25.0–29.9) or obese (BMI ≥30)
- Before giving a drug that can cause weight gain to an overweight or obese patient, consider determining whether the patient already has pre-diabetes (fasting plasma glucose 100–125 mg/dL), diabetes (fasting plasma glucose >126 mg/dL), or dyslipidemia (increased total cholesterol, LDL cholesterol, and triglycerides; decreased HDL cholesterol), and treat or refer such patients for treatment, including nutrition and weight management, physical activity counseling, smoking cessation, and medical management
- ✻ Monitor weight and BMI during treatment
- ✻ Consider monitoring fasting triglycerides monthly for several months in patients at high risk for metabolic complications and when initiating or switching antipsychotics
- ✻ While giving a drug to a patient who has gained >5% of initial weight, consider evaluating for the presence of pre-diabetes, diabetes, or dyslipidemia, or consider switching to a different antipsychotic
- Should check blood pressure in the elderly before starting and for the first few weeks of treatment
- Monitoring elevated prolactin levels of dubious clinical benefit
- Phenothiazines may cause false-positive phenylketonuria results
- Patients with low white blood cell count (WBC) or history of drug-induced leucopenia/neutropenia should have complete blood count (CBC) monitored frequently during the first few months and mesoridazine should be discontinued at the first sign of decline of WBC in the absence of other causative factors

SIDE EFFECTS

How Drug Causes Side Effects

- By blocking dopamine 2 receptors in the striatum, it can cause motor side effects
- By blocking dopamine 2 receptors in the pituitary, it can cause elevations in prolactin
- By blocking dopamine 2 receptors excessively in the mesocortical and mesolimbic dopamine pathways, especially at high doses, it can cause worsening of negative and cognitive symptoms (neuroleptic-induced deficit syndrome)
- Anticholinergic actions may cause sedation, blurred vision, constipation, dry mouth
- Antihistaminic actions may cause sedation, weight gain
- By blocking alpha 1 adrenergic receptors, it can cause dizziness, sedation, and hypotension
- Mechanism of weight gain and any possible increased incidence of diabetes or dyslipidemia with conventional antipsychotics is unknown

✻ Mechanism of potentially dangerous QTc prolongation may be related to actions at ion channels

Notable Side Effects

✻ Neuroleptic-induced deficit syndrome
✻ Akathisia
✻ Priapism
✻ Extrapyramidal symptoms, parkinsonism, tardive dyskinesia
✻ Galactorrhea, amenorrhea
✻ Pigmentary retinopathy at high doses

- Dizziness, sedation
- Dry mouth, constipation, blurred vision
- Decreased sweating
- Sexual dysfunction
- Hypotension
- Weight gain

Life-Threatening or Dangerous Side Effects

- Rare neuroleptic malignant syndrome
- Rare jaundice, agranulocytosis
- Rare seizures

✻ Dose-dependent QTc prolongation

- Ventricular arrhythmias and sudden death
- Increased risk of death and cerebrovascular events in elderly patients with dementia-related psychosis

Weight Gain

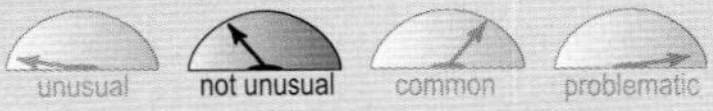

- Occurs in significant minority

Sedation

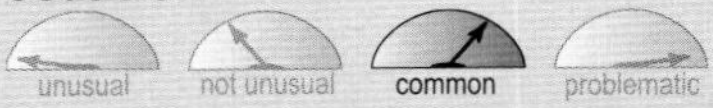

- Many experience and/or can be significant in amount
- Sedation is usually transient

What to Do About Side Effects

- Wait
- Wait
- Wait
- For motor symptoms, add an anticholinergic agent
- Reduce the dose
- For sedation, give at night
- Switch to an atypical antipsychotic
- Weight loss, exercise programs, and medical management for high BMIs, diabetes, dyslipidemia

Best Augmenting Agents for Side Effects

- Augmentation of mesoridazine has not been systematically studied and can be dangerous

DOSING AND USE

Usual Dosage Range

- Oral: 100–400 mg/day
- Injection: 25–200 mg/day

Dosage Forms

- Tablet 10 mg, 25 mg, 50 mg, 100 mg
- Ampul 25 mg/mL, 1 mL
- Concentrate 25 mg/mL

How to Dose

- Oral: initial 50 mg 3 times a day; increase dose cautiously as needed
- Injection: initial 25 mg; repeat after 30–60 minutes if needed
- Take liquid formulation in water, orange juice, or grapefruit juice

Dosing Tips

* ✻ The effects of mesoridazine on the QTc interval are dose-dependent, so start low and go slow while carefully monitoring QTc interval
* Treatment should be suspended if absolute neutrophil count falls below 1,000/mm^3

Overdose

* Deaths have occurred; sedation, confusion, agitation, respiratory depression, cardiac disturbances, coma

Long-Term Use

* Some side effects may be irreversible (e.g., tardive dyskinesia)

Habit Forming

* No

How to Stop

* Slow down-titration of oral formulation (over 6–8 weeks), especially when simultaneously beginning a new antipsychotic while switching (i.e., cross-titration)
* Rapid oral discontinuation may lead to rebound psychosis and worsening of symptoms
* If antiparkinson agents are being used, they should be continued for a few weeks after mesoridazine is discontinued

Pharmacokinetics

* Half-life approximately 2–9 hours

Drug Interactions

* May decrease the effects of levodopa, dopamine agonists
* May increase the effects of antihypertensive drugs
* May enhance QTc prolongation of other drugs capable of prolonging QTc interval
* Additive effects may occur if used with CNS depressants
* Respiratory depression or respiratory arrest may occur if mesoridazine is used with a barbiturate
* Some patients taking a neuroleptic and lithium have developed an encephalopathic syndrome similar to neuroleptic malignant syndrome
* Combined use with epinephrine may lower blood pressure

Other Warnings/ Precautions

* If signs of neuroleptic malignant syndrome develop, treatment should be immediately discontinued
* Use with caution in patients with respiratory disorders, glaucoma, or urinary retention
* Use cautiously in patients with alcohol withdrawal or convulsive disorders because of possible lowering of seizure threshold
* Use with caution if at all in Parkinson's disease or Lewy body dementia
* Avoid extreme heat exposure
* Antiemetic effect can mask signs of other disorders or overdose
* Do not use epinephrine in event of overdose as interaction with some pressor agents may lower blood pressure
* Because mesoridazine may dose-dependently prolong QTc interval, use with caution in patients who have bradycardia or who are taking drugs that can induce bradycardia (e.g., beta blockers, calcium channel blockers, clonidine, digitalis)
* Because mesoridazine may dose-dependently prolong QTc interval, use with caution in patients who have hypokalemia and/or hypomagnesemia or who are taking drugs that can induce hypokalemia and/or magnesemia (e.g., diuretics, stimulant laxatives, intravenous amphotericin B, glucocorticoids, tetracosactide)
* Mesoridazine can increase the QTc interval, potentially causing torsades de pointes-type arrhythmia or sudden death

Do Not Use

* If there is a history of QTc prolongation or cardiac arrhythmia, recent acute myocardial infarction, uncompensated heart failure
* ✻ If QTc interval greater than 450 msec or if taking an agent capable of prolonging the QTc interval
* If patient is in a comatose state or has CNS depression
* If there is a proven allergy to mesoridazine
* If there is a known sensitivity to any phenothiazine

SPECIAL POPULATIONS

Renal Impairment
- Use with caution

Hepatic Impairment
- Use with caution

Cardiac Impairment
- Mesoridazine produces a dose-dependent prolongation of QTc interval, which may be enhanced by the existence of bradycardia, hypokalemia, congenital, or acquired long QTc interval, which should be evaluated prior to administering mesoridazine
- Use with caution if treating concomitantly with a medication likely to produce prolonged bradycardia, hypokalemia, slowing of intracardiac conduction, or prolongation of the QTc interval
- Avoid mesoridazine in patients with a known history of QTc prolongation, recent acute myocardial infarction, and uncompensated heart failure
- ✻ Risk/benefit ratio may not justify use in cardiac impairment

Elderly
- Lower doses should be used and patient should be monitored closely
- Although conventional antipsychotics are commonly used for behavioral disturbances in dementia, no agent has been approved for treatment of elderly patients with dementia-related psychosis
- Elderly patients with dementia-related psychosis treated with antipsychotics are at an increased risk of death compared to placebo, and also have an increased risk of cerebrovascular events

Children and Adolescents
- Safety and efficacy not established

Pregnancy
- Effective June 30, 2015, the US FDA requires changes to the content and format of pregnancy and lactation information in prescription drug labels, including the elimination of the pregnancy letter categories; the Pregnancy and Lactation Labeling Rule (PLLR or final rule) applies only to prescription drugs and will be phased in gradually for drugs approved on or after June 30, 2001
- Controlled studies have not been conducted in pregnant women
- There is a risk of abnormal muscle movements and withdrawal symptoms in newborns whose mothers took an antipsychotic during the third trimester; symptoms may include agitation, abnormally increased or decreased muscle tone, tremor, sleepiness, severe difficulty breathing, and difficulty feeding
- Reports of extrapyramidal symptoms, jaundice, hyperreflexia, hyporeflexia in infants whose mothers took a phenothiazine during pregnancy
- Psychotic symptoms may worsen during pregnancy and some form of treatment may be necessary
- Atypical antipsychotics may be preferable to conventional antipsychotics or anticonvulsant mood stabilizers if treatment is required during pregnancy
- Mesoridazine should generally not be used during the first trimester
- Should evaluate for an antipsychotic with a better risk/benefit ratio if treatment is required during pregnancy

Breast Feeding
- Some drug is found in mother's breast milk
- Effects on infant have been observed (dystonia, tardive dyskinesia, sedation)
- ✻ Recommended either to discontinue drug or bottle feed

THE ART OF PSYCHOPHARMACOLOGY

Potential Advantages
- Only for patients who respond to this agent and not other antipsychotics

Potential Disadvantages
- Vulnerable populations such as children or elderly
- Patients on other drugs

Primary Target Symptoms
- Positive symptoms of psychosis in patients who fail to respond to treatment with other antipsychotics

- Motor and autonomic hyperactivity in patients who fail to respond to treatment with other antipsychotics
- Violent or aggressive behavior in patients who fail to respond to treatment with other antipsychotics

Pearls

✱ Generally, the benefits of mesoridazine do not outweigh its risks for most patients

✱ Because of its effects on the QTc interval, mesoridazine is not intended for use unless other options (at least 2 antipsychotics) have failed

- Mesoridazine has not been systematically studied in treatment-refractory schizophrenia
- Patients with inadequate responses to atypical antipsychotics may benefit from a trial of augmentation with a conventional antipsychotic or switching to a conventional antipsychotic
- However, long-term polypharmacy with a combination of a conventional antipsychotic with an atypical antipsychotic may combine their side effects without clearly augmenting the efficacy of either
- For treatment-resistant patients, especially those with impulsivity, aggression, violence, and self-harm, long-term polypharmacy with 2 atypical antipsychotics or with 1 atypical antipsychotic and 1 conventional antipsychotic may be useful or even necessary while closely monitoring
- In such cases, it may be beneficial to combine 1 depot antipsychotic with 1 oral antipsychotic
- Although a frequent practice by some prescribers, adding 2 conventional antipsychotics together has little rationale and may reduce tolerability without clearly enhancing efficacy

Suggested Reading

Frankenburg FR. Choices in antipsychotic therapy in schizophrenia. Harv Rev Psychiatry 1999;6:241–9.

Gardos G, Tecce JJ, Hartmann E, Bowers P, Cole JO. Treatment with mesoridazine and thioridazine in chronic schizophrenia: II. Potential predictors of drug response. Compr Psychiatry 1978;19:527–32.

Gershon S, Sakalis G, Bowers PA. Mesoridazine – a pharmacodynamic and pharmacokinetic profile. J Clin Psychiatry 1981;42:463–9.

THERAPEUTICS

Brands • Deplin

see index for additional brand names

Generic? No

Class

- Medical food (bioavailable form of folate)
- Trimonoamine modulator

Commonly Prescribed for

(bold for FDA approved as medical food indications)

- **Suboptimal folate levels in depressed patients (adjunct to antidepressant)**
- **Hyperhomocysteinemia in schizophrenia patients (adjunct to antipsychotic)**
- Enhancement of antidepressant response at the initiation of treatment
- Cognitive or mood symptoms in patients with MTHFR (methylene tetrahydrofolate) deficiency

How the Drug Works

- Folate is a water-soluble B vitamin (B9) that is essential for cell growth/ reproduction, breakdown/utilization of proteins, formation of nucleic acids, and other functions
- L-methylfolate, or 6-(S)-5-methyl-tetrahydrofolate, is derived from folate and is the form that enters the brain and works directly as a methyl donor and monoamine synthesis modulator
- That is, it regulates tetrahydrobiopterin (BH4), a critical enzyme cofactor for trimonoamine neurotransmitter synthesis
- Methyl donor for DNA methylation and thus an epigenetic regulator

How Long Until It Works

- Onset of therapeutic actions in depression is usually not immediate, but often delayed 2–4 weeks
- If it is not working within 6–8 weeks for depression, it may require a dosage increase or it may not work at all
- May continue to work for many years to prevent relapse of symptoms

If It Works

- The goal of treatment for depression is complete remission of current symptoms as well as prevention of future relapses
- Treatment most often reduces or even eliminates symptoms, but not a cure since symptoms can recur after medicine is stopped
- Continue treatment until all symptoms are gone (remission)
- Once symptoms gone, continue treating for 1 year for the first episode of depression
- For second and subsequent episodes of depression, treatment may need to be indefinite

If It Doesn't Work

- Many patients with depression have only a partial response where some symptoms are improved but others persist (especially insomnia, fatigue, and problems concentrating)
- Other patients may be nonresponders, sometimes called treatment-resistant or treatment-refractory
- Consider increasing dose, switching to another agent or adding an appropriate augmenting agent
- Consider psychotherapy
- Consider evaluation for another diagnosis or for a comorbid condition (e.g., medical illness, substance abuse, etc.)
- Some patients may experience apparent lack of consistent efficacy due to activation of latent or underlying bipolar disorder, and require antidepressant discontinuation and a switch to a mood stabilizer

Best Augmenting Combos for Partial Response or Treatment Resistance

- L-methylfolate is itself an adjunct to standard treatments for depression or schizophrenia at the initiation of treatment or to augment a partial response

Tests

- Baseline folate levels (serum levels for recent folate intake; red blood cell or CSF levels for long-term folate levels)
- Baseline homocysteine levels (reciprocal relationship with folate levels; high homocysteine levels may be more sensitive in detected folate deficiency than folate levels themselves in some patients)

- May monitor folate levels for patients taking an agent capable of affecting folate metabolism, absorption, or degradation
- May consider genotyping for deficient folate synthesis via MTHFR T alleles or MTHFD1 A alleles

SIDE EFFECTS

How Drug Causes Side Effects
- L-methylfolate does not typically cause side effects

Notable Side Effects
- L-methylfolate does not typically cause side effects

Life-Threatening or Dangerous Side Effects
- Theoretically, rare induction of mania or suicidal ideation and behavior (suicidality)

Weight Gain

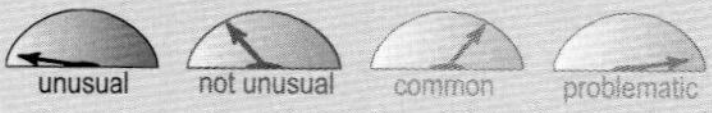

- Reported but not expected

Sedation

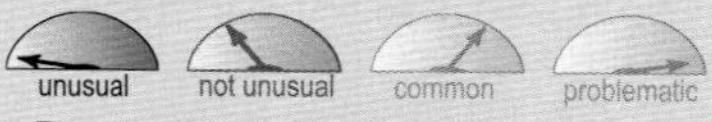

- Reported but not expected

What to Do About Side Effects
- Wait
- Lower the dose or administer in divided doses
- Switch to another drug

Best Augmenting Agents for Side Effects
- Many side effects cannot be improved with an augmenting agent
- Activation and agitation may represent the induction of a bipolar state, especially a mixed dysphoric bipolar II condition sometimes associated with suicidal ideation, and require the addition of lithium, a mood stabilizer or an atypical antipsychotic, and/or discontinuation of l-methylfolate or the primary antidepressant

DOSING AND USE

Usual Dosage Range
- 7.5–15 mg/day

Dosage Forms
- Tablet 7.5 mg, 15 mg

How to Dose
- Initial 7.5–15 mg/day
- Doses above 15 mg/day should be administered in divided doses

Dosing Tips
- Can be taken with or without food
- L-methyltetrahydrofolate was shown to be 7 times more bioavailable than folic acid
- That means 7.5 mg of the active l enantiomer of methylfolate may be equivalent to 52 mg of folate (usual dose of folate is 100 ug to 1.0 mg)
- If intolerable anxiety, insomnia, agitation, akathisia, or activation occur either upon dosing initiation or discontinuation, consider the possibility of activated bipolar disorder and switch to a mood stabilizer or an atypical antipsychotic

Overdose
- Doses up to 90 mg/day of methylfolate (45 mg l-methylfolate) have been studied without any additional adverse events
- L-methylfolate is generally regarded as safe
- A toxic dose of l-methylfolate is not known at this time

Long-Term Use
- Safe

Habit Forming
- No

How to Stop
- Taper not necessary

Pharmacokinetics
- Mean elimination half-life approximately 3 hours for d,l-methylfolate
- L-methylfolate is naturally stored in most cells and used by the body when needed; therefore, l-methylfolate may not follow typical drug pharmacokinetic patterns

Drug Interactions

- L-methylfolate may reduce plasma levels of certain anticonvulsants, including phenytoin, carbamazepine, fosphenytoin, phenobarbital, primidone, or valproate
- L-methylfolate may reduce plasma levels of pyrimethamine
- Patients taking folate-lowering drugs (e.g., anticonvulsants, cholestyramine, colestipol, cycloserine, aminopterin, methotrexate, sulfasalazine, pyrimethamine, triamterene, trimethoprim, isotretinoin, fluoxetine, nonsteroidal anti-inflammatory drugs (NSAIDs), methylprednisolone, pentamidine, or who smoke or drink heavily may require higher doses of l-methylfolate

Other Warnings/ Precautions

- Folic acid may mask symptoms of B12 deficiency (e.g., pernicious anemia), although this may be less likely with l-methylfolate
- Use with caution in patients with bipolar disorder unless treated with concomitant mood-stabilizing agent
- Monitor patients for activation of suicidal ideation, especially children and adolescents
- Folic acid, when administered in doses above 800 mcg, may increase the amount of unmetabolized folic acid, which has been linked to accelerated growth of existing neoplasms in the colon; l-methylfolate may be less likely than folic acid to accelerate the growth of existing neoplasms

Do Not Use

- If there is a proven allergy to folate or folic acid

SPECIAL POPULATIONS

Renal Impairment

- Dose adjustment not necessary

Hepatic Impairment

- Dose adjustment not necessary

Cardiac Impairment

- Dose adjustment not necessary

Elderly

- Dose adjustment not necessary

Children and Adolescents

- Use with caution, observing for activation of known or unknown bipolar disorder and/ or suicidal ideation, and inform parents or guardians of this risk so they can help observe child or adolescent patients
- Safety and efficacy have not been established

Pregnancy

- No controlled studies in humans or animals
- Controlled studies of folic acid at recommended doses have failed to demonstrate risk to the fetus
- There are no studies of folic acid at high doses
- Because pregnant women are advised to take folic acid or prenatal vitamins that contain folic acid, it is important to ask the patient about any supplements or vitamins she may be taking and consider this when deciding whether to prescribe l-methylfolate

Breast Feeding

- Some drug is found in mother's breast milk

THE ART OF PSYCHOPHARMACOLOGY

Potential Advantages

- Patients who need efficacy greater than an antidepressant alone at the initiation of treatment
- Patients with partial or inadequate response to antidepressants
- Patients who cannot tolerate other antidepressants

Potential Disadvantages

- Patients with adequate folate levels

Primary Target Symptoms

- Depressed mood
- Cognitive symptoms

Pearls

- Numerous studies suggest that low plasma, red blood cell, and/or CSF levels of folate may be associated with depression in some patients
- Treatment with l-methylfolate seems to be safe, has few if any side effects, and is generally less expensive than augmenting with a second branded antidepressant or atypical antipsychotic
- L-methylfolate is able to cross the blood-brain barrier and support the synthesis of monoamines
- Early studies suggest that those with obesity may be better responders
- Early studies suggest that those with genetic polymorphisms reducing the formation of l-methylfolate may be better responders

Suggested Reading

Bottiglieri T. Homocysteine and folate metabolism in depression. Prog Neuropsychopharmacology Biol Psychiatry 2005;29:1103–12.

Fava M, Mischoulon D. Folate in depression: efficacy, safety, differences in formulations, and clinical issues. J Clin Psychiatry 2009;70 (Suppl 5):S12–17.

Miller AL. The methylation, neurotransmitter, and antioxidant connections between folate and depression. Altern Med Rev 2008;13(3):216–26.

Stahl SM. L-methylfolate: A vitamin for your monoamines. J Clin Psychiatry 2008;69(9):1352–3.

THERAPEUTICS

Brands • Focalin
• Focalin XR

see index for additional brand names

Generic? Yes

Class

- Neuroscience-based Nomenclature: dopamine, norepinephrine reuptake inhibitor and releaser (DN-RIRe)
- Stimulant

Commonly Prescribed for

(bold for FDA approved)

- **Attention deficit hyperactivity disorder (ADHD) in children ages 6–17 (Focalin, Focalin XR) and in adults (Focalin XR)**
- Narcolepsy
- Treatment-resistant depression

How the Drug Works

✱ Increases norepinephrine and especially dopamine actions by blocking their reuptake

- Enhancement of dopamine and norepinephrine actions in certain brain regions (e.g., dorsolateral prefrontal cortex) may improve attention, concentration, executive function, and wakefulness
- Enhancement of dopamine actions in other brain regions (e.g., basal ganglia) may improve hyperactivity
- Enhancement of dopamine and norepinephrine in yet other brain regions (e.g., medial prefrontal cortex, hypothalamus) may improve depression, fatigue, and sleepiness

How Long Until It Works

- Onset of action can occur 30 minutes post-administration
- Can take several weeks to attain maximum therapeutic benefit

If It Works (for ADHD)

- The goal of treatment of ADHD is reduction of symptoms of inattentiveness, motor hyperactivity, and/or impulsiveness that disrupt social, school, and/or occupational functioning
- Continue treatment until all symptoms are under control or improvement is stable and then continue treatment indefinitely as long as improvement persists
- Reevaluate the need for treatment periodically
- Treatment for ADHD begun in childhood may need to be continued into adolescence and adulthood if continued benefit is documented

If It Doesn't Work (for ADHD)

- Consider adjusting dose or switching to a formulation of d,l-methylphenidate or to another agent
- Consider behavioral therapy
- Consider the presence of noncompliance and counsel patient and parents
- Consider evaluation for another diagnosis or for a comorbid condition (e.g., bipolar disorder, substance abuse, medical illness, etc.)

✱ Some ADHD patients and some depressed patients may experience lack of consistent efficacy due to activation of latent or underlying bipolar disorder, and require either augmenting with a mood stabilizer or switching to a mood stabilizer

Best Augmenting Combos for Partial Response or Treatment Resistance

✱ Best to attempt other monotherapies prior to augmenting

- For the expert, can combine immediate-release formulation of d-methylphenidate with a sustained-release formulation of d-methylphenidate for ADHD
- For the expert, can combine with modafinil or atomoxetine for ADHD
- For the expert, can occasionally combine with atypical antipsychotics in highly treatment-resistant cases of bipolar disorder or ADHD
- For the expert, can combine with antidepressants to boost antidepressant efficacy in highly treatment-resistant cases of depression while carefully monitoring patient

Tests

- Before treatment, assess for presence of cardiac disease (history, family history, physical exam)
- Blood pressure should be monitored regularly
- In children, monitor weight and height
- Periodic complete blood cell and platelet counts may be considered during prolonged therapy (rare leukopenia and/or anemia)

SIDE EFFECTS

How Drug Causes Side Effects
- Increases in norepinephrine peripherally can cause autonomic side effects, including tremor, tachycardia, hypertension, and cardiac arrhythmias
- Increases in norepinephrine and dopamine centrally can cause CNS side effects such as insomnia, agitation, psychosis, and substance abuse

Notable Side Effects
✻ Insomnia, headache, exacerbation of tics, nervousness, irritability, overstimulation, tremor, dizziness
- Anorexia, nausea, abdominal pain, weight loss
- Can temporarily slow normal growth in children (controversial)
- Blurred vision

Life-Threatening or Dangerous Side Effects
- Psychotic episodes, especially with parenteral abuse

✻ Rare priapism
- Seizures
- Palpitations, tachycardia, hypertension
- Rare neuroleptic malignant syndrome
- Rare activation of hypomania, mania, or suicidal ideation (controversial)
- Cardiovascular adverse effects, sudden death in patients with preexisting cardiac structural abnormalities

Weight Gain
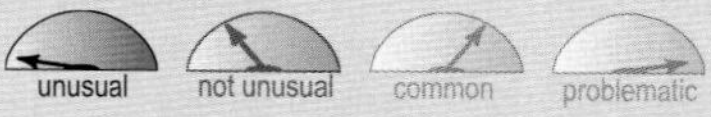

- Reported but not expected
- Some patients may experience weight loss

Sedation
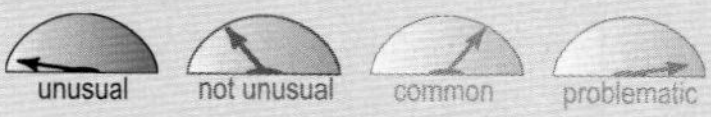

- Reported but not expected
- Activation much more common than sedation

What to Do About Side Effects
- Wait
- Adjust dose
- Switch to a formulation of d,l-methylphenidate
- Switch to another agent
- For insomnia, avoid dosing in afternoon/evening

Best Augmenting Agents for Side Effects
- Beta blockers for peripheral autonomic side effects
- Dose reduction or switching to another agent may be more effective since most side effects cannot be improved with an augmenting agent

DOSING AND USE

Usual Dosage Range
- 2.5–10 mg twice per day

Dosage Forms
- Immediate-release tablet 2.5 mg, 5 mg, 10 mg
- Extended-release capsule 5 mg, 10 mg, 15 mg, 20 mg, 25 mg, 30 mg, 35 mg, 40 mg

How to Dose
- Immediate-release: for patients who are not taking racemic d,l-methylphenidate, initial 2.5 mg twice per day in 4-hour intervals; may adjust dose in weekly intervals by 2.5–5 mg/day; maximum dose generally 10 mg twice per day
- Immediate-release: for patients currently taking racemic d,l-methylphenidate, initial dose should be half the current dose of racemic d,l-methylphenidate; maximum dose generally 10 mg twice per day
- Extended-release: for children, same titration schedule as immediate-release but dosed once in the morning; maximum dose 30 mg/day
- Extended-release: for adults not taking racemic d,l-methylphenidate, initial 10 mg/day in the morning; may adjust dose in weekly intervals by 10 mg/day; maximum dose generally 40 mg/day

Dosing Tips
✻ Immediate-release d-methylphenidate has the same onset of action and duration of action as immediate-release racemic d,l-methylphenidate (i.e., 2–4 hours) but at half the dose

- Extended-release d-methylphenidate contains half the dose as immediate-release beads and half as delayed-release beads, so the dose is released in 2 pulses
- Although d-methylphenidate is generally considered to be twice as potent as racemic d,l-methylphenidate, some studies suggest that the d-isomer is actually more than twice as effective as racemic d,l-methylphenidate
- Side effects are generally dose-related
- Off-label uses are dosed the same as for ADHD

✽ May be possible to dose only during the school week for some ADHD patients

✽ May be able to give drug holidays over the summer in order to reassess therapeutic utility and effects on growth and to allow catch-up from any growth suppression as well as to assess any other side effects and the need to reinstitute stimulant treatment for the next school term

- Avoid dosing late in the day because of the risk of insomnia
- Taking with food may delay peak actions for 2–3 hours

Overdose
- Vomiting, tremor, coma, convulsion, hyperreflexia, euphoria, confusion, hallucination, tachycardia, flushing, palpitations, sweating, hyperpyrexia, hypertension, arrhythmia, mydriasis, agitation, delirium, headache

Long-Term Use
- Often used long-term for ADHD when ongoing monitoring documents continued efficacy
- Dependence and/or abuse may develop
- Tolerance to therapeutic effects may develop in some patients
- Long-term stimulant use may be associated with growth suppression in children (controversial)
- Periodic monitoring of weight, blood pressure, CBC, platelet counts, and liver function may be prudent

Habit Forming
- High abuse potential, Schedule II drug
- Patients may develop tolerance, psychological dependence

How to Stop
- Taper to avoid withdrawal effects
- Withdrawal following chronic therapeutic use may unmask symptoms of the underlying disorder and may require follow-up and reinstitution of treatment
- Careful supervision is required during withdrawal from abusive use since severe depression may occur

Pharmacokinetics
- d-*threo*-enantiomer of racemic d,l-methylphenidate
- Mean plasma elimination half-life approximately 2.2 hours (same as d,l-methylphenidate)
- Does not inhibit CYP450 enzymes

Drug Interactions
- May affect blood pressure and should be used cautiously with agents used to control blood pressure
- May inhibit metabolism of SSRIs, anticonvulsants (phenobarbital, phenytoin, primidone), TCAs, and coumarin anticoagulants, requiring downward dosage adjustments of these drugs
- Serious adverse effects may occur if combined with clonidine (controversial)
- Use with MAOIs, including within 14 days of MAOI use, is not advised, but this can sometimes be considered by experts who monitor depressed patients closely when other treatment options for depression fail
- CNS and cardiovascular actions of d-methylphenidate could theoretically be enhanced by combination with agents that block norepinephrine reuptake, such as the TCAs desipramine or protriptyline, venlafaxine, duloxetine, atomoxetine, milnacipran, and reboxetine
- Theoretically, antipsychotics should inhibit the stimulatory effects of d-methylphenidate
- Theoretically, d-methylphenidate could inhibit the antipsychotic actions of antipsychotics
- Theoretically, d-methylphenidate could inhibit the mood-stabilizing actions of atypical antipsychotics in some patients
- Combinations of d-methylphenidate with mood stabilizers (lithium, anticonvulsants,

atypical antipsychotics) is generally something for experts only, when monitoring patients closely and when other options fail
- Antacids or acid suppressants could alter the release of extended-release formulation

Other Warnings/ Precautions

- Use with caution in patients with any degree of hypertension, hyperthyroidism, or history of drug abuse
- Children who are not growing or gaining weight should stop treatment, at least temporarily
- May worsen motor and phonic tics
- May worsen symptoms of thought disorder and behavioral disturbance in psychotic patients
- Stimulants have a high potential for abuse and must be used with caution in anyone with a current or past history of substance abuse or alcoholism or in emotionally unstable patients
- Administration of stimulants for prolonged periods of time should be avoided whenever possible or done only with close monitoring, as it may lead to marked tolerance and drug dependence, including psychological dependence with varying degrees of abnormal behavior
- Particular attention should be paid to the possibility of subjects obtaining stimulants for nontherapeutic use or distribution to others and the drugs should in general be prescribed sparingly with documentation of appropriate use
- Usual dosing has been associated with sudden death in children with structural cardiac abnormalities
- Not an appropriate first-line treatment for depression or for normal fatigue
- May lower the seizure threshold
- Emergence or worsening of activation and agitation may represent the induction of a bipolar state, especially a mixed dysphoric bipolar II condition sometimes associated with suicidal ideation, and require the addition of a mood stabilizer and/or discontinuation of d-methylphenidate

Do Not Use

- If patient has extreme anxiety or agitation
- If patient has motor tics or Tourette's syndrome or if there is a family history of Tourette's, unless administered by an expert in cases when the potential benefits for ADHD outweigh the risks of worsening tics
- Should generally not be administered with an MAOI, including within 14 days of MAOI use, except in heroic circumstances and by an expert
- If patient has glaucoma
- If patient has structural cardiac abnormalities
- If patient has angioedema or anaphylaxis
- If there is a proven allergy to methylphenidate

SPECIAL POPULATIONS

Renal Impairment

- No dose adjustment necessary

Hepatic Impairment

- No dose adjustment necessary

Cardiac Impairment

- Use with caution, particularly in patients with recent myocardial infarction or other conditions that could be negatively affected by increased blood pressure
- Do not use in patients with structural cardiac abnormalities

Elderly

- Some patients may tolerate lower doses better

Children and Adolescents

- Safety and efficacy not established in children under age 6
- Use in young children should be reserved for the expert
- Methylphenidate has acute effects on growth hormone; long-term effects are unknown but weight and height should be monitored during long-term treatment
- Sudden death in children and adolescents with serious heart problems has been reported
- American Heart Association recommends EKG prior to initiating stimulant treatment in children, although not all experts agree

Pregnancy

- Effective June 30, 2015, the US FDA requires changes to the content and format of pregnancy and lactation information in prescription drug labels, including the elimination of the pregnancy letter categories; the Pregnancy and Lactation Labeling Rule (PLLR or final rule) applies only to prescription drugs and will be phased in gradually for drugs approved on or after June 30, 2001
- Controlled studies have not been conducted in pregnant women
- Infants whose mothers took methylphenidate during pregnancy may experience withdrawal symptoms
- Racemic methylphenidate has been shown to have teratogenic effects in rabbits when given in doses of 200 mg/kg/day throughout organogenesis
- Use in women of childbearing potential requires weighing potential benefits to the mother against potential risks to the fetus
- ❋ For ADHD patients, methylphenidate should generally be discontinued before anticipated pregnancies

Breast Feeding

- Unknown if methylphenidate is secreted in human breast milk, but all psychotropics assumed to be secreted in breast milk
- ❋ Recommended either to discontinue drug or bottle feed
- If infant shows signs of irritability, drug may need to be discontinued

THE ART OF PSYCHOPHARMACOLOGY

Potential Advantages

- The active d enantiomer of methylphenidate may be slightly more than twice as efficacious as racemic d,l-methylphenidate

Potential Disadvantages

- Patients with current or past substance abuse, bipolar disorder, or psychosis

Primary Target Symptoms

- Concentration, attention span
- Motor hyperactivity
- Impulsiveness
- Physical and mental fatigue
- Daytime sleepiness
- Depression

Pearls

- May be useful for treatment of depressive symptoms in medically ill elderly patients
- May be useful for treatment of post-stroke depression
- A classical augmentation strategy for treatment-refractory depression
- Specifically, may be useful for treatment of cognitive dysfunction and fatigue as residual symptoms of major depressive disorder unresponsive to multiple prior treatments
- May also be useful for the treatment of cognitive impairment, depressive symptoms, and severe fatigue in patients with HIV infection and in cancer patients
- Can be used to potentiate opioid analgesia and reduce sedation, particularly in end-of-life management
- Atypical antipsychotics may be useful in treating stimulant or psychotic consequences of overdose
- Some patients respond to or tolerate methylphenidate better than amphetamine, and vice versa
- Taking with food may delay peak actions of immediate-release d-methylphenidate for 2–3 hours
- Half-life and duration of clinical action tend to be shorter in younger children
- Drug abuse may actually be lower in ADHD adolescents treated with stimulants than in ADHD adolescents who are not treated
- New extended-release formulation is truly a once daily dose
- Extended-release capsule can be sprinkled over applesauce for patients unable to swallow the capsule
- Some patients may benefit from an occasional addition of an immediate-release dose of d-methylphenidate to the daily base dose of extended-release d-methylphenidate

Suggested Reading

Dexmethylphenidate – Novartis/Celgene. Focalin, D-MPH, D-methylphenidate hydrochloride, D-methylphenidate, dexmethylphenidate, dexmethylphenidate hydrochloride. Drugs R D 2002;3(4):279–82.

Keating GM, Figgitt DP. Dexmethylphenidate. Drugs 2002;62(13):1899–904.

THERAPEUTICS

Brands
- Concerta
- Metadate CD
- Ritalin
- Ritalin LA
- Methylin
- QuilliChew ER
- Quillivant XR
- Aptensio XR
- Daytrana

see index for additional brand names

Generic? Yes

Class
- Neuroscience-based Nomenclature: dopamine, norepinephrine reuptake inhibitor and releaser (DN-RIRe)
- Stimulant

Commonly Prescribed for
(bold for FDA approved)
- **Attention deficit hyperactivity disorder (ADHD) in children and adults (approved ages vary based on formulation)**
- **Narcolepsy (Metadate ER, Methylin ER, Ritalin, Ritalin SR)**
- Treatment-resistant depression

How the Drug Works
* Increases norepinephrine and especially dopamine actions by blocking their reuptake
- Enhancement of dopamine and norepinephrine actions in certain brain regions (e.g., dorsolateral prefrontal cortex) may improve attention, concentration, executive function, and wakefulness
- Enhancement of dopamine actions in other brain regions (e.g., basal ganglia) may improve hyperactivity
- Enhancement of dopamine and norepinephrine in yet other brain regions (e.g., medial prefrontal cortex, hypothalamus) may improve depression, fatigue, and sleepiness

How Long Until It Works
- Some immediate effects can be seen with first dosing
- Can take several weeks to attain maximum therapeutic benefit

If It Works (for ADHD)
- The goal of treatment of ADHD is reduction of symptoms of inattentiveness, motor hyperactivity, and/or impulsiveness that disrupt social, school, and/or occupational functioning
- Continue treatment until all symptoms are under control or improvement is stable and then continue treatment indefinitely as long as improvement persists
- Reevaluate the need for treatment periodically
- Treatment for ADHD begun in childhood may need to be continued into adolescence and adulthood if continued benefit is documented

If It Doesn't Work (for ADHD)
- Consider adjusting dose or switching to another formulation of d,l-methylphenidate or to another agent
- Consider behavioral therapy
- Consider the presence of noncompliance and counsel patient and parents
- Consider evaluation for another diagnosis or for a comorbid condition (e.g., bipolar disorder, substance abuse, medical illness, etc.)

* Some ADHD patients and some depressed patients may experience lack of consistent efficacy due to activation of latent or underlying bipolar disorder, and require either augmenting with a mood stabilizer or switching to a mood stabilizer

Best Augmenting Combos for Partial Response or Treatment Resistance
* Best to attempt other monotherapies prior to augmenting
- For the expert, can combine immediate-release formulation with a sustained-release formulation of d,l-methylphenidate for ADHD
- For the expert, can combine with modafinil or atomoxetine for ADHD
- For the expert, can occasionally combine with atypical antipsychotics in highly treatment-resistant cases of bipolar disorder or ADHD
- For the expert, can combine with antidepressants to boost antidepressant efficacy in highly treatment-resistant cases of depression while carefully monitoring patient

Tests
- Before treatment, assess for presence of cardiac disease (history, family history, physical exam)
- Blood pressure should be monitored regularly
- In children, monitor weight and height
- Periodic complete blood cell and platelet counts may be considered during prolonged therapy (rare leukopenia and/or anemia)

SIDE EFFECTS

How Drug Causes Side Effects
- Increases in norepinephrine peripherally can cause autonomic side effects, including tremor, tachycardia, hypertension, and cardiac arrhythmias
- Increases in norepinephrine and dopamine centrally can cause CNS side effects such as insomnia, agitation, psychosis, and substance abuse

Notable Side Effects
✻ Insomnia, headache, exacerbation of tics, nervousness, irritability, overstimulation, tremor, dizziness
- Anorexia, nausea, abdominal pain, weight loss
- Can temporarily slow normal growth in children (controversial)
- Blurred vision
- Transdermal: application site reactions, including contact sensitization (erythema, edema, papules, vesicles) and chemical leukoderma

Life-Threatening or Dangerous Side Effects
✻ Rare priapism
- Psychotic episodes, especially with parenteral abuse
- Seizures
- Palpitations, tachycardia, hypertension
- Rare neuroleptic malignant syndrome
- Rare activation of hypomania, mania, or suicidal ideation (controversial)
- Cardiovascular adverse effects, sudden death in patients with preexisting cardiac structural abnormalities

Weight Gain
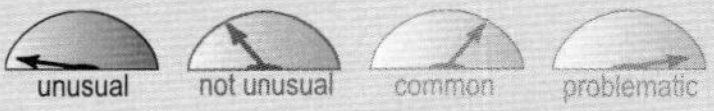

- Reported but not expected
- Some patients may experience weight loss

Sedation
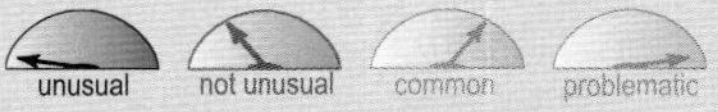

- Reported but not expected
- Activation much more common than sedation

What to Do About Side Effects
- Wait
- Adjust dose
- Switch to another formulation of d,l-methylphenidate
- Switch to another agent
- For insomnia, avoid dosing in afternoon/evening

Best Augmenting Agents for Side Effects
- Beta blockers for peripheral autonomic side effects
- Dose reduction or switching to another agent may be more effective since most side effects cannot be improved with an augmenting agent

DOSING AND USE

Usual Dosage Range
- ADHD (oral): up to 2 mg/kg per day in children 6 years and older, with a maximum daily dose of 60 mg/day; in adults usually 20–30 mg/day, but may use up to 40–60 mg/day
- ADHD (transdermal): 10–30 mg/9 hours
- Narcolepsy: 20–60 mg/day in 2–3 divided doses

Dosage Forms
- Immediate-release tablets 5 mg, 10 mg, 20 mg (Ritalin, generic methylphenidate)
- Oral solution 5 mg/mL, 10 mg/5 mL (Methylin)
- Older sustained-release tablets 10 mg, 20 mg (Methylin ER); 20 mg (Ritalin SR, Metadate ER)

✻ Newer sustained-release capsules 10 mg, 20 mg, 30 mg, 40 mg, 60 mg (Ritalin LA);

10 mg, 20 mg, 30 mg, 40 mg, 50 mg, 60 mg (Metadate CD)

✻ Newer sustained-release tablets 18 mg, 27 mg, 36 mg, 54 mg (Concerta)

- Sustained-release chewable tablets 20 mg scored, 30 mg, 40 mg (QuilliChew ER)
- Extended-release capsule, multi-layer release (Aptensio XR) 10 mg, 15 mg, 20 mg, 30 mg, 40 mg, 50 mg, 60 mg
- Extended-release oral suspension 5 mg/mL (Quillivant XR)
- Transdermal patch 27 mg/12.5 cm^2, (10 mg/9 hr; 1.1 mg/hr), 41.3 mg/18.75 cm^2 (15 mg/9 hr; 1.6 mg/hr), 55 mg/25 cm^2 (20 mg/9 hr; 2.2 mg/hr), 82.5 mg/37.5 cm^2 (30 mg/9 hr; 3.3 mg/hr)

How to Dose

- Immediate-release Ritalin, generic methylphenidate (2–4 hour duration of action)
  - ADHD: initial 5 mg in morning, 5 mg at lunch; can increase by 5–10 mg each week; maximum dose generally 60 mg/day
  - Narcolepsy: give each dose 30–45 minutes before meals; maximum dose generally 60 mg/day
- Older extended-release Ritalin SR, Methylin SR, and Metadate ER
  - These formulations have a duration of action of approximately 4–6 hours; therefore, these formulations may be used in place of immediate-release formulations when the 4–6 hour dosage of these sustained-release formulations corresponds to the titrated 4–6 hour dosage of the immediate-release formulation
  - Average dose is 20–30 mg/day, usually in 2 divided doses
- ✻ Newer sustained-release formulations for ADHD
  - Concerta (up to 12 hours duration of action): initial 18 mg/day in morning; can increase by 18 mg each week; maximum dose generally 72 mg/day
  - Ritalin LA, Metadate CD, QuilliChew ER (up to 8 hours duration of action): initial 20 mg once daily; dosage may be adjusted in weekly increments of 10 mg or 20 mg (QuilliChew ER only) to a maximum of 60 mg/day taken in the morning
  - Quillivant XR (up to 12-hour duration): initial 20 mg once daily; dosage may be adjusted in weekly increments of 10–20 mg to a maximum of 60 mg/day taken in the morning
  - Aptensio XR (up to 12-hour duration): initial 10 mg once daily; dosage may be adjusted in weekly increments of 10 mg to a maximum of 60 mg/day taken in the morning
- ✻ Transdermal formulation for ADHD
  - Initial 10 mg/9 hours; can increase by 5 mg/9 hours every week; maximum dose generally 30 mg/9 hours
  - Patch should be applied 2 hours before effect is needed and should be worn for 9 hours
  - Patients should follow the same titration schedule when they are naive to methylphenidate or are switching from another formulation

Dosing Tips

- Clinical duration of action often differs from pharmacokinetic half-life
- Taking oral formulations with food may delay peak actions for 2–3 hours

✻ Immediate-release formulations (Ritalin, Methylin, generic methylphenidate) have 2–4 hour durations of clinical action

✻ Older sustained-release formulations such as Methylin ER, Ritalin SR, Metadate ER, and generic methylphenidate sustained-release all have approximately 4–6 hour durations of clinical action, which for most patients is generally not long enough for once daily dosing in the morning and thus generally requires lunchtime dosing at school

✻ The newer sustained-release Metadate CD has an early peak and an 8-hour duration of action

✻ The newer sustained-release Ritalin LA also has an early peak and an 8-hour duration of action, with 2 pulses (immediate and after 4 hours)

✻ The newer sustained-release Concerta trilayer tablet has longest duration of action (12 hours)

- Most sustained-release formulations (especially Concerta, Metadate CD, and Ritalin LA) should not be chewed but rather should only be swallowed whole

- QuilliChew ER is a chewable tablet and can be taken with or without food
- ✻ Newer sustained-release formulations have a sufficiently long duration of clinical action to eliminate the need for a lunchtime dosing if taken in the morning
- ✻ This innovation can be an important practical element in stimulant utilization, eliminating the hassle and pragmatic difficulties of lunchtime dosing at school, including storage problems, potential diversion, and the need for a medical professional to supervise dosing away from home
- Off-label uses are dosed the same as for ADHD
- ✻ May be possible to dose only during the school week for some ADHD patients
- ✻ May be able to give drug holidays over the summer in order to reassess therapeutic utility and effects on growth and to allow catch-up from any growth suppression as well as to assess any other side effects and the need to reinstitute stimulant treatment for the next school term
- Avoid dosing late in the day because of the risk of insomnia
- Concerta tablet does not change shape in the gastrointestinal tract and generally should not be used in patients with gastrointestinal narrowing because of the risk of intestinal obstruction
- Side effects are generally dose-related
- Transdermal patch should be applied to dry, intact skin on the hip
- New application site should be selected for each day; only one patch should be applied at a time; patches should not be cut
- Avoid touching the exposed (sticky) side of the patch, and after application, wash hands with soap and water; do not touch eyes until after hands have been washed
- Heat can increase the amount of methylphenidate absorbed from the transdermal patch, so patients should avoid exposing the application site to external source of direct heat (e.g., heating pads, prolonged direct sunlight)
- If a patch comes off a new patch may be applied at a different site; total daily wear time should remain 9 hours regardless of number of patches used
- Early removal of transdermal patch can be useful to terminate drug action when desired

Overdose

- Vomiting, tremor, coma, convulsion, hyperreflexia, euphoria, confusion, hallucination, tachycardia, flushing, palpitations, sweating, hyperprexia, hypertension, arrhythmia, mydriasis

Long-Term Use

- Often used long-term for ADHD when ongoing monitoring documents continued efficacy
- Dependence and/or abuse may develop
- Tolerance to therapeutic effects may develop in some patients
- Long-term stimulant use may be associated with growth suppression in children (controversial)
- Periodic monitoring of weight, blood pressure, CBC, platelet counts, and liver function may be prudent

Habit Forming

- High abuse potential, Schedule II drug
- Patients may develop tolerance, psychological dependence

How to Stop

- Taper to avoid withdrawal effects
- Withdrawal following chronic therapeutic use may unmask symptoms of the underlying disorder and may require follow-up and reinstitution of treatment
- Careful supervision is required during withdrawal from abusive use since severe depression may occur

Pharmacokinetics

- Average half-life in adults is 3.5 hours (1.3–7.7 hours)
- Average half-life in children is 2.5 hours (1.5–5 hours)
- First-pass metabolism is not extensive with transdermal dosing, thus resulting in notably higher exposure to methylphenidate and lower exposure to metabolites as compared to oral dosing

Drug Interactions

- May affect blood pressure and should be used cautiously with agents used to control blood pressure
- May inhibit metabolism of SSRIs, anticonvulsants (phenobarbital, phenytoin, primidone), TCAs, and coumarin

anticoagulants, requiring downward dosage adjustments of these drugs
- Serious adverse effects may occur if combined with clonidine (controversial)
- Use with MAOIs, including within 14 days of MAOI use, is not advised, but this can sometimes be considered by experts who monitor depressed patients closely when other treatment options for depression fail
- CNS and cardiovascular actions of d,l-methylphenidate could theoretically be enhanced by combination with agents that block norepinephrine reuptake, such as the TCAs desipramine or protriptyline, venlafaxine, duloxetine, atomoxetine, milnacipran, and reboxetine
- Theoretically, antipsychotics should inhibit the stimulatory effects of d,l-methylphenidate
- Theoretically, d,l-methylphenidate could inhibit the antipsychotic actions of antipsychotics
- Theoretically, d,l-methylphenidate could inhibit the mood-stabilizing actions of atypical antipsychotics in some patients
- Combination of d,l-methylphenidate with mood stabilizers (lithium, anticonvulsants, atypical antipsychotics) is generally something for experts only, when monitoring patients closely and when other options fail

Other Warnings/ Precautions

- Use with caution in patients with any degree of hypertension, hyperthyroidism, or history of drug abuse
- Children who are not growing or gaining weight should stop treatment, at least temporarily
- May worsen motor and phonic tics
- May worsen symptoms of thought disorder and behavioral disturbance in psychotic patients
- Stimulants have a high potential for abuse and must be used with caution in anyone with a current or past history of substance abuse or alcoholism or in emotionally unstable patients
- Administration of stimulants for prolonged periods of time should be avoided whenever possible or done only with close monitoring, as it may lead to marked tolerance and drug dependence, including psychological dependence with varying degrees of abnormal behavior
- Particular attention should be paid to the possibility of subjects obtaining stimulants for nontherapeutic use or distribution to others and the drugs should in general be prescribed sparingly with documentation of appropriate use
- Usual dosing has been associated with sudden death in children with structural cardiac abnormalities
- Not an appropriate first-line treatment for depression or for normal fatigue
- May lower the seizure threshold
- Emergence or worsening of activation and agitation may represent the induction of a bipolar state, especially a mixed dysphoric bipolar II condition sometimes associated with suicidal ideation, and require the addition of a mood stabilizer and/or discontinuation of d,l-methylphenidate
- Permanent skin color loss, known as chemical leukoderma, may occur with use of the transdermal Daytrana patch; patients should be advised to watch for signs of skin color changes and if they occur alternative treatment options should be considered
- Certain transdermal patches containing even small traces of aluminum or other metals in the adhesive backing can cause skin burns if worn during MRI, so warn patients taking the transdermal formulation about this possibility and advise them to disclose this information if they need an MRI

Do Not Use

- If patient has extreme anxiety or agitation
- If patient has motor tics or Tourette's syndrome or if there is a family history of Tourette's, unless administered by an expert in cases when the potential benefits for ADHD outweigh the risks of worsening tics
- Should generally not be administered with an MAOI, including within 14 days of MAOI use, except in heroic circumstances and by an expert
- If patient has glaucoma
- If patient has structural cardiac abnormalities
- If there is a proven allergy to methylphenidate

SPECIAL POPULATIONS

Renal Impairment
- No dose adjustment necessary

Hepatic Impairment
- No dose adjustment necessary

Cardiac Impairment
- Use with caution, particularly in patients with recent myocardial infarction or other conditions that could be negatively affected by increased blood pressure
- Do not use in patients with structural cardiac abnormalities

Elderly
- Some patients may tolerate lower doses better

Children and Adolescents
- Safety and efficacy not established in children under age 6
- Use in young children should be reserved for the expert
- Methylphenidate has acute effects on growth hormone; long-term effects are unknown but weight and height should be monitored during long-term treatment
- Sudden death in children and adolescents with serious heart problems has been reported
- American Heart Association recommends EKG prior to initiating stimulant treatment in children, although not all experts agree

Pregnancy
- Effective June 30, 2015, the US FDA requires changes to the content and format of pregnancy and lactation information in prescription drug labels, including the elimination of the pregnancy letter categories; the Pregnancy and Lactation Labeling Rule (PLLR or final rule) applies only to prescription drugs and will be phased in gradually for drugs approved on or after June 30, 2001
- Controlled studies have not been conducted in pregnant women
- Infants whose mothers took methylphenidate during pregnancy may experience withdrawal symptoms
- Racemic methylphenidate has been shown to have teratogenic effects in rabbits when given in doses of 200 mg/kg/day throughout organogenesis
- Use in women of childbearing potential requires weighing potential benefits to the mother against potential risks to the fetus

✻ For ADHD patients, methylphenidate should generally be discontinued before anticipated pregnancies

Breast Feeding
- Unknown if methylphenidate is secreted in human breast milk, but all psychotropics assumed to be secreted in breast milk

✻ Recommended either to discontinue drug or bottle feed

- If infant shows signs of irritability, drug may need to be discontinued

THE ART OF PSYCHOPHARMACOLOGY

Potential Advantages
- Established long-term efficacy as a first-line treatment for ADHD
- Multiple options for drug delivery, peak actions, and duration of action

Potential Disadvantages
- Patients with current or past substance abuse
- Patients with current or past bipolar disorder or psychosis

Primary Target Symptoms
- Concentration, attention span
- Motor hyperactivity
- Impulsiveness
- Physical and mental fatigue
- Daytime sleepiness
- Depression

Pearls
✻ May be useful for treatment of depressive symptoms in medically ill elderly patients

✻ May be useful for treatment of post-stroke depression

✻ A classical augmentation strategy for treatment-refractory depression

✻ Specifically, may be useful for treatment of cognitive dysfunction and fatigue as residual symptoms of major depressive

disorder unresponsive to multiple prior treatments
- ✻ May also be useful for the treatment of cognitive impairment, depressive symptoms, and severe fatigue in patients with HIV infection and in cancer patients
- Can be used to potentiate opioid analgesia and reduce sedation, particularly in end-of-life management
- Atypical antipsychotics may be useful in treating stimulant or psychotic consequences of overdose
- Some patients respond to or tolerate methylphenidate better than amphetamine and vice versa
- Taking with food may delay peak actions of oral formulations for 2–3 hours
- Half-life and duration of clinical action tend to be shorter in younger children
- Drug abuse may actually be lower in ADHD adolescents treated with stimulants than in ADHD adolescents who are not treated
- Older sustained-release technologies for methylphenidate were not significant advances over immediate-release methylphenidate because they did not eliminate the need for lunchtime dosing or allow once daily administration
- ✻ Newer sustained-release technologies are truly once a day dosing systems
- ✻ Metadate CD and Ritalin LA are somewhat similar to each other, both with an early peak and duration of action of about 8 hours
- ✻ Concerta has less of an early peak but a longer duration of action (up to 12 hours)
- ✻ Concerta trilayer tablet consists of 3 compartments (2 containing drug, 1 a "push" compartment) and an orifice at the head of the first drug compartment; water fills the push compartment and gradually pushes drug up and out of the tablet through the orifice
- ✻ Concerta may be preferable for those ADHD patients who work in the evening or do homework up to 12 hours after morning dosing
- ✻ Metadate CD and Ritalin LA may be preferable for those ADHD patients who lose their appetite for dinner or have insomnia with Concerta
- Some patients may benefit from an occasional addition of 5–10 mg of immediate-release methylphenidate to their daily base of sustained-release methylphenidate
- Transdermal formulation may confer lower abuse potential than oral formulations
- Transdermal formulation may enhance adherence to treatment compared to some oral formulations because it allows once daily application with all day efficacy, has a smoother absorption curve, and allows for daily customization of treatment (i.e., it can be removed early if desired)
- On the other hand, transdermal formulation has slower onset than oral formulations, requires a specific removal time, can cause skin sensitization, can be large depending on dose, and may lead to reduced efficacy if removed prematurely

Suggested Reading

Challman TD, Lipsky JJ. Methylphenidate: its pharmacology and uses. Mayo Clin Proc 2000;75:711–21.

Kimko HC, Cross JT, Abemethy DR. Pharmacokinetics and clinical effectiveness of methylphenidate. Clin Pharmacokinet 1999;37:457–70.

Wolraich ML, Greenhill LL, Pelham W, et al. Randomized, controlled trial of oros methylphenidate once a day in children with attention-deficit/hyperactivity disorder. Pediatrics 2001;108:883–92.

THERAPEUTICS

Brands • Lerivon

see index for additional brand names

Generic? Yes

Class

- Neuroscience-based Nomenclature: norepinephrine multi-modal (N-MM)
- Tetracyclic antidepressant
- Noradrenergic agent

Commonly Prescribed for

(bold for FDA approved)

- Depression
- Anxiety
- Insomnia
- Treatment-resistant depression

How the Drug Works

- Blocks alpha 2 adrenergic presynaptic receptor, thereby increasing norepinephrine neurotransmission
- This is a novel mechanism independent of norepinephrine reuptake blockade
- Blocks alpha 2 adrenergic presynaptic receptors but also alpha 1 adrenergic receptors on serotonin neurons, thereby causing little increase in serotonin neurotransmission
- Blocks 5HT2A, 5HT2C, and 5HT3 serotonin receptors
- Blocks H1 histamine receptors

How Long Until It Works

* Actions on insomnia and anxiety can start shortly after initiation of dosing
- Onset of therapeutic actions in depression, however, is usually not immediate, but often delayed 2–4 weeks
- If it is not working within 6–8 weeks for depression, it may require a dosage increase or it may not work at all
- May continue to work for many years to prevent relapse of symptoms

If It Works

- The goal of treatment is complete remission of current symptoms as well as prevention of future relapses
- Treatment most often reduces or even eliminates symptoms, but not a cure since symptoms can recur after medicine is stopped
- Continue treatment until all symptoms are gone (remission)
- Once symptoms gone, continue treating for 1 year for the first episode of depression
- For second and subsequent episodes of depression, treatment may need to be indefinite
- Use in anxiety disorders may also need to be indefinite

If It Doesn't Work

- Many patients have only a partial response where some symptoms are improved but others persist (especially insomnia, fatigue, and problems concentrating)
- Other patients may be nonresponders, sometimes called treatment-resistant or treatment-refractory
- Consider increasing dose, switching to another agent or adding an appropriate augmenting agent
- Consider psychotherapy
- Consider evaluation for another diagnosis or for a comorbid condition (e.g., medical illness, substance abuse, etc.)
- Some patients may experience apparent lack of consistent efficacy due to activation of latent or underlying bipolar disorder, and require antidepressant discontinuation and a switch to a mood stabilizer

Best Augmenting Combos for Partial Response or Treatment Resistance

- SSRIs, SNRIs, bupropion, reboxetine, atomoxetine (use combinations of antidepressant with caution as this may activate bipolar disorder and suicidal ideation)
- Modafinil, especially for fatigue, sleepiness, and lack of concentration
- Mood stabilizers or atypical antipsychotics for bipolar depression, psychotic depression, or treatment-resistant depression
- Benzodiazepines

Tests

- Baseline ECG is recommended for patients over age 50

- May need to monitor blood count during treatment for those with blood dyscrasias, leucopenia, or granylocytopenia
- Since some antidepressants such as mianserin can be associated with weight gain, before starting treatment, weigh all patients and determine if the patient is already overweight (BMI 25.0–29.9) or obese (BMI ≥30)
- Before giving a drug that can cause weight gain to an overweight or obese patient, consider determining whether the patient already has pre-diabetes (fasting plasma glucose 100–125 mg/dL), diabetes (fasting plasma glucose >126 mg/dL), or dyslipidemia (increased total cholesterol, LDL cholesterol, and triglycerides; decreased HDL cholesterol), and treat or refer such patients for treatment, including nutrition and weight management, physical activity counseling, smoking cessation, and medical management

✻ Monitor weight and BMI during treatment

✻ While giving a drug to a patient who has gained >5% of initial weight, consider evaluating for the presence of pre-diabetes, diabetes, or dyslipidemia, or consider switching to a different antidepressant

SIDE EFFECTS

How Drug Causes Side Effects

- Most side effects are immediate but often go away with time

✻ Histamine 1 receptor antagonism may explain sedative effects

✻ Histamine 1 receptor antagonism plus 5HT2C antagonism may explain some aspects of weight gain

Notable Side Effects

- Sedation
- Increased appetite, weight gain

Life-Threatening or Dangerous Side Effects

- Rare seizures
- Rare blood dyscrasias
- Rare induction of mania
- Rare activation of suicidal ideation and behavior (suicidality) (short-term studies did not show an increase in the risk of suicidality with antidepressants compared to placebo beyond age 24)

Weight Gain

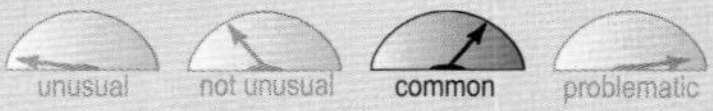

- Many experience and/or can be significant in amount

Sedation

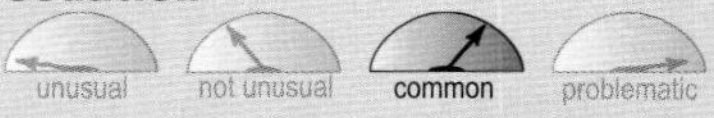

- Many experience and/or can be significant in amount
- Generally transient

What to Do About Side Effects

- Wait
- Wait
- Wait
- Switch to another drug

Best Augmenting Agents for Side Effects

- Often best to try another antidepressant monotherapy prior to resorting to augmentation strategies to treat side effects
- Many side effects are dose-dependent (i.e., they increase as dose increases, or they reemerge until tolerance redevelops)
- Many side effects are time-dependent (i.e., they start immediately upon dosing and upon each dose increase, but go away with time)
- Many side effects cannot be improved with an augmenting agent
- Activation and agitation may represent the induction of a bipolar state, especially a mixed dysphoric bipolar II condition sometimes associated with suicidal ideation, and require the addition of lithium, a mood stabilizer or an atypical antipsychotic, and/or discontinuation of mianserin

DOSING AND USE

Usual Dosage Range

- 30–60 mg/day

Dosage Forms

- Tablet 10 mg, 30 mg, 60 mg

How to Dose

- Initial 30 mg/day; maximum usually 90 mg/day

Dosing Tips
- Can be dosed once or twice daily
- If intolerable anxiety, insomnia, agitation, akathisia, or activation occur either upon dosing initiation or discontinuation, consider the possibility of activated bipolar disorder and switch to a mood stabilizer or an atypical antipsychotic

Overdose
- Relatively safe in overdose; sedation, hypertension, or hypotension

Long-Term Use
- Safe

Habit Forming
- Not expected

How to Stop
- Taper is prudent to avoid withdrawal effects, but tolerance, dependence, and withdrawal effects not reliably reported

Pharmacokinetics
- Half-life 12–29 hours

Drug Interactions
- Tramadol increases the risk of seizures in patients taking an antidepressant
- Carbamazepine and phenytoin may reduce mianserin levels
- Theoretically could cause a fatal "serotonin syndrome" when combined with MAOIs, so do not use with MAOIs or for at least 14 days after MAOIs are stopped unless you are an expert and only for treatment-resistant cases that may justify the risk
- Do not start an MAOI for at least 5 half-lives (5 to 7 days for most drugs) after discontinuing mianserin

Other Warnings/ Precautions
- Drug may lower white blood cell count (rare; may not be increased compared to other antidepressants but controlled studies lacking)
- Avoid alcohol, which may increase sedation and cognitive and motor effects
- Use with caution in patients with history of seizures
- Use with caution in patients with bipolar disorder unless treated with concomitant mood-stabilizing agent
- When treating children, carefully weigh the risks and benefits of pharmacological treatment against the risks and benefits of nontreatment with antidepressants and make sure to document this in the patient's chart
- Warn patients and their caregivers about the possibility of activating side effects and advise them to report such symptoms immediately
- Monitor patients for activation of suicidal ideation, especially children and adolescents

Do Not Use
- If patient is taking an MAOI
- If there is a proven allergy to mianserin

SPECIAL POPULATIONS

Renal Impairment
- Dose adjustment not necessary

Hepatic Impairment
- Dose adjustment not necessary

Cardiac Impairment
- Baseline ECG is recommended
- Drug should be used with caution

Elderly
- Baseline ECG is recommended for patients over age 50
- Some patients may tolerate lower doses better
- Blood dyscrasias, though still rare, may be more common in the elderly

Children and Adolescents
- Carefully weigh the risks and benefits of pharmacological treatment against the risks and benefits of nontreatment with antidepressants and make sure to document this in the patient's chart
- Monitor patients face-to-face regularly, particularly during the first several weeks of treatment

- Use with caution, observing for activation of known or unknown bipolar disorder and/or suicidal ideation, and inform parents or guardians of this risk so they can help observe child or adolescent patients
- Safety and efficacy have not been established

Pregnancy
- Controlled studies have not been conducted in pregnant women
- Not generally recommended for use during pregnancy, especially during first trimester
- Must weigh the risk of treatment (first trimester fetal development, third trimester newborn delivery) to the child against the risk of no treatment (recurrence of depression, maternal health, infant bonding) to the mother and child
- For many patients this may mean continuing treatment during pregnancy

Breast Feeding
- Some drug is found in mother's breast milk
- If child becomes irritable or sedated, breast feeding or drug may need to be discontinued
- Immediate postpartum period is a high-risk time for depression, especially in women who have had prior depressive episodes, so drug may need to be reinstituted late in the third trimester or shortly after childbirth to prevent a recurrence during the postpartum period
- Must weigh benefits of breast feeding with risks and benefits of antidepressant treatment versus nontreatment to both the infant and the mother
- For many patients, this may mean continuing treatment during breast feeding

THE ART OF PSYCHOPHARMACOLOGY

Potential Advantages
- Patients particularly concerned about sexual side effects
- Patients with symptoms of anxiety
- As an augmenting agent to boost the efficacy of other antidepressants
- Patients with cardiovascular disease

Potential Disadvantages
- Patients particularly concerned about gaining weight
- Patients with low energy

Primary Target Symptoms
- Depressed mood
- Sleep disturbance
- Anxiety

Pearls
✻ Adding alpha 2 antagonism to agents that block serotonin and/or norepinephrine reuptake may be synergistic for severe depression
- Adding mianserin to venlafaxine or SSRIs may reverse drug-induced anxiety and insomnia
- Efficacy of mianserin for depression in cancer patients has been shown in small controlled studies

✻ Only causes sexual dysfunction infrequently
- Generally better tolerated than TCAs, including safer in overdose
- General lack of cardiovascular toxicity

Suggested Reading

Brogden RN, Heel RC, Speight TM, Avery GS. Mianserin: a review of its pharmacological properties and therapeutic efficacy in depressive illness. Drugs 1978;16(4):273–301.

De Ridder JJ. Mianserin: result of a decade of antidepressant research. Pharm Weekbl Sci 1982;4(5):139–45.

Leinonen E, Koponen H, Lepola U. Serum mianserin and ageing. Prog Neuropsychopharmacol Biol Psychiatry 1994;18(5):833–45.

Rotzinger S, Bourin M, Akimoto Y, Coutts RT, Baker GB. Metabolism of some "second-" and "fourth-"generation antidepressants: iprindole, viloxazine, bupropion, mianserin, maprotiline, trazodone, nefazodone, and venlafaxine. Cell Mol Neurobiol 1999;19(4):427–42.

Wakeling A. Efficacy and side effects of mianserin, a tetracyclic antidepressant. Postgrad Med J 1983;59(690):229–31.

THERAPEUTICS

Brands • Versed

see index for additional brand names

Generic? Yes

Class

- Neuroscience-based Nomenclature: GABA positive allosteric modulator (GABA-PAM)
- Benzodiazepine (hypnotic)

Commonly Prescribed for

(bold for FDA approved)

- **Sedation in pediatric patients**
- **Sedation (adjunct to anesthesia)**
- **Preoperative anxiolytic**
- **Drug-induced amnesia**
- Catatonia

How the Drug Works

- Binds to benzodiazepine receptors at the GABA-A ligand-gated chloride channel complex
- Enhances the inhibitory effects of GABA
- Boosts chloride conductance through GABA-regulated channels
- Inhibitory actions in sleep centers may provide sedative hypnotic effects

How Long Until It Works

- Intravenous injection: onset 3–5 minutes
- Intramuscular injection: onset 15 minutes, peak 30–60 minutes

If It Works

- Patients generally recover 2–6 hours after awakening

If It Doesn't Work

- Increase the dose
- Switch to another agent

Best Augmenting Combos for Partial Response or Treatment Resistance

- Augmenting agents have not been adequately studied

Tests

- None for healthy individuals

SIDE EFFECTS

How Drug Causes Side Effects

- Actions at benzodiazepine receptors that carry over to next day can cause daytime sedation, amnesia, and ataxia

Notable Side Effects

- Oversedation, impaired recall, agitation, involuntary movements, headache
- Nausea, vomiting
- Hiccups, fluctuation in vital signs, irritation/ pain at site of injection
- Hypotension

Life-Threatening or Dangerous Side Effects

- Respiratory depression, apnea, respiratory arrest
- Cardiac arrest

Weight Gain

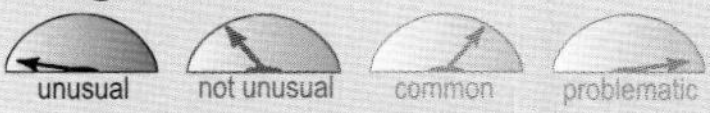

- Reported but not expected

Sedation

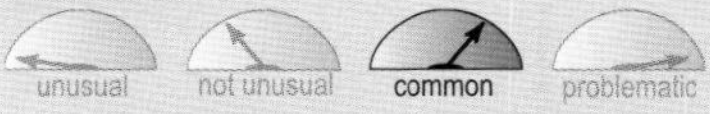

- Many experience and/or can be significant in amount

What to Do About Side Effects

- Wait
- Switch to another agent
- Administer flumazenil if side effects are severe or life-threatening

Best Augmenting Agents for Side Effects

- Many side effects cannot be improved with an augmenting agent

DOSING AND USE

Usual Dosage Range

- Intravenous (adults): 1–2.5 mg
- Liquid (age 16 and under): 0.25–1.0 mg/kg

Dosage Forms

- Intravenous: 5 mg/mL – 1 mL vial, 2 mL vial, 5 mL vial, 10 mL vial
- Liquid: 2 mg/mL – 118 mL bottle

How to Dose
- Liquid single dose: 0.25–1.0 mg/kg; maximum dose generally 20 mg
- Intravenous (adults): administer over 2 minutes; monitor patient over the next 2 or more minutes to determine effects; allow 3–5 minutes between administrations; maximum 2.5 mg within 2 minutes

Dosing Tips
- Better to underdose, observe for effects, and then prudently raise dose while monitoring carefully

Overdose
- Sedation, confusion, poor coordination, respiratory depression, coma

Long-Term Use
- Not generally intended for long-term use

Habit Forming
- Some patients may develop dependence and/or tolerance; risk may be greater with higher doses
- History of drug addiction may increase risk of dependence

How to Stop
- If administration was prolonged, do not stop abruptly

Pharmacokinetics
- Elimination half-life 1.8–6.4 hours
- Active metabolite

Drug Interactions
- If CNS depressants are used concomitantly, midazolam dose should be reduced by half or more
- Increased depressive effects when taken with other CNS depressants (see Warnings below)
- Drugs that inhibit CYP450 3A4, such as nefazodone and fluvoxamine, may reduce midazolam clearance and thus raise midazolam levels
- Midazolam decreases the minimum alveolar concentration of halothane needed for general anesthesia

Other Warnings/ Precautions
- Boxed warning regarding the increased risk of CNS depressant effects when benzodiazepines and opioid medications are used together, including specifically the risk of slowed or difficulty breathing and death
- Midazolam should be used only in an environment in which the patient can be closely monitored (e.g., hospital) because of the risk of respiratory depression and respiratory arrest
- Sedated pediatric patients should be monitored throughout the procedure
- Patients with COPD should receive lower doses
- Use with caution in patients with impaired respiratory function

Do Not Use
- If patient has angle-closure glaucoma
- If there is a proven allergy to midazolam or any benzodiazepine

SPECIAL POPULATIONS

Renal Impairment
- May have longer elimination half-life, prolonging time to recovery

Hepatic Impairment
- Longer elimination half-life; clearance is reduced

Cardiac Impairment
- Longer elimination half-life; clearance is reduced

Elderly
- Longer elimination half-life; clearance is reduced
- Intravenous: 1–3.5 mg; maximum 1.5 mg within 2 minutes

Children and Adolescents
- In most pediatric populations, pharmacokinetic properties are similar to those in adults

- Seriously ill neonates have reduced clearance and longer elimination half-life
- Hypotension has occurred in neonates given midazolam and fentanyl
- Intravenous dose: dependent on age, weight, route, procedure

Pregnancy

- Effective June 30, 2015, the US FDA requires changes to the content and format of pregnancy and lactation information in prescription drug labels, including the elimination of the pregnancy letter categories; the Pregnancy and Lactation Labeling Rule (PLLR or final rule) applies only to prescription drugs and will be phased in gradually for drugs approved on or after June 30, 2001
- Controlled studies have not been conducted in pregnant women
- Midazolam crosses the placenta
- Neonatal flaccidity has been reported in infants whose mother took a benzodiazepine during pregnancy

Breast Feeding

- Some drug is found in mother's breast milk
- Effects on infant have been observed and include feeding difficulties, sedation, and weight loss
- Midazolam can be used to relieve postoperative pain after cesarean section

THE ART OF PSYCHOPHARMACOLOGY

Potential Advantages

- Fast onset
- Parenteral dosage forms

Potential Disadvantages

- Can be oversedating

Primary Target Symptoms

- Anxiety

Pearls

- Recovery (e.g., ability to stand/walk) generally takes from 2–6 hours after wakening
- Half-life may be longer in obese patients
- Patients with premenstrual syndrome may be less sensitive to midazolam than healthy women throughout the cycle
- Midazolam clearance may be reduced in postmenopausal women compared to premenopausal women
- Though not systematically studied, benzodiazepines have been used effectively to treat catatonia and are the initial recommended treatment

Suggested Reading

Blumer JL. Clinical pharmacology of midazolam in infants and children. Clin Pharmacokinet 1998;35:37–47.

Fountain NB, Adams RE. Midazolam treatment of acute and refractory status epilepticus. Clin Neuropharmacol 1999;22:261–7.

Shafer A. Complications of sedation with midazolam in the intensive care unit and a comparison with other sedative regimens. Crit Care Med 1998;26:947–56.

Yuan R, Flockhart DA, Balian JD. Pharmacokinetic and pharmacodynamic consequences of metabolism-based drug interactions with alprazolam, midazolam, and triazolam. J Clin Pharmacol 1999;39:1109–25.

MILNACIPRAN

THERAPEUTICS

Brands
- Toledomin
- Ixel
- Savella

see index for additional brand names

Generic? No

Class

- Neuroscience-based Nomenclature: serotonin, norepinephrine reuptake inhibitor (SN-RI)
- SNRI (dual serotonin and norepinephrine reuptake inhibitor); antidepressant; chronic pain treatment

Commonly Prescribed for

(bold for FDA approved)
- **Fibromyalgia**
- Major depressive disorder
- Neuropathic pain/chronic pain

How the Drug Works

- Boosts neurotransmitters serotonin, norepinephrine/noradrenaline, and dopamine
- Blocks serotonin reuptake pump (serotonin transporter), presumably increasing serotonergic neurotransmission
- Blocks norepinephrine reuptake pump (norepinephrine transporter), presumably increasing noradrenergic neurotransmission
- Presumably desensitizes both serotonin 1A receptors and beta adrenergic receptors
- ✽ Weak noncompetitive NMDA-receptor antagonist (high doses), which may contribute to actions in chronic pain
- Since dopamine is inactivated by norepinephrine reuptake in frontal cortex, which largely lacks dopamine transporters, milnacipran can increase dopamine neurotransmission in this part of the brain

How Long Until It Works

- Onset of therapeutic actions usually not immediate, but often delayed 2–4 weeks
- If it is not working within 6–8 weeks, it may require a dosage increase or it may not work at all
- May continue to work for many years to prevent relapse of symptoms in depression

If It Works

- The goal of treatment of depression is complete remission of current symptoms as well as prevention of future relapses
- The goal of treatment of fibromyalgia and chronic neuropathic pain is to reduce symptoms as much as possible, especially in combination with other treatments
- Treatment of depression most often reduces or even eliminates symptoms, but is not a cure since symptoms can recur after medicine stopped
- Treatment of fibromyalgia and chronic neuropathic pain may reduce symptoms, but rarely eliminates them completely, and is not a cure since symptoms can recur after medicine is stopped
- Continue treatment of depression until all symptoms are gone (remission)
- Once symptoms of depression are gone, continue treating for 1 year for the first episode of depression
- For second and subsequent episodes of depression, treatment may need to be indefinite
- Use in fibromyalgia and chronic neuropathic pain may also need to be indefinite, but long-term treatment is not well studied in these conditions

If It Doesn't Work

- Many depressed patients have only a partial response where some symptoms are improved but others persist (especially insomnia, fatigue, and problems concentrating)
- Other depressed patients may be nonresponders, sometimes called treatment-resistant or treatment-refractory
- Some depressed patients who have an initial response may relapse even though they continue treatment, sometimes called "poop-out"
- Consider increasing dose, switching to another agent or adding an appropriate augmenting agent
- Consider psychotherapy
- Consider evaluation for another diagnosis or for a comorbid condition (e.g., medical illness, substance abuse, etc.)
- Some patients may experience apparent lack of consistent efficacy due to activation of latent or underlying bipolar disorder, and require antidepressant discontinuation and switch to a mood stabilizer

Best Augmenting Combos for Partial Response or Treatment Resistance

- Augmentation experience is limited compared to other antidepressants
- Benzodiazepines can reduce insomnia and anxiety
- Adding other agents to milnacipran for treating depression could follow the same practice for augmenting SSRIs or other SNRIs if done by experts while monitoring carefully in difficult cases
- Although no controlled studies and little clinical experience, adding other agents for treating fibromyalgia and chronic neuropathic pain could theoretically include gabapentin, tiagabine, other anticonvulsants, or even opiates if done by experts while monitoring carefully in difficult cases
- Mirtazapine, bupropion, reboxetine, atomoxetine (use combinations of antidepressants with caution as this may activate bipolar disorder and suicidal ideation)
- Modafinil, especially for fatigue, sleepiness, and lack of concentration
- Mood stabilizers or atypical antipsychotics for bipolar depression, psychotic depression, or treatment-resistant depression
- Hypnotics or trazodone for insomnia
- Classically, lithium, buspirone, or thyroid hormone

Tests

- Check blood pressure before initiating treatment and regularly during treatment

SIDE EFFECTS

How Drug Causes Side Effects

- Theoretically due to increases in serotonin and norepinephrine concentrations at receptors in parts of the brain and body other than those that cause therapeutic actions (e.g., unwanted actions of serotonin in sleep centers causing insomnia, unwanted actions of norepinephrine on acetylcholine release causing urinary retention or constipation)
- Most side effects are immediate but often go away with time

Notable Side Effects

- Most side effects increase with higher doses, at least transiently
- Headache, nervousness, insomnia, sedation
- Nausea, diarrhea, decreased appetite
- Sexual dysfunction (abnormal ejaculation/orgasm, impotence)
- Asthenia, sweating
- SIADH (syndrome of inappropriate antidiuretic hormone secretion)
- Dose-dependent increased blood pressure
- Dry mouth, constipation
- Dysuria, urological complaints, urinary hesitancy, urinary retention
- Increase in heart rate
- Palpitations

Life-Threatening or Dangerous Side Effects

- Rare induction of mania
- Rare activation of suicidal ideation and behavior (suicidality) (short-term studies did not show an increase in the risk of suicidality with antidepressants compared to placebo beyond age 24)
- Rare seizures

Weight Gain

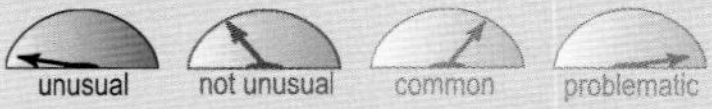

- Reported but not expected

Sedation

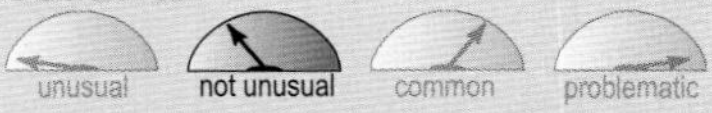

- Occurs in significant minority

What to Do About Side Effects

- Wait
- Wait
- Wait
- Lower the dose
- In a few weeks, switch or add other drugs

Best Augmenting Agents for Side Effects

* For urinary hesitancy, give an alpha 1 blocker such as tamsulosin or naftopidil
- Often best to try another antidepressant monotherapy prior to resorting to augmentation strategies to treat side effects
- Trazodone or a hypnotic for insomnia

- Bupropion, sildenafil, vardenafil, or tadalafil for sexual dysfunction
- Benzodiazepines for anxiety, agitation
- Mirtazapine for insomnia, agitation, and gastrointestinal side effects
- Many side effects are dose-dependent (i.e., they increase as dose increases, or they reemerge until tolerance redevelops)
- Many side effects are time-dependent (i.e., they start immediately upon dosing and upon each dose increase, but go away with time)
- Activation and agitation may represent the induction of a bipolar state, especially a mixed dysphoric bipolar II condition sometimes associated with suicidal ideation, and require the addition of lithium, a mood stabilizer or an atypical antipsychotic, and/or discontinuation of milnacipran

DOSING AND USE

Usual Dosage Range
- 30–200 mg/day in 2 doses

Dosage Forms
- Capsule 25 mg, 50 mg (France, other European countries, and worldwide markets)
- Capsule 15 mg, 25 mg, 50 mg (Japan)
- Tablet 12.5 mg, 25 mg, 50 mg, 100 mg

How to Dose
- Should be administered in 2 divided doses
- Initial 12.5 mg once daily; increase to 25 mg/day in 2 divided doses on day 2; increase to 50 mg/day in 2 divided doses on day 4; increase to 100 mg/day in 2 divided doses on day 7; maximum dose generally 200 mg/day

Dosing Tips
- Preferred dose for fibromyalgia may be 100 mg twice daily
- Higher doses usually well tolerated in fibromyalgia patients
- * Once daily dosing has far less consistent efficacy, so only give as twice daily
- Higher doses (>200 mg/day) not consistently effective in all studies of depression
- Nevertheless, some patients respond better to higher doses (200–300 mg/day) than to lower doses
- Different doses in different countries
- Different doses in different indications and different populations
- Preferred dose for depression may be 50 mg twice daily to 100 mg twice daily in France
- Preferred dose for depression in the elderly may be 15 mg twice daily to 25 mg twice daily in Japan
- Preferred dosing for depression in other adults may be 25 mg twice daily to 50 mg twice daily in Japan
- * Thus, clinicians must be aware that titration of twice daily dosing across a 10-fold range (30 mg–300 mg total daily dose) can optimize milnacipran's efficacy in broad clinical use
- Patients with agitation or anxiety may require slower titration to optimize tolerability
- No pharmacokinetic drug interactions (not an inhibitor of CYP450 2D6 or 3A4)
- As milnacipran is a more potent norepinephrine reuptake inhibitor than a serotonin reuptake inhibitor, some patients may require dosing at the higher end of the dosing range to obtain robust dual SNRI actions
- At high doses, NMDA glutamate antagonist actions may be a factor

Overdose
- Vomiting, hypertension, sedation, tachycardia
- The emetic effect of high doses of milnacipran may reduce the risk of serious adverse effects

Long-Term Use
- Safe

Habit Forming
- No

How to Stop
- Taper is prudent, but usually not necessary

Pharmacokinetics
- Half-life 8 hours
- No active metabolite

Drug Interactions

- Tramadol increases the risk of seizures in patients taking an antidepressant
- Can cause a fatal "serotonin syndrome" when combined with MAOIs, so do not use with MAOIs or for at least 14 days after MAOIs are stopped
- Do not start an MAOI for at least 5 half-lives (5 to 7 days for most drugs) after discontinuing milnacipran
- Possible increased risk of bleeding, especially when combined with anticoagulants (e.g., warfarin, NSAIDs)
- Switching from or addition of other norepinephrine reuptake inhibitors should be done with caution, as the additive pro-noradrenergic effects may enhance therapeutic actions in depression, but also enhance noradrenergically mediated side effects
- Few known adverse pharmacokinetic drug interactions

Other Warnings/ Precautions

- Use with caution in patients with history of seizures
- Use with caution in patients with bipolar disorder unless treated with concomitant mood-stabilizing agent
- Can cause mild elevations in ALT/AST, so avoid use with alcohol or in cases of chronic liver disease
- When treating children, carefully weigh the risks and benefits of pharmacological treatment against the risks and benefits of nontreatment with antidepressants and make sure to document this in the patient's chart
- Distribute the brochures provided by the FDA and the drug companies
- Warn patients and their caregivers about the possibility of activating side effects and advise them to report such symptoms immediately
- Monitor patients for activation of suicidal ideation, especially children and adolescents

Do Not Use

- If patient has uncontrolled angle-closure glaucoma
- If patient is taking an MAOI
- If there is a proven allergy to milnacipran

SPECIAL POPULATIONS

Renal Impairment

- Use caution for moderate impairment
- For severe impairment, 50 mg/day; can increase to 100 mg/day if needed
- Not recommended for patients with end-stage renal disease

Hepatic Impairment

- No dose adjustment necessary
- Not recommended for us in chronic liver disease

Cardiac Impairment

- Drug should be used with caution

Elderly

- Some patients may tolerate lower doses better
- Reduction in the risk of suicidality with antidepressants compared to placebo in adults age 65 and older

Children and Adolescents

- Carefully weigh the risks and benefits of pharmacological treatment against the risks and benefits of nontreatment with antidepressants and make sure to document this in the patient's chart
- Monitor patients face-to-face regularly, particularly during the first several weeks of treatment
- Use with caution, observing for activation of known or unknown bipolar disorder and/ or suicidal ideation, and inform parents or guardians of this risk so they can help observe child or adolescent patients
- Not well studied

Pregnancy

- Effective June 30, 2015, the US FDA requires changes to the content and format of pregnancy and lactation information in prescription drug labels, including the elimination of the pregnancy letter categories; the Pregnancy and Lactation Labeling Rule (PLLR or final rule) applies only to prescription drugs and will be phased in gradually for drugs approved on or after June 30, 2001

- Controlled studies have not been conducted in pregnant women
- Not generally recommended for use during pregnancy, especially during first trimester
- Nonetheless, continuous treatment during pregnancy may be necessary and has not been proven to be harmful to the fetus
- Must weigh the risk of treatment (first trimester fetal development, third trimester newborn delivery) to the child against the risk of no treatment (recurrence of depression, maternal health, infant bonding) to the mother and child
- For many patients this may mean continuing treatment during pregnancy
- Neonates exposed to SSRIs or SNRIs late in the third trimester have developed complications requiring prolonged hospitalization, respiratory support, and tube feeding; reported symptoms are consistent with either a direct toxic effect of SSRIs and SNRIs or, possibly, a drug discontinuation syndrome, and include respiratory distress, cyanosis, apnea, seizures, temperature instability, feeding difficulty, vomiting, hypoglycemia, hypotonia, hypertonia, hyperreflexia, tremor, jitteriness, irritability, and constant crying

Breast Feeding

- Some drug is found in mother's breast milk
- Immediate postpartum period is a high-risk time for depression, especially in women who have had prior depressive episodes, so drug may need to be reinstituted late in the third trimester or shortly after childbirth to prevent a recurrence during the postpartum period
- Must weigh benefits of breast feeding with risks and benefits of antidepressant treatment versus nontreatment to both the infant and the mother
- For many patients, this may mean continuing treatment during breast feeding

THE ART OF PSYCHOPHARMACOLOGY

Potential Advantages

- Fibromyalgia, chronic pain syndrome
- Patients with retarded depression
- Patients with hypersomnia
- Patients with atypical depression
- Patients with depression may have higher remission rates on SNRIs than on SSRIs
- Depressed patients with somatic symptoms, fatigue, and pain

Potential Disadvantages

- Patients with urologic disorders, prostate disorders
- Patients with borderline or uncontrolled hypertension
- Patients with agitation and anxiety (short-term)

Primary Target Symptoms

- Pain
- Physical symptoms
- Depressed mood
- Energy, motivation, and interest
- Sleep disturbance

Pearls

- Approved in the USA. for use in pain and fibromyalgia
- Not studied in stress urinary incontinence
- Not well studied in ADHD or anxiety disorders, but may be effective

✻ Has greater potency for norepinephrine reuptake blockade than for serotonin reuptake blockade, but this is of unclear clinical significance as a differentiating feature from other SNRIs, although it might contribute to its therapeutic activity in fibromyalgia and chronic pain

✻ Onset of action in fibromyalgia may be somewhat faster than depression (i.e., 2 weeks rather than 2–8 weeks)

- Therapeutic actions in fibromyalgia are partial, with symptom reduction but not necessarily remission of painful symptoms in many patients

✻ Potent noradrenergic actions may account for possibly higher incidence of sweating and urinary hesitancy than other SNRIs

- Urinary hesitancy more common in men than women and in older men than in younger men
- Alpha 1 antagonists such as tamsulosin or naftopidil can reverse urinary hesitancy or retention
- Alpha 1 antagonists given prophylactically may prevent urinary hesitancy or retention

in patients at higher risk, such as elderly men with borderline urine flow
- May be better tolerated than tricyclic or tetracyclic antidepressants in the treatment of fibromyalgia or other chronic pain syndromes
- No pharmacokinetic interactions or elevations in plasma drug levels of tricyclic or tetracyclic antidepressants when adding or switching to or from milnacipran

Suggested Reading

Bisserbe JC. Clinical utility of milnacipran in comparison with other antidepressants. Int Clin Psychopharmacol 2002;17(Suppl 1):S43–50.

Derry S, Gill D, Phillips T, Moore RA. Milnacipran for neuropathic pain and fibromyalgia in adults. Cochrane Database Syst Rev 2012;14(3):CD008244.

Leo RJ, Brooks VL. Clinical potential of milnacipran, a serotonin and norepinephrine reuptake inhibitor in pain. Curr Opin Investig Drugs 2006;7(7):637–42.

Puozzo C, Panconi E, Deprez D. Pharmacology and pharmacokinetics of milnacipran. Int Clin Psychopharmacol 2002;17(Suppl 1):S25–35.

THERAPEUTICS

Brands • Remeron

see index for additional brand names

Generic? Yes

Class

- Neuroscience-based Nomenclature: serotonin, norepinephrine receptor antagonist (SN-RAn)
- Alpha 2 antagonist; NaSSA (noradrenaline and specific serotonergic agent); dual serotonin and norepinephrine agent; antidepressant

Commonly Prescribed for

(bold for FDA approved)

- **Major depressive disorder**
- Panic disorder
- Generalized anxiety disorder
- Posttraumatic stress disorder

How the Drug Works

- Boost neurotransmitters serotonin and norepinephrine/noradrenaline
- Blocks alpha 2 adrenergic presynaptic receptor, thereby increasing norepinephrine neurotransmission
- Blocks alpha 2 adrenergic presynaptic receptor on serotonin neurons (heteroreceptors), thereby increasing serotonin neurotransmission
- This is a novel mechanism independent of norepinephrine and serotonin reuptake blockade
- Blocks 5HT2A, 5HT2C, and 5HT3 serotonin receptors
- Blocks H1 histamine receptors

How Long Until It Works

✻ Actions on insomnia and anxiety can start shortly after initiation of dosing

- Onset of therapeutic actions in depression, however, is usually not immediate, but often delayed 2–4 weeks
- If it is not working within 6–8 weeks for depression, it may require a dosage increase or it may not work at all
- May continue to work for many years to prevent relapse of symptoms

If It Works

- The goal of treatment is complete remission of current symptoms as well as prevention of future relapses
- Treatment most often reduces or even eliminates symptoms, but not a cure since symptoms can recur after medicine stopped
- Continue treatment until all symptoms are gone (remission)
- Once symptoms are gone, continue treating for 1 year for the first episode of depression
- For second and subsequent episodes of depression, treatment may need to be indefinite
- Use in anxiety disorders may also need to be indefinite

If It Doesn't Work

- Many patients have only a partial response where some symptoms are improved but others persist (especially insomnia, fatigue, and problems concentrating)
- Other patients may be nonresponders, sometimes called treatment-resistant or treatment-refractory
- Consider increasing dose, switching to another agent or adding an appropriate augmenting agent
- Consider psychotherapy
- Consider evaluation for another diagnosis or for a comorbid condition (e.g., medical illness, substance abuse, etc.)
- Some patients may experience apparent lack of consistent efficacy due to activation of latent or underlying bipolar disorder, and require antidepressant discontinuation and a switch to a mood stabilizer

Best Augmenting Combos for Partial Response or Treatment Resistance

- SSRIs, bupropion, reboxetine, atomoxetine (use combinations of antidepressants with caution as this may activate bipolar disorder and suicidal ideation)

✻ Venlafaxine ("California rocket fuel"; a potentially powerful dual serotonin and norepinephrine combination, but observe for activation of bipolar disorder and suicidal ideation)

- Modafinil, especially for fatigue, sleepiness, and lack of concentration

- Mood stabilizers or atypical antipsychotics for bipolar depression, psychotic depression or treatment-resistant depression
- Benzodiazepines
- Hypnotics or trazodone for insomnia

Tests

- None for healthy individuals
- May need liver function tests for those with hepatic abnormalities before initiating treatment
- May need to monitor blood count during treatment for those with blood dyscrasias, leucopenia, or granulocytopenia
- Since some antidepressants such as mirtazapine can be associated with significant weight gain, before starting treatment, weigh all patients and determine if the patient is already overweight (BMI >25.0–29.9) or obese (BMI ≥30)
- Before giving a drug that can cause weight gain to an overweight or obese patient, consider determining whether the patient already has pre-diabetes (fasting plasma glucose 100–125 mg/dL), diabetes (fasting plasma glucose >126 mg/dL), or dyslipidemia (increased total cholesterol, LDL cholesterol, and triglycerides; decreased HDL cholesterol), and treat or refer such patients for treatment, including nutrition and weight management, physical activity counseling, smoking cessation, and medical management

✻ Monitor weight and BMI during treatment

✻ While giving a drug to a patient who has gained >5% of initial weight, consider evaluating for the presence of pre-diabetes, diabetes, or dyslipidemia, or consider switching to a different antidepressant

SIDE EFFECTS

How Drug Causes Side Effects

- Most side effects are immediate but often go away with time

✻ Histamine 1 receptor antagonism may explain sedative effects

✻ Histamine 1 receptor antagonism plus 5HT2C antagonism may explain some aspects of weight gain

Notable Side Effects

- Dry mouth, constipation, increased appetite, weight gain
- Sedation, dizziness, abnormal dreams, confusion
- Flu-like symptoms (may indicate low white blood cell or granulocyte count)
- Change in urinary function
- Hypotension

Life-Threatening or Dangerous Side Effects

- Rare seizures
- Rare induction of mania
- Rare activation of suicidal ideation and behavior (suicidality) (short-term studies did not show an increase in the risk of suicidality with antidepressants compared to placebo beyond age 24)

Weight Gain

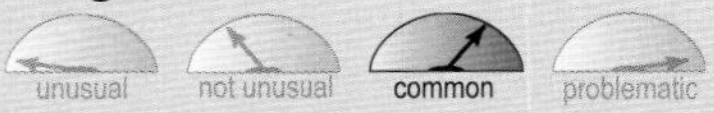

- Many experience and/or can be significant in amount

Sedation

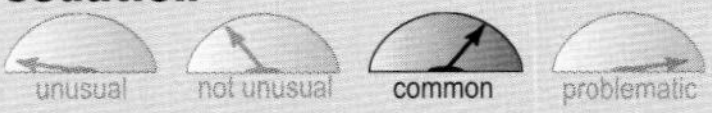

- Many experience and/or can be significant in amount

What to Do About Side Effects

- Wait
- Wait
- Wait
- Switch to another drug

Best Augmenting Agents for Side Effects

- Often best to try another antidepressant monotherapy prior to resorting to augmentation strategies to treat side effects
- Many side effects are dose-dependent (i.e., they increase as dose increases, or they reemerge until tolerance redevelops)
- Many side effects are time-dependent (i.e., they start immediately upon dosing and upon each dose increase, but go away with time)
- Trazodone or a hypnotic for insomnia
- Many side effects cannot be improved with an augmenting agent

- Activation and agitation may represent the induction of a bipolar state, especially a mixed dysphoric bipolar II condition sometimes associated with suicidal ideation, and require the addition of lithium, a mood stabilizer or an atypical antipsychotic, and/or discontinuation of mirtazapine

DOSING AND USE

Usual Dosage Range
- 15–45 mg at night

Dosage Forms
- Tablet 15 mg scored, 30 mg scored, 45 mg
- SolTab disintegrating tablet 15 mg, 30 mg, 45 mg

How to Dose
- Initial 15 mg/day in the evening; increase every 1–2 weeks until desired efficacy is reached; maximum generally 45 mg/day

Dosing Tips
- Sedation may not worsen as dose increases
- * Breaking a 15-mg tablet in half and administering 7.5 mg dose may actually increase sedation
- Some patients require more than 45 mg daily, including up to 90 mg in difficult patients who tolerate these doses
- If intolerable anxiety, insomnia, agitation, akathisia, or activation occur either upon dosing initiation or discontinuation, consider the possibility of activated bipolar disorder and switch to a mood stabilizer or an atypical antipsychotic

Overdose
- Rarely lethal; all fatalities have involved other medications; symptoms include sedation, disorientation, memory impairment, rapid heartbeat

Long-Term Use
- Safe

Habit Forming
- Not expected

How to Stop
- Taper is prudent to avoid withdrawal effects, but tolerance, dependence, and withdrawal effects not reliably reported

Pharmacokinetics
- Half-life 20–40 hours
- Substrate for CYP450 2D6, 3A4, and possibly also CYP450 1A2
- Food does not affect absorption

Drug Interactions
- Tramadol increases the risk of seizures in patients taking an antidepressant
- No significant pharmacokinetic drug interactions
- Can cause a fatal "serotonin syndrome" when combined with MAOIs, so do not use with MAOIs or for at least 14 days after MAOIs are stopped
- Do not start an MAOI for at least 5 half-lives (5 to 7 days for most drugs) after discontinuing mirtazapine

Other Warnings/ Precautions
- Drug may lower white blood cell count (rare; may not be increased compared to other antidepressants but controlled studies lacking; not a common problem reported in postmarketing surveillance)
- Drug may increase cholesterol
- May cause photosensitivity
- Avoid alcohol, which may increase sedation and cognitive and motor effects
- Use with caution in patients with history of seizures
- Use with caution in patients with bipolar disorder unless treated with concomitant mood-stabilizing agent
- When treating children, carefully weigh the risks and benefits of pharmacological treatment against the risks and benefits of nontreatment with antidepressants and make sure to document this in the patient's chart
- Distribute the brochures provided by the FDA and the drug companies
- Warn patients and their caregivers about the possibility of activating side effects and advise them to report such symptoms immediately

- Monitor patients for activation of suicidal ideation, especially children and adolescents

Do Not Use

- If patient is taking an MAOI
- If there is a proven allergy to mirtazapine

SPECIAL POPULATIONS

Renal Impairment

- Drug should be used with caution

Hepatic Impairment

- Drug should be used with caution
- May require lower dose

Cardiac Impairment

- Drug should be used with caution
- The potential risk of hypotension should be considered

Elderly

- Some patients may tolerate lower doses better
- Reduction in the risk of suicidality with antidepressants compared to placebo in adults age 65 and older

Children and Adolescents

- Carefully weigh the risks and benefits of pharmacological treatment against the risks and benefits of nontreatment with antidepressants and make sure to document this in the patient's chart
- Monitor patients face-to-face regularly, particularly during the first several weeks of treatment
- Use with caution, observing for activation of known or unknown bipolar disorder and/or suicidal ideation, and inform parents or guardians of this risk so they can help observe child or adolescent patients
- Safety and efficacy have not been established

Pregnancy

- Effective June 30, 2015, the US FDA requires changes to the content and format of pregnancy and lactation information in prescription drug labels, including the elimination of the pregnancy letter categories; the Pregnancy and Lactation Labeling Rule (PLLR or final rule) applies only to prescription drugs and will be phased in gradually for drugs approved on or after June 30, 2001
- Controlled studies have not been conducted in pregnant women
- Not generally recommended for use during pregnancy, especially during first trimester
- Must weigh the risk of treatment (first trimester fetal development, third trimester newborn delivery) to the child against the risk of no treatment (recurrence of depression, maternal health, infant bonding) to the mother and child
- For many patients this may mean continuing treatment during pregnancy

Breast Feeding

- Unknown if mirtazapine is secreted in human breast milk, but all psychotropics assumed to be secreted in breast milk
- If child becomes irritable or sedated, breast feeding or drug may need to be discontinued
- Immediate postpartum period is a high-risk time for depression, especially in women who have had prior depressive episodes, so drug may need to be reinstituted late in the third trimester or shortly after childbirth to prevent a recurrence during the postpartum period
- Must weigh benefits of breast feeding with risks and benefits of antidepressant treatment versus nontreatment to both the infant and the mother
- For many patients, this may mean continuing treatment during breast feeding

THE ART OF PSYCHOPHARMACOLOGY

Potential Advantages

- Patients particularly concerned about sexual side effects
- Patients with symptoms of anxiety
- Patients on concomitant medications
- As an augmenting agent to boost the efficacy of other antidepressants

Potential Disadvantages

- Patients particularly concerned about gaining weight
- Patients with low energy

Primary Target Symptoms

- Depressed mood
- Sleep disturbance
- Anxiety

Pearls

✻ Adding alpha 2 antagonism to agents that block serotonin and/or norepinephrine reuptake may be synergistic for severe depression
- Adding mirtazapine to venlafaxine or SSRIs may reverse drug-induced anxiety and insomnia
- Adding mirtazapine's 5HT3 antagonism to venlafaxine or SSRIs may reverse drug-induced nausea, diarrhea, stomach cramps, and gastrointestinal side effects
- SSRIs, venlafaxine, bupropion, phentermine, or stimulants may mitigate mirtazapine-induced weight gain
- If weight gain has not occurred by week 6 of treatment, it is less likely for there to be significant weight gain
- Has been demonstrated to have an earlier onset of action than SSRIs

✻ Does not affect the CYP450 system, and so may be preferable in patients requiring concomitant medications
- Preliminary evidence suggests efficacy as an augmenting agent to haloperidol in treating negative symptoms of schizophrenia
- Anecdotal reports of efficacy in recurrent brief depression
- Weight gain as a result of mirtazapine treatment is more likely in women than in men, and before menopause rather than after

✻ May cause sexual dysfunction only infrequently
- Patients can have carryover sedation and intoxicated-like feeling if particularly sensitive to sedative side effects when initiating dosing
- Rarely, patients may complain of visual "trails" or after-images on mirtazapine

Suggested Reading

Anttila SA, Leinonen EV. A review of the pharmacological and clinical profile of mirtazapine. CNS Drug Rev 2001;7(3):249–64.

Benkert O, Muller M, Szegedi A. An overview of the clinical efficacy of mirtazapine. Hum Psychopharmacol 2002;17(Suppl 1):S23–6.

Falkai P. Mirtazapine: other indications. J Clin Psychiatry 1999;60(Suppl 17):S36–40.

Fawcett J, Barkin RL. A meta-analysis of eight randomized, double-blind, controlled clinical trials of mirtazapine for the treatment of patients with major depression and symptoms of anxiety. J Clin Psychiatry 1998;59:123–7.

Masand PS, Gupta S. Long-term side effects of newer-generation antidepressants: SSRIS, venlafaxine, nefazodone, bupropion, and mirtazapine. Ann Clin Psychiatry 2002;14:175–82.

Watanabe N, Omori IM, Nakagawa A, et al. Mirtazapine versus other antidepressive agents for depression. Cochrane Database Syst Rev 2011;7(12):CD006528.

THERAPEUTICS

Brands
- Aurorix
- Arima
- Manerix

see index for additional brand names

Generic? No

Class
- Neuroscience-based Nomenclature: serotonin, norepinephrine, dopamine reversible enzyme inhibitor (SN-RevEI)
- Reversible inhibitor of monoamine oxidase A (MAO-A) (RIMA)

Commonly Prescribed for
(bold for FDA approved)
- Depression
- Social anxiety disorder

How the Drug Works
- Reversibly blocks MAO-A from breaking down norepinephrine, dopamine, and serotonin
- This presumably boosts noradrenergic, serotonergic, and dopaminergic neurotransmission
- MAO-A inhibition predominates unless significant concentrations of monoamines build up (e.g., due to dietary tyramine), in which case MAO-A inhibition is theoretically reversed

How Long Until It Works
- Onset of therapeutic actions usually not immediate, but often delayed 2–4 weeks
- If it is not working within 6–8 weeks, it may require a dosage increase or it may not work at all
- May continue to work for many years to prevent relapse of symptoms

If It Works
- The goal of treatment is complete remission of current symptoms as well as prevention of future relapses
- Treatment most often reduces or even eliminates symptoms, but not a cure since symptoms can recur after medicine stopped
- Continue treatment until all symptoms are gone (remission)
- Once symptoms gone, continue treating for 1 year for the first episode of depression
- For second and subsequent episodes of depression, treatment may need to be indefinite
- Use in anxiety disorders may also need to be indefinite

If It Doesn't Work
- Many patients have only a partial response where some symptoms are improved but others persist (especially insomnia, fatigue, and problems concentrating)
- Other patients may be nonresponders, sometimes called treatment-resistant or treatment-refractory
- Consider increasing dose, switching to another agent, or adding an appropriate augmenting agent
- Consider psychotherapy
- Consider evaluation for another diagnosis or for a comorbid condition (e.g., medical illness, substance abuse, etc.)
- Some patients may experience apparent lack of consistent efficacy due to activation of latent or underlying bipolar disorder, and require antidepressant discontinuation and a switch to a mood stabilizer

Best Augmenting Combos for Partial Response or Treatment Resistance
* Augmentation of MAOIs has not been systematically studied, and this is something for the expert, to be done with caution and with careful monitoring, but may be somewhat less risky with moclobemide than with other MAOIs
* A stimulant such as d-amphetamine or methylphenidate (with caution; may activate bipolar disorder and suicidal ideation)
- Lithium
- Mood-stabilizing anticonvulsants
- Atypical antipsychotics (with special caution for those agents with monoamine reuptake blocking properties, such as ziprasidone and zotepine)

Tests
- Patients should be monitored for changes in blood pressure

SIDE EFFECTS

How Drug Causes Side Effects

- Theoretically due to increases in monoamines in parts of the brain and body and at receptors other than those that cause therapeutic actions (e.g., unwanted actions of serotonin in sleep centers causing insomnia, unwanted actions of norepinephrine on vascular smooth muscle causing changes in blood pressure)
- Side effects are generally immediate, but immediate side effects often disappear in time

Notable Side Effects

- Insomnia, dizziness, agitation, anxiety, restlessness
- Dry mouth, diarrhea, constipation, nausea, vomiting
- Galactorrhea
- Rare hypertension

Life-Threatening or Dangerous Side Effects

- Hypertensive crisis (especially when MAOIs are used with certain tyramine containing foods – reduced risk compared to irreversible MAOIs)
- Induction of mania
- Rare activation of suicidal ideation and behavior (suicidality) (short-term studies did not show an increase in the risk of suicidality with antidepressants compared to placebo beyond age 24)
- Seizures

Weight Gain

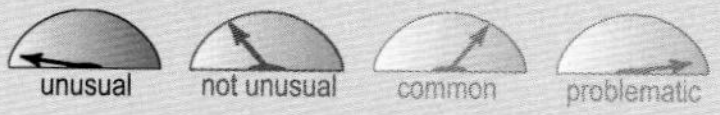

- Reported but not expected

Sedation

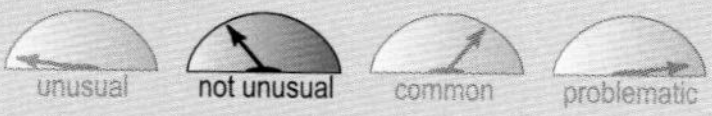

- Occurs in significant minority

What to Do About Side Effects

- Wait
- Wait
- Wait
- Lower the dose
- Switch to an SSRI or newer antidepressant

Best Augmenting Agents for Side Effects

- Trazodone (with caution) for insomnia
- Benzodiazepines for insomnia
- ✻ Single oral or sublingual dose of a calcium channel blocker (e.g., nifedipine) for urgent treatment of hypertension due to drug interaction or dietary tyramine
- Many side effects cannot be improved with an augmenting agent

DOSING AND USE

Usual Dosage Range

- 300–600 mg/day

Dosage Forms

- Tablet 100 mg scored, 150 mg scored

How to Dose

- Initial 300 mg/day in 3 divided doses after a meal; increase dose gradually; maximum dose generally 600 mg/day; minimum dose generally 150 mg/day

Dosing Tips

- ✻ At higher doses, moclobemide also inhibits MAO-B and thereby loses its selectivity for MAO-A, with uncertain clinical consequences
- ✻ Taking moclobemide after meals as opposed to before may minimize the chances of interactions with tyramine
- May be less toxic in overdose than TCAs and older MAOIs
- Clinical duration of action may be longer than biological half-life and allow twice daily dosing in some patients, or even once daily dosing, especially at lower doses

Overdose

- Agitation, aggression, behavioral disturbances, gastrointestinal irritation

Long-Term Use

- MAOIs may lose efficacy long-term

Habit Forming

- Some patients have developed dependence to MAOIs

How to Stop

- Taper not generally necessary

Pharmacokinetics

- Partially metabolized by CYP450 2C19 and 2D6
- Inactive metabolites
- Elimination half-life approximately 1–4 hours
- Clinical duration of action at least 24 hours

Drug Interactions

- Tramadol may increase the risk of seizures in patients taking an MAOI
- Can cause a fatal "serotonin syndrome" when combined with drugs that block serotonin reuptake, so do not use with a serotonin reuptake inhibitor or for 5 half-lives after stopping the serotonin reuptake inhibitor (see Table 1 after Pearls)
- Hypertensive crisis with headache, intracranial bleeding, and death may result from combining MAOIs with sympathomimetic drugs (e.g., amphetamines, methylphenidate, cocaine, dopamine, epinephrine, norepinephrine, and related compounds methyldopa, levodopa, L-tryptophan, L-tyrosine, and phenylalanine)
- Do not combine with another MAOI, alcohol, or guanethidine
- Adverse drug reactions can result from combining MAOIs with tricyclic/tetracyclic antidepressants and related compounds, including carbamazepine, cyclobenzaprine, and mirtazapine, and should be avoided except by experts to treat difficult cases
- MAOIs in combination with spinal anesthesia may cause combined hypotensive effects
- Combination of MAOIs and CNS depressants may enhance sedation and hypotension
- Cimetidine may increase plasma concentrations of moclobemide
- Moclobemide may enhance the effects of NSAIDs such as ibuprofen
- Risk of hypertensive crisis may be increased if moclobemide is used concurrently with levodopa or other dopaminergic agents

Other Warnings/ Precautions

- Use still requires low tyramine diet, although more tyramine may be tolerated with moclobemide than with other MAOIs before eliciting a hypertensive reaction (see Table 2 after Pearls)
- Patient and prescriber must be vigilant to potential interactions with any drug, including antihypertensives and over-the-counter cough/cold preparations
- Over-the-counter medications to avoid include cough and cold preparations, including those containing dextromethorphan, nasal decongestants (tablets, drops, or spray), hay-fever medications, sinus medications, asthma inhalant medications, anti-appetite medications, weight reducing preparations, "pep" pills (see Table 3 after Pearls)
- Use cautiously in hypertensive patients
- Moclobemide is not recommended for use in patients who cannot be monitored closely
- When treating children, carefully weigh the risks and benefits of pharmacological treatment against the risks and benefits of nontreatment with antidepressants and make sure to document this in the patient's chart
- Distribute the brochures provided by the FDA and the drug companies
- Warn patients and their caregivers about the possibility of activating side effects and advise them to report such symptoms immediately
- Monitor patients for activation of suicidal ideation, especially children and adolescents

Do Not Use

- If patient is taking meperidine (pethidine)
- If patient is taking a sympathomimetic agent or taking guanethidine
- If patient is taking another MAOI
- If patient is taking any agent that can inhibit serotonin reuptake (e.g., SSRIs, sibutramine, tramadol, milnacipran, duloxetine, venlafaxine, clomipramine, etc.)
- If patient is in an acute confusional state
- If patient has pheochromocytoma or thyrotoxicosis
- If patient has frequent or severe headaches

- If patient is undergoing elective surgery and requires general anesthesia
- If there is a proven allergy to moclobemide

SPECIAL POPULATIONS

Renal Impairment
- Use with caution

Hepatic Impairment
- Plasma concentrations are increased
- May require one-half to one-third of usual adult dose

Cardiac Impairment
- Cardiac impairment may require lower than usual adult dose
- Patients with angina pectoris or coronary artery disease should limit their exertion

Elderly
- Elderly patients may have greater sensitivity to adverse effects
- Reduction in the risk of suicidality with antidepressants compared to placebo in adults age 65 and older

Children and Adolescents
- Not recommended for use in children under age 18
- Carefully weigh the risks and benefits of pharmacological treatment against the risks and benefits of nontreatment with antidepressants and make sure to document this in the patient's chart
- Monitor patients face-to-face regularly, particularly during the first several weeks of treatment
- Use with caution, observing for activation of known or unknown bipolar disorder and/or suicidal ideation, and inform parents or guardians of this risk so they can help observe child or adolescent patients

Pregnancy
- Not generally recommended for use during pregnancy, especially during first trimester
- Should evaluate patient for treatment with an antidepressant with a better risk/benefit ratio

Breast Feeding
- Some drug is found in mother's breast milk
- Effects on infant are unknown
- Immediate postpartum period is a high-risk time for depression, especially in women who have had prior depressive episodes, so drug may need to be reinstituted late in the third trimester or shortly after childbirth to prevent a recurrence during the postpartum period
- Should evaluate patient for treatment with an antidepressant with a better risk/benefit ratio

THE ART OF PSYCHOPHARMACOLOGY

Potential Advantages
- Atypical depression
- Severe depression
- Treatment-resistant depression or anxiety disorders

Potential Disadvantages
- Patients noncompliant with dietary restrictions, concomitant drug restrictions, and twice daily dosing after meals

Primary Target Symptoms
- Depressed mood

Pearls
- MAOIs are generally reserved for second-line use after SSRIs, SNRIs, and combinations of newer antidepressants have failed
- Patient should be advised not to take any prescription or over-the-counter drugs without consulting his/her doctor because of possible drug interactions with the MAOI
- Headache is often the first symptom of hypertensive crisis
- Moclobemide has a much reduced risk of interactions with tyramine than nonselective MAOIs

- Especially at higher doses of moclobemide, foods with high tyramine need to be avoided (see Table 2)
- The rigid dietary restrictions may reduce compliance
- ✻ May be a safer alternative to classical irreversible nonselective MAO-A and MAO-B inhibitors with less propensity for tyramine and drug interactions and hepatotoxicity (although not entirely free of interactions)
- May not be as effective at low doses, and may have more side effects at higher doses
- Moclobemide's profile at higher doses may be more similar to classical MAOIs
- MAOIs are a viable second-line treatment option in depression, but are not frequently used
- ✻ Myths about the danger of dietary tyramine can be exaggerated, but prohibitions against concomitant drugs often not followed closely enough
- Orthostatic hypotension, insomnia, and sexual dysfunction are often the most troublesome common side effects
- ✻ MAOIs should be for the expert, especially if combining with agents of potential risk (e.g., stimulants, trazodone, TCAs)
- ✻ MAOIs should not be neglected as therapeutic agents for the treatment-resistant
- Although generally prohibited, a heroic but potentially dangerous treatment for severely treatment-resistant patients is for an expert to give a tricyclic/tetracyclic antidepressant other than clomipramine simultaneously with an MAOI for patients who fail to respond to numerous other antidepressants
- Use of MAOIs with clomipramine is always prohibited because of the risk of serotonin syndrome and death
- Amoxapine may be the preferred trycyclic/tetracyclic antidepressant to combine with an MAOI in heroic cases due to its theoretically protective 5HT2A antagonist properties
- If this option is elected, start the MAOI with the tricyclic/tetracyclic antidepressant simultaneously at low doses after appropriate drug washout, then alternately increase doses of these agents every few days to a week as tolerated
- Although very strict dietary and concomitant drug restrictions must be observed to prevent hypertensive crises and serotonin syndrome, the most common side effects of MAOI and tricyclic/tetracyclic combinations may be weight gain and orthostatic hypotension

Table 1. Drugs contraindicated due to risk of serotonin syndrome/toxicity

Do Not Use:			
Antidepressants	**Drugs of Abuse**	**Opioids**	**Other**
SSRIs	MDMA (ecstasy)	Meperidine	Non-subcutaneous sumatriptan
SNRIs	Cocaine	Tramadol	Chlorpheniramine
Clomipramine	Methamphetamine	Methadone	Brompheniramine
St. John's wort	High-dose or injected amphetamine	Fentanyl	Dextromethorphan
			Procarbazine?

Table 2. Dietary guidelines for patients taking MAOIs

Foods to avoid*	**Foods allowed**
Dried, aged, smoked, fermented, spoiled, or improperly stored meat, poultry, and fish	Fresh or processed meat, poultry, and fish; properly stored pickled or smoked fish
Broad bean pods	All other vegetables
Aged cheeses	Processed cheese slices, cottage cheese, ricotta cheese, yogurt, cream cheese
Tap and unpasteurized beer	Canned or bottled beer and alcohol
Marmite	Brewer's and baker's yeast
Sauerkraut, kimchee	
Soy products/tofu	Peanuts
Banana peel	Bananas, avocados, raspberries
Tyramine-containing nutritional supplement	

*Not necessary for 6-mg transdermal or low-dose oral selegiline

Table 3. Drugs that boost norepinephrine: should only be used with caution with MAOIs

Use With Caution:			
Decongestants	**Stimulants**	**Antidepressants with norepinephrine reuptake inhibition**	**Other**
Phenylephrine	Amphetamines	Most tricyclics	Phentermine
Pseudoephedrine	Methylphenidate	NRIs	Local anesthetics containing vasoconstrictors
	Cocaine	NDRIs	
	Methamphetamine		
	Modafinil		Tapentadol
	Armodafinil		

Suggested Reading

Amrein R, Martin JR, Cameron AM. Moclobemide in patients with dementia and depression. Adv Neurol 1999;80:509–19.

Fulton B, Benfield P. Moclobemide. An update of its pharmacological properties and therapeutic use. Drugs 1996;52:450–74.

Kennedy SH. Continuation and maintenance treatments in major depression: the neglected role of monoamine oxidase inhibitors. J Psychiatry Neurosci 1997;22:127–31.

Lippman SB, Nash K. Monoamine oxidase inhibitor update. Potential adverse food and drug interactions. Drug Saf 1990;5:195–204.

Nutt D, Montgomery SA. Moclobemide in the treatment of social phobia. Int Clin Psychopharmacol 1996;11(Suppl 3):S77–82.

THERAPEUTICS

Brands
- Provigil
- Alertec
- Modiodal

see index for additional brand names

Generic? Yes

Class
- Neuroscience-based Nomenclature: dopamine reuptake inhibitor (D-RI)
- Wake-promoting

Commonly Prescribed for
(bold for FDA approved)
- **Reducing excessive sleepiness in patients with narcolepsy and shift work sleep disorder**
- **Reducing excessive sleepiness in patients with obstructive sleep apnea/hypopnea syndrome (OSAHS) (adjunct to standard treatment for underlying airway obstruction)**
- Attention deficit hyperactivity disorder (ADHD)
- Fatigue and sleepiness in depression
- Fatigue in multiple sclerosis
- Bipolar depression

How the Drug Works
- Unknown, but clearly different from classical stimulants such as methylphenidate and amphetamine
- Binds to and requires the presence of the dopamine transporter; also requires the presence of alpha adrenergic receptors
- Hypothetically acts as an inhibitor of the dopamine transporter
- Increases neuronal activity selectively in the hypothalamus
- ✻ Presumably enhances activity in hypothalamic wakefulness center (TMN, tuberomammillary nucleus) within the hypothalamic sleep-wake switch by an unknown mechanism
- ✻ Activates TMN neurons that release histamine
- ✻ Activates other hypothalamic neurons that release orexin/hypocretin

How Long Until It Works
- Can immediately reduce daytime sleepiness and improve cognitive task performance within 2 hours of first dosing
- Can take several days to optimize dosing and clinical improvement

If It Works
- ✻ Improves daytime sleepiness and may improve attention as well as fatigue
- ✻ Does not generally prevent one from falling asleep when needed
- May not completely normalize wakefulness
- Treat until improvement stabilizes and then continue treatment indefinitely as long as improvement persists (studies support at least 12 weeks of treatment)

If It Doesn't Work
- ✻ Change dose; some patients do better with an increased dose but some actually do better with a decreased dose
- Augment or consider an alternative treatment for daytime sleepiness, fatigue, or ADHD

Best Augmenting Combos for Partial Response or Treatment Resistance
- ✻ Modafinil is itself an adjunct to standard treatments for obstructive sleep apnea/hypopnea syndrome (OSAHS); if continuous positive airway pressure (CPAP) is the treatment of choice, a maximal effort to treat first with CPAP should be made prior to initiating modafinil and CPAP should be continued after initiation of modafinil
- ✻ Modafinil is itself an augmenting therapy to antidepressants for residual sleepiness and fatigue in major depressive disorder
- Best to attempt another monotherapy prior to augmenting with other drugs in the treatment of sleepiness associated with sleep disorders or problems concentrating in ADHD
- Combination of modafinil with stimulants such as methylphenidate or amphetamine or with atomoxetine for ADHD has not been systematically studied
- However, such combinations may be useful options for experts, with close monitoring, when numerous monotherapies for sleepiness or ADHD have failed

Tests
- None for healthy individuals

SIDE EFFECTS

How Drug Causes Side Effects
- Unknown
- CNS side effects presumably due to excessive CNS actions on various neurotransmitter systems

Notable Side Effects
✻ Headache (dose-dependent)
- Anxiety, nervousness, insomnia
- Dry mouth, diarrhea, nausea, anorexia
- Pharyngitis, rhinitis, infection
- Hypertension
- Palpitations

Life-Threatening or Dangerous Side Effects
- Transient EKG ischemic changes in patients with mitral valve prolapse or left ventricular hypertrophy have been reported (rare)
- Rare activation of (hypo)mania, anxiety, hallucinations, or suicidal ideation
- Rare severe dermatologic reactions (Stevens-Johnson syndrome and others)
- Angioedema, anaphylactoid reactions, and multi-organ hypersensitivity reactions have been reported

Weight Gain
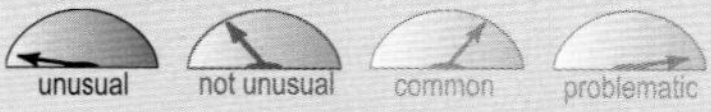

- Reported but not expected

Sedation
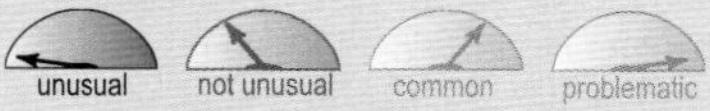

- Reported but not expected
- Patients are usually awakened and some may be activated

What to Do About Side Effects
- Wait
- Lower the dose
- Give only once daily
- Give smaller split doses 2 or more times daily
- For activation or insomnia, do not give in the evening
- If unacceptable side effects persist, discontinue use
- For life-threatening or dangerous side effects, discontinue immediately (e.g., at first sign of a drug-related rash)

Best Augmenting Agents for Side Effects
- Many side effects cannot be improved with an augmenting agent

DOSING AND USE

Usual Dosage Range
- 200 mg/day in the morning

Dosage Forms
- Tablet 100 mg, 200 mg (scored)

How to Dose
- Titration up or down only necessary if not optimally efficacious at the standard starting dose of 200 mg once a day in the morning

Dosing Tips
✻ For sleepiness, <u>more may be more</u>: higher doses (200–800 mg/day) may be better than lower doses (50–200 mg/day) in patients with daytime sleepiness in sleep disorders
✻ For problems concentrating and fatigue, <u>less may be more</u>: lower doses (50–200 mg/day) may be paradoxically better than higher doses (200–800 mg/day) in some patients
- At high doses, may slightly induce its own metabolism, possibly by actions of inducing CYP450 3A4
- Dose may creep upward in some patients with long-term treatment due to autoinduction; drug holiday may restore efficacy at original dose

Overdose
- No fatalities; agitation, insomnia, increase in hemodynamic parameters
- Postmarketing experience includes CNS symptoms, such as restlessness, disorientation, confusion, excitation, and hallucinations; digestive changes, such as nausea and diarrhea; and cardiovascular changes, such as tachycardia, bradycardia, hypertension, and chest pain

Long-Term Use
- Efficacy in reducing excessive sleepiness in sleep disorders has been demonstrated in 9- to 12-week trials
- Unpublished data show safety for up to 136 weeks

- The need for continued treatment should be reevaluated periodically

Habit Forming

- Schedule IV; may have some potential for abuse but unusual in clinical practice

How to Stop

- Taper not necessary; patients may have sleepiness on discontinuation

Pharmacokinetics

- Metabolized by the liver
- Excreted renally
- Elimination half-life 10–12 hours
- Inhibits CYP450 2C19 (and perhaps 2C9)
- Induces CYP450 3A4 (and slightly 1A2 and 2B6)

Drug Interactions

- May increase plasma levels of drugs metabolized by CYP450 2C19 (e.g., diazepam, phenytoin, propranolol)
- Modafinil may increase plasma levels of CYP450 2D6 substrates such as TCAs and SSRIs, perhaps requiring downward dose adjustments of these agents
- Modafinil may decrease plasma levels of CYP450 3A4 substrates such as ethinyl estradiol and triazolam
- Due to induction of CYP450 3A4, effectiveness of steroidal contraceptives may be reduced by modafinil, including 1 month after discontinuation
- Inducers or inhibitors of CYP450 3A4 may affect levels of modafinil (e.g., carbamazepine may lower modafinil plasma levels; fluvoxamine and fluoxetine may raise modafinil plasma levels)
- Modafinil may slightly reduce its own levels by autoinduction of CYP450 3A4
- Modafinil may increase clearance of drugs dependent on CYP450 1A2 and reduce their plasma levels
- Patients on modafinil and warfarin should have prothrombin times monitored
- Methylphenidate may delay absorption of modafinil by an hour

✽ However, coadministration with methylphenidate does not significantly change the pharmacokinetics of either modafinil or methylphenidate

✽ Coadministration with dextroamphetamine also does not significantly change the pharmacokinetics of either modafinil or dextroamphetamine

- Interaction studies with MAOIs have not been performed, but MAOIs can be given with modafinil by experts with cautious monitoring

Other Warnings/ Precautions

- Patients with history of drug abuse should be monitored closely
- Modafinil may cause CNS effects similar to those caused by other CNS agents (e.g., changes in mood and, theoretically, activation of psychosis, mania, or suicidal ideation)
- Modafinil should be used in patients with sleep disorders that have been completely evaluated for narcolepsy, obstructive sleep apnea/hypopnea syndrome (OSAHS), and shift work sleep disorder
- In OSAHS patients for whom continuous positive airway pressure (CPAP) is the treatment of choice, a maximal effort to treat first with CPAP should be made prior to initiating modafinil, and then CPAP should be continued after initiating modafinil
- The effectiveness of steroidal contraceptives may be reduced when used with modafinil and for 1 month after discontinuation of modafinil
- Modafinil is not a replacement for sleep

Do Not Use

- If patient has severe hypertension
- If patient has cardiac arrhythmias
- If there is a proven allergy to modafinil

SPECIAL POPULATIONS

Renal Impairment

- Use with caution; dose reduction is recommended

Hepatic Impairment

- Reduce dose by half in severely impaired patients

Cardiac Impairment

- Use with caution

- Not recommended for use in patients with a history of left ventricular hypertrophy, ischemic EKG changes, chest pain, arrhythmias, or recent myocardial infarction

Elderly

- Limited experience in patients over 65
- Clearance of modafinil may be reduced in elderly patients

Children and Adolescents

- Safety and efficacy not established under age 16
- Can be used cautiously by experts for children and adolescents

Pregnancy

- Effective June 30, 2015, the US FDA requires changes to the content and format of pregnancy and lactation information in prescription drug labels, including the elimination of the pregnancy letter categories; the Pregnancy and Lactation Labeling Rule (PLLR or final rule) applies only to prescription drugs and will be phased in gradually for drugs approved on or after June 30, 2001
- Controlled studies have not been conducted in pregnant women
- Intrauterine growth restriction and spontaneous abortion have been reported with armodafinil and modafinil
- In animal studies, developmental toxicity was observed at clinically relevant plasma exposures of armodafinil and modafinil
- Use in women of childbearing potential requires weighing potential benefits to the mother against potential risks to the fetus

✽ Generally, modafinil should be discontinued prior to anticipated pregnancies

Breast Feeding

- Unknown if modafinil is secreted in human breast milk, but all psychotropics assumed to be secreted in breast milk

✽ Recommended either to discontinue drug or bottle feed

THE ART OF PSYCHOPHARMACOLOGY

Potential Advantages

- Selective for areas of brain involved in sleep/wake promotion
- Less activating and less abuse potential than stimulants

Potential Disadvantages

- May not work as well as stimulants in some patients

Primary Target Symptoms

- Sleepiness
- Concentration
- Physical and mental fatigue

Pearls

✽ Anecdotal usefulness for jet lag short-term (off label)

✽ Modafinil is not a replacement for sleep

✽ The treatment for sleep deprivation is sleep, not modafinil

- Controlled studies suggest modafinil improves <u>attention</u> in OSAHS, shift work sleep disorder, and ADHD (both children and adults), but controlled studies of attention have not been performed in major depressive disorder

✽ May be useful to treat <u>fatigue</u> in patients with depression as well as other disorders, such as multiple sclerosis, myotonic dystrophy, HIV/AIDS

- In depression, modafinil's actions on <u>fatigue</u> appear to be independent of actions (if any) on mood
- In depression, modafinil's actions on <u>sleepiness</u> also appear to be independent of actions (if any) on mood but may be linked to actions on fatigue or on global functioning
- Several controlled studies in depression show improvement in <u>sleepiness or global functioning</u>, especially for depressed patients with sleepiness and fatigue
- May be useful adjunct to mood stabilizers for bipolar depression
- May be useful in treating <u>sleepiness</u> associated with opioid analgesia, particularly in end-of-life management
- Subjective sensation associated with modafinil is usually one of normal

wakefulness, not of stimulation, although jitteriness can rarely occur

- Anecdotally, some patients may experience wearing off of efficacy over time, especially for off-label uses, with restoration of efficacy after a drug holiday; such wearing off is less likely with intermittent dosing

* Compared to stimulants, modafinil has a novel mechanism of action, novel therapeutic uses, and less abuse potential, but is often inaccurately classified as a stimulant

- Alpha 1 antagonists such as prazosin may block the therapeutic actions of modafinil
- The active R enantiomer of modafinil, called armodafinil, is also available

Suggested Reading

Batejat DM, Lagarde DP. Naps and modafinil as countermeasures for the effects of sleep deprivation on cognitive performance. Aviat Space Environ Med 1999;70:493–8.

Bourdon L, Jacobs I, Bateman WA, Vallerand AL. Effect of modafinil on heat production and regulation of body temperatures in cold-exposed humans. Aviat Space Environ Med 1994;65:999–1004.

Cox JM, Pappagallo M. Modafinil: a gift to portmanteau. Am J Hosp Palliat Care 2001;18:408–10.

Jasinski DR, Koyacevic-Ristanovic. Evaluation of the abuse liability of modafinil and other drugs for excessive daytime sleepiness associated with narcolepsy. Clin Neuropharmacol 2000;23:149–56.

Kumar R. Approved and investigational uses of modafinil: an evidence-based review. Drugs 2008;68(13):1803–39.

Wesensten NJ, Belenky G, Kautz MA, et al. Maintaining alertness and performance during sleep deprivation: modafinil versus caffeine. Psychopharmacology (Berl) 2002;159:238–47.

THERAPEUTICS

Brands • Moban

see index for additional brand names

Generic? Yes

Class

- Conventional antipsychotic (neuroleptic, dopamine 2 antagonist)

Commonly Prescribed for

(bold for FDA approved)

- **Schizophrenia (no longer available in the USA)**
- Other psychotic disorders
- Bipolar disorder

How the Drug Works

- Blocks dopamine 2 receptors, reducing positive symptoms of psychosis

How Long Until It Works

- Psychotic symptoms can improve within 1 week, but it may take several weeks for full effect on behavior

If It Works

- Most often reduces positive symptoms in schizophrenia but does not eliminate them
- Most schizophrenic patients do not have a total remission of symptoms but rather a reduction of symptoms by about a third
- Continue treatment in schizophrenia until reaching a plateau of improvement
- After reaching a satisfactory plateau, continue treatment for at least a year after first episode of psychosis in schizophrenia
- For second and subsequent episodes of psychosis in schizophrenia, treatment may need to be indefinite
- Reduces symptoms of acute psychotic mania but not proven as a mood stabilizer or as an effective maintenance treatment in bipolar disorder
- After reducing acute psychotic symptoms in mania, switch to a mood stabilizer and/or an atypical antipsychotic for mood stabilization and maintenance

If It Doesn't Work

- Consider trying one of the first-line atypical antipsychotics (risperidone, olanzapine, quetiapine, ziprasidone, aripiprazole, paliperidone, asenapine, iloperidone, lurasidone, amisulpride)
- Consider trying another conventional antipsychotic
- If 2 or more antipsychotic monotherapies do not work, consider clozapine

Best Augmenting Combos for Partial Response or Treatment Resistance

- Augmentation of conventional antipsychotics has not been systematically studied
- Addition of a mood-stabilizing anticonvulsant such as valproate, carbamazepine, or lamotrigine may be helpful in both schizophrenia and bipolar mania
- Augmentation with lithium in bipolar mania may be helpful
- Addition of a benzodiazepine, especially short-term for agitation

Tests

❋ Since conventional antipsychotics are frequently associated with weight gain, before starting treatment, weigh all patients and determine if the patient is already overweight (BMI 25.0–29.9) or obese (BMI ≥30)

- Before giving a drug that can cause weight gain to an overweight or obese patient, consider determining whether the patient already has pre-diabetes (fasting plasma glucose 100–125 mg/dL), diabetes (fasting plasma glucose >126 mg/dL), or dyslipidemia (increased total cholesterol, LDL cholesterol, and triglycerides; decreased HDL cholesterol), and treat or refer such patients for treatment, including nutrition and weight management, physical activity counseling, smoking cessation, and medical management

❋ Monitor weight and BMI during treatment

❋ Consider monitoring fasting triglycerides monthly for several months in patients at high risk for metabolic complications and when initiating or switching antipsychotics

❋ While giving a drug to a patient who has gained >5% of initial weight, consider evaluating for the presence of pre-diabetes, diabetes, or dyslipidemia, or consider switching to a different antipsychotic

- Should check blood pressure in the elderly before starting and for the first few weeks of treatment

- Monitoring elevated prolactin levels of dubious clinical benefit
- Patients with low white blood cell count (WBC) or history of drug-induced leucopenia/neutropenia should have complete blood count (CBC) monitored frequently during the first few months and molindone should be discontinued at the first sign of decline of WBC in the absence of other causative factors

SIDE EFFECTS

How Drug Causes Side Effects

- By blocking dopamine 2 receptors in the striatum, it can cause motor side effects
- By blocking dopamine 2 receptors in the pituitary, it can cause elevations in prolactin
- By blocking dopamine 2 receptors excessively in the mesocortical and mesolimbic dopamine pathways, especially at high doses, it can cause worsening of negative and cognitive symptoms (neuroleptic-induced deficit syndrome)
- Anticholinergic actions may cause sedation, blurred vision, constipation, dry mouth
- Antihistaminic actions may cause sedation, weight gain
- By blocking alpha 1 adrenergic receptors, it can cause dizziness, sedation, and hypotension
- Mechanism of weight gain and any possible increased incidence of diabetes or dyslipidemia with conventional antipsychotics is unknown

Notable Side Effects

* Neuroleptic-induced deficit syndrome
* Akathisia
* Extrapyramidal symptoms, parkinsonism, tardive dyskinesia
* Galactorrhea, amenorrhea
- Sedation
- Dry mouth, constipation, vision disturbance, urninary retention
- Hypotension, tachycardia

Life-Threatening or Dangerous Side Effects

- Rare neuroleptic malignant syndrome
- Rare leukopenia
- Rare seizures
- Increased risk of death and cerebrovascular events in elderly patients with dementia-related psychosis

Weight Gain

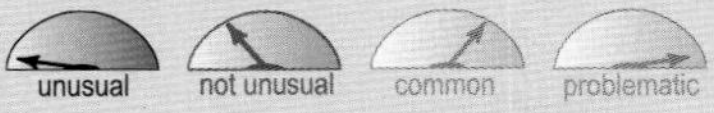

* Reported but not expected

Sedation

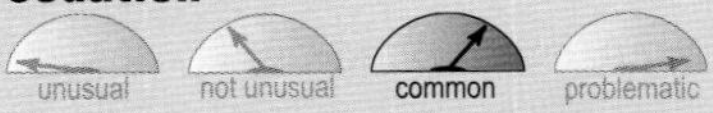

- Many experience and/or can be significant in amount
- Sedation is usually transient

What to Do About Side Effects

- Wait
- Wait
- Wait
- For motor symptoms, add an anticholinergic agent
- Reduce the dose
- For sedation, give at night
- Switch to an atypical antipsychotic
- Weight loss, exercise programs, and medical management for high BMIs, diabetes, dyslipidemia

Best Augmenting Agents for Side Effects

- Benztropine or trihexyphenidyl for motor side effects
- Sometimes amantadine can be helpful for motor side effects
- Benzodiazepines may be helpful for akathisia
- Many side effects cannot be improved with an augmenting agent

DOSING AND USE

Usual Dosage Range

- 40–100 mg/day in divided doses

Dosage Forms

- Tablet 5 mg, 10 mg, 25 mg scored, 50 mg scored, 100 mg scored
- Liquid 20 mg/mL

How to Dose

- Initial 50–75 mg/day; increase to 100 mg/day after 3–4 days; maximum 225 mg/day

Dosing Tips

- Very short half-life, but some patients may only require once daily dosing
- Other patients may do better with 3 or 4 divided doses daily
- Patients receiving atypical antipsychotics may occasionally require a "top up" of a conventional antipsychotic to control aggression or violent behavior
- Treatment should be suspended if absolute neutrophil count falls below 1,000/mm^3

Overdose

- Deaths have occurred; extrapyramidal symptoms, sedation, hypotension, respiratory depression, coma

Long-Term Use

- Some side effects may be irreversible (e.g., tardive dyskinesia)

Habit Forming

- No

How to Stop

- Slow down-titration (over 6–8 weeks), especially when simultaneously beginning a new antipsychotic while switching (i.e., cross-titration)
- Rapid discontinuation may lead to rebound psychosis and worsening of symptoms
- If antiparkinson agents are being used, they should be continued for a few weeks after molindone is discontinued

Pharmacokinetics

- Half-life approximately 1.5 hours

Drug Interactions

- Additive effects may occur if used with CNS depressants
- Some patients taking a neuroleptic and lithium have developed an encephalopathic syndrome similar to neuroleptic malignant syndrome
- Molindone tablets contain calcium sulfate, which may interfere with absorption of phenytoin sodium or tetracyclines
- Combined use with epinephrine may lower blood pressure
- May increase the effects of antihypertensive drugs

Other Warnings/ Precautions

- If signs of neuroleptic malignant syndrome develop, treatment should be immediately discontinued
- Liquid molindone contains sodium metabisulfite, which may cause allergic reactions in some people, especially in asthmatic people
- Use cautiously in patients with alcohol withdrawal or convulsive disorders because of possible lowering of seizure threshold
- Antiemetic effect can mask signs of other disorders or overdose
- Do not use epinephrine in event of overdose as interaction with some pressor agents may lower blood pressure
- Use cautiously in patients with glaucoma, urinary retention
- Observe for signs of ocular toxicity (pigmentary retinopathy, lenticular pigmentation)
- Use only with caution if at all in Parkinson's disease or Lewy body dementia

Do Not Use

- If patient is in a comatose state or has CNS depression
- If there is a proven allergy to molindone

SPECIAL POPULATIONS

Renal Impairment

- Should receive initial lower dose

Hepatic Impairment

- Should receive initial lower dose

Cardiac Impairment

- Use with caution

Elderly

- Should receive initial lower dose
- Although conventional antipsychotics are commonly used for behavioral disturbances in dementia, no agent has been approved for treatment of elderly patients with dementia-related psychosis
- Elderly patients with dementia-related psychosis treated with antipsychotics are at an increased risk of death compared to placebo, and also have an increased risk of cerebrovascular events

Children and Adolescents
- Safety and efficacy not well established
- Generally consider second-line after atypical antipsychotics

Pregnancy
- Controlled studies have not been conducted in pregnant women
- Animal studies have not shown adverse effects
- There is a risk of abnormal muscle movements and withdrawal symptoms in newborns whose mothers took an antipsychotic during the third trimester; symptoms may include agitation, abnormally increased or decreased muscle tone, tremor, sleepiness, severe difficulty breathing, and difficulty feeding
- Psychotic symptoms may worsen during pregnancy and some form of treatment may be necessary
- Atypical antipsychotics may be preferable to conventional antipsychotics or anticonvulsant mood stabilizers if treatment is required during pregnancy

Breast Feeding
- Unknown if molindone is secreted in human breast milk, but all psychotropics assumed to be secreted in breast milk
- ✽ Recommended either to discontinue drug or bottle feed

THE ART OF PSYCHOPHARMACOLOGY

Potential Advantages
- Some patients benefit from molindone's sedative properties

Potential Disadvantages
- Patients with tardive dyskinesia

Primary Target Symptoms
- Positive symptoms of psychosis
- Motor and autonomic hyperactivity
- Violent or aggressive behavior

Pearls
- No longer available in the USA
- ✽ May cause less weight gain than some other antipsychotics
- Not shown to be effective for behavioral problems in mental retardation
- Patients have very similar antipsychotic responses to any conventional antipsychotic, which is different from atypical antipsychotics where antipsychotic responses of individual patients can occasionally vary greatly from one atypical antipsychotic to another
- Patients with inadequate responses to atypical antipsychotics may benefit from a trial of augmentation with a conventional antipsychotic such as molindone or from switching to a conventional antipsychotic such as molindone
- However, long-term polypharmacy with a combination of a conventional antipsychotic such as molindone with an atypical antipsychotic may combine their side effects without clearly augmenting the efficacy of either
- Although a frequent practice by some prescribers, adding two conventional antipsychotics together has little rationale and may reduce tolerability without clearly enhancing efficacy

Suggested Reading

Bagnall A, Fenton M, Kleijnen J, Lewis R. Molindone for schizophrenia and severe mental illness. Cochrane Database Syst Rev 2007;24(1):CD002083.

Owen RR Jr, Cole JO. Molindone hydrochloride: a review of laboratory and clinical findings. J Clin Psychopharmacol 1989;9(4):268–76.

NALMEFENE

THERAPEUTICS

Brands
- Selincro

see index for additional brand names

Generic?
Yes (not for oral)

Class
- Neuroscience-based Nomenclature: opioid receptor antagonist (O-RAn)
- Alcohol dependence treatment; mu and delta opioid receptor antagonist and kappa opioid receptor partial agonist

Commonly Prescribed for
(bold for FDA approved)
- Reduction of alcohol consumption in patients with alcohol dependence who have a high drinking risk level

How the Drug Works
- Reduces alcohol consumption through modulation of opioid systems, thereby reducing the reinforcing effects of alcohol
- Blockade of mu opioid receptors prevents the pleasurable effects of alcohol, whereas modulation of the kappa opioid receptors may reduce dysphoria associated with alcohol withdrawal

How Long Until It Works
- Can begin working immediately and can be used as needed

If It Works
- Reduces alcohol consumption by diminishing reinforcing properties of alcohol (rewarding effects, cravings)

If It Doesn't Work
- Evaluate for and address contributing factors
- Consider switching to another agent

Best Augmenting Combos for Partial Response or Treatment Resistance
- Augmentation with behavioral, educational, and/or supportive therapy in groups or as an individual is key to successful treatment

Tests
- None for healthy individuals, although baseline liver function testing, usually obtained anyway for managing alcohol dependence, may be useful

SIDE EFFECTS

How Drug Causes Side Effects
- Blockade of mu opioid receptors

Notable Side Effects
- Nausea, vomiting
- Dizziness, insomnia, headache

Life-Threatening or Dangerous Side Effects
- Confusion, rare hallucinations

Weight Gain
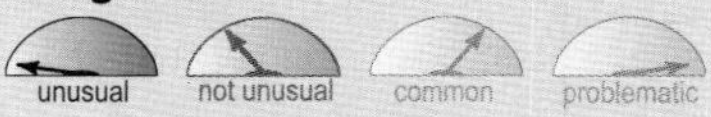

- Reported but not expected
- May cause weight loss

Sedation
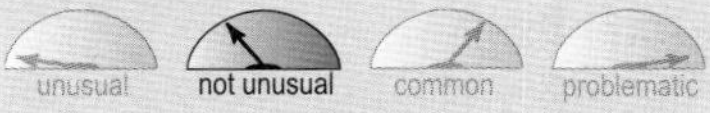

- Occurs in significant minority

What to Do About Side Effects
- Wait
- Switch to another agent

Best Augmenting Agents for Side Effects
- Switching to another agent may be more effective since most side effects cannot be improved with an augmenting agent

DOSING AND USE

Usual Dosage Range
- 18 mg/day as needed

Dosage Forms
- Tablet 18 mg

How to Dose
- After an initial visit, patient should keep a record of alcohol consumption for 2 weeks;

patients who continue to have a high drinking risk level during those 2 weeks can be initiated on nalmefene
- Nalmefene is taken as needed: on each day the patient perceives a risk of drinking alcohol, 18 mg should be taken 1–2 hours before the anticipated time of drinking
- If the patient has already begun drinking, 18 mg should be taken as soon as possible
- Maximum dose is 18 mg/day
- Patient should be opioid free for 7–10 days prior to initiating treatment

Dosing Tips
- Can be taken with or without food
- Providing educational materials and counseling in combination with nalmefene treatment can increase the chances of success
- Nalmefene tablet should not be chewed or crushed, as nalmefene may cause skin sensitization when in direct contact with skin

Overdose
- Limited experience

Long-Term Use
- Has been evaluated in trials for up to 1 year

Habit Forming
- No

How to Stop
- Taper not necessary

Pharmacokinetics
- Extensively metabolized by the liver
- Terminal half-life is 12.5 hours

Drug Interactions
- Increased depressive effects, particularly respiratory depression, have occurred when taken with other CNS depressants; consider dose reduction of either or both when taken concomitantly
- UGT2B7 inhibitors (e.g., diclofenac, fluconazole, medroxyprogesterone acetate, meclofenamic acid) may increase nalmefene levels
- UGT2B7 inducers (e.g., dexamethasone, phenobarbital, rifampicin, omeprazole) may decrease nalmefene levels

Other Warnings/ Precautions
- To prevent withdrawal in patients dependent on opioids, patients must be opioid free for at least 7–10 days prior to initiating treatment
- Individuals receiving nalmefene who require pain management with opioid analgesia may need a higher dose than usual and may experience deeper and more prolonged respiratory depression; pain management with non-opioid or rapid-acting opioid analgesics is recommended if possible
- Nalmefene should be temporarily discontinued 1 week prior to anticipated use of opioids (e.g., opioid analgesia during elective surgery)
- Use caution when using products containing opioids (e.g., cough medicines)
- Risk of respiratory depression is increased with concomitant use of CNS depressants

Do Not Use
- If patient is taking opioid analgesics
- If patient is currently dependent on opioids or is in acute opiate withdrawal
- If patient has severe renal or hepatic impairment
- If patient has a recent history of acute alcohol withdrawal syndrome
- If patient has galactose intolerance, Lapp lactase deficiency, or glucose-galactose malabsorption
- If there is a proven allergy to nalmefene

SPECIAL POPULATIONS

Renal Impairment
- Dose adjustment not necessary for mild to moderate impairment
- Not recommended for use in severe impairment

Hepatic Impairment
- Dose adjustment not necessary for mild to moderate impairment
- Not recommended for use in severe impairment

Cardiac Impairment
- Not studied

Elderly
- Limited data available

Children and Adolescents
- Safety and efficacy have not been established

Pregnancy
- Controlled studies have not been conducted in pregnant women
- Some animal studies have shown adverse effects
- Pregnant women needing to stop drinking may consider behavioral therapy before pharmacotherapy
- Not generally recommended for use during pregnancy, especially during first trimester

Breast Feeding
- Unknown if nalmefene is secreted in human breast milk, but all psychotropics assumed to be secreted in breast milk
- ✻ Recommended either to discontinue drug or bottle feed

THE ART OF PSYCHOPHARMACOLOGY

Potential Advantages
- Individuals who are not ready to abstain completely from alcohol

Potential Disadvantages
- Individuals whose goal is immediate abstinence

Primary Target Symptoms
- Alcohol dependence

Pearls
- Nalmefene was originally used as a parenteral agent to reverse the opioid agonist effects of opioid anesthesia or in opioid overdose
- In Europe, nalmefene is approved for reduction of alcohol consumption without previous detoxification
- Nalmefene is intended for patients with the goal of reduced-risk drinking (i.e., 3–4 drinks per day in men, maximum 16 drinks per week; 2–3 drinks per day in women, maximum 12 drinks per week); it has been shown to reduce alcohol consumption on average by 60%
- Reduction in alcohol consumption has been shown to be maintained for 12 years
- There is no clinically reported dose-dependent hepatotoxicity
- Like naltrexone, nalmefene is a mu opioid receptor antagonist; however, nalmefene is also a partial agonist at kappa opioid receptors, which are thought to contribute to the dysphoria and anxiety experienced during alcohol withdrawal
- Nalmefene is unique in that it is taken as needed when the patient perceives a risk of drinking alcohol

Suggested Reading

Gual A, He Y, Torup L, et al. A randomized, double-blind, placebo-controlled, efficacy study of nalmefene, as-needed use, in patients with alcohol dependence. Eur Neuropsychopharmacol 2013;23:1432–42.

Keating GM. Nalmefene: a review of its use in the treatment of alcohol dependence. CNS Drugs 2013;27:761–72.

Mann K, Bladstrom A, Torup L, Gual A, van den Brink W. Extending the treatment options in alcohol dependence: a randomized controlled study of as-needed nalmefene. Biol Psychiatry 2013;73(8):706–13.

Rosner S, Hackl-Herrwerth A, Leucht S, et al. Opioid antagonists for alcohol dependence. Cochrane Database Syst Rev 2010 Dec;8(12):CD001867.

van den Brink W, Aubin HJ, Bladstrom A, et al. Efficacy of as-needed nalmefene in alcohol-dependent patients with at least a high drinking risk level: results from a subgroup analysis of two randomized controlled 6-month studies. Alcohol Alcohol 2013;48(5):570–8.

NALTREXONE

THERAPEUTICS

Brands • Revia (oral)
• Vivitrol (injection)

see index for additional brand names

Generic? Yes (not injection or solution)

Class

- Neuroscience-based Nomenclature: opioid receptor antagonist (O-RAn)
- Alcohol dependence treatment; mu opioid receptor antagonist

Commonly Prescribed for

(bold for FDA approved)

- **Alcohol dependence**
- **Blockade of effects of exogenously administered opioids (oral)**
- **Prevention of relapse to opioid dependence (injection)**

How the Drug Works

- Blocks mu opioid receptors, preventing exogenous opioids from binding there and thus preventing the pleasurable effects of opioid consumption
- Reduces alcohol consumption through modulation of opioid systems, thereby reducing the reinforcing effects of alcohol

How Long Until It Works

- Can begin working within a few days but maximum effects may not be seen for a few weeks

If It Works

- Reduces alcohol and opioid consumption by diminishing their reinforcing properties (rewarding effects, cravings)

If It Doesn't Work

- Evaluate for and address contributing factors
- Consider switching to another agent
- Consider augmenting with acamprosate

Best Augmenting Combos for Partial Response or Treatment Resistance

- Acamprosate
- Augmentation therapy may be more effective than monotherapy
- Augmentation with behavioral, education, and/or supportive therapy in groups or as an individual is probably key to successful treatment

Tests

- Urine screen for opioids and/or naloxone challenge test prior to initiating treatment for opioid use
- None for use in treating alcohol dependence, although baseline liver function testing, usually obtained anyway for managing alcohol dependence, may be useful

SIDE EFFECTS

How Drug Causes Side Effects

- Blockade of mu opioid receptors

Notable Side Effects

- Nausea, vomiting, decreased appetite
- Dizziness, dysphoria, anxiety
- Injection site reactions (pain, tenderness, pruritis, induration, swelling, erythema, or bruising); in some cases injection site reactions may be very severe

Life-Threatening or Dangerous Side Effects

- Eosinophilic pneumonia
- Hepatocellular injury (at excessive doses)
- Severe injection site reactions requiring surgery

Weight Gain

unusual not unusual common problematic

- Reported but not expected

Sedation

unusual **not unusual** common problematic

- Occurs in significant minority

What to Do About Side Effects

- Wait
- Adjust dose
- If side effects persist, discontinue use

Best Augmenting Agents for Side Effects

- Dose reduction or switching to another agent may be more effective since most side effects cannot be improved with an augmenting agent

DOSING AND USE

Usual Dosage Range
- Oral: 50 mg/day or 100 mg on Mon and Wed and 150 mg on Fri
- Injection: 380 mg every 4 weeks

Dosage Forms
- Tablet 25 mg, 50 mg, 100 mg
- Oral solution 12 mg/0.6 mL
- Intramuscular formulation 380 mg/vial

How to Dose
- For treating alcohol dependence (oral): recommended dose is 50 mg/day; titration is not required
- For treating alcohol dependence (injection): 380 mg delivered intramuscularly in the gluteal region every 4 weeks; alternate buttocks; must be administered by health-care professional
- Patient should be opioid free for 7–10 days prior to initiating treatment, as confirmed by negative urine screen and/or naloxone challenge test
- Opioid dependence (oral): initial 25 mg/day; day 2 can increase to 50 mg/day

Dosing Tips
- Providing educational materials and counseling in combination with naltrexone treatment can increase the chances of success
- Individuals who abstain from alcohol for several days prior to initiating treatment with naltrexone may have greater reductions in the number of drinking days as well as number of heavy drinking days, and may also be more likely to abstain completely throughout treatment
- Long-acting naltrexone (injection) must be kept refrigerated
- For long-acting naltrexone (injection), the suspension should be administered immediately after mixing
- Adherence greatly enhanced and assured for 30 days at a time when administering by once monthly depot injection; oral treatment requires 30 decisions to comply in 30 days whereas long-acting injection requires only one decision every 30 days to comply
- Patients must be completely withdrawn and abstinent from opioids for 5 days (short-acting opioids) to 7 days (long-acting opioids) before starting naltrexone

Overdose
- Nausea, abdominal pain, sedation, dizziness, injection site reactions

Long-Term Use
- Has been studied in trials up to 1 year

Habit Forming
- No

How to Stop
- Taper not necessary

Pharmacokinetics
- Elimination half-life of oral naltrexone is approximately 13 hours
- Elimination half-life of naltrexone via injection is 5–10 days

Drug Interactions
- Is hepatically metabolized by dihydrodiol dehydrogenase and not by the CYP450 enzyme system, and thus is unlikely to be affected by drugs that induce or inhibit CYP450 enzymes
- Can block the effects of opioid-containing medications (e.g., some cough and cold remedies, antidiarrheal preparations, opioid analgesics)
- Concomitant administration with acamprosate may increase plasma levels of acamprosate, but this does not appear to be clinically significant and dose adjustment is not recommended

Other Warnings/ Precautions
- Can cause hepatocellular injury when given in excessive doses
- To prevent withdrawal in patients dependent on opioids, patients must be opioid free for at least 7–10 days prior to initiating treatment
- Attempts by patients to overcome blockade of opioid receptors by taking large amounts of exogenous opioids could lead to opioid intoxication or even fatal overdose
- Individuals who have been previously treated with naltrexone should be warned that they may respond to lower doses of

opioids than previously used, and thus previous doses may also lead to opioid intoxication
- Individuals receiving naltrexone who require pain management with opioid analgesia may need a higher dose than usual and may experience deeper and more prolonged respiratory depression; pain management with non-opioid or rapid-acting opioid analgesics is recommended if possible
- Monitor patients for emergence of depressed mood or suicidality
- Use cautiously in individuals with known psychiatric illness
- Injection should be used cautiously in individuals with thrombocytopenia or any coagulation disorder

Do Not Use
- If patient is taking opioid analgesics
- If patient is currently dependent on opioids or is in acute opiate withdrawal
- If patient has failed the naloxone challenge test or has a positive urine screen for opioids
- If patient has acute hepatitis or liver failure
- If there is a proven allergy to naltrexone
- If there is a proven allergy to polylactideco-glycolide (PLG), arboxymethylcellulose, or any other components of the diluent (injection)

SPECIAL POPULATIONS

Renal Impairment
- Dose adjustment not generally necessary for mild impairment
- Not studied in moderate to severe renal impairment

Hepatic Impairment
- Has the potential to cause hepatocellular injury when given in excessive doses
- Dose adjustment not generally necessary for mild impairment
- Not studied in severe hepatic impairment
- Contraindicated in acute hepatitis or liver failure

Cardiac Impairment
- Limited available data

Elderly
- Safety and efficacy have not been established
- Some patients may tolerate lower doses better

Children and Adolescents
- Safety and efficacy have not been established

Pregnancy
- Effective June 30, 2015, the US FDA requires changes to the content and format of pregnancy and lactation information in prescription drug labels, including the elimination of the pregnancy letter categories; the Pregnancy and Lactation Labeling Rule (PLLR or final rule) applies only to prescription drugs and will be phased in gradually for drugs approved on or after June 30, 2001
- Controlled studies have not been conducted in pregnant women
- Pregnant women needing to stop drinking may consider behavioral therapy before pharmacotherapy
- Not generally recommended for use during pregnancy, especially during first trimester

Breast Feeding
- Some drug is found in mother's breast milk
- Recommended either to discontinue drug or bottle feed

THE ART OF PSYCHOPHARMACOLOGY

Potential Advantages
- Individuals who are not ready to abstain completely from alcohol
- For binge drinkers

Potential Disadvantages
- Patients who "drink over" their treatment, including their long-acting injection
- Less effective in patients who are not abstinent at the time of treatment initation

Primary Target Symptoms
- Alcohol dependence

Pearls

- Not only increases total abstinence, but also can reduce days of heavy drinking
- May be a preferred treatment if the goal is reduced-risk drinking (i.e., 3–4 drinks per day in men, maximum 16 drinks per week; 2–3 drinks per day in women, maximum 12 drinks per week)
- Less effective in patients who are not abstinent at the time of treatment initiation
- Some patients complain of apathy or loss of pleasure with chronic treatment
- The combination of naltrexone and bupropion has demonstrated efficacy as treatment for obesity and is currently being evaluated in a long-term study to assess the cardiovascular health outcomes of this treatment

Suggested Reading

Anton RF, O'Malley SS, Ciraulo DA, et al. Combined pharmacotherapies and behavioral interventions for alcohol dependence: the COMBINE study: a randomized controlled trial. JAMA 2006;295(17):2003–17.

Johansson BA, Berglund M, Lindregn A. Efficacy of maintenance treatment with naltrexone for opioid dependence: a meta-analytical review. Addiction 2006;101(4):491–503.

Mannelli P, Peindl K, Masand PS, Patkar SS. Long-acting injectable naltrexone for the treatment of alcohol dependence. Expert Rev Neurother 2007;7(10):1265–77.

Rosner S, Leucht S, Lehert P, Soyka M. Acamprosate supports abstinence, naltrexone prevents excessive drinking: evidence from a meta-analysis with unreported outcomes. J Psychopharmacol 2008;22:11–23.

THERAPEUTICS

Brands • Contrave

Generic? No

Class

- Neuroscience-based Nomenclature: opioid receptor antagonist (naltrexone, O-RAn) and dopamine reuptake inhibitor and releaser (bupropion, D-RIRe)
- Opioid antagonist (naltrexone) combined with a norepinephrine dopamine reuptake inhibitor (bupropion); weight management medication

Commonly prescribed for

(bold for FDA approved)

- **Chronic weight management (adjunct to reduced-calorie diet and increased physical activity) in adults with an initial BMI of at least 30 kg/m^2 (obese) or at least 27 kg/m^2 (overweight) in the presence of at least 1 weight-related comorbid condition**

How the Drug Works

- Bupropion increases dopamine and norepinephrine by blocking both the dopamine and the norepinephrine transporters. In the hypothalamus, these 2 neurotransmitters activate POMC neurons, causing the release of proopiomelanocortin (POMC). POMC is then broken down into alpha-melanocyte stimulating hormone, which binds to melanocortin 4 receptors to suppress appetite. However, stimulation of POMC neurons also activates an endogenous opioid-mediated negative feedback loop, which mitigates the appetite-suppressing effects.
- Naltrexone can block mu opioid receptors, thus preventing opioid-mediated negative feedback. Such an action would synergize with simultaneous activation of the appetite-suppressing pathway by bupropion. This results in more robust and long-lasting appetite suppression than with either drug alone.

How Long Until It Works

- At least 5% weight loss is generally achieved after 12 weeks on maximum daily dose

If It Works

- Patients may achieve 5–10% reduction from baseline in body weight

If It Doesn't Work

- Discontinue if 5% weight loss is not achieved after 12 weeks on maximum daily dose

Best Augmenting Combos for Partial Response or Treatment Resistance

- Naltrexone-bupropion itself should be administered in conjunction with reduced-calorie diet and increased physical activity
- Often best to try another strategy prior to resorting to augmentation

Tests

- Measurement of blood glucose levels before and during treatment is recommended for patients with type 2 diabetes
- Measurement of blood pressure and heart rate prior to starting naltrexone-bupropion and during treatment is recommended, particularly in patients with cardiac or cerebrovascular disease

SIDE EFFECTS

How Drug Causes Side Effects

- CNS side effects theoretically due to excessive actions at mu opioid receptors or excessive actions on norepinephrine and dopamine

Notable Side Effects

- Nausea, constipation, vomiting, diarrhea, dry mouth
- Headache, dizziness, insomnia

Life-Threatening or Dangerous Side Effects

- Increased blood pressure or heart rate
- Rare seizures (risk increases with doses above the recommended maximums; risk increases for patients with predisposing factors)
- Hepatocellular injury (at excessive doses)

- Rare induction of mania
- Rare activation of suicidal ideation and behavior (suicidality) (short-term studies did not show an increase in the risk of suicidality with antidepressants compared to placebo beyond age 24)

Weight Gain

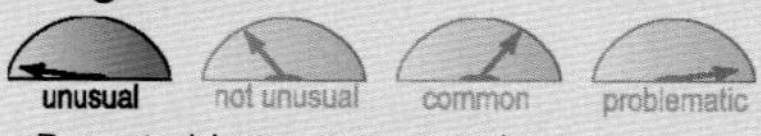

- Reported but not expected

Sedation

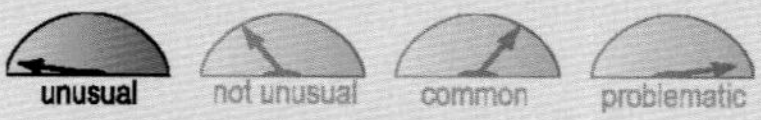

- Reported but not expected

What to Do About Side Effects

- Wait
- In a few weeks, switch to another agent

Best Augmenting Agents for Side Effects

- Often best to try another treatment prior to resorting to augmentation strategies to treat side effects
- Activation and agitation may represent the induction of a bipolar state, especially a mixed dysphoric bipolar II condition sometimes associated with suicidal ideation, and require discontinuation of bupropion

DOSING AND USE

Usual Dosage Range

- 16 mg naltrexone/180 mg bupropion twice per day

Dosage Forms

- Extended-release tablet (naltrexone/bupropion) 8 mg/90 mg

How to Dose

- Week 1: 8 mg/90 mg in the morning; week 2: increase to 8 mg/90 mg twice per day; week 3: increase to 16 mg/180 mg in the morning and 8 mg/90 mg in the evening; week 4: increase to 16 mg/180 mg twice per day (maximum recommended dose)
- Discontinue if at least 5% weight loss is not achieved after 12 weeks on 16 mg/180 mg twice per day

Dosing Tips

- Do not break or chew tablets as this will alter controlled-release properties
- Can be taken with food, but should not be taken with a high-fat meal because this may increase bupropion and naltrexone systemic exposure
- Patients must be completely withdrawn and abstinent from opioids for 5 days (short-acting opioids) to 7 days (long-acting opioids) before starting naltrexone-bupropion; if patients require intermittent opioid treatment, naltrexone-bupropion should be temporarily discontinued and lower doses of opioids may be needed
- If intolerable anxiety, insomnia, agitation, akathisia, or activation occur upon either dosing initiation or discontinuation, consider the possibility of activated bipolar disorder and switch to a mood stabilizer or an atypical antipsychotic

Overdose

- Naltrexone: nausea, abdominal pain, sedation, dizziness
- Bupropion: rarely lethal; seizures, cardiac disturbances, hallucinations, loss of consciousness

Long-Term Use

- Has been evaluated in controlled studies up to 56 weeks

Habit Forming

- No

How to Stop

- Tapering is prudent

Pharmacokinetics

- Mean elimination half-life following a single dose of naltrexone-bupropion to healthy subjects was approximately 5 hours for naltrexone and 21 hours for bupropion
- Bupropion inhibits CYP450 2D6

Drug Interactions

- Do not use with MAOIs, including 14 days after MAOIs are stopped
- Via CYP450 2D6 inhibition, bupropion-naltrexone could increase concentrations of drugs metabolized by CYP450 2D6 (e.g.,

TCAs, thioridazine); this may require lower doses of the concomitant medication
- Via CYP450 2D6 inhibition, bupropion could theoretically interfere with the analgesic actions of codeine, and increase the plasma levels of some beta blockers and of atomoxetine
- Bupropion is metabolized by CYP450 2B6; the maximum dose of naltrexone-bupropion in patients receiving a concomitant CYP450 2B6 inhibitor (ticlopidine, clopidogrel) is 8 mg/90 mg twice per day; coadministration of naltrexone-bupropion with CYP450 2B6 inducers (e.g., ritonavir, lopinavir, efavirenz) is not recommended
- Bupropion should be used with caution in patients taking levodopa or amantadine, as these agents can potentially enhance dopamine neurotransmission and be activating
- Can block the effects of opioid-containing medications (e.g., some cough and cold remedies, antidiarrheal preparations, opioid analgesics)
- False-positive urine immunoassay screening tests for amphetamines have been reported in patients taking bupropion due to a lack of specificity of the screening tests
- False-positive results may be expected even following discontinuation of bupropion
- Naltrexone is hepatically metabolized by dihydrodiol dehydrogenase and not by the CYP450 enzyme system, and thus is unlikely to be affected by drugs that induce or inhibit CYP450 enzymes

Other Warnings/ Precautions

- Naltrexone–bupropion can increase blood pressure or heart rate, particularly during the first 3 months of treatment
- Use cautiously with other drugs that increase seizure risk (TCAs, lithium, phenothiazines, thioxanthenes, some antipsychotics) or in patients with predisposing factors that may increase the risk of seizures (e.g., history of head trauma)
- To prevent withdrawal in patients dependent on opioids, patients must be opioid free (including tramadol) for at least 7–10 days prior to initiating treatment
- Attempts by patients to overcome blockade of opioid receptors by taking large amounts of exogenous opioids could lead to opioid intoxication or even fatal overdose
- Individuals who have previously been treated with naltrexone should be warned that they may respond to lower doses of opioids than previously used, and thus previous doses may also lead to opioid intoxication
- Weight loss may increase the risk of hypoglycemia in patients with type 2 diabetes mellitus treated with insulin and/or insulin secretagogues, and medication adjustments may be necessary
- Use with caution in patients with bipolar disorder unless treated with concomitant mood-stabilizing agent
- Warn patients about the possibility of activation of suicidal ideation and advise them to report such side effects immediately

Do Not Use

- If patient has uncontrolled hypertension
- If patient is pregnant
- If patient has history of seizures
- If patient is anorexic or bulimic, either currently or in the past
- If patient has acute hepatitis or liver failure
- If patient is abruptly discontinuing alcohol or sedative use
- If patient is taking opioid analgesics, is currently dependent on opioids, or is in acute opiate withdrawal
- If patient is taking an MAOI
- If patient is taking Wellbutrin, Zyban, Aplenzin, or any other formulation that contains bupropion
- If patient is taking Revia, Vivitrol, or any other formulation that contains naltrexone
- If there is a proven allergy to naltrexone or bupropion

SPECIAL POPULATIONS

Renal Impairment

- Maximum dose is 8 mg/90 mg twice per day in patients with moderate to severe impairment
- Not studied or recommended for use in patients with end-stage renal disease

Hepatic Impairment
- Maximum dose is 8 mg/90 mg once per day in the morning

Cardiac Impairment
- Not systematically evaluated in patients with cardiac impairment
- Measure blood pressure and heart rate before and during treatment

Elderly
- Some patients may tolerate lower doses better

Children and Adolescents
- Safety and efficacy have not been established
- Not recommended for use in children or adolescents

Pregnancy
- Contraindicated
- Effective June 30, 2015, the US FDA requires changes to the content and format of pregnancy and lactation information in prescription drug labels, including the elimination of the pregnancy letter categories; the Pregnancy and Lactation Labeling Rule (PLLR or final rule) applies only to prescription drugs and will be phased in gradually for drugs approved on or after June 30, 2001

Breast Feeding
- Some drug is found in mother's breast milk
- Recommended to discontinue drug or bottle feed

THE ART OF PSYCHOPHARMACOLOGY

Potential Advantages
- Patients who have had past weight loss on either active compound alone may experience a more robust weight loss effect and better tolerability on the combination of naltrexone with bupropion than with administration of either drug alone

Potential Disadvantages
- Women who are pregnant or wish to become pregnant

Primary Target Symptoms
- Excess weight

Pearls
- No head-to-head studies with other drugs approved for weight management, including lorcaserin or phentermine–topiramate, so comparative efficacy to these agents is unknown; however, some patients who do not respond to these other agents may respond to Contrave
- Unlike lorcaserin and phentermine–topiramate, naltrexone-bupropion does not have abuse potential
- Could theoretically be effective in binge eating disorder
- May be useful in antipsychotic-induced weight gain, especially for nonpsychotic patients taking antipsychotic agents for depression
- Contrave could theoretically exacerbate psychosis in patients with a psychotic disorder; however, no controlled studies of this use yet

Suggested Reading

Caixas A, Albert L, Capel I, Rigla M. Naltrexone sustained-release/bupropion sustained-release for the management of obesity: review of the data to date. Drug Des Devel Ther 2014;8:1419–1427.

Verpeut JL, Bello NT. Drug safety evaluation of naltrexone/bupropion for the treatment of obesity. Expert Opin Drug Saf 2014;13(6):831–41.

Wang GJ, Tomasi D, Volkow ND, et al. Effect of combined naltrexone and bupropion therapy on the brain's reactivity to food cues. Int J Obes (Lond) 2014;38(5):682–8.

THERAPEUTICS

Brands • Dutonin

see index for additional brand names

Generic? Yes

Class

- Neuroscience-based Nomenclature: serotonin receptor antagonist
- SARI (serotonin 2 antagonist/reuptake inhibitor); antidepressant

Commonly Prescribed for

(bold for FDA approved)

- **Depression**
- **Relapse prevention in major depressive disorder**
- Panic disorder
- Posttraumatic stress disorder (PTSD)

How the Drug Works

- Blocks serotonin 2A receptors potently
- Blocks serotonin reuptake pump (serotonin transporter) and norepinephrine reuptake pump (norepinephrine transporter) less potently

How Long Until It Works

- Can improve insomnia and anxiety early after initiating dosing
- Onset of therapeutic actions usually not immediate, but often delayed 2–4 weeks
- If it is not working within 6–8 weeks for depression, it may require a dosage increase or it may not work at all
- May continue to work for many years to prevent relapse of symptoms

If It Works

- The goal of treatment is complete remission of current symptoms as well as prevention of future relapses
- Treatment most often reduces or even eliminates symptoms, but not a cure since symptoms can recur after medicine stopped
- Continue treatment until all symptoms are gone (remission)
- Once symptoms gone, continue treating for 1 year for the first episode of depression
- For second and subsequent episodes of depression, treatment may need to be indefinite
- Use in anxiety disorders may also need to be indefinite

If It Doesn't Work

- Many patients have only a partial response where some symptoms are improved but others persist (especially insomnia, fatigue, and problems concentrating)
- Other patients may be nonresponders, sometimes called treatment-resistant or treatment-refractory
- Some patients who have an initial response may relapse even though they continue treatment, sometimes called "poop-out"
- Consider increasing dose, switching to another agent, or adding an appropriate augmenting agent
- Consider psychotherapy, especially cognitive-behavioral psychotherapies, which have been specifically shown to enhance nefazodone's antidepressant actions
- Consider evaluation for another diagnosis or for a comorbid condition (e.g., medical illness, substance abuse, etc.)
- Some patients may experience apparent lack of consistent efficacy due to activation of latent or underlying bipolar disorder, and require antidepressant discontinuation and a switch to a mood stabilizer

Best Augmenting Combos for Partial Response or Treatment Resistance

- ✻ Venlafaxine and escitalopram may be the best tolerated when switching or augmenting with a serotonin reuptake inhibitor, as neither is a potent CYP450 2D6 inhibitor (use combinations of antidepressants with caution as this may activate bipolar disorder and suicidal ideation)
- Modafinil, especially for fatigue, sleepiness, and lack of concentration
- Mood stabilizers or atypical antipsychotics for bipolar depression, psychotic depression, or treatment-resistant depression
- Benzodiazepines for anxiety, but give alprazolam cautiously with nefazodone as alprazolam levels can be much higher in the presence of nefazodone
- Classically, lithium, buspirone, or thyroid hormone

Tests

- ✱ Liver function testing is not required but is often prudent given the small but finite risk of serious hepatotoxicity
- ✱ However, to date no clinical strategy, including routine liver function tests, has been identified to reduce the risk of irreversible liver failure

SIDE EFFECTS

How Drug Causes Side Effects

- Blockade of alpha adrenergic 1 receptors may explain dizziness, sedation, and hypotension
- A metabolite of nefazodone, mCPP (meta-chloro-phenyl-piperazine), can cause side effects if its levels rise significantly
- ✱ If CYP450 2D6 is absent (7% of Caucasians lack CYP450 2D6) or inhibited (concomitant treatment with CYP450 2D6 inhibitors such as fluoxetine or paroxetine), increased levels of mCPP can form, leading to stimulation of 5HT2C receptors and causing dizziness, insomnia, and agitation
- Most side effects are immediate but often go away with time

Notable Side Effects

- Nausea, dry mouth, constipation, dyspepsia, increased appetite
- Headache, dizziness, vision changes, sedation, insomnia, agitation, confusion, memory impairment
- Ataxia, paresthesia, asthenia
- Cough increased
- Rare postural hypotension

Life-Threatening or Dangerous Side Effects

- Rare seizures
- Rare induction of mania
- Rare activation of suicidal ideation and behavior (suicidality) (short-term studies did not show an increase in the risk of suicidality with antidepressants compared to placebo beyond age 24)
- Rare priapism (no causal relationship established)
- Hepatic failure requiring liver transplant and/or fatal

Weight Gain

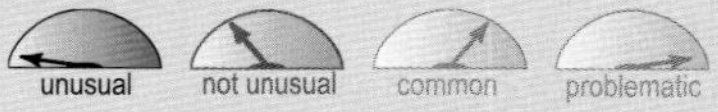

- Reported but not expected

Sedation

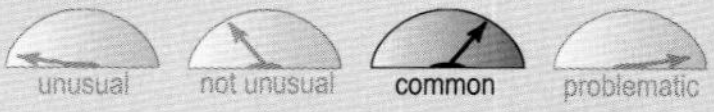

- Many experience and/or can be significant in amount

What to Do About Side Effects

- Wait
- Wait
- Wait
- Take once daily at night to reduce daytime sedation
- Lower the dose and try titrating again more slowly as tolerated
- Switch to another agent

Best Augmenting Agents for Side Effects

- Often best to try another antidepressant monotherapy prior to resorting to augmentation strategies to treat side effects
- Many side effects cannot be improved with an augmenting agent
- Many side effects are dose-dependent (i.e., they increase as dose increases, or they reemerge until tolerance redevelops)
- Many side effects are time-dependent (i.e., they start immediately upon dosing and upon each dose increase, but go away with time)
- Activation and agitation may represent the induction of a bipolar state, especially a mixed dysphoric bipolar II condition sometimes associated with suicidal ideation, and require the addition of lithium, a mood stabilizer or an atypical antipsychotic, and/or discontinuation of nefazodone

DOSING AND USE

Usual Dosage Range

- 300–600 mg/day

Dosage Forms

- Tablet 50 mg, 100 mg scored, 150 mg scored, 200 mg, 250 mg

How to Dose

- Initial dose 100 mg twice a day; increase by 100–200 mg/day each week until desired efficacy is reached; maximum dose 600 mg twice a day

Dosing Tips

- Take care switching from or adding to SSRIs (especially fluoxetine or paroxetine) because of side effects due to the drug interaction
- Do not underdose the elderly
- Normally twice daily dosing, especially when initiating treatment
- Patients may tolerate all dosing once daily at night once titrated
- Often much more effective at 400–600 mg/day than at lower doses if tolerated
- Slow titration can enhance tolerability when initiating dosing

Overdose

- Rarely lethal; sedation, nausea, vomiting, low blood pressure

Long-Term Use

- Safe

Habit Forming

- No

How to Stop

- Taper is prudent to avoid withdrawal effects, but problems in withdrawal not common

Pharmacokinetics

- Half-life of parent compound is 2–4 hours
- Half-life of active mebatolites up to 12 hours
- Inhibits CYP450 3A4

Drug Interactions

- Tramadol increases the risk of seizures in patients taking an antidepressant
- May interact with SSRIs such as paroxetine, fluoxetine, and others that inhibit CYP450 2D6

✱ Since a metabolite of nefazodone, mCPP, is a substrate of CYP450 2D6, combination of 2D6 inhibitors with nefazodone will raise mCPP levels, leading to stimulation of 5HT2C receptors and causing dizziness and agitation

- Can cause a fatal "serotonin syndrome" when combined with MAOIs, so do not use with MAOIs or for at least 14 days after MAOIs are stopped
- Do not start an MAOI for at least 5 half-lives (5 to 7 days for most drugs) after discontinuing nefazodone
- Via CYP450 3A4 inhibition, nefazodone may increase the half-life of alprazolam and triazolam, so their dosing may need to be reduced by half or more
- Via CYP450 3A4, nefazodone may increase plasma concentrations of buspirone, so buspirone dose may need to be reduced
- Via CYP450 3A4 inhibition, nefazodone could theoretically increase concentrations of certain cholesterol lowering HMG CoA reductase inhibitors, especially simvastatin, atorvastatin, and lovastatin, but not pravastatin or fluvastatin, which would increase the risk of rhabdomyolysis; thus, coadministration of nefazodone with certain HMG CoA reductase inhibitors should proceed with caution
- Via CYP450 3A4 inhibition, nefazodone could theoretically increase the concentrations of pimozide, and cause QTc prolongation and dangerous cardiac arrhythmias
- Nefazodone may reduce clearance of haloperidol, so haloperidol dose may need to be reduced
- It is recommended to discontinue nefazodone prior to elective surgery because of the potential for interaction with general anesthetics

Other Warnings/ Precautions

✱ Hepatotoxicity, sometimes requiring liver transplant and/or fatal, has occurred with nefazodone use. Risk may be one in every 250,000 to 300,000 patient years. Patients should be advised to report symptoms such as jaundice, dark urine, loss of appetite, nausea, and abdominal pain to prescriber immediately. If patient develops signs of hepatocellular injury, such as increased serum AST or serum ALPT levels >3 times the upper limit of normal, nefazodone treatment should be discontinued.

- ✽ No risk factor yet predicts who will develop irreversible liver failure with nefazodone and no clinical strategy, including routine monitoring of liver function tests, is known to reduce the risk of liver failure
- Use with caution in patients with history of seizures
- Use with caution in patients with bipolar disorder unless treated with concomitant mood-stabilizing agent
- When treating children, carefully weigh the risks and benefits of pharmacological treatment against the risks and benefits of nontreatment with antidepressants and make sure to document this in the patient's chart
- Distribute the brochures provided by the FDA and the drug companies
- Warn patients and their caregivers about the possibility of activating side effects and advise them to report such symptoms immediately
- Monitor patients for activation of suicidal ideation, especially children and adolescents

Do Not Use

- If patient is taking an MAOI
- If patient has acute hepatic impairment or elevated baseline serum transaminases
- If patient was previously withdrawn from nefazodone treatment due to hepatic injury
- If patient is taking pimozide, as nefazodone could raise pimozide levels and increase QTc interval, perhaps causing dangerous arrhythmia
- If patient is taking carbamazepine, as this agent can dramatically reduce nefazodone levels and thus interfere with its antidepressant actions
- If there is a proven allergy to nefazodone

SPECIAL POPULATIONS

Renal Impairment

- No dose adjustment necessary

Hepatic Impairment

- Contraindicated in patients with known hepatic impairment

Cardiac Impairment

- Use in patients with cardiac impairment has not been studied, so use with caution because of risk of orthostatic hypotension

Elderly

- Recommended to initiate treatment at half the usual adult dose, but to follow the same titration schedule as with younger patients, including same ultimate dose
- Reduction in the risk of suicidality with antidepressants compared to placebo in adults age 65 and older.

Children and Adolescents

- Carefully weigh the risks and benefits of pharmacological treatment against the risks and benefits of nontreatment with antidepressants and make sure to document this in the patient's chart
- Monitor patients face-to-face regularly, particularly during the first several weeks of treatment
- Use with caution, observing for activation of known or unknown bipolar disorder and/or suicidal ideation, and inform parents or guardians of this risk so they can help observe child or adolescent patients
- Safety and efficacy have not been established
- Preliminary research indicates efficacy and tolerability of nefazodone in children and adolescents with depression

Pregnancy

- Effective June 30, 2015, the US FDA requires changes to the content and format of pregnancy and lactation information in prescription drug labels, including the elimination of the pregnancy letter categories; the Pregnancy and Lactation Labeling Rule (PLLR or final rule) applies only to prescription drugs and will be phased in gradually for drugs approved on or after June 30, 2001
- Controlled studies have not been conducted in pregnant women
- Not generally recommended for use during pregnancy, especially during first trimester
- Must weigh the risk of treatment (first trimester fetal development, third trimester

newborn delivery) to the child against the risk of no treatment (recurrence of depression, maternal health, infant bonding) to the mother and child
- For many patients this may mean continuing treatment during pregnancy

Breast Feeding
- Unknown if nefazodone is secreted in human breast milk, but all psychotropics assumed to be secreted in breast milk
- Trace amounts may be present in nursing children whose mothers are on nefazodone
- If child becomes irritable or sedated, breast feeding or drug may need to be discontinued
- Immediate postpartum period is a high-risk time for depression, especially in women who have had prior depressive episodes, so drug may need to be reinstituted late in the third trimester or shortly after childbirth to prevent a recurrence during the postpartum period
- Must weigh benefits of breast feeding with risks and benefits of antidepressant treatment versus nontreatment to both the infant and the mother
- For many patients, this may mean continuing treatment during breast feeding

THE ART OF PSYCHOPHARMACOLOGY

Potential Advantages
- Depressed patients with anxiety or insomnia who do not respond to other antidepressants
- Patients with SSRI-induced sexual dysfunction

Potential Disadvantages
- Patients who have difficulty with a long titration period or twice daily dosing
- Patients with hepatic impairment

Primary Target Symptoms
- Depressed mood
- Sleep disturbance
- Anxiety

Pearls
- Preliminary data for efficacy in panic disorder and PTSD
- Fluoxetine and paroxetine may not be tolerated when switching or augmenting
- For elderly patients with early dementia and agitated depression, consider nefazodone in the morning and additional trazodone at night
- Anecdotal reports suggest that nefazodone may be effective in treating PMDD
- ✻ Studies suggest that cognitive behavioral psychotherapy enhances the efficacy of nefazodone in chronic depression
- ✻ Risk of hepatotoxicity makes this agent a second-line choice and has led to its withdrawal from some markets, including the withdrawal of Serzone from the US market
- Rarely, patients may complain of visual "trails" or after-images on nefazodone

Suggested Reading

DeVane CL, Grothe DR, Smith SL. Pharmacology of antidepressants: focus on nefazodone. J Clin Psychiatry 2002;63(1):10–17.

Dunner DL, Laird LK, Zajecka J, et al. Six-year perspectives on the safety and tolerability of nefazodone. J Clin Psychiatry 2002;63(1):32–41.

Khouzam HR. The antidepressant nefazodone. A review of its pharmacology, clinical efficacy, adverse effects, dosage, and administration. J Psychosocial Nursing Ment Health Serv 2000;38:20–5.

Masand PS, Gupta S. Long-term side effects of newer-generation antidepressants: SSRIs, venlafaxine, nefazodone, bupropion, and mirtazapine. Ann Clin Psychiatry 2002;14:175–82.

Schatzberg AF, Prather MR, Keller MB, et al. Clinical use of nefazodone in major depression: a 6-year perspective. J Clin Psychiatry 2002;63(1):18–31.

NORTRIPTYLINE

THERAPEUTICS

Brands • Pamelor

see index for additional brand names

Generic? Yes

Class

- Neuroscience-based Nomenclature: serotonin, norepinephrine reuptake inhibitor (SN-RI)
- Tricyclic antidepressant (TCA)
- Predominantly a norepinephrine/noradrenaline reuptake inhibitor

Commonly Prescribed for

(bold for FDA approved)

- **Major depressive disorder**
- Anxiety
- Insomnia
- Neuropathic pain/chronic pain
- Treatment-resistant depression

How the Drug Works

- Boosts neurotransmitter norepinephrine/noradrenaline
- Blocks norepinephrine reuptake pump (norepinephrine transporter), presumably increasing noradrenergic neurotransmission
- Since dopamine is inactivated by norepinephrine reuptake in frontal cortex, which largely lacks dopamine transporters, nortriptyline can increase dopamine neurotransmission in this part of the brain
- A more potent inhibitor of norepinephrine reuptake pump than serotonin reuptake pump (serotonin transporter)
- At high doses may also boost neurotransmitter serotonin and presumably increase serotonergic neurotransmission

How Long Until It Works

- May have immediate effects in treating insomnia or anxiety
- Onset of therapeutic actions usually not immediate, but often delayed 2 to 4 weeks
- If it is not working within 6 to 8 weeks for depression, it may require a dosage increase or it may not work at all
- May continue to work for many years to prevent relapse of symptoms

If It Works

- The goal of treatment of depression is complete remission of current symptoms as well as prevention of future relapses
- The goal of treatment of chronic neuropathic pain is to reduce symptoms as much as possible, especially in combination with other treatments
- Treatment of depression most often reduces or even eliminates symptoms, but not a cure since symptoms can recur after medicine stopped
- Treatment of chronic neuropathic pain may reduce symptoms, but rarely eliminates them completely, and is not a cure since symptoms can recur after medicine is stopped
- Continue treatment of depression until all symptoms are gone (remission)
- Once symptoms of depression are gone, continue treating for 1 year for the first episode of depression
- For second and subsequent episodes of depression, treatment may need to be indefinite
- Use in anxiety disorders and chronic pain may also need to be indefinite, but long-term treatment is not well studied in these conditions

If It Doesn't Work

- Many depressed patients have only a partial response where some symptoms are improved but others persist (especially insomnia, fatigue, and problems concentrating)
- Other depressed patients may be nonresponders, sometimes called treatment-resistant or treatment-refractory
- Consider increasing dose, switching to another agent or adding an appropriate augmenting agent
- Consider psychotherapy
- Consider evaluation for another diagnosis or for a comorbid condition (e.g., medical illness, substance abuse, etc.)
- Some patients may experience apparent lack of consistent efficacy due to activation of latent or underlying bipolar disorder, and require antidepressant discontinuation and a switch to a mood stabilizer

Best Augmenting Combos for Partial Response or Treatment Resistance

- Lithium, buspirone, thyroid hormone (for depression)
- Gabapentin, tiagabine, other anticonvulsants, even opiates if done by experts while monitoring carefully in difficult cases (for chronic pain)

Tests

- Baseline ECG is recommended for patients over age 50

✽ Monitoring of plasma drug levels is available

✽ Since tricyclic and tetracyclic antidepressants are frequently associated with weight gain, before starting treatment, weigh all patients and determine if the patient is already overweight (BMI 25.0–29.9) or obese (BMI ≥30)

- Before giving a drug that can cause weight gain to an overweight or obese patient, consider determining whether the patient already has pre-diabetes (fasting plasma glucose 100–125 mg/dL), diabetes (fasting plasma glucose >126 mg/dL), or dyslipidemia (increased total cholesterol, LDL cholesterol, and triglycerides; decreased HDL cholesterol), and treat or refer such patients for treatment, including nutrition and weight management, physical activity counseling, smoking cessation, and medical management

✽ Monitor weight and BMI during treatment

✽ While giving a drug to a patient who has gained >5% of initial weight, consider evaluating for the presence of pre-diabetes, diabetes, or dyslipidemia, or consider switching to a different antidepressant

- EKGs may be useful for selected patients (e.g., those with personal or family history of QTc prolongation; cardiac arrhythmia; recent myocardial infarction; uncompensated heart failure; or taking agents that prolong QTc interval such as pimozide, thioridazine, selected antiarrhythmics, moxifloxacin, sparfloxacin, etc.)
- Patients at risk for electrolyte disturbances (e.g., patients on diuretic therapy) should have baseline and periodic serum potassium and magnesium measurements

SIDE EFFECTS

How Drug Causes Side Effects

- Anticholinergic activity may explain sedative effects, dry mouth, constipation, and blurred vision
- Sedative effects and weight gain may be due to antihistamine properties
- Blockade of alpha adrenergic 1 receptors may explain dizziness, sedation, and hypotension
- Cardiac arrhythmias and seizures, especially in overdose, may be caused by blockade of ion channels

Notable Side Effects

- Blurred vision, constipation, urinary retention, increased appetite, dry mouth, nausea, diarrhea, heartburn, unusual taste in mouth, weight gain
- Fatigue, weakness, dizziness, sedation, headache, anxiety, nervousness, restlessness
- Sexual dysfunction (impotence, change in libido)
- Sweating, rash, itching

Life-Threatening or Dangerous Side Effects

- Paralytic ileus, hyperthermia (TCAs + anticholinergic agents)
- Lowered seizure threshold and rare seizures
- Orthostatic hypotension, sudden death, arrhythmias, tachycardia
- QTc prolongation
- Hepatic failure, extrapyramidal symptoms
- Increased intraocular pressure
- Rare induction of mania
- Rare activation of suicidal ideation and behavior (suicidality) (short-term studies did not show an increase in the risk of suicidality with antidepressants compared to placebo beyond age 24)

Weight Gain

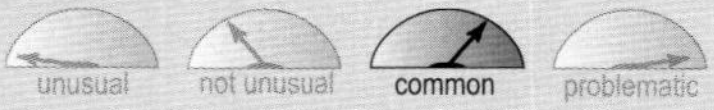

- Many experience and/or can be significant in amount
- Can increase appetite and carbohydrate craving

Sedation

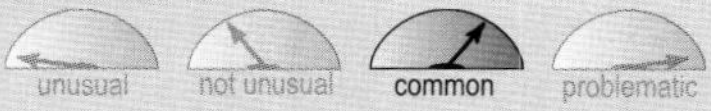

- Many experience and/or can be significant in amount
- Tolerance to sedative effect may develop with long-term use

What to Do About Side Effects

- Wait
- Wait
- Wait
- Lower the dose
- Switch to an SSRI or newer antidepressant

Best Augmenting Agents for Side Effects

- Many side effects cannot be improved with an augmenting agent

DOSING AND USE

Usual Dosage Range

- 75–150 mg/day once daily or in up to 4 divided doses (for depression)
- 50–150 mg/day (for chronic pain)

Dosage Forms

- Capsule 10 mg, 25 mg, 50 mg, 75 mg
- Liquid 10 mg/5mL

How to Dose

- Initial 10–25 mg/day at bedtime; increase by 25 mg every 3–7 days; can be dosed once daily or in divided doses; maximum dose 300 mg/day
- When treating nicotine dependence, nortriptyline should be initiated 10–28 days before cessation of smoking to achieve steady drug states

Dosing Tips

- If given in a single dose, should generally be administered at bedtime because of its sedative properties
- If given in split doses, largest dose should generally be given at bedtime because of its sedative properties
- If patients experience nightmares, split dose and do not give large dose at bedtime
- Patients treated for chronic pain may require only lower doses
- Risk of seizure increases with dose
- ❋ Monitoring plasma levels of nortriptyline is recommended in patients who do not respond to the usual dose or whose treatment is regarded as urgent
- Some formulations of nortriptyline contain sodium bisulphate, which may cause allergic reactions in some patients, perhaps more frequently in asthmatics
- If intolerable anxiety, insomnia, agitation, akathisia, or activation occur either upon dosing initiation or discontinuation, consider the possibility of activated bipolar disorder, and switch to a mood stabilizer or an atypical antipsychotic

Overdose

- Death may occur; CNS depression, convulsions, cardiac dysrhythmias, severe hypotension, EKG changes, coma

Long-Term Use

- Safe

Habit Forming

- No

How to Stop

- Taper to avoid withdrawal effects
- Even with gradual dose reduction some withdrawal symptoms may appear within the first 2 weeks
- Many patients tolerate 50% dose reduction for 3 days, then another 50% reduction for 3 days, then discontinuation
- If withdrawal symptoms emerge during discontinuation, raise dose to stop symptoms and then restart withdrawal much more slowly

Pharmacokinetics

- Substrate for CYP450 2D6 and 3A4
- Nortriptyline is the active metabolite of amitriptyline, formed by demethylation via CYP450 1A2
- Half-life approximately 36 hours
- Food does not affect absorption

Drug Interactions

- Tramadol increases the risk of seizures in patients taking TCAs
- Use of TCAs with anticholinergic drugs may result in paralytic ileus or hyperthermia

- Fluoxetine, paroxetine, bupropion, duloxetine, and other CYP450 2D6 inhibitors may increase TCA concentrations and cause side effects including dangerous arrhythmias
- Cimetidine may increase plasma concentrations of TCAs and cause anticholinergic symptoms
- Phenothiazines or haloperidol may raise TCA blood concentrations
- May alter effects of antihypertensive drugs; may inhibit hypotensive effects of clonidine
- Use of TCAs with sympathomimetic agents may increase sympathetic activity
- Methylphenidate may inhibit metabolism of TCAs
- Nortriptyline may raise plasma levels of dicumarol
- Activation and agitation, especially following switching or adding antidepressants, may represent the induction of a bipolar state, especially a mixed dysphoric bipolar II condition sometimes associated with suicidal ideation, and require the addition of lithium, a mood stabilizer or an atypical antipsychotic, and/or discontinuation of nortriptyline

Other Warnings/ Precautions

- Add or initiate other antidepressants with caution for up to 2 weeks after discontinuing nortriptyline
- Generally, do not use with MAOIs, including 14 days after MAOIs are stopped; do not start an MAOI for at least 5 half-lives (5 to 7 days for most drugs) after discontinuing nortriptyline, but see Pearls
- Use with caution in patients with history of seizures, urinary retention, angle-closure glaucoma, hyperthyroidism
- TCAs can increase QTc interval, especially at toxic doses, which can be attained not only by overdose but also by combining with drugs that inhibit TCA metabolism via CYP450 2D6, potentially causing torsade de pointes-type arrhythmia or sudden death
- Because TCAs can prolong QTc interval, use with caution in patients who have bradycardia or who are taking drugs that can induce bradycardia (e.g., beta blockers, calcium channel blockers, clonidine, digitalis)
- Because TCAs can prolong QTc interval, use with caution in patients who have hypokalemia and/or hypomagnesemia or who are taking drugs that can induce hypokalemia and/or magnesemia (e.g., diuretics, stimulant laxatives, intravenous amphotericin B, glucocorticoids, tetracosactide)
- When treating children, carefully weigh the risks and benefits of pharmacological treatment against the risks and benefits of nontreatment with antidepressants and make sure to document this in the patient's chart
- Distribute the brochures provided by the FDA and the drug companies
- Warn patients and their caregivers about the possibility of activating side effects and advise them to report such symptoms immediately
- Monitor patients for activation of suicidal ideation, especially children and adolescents

Do Not Use

- If patient is recovering from myocardial infarction
- If patient is taking agents capable of significantly prolonging QTc interval (e.g., pimozide, thioridazine, selected antiarrhythmics, moxifloxacin, sparfloxacin)
- If there is a history of QTc prolongation or cardiac arrhythmia, recent acute myocardial infarction, uncompensated heart failure
- If patient is taking drugs that inhibit TCA metabolism, including CYP450 2D6 inhibitors, except by an expert
- If there is reduced CYP450 2D6 function, such as patients who are poor 2D6 metabolizers, except by an expert and at low doses
- If there is a proven allergy to nortriptyline or amitriptyline

SPECIAL POPULATIONS

Renal Impairment

- Use with caution; may need to lower dose
- May need to monitor plasma levels

Hepatic Impairment

- Use with caution
- May need to monitor plasma levels
- May require a lower dose with slower titration

Cardiac Impairment

- Baseline ECG is recommended
- TCAs have been reported to cause arrhythmias, prolongation of conduction time, orthostatic hypotension, sinus tachycardia, and heart failure, especially in the diseased heart
- Myocardial infarction and stroke have been reported with TCAs
- TCAs produce QTc prolongation, which may be enhanced by the existence of bradycardia, hypokalemia, congenital or acquired long QTc interval, which should be evaluated prior to administering nortriptyline
- Use with caution if treating concomitantly with a medication likely to produce prolonged bradycardia, hypokalemia, slowing of intracardiac conduction, or prolongation of the QTc interval
- Avoid TCAs in patients with a known history of QTc prolongation, recent acute myocardial infarction, and uncompensated heart failure
- TCAs may cause a sustained increase in heart rate in patients with ischemic heart disease and may worsen (decrease) heart rate variability, an independent risk of mortality in cardiac populations
- Since SSRIs may improve (increase) heart rate variability in patients following a myocardial infarct and may improve survival as well as mood in patients with acute angina or following a myocardial infarction, these are more appropriate agents for cardiac population than tricyclic/tetracyclic antidepressants

✻ Risk/benefit ratio may not justify use of TCAs in cardiac impairment

Elderly

- Baseline ECG is recommended for patients over age 50
- May be more sensitive to anticholinergic, cardiovascular, hypotensive, and sedative effects
- May require lower dose; it may be useful to monitor plasma levels in elderly patients
- Reduction in the risk of suicidality with antidepressants compared to placebo in adults age 65 and older

Children and Adolescents

- Carefully weigh the risks and benefits of pharmacological treatment against the risks and benefits of nontreatment with antidepressants and make sure to document this in the patient's chart
- Monitor patients face-to-face regularly, particularly during the first several weeks of treatment
- Use with caution, observing for activation of known or unknown bipolar disorder and/ or suicidal ideation, and inform parents or guardians of this risk so they can help observe child or adolescent patients
- Not recommended for use in children under age 12
- Not intended for use in children under age 6
- Several studies show lack of efficacy of TCAs for depression
- May be used to treat enuresis or hyperactive/impulsive behaviors
- Some cases of sudden death have occurred in children taking TCAs
- Plasma levels may need to be monitored
- Dose in children generally less than 50 mg/ day
- May be useful to monitor plasma levels in children and adolescents

Pregnancy

- Effective June 30, 2015, the US FDA requires changes to the content and format of pregnancy and lactation information in prescription drug labels, including the elimination of the pregnancy letter categories; the Pregnancy and Lactation Labeling Rule (PLLR or final rule) applies only to prescription drugs and will be phased in gradually for drugs approved on or after June 30, 2001
- Crosses the placenta
- Should be used only if potential benefits outweigh potential risks
- Adverse effects have been reported in infants whose mothers took a TCA (lethargy, withdrawal symptoms, fetal malformations)
- Evaluate for treatment with an antidepressant with a better risk/benefit ratio

Breast Feeding

- Some drug is found in mother's breast milk

❋ Recommended either to discontinue drug or bottle feed

- Immediate postpartum period is a high-risk time for depression, especially in women who have had prior depressive episodes, so drug may need to be reinstituted late in the third trimester or shortly after childbirth to prevent a recurrence during the postpartum period
- Must weigh benefits of breast feeding with risks and benefits of antidepressant treatment versus nontreatment to both the infant and the mother
- For many patients this may mean continuing treatment during breast feeding

THE ART OF PSYCHOPHARMACOLOGY

Potential Advantages

- Patients with insomnia
- Severe or treatment-resistant depression
- Patients for whom therapeutic drug monitoring is desirable

Potential Disadvantages

- Pediatric and geriatric patients
- Patients concerned with weight gain
- Cardiac patients

Primary Target Symptoms

- Depressed mood
- Chronic pain

Pearls

- TCAs are often a first-line treatment option for chronic pain
- TCAs are no longer generally considered a first-line option for depression because of their side effect profile
- TCAs continue to be useful for severe or treatment-resistant depression
- Noradrenergic reuptake inhibitors such as nortriptyline can be used as a second-line treatment for smoking cessation, cocaine dependence, and attention deficit disorder
- TCAs may aggravate psychotic symptoms
- Alcohol should be avoided because of additive CNS effects
- Underweight patients may be more susceptible to adverse cardiovascular effects
- Children, patients with inadequate hydration, and patients with cardiac disease may be more susceptible to TCA-induced cardiotoxicity than healthy adults
- For the expert only: although generally prohibited, a heroic but potentially dangerous treatment for severely treatment-resistant patients is for an expert to give a tricyclic/tetracyclic antidepressant other than clomipramine simultaneously with an MAOI for patients who fail to respond to numerous other antidepressants
- If this option is elected, start the MAOI with the tricyclic/tetracyclic antidepressant simultaneously at low doses after appropriate drug washout, then alternately increase doses of these agents every few days to a week as tolerated
- Although very strict dietary and concomitant drug restrictions must be observed to prevent hypertensive crises and serotonin syndrome, the most common side effects of MAOI and tricyclic/tetracyclic antidepressant combinations may be weight gain and orthostatic hypotension
- Patients on TCAs should be aware that they may experience symptoms such as photosensitivity or blue-green urine
- SSRIs may be more effective than TCAs in women, and TCAs may be more effective than SSRIs in men
- Not recommended for first-line use in children with ADHD because of the availability of safer treatments with better documented efficacy and because of nortriptyline's potential for sudden death in children

❋ Nortriptyline is one of the few TCAs where monitoring of plasma drug levels has been well studied

- Since tricyclic/tetracyclic antidepressants are substrates for CYP450 2D6, and 7% of the population (especially Caucasians) may have a genetic variant leading to reduced activity of 2D6, such patients may not safely tolerate normal doses of tricyclic/tetracyclic antidepressants and may require dose reduction

- Phenotypic testing may be necessary to detect this genetic variant prior to dosing with a tricyclic/tetracyclic antidepressant, especially in vulnerable populations such as children, elderly, cardiac populations, and those on concomitant medications
- Patients who seem to have extraordinarily severe side effects at normal or low doses may have this phenotypic CYP450 2D6 variant and require low doses or switching to another antidepressant not metabolized by 2D6

Suggested Reading

Anderson IM. Meta-analytical studies on new antidepressants. Br Med Bull 2001;57:161–78.

Anderson IM. Selective serotonin reuptake inhibitors versus tricyclic antidepressants: a meta-analysis of efficacy and tolerability. J Aff Disorders 2000;58:19–36.

Hughes JR, Stead LF, Lancaster T. Antidepressants for smoking cessation. Cochrane Database Syst Rev 2000;4:CD000031.

Wilens TE, Biederman J, Baldessarini RJ, et al. Cardiovascular effects of therapeutic doses of tricyclic antidepressants in children and adolescents. J Am Acad Child Adolesc Psychiatry 1996;35(11):1491–501.

THERAPEUTICS

Brands
- Zyprexa
- Symbyax (olanzapine-fluoxetine combination)
- Relprevv

see index for additional brand names

Generic? Yes

Class
- Neuroscience-based Nomenclature: dopamine and serotonin receptor antagonist (DS-RAn)
- Atypical antipsychotic (serotonin-dopamine antagonist; second-generation antipsychotic; also a mood stabilizer)

Commonly Prescribed for
(bold for FDA approved)
- **Schizophrenia (ages 13 and older)**
- **Maintaining response in schizophrenia**
- **Acute agitation associated with schizophrenia (intramuscular)**
- **Acute mania/mixed mania (monotherapy and adjunct to lithium or valproate) (ages 13 and older)**
- **Bipolar maintenance**
- **Acute agitation associated with bipolar I mania (intramuscular)**
- **Bipolar depression [in combination with fluoxetine (Symbyax)]**
- **Treatment-resistant depression [in combination with fluoxetine (Symbyax)]**
- Other psychotic disorders
- Behavioral disturbances in dementias
- Behavioral disturbances in children and adolescents
- Disorders associated with problems with impulse control
- Borderline personality disorder

How the Drug Works
- Blocks dopamine 2 receptors, reducing positive symptoms of psychosis and stabilizing affective symptoms
- Blocks serotonin 2A receptors, causing enhancement of dopamine release in certain brain regions and thus reducing motor side effects and possibly improving cognitive and affective symptoms
- Interactions at a myriad of other neurotransmitter receptors may contribute to olanzapine's efficacy

✻ Specifically, antagonist actions at 5HT2C receptors may contribute to efficacy for cognitive and affective symptoms in some patients

✻ 5HT2C antagonist actions plus serotonin reuptake blockade of fluoxetine add to the actions of olanzapine when given as Symbyax (olanzapine-fluoxetine combination)

How Long Until It Works
- Psychotic and manic symptoms can improve within 1 week, but it may take several weeks for full effect on behavior as well as on cognition and affective stabilization
- Classically recommended to wait at least 4–6 weeks to determine efficacy of drug, but in practice some patients require up to 16–20 weeks to show a good response, especially on cognitive symptoms
- IM formulation can reduce agitation in 15–30 minutes

If It Works
- Most often reduces positive symptoms in schizophrenia but does not eliminate them
- Can improve negative symptoms, as well as aggressive, cognitive, and affective symptoms in schizophrenia
- Most schizophrenic patients do not have a total remission of symptoms but rather a reduction of symptoms by about a third
- Perhaps 5–15% of schizophrenic patients can experience an overall improvement of greater than 50–60%, especially when receiving stable treatment for more than a year
- Such patients are considered super-responders or "awakeners" since they may be well enough to be employed, live independently, and sustain long-term relationships
- Many bipolar patients may experience a reduction of symptoms by half or more
- Continue treatment until reaching a plateau of improvement
- After reaching a satisfactory plateau, continue treatment for at least a year after first episode of psychosis

- For second and subsequent episodes of psychosis, treatment may need to be indefinite
- Even for first episodes of psychosis, it may be preferable to continue treatment indefinitely to avoid subsequent episodes
- Treatment may not only reduce mania but also prevent recurrences of mania in bipolar disorder

If It Doesn't Work

- Try one of the other atypical antipsychotics (risperidone, quetiapine, ziprasidone, aripiprazole, paliperidone, amisulpride, asenapine, iloperidone, lurasidone)
- If 2 or more antipsychotic monotherapies do not work, consider clozapine
- Some patients may require treatment with a conventional antipsychotic
- If no first-line atypical antipsychotic is effective, consider higher doses or augmentation with valproate or lamotrigine
- Consider noncompliance and switch to another antipsychotic with fewer side effects or to an antipsychotic that can be given by depot injection
- Consider initiating rehabilitation and psychotherapy such as cognitive remediation
- Consider presence of concomitant drug abuse

Best Augmenting Combos for Partial Response or Treatment Resistance

- Valproic acid (valproate, divalproex, divalproex ER)
- Other mood-stabilizing anticonvulsants (carbamazepine, oxcarbazepine, lamotrigine)
- Lithium
- Benzodiazepines
- Fluoxetine and other antidepressants may be effective augmenting agents to olanzapine for bipolar depression, psychotic depression, and for unipolar depression not responsive to antidepressants alone (e.g., olanzapine-fluoxetine combination)

Tests

Before starting an atypical antipsychotic

✽ Weigh all patients and track BMI during treatment
- Get baseline personal and family history of diabetes, obesity, dyslipidemia, hypertension, and cardiovascular disease

✽ Get waist circumference (at umbilicus), blood pressure, fasting plasma glucose, and fasting lipid profile
- Determine if the patient is
  - overweight (BMI 25.0–29.9)
  - obese (BMI ≥30)
  - has pre-diabetes (fasting plasma glucose 100–125 mg/dL)
  - has diabetes (fasting plasma glucose >126 mg/dL)
  - has hypertension (BP >140/90 mm Hg)
  - has dyslipidemia (increased total cholesterol, LDL cholesterol, and triglycerides; decreased HDL cholesterol)
- Treat or refer such patients for treatment, including nutrition and weight management, physical activity counseling, smoking cessation, and medical management

Monitoring after starting an atypical antipsychotic

✽ BMI monthly for 3 months, then quarterly

✽ Consider monitoring fasting triglycerides monthly for several months in patients at high risk for metabolic complications and when initiating or switching antipsychotics

✽ Blood pressure, fasting plasma glucose, fasting lipids within 3 months and then annually, but earlier and more frequently for patients with diabetes or who have gained >5% of initial weight
- Treat or refer for treatment and consider switching to another atypical antipsychotic for patients who become overweight, obese, pre-diabetic, diabetic, hypertensive, or dyslipidemic while receiving an atypical antipsychotic

✽ Even in patients without known diabetes, be vigilant for the rare but life-threatening onset of diabetic ketoacidosis, which always requires immediate treatment, by monitoring for the rapid onset of polyuria, polydipsia, weight loss, nausea, vomiting, dehydration, rapid respiration, weakness, and clouding of sensorium, even coma
- Patients with liver disease should have blood tests a few times a year
- Patients with low white blood cell count (WBC) or history of drug-induced leucopenia/neutropenia should have complete blood count (CBC) monitored frequently during the first few months and olanzapine should be discontinued at the first sign of decline of WBC in the absence of other causative factors

SIDE EFFECTS

How Drug Causes Side Effects

- By blocking histamine 1 receptors in the brain, it can cause sedation and possibly weight gain
- By blocking alpha 1 adrenergic receptors, it can cause dizziness, sedation, and hypotension
- By blocking muscarinic 1 receptors, it can cause dry mouth, constipation, and sedation
- By blocking dopamine 2 receptors in the striatum, it can cause motor side effects (unusual)
- Mechanism of weight gain and increased incidence of diabetes and dyslipidemia with atypical antipsychotics is unknown but insulin regulation may be impaired by blocking pancreatic M3 muscarinic receptors

Notable Side Effects

- * Probably increases risk for diabetes mellitus and dyslipidemia
- Dizziness, sedation
- Dry mouth, constipation, dyspepsia, weight gain
- Peripheral edema
- Joint pain, back pain, chest pain, extremity pain, abnormal gait, ecchymosis
- Tachycardia
- Orthostatic hypotension, usually during initial dose titration
- Rare tardive dyskinesia (much reduced risk compared to conventional antipsychotics)
- Rare rash on exposure to sunlight

Life-Threatening or Dangerous Side Effects

- Hyperglycemia, in some cases extreme and associated with ketoacidosis or hyperosmolar coma or death, has been reported in patients taking atypical antipsychotics
- Rare but serious skin condition known as Drug Reaction with Eosinophilia (DRESS)
- Rare neuroleptic malignant syndrome (much reduced risk compared to conventional antipsychotics)
- Rare seizures
- Increased risk of death and cerebrovascular events in elderly patients with dementia-related psychosis

Weight Gain

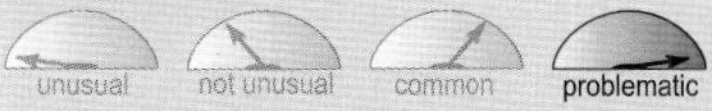

- Frequent and can be significant in amount
- Can become a health problem in some
- More than for some other antipsychotics, but never say always as not a problem in everyone

Sedation

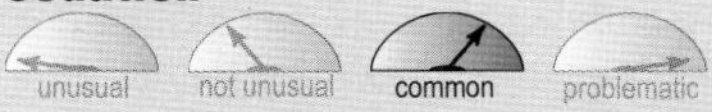

- Many patients experience and/or can be significant in amount
- Usually transient
- May be less than for some antipsychotics, more than for others

What to Do About Side Effects

- Wait
- Wait
- Wait
- Take at bedtime to help reduce daytime sedation
- Anticholinergics may reduce motor side effects such as akathisia when present, but rarely necessary
- Weight loss, exercise programs, and medical management for high BMIs, diabetes, dyslipidemia
- Switch to another atypical antipsychotic

Best Augmenting Agents for Side Effects

- Benztropine or trihexyphenidyl for motor side effects
- Many side effects cannot be improved with an augmenting agent

DOSING AND USE

Usual Dosage Range

- 10–20 mg/day (oral or intramuscular)
- 6–12 mg olanzapine/25–50 mg fluoxetine (olanzapine-fluoxetine combination)
- 150–300 mg/2 weeks or 300–405 mg/4 weeks (see Olanzapine Pamoate after Pearls for dosing and use)

Dosage Forms

- Tablets 2.5 mg, 5 mg, 7.5 mg, 10 mg, 15 mg, 20 mg
- Orally disintegrating tablets 5 mg, 10 mg, 15 mg, 20 mg

- Intramuscular formulation 5 mg/mL, each vial contains 10 mg (available in some countries)
- Depot 210 mg, 300 mg, 405 mg
- Olanzapine-fluoxetine combination capsule (mg equivalent olanzapine/mg equivalent fluoxetine) 6 mg/25 mg, 6 mg/50 mg, 12 mg/25 mg, 12 mg/50 mg

How to Dose

- Initial 5–10 mg once daily orally; increase by 5 mg/day once a week until desired efficacy is reached; maximum approved dose is 20 mg/day
- For intramuscular formulation, recommended initial dose 10 mg; second injection of 5–10 mg may be administered 2 hours after first injection; maximum daily dose of olanzapine is 20 mg, with no more than 3 injections per 24 hours
- For olanzapine-fluoxetine combination, recommended initial dose 6 mg/25 mg once daily in evening; increase dose based on efficacy and tolerability; maximum generally 18 mg/75 mg

Dosing Tips – Oral

✽ **More may be more:** raising usual dose above 15 mg/day can be useful for acutely ill and agitated patients and some treatment-resistant patients, gaining efficacy without many more side effects

✽ Some heroic uses for patients who do not respond to other antipsychotics can occasionally justify dosing over 30 mg/day and short-term up to 90 mg/day

- For high doses in treatment-resistant or violent patients, monitor therapeutic drug levels and target generally higher than the usual range of 5–75 mg/mL (i.e., greater than 125 mg/mL), but keep below the toxic range associated with QTc prolongation (700–800 mg/mL)
- See also the Switching section, after Pearls, for initiating both oral and long-acting injectable
- Rather than raise the dose above these levels in acutely agitated patients requiring acute antipsychotic actions, consider augmentation with a benzodiazepine or conventional antipsychotic, either orally or intramuscularly
- Rather than raise the dose above these levels in partial responders, consider augmentation with a mood-stabilizing anticonvulsant, such as valproate or lamotrigine
- Clearance of olanzapine is slightly reduced in women compared to men, so women may need lower doses than men
- Children and elderly should generally be dosed at the lower end of the dosage spectrum

✽ Olanzapine intramuscularly can be given short-term, both to initiate dosing with oral olanzapine or another oral antipsychotic and to treat breakthrough agitation in patients maintained on oral antipsychotics

- Treatment should be suspended if absolute neutrophil count falls below 1,000/mm^3

Overdose

- Rarely lethal in monotherapy overdose; sedation, slurred speech

Long-Term Use

- Approved to maintain response in long-term treatment of schizophrenia
- Approved for long-term maintenance in bipolar disorder
- Often used for long-term maintenance in various behavioral disorders

Habit Forming

- No

How to Stop

- See Switching section of individual agents for how to stop olanzapine
- Rapid oral discontinuation may lead to rebound psychosis and worsening of symptoms

Pharmacokinetics

- Metabolites are inactive
- Parent drug has 21–54 hour half-life
- Substrate for CYP450 1A2 and 2D6
- Food does not affect absorption

Drug Interactions

- May increase effect of antihypertensive agents
- May antagonize levodopa, dopamine agonists
- Dose may need to be lowered if given with CYP450 1A2 inhibitors (e.g., fluvoxamine); raised if given in conjunction with CYP450 1A2 inducers (e.g., cigarette smoke, carbamazepine)

Other Warnings/ Precautions

- Olanzapine is associated with a rare but serious skin condition known as Drug Reaction with Eosinophilia (DRESS). DRESS may begin as a rash but can progress to others parts of the body and can include symptoms such as fever, swollen lymph nodes, swollen face, inflammation of organs, and an increase in white blood cells known as eosinophilia. In some cases, DRESS can lead to death. Clinicians prescribing olanzapine should inform patients about the risk of DRESS; patients who develop a fever with rash and swollen lymph nodes or swollen face should seek medical care. Patients are not advised to stop their medication without consulting their prescribing clinician.
- Use with caution in patients with conditions that predispose to hypotension (dehydration, overheating)
- Use with caution in patients with prostatic hypertrophy, angle-closure glaucoma, paralytic ileus
- Patients receiving the intramuscular formulation of olanzapine should be observed closely for hypotension
- Intramuscular formulation is not generally recommended to be administered with parenteral benzodiazepines; if patient requires a parenteral benzodiazepine it should be given at least 1 hour after intramuscular olanzapine
- Olanzapine should be used cautiously in patients at risk for aspiration pneumonia, as dysphagia has been reported

Do Not Use

- If there is a known risk of angle-closure glaucoma (intramuscular formulation)
- If patient has unstable medical condition (e.g., acute myocardial infarction, unstable angina pectoris, severe hypotension and/or bradycardia, sick sinus syndrome, recent heart surgery) (intramuscular formulation)
- If there is a proven allergy to olanzapine

SPECIAL POPULATIONS

Renal Impairment

- No dose adjustment required for oral formulation
- Not removed by hemodialysis
- For intramuscular formulation, consider lower starting dose (5 mg)

Hepatic Impairment

- May need to lower dose
- Patients with liver disease should have liver function tests a few times a year
- For moderate to severe hepatic impairment, starting oral dose 5 mg; increase with caution
- For intramuscuar formulation, consider lower starting dose (5 mg)

Cardiac Impairment

- Drug should be used with caution because of risk of orthostatic hypotension

Elderly

- Some patients may tolerate lower doses better
- Increased incidence of stroke
- For intramuscular formulation, recommended starting dose is 2.5–5 mg; a second injection of 2.5–5 mg may be administered 2 hours after first injection; no more than 3 injections should be administered within 24 hours
- Although atypical antipsychotics are commonly used for behavioral disturbances in dementia, no agent has been approved for treatment of elderly patients with dementia-related psychosis
- Elderly patients with dementia-related psychosis treated with atypical antipsychotics are at an increased risk of death compared to placebo, and also have an increased risk of cerebrovascular events

Children and Adolescents

- Approved for use in schizophrenia and manic/mixed episodes (ages 13 and older for both)
- Clinical experience and early data suggest olanzapine is probably safe and effective for behavioral disturbances in children and adolescents

- Children and adolescents using olanzapine may need to be monitored more often than adults
- Intramuscular formulation has not been studied in patients under 18 and is not recommended for use in this population

Pregnancy

- Effective June 30, 2015, the US FDA requires changes to the content and format of pregnancy and lactation information in prescription drug labels, including the elimination of the pregnancy letter categories; the Pregnancy and Lactation Labeling Rule (PLLR or final rule) applies only to prescription drugs and will be phased in gradually for drugs approved on or after June 30, 2001
- Controlled studies have not been conducted in pregnant women
- There is a risk of abnormal muscle movements and withdrawal symptoms in newborns whose mothers took an antipsychotic during the third trimester; symptoms may include agitation, abnormally increased or decreased muscle tone, tremor, sleepiness, severe difficulty breathing, and difficulty feeding
- Psychotic symptoms may worsen during pregnancy, and some form of treatment may be necessary
- Early findings of infants exposed to olanzapine in utero currently do not show adverse consequences
- Olanzapine may be preferable to anticonvulsant mood stabilizers if treatment is required during pregnancy
- National Pregnancy Registry for Atypical Antipsychotics: 1-866-961-2388 or http://womensmentalhealth.org/clinical-and-research-programs/pregnancyregistry/

Breast Feeding

- Unknown if olanzapine is secreted in human breast milk, but all psychotropics assumed to be secreted in breast milk
- ✻ Recommended either to discontinue drug or bottle feed
- Infants of women who choose to breast feed while on olanzapine should be monitored for possible adverse effects

THE ART OF PSYCHOPHARMACOLOGY

Potential Advantages

- ✻ Some cases of psychosis and bipolar disorder refractory to treatment with other antipsychotics
- ✻ Often a preferred augmenting agent in bipolar depression or treatment-resistant unipolar depression
- ✻ Patients needing rapid onset of antipsychotic action without drug titration
- Patients switching from intramuscular olanzapine to an oral preparation

Potential Disadvantages

- Patients concerned about gaining weight
- ✻ Patients with diabetes mellitus, obesity, and/or dyslipidemia

Primary Target Symptoms

- Positive symptoms of psychosis
- Negative symptoms of psychosis
- Cognitive symptoms
- Unstable mood (both depressed mood and mania)
- Aggressive symptoms

Pearls

- Recent landmark head-to-head study in schizophrenia suggests greater effectiveness (i.e., lower dropouts of all causes) at moderately high doses compared to some other atypical and conventional antipsychotics at moderate doses
- Same recent head-to-head study in schizophrenia suggests greater efficacy but greater metabolic side effects compared to some other atypical and conventional antipsychotics
- Well accepted for use in schizophrenia and bipolar disorder, including difficult cases
- ✻ Documented utility in treatment-refractory cases, especially at higher doses
- ✻ Documented efficacy as augmenting agent to SSRIs (fluoxetine) in nonpsychotic treatment-resistant major depressive disorder
- ✻ Documented efficacy in bipolar depression, especially in combination with fluoxetine
- More weight gain than many other antipsychotics – does not mean every patient gains weight
- Motor side effects unusual at low- to mid-doses
- Less sedation than for some other antipsychotics, more than for others

* Controversial as to whether olanzapine has more risk of diabetes and dyslipidemia than other antipsychotics
* Cigarette smoke can decrease olanzapine levels and patients may require a dose increase if they begin or increase smoking
* A short-acting intramuscular dosage formulation is available
* Long-acting intramuscular dosage formulation is also approved
* Patients with inadequate responses to atypical antipsychotics may benefit from determination of plasma drug levels and, if low, a dosage increase even beyond the usual prescribing limits
* Patients with inadequate responses to atypical antipsychotics may also benefit from a trial of augmentation with a conventional antipsychotic or switching to a conventional antipsychotic
* However, long-term polypharmacy with a combination of a conventional antipsychotic with an atypical antipsychotic may combine their side effects without clearly augmenting the efficacy of either
* For treatment-resistant patients, especially those with impulsivity, aggression, violence, and self-harm, long-term polypharmacy with 2 atypical antipsychotics or with 1 atypical antipsychotic and 1 conventional antipsychotic may be useful or even necessary while closely monitoring
* In such cases, it may be beneficial to combine 1 depot antipsychotic with 1 oral antipsychotic
* Although a frequent practice by some prescribers, adding 2 conventional antipsychotics together has little rationale and may reduce tolerability without clearly enhancing efficacy

PAMOATE

Vehicle	Water
Tmax	3–4 days
T1/2 with multiple dosing	30 days
Time to reach steady state	3 months
Able to be loaded	Yes
Dosing schedule (maintenance)	2 weeks or 4 weeks
Injection site	Intramuscular gluteal
Needle gauge	19
Dosage forms	210 mg, 300 mg, 405 mg
Injection volume	150 mg/mL (range 1.0–2.7 mL)

Usual Dosage Range
* 150–300 mg/2 weeks or 300–405 mg/4 weeks

How to Dose
* Conversion from oral: dose should be loaded during the initial 8 weeks based on the prior stable oral dose of olanzapine

Daily oral olanzapine dose	LAI dose: first 8 weeks	LAI dose: after 8 weeks
10 mg	210 mg/2 weeks OR 405 mg/4 weeks	150 mg/2 weeks OR 300 mg/4 weeks
15 mg	300 mg/2 weeks	210 mg/2 weeks OR 405 mg/4 weeks
20 mg	300 mg/2 weeks	300 mg/2 weeks

* Oral supplementation may be needed if adequate loading is not used
* Maximum dose 300 mg/2 weeks

Dosing Tips
* With LAIs, the absorption rate constant is slower than the elimination rate constant, thus resulting in "flip-flop" kinetics—i.e., time to steady-state is a function of absorption rate, while concentration at steady-state is a function of elimination rate
* The rate-limiting step for plasma drug levels for LAIs is not drug metabolism, but rather slow absorption from the injection site
* In general, 5 half-lives of any medication are needed to achieve 97% of steady-state levels
* The long half-lives of depot antipsychotics mean that one must either adequately load the dose (if possible) or provide oral supplementation
* The failure to adequately load the dose leads either to prolonged cross-titration

from oral antipsychotic or to sub-therapeutic antipsychotic plasma levels for weeks or months in patients who are not receiving (or adhering to) oral supplementation

- Because plasma antipsychotic levels increase gradually over time, dose requirements may ultimately decrease from initial; obtaining periodic plasma levels can be beneficial to prevent unnecessary plasma level creep
- The time to get a blood level for patients receiving LAI is the morning of the day they will receive their next injection
- Advantages: efficacy advantage of oral olanzapine
- Disadvantages: 3-hour post-injection monitoring required due to risk (0.2%) of post-injection delirium from vascular breach
- Response threshold is generally 21 ng/mL; plasma levels greater than 176 ng/mL are generally not well tolerated

SWITCHING FROM ORAL ANTIPSYCHOTICS TO OLANZAPINE PAMOATE

Expected Olanzapine Levels Without Oral Coverage

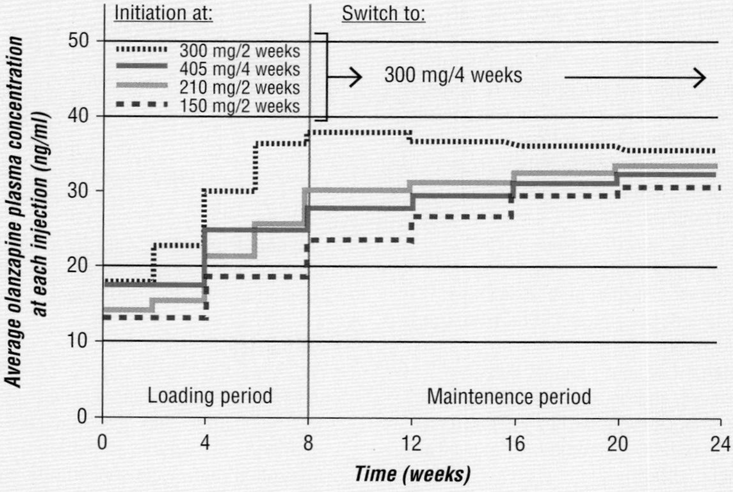

- Discontinuation of oral antipsychotic can begin immediately if adequate loading is pursued
- How to discontinue oral formulations
  - Down-titration is not required for: amisulpride, aripiprazole, brexpiprazole, cariprazine, olanzapine, paliperidone ER
  - 1-week down-titration is required for: iloperidone, lurasidone, risperidone, ziprasidone, asenapine, quetiapine
  - 4+-week down-titration may be required for: clozapine

THE ART OF SWITCHING

Switching from Oral Antipsychotics to Oral Olanzapine

- With aripiprazole, amisulpride, and paliperidone ER, immediate stop is possible; begin olanzapine at middle dose
- With risperidone, ziprasidone, iloperidone, and luasidone, begin olanzapine gradually, titrating over at least 2 weeks to allow patients to become tolerant to the sedating effect

*May need to taper clozapine slowly over 4 weeks or longer

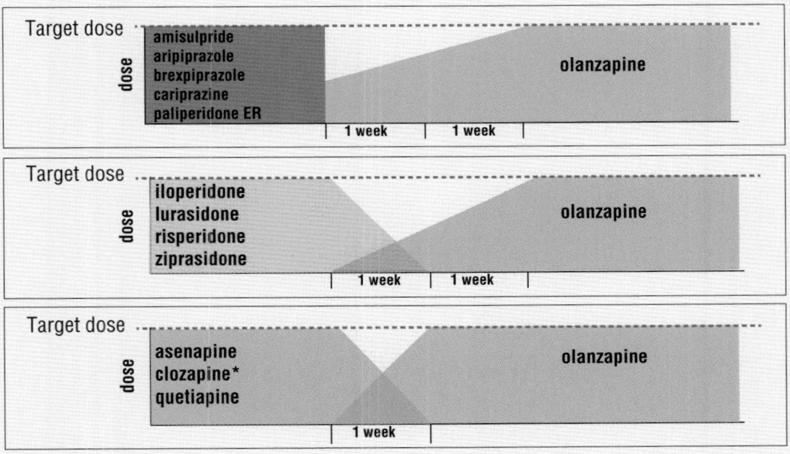

Suggested Reading

Citrome L. Adjunctive aripiprazole, olanzapine, or quetiapine for major depressive disorder: an analysis of number needed to treat, number needed to harm, and likelihood to be helped or harmed. Postgrad Med 2010;122(4):39–48.

Detke HC, Zhao F, Garhyan P, Carlson J, McDonnell D. Dose correspondence between olanzapine long-acting injection and oral olanzapine: recommendations for switching. Int Clin Psychopharmacol 2011;26:35–42.

Komossa K, Rummel-Kluge C, Hunger H, et al. Olanzapine versus other atypical antipsychotics for schizophrenia. Cochrane Database Syst Rev 2010;17(3):CD006654.

Nasrallah HA. Atypical antipsychotic-induced metabolic side effects: insights from receptor-binding profiles. Mol Psychiatry 2008;13(1):27–35.

Smith LA, Cornelius V, Warnock A, Tacchi MJ, Taylor D. Pharmacological interventions for acute bipolar mania: a systematic review of randomized placebo-controlled trials. Bipolar Disord 2007;9(6):551–60.

OXAZEPAM

THERAPEUTICS

Brands • Serax
see index for additional brand names

Generic? Yes

Class
- Neuroscience-based Nomenclature: GABA positive allosteric modulator (GABA-PAM)
- Benzodiazepine (anxiolytic)

Commonly Prescribed for
(bold for FDA approved)
- **Anxiety**
- **Anxiety associated with depression**
- **Alcohol withdrawal**
- Catatonia

How the Drug Works
- Binds to benzodiazepine receptors at the GABA-A ligand-gated chloride channel complex
- Enhances the inhibitory effects of GABA
- Boosts chloride conductance through GABA-regulated channels
- Inhibits neuronal activity presumably in amygdala-centered fear circuits to provide therapeutic benefits in anxiety disorders

How Long Until It Works
- Some immediate relief with first dosing is common; can take several weeks with daily dosing for maximal therapeutic benefit

If It Works
- For short-term symptoms of anxiety – after a few weeks, discontinue use or use on an "as-needed" basis
- For chronic anxiety disorders, the goal of treatment is complete remission of symptoms as well as prevention of future relapses
- For chronic anxiety disorders, treatment most often reduces or even eliminates symptoms, but not a cure since symptoms can recur after medicine stopped
- For long-term symptoms of anxiety, consider switching to an SSRI or SNRI for long-term maintenance
- If long-term maintenance with a benzodiazepine is necessary, continue treatment for 6 months after symptoms resolve, and then taper dose slowly
- If symptoms reemerge, consider treatment with an SSRI or SNRI, or consider restarting the benzodiazepine; sometimes benzodiazepines have to be used in combination with SSRIs or SNRIs for best results

If It Doesn't Work
- Consider switching to another agent or adding an appropriate augmenting agent
- Consider psychotherapy, especially cognitive behavioral psychotherapy
- Consider presence of concomitant substance abuse
- Consider presence of oxazepam abuse
- Consider another diagnosis, such as a comorbid medical condition

Best Augmenting Combos for Partial Response or Treatment Resistance
- Benzodiazepines are frequently used as augmenting agents for antipsychotics and mood stabilizers in the treatment of psychotic and bipolar disorders
- Benzodiazepines are frequently used as augmenting agents for SSRIs and SNRIs in the treatment of anxiety disorders
- Not generally rational to combine with other benzodiazepines
- Caution if using as an anxiolytic concomitantly with other sedative hypnotics for sleep

Tests
- In patients with seizure disorders, concomitant medical illness, and/or those with multiple concomitant long-term medications, periodic liver tests and blood counts may be prudent

SIDE EFFECTS

How Drug Causes Side Effects
- Same mechanism for side effects as for therapeutic effects – namely due to excessive actions at benzodiazepine receptors
- Long-term adaptations in benzodiazepine receptors may explain the development of dependence, tolerance, and withdrawal
- Side effects are generally immediate, but immediate side effects often disappear in time

Notable Side Effects

- ✽ Sedation, fatigue, depression
- ✽ Dizziness, ataxia, slurred speech, weakness
- ✽ Forgetfulness, confusion
- ✽ Hyperexcitability, nervousness
- Rare hallucinations, mania
- Rare hypotension
- Hypersalivation, dry mouth

Life-Threatening or Dangerous Side Effects

- Respiratory depression, especially when taken with CNS depressants in overdose
- Rare hepatic dysfunction, renal dysfunction, blood dyscrasias

Weight Gain

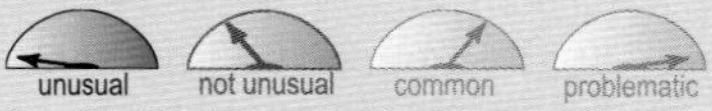

- Reported but not expected

Sedation

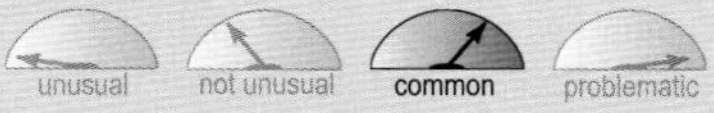

- Many experience and/or can be significant in amount
- Especially at initiation of treatment or when dose increases
- Tolerance often develops over time

What to Do About Side Effects

- Wait
- Wait
- Wait
- Lower the dose
- Take largest dose at bedtime to avoid sedative effects during the day
- Switch to another agent
- Administer flumazenil if side effects are severe or life-threatening

Best Augmenting Agents for Side Effects

- Many side effects cannot be improved with an augmenting agent

DOSING AND USE

Usual Dosage Range

- Mild to moderate anxiety: 30–60 mg/day in 3–4 divided doses
- Severe anxiety, anxiety associated with alcohol withdrawal: 45–120 mg/day in 3–4 divided doses

Dosage Forms

- Capsule 10 mg, 15 mg, 30 mg
- Tablet 15 mg

How to Dose

- Titration generally not necessary

Dosing Tips

- Use lowest possible effective dose for the shortest possible period of time (a benzodiazepine-sparing strategy)
- 15-mg tablet contains tartrazine, which may cause allergic reactions in certain patients, particularly those who are sensitive to aspirin
- For interdose symptoms of anxiety, can either increase dose or maintain same total daily dose but divide into more frequent doses
- Can also use an as-needed occasional "top up" dose for interdose anxiety
- Because anxiety disorders can require higher doses, the risk of dependence may be greater in these patients
- Some severely ill patients may require doses higher than the generally recommended maximum dose
- Frequency of dosing in practice is often greater than predicted from half-life, as duration of biological activity is often shorter than pharmacokinetic terminal half-life

Overdose

- Fatalities can occur; hypotension, tiredness, ataxia, confusion, coma

Long-Term Use

- Risk of dependence, particularly for treatment periods longer than 12 weeks and especially in patients with past or current polysubstance abuse

Habit Forming

- Oxazepam is a Schedule IV drug
- Patients may develop dependence and/or tolerance with long-term use

How to Stop
- Patients with history of seizure may seize upon withdrawal, especially if withdrawal is abrupt
- Taper by 15 mg every 3 days to reduce chances of withdrawal effects
- For difficult to taper cases, consider reducing dose much more slowly once reaching 45 mg/day, perhaps by as little as 10 mg per week or less
- For other patients with severe problems discontinuing a benzodiazepine, dosing may need to be tapered over many months (i.e., reduce dose by 1% every 3 days by crushing tablet and suspending or dissolving in 100 mL of fruit juice and then disposing of 1 mL while drinking the rest; 3–7 days later, dispose of 2 mL, and so on). This is both a form of very slow biological tapering and a form of behavioral desensitization
- Be sure to differentiate reemergence of symptoms requiring reinstitution of treatment from withdrawal symptoms
- Benzodiazepine-dependent anxiety patients and insulin-dependent diabetics are not addicted to their medications. When benzodiazepine-dependent patients stop their medication, disease symptoms can reemerge, disease symptoms can worsen (rebound), and/or withdrawal symptoms can emerge

Pharmacokinetics
- Elimination half-life 3–21 hours
- No active metabolites

Drug Interactions
- Increased depressive effects when taken with other CNS depressants (see Warnings below)

Other Warnings/ Precautions
- Boxed warning regarding the increased risk of CNS depressant effects when benzodiazepines and opioid medications are used together, including specifically the risk of slowed or difficulty breathing and death
- If alternatives to the combined use of benzodiazepines and opioids are not available, clinicians should limit the dosage and duration of each drug to the minimum possible while still achieving therapeutic efficacy
- Patients and their caregivers should be warned to seek medical attention if unusual dizziness, lightheadedness, sedation, slowed or difficulty breathing, or unresponsiveness occur
- Dosage changes should be made in collaboration with prescriber
- Use with caution in patients with pulmonary disease; rare reports of death after initiation of benzodiazepines in patients with severe pulmonary impairment
- History of drug or alcohol abuse often creates greater risk for dependency
- Some depressed patients may experience a worsening of suicidal ideation
- Some patients may exhibit abnormal thinking or behavioral changes similar to those caused by other CNS depressants (i.e., either depressant actions or disinhibiting actions)

Do Not Use
- If patient has angle-closure glaucoma
- If there is a proven allergy to oxazepam or any benzodiazepine

SPECIAL POPULATIONS

Renal Impairment
- Use with caution; oxazepam levels may be increased

Hepatic Impairment
- Use with caution; oxazepam levels may be increased
- Because of its short half-life and inactive metabolites, oxazepam may be a preferred benzodiazepine in some patients with liver disease

Cardiac Impairment
- Benzodiazepines have been used to treat anxiety associated with acute myocardial infarction

Elderly
- Initial 30 mg in 3 divided doses; can be increased to 30–60 mg/day in 3–4 divided doses

Children and Adolescents

- Safety and efficacy not established under age 6
- No clear dosing guidelines for children ages 6–12
- Long-term effects of oxazepam in children/adolescents are unknown
- Should generally receive lower doses and be more closely monitored

Pregnancy

- Effective June 30, 2015, the US FDA requires changes to the content and format of pregnancy and lactation information in prescription drug labels, including the elimination of the pregnancy letter categories; the Pregnancy and Lactation Labeling Rule (PLLR or final rule) applies only to prescription drugs and will be phased in gradually for drugs approved on or after June 30, 2001
- Possible increased risk of birth defects when benzodiazepines taken during pregnancy
- Because of the potential risks, oxazepam is not generally recommended as treatment for anxiety during pregnancy, especially during the first trimester
- Drug should be tapered if discontinued
- Infants whose mothers received a benzodiazepine late in pregnancy may experience withdrawal effects
- Neonatal flaccidity has been reported in infants whose mothers took a benzodiazepine during pregnancy
- Seizures, even mild seizures, may cause harm to the embryo/fetus

Breast Feeding

- Some drug is found in mother's breast milk

✻ Recommended either to discontinue drug or bottle feed

- Effects on infant have been observed and include feeding difficulties, sedation, and weight loss

THE ART OF PSYCHOPHARMACOLOGY

Potential Advantages

- Rapid onset of action

Potential Disadvantages

- Euphoria may lead to abuse
- Abuse especially risky in past or present substance abusers

Primary Target Symptoms

- Panic attacks
- Anxiety
- Agitation

Pearls

- Can be a very useful adjunct to SSRIs and SNRIs in the treatment of numerous anxiety disorders
- Not effective for treating psychosis as a monotherapy, but can be used as an adjunct to antipsychotics
- Not effective for treating bipolar disorder as a monotherapy, but can be used as an adjunct to mood stabilizers and antipsychotics

✻ Because of its short half-life and inactive metabolites, oxazepam may be preferred over some benzodiazepines for patients with liver disease

- Oxazepam may be preferred over some other benzodiazepines for the treatment of delirium
- Can both cause and treat depression in different patients
- When using to treat insomnia, remember that insomnia may be a symptom of some other primary disorder itself, and thus warrant evaluation for comorbid psychiatric and/or medical conditions
- Though not systematically studied, benzodiazepines have been used effectively to treat catatonia and are the initial recommended treatment

Suggested Reading

Ayd FJ Jr. Oxazepam: update 1989. Int Clin Psychopharmacol 1990;5:1–15.

Garattini S. Biochemical and pharmacological properties of oxazepam. Acta Psychiatr Scand Suppl 1978;274:9–18.

Greenblatt DJ. Clinical pharmacokinetics of oxazepam and lorazepam. Clin Pharmacokinet 1981;6:89–105.

OXCARBAZEPINE

THERAPEUTICS

Brands • Trileptal

see index for additional brand names

Generic? Yes

Class

• Anticonvulsant, voltage-sensitive sodium channel antagonist

Commonly Prescribed for

(bold for FDA approved)

• **Partial seizures in adults with epilepsy (monotherapy or adjunctive)**
• **Partial seizures in children ages 4–16 with epilepsy (monotherapy or adjunctive)**
• Bipolar disorder

How the Drug Works

✽ Acts as a use-dependent blocker of voltage-sensitive sodium channels
✽ Interacts with the open channel conformation of voltage-sensitive sodium channels
✽ Interacts at a specific site of the alpha pore-forming subunit of voltage-sensitive sodium channels
• Inhibits release of glutamate

How Long Until It Works

• For acute mania, effects should occur within a few weeks
• May take several weeks to months to optimize an effect on mood stabilization
• Should reduce seizures by 2 weeks

If It Works

• The goal of treatment is complete remission of symptoms (e.g., seizures, mania)
• Continue treatment until all symptoms are gone or until improvement is stable and then continue treating indefinitely as long as improvement persists
• Continue treatment indefinitely to avoid recurrence of mania and seizures

If It Doesn't Work (for bipolar disorder)

✽ Many patients have only a partial response where some symptoms are improved but others persist or continue to wax and wane without stabilization of mood
• Other patients may be nonresponders, sometimes called treatment-resistant or treatment-refractory
• Consider increasing dose, switching to another agent, or adding an appropriate augmenting agent
• Consider adding psychotherapy
• For bipolar disorder, consider the presence of noncompliance and counsel patient
• Switch to another mood stabilizer with fewer side effects
• Consider evaluation for another diagnosis or for a comorbid condition (e.g., medical illness, substance abuse, etc.)

Best Augmenting Combos for Partial Response or Treatment Resistance

• Oxcarbazepine is itself a second-line augmenting agent for numerous other anticonvulsants, lithium, and atypical antipsychotics in treating bipolar disorder, although its use in bipolar disorder is not yet well studied
• Oxcarbazepine may be a second- or third-line augmenting agent for antipsychotics in treating schizophrenia, although its use in schizophrenia is also not yet well studied

Tests

• Consider monitoring sodium levels because of possibility of hyponatremia, especially during the first 3 months

SIDE EFFECTS

How Drug Causes Side Effects

• CNS side effects theoretically due to excessive actions at voltage-sensitive sodium channels

Notable Side Effects

✽ Sedation (dose-dependent), dizziness (dose-dependent), headache, ataxia (dose-dependent), nystagmus, abnormal gait, confusion, nervousness, fatigue
✽ Nausea (dose-dependent), vomiting, abdominal pain, dyspepsia
• Diplopia (dose-dependent), vertigo, abnormal vision
✽ Rash

Life-Threatening or Dangerous Side Effects

- Hyponatremia
- Rare activation of suicidal ideation and behavior (suicidality)

Weight Gain

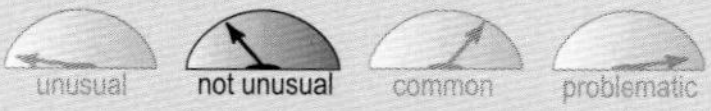

- Occurs in significant minority
- Some patients experience increased appetite

Sedation

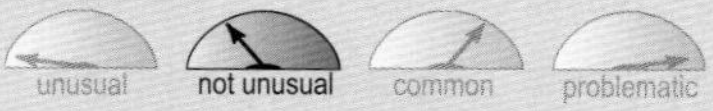

- Occurs in significant minority
- Dose-related
- Less than carbamazepine
- More when combined with other anticonvulsants
- Can wear off with time, but may not wear off at high doses

What to Do About Side Effects

- Wait
- Wait
- Wait
- Switch to another agent

Best Augmenting Agents for Side Effects

- Many side effects cannot be improved with an augmenting agent

DOSING AND USE

Usual Dosage Range

- 1,200–2,400 mg/day

Dosage Forms

- Tablet 150 mg, 300 mg, 600 mg
- Liquid 300 mg/5 mL

How to Dose

- Monotherapy for seizures or bipolar disorder: initial 600 mg/day in 2 doses; increase every 3 days by 300 mg/day; maximum dose generally 2,400 mg/day
- Adjunctive: initial 600 mg/day in 2 doses; each week can increase by 600 mg/day; recommended dose 1,200 mg/day; maximum dose generally 2,400 mg/day
- When converting from adjunctive to monotherapy in the treatment of epilepsy, titrate concomitant drug down over 3–6 weeks while titrating oxcarbazepine up over 2–4 weeks, with an initial daily oxcarbazepine dose of 600 mg divided in 2 doses

Dosing Tips

✻ Doses of oxcarbazepine need to be about one-third higher than those of carbamazepine for similar results
- Usually administered as adjunctive medication to other anticonvulsants, lithium, or atypical antipsychotics for bipolar disorder
- Side effects may increase with dose
- Although increased efficacy for seizures is seen at 2,400 mg/day compared to 1,200 mg/day, CNS side effects may be intolerable at the higher dose
- Liquid formulation can be administered mixed in a glass of water or directly from the oral dosing syringe supplied
- Slow dose titration may delay onset of therapeutic action but enhance tolerability to sedating side effects
- Should titrate slowly in the presence of other sedating agents, such as other anticonvulsants, in order to best tolerate additive sedative side effects

Overdose

- No fatalities reported

Long-Term Use

- Safe
- Monitoring of sodium may be required, especially during the first 3 months

Habit Forming

- No

How to Stop

- Taper
- Epilepsy patients may seize upon withdrawal, especially if withdrawal is abrupt

✻ Rapid discontinuation may increase the risk of relapse in bipolar disorder
- Discontinuation symptoms uncommon

Pharmacokinetics

- Metabolized in the liver
- Renally excreted
- Inhibits CYP450 2C19

✻ Oxcarbazepine is a prodrug for 10-hydroxy carbazepine

✻ This main active metabolite is sometimes called the monohydroxy derivative or MHD, and is also known as licarbazepine

✻ Half-life of parent drug is approximately 2 hours; half-life of MHD is approximately 9 hours; thus oxcarbazepine is essentially a prodrug rapidly converted to its MHD, licarbazepine

- A mild inducer of CYP450 3A4
- Food does not affect absorption

Drug Interactions

- Depressive effects may be increased by other CNS depressants (alcohol, MAOIs, other anticonvulsants, etc.)
- Strong inducers of CYP450 cytochromes (e.g., carbamazepine, phenobarbital, phenytoin, and primidone) can decrease plasma levels of the active metabolite MHD
- Verapamil may decrease plasma levels of the active metabolite MHD
- Oxcarbazepine can decrease plasma levels of hormonal contraceptives and dihydropyridine calcium antagonists
- Oxcarbazepine at doses greater than 1,200 mg/day may increase plasma levels of phenytoin, possibly requiring dose reduction of phenytoin

Other Warnings/ Precautions

- Because oxcarbazepine has a tricyclic chemical structure, it is not recommended to be taken with MAOIs, including 14 days after MAOIs are stopped; do not start an MAOI until 2 weeks after discontinuing oxcarbazepine
- Because oxcarbazepine can lower plasma levels of hormonal contraceptives, it may also reduce their effectiveness
- May exacerbate angle-closure glaucoma
- May need to restrict fluids and/or monitor sodium because of risk of hyponatremia
- Use cautiously in patients who have demonstrated hypersensitivity to carbamazepine
- Warn patients and their caregivers about the possibility of activation of suicidal ideation and advise them to report such side effects immediately

Do Not Use

- If patient is taking an MAOI
- If there is a proven allergy to any tricyclic compound
- If there is a proven allergy to oxcarbazepine

SPECIAL POPULATIONS

Renal Impairment

- Oxcarbazepine is renally excreted
- Elimination half-life of active metabolite MHD is increased
- Reduce initial dose by half; may need to use slower titration

Hepatic Impairment

- No dose adjustment recommended for mild to moderate hepatic impairment
- Use with caution in patients with severe impairment

Cardiac Impairment

- No dose adjustment recommended

Elderly

- Older patients may have reduced creatinine clearance and require reduced dosing
- Elderly patients may be more susceptible to adverse effects
- Some patients may tolerate lower doses better

Children and Adolescents

- Approved as adjunctive therapy or monotherapy for partial seizures in children 4 and older
- Ages 4–16 (adjunctive): initial 8–10 mg/kg per day or less than 600 mg/day in 2 doses; increase over 2 weeks to 900 mg/day (20–29 kg), 1,200 mg/day (29.1–39 kg), or 1,800 mg/day (>39 kg)
- When converting from adjunctive to monotherapy, titrate concomitant drug down over 3–6 weeks while titrating oxcarbazepine up by no more than 10 mg/kg per day each week, with an initial daily

oxcarbazepine dose of 8–10 mg/kg per day divided in 2 doses

- Monotherapy: initial 8–10 mg/kg per day in 2 doses; increase every 3 days by 5 mg/kg per day; recommended maintenance dose dependent on weight
- 0–20 kg (600–900 mg/day);
  21–30 kg (900–1,200 mg/day);
  31–40 kg (900–1,500 mg/day);
  41–45 kg (1,200–1,500 mg/day);
  46–55 kg (1,200–1,800 mg/day);
  56–65 kg (1,200–2,100 mg/day);
  over 65 kg (1,500–2,100 mg)
- Children below age 8 may have increased clearance compared to adults

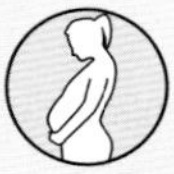

Pregnancy

- Effective June 30, 2015, the US FDA requires changes to the content and format of pregnancy and lactation information in prescription drug labels, including the elimination of the pregnancy letter categories; the Pregnancy and Lactation Labeling Rule (PLLR or final rule) applies only to prescription drugs and will be phased in gradually for drugs approved on or after June 30, 2001
- Controlled studies have not been conducted in pregnant women
- ✱ Oxcarbazepine is structurally similar to carbamazepine, which is thought to be teratogenic in humans
- ✱ Use during first trimester may raise risk of neural tube defects (e.g., spina bifida) or other congenital anomalies
- Use in women of childbearing potential requires weighing potential benefits to the mother against the risks to the fetus
- ✱ If drug is continued, perform tests to detect birth defects
- ✱ If drug is continued, start on folate 1 mg/day to reduce risk of neural tube defects
- Antiepileptic Drug Pregnancy Registry: (888) 233–2334
- Taper drug if discontinuing
- ✱ For bipolar patients, oxcarbazepine should generally be discontinued before anticipated pregnancies
- Seizures, even mild seizures, may cause harm to the embryo/fetus
- Recurrent bipolar illness during pregnancy can be quite disruptive
- ✱ For bipolar patients, given the risk of relapse in the postpartum period, some form of mood stabilizer treatment may need to be restarted immediately after delivery if patient is unmedicated during pregnancy
- ✱ Atypical antipsychotics may be preferable to lithium or anticonvulsants such as oxcarbazepine if treatment of bipolar disorder is required during pregnancy
- Bipolar symptoms may recur or worsen during pregnancy and some form of treatment may be necessary

Breast Feeding

- Some drug is found in mother's breast milk
- ✱ Recommended either to discontinue drug or bottle feed
- If drug is continued while breast feeding, infant should be monitored for possible adverse effects
- If infant shows signs of irritability or sedation, drug may need to be discontinued
- Bipolar disorder may recur during the postpartum period, particularly if there is a history of prior postpartum episodes of either depression or psychosis
- ✱ Relapse rates may be lower in women who receive prophylactic treatment for postpartum episodes of bipolar disorder
- Atypical antipsychotics and anticonvulsants such as valproate may be safer than oxcarbazepine during the postpartum period when breast feeding

THE ART OF PSYCHOPHARMACOLOGY

Potential Advantages

- Treatment-resistant bipolar and psychotic disorders
- Those unable to tolerate carbamazepine but who respond to carbamazepine

Potential Disadvantages

- Patients at risk for hyponatremia

Primary Target Symptoms

- Incidence of seizures
- Severity of seizures
- Unstable mood, especially mania

Pearls

- ✻ Some evidence of effectiveness in treating acute mania; included in American Psychiatric Association's bipolar treatment guidelines as an option for acute treatment and maintenance treatment of bipolar disorder
- Some evidence of effectiveness as adjunctive treatment in schizophrenia and schizoaffective disorders
- Oxcarbazepine is the 10-keto analog of carbamazepine, but not a metabolite of carbamazepine
- Less well investigated in bipolar disorder than carbamazepine
- ✻ Oxcarbazepine seems to have the same mechanism of therapeutic action as carbamazepine but with fewer side effects
- ✻ Specifically, risk of leukopenia, aplastic anemia, agranulocytosis, elevated liver enzymes, or Stevens-Johnson syndrome and serious rash associated with carbamazepine does not seem to be associated with oxcarbazepine
- Skin rash reactions to carbamazepine may resolve in 75% of patients with epilepsy when switched to oxcarbazepine; thus, 25% of patients who experience rash with carbamazepine may also experience it with oxcarbazepine
- Oxcarbazepine has much less prominent actions on CYP 450 enzyme systems than carbamazepine, and thus fewer drug-drug interactions
- Specifically, oxcarbazepine and its active metabolite, the monohydroxy derivative (MHD), cause less enzyme induction of CYP450 3A4 than the structurally related carbamazepine
- The active metabolite MHD, also called licarbazepine, is a racemic mixture of 80% S-MHD (active) and 20% R-MHD (inactive)
- A related compound, APTIOM, is a dibenz[b,f]azepine-5-carboxamide derivative of eslicarbazepine and is also extensively converted to eslicarbazepine
- APTIOM is now approved as an anticonvulsant, but adequate studies have not been conducted on its potential use as a mood stabilizer
- ✻ Most significant risk of oxcarbazepine may be clinically significant hyponatremia (sodium level <125 m mol/L), most likely occurring within the first 3 months of treatment, and occurring in 2–3% of patients
- Unknown if this risk is higher than for carbamazepine
- ✻ Since SSRIs can sometimes also reduce sodium due to SIADH (syndrome of inappropriate antidiuretic hormone production), patients treated with combinations of oxcarbazepine and SSRIs should be carefully monitored, especially in the early stages of treatment
- By analogy with carbamazepine, could theoretically be useful in chronic neuropathic pain

Suggested Reading

Beydoun A. Safety and efficacy of oxcarbazepine: results of randomized, double-blind trials. Pharmacotherapy 2000;20(8 Pt 2):152S–158S.

Centorrino F, Albert MJ, Berry JM, et al. Oxcarbazepine: clinical experience with hospitalized psychiatric patients. Bipolar Disord 2003;5:370–4.

Dietrich DE, Kropp S, Emrich HM. Oxcarbazepine in affective and schizoaffective disorders. Pharmacopsychiatry 2001;34:242–50.

Glauser TA. Oxcarbazepine in the treatment of epilepsy. Pharmacotherapy 2001;21:904–19.

Vasudev A, Macritchie K, Vasudev K, et al. Oxcarbazepine for acute affective episodes in bipolar disorder. Cochrane Database Syst Rev 2011;7(12):CD004857.

PALIPERIDONE

THERAPEUTICS

Brands • INVEGA
• INVEGA SUSTENNA
• INVEGA TRINZA

see index for additional brand names

Generic? No

Class

- Neuroscience-based Nomenclature: dopamine, serotonin receptor antagonist (DS-RAn)
- Atypical antipsychotic (serotonin-dopamine antagonist; second generation antipsychotics; also a mood stabilizer)

Commonly Prescribed for

(bold for FDA approved)

- **Schizophrenia (ages 12 and older)**
- **Maintaining response in schizophrenia**
- **Schizoaffective disorder**
- Other psychotic disorders
- Bipolar disorder
- Behavioral disturbances in dementia
- Behavioral disturbances in children and adolescents
- Disorders associated with problems with impulse control

How the Drug Works

- Blocks dopamine 2 receptors, reducing positive symptoms of psychosis and stabilizing affective symptoms
- Blocks serotonin 2A receptors, causing enhancement of dopamine release in certain brain regions and thus reducing motor side effects and possibly improving cognitive and affective symptoms

✻ Serotonin 7 antagonist properties may contribute to antidepressant actions

How Long Until It Works

- Psychotic symptoms can improve within 1 week, but it may take several weeks for full effect on behavior as well as on cognition
- Classically recommended to wait at least 4–6 weeks to determine efficacy of drug, but in practice some patients may require up to 16–20 weeks to show a good response, especially on cognitive symptoms

If It Works

- Most often reduces positive symptoms but does not eliminate them
- Can improve negative symptoms, as well as aggressive, cognitive, and affective symptoms in schizophrenia
- Most schizophrenia patients do not have a total remission of symptoms but rather a reduction of symptoms by about a third
- Perhaps 5–15% of schizophrenia patients can experience an overall improvement of greater than 50–60%, especially when receiving stable treatment for more than a year
- Such patients are considered superresponders or "awakeners" since they may be well enough to be employed, live independently, and sustain long-term relationships
- Continue treatment until reaching a plateau of improvement
- After reaching a satisfactory plateau, continue treatment for at least a year after first episode of psychosis
- For second and subsequent episodes of psychosis, treatment may need to be indefinite
- Even for first episodes of psychosis, it may be preferable to continue treatment

If It Doesn't Work

- Try one of the other atypical antipsychotics (risperidone, olanzapine, quetiapine, ziprasidone, aripiprazole, amisulpride, asenapine, iloperidone, lurasidone)
- If 2 or more antipsychotic monotherapies do not work, consider clozapine
- Some patients may require treatment with a conventional antipsychotic
- If no first-line atypical antipsychotic is effective, consider higher doses or augmentation with valproate or lamotrigine
- Consider noncompliance and switch to another antipsychotic with fewer side effects or to an antipsychotic that can be given by depot injection (a depot formulation of paliperidone is in development)
- Consider initiating rehabilitation and psychotherapy such as cognitive remediation
- Consider presence of concomitant drug abuse

Best Augmenting Combos for Partial Response or Treatment Resistance

- Valproic acid (valproate, divalproex, divalproex ER)

- Other mood-stabilizing anticonvulsants (carbamazepine, oxcarbazepine, lamotrigine)
- Lithium
- Benzodiazepines

Tests

Before starting an atypical antipsychotic:

✻ Weigh all patients and track BMI during treatment

- Get baseline personal and family history of diabetes, obesity, dyslipidemia, hypertension, and cardiovascular disease

✻ Get waist circumference (at umbilicus), blood pressure, fasting plasma glucose, and fasting lipid profile

- Determine if the patient is
  - overweight (BMI 25.0–29.9)
  - obese (BMI >30)
  - has pre-diabetes (fasting plasma glucose 100–125 mg/dL)
  - has diabetes (fasting plasma glucose >126 mg/dL)
  - has hypertension (BP >140/90 mm Hg)
  - has dyslipidemia (increased total cholesterol, LDL cholesterol, and triglycerides; decreased HDL cholesterol)
- Treat or refer such patients for treatment, including nutrition and weight management, physical activity counseling, smoking cessation, and medical management

Monitoring after starting an atypical antipsychotic:

✻ BMI monthly for 3 months, then quarterly

✻ Consider monitoring fasting triglycerides monthly for several months in patients at high risk for metabolic complications and when initiating or switching antipsychotics

✻ Blood pressure, fasting plasma glucose, fasting lipids within 3 months and then annually, but earlier and more frequently for patients with diabetes or who have gained >5% of initial weight

- Treat or refer for treatment and consider switching to another atypical antipsychotic for patients who become overweight, obese, pre-diabetic, diabetic, hypertensive, or dyslipidemic while receiving an atypical antipsychotic

✻ Even in patients without known diabetes, be vigilant for the rare but life-threatening onset of diabetic ketoacidosis, which always requires immediate treatment, by monitoring for the rapid onset of polyuria, polydipsia, weight loss, nausea, vomiting, dehydration, rapid respiration, weakness, and clouding of sensorium, even coma

- Should check blood pressure in the elderly before starting and for the first few weeks of treatment
- Monitoring elevated prolactin levels of dubious clinical benefit
- Patients with low white blood cell count (WBC) or history of drug-induced leucopenia/neutropenia should have complete blood count (CBC) monitored frequently during the first few months and paliperidone should be discontinued at the first sign of decline of WBC in the absence of other causative factors

SIDE EFFECTS

How Drug Causes Side Effects

- By blocking alpha 1 adrenergic receptors, it can cause dizziness, sedation, and hypotension
- By blocking dopamine 2 receptors in the striatum, it can cause motor side effects, especially at high doses
- By blocking dopamine 2 receptors in the pituitary, it can cause elevations in prolactin
- Mechanism of weight gain and increased incidence of diabetes and dyslipidemia with atypical antipsychotics is unknown

Notable Side Effects

✻ Dose-dependent extrapyramidal symptoms

✻ Hyperprolactinemia

✻ May increase risk for diabetes and dyslipidemia

- Rare tardive dyskinesia (much reduced risk compared to conventional antipsychotics)
- Sedation, hypersalivation
- Dose-dependent orthostatic hypotension
- Tachycardia
- Injection site reactions

Life-Threatening or Dangerous Side Effects

- Hyperglycemia, in some cases extreme and associated with ketoacidosis or hyperosmolar coma or death, has been reported in patients taking atypical antipsychotics
- Increased risk of death and cerebrovascular events in elderly patients with dementia-related psychosis
- Rare neuroleptic malignant syndrome (much reduced risk compared to conventional antipsychotics)
- Rare seizures

Weight Gain

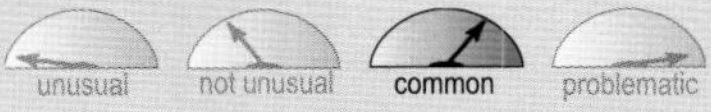

- Many patients experience and/or can be significant in amount
- May be dose-dependent
- May be less than for some antipsychotics, more than for others

Sedation

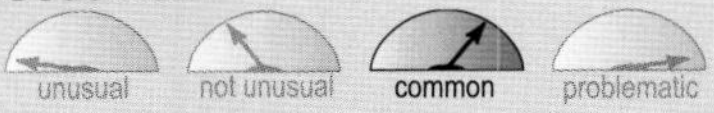

- Many experience and/or can be significant in amount
- May be dose-dependent
- May be less than for some antipsychotics, more than for others

What to Do About Side Effects

- Wait
- Wait
- Wait
- Anticholinergics may reduce motor side effects when present
- Weight loss, exercise programs, and medical management for high BMIs, diabetes, dyslipidemia
- Switch to another atypical antipsychotic

Best Augmenting Agents for Side Effects

- Benztropine or trihexyphenidyl for motor side effects
- Many side effects cannot be improved with an augmenting agent

DOSING AND USE

Usual Dosage Range

- 6 mg/day (oral)
- 39–234 mg/month (Sustenna; see Paliperidone Palmitate section after Pearls for dosing and use)
- 273–819 mg/3 months (Trinza; see Paliperidone Palmitate section after Pearls for dosing and use)

Dosage Forms

- Tablet (extended-release) 1.5 mg, 3 mg, 6 mg, 9 mg
- 1-month injection 39 mg, 78 mg, 117 mg, 156 mg, 234 mg
- 3-month injection 273 mg, 410 mg, 546 mg, 819 mg

How to Dose

- Initial dose 6 mg/day taken in the morning
- Can increase by 3 mg/day every 5 days; maximum dose generally 12 mg/day
- LAI paliperidone is not recommended for patients who have not first demonstrated tolerability to oral paliperidone or risperidone
- See also the Switching section, after Pearls

Dosing Tips – Oral

- Tablet should not be divided or chewed, but rather should only be swallowed whole
- Tablet does not change shape in the gastrointestinal tract and generally should not be used in patients with gastrointestinal narrowing because of the risk of intestinal obstruction
- Some patients may benefit from doses above 6 mg/day; alternatively, for some patients 3 mg/day may be sufficient
- A common dosage error is to assume the paliperidone ER oral dose is the same as the risperidone oral dose in mg, and that paliperidone should be titrated. However, many patients do well initiating a dose of 6 mg orally of paliperidone ER without titration
- There is a dose-dependent increase in some side effects, including extrapyramidal symptoms and weight gain, above 6 mg/day

- Rather than raise the dose above these levels in acutely agitated patients requiring acute antipsychotic actions, consider augmentation with a benzodiazepine or conventional antipsychotic, either orally or intramuscularly
- Rather than raise the dose above these levels in partial responders, consider augmentation with a mood-stabilizing anticonvulsant, such as valproate or lamotrigine
- Children and elderly should generally be dosed at the lower end of the dosage spectrum
- Treatment should be suspended if absolute neutrophil count falls below 1,000/mm^3
- Oral doses correspond to injection doses as follows: 3 mg oral to 39–78 mg injection, 6 mg oral to 117 mg injection, 12 mg oral to 234 mg injection

Overdose
- Extrapyramidal symptoms, gait unsteadiness, sedation, tachycardia, hypotension, QT prolongation

Long-Term Use
- Approved for maintenance in schizophrenia

Habit Forming
- No

How to Stop
- See Switching section of individual agents for how to stop paliperidone ER and LAI
- Rapid oral discontinuation may lead to rebound psychosis and worsening of symptoms

Pharmacokinetics
- Active metabolite of risperidone
- Half-life approximately 23 hours
- Absorption is reduced if taken on an empty stomach

Drug Interactions
- May increase effects of antihypertensive agents
- May antagonize levodopa, dopamine agonists
- May enhance QTc prolongation of other drugs capable of prolonging QTc interval

Other Warnings/ Precautions
- Use with caution in patients with conditions that predispose to hypotension (dehydration, overheating)
- Dysphagia has been associated with antipsychotic use, and paliperidone should be used cautiously in patients at risk for aspiration pneumonia
- Paliperidone prolongs QTc interval more than some other antipsychotics
- Priapism has been reported with other antipsychotics, including risperidone

Do Not Use
- If patient is taking agents capable of significantly prolonging QTc interval (e.g., pimozide, thioridazine, selected antiarrhythmics, moxifloxacin, sparfloxacin)
- If there is a history of QTc prolongation or cardiac arrhythmia, recent acute myocardial infarction, uncompensated heart failure
- If patient has a preexisting severe gastrointestinal narrowing
- If there is a proven allergy to paliperidone or risperidone

SPECIAL POPULATIONS

Renal Impairment
- For mild impairment, maximum recommended dose 6 mg/day
- For moderate impairment, initial and maximum recommended dose 3 mg/day
- For severe impairment, initial dose 1.5 mg/day; maximum recommended dose 3 mg/day

Hepatic Impairment
- No dose adjustment necessary for mild to moderate impairment
- Use in individuals with severe hepatic impairment has not been studied

Cardiac Impairment
- Drug should be used with caution because of risk of orthostatic hypotension

Elderly
- Some patients may tolerate lower doses better

- Although atypical antipsychotics are commonly used for behavioral disturbances in dementia, no agent has been approved for treatment of elderly patients with dementia-related psychosis
- Elderly patients with dementia-related psychosis treated with atypical antipsychotics are at an increased risk of death compared to placebo, and also have an increased risk of cerebrovascular events

Children and Adolescents

- Safety and efficacy have not been established under age 12
- Adolescents <51 kg: initial 3 mg/day; recommended 3–6 mg/day; maximum 6 mg/day
- Adolescents >51 kg: initial 3 mg/day; recommended 3–12 mg/day; maximum 12 mg/day
- Children and adolescents using paliperidone may need to be monitored more often than adults

Pregnancy

- Effective June 30, 2015, the US FDA requires changes to the content and format of pregnancy and lactation information in prescription drug labels, including the elimination of the pregnancy letter categories; the Pregnancy and Lactation Labeling Rule (PLLR or final rule) applies only to prescription drugs and will be phased in gradually for drugs approved on or after June 30, 2001
- Controlled studies have not been conducted in pregnant women
- There is a risk of abnormal muscle movements and withdrawal symptoms in newborns whose mothers took an antipsychotic during the third trimester; symptoms may include agitation, abnormally increased or decreased muscle tone, tremor, sleepiness, severe difficulty breathing, and difficulty feeding
- Psychotic symptoms may worsen during pregnancy and some form of treatment may be necessary
- Paliperidone may be preferable to anticonvulsant mood stabilizers if treatment is required during pregnancy
- Effects of hyperprolactinemia on the fetus are unknown
- National Pregnancy Registry for Atypical Antipsychotics: 1-866-961-2388 or http://womensmentalhealth.org/clinical-and-research-programs/pregnancyregistry/

Breast Feeding

- Some drug is found in mother's breast milk
- Recommended either to discontinue drug or bottle feed
- Infants of women who choose to breast feed while on paliperidone should be monitored for possible adverse effects

THE ART OF PSYCHOPHARMACOLOGY

Potential Advantages

- Some cases of psychosis and bipolar disorder refractory to treatment with other antipsychotics
- Patients requiring rapid onset of antipsychotic action without dosage titration

Potential Disadvantages

- Patients for whom elevated prolactin may not be desired (e.g., possibly pregnant patients; pubescent girls with amenorrhea; postmenopausal women with low estrogen who do not take estrogen replacement therapy)

Primary Target Symptoms

- Positive symptoms of psychosis
- Negative symptoms of psychosis
- Cognitive symptoms
- Unstable mood (both depression and mania)
- Aggressive symptoms

Pearls

- Some patients respond to paliperidone or tolerate paliperidone better than the parent drug risperidone
- Hyperprolactinemia in women with low estrogen may accelerate osteoporosis
- Less weight gain than some antipsychotics, more than others
- May cause more motor side effects than some other atypical antipsychotics,

especially when administered to patients with Parkinson's disease or Lewy body dementia
- Trilayer tablet consists of 3 compartments (2 containing drug, 1 a "push" compartment) and an orifice at the head of the first drug compartment; water fills the push compartment and gradually pushes drug up and out of the tablet through the orifice
- LAI does not require simultaneous oral medication
- LAI may work better and better after a few weeks of treatment in some patients
- LAI may be very well tolerated
- LAI may be combined with a second antipsychotic administered orally for difficult cases
- Patients with inadequate responses to atypical antipsychotics may benefit from determination of plasma drug levels and, if low, a dosage increase even beyond the usual prescribing limits
- For treatment-resistant patients, especially those with impulsivity, aggression, violence, and self-harm, long-term polypharmacy with 2 atypical antipsychotics or with 1 atypical antipsychotic and 1 conventional antipsychotic may be useful or even necessary while closely monitoring
- In such cases, it may be beneficial to combine 1 depot antipsychotic with 1 oral antipsychotic
- Patients with inadequate responses to atypical antipsychotics may also benefit from a trial of augmentation with a conventional antipsychotic or switching to a conventional antipsychotic
- However, long-term polypharmacy with a combination of a conventional antipsychotic with an atypical antipsychotic may combine their side effects without clearly augmenting the efficacy of either
- Although a frequent practice by some prescribers, adding 2 conventional antipsychotics together has little rationale and may reduce tolerability without clearly enhancing efficacy

PALMITATE

	1-month (Sustenna)	3-month (Trinza)
Vehicle	Water	Water
Tmax	13 days	30–33 days
T1/2 with multiple dosing	25–49 days	84–95 days (deltoid) 118–139 days (gluteal)
Time to reach steady state	1 week	
Able to be loaded	Yes	N/A
Dosing schedule (maintenance)	4 weeks	12 weeks
Injection site	Intramuscular (deltoid at initiation, then either deltoid or gluteal)	Intramuscular (deltoid or gluteal)
Needle gauge	22 or 23	22
Dosage forms	39 mg, 78 mg, 117 mg, 156 mg, 234 mg	273 mg, 410 mg, 546 mg, 819 mg
Injection volume	156 mg/mL; range 0.25–1.5 mL	0.875–2.625 mL

Usual Dosage Range

- 1-month injectable maintenance dose: 117 mg/month (range 39–234 mg/month)
- 3-month injectable maintenance dose: 273–819 mg/3 months

How to Dose – 1-month Injectable

- Not recommended for patients who have not first demonstrated tolerability to oral paliperidone or risperidone (in clinical trials, 2 oral or short-acting IM doses are generally used to establish tolerability)
- Conversion from oral: 234 mg delivered intramuscularly in the deltoid on Day 1; 156 mg delivered intramuscularly in the deltoid on Day 8; maintenance dose should start 4 weeks after the 2nd loading injection

Oral Equivalence (Approximate)	
Oral paliperidone	**1-month Sustenna**
3 mg	39–78 mg
6 mg	117 mg
9 mg	156 mg
12 mg	234 mg

How to Dose – 3-month Injectable

- Only for patients who have received adequate treatment with paliperidone Sustenna for at least 4 months
- The last 2 doses of paliperidone Sustenna should ideally be the same dosage strength, so that a consistent maintenance dose is established prior to starting paliperidone Trinza
- Conversion from 1-month injectable: initiate 3-month LAI when the next 1-month LAI injection is scheduled; dosing is based on the previous 1-month injection dose

1-month Sustenna	3-month Trinza
78 mg	273 mg
117 mg	410 mg
156 mg	546 mg
234 mg	819 mg

- Dose adjustments can be made every 3 months if needed; the long-acting nature of paliperidone Trinza means that a patient's response to an adjusted dose may not be apparent for multiple months
- Injection can be given up to 2 weeks before or after the 3-month time point
- If dose has been missed for 4–9 months, the following re-initiation schedule must be followed:

Last Trinza Dose	Day 1	Day 8	1 Month After Day 8
273 mg	78 mg Sustenna (deltoid)	78 mg Sustenna (deltoid)	273 mg Trinza (deltoid or gluteal)
410 mg	117 mg Sustenna (deltoid)	117 mg Sustenna (deltoid)	410 mg Trinza (deltoid or gluteal)
546 mg	156 mg Sustenna (deltoid)	156 mg Sustenna (deltoid)	546 mg Trinza (deltoid or gluteal)
819 mg	156 mg Sustenna (deltoid)	156 mg Sustenna (deltoid)	819 mg Trinza (deltoid or gluteal)

- If dose has been missed for more than 9 months, re-initiate treatment with paliperidone Sustenna according to its prescribing information; paliperidone Trinza can be used after the patient has been adequately treated with paliperidone Sustenna for at least 4 months

Dosing Tips

- With LAIs, the absorption rate constant is slower than the elimination rate constant, thus resulting in "flip-flop" kinetics—i.e., time to steady-state is a function of absorption rate, while concentration at steady-state is a function of elimination rate
- The rate-limiting step for plasma drug levels for LAIs is not drug metabolism, but rather slow absorption from the injection site

- In general, 5 half-lives of any medication are needed to achieve 97% of steady-state levels
- The long half-lives of depot antipsychotics mean that one must either adequately load the dose (if possible) or provide oral supplementation
- The failure to adequately load the dose leads either to prolonged cross-titration from oral antipsychotic or to sub-therapeutic antipsychotic plasma levels for weeks or months in patients who are not receiving (or adhering to) oral supplementation
- Because plasma antipsychotic levels increase gradually over time, dose requirements may ultimately decrease from initial; obtaining periodic plasma levels can be beneficial to prevent unnecessary plasma level creep
- The time to get a blood level for patients receiving LAI is the morning of the day they will receive their next injection
- Kinetics for paliperidone palmitate are determined by particle size: smaller particles (1-month) vs. larger particles (3-month)
- Advantages: no need for oral coverage; 3-month injection schedule with Trinza
- Disadvantages: plasma levels have limited value in guiding treatment

THE ART OF SWITCHING

Switching from Oral Antipsychotics to Paliperidone palmitate (1-Month)

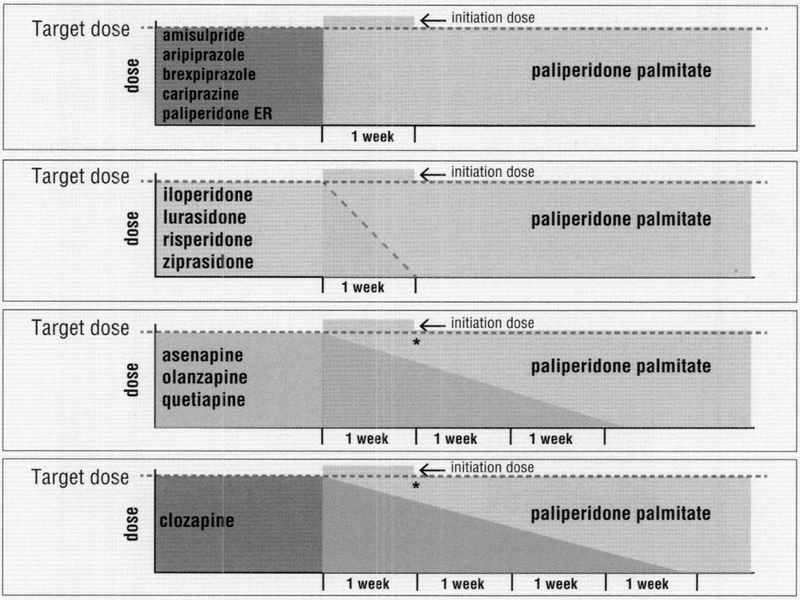

- Discontinuation of oral antipsychotic can begin immediately if adequate loading is pursued
- How to discontinue oral formulations
  - Down-titration is not required for: amisulpride, aripiprazole, brexpiprazole, cariprazine, paliperidone ER
  - 1-week down-titration is required for: iloperidone, lurasidone, risperidone, ziprasidone
  - 3–4-week down-titration is required for: asenapine, olanzapine, quetiapine
  - 4+-week down-titration is required for: clozapine
  - For patients taking benzodiazepine or anticholinergic medication, this can be continued during cross-titration to help alleviate side effects such as insomnia, agitation, and/or psychosis. Once the patient is stable on LAI, these can be tapered one at a time as appropriate.

THE ART OF SWITCHING

Switching from Oral Antipsychotics to Paliperidone ER

- Due to OROS technology, paliperidone ER can be initiated at full desired dose; however, titration over 1–2 weeks may be appropriate for some patients
- With aripiprazole and amisulpride, immediate stop is possible; begin paliperidone ER at an intermediate, or if needed, effective dose
- Risperidone, ziprasidone, iloperidone, and lurasidone can be tapered off over a period of 1 week due to the risk of withdrawal symptoms such as insomnia
- Clinical experience has shown that quetiapine, olanzapine, and asenapine should be tapered off slowly over a period of 3–4 weeks, to allow patients to readapt to the withdrawal of blocking cholinergic, histaminergic, and alpha 1 receptors
- Clozapine should always be tapered off slowly, over a period of 4 weeks or more

* Benzodiazepine or anticholinergic medication can be administered during cross-titration to help alleviate side effects such as insomnia, agitation, and/or psychosis

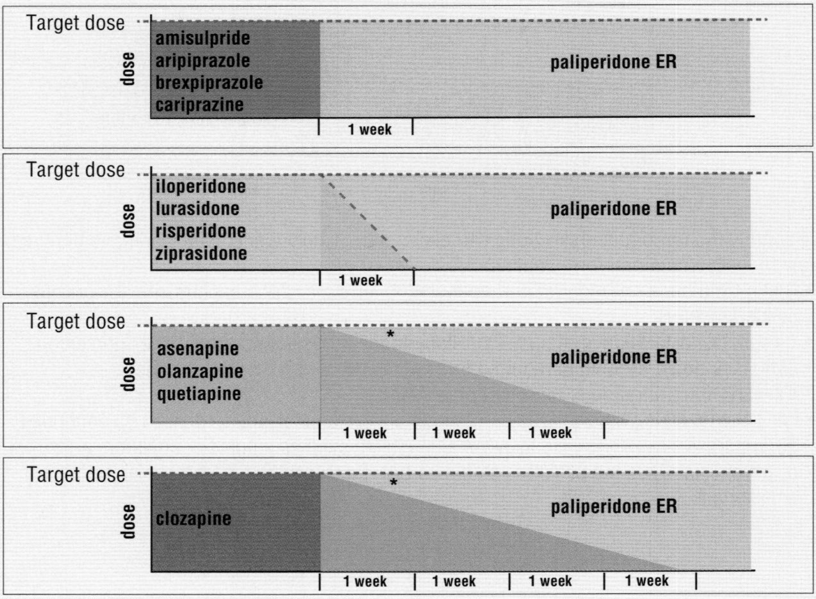

Suggested Reading

Meltzer HY, Bobo WV, Nuamah IF, et al. Efficacy and tolerability of oral paliperidone extended-release tablets in the treatment of acute schizophrenia: pooled data from three 6-week, placebo-controlled studies. J Clin Psychiatry 2008 May;6 e1–e13. [Epub ahead of print]

Nasrallah HA. Atypical antipsychotic-induced metabolic side effects: insights from receptor-binding profiles. Mol Psychiatry 2008;13(1): 27–35.

Nussbaum A, Stroup TS. Paliperidone for schizophrenia. Cochrane Database Syst Rev 2008;16(2):CD006369.

THERAPEUTICS

Brands • Paxil
• Paxil CR

see index for additional brand names

Generic? Yes

Class

- Neuroscience-based Nomenclature: serotonin reuptake inhibitor (S-RI)
- SSRI (selective serotonin reuptake inhibitor); often classified as an antidepressant, but it is not just an antidepressant

Commonly Prescribed for

(bold for FDA approved)

- **Major depressive disorder (paroxetine and paroxetine CR)**
- **Obsessive-compulsive disorder (OCD)**
- **Panic disorder (paroxetine and paroxetine CR)**
- **Social anxiety disorder (social phobia) (paroxetine and paroxetine CR)**
- **Posttraumatic stress disorder (PTSD)**
- **Generalized anxiety disorder (GAD)**
- **Premenstrual dysphoric disorder (PMDD) (paroxetine CR)**
- **Vasomotor symptoms (Brisdelle)**

How the Drug Works

- Boosts neurotransmitter serotonin
- Blocks serotonin reuptake pump (serotonin transporter)
- Desensitizes serotonin receptors, especially serotonin 1A autoreceptors
- Presumably increases serotonergic neurotransmission
- Paroxetine also has mild anticholinergic actions
- Paroxetine may have mild norepinephrine reuptake blocking actions

How Long Until It Works

✻ Some patients may experience relief of insomnia or anxiety early after initiation of treatment

- Onset of therapeutic actions usually not immediate, but often delayed 2–4 weeks
- If it is not working within 6–8 weeks for depression, it may require a dosage increase or it may not work at all
- By contrast, for generalized anxiety, onset of response and increases in remission rates may still occur after 8 weeks of treatment and for up to 6 months after initiating dosing
- May continue to work for many years to prevent relapse of symptoms

If It Works

- The goal of treatment is complete remission of current symptoms as well as prevention of future relapses
- Treatment most often reduces or even eliminates symptoms, but not a cure since symptoms can recur after medicine stopped
- Continue treatment until all symptoms are gone (remission) or significantly reduced (e.g., OCD, PTSD)
- Once symptoms are gone, continue treating for 1 year for the first episode of depression
- For second and subsequent episodes of depression, treatment may need to be indefinite
- Use in anxiety disorders may also need to be indefinite

If It Doesn't Work

- Many patients have only a partial response where some symptoms are improved but others persist (especially insomnia, fatigue, and problems concentrating in depression)
- Other patients may be nonresponders, sometimes called treatment-resistant or treatment-refractory
- Some patients who have an initial response may relapse even though they continue treatment, sometimes called "poop-out"
- Consider increasing dose, switching to another agent or adding an appropriate augmenting agent
- Consider psychotherapy
- Consider evaluation for another diagnosis or for a comorbid condition (e.g., medical illness, substance abuse, etc.)
- Some patients may experience apparent lack of consistent efficacy due to activation of latent or underlying bipolar disorder, and require antidepressant discontinuation and a switch to a mood stabilizer

Best Augmenting Combos for Partial Response or Treatment Resistance

- Trazodone, especially for insomnia
- Bupropion, mirtazapine, reboxetine, or atomoxetine (add with caution and at lower

doses since paroxetine could theoretically raise atomoxetine levels); use combinations of antidepressants with caution as this may activate bipolar disorder and suicidal ideation
- Modafinil, especially for fatigue, sleepiness, and lack of concentration
- Mood stabilizers or atypical antipsychotics for bipolar depression, psychotic depression, treatment-resistant depression, or treatment-resistant anxiety disorders
- Benzodiazepines
- If all else fails for anxiety disorders, consider gabapentin or tiagabine
- Hypnotics for insomnia
- Classically, lithium, buspirone, or thyroid hormone

Tests
- None for healthy individuals

SIDE EFFECTS

How Drug Causes Side Effects
- Theoretically due to increases in serotonin concentrations at serotonin receptors in parts of the brain and body other than those that cause therapeutic actions (e.g., unwanted actions of serotonin in sleep centers causing insomnia, unwanted actions of serotonin in the gut causing diarrhea, etc.)
- Increasing serotonin can cause diminished dopamine release and might contribute to emotional flattening, cognitive slowing, and apathy in some patients
- Most side effects are immediate but often go away with time, in contrast to most therapeutic effects, which are delayed and are enhanced over time

* Paroxetine's weak antimuscarinic properties can cause constipation, dry mouth, sedation

Notable Side Effects
- Sexual dysfunction (dose-dependent; men: delayed ejaculation, erectile dysfunction; men and women: decreased sexual desire, anorgasmia)
- Gastrointestinal (decreased appetite, nausea, diarrhea, constipation, dry mouth)
- Mostly CNS (insomnia but also sedation, agitation, dose-dependent tremors, headache, dizziness)
- Weight gain
- Activation (short-term; patients with diagnosed or undiagnosed bipolar or psychotic disorders may be more vulnerable to CNS-activating actions of SSRIs
- Autonomic (dose-dependent sweating)
- Bruising and rare bleeding
- SIADH (syndrome of inappropriate antidiuretic hormone secretion)

Life-Threatening or Dangerous Side Effects
- Rare seizures
- Rare induction of mania
- Rare activation of suicidal ideation and behavior (suicidality) (short-term studies did not show an increase in the risk of suicidality with antidepressants compared to placebo beyond age 24)

Weight Gain
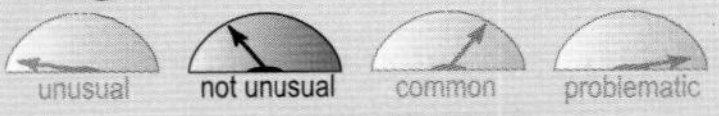

- Occurs in significant minority

Sedation
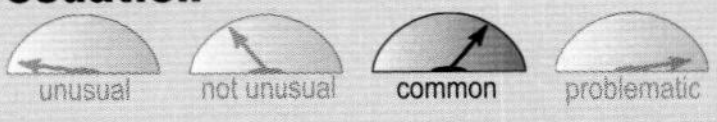

- Many experience and/or can be significant in amount
- Generally transient

What to Do About Side Effects
- Wait
- Wait
- Wait
- If paroxetine is sedating, take at night to reduce daytime drowsiness
- Reduce dose to 5–10 mg (12.5 mg for CR) until side effects abate, then increase as tolerated, usually to at least 20 mg (25 mg CR)
- In a few weeks, switch or add other drugs

Best Augmenting Agents for Side Effects
- Often best to try another SSRI or another antidepressant monotherapy prior to resorting to augmentation strategies to treat side effects
- Trazodone or a hypnotic for insomnia
- Bupropion, sildenafil, vardenafil, or tadalafil for sexual dysfunction

- Bupropion for emotional flattening, cognitive slowing, or apathy
- Mirtazapine for insomnia, agitation, and gastrointestinal side effects
- Benzodiazepines for jitteriness and anxiety, especially at initiation of treatment and especially for anxious patients
- Many side effects are dose-dependent (i.e., they increase as dose increases, or they reemerge until tolerance redevelops)
- Many side effects are time-dependent (i.e., they start immediately upon dosing and upon each dose increase, but go away with time)
- Activation and agitation may represent the induction of a bipolar state, especially a mixed dysphoric bipolar II condition sometimes associated with suicidal ideation, and require the addition of lithium, a mood stabilizer or an atypical antipsychotic, and/or discontinuation of paroxetine

DOSING AND USE

Usual Dosage Range

- Depression: 20–50 mg (25–62.5 mg CR)
- Vasomotor symptoms: 7.5 mg at bedtime

Dosage Forms

- Tablets 10 mg scored, 20 mg scored, 30 mg, 40 mg
- Controlled-release tablets 12.5 mg, 25 mg
- Liquid 10 mg/5mL – 250 mL bottle

How to Dose

- Depression: initial 20 mg (25 mg CR); usually wait a few weeks to assess drug effects before increasing dose, but can increase by 10 mg/day (12.5 mg/day CR) once a week; maximum generally 50 mg/day (62.5 mg/day CR); single dose
- Panic disorder: initial 10 mg/day (12.5 mg/day CR); usually wait a few weeks to assess drug effects before increasing dose, but can increase by 10 mg/day (12.5 mg/day CR) once a week; maximum generally 60 mg/day (75 mg/day CR); single dose
- Social anxiety disorder: initial 20 mg/day (25 mg/day CR); usually wait a few weeks to assess drug effects before increasing dose, but can increase by 10 mg/day (12.5 mg/day CR) once a week; maximum 60 mg/day (75 mg/day CR); single dose
- Other anxiety disorders: initial 20 mg/day (25 mg/day CR); usually wait a few weeks to assess drug effects before increasing dose, but can increase by 10 mg/day (12.5 mg/day CR) once a week; maximum 60 mg/day (75 mg/day CR); single dose

Dosing Tips

- 20-mg tablet is scored, so to save costs, give 10 mg as half of 20-mg tablet, since 10-mg and 20-mg tablets cost about the same in many markets
- Given once daily, often at bedtime, but any time of day tolerated
- 20 mg/day (25 mg/day CR) is often sufficient for patients with social anxiety disorder and depression
- Other anxiety disorders, as well as difficult cases in general, may require higher dosing
- Occasional patients are dosed above 60 mg/day (75 mg/day CR), but this is for experts and requires caution
- If intolerable anxiety, insomnia, agitation, akathisia, or activation occur either upon dosing initiation or discontinuation, consider the possibility of activated bipolar disorder and switch to a mood stabilizer or an atypical antipsychotic
- Liquid formulation easiest for doses below 10 mg when used for cases that are very intolerant to paroxetine or especially for very slow down-titration during discontinuation for patients with withdrawal symptoms
- Paroxetine CR tablets not scored, so chewing or cutting in half can destroy controlled-release properties
- Unlike other SSRIs and antidepressants where dosage increments can be double and triple the starting dose, paroxetine's dosing increments are in 50% increments (i.e., 20, 30, 40; or 25, 37.5, 50 CR)
- Paroxetine inhibits its own metabolism and thus plasma concentrations can double when oral doses increase by 50%; plasma concentrations can increase 2–7-fold when oral doses are doubled

✻ Main advantage of CR is reduced side effects, especially nausea and perhaps sedation, sexual dysfunction, and withdrawal

✻ For patients with severe problems discontinuing paroxetine, dosing may need to be tapered over many months (i.e., reduce dose by 1% every 3 days by crushing tablet and suspending or dissolving in 100 mL of fruit juice and then disposing of 1 mL while drinking the rest; 3–7 days later, dispose of 2 mL, and so on). This is both a form of very slow biological tapering and a form of behavioral desensitization (not for CR)
- For some patients with severe problems discontinuing paroxetine, it may be useful to add an SSRI with a long half-life, especially fluoxetine, prior to taper of paroxetine; while maintaining fluoxetine dosing, first slowly taper paroxetine and then taper fluoxetine
- Be sure to differentiate between reemergence of symptoms requiring reinstitution of treatment and withdrawal symptoms

Overdose
- Rarely lethal in monotherapy overdose; vomiting, sedation, heart rhythm disturbances, dilated pupils, dry mouth

Long-Term Use
- Safe

Habit Forming
- No

How to Stop
- Taper to avoid withdrawal effects (dizziness, nausea, stomach cramps, sweating, tingling, dysesthesias)
- Many patients tolerate 50% dose reduction for 3 days, then another 50% reduction for 3 days, then discontinuation
- If withdrawal symptoms emerge during discontinuation, raise dose to stop symptoms and then restart withdrawal much more slowly

✻ Withdrawal effects can be more common or more severe with paroxetine than with some other SSRIs
- Paroxetine's withdrawal effects may be related in part to the fact that it inhibits its own metabolism
- Thus, when paroxetine is withdrawn, the rate of its decline can be faster as it stops inhibiting its metabolism
- Controlled-release paroxetine may slow the rate of decline and thus reduce withdrawal reactions in some patients
- Readaptation of cholinergic receptors after prolonged blockade may contribute to withdrawal effects of paroxetine

Pharmacokinetics
- Inactive metabolites
- Half-life approximately 24 hours
- Inhibits CYP450 2D6

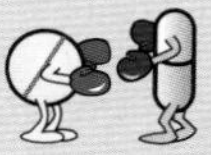

Drug Interactions
- Tramadol increases the risk of seizures in patients taking an antidepressant
- Can increase TCA levels; use with caution with TCAs or when switching from a TCA to paroxetine
- Can cause a fatal "serotonin syndrome" when combined with MAOIs, so do not use with MAOIs or for at least 14 days after MAOIs are stopped
- Do not start an MAOI for at least 5 half-lives (5 to 7 days for most drugs) after discontinuing paroxetine
- May displace highly protein bound drugs (e.g., warfarin)
- There are reports of elevated theophylline levels associated with paroxetine treatment, so it is recommended that theophylline levels be monitored when these drugs are administered together
- May increase anticholinergic effects of procyclidine and other drugs with anticholinergic properties
- Can rarely cause weakness, hyperreflexia, and incoordination when combined with sumatriptan or possibly with other triptans, requiring careful monitoring of patient
- Possible increased risk of bleeding, especially when combined with anticoagulants (e.g., warfarin, NSAIDs)
- NSAIDs may impair effectiveness of SSRIs
- Via CYP450 2D6 inhibition, paroxetine could theoretically interfere with the analgesic actions of codeine, and increase the plasma levels of some beta blockers and of atomoxetine
- Via CYP450 2D6 inhibition, paroxetine could theoretically increase concentrations of thioridazine and cause dangerous cardiac arrhythmias

- Paroxetine increases pimozide levels, and pimozide prolongs QT interval, so concomitant use of pimozide and paroxetine is contraindicated

Other Warnings/ Precautions

- Add or initiate other antidepressants with caution for up to 2 weeks after discontinuing paroxetine
- Use with caution in patients with history of seizures
- Use with caution in patients with bipolar disorder unless treated with concomitant mood-stabilizing agent
- When treating children, carefully weigh the risks and benefits of pharmacological treatment against the risks and benefits of nontreatment with antidepressants and make sure to document this in the patient's chart
- Distribute the brochures provided by the FDA and the drug companies
- Warn patients and their caregivers about the possibility of activating side effects and advise them to report such symptoms immediately
- Monitor patients for activation of suicidal ideation, especially children and adolescents

Do Not Use

- If patient is taking an MAOI
- If patient is taking thioridazine
- If patient is taking pimozide
- If patient is taking tamoxifen
- If there is a proven allergy to paroxetine

SPECIAL POPULATIONS

Renal Impairment

- Lower dose [initial 10 mg/day (12.5 mg CR), maximum 40 mg/day (50 mg/day CR)]

Hepatic Impairment

- Lower dose [initial 10 mg/day (12.5 mg CR), maximum 40 mg/day (50 mg/day CR)]

Cardiac Impairment

- Preliminary research suggests that paroxetine is safe in these patients
- Treating depression with SSRIs in patients with acute angina or following myocardial infarction may reduce cardiac events and improve survival as well as mood

Elderly

- Lower dose [initial 10 mg/day (12.5 mg CR), maximum 40 mg/day (50 mg/day CR)]
- Risk of SIADH with SSRIs is higher in the elderly
- Reduction in the risk of suicidality with antidepressants compared to placebo in adults age 65 and older

Children and Adolescents

- Carefully weigh the risks and benefits of pharmacological treatment against the risks and benefits of nontreatment with antidepressants and make sure to document this in the patient's chart
- Monitor patients face-to-face regularly, particularly during the first several weeks of treatment
- Use with caution, observing for activation of known or unknown bipolar disorder and/or suicidal ideation, and inform parents or guardians of this risk so they can help observe child or adolescent patients
- Not specifically approved, but preliminary evidence suggests efficacy in children and adolescents with OCD, social phobia, or depression

Pregnancy

- Effective June 30, 2015, the US FDA requires changes to the content and format of pregnancy and lactation information in prescription drug labels, including the elimination of the pregnancy letter categories; the Pregnancy and Lactation Labeling Rule (PLLR or final rule) applies only to prescription drugs and will be phased in gradually for drugs approved on or after June 30, 2001
- Not generally recommended for use during pregnancy, especially during first trimester
- Epidemiological data have shown an increased risk of cardiovascular malformations (primarily ventricular and atrial septal defects) in infants born to women who took paroxetine during the first trimester (absolute risk is small)

- Unless the benefits of paroxetine to the mother justify continuing treatment, consider discontinuing paroxetine or switching to another antidepressant
- Paroxetine use late in pregnancy may be associated with higher risk of neonatal complications, including respiratory distress
- At delivery there may be more bleeding in the mother and transient irritability or sedation in the newborn
- Must weigh the risk of treatment (first trimester fetal development, third trimester newborn delivery) to the child against the risk of no treatment (recurrence of depression, maternal health, infant bonding) to the mother and child
- For many patients this may mean continuing treatment during pregnancy
- SSRI use beyond the 20th week of pregnancy may be associated with increased risk of pulmonary hypertension in newborns, although this is not proven
- Exposure to SSRIs late in pregnancy may be associated with increased risk of gestational hypertension and preeclampsia
- Neonates exposed to SSRIs or SNRIs late in the third trimester have developed complications requiring prolonged hospitalization, respiratory support, and tube feeding; reported symptoms are consistent with either a direct toxic effect of SSRIs and SNRIs or, possibly, a drug discontinuation syndrome, and include respiratory distress, cyanosis, apnea, seizures, temperature instability, feeding difficulty, vomiting, hypoglycemia, hypotonia, hypertonia, hyperreflexia, tremor, jitteriness, irritability, and constant crying

Breast Feeding

- Some drug is found in mother's breast milk
- Trace amounts may be present in nursing children whose mothers are on paroxetine
- If child becomes irritable or sedated, breast feeding or drug may need to be discontinued
- Immediate postpartum period is a high-risk time for depression, especially in women who have had prior depressive episodes, so drug may need to be reinstituted late in the third trimester or shortly after childbirth to prevent a recurrence during the postpartum period
- Must weigh benefits of breast feeding with risks and benefits of antidepressant treatment versus nontreatment to both the infant and the mother
- For many patients, this may mean continuing treatment during breast feeding

THE ART OF PSYCHOPHARMACOLOGY

Potential Advantages

- Patients with anxiety disorders and insomnia
- Patients with mixed anxiety/depression

Potential Disadvantages

- Patients with hypersomnia
- Alzheimer/cognitive disorders
- Patients with psychomotor retardation, fatigue, and low energy

Primary Target Symptoms

- Depressed mood
- Anxiety
- Sleep disturbance, especially insomnia
- Panic attacks, avoidant behavior, re-experiencing, hyperarousal

Pearls

✱ Often a preferred treatment of anxious depression as well as major depressive disorder comorbid with anxiety disorders

✱ Withdrawal effects may be more likely than for some other SSRIs when discontinued (especially akathisia, restlessness, gastrointestinal symptoms, dizziness, tingling, dysesthesias, nausea, stomach cramps, restlessness)

- Inhibits own metabolism, so dosing is not linear

✱ Paroxetine has mild anticholinergic actions that can enhance the rapid onset of anxiolytic and hypnotic efficacy but also cause mild anticholinergic side effects

- Can cause cognitive and affective "flattening"
- May be less activating than other SSRIs
- Paroxetine is a potent CYP450 2D6 inhibitor
- SSRIs may be less effective in women over 50, especially if they are not taking estrogen

- SSRIs may be useful for hot flushes in perimenopausal women
- Some anecdotal reports suggest greater weight gain and sexual dysfunction than some other SSRIs, but the clinical significance of this is unknown
- For sexual dysfunction, can augment with bupropion, sildenafil, tadalafil, or switch to a non-SSRI such as bupropion or mirtazapine
- Some postmenopausal women's depression will respond better to paroxetine plus estrogen augmentation than to paroxetine alone
- Nonresponse to paroxetine in elderly may require consideration of mild cognitive impairment or Alzheimer disease
- CR formulation may enhance tolerability, especially for nausea
- Can be better tolerated than some SSRIs for patients with anxiety and insomnia and can reduce these symptoms early in dosing

Suggested Reading

Bourin M, Chue P, Guillon Y. Paroxetine: a review. CNS Drug Rev 2001;7:25–47.

Gibiino S, Serretti A. Paroxetine for the treatment of depression: a critical update. Expert Opin Pharmacother 2012;13(3):421–31.

Green B. Focus on paroxetine. Curr Med Res Opin 2003;19:13–21.

Wagstaff AJ, Cheer SM, Matheson AJ, Ormrod D, Goa KL. Paroxetine: an update of its use in psychiatric disorders in adults. Drugs 2002;62:655–703.

PEROSPIRONE

THERAPEUTICS

Brands • Lullan

see index for additional brand names

Generic? No

Class

- Neuroscience-based Nomenclature: dopamine and serotonin receptor antagonist (DS-RAn)
- Atypical antipsychotic (serotonin-dopamine antagonist, second generation antipsychotic)

Commonly Prescribed for

(bold for FDA approved)

- Schizophrenia (Japan)

How the Drug Works

- Blocks dopamine 2 receptors, reducing positive symptoms of psychosis
- Blocks serotonin 2A receptors, causing enhancement of dopamine release in certain brain regions and thus reducing motor side effects and possibly improving cognitive and affective symptoms

✻ Interactions at 5HT1A receptors may contribute to efficacy for cognitive and affective symptoms in some patients

How Long Until It Works

- Psychotic symptoms can improve within 1 week, but it may take several weeks for full effect on behavior as well as on cognition and affective stabilization
- Classically recommended to wait at least 4–6 weeks to determine efficacy of drug, but in practice some patients require up to 16–20 weeks to show a good response, especially on cognitive symptoms

If It Works

- Most often reduces positive symptoms in schizophrenia but does not eliminate them
- Can improve negative symptoms, as well as aggressive, cognitive, and affective symptoms in schizophrenia
- Most schizophrenic patients do not have a total remission of symptoms but rather a reduction of symptoms by about a third
- Perhaps 5–15% of schizophrenic patients can experience an overall improvement of greater than 50–60%, especially when receiving stable treatment for more than a year
- Such patients are considered super-responders or "awakeners" since they may be well enough to be employed, live independently, and sustain long-term relationships
- Continue treatment until reaching a plateau of improvement
- After reaching a satisfactory plateau, continue treatment for at least a year after first episode of psychosis
- For second and subsequent episodes of psychosis, treatment may need to be indefinite
- Even for first episodes of psychosis, it may be preferable to continue treatment

If It Doesn't Work

- Consider trying one of the first-line atypical antipsychotics (e.g., risperidone, olanzapine, quetiapine, aripiprazole, paliperidone, asenapine, iloperidone, lurasidone)
- If 2 or more antipsychotic monotherapies do not work, consider clozapine
- If no first-line atypical antipsychotic is effective, consider higher doses or augmentation with valproate or lamotrigine
- Some patients may require treatment with a conventional antipsychotic
- Consider noncompliance and switch to another antipsychotic with fewer side effects or to an antipsychotic that can be given by depot injection
- Consider initiating rehabilitation and psychotherapy such as cognitive remediation
- Consider presence of concomitant drug abuse

Best Augmenting Combos for Partial Response or Treatment Resistance

- Augmentation of perospirone has not been systematically studied
- Addition of a benzodiazepine, especially short-term for agitation
- Addition of a mood-stabilizing anticonvulsant such as valproate, carbamazepine, or lamotrigine may theoretically be helpful in both schizophrenia and bipolar mania
- Augmentation with lithium in bipolar mania may be helpful

Tests

✱ Potential of weight gain, diabetes, and dyslipidemia associated with perospirone has not been systematically studied, but patients should be monitored the same as for other atypical antipsychotics

Before starting an atypical antipsychotic

✱ Weigh all patients and track BMI during treatment
- Get baseline personal and family history of diabetes, obesity, dyslipidemia, hypertension, and cardiovascular disease

✱ Get waist circumference (at umbilicus), blood pressure, fasting plasma glucose, and fasting lipid profile
- Determine if patient is
  - overweight (BMI 25.0–29.9)
  - obese (BMI ≥30)
  - has pre-diabetes (fasting plasma glucose 100–125 mg/dL)
  - has diabetes (fasting plasma glucose >126 mg/dL)
  - has hypertension (BP >140/90 mm Hg)
  - has dyslipidemia (increased total cholesterol, LDL cholesterol, and triglycerides; decreased HDL cholesterol)
- Treat or refer such patients for treatment, including nutrition and weight management, physical activity counseling, smoking cessation, and medical management

Monitoring after starting an atypical antipsychotic

✱ BMI monthly for 3 months, then quarterly

✱ Consider monitoring fasting triglycerides monthly for several months in patients at high risk for metabolic complications and when initiating or switching antipsychotics

✱ Blood pressure, fasting plasma glucose, fasting lipids within 3 months and then annually, but earlier and more frequently for patients with diabetes or who have gained >5% of initial weight
- Treat or refer for treatment and consider switching to another atypical antipsychotic for patients who become overweight, obese, pre-diabetic, diabetic, hypertensive, or dyslipidemic while receiving an atypical antipsychotic

✱ Even in patients without known diabetes, be vigilant for the rare but life-threatening onset of diabetic ketoacidosis, which always requires immediate treatment, by monitoring for the rapid onset of polyuria, polydipsia, weight loss, nausea, vomiting, dehydration, rapid respiration, weakness, and clouding of sensorium, even coma
- Should check blood pressure in the elderly before starting and for the first few weeks of treatment
- Patients with low white blood cell count (WBC) or history of drug-induced leucopenia/neutropenia should have complete blood count (CBC) monitored frequently during the first few months and perospirone should be discontinued at the first sign of decline of WBC in the absence of other causative factors

SIDE EFFECTS

How Drug Causes Side Effects

- By blocking dopamine 2 receptors in the striatum, it can cause motor side effects
- By blocking dopamine 2 receptors in the pituitary, it can cause increased prolactin (unusual)
- Mechanism of weight gain and increased incidence of diabetes and dyslipidemia with some atypical antipsychotics is unknown
- Receptor binding portfolio of perospirone is not well characterized

Notable Side Effects

✱ Extrapyramidal symptoms, akathisia

✱ Insomnia
- Sedation, anxiety, weakness, headache, anorexia, constipation
- Theoretically, tardive dyskinesia (should be reduced risk compared to conventional antipsychotics)
- Elevated creatine phosphokinase levels

Life-Threatening or Dangerous Side Effects

- Rare neuroleptic malignant syndrome
- Theoretically, seizures are rarely associated with atypical antipsychotics
- Increased risk of death and cerebrovascular events in elderly patients with dementia-related psychosis

Weight Gain

✱ Not well characterized

Sedation

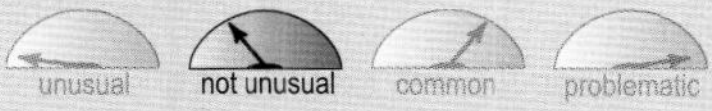

- Occurs in significant minority

What to Do About Side Effects

- Wait
- Wait
- Wait
- For motor symptoms, add an anticholinergic agent
- Reduce the dose
- Switch to another atypical antipsychotic

Best Augmenting Agents for Side Effects

- Benztropine or trihexyphenidyl for motor side effects
- Sometimes amantadine can be helpful for motor side effects
- Benzodiazepines may be helpful for akathisia
- Many side effects cannot be improved with an augmenting agent

DOSING AND USE

Usual Dosage Range

- 8–48 mg/day in 3 divided doses

Dosage Forms

- Tablet 4 mg, 8 mg

How to Dose

- Begin at 4 mg 3 times a day, increasing as tolerated up to 16 mg 3 times a day

Dosing Tips

- Some patients have been treated with up to 96 mg/day in 3 divided doses
- Unknown whether dosing frequency can be reduced to once or twice daily, but by analogy with other agents in this class with half-lives shorter than 24 hours, this may be possible
- Treatment should be suspended if absolute neutrophil count falls below 1,000/mm^3

Overdose

- Not reported

Long-Term Use

- Long-term studies not reported, but as for other atypical antipsychotics, long-term use for treatment of schizophrenia is common

Habit Forming

- No

How to Stop

- Slow down-titration (over 6–8 weeks), especially when simultaneously beginning a new antipsychotic while switching (i.e., cross-titration)
- Rapid discontinuation may lead to rebound psychosis and worsening of symptoms
- If antiparkinson agents are being used, they should be continued for a few weeks after perospirone is discontinued

Pharmacokinetics

- Metabolized primarily by CYP450 3A4
- No active metabolites

Drug Interactions

- Ketaconazole and possibly other CYP450 3A4 inhibitors such as nefazodone, fluvoxamine, and fluoxetine may increase plasma levels of perospirone
- Carbamazepine and possibly other inducers of CYP450 3A4 may decrease plasma levels of perospirone

Other Warnings/ Precautions

- Not reported

Do Not Use

- If there is a proven allergy to perospirone

SPECIAL POPULATIONS

Renal Impairment

- Use with caution

Hepatic Impairment

- Use with caution

Cardiac Impairment

- Use with caution

Elderly
- Some patients may tolerate lower doses better
- Although atypical antipsychotics are commonly used for behavioral disturbances in dementia, no agent has been approved for treatment of elderly patients with dementia-related psychosis
- Elderly patients with dementia-related psychosis treated with atypical antipsychotics are at an increased risk of death compared to placebo, and also have an increased risk of cerebrovascular events

Children and Adolescents
- Use with caution

Pregnancy
- There is a risk of abnormal muscle movements and withdrawal symptoms in newborns whose mothers took an antipsychotic during the third trimester; symptoms may include agitation, abnormally increased or decreased muscle tone, tremor, sleepiness, severe difficulty breathing, and difficulty feeding
- Psychotic symptoms may worsen during pregnancy and some form of treatment may be necessary

Breast Feeding
- Unknown if perospirone is secreted in human breast milk, but all psychotropics assumed to be secreted in breast milk
- * Recommended either to discontinue drug or bottle feed
- Infants of women who choose to breast feed should be monitored for possible adverse effects

THE ART OF PSYCHOPHARMACOLOGY

Potential Advantages
- In Japan, studies suggest efficacy for negative symptoms of schizophrenia

Potential Disadvantages
- Patients who have difficulty complying with three times daily administration

Primary Target Symptoms
- Positive symptoms of psychosis
- Negative symptoms of psychosis
- Affective symptoms (depression, anxiety)
- Cognitive symptoms

Pearls
- Extrapyramidal symptoms may be more frequent than with some other atypical antipsychotics
- Potent 5HT1A binding properties may be helpful for improving cognitive symptoms of schizophrenia in long-term treatment
- Theoretically, should be effective in acute bipolar mania

Suggested Reading
Ohno Y. Pharmacological characteristics of perospirone hydrochloride, a novel antipsychotic agent. Nippon Yakurigaku Zasshi 2000;116(4):225–31.

THERAPEUTICS

Brands • Trilafon

see index for additional brand names

Generic? Yes

Class

- Neuroscience-based Nomenclature: dopamine receptor antagonist (D-RAn)
- Conventional antipsychotic (neuroleptic, phenothiazine, dopamine 2 antagonist, antiemetic)

Commonly Prescribed for

(bold for FDA approved)

- **Schizophrenia**
- **Nausea, vomiting**
- Other psychotic disorders
- Bipolar disorder

How the Drug Works

- Blocks dopamine 2 receptors, reducing positive symptoms of psychosis
- Combination of dopamine D2, histamine H1, and cholinergic M1 blockade in the vomiting center may reduce nausea and vomiting

How Long Until It Works

- Psychotic symptoms can improve within 1 week, but may take several weeks for full effect on behavior
- Injection: initial effect after 10 minutes, peak after 1–2 hours
- Actions on nausea and vomiting are immediate

If It Works

- Most often reduces positive symptoms in schizophrenia but does not eliminate them
- Most schizophrenic patients do not have a total remission of symptoms but rather a reduction of symptoms by about a third
- Continue treatment in schizophrenia until reaching a plateau of improvement
- After reaching a satisfactory plateau, continue treatment for at least a year after first episode of psychosis in schizophrenia
- For second and subsequent episodes of psychosis in schizophrenia, treatment may need to be indefinite
- Reduces symptoms of acute psychotic mania but not proven as a mood stabilizer or as an effective maintenance treatment in bipolar disorder
- After reducing acute psychotic symptoms in mania, switch to a mood stabilizer and/or an atypical antipsychotic for mood stabilization and maintenance

If It Doesn't Work

- Consider trying one of the first-line atypical antipsychotics (risperidone, olanzapine, quetiapine, ziprasidone, aripiprazole, paliperidone, amisulpride, asenapine, iloperidone, lurasidone)
- Consider trying another conventional antipsychotic
- If 2 or more antipsychotic monotherapies do not work, consider clozapine

Best Augmenting Combos for Partial Response or Treatment Resistance

- Augmentation of conventional antipsychotics has not been systematically studied
- Addition of a mood-stabilizing anticonvulsant such as valproate, carbamazepine, or lamotrigine may be helpful in both schizophrenia and bipolar mania
- Augmentation with lithium in bipolar mania may be helpful
- Addition of a benzodiazepine, especially short-term for agitation

Tests

❋ Since conventional antipsychotics are frequently associated with weight gain, before starting treatment, weigh all patients and determine if the patient is already overweight (BMI 25.0–29.9) or obese (BMI ≥30)

- Before giving a drug that can cause weight gain to an overweight or obese patient, consider determining whether the patient already has pre-diabetes (fasting plasma glucose 100–125 mg/dL), diabetes (fasting plasma glucose >126 mg/dL), or dyslipidemia (increased total cholesterol, LDL cholesterol, and triglycerides; decreased HDL cholesterol), and treat or refer such patients for treatment, including nutrition and weight management, physical activity counseling, smoking cessation, and medical management

❋ Monitor weight and BMI during treatment

* Consider monitoring fasting triglycerides monthly for several months in patients at high risk for metabolic complications and when initiating or switching antipsychotics
* While giving a drug to a patient who has gained >5% of initial weight, consider evaluating for the presence of pre-diabetes, diabetes, or dyslipidemia, or consider switching to a different antipsychotic
- Should check blood pressure in the elderly before starting and for the first few weeks of treatment
- Monitoring elevated prolactin levels of dubious clinical benefit
- Phenothiazines may cause false-positive phenylketonuria results
- Patients with low white blood cell count (WBC) or history of drug-induced leucopenia/neutropenia should have complete blood count (CBC) monitored frequently during the first few months and perphenazine should be discontinued at the first sign of decline of WBC in the absence of other causative factors

SIDE EFFECTS

How Drug Causes Side Effects

- By blocking dopamine 2 receptors in the striatum, it can cause motor side effects
- By blocking dopamine 2 receptors in the pituitary, it can cause elevations in prolactin
- By blocking dopamine 2 receptors excessively in the mesocortical and mesolimbic dopamine pathways, especially at high doses, it can cause worsening of negative and cognitive symptoms (neuroleptic-induced deficit syndrome)
- Anticholinergic actions may cause sedation, blurred vision, constipation, dry mouth
- Antihistaminic actions may cause sedation, weight gain
- By blocking alpha 1 adrenergic receptors, it can cause dizziness, sedation, and hypotension
- Mechanism of weight gain and any possible increased incidence of diabetes or dyslipidemia with conventional antipsychotics is unknown

Notable Side Effects

* Neuroleptic-induced deficit syndrome
* Akathisia
* Extrapyramidal symptoms, parkinsonism, tardive dyskinesia
* Galactorrhea, amenorrhea
- Dizziness, sedation
- Dry mouth, constipation, urinary retention, blurred vision
- Decreased sweating
- Sexual dysfunction
- Hypotension, tachycardia, syncope
- Weight gain

Life-Threatening or Dangerous Side Effects

- Rare neuroleptic malignant syndrome
- Rare jaundice, agranulocytosis
- Rare seizures
- Increased risk of death and cerebrovascular events in elderly patients with dementia-related psychosis

Weight Gain

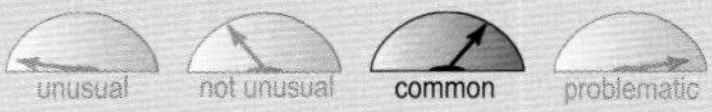

- Many experience and/or can be significant in amount

Sedation

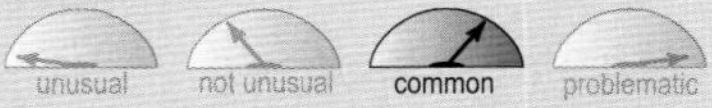

- Many experience and/or can be significant in amount
- Sedation is usually transient

What to Do About Side Effects

- Wait
- Wait
- Wait
- For motor symptoms, add an anticholinergic agent
- Reduce the dose
- For sedation, give at night
- Switch to an atypical antipsychotic
- Weight loss, exercise programs, and medical management for high BMIs, diabetes, dyslipidemia

Best Augmenting Agents for Side Effects

- Benztropine or trihexyphenidyl for motor side effects
- Sometimes amantadine can be helpful for motor side effects

- Benzodiazepines may be helpful for akathisia
- Many side effects cannot be improved with an augmenting agent

DOSING AND USE

Usual Dosage Range

- Psychosis: oral: 12–24 mg/day; 16–64 mg/day in hospitalized patients
- Nausea/vomiting: 8–16 mg/day oral, 5 mg intramuscularly

Dosage Forms

- Tablet 2 mg, 4 mg, 8 mg, 16 mg
- Injection 5 mg/mL

How to Dose

- Oral: psychosis: 4–8 mg 3 times a day; 8–16 mg 2 times a day to 4 times a day in hospitalized patients; maximum 64 mg/day
- Oral: nausea/vomiting: 8–16 mg/day in divided doses; maximum 24 mg/day
- Intramuscular: psychosis: initial 5 mg; can repeat every 6 hours; maximum 15 mg/day (30 mg/day in hospitalized patients)

Dosing Tips

- Injection contains sulfites that may cause allergic reactions, particularly in patients with asthma
- Oral perphenazine is less potent than the injection, so patients should receive equal or higher dosage when switched from injection to tablet
- Treatment should be suspended if absolute neutrophil count falls below 1,000/mm^3

Overdose

- Extrapyramidal symptoms, coma, hypotension, sedation, seizures, respiratory depression

Long-Term Use

- Some side effects may be irreversible (e.g., tardive dyskinesia)

Habit Forming

- No

How to Stop

- Slow down-titration of oral formulation (over 6–8 weeks), especially when simultaneously beginning a new antipsychotic while switching (i.e., cross-titration)
- Rapid oral discontinuation may lead to rebound psychosis and worsening of symptoms
- If antiparkinson agents are being used, they should be continued for a few weeks after perphenazine is discontinued

Pharmacokinetics

- Half-life approximately 9.5 hours

Drug Interactions

- May decrease the effects of levodopa, dopamine agonists
- May increase the effects of antihypertensive drugs except for guanethidine, whose antihypertensive actions perphenazine may antagonize
- Additive effects may occur if used with CNS depressants
- Anticholinergic effects may occur if used with atropine or related compounds
- Some patients taking a neuroleptic and lithium have developed an encephalopathic syndrome similar to neuroleptic malignant syndrome
- Epinephrine may lower blood pressure; diuretics and alcohol may increase risk of hypotension

Other Warnings/ Precautions

- If signs of neuroleptic malignant syndrome develop, treatment should be immediately discontinued
- Use cautiously in patients with respiratory disorders
- Use cautiously in patients with alcohol withdrawal or convulsive disorders because of possible lowering of seizure threshold
- Do not use epinephrine in event of overdose as interaction with some pressor agents may lower blood pressure
- Avoid undue exposure to sunlight
- Avoid extreme heat exposure
- Use with caution in patients with respiratory disorders, glaucoma, or urinary retention
- Antiemetic effect of perphenazine may mask signs of other disorders or overdose;

suppression of cough reflex may cause asphyxia
- Observe for signs of ocular toxicity (corneal and lenticular deposits)
- Use only with caution if at all in Parkinson's disease or Lewy body dementia

Do Not Use
- If patient is in a comatose state or has CNS depression
- If there is the presence of blood dyscrasias, subcortical brain damage, bone marrow depression, or liver disease
- If there is a proven allergy to perphenazine
- If there is a known sensitivity to any phenothiazine

SPECIAL POPULATIONS

Renal Impairment
- Use with caution

Hepatic Impairment
- Use with caution; may not be recommended as long-term treatment because perphenazine may increase risk of further liver damage

Cardiac Impairment
- Cardiovascular toxicity can occur, especially orthostatic hypotension

Elderly
- Lower doses should be used and patient should be monitored closely
- Although conventional antipsychotics are commonly used for behavioral disturbances in dementia, no agent has been approved for treatment of elderly patients with dementia-related psychosis
- Elderly patients with dementia-related psychosis treated with antipsychotics are at an increased risk of death compared to placebo, and also have an increased risk of cerebrovascular events

Children and Adolescents
- Not recommended for use in children under age 12
- Over age 12: if given intramuscularly, should receive lowest adult dose
- Generally consider second-line after atypical antipsychotics

Pregnancy
- Effective June 30, 2015, the US FDA requires changes to the content and format of pregnancy and lactation information in prescription drug labels, including the elimination of the pregnancy letter categories; the Pregnancy and Lactation Labeling Rule (PLLR or final rule) applies only to prescription drugs and will be phased in gradually for drugs approved on or after June 30, 2001
- Controlled studies have not been conducted in pregnant women
- There is a risk of abnormal muscle movements and withdrawal symptoms in newborns whose mothers took an antipsychotic during the third trimester; symptoms may include agitation, abnormally increased or decreased muscle tone, tremor, sleepiness, severe difficulty breathing, and difficulty feeding
- Reports of extrapyramidal symptoms, jaundice, hyperreflexia, hyporeflexia in infants whose mothers took a phenothiazine during pregnancy
- Perphenazine should only be used during pregnancy if clearly needed
- Psychotic symptoms may worsen during pregnancy and some form of treatment may be necessary
- Atypical antipsychotics may be preferable to conventional antipsychotics or anticonvulsant mood stabilizers if treatment is required during pregnancy

Breast Feeding
- Unknown if perphenazine is secreted in human breast milk, but all psychotropics assumed to be secreted in breast milk

✻ Recommended either to discontinue drug or bottle feed

THE ART OF PSYCHOPHARMACOLOGY

Potential Advantages
- Intramuscular formulation for emergency use

Potential Disadvantages
- Patients with tardive dyskinesia
- Children
- Elderly

Primary Target Symptoms

- Positive symptoms of psychosis
- Motor and autonomic hyperactivity
- Violent or aggressive behavior

Pearls

- Recent landmark head-to-head study in schizophrenia suggests comparable effectiveness with some atypical antipsychotics
- Perphenazine is a higher potency phenothiazine
- Less risk of sedation and orthostatic hypotension but greater risk of extrapyramidal symptoms than with low potency phenothiazines
- Patients have very similar antipsychotic responses to any conventional antipsychotic, which is different from atypical antipsychotics where antipsychotic responses of individual patients can occasionally vary greatly from one atypical antipsychotic to another
- Patients with inadequate responses to atypical antipsychotics may benefit from a trial of augmentation with a conventional antipsychotic such as perphenazine or from switching to a conventional antipsychotic such as perphenazine
- However, long-term polypharmacy with a combination of a conventional antipsychotic such as perphenazine with an atypical antipsychotic may combine their side effects without clearly augmenting the efficacy of either
- For treatment-resistant patients, especially those with impulsivity, aggression, violence, and self-harm, long-term polypharmacy with 2 atypical antipsychotics or with 1 atypical antipsychotic and 1 conventional antipsychotic may be useful or even necessary while closely monitoring
- In such cases, it may be beneficial to combine 1 depot antipsychotic with 1 oral antipsychotic
- Although a frequent practice by some prescribers, adding 2 conventional antipsychotics together has little rationale and may reduce tolerability without clearly enhancing efficacy
- Availability of alternative treatments and risk of tardive dyskinesia make utilization of perphenazine for nausea and vomiting a short-term and second-line treatment option

Suggested Reading

David A, Quraishi S, Rathbone J. Depot perphenazine decanoate and enanthate for schizophrenia. Cochrane Database Syst Rev 2005;20(3):CD001717.

Dencker SJ, Gios I, Martensson E, et al. A long-term cross-over pharmacokinetic study comparing perphenazine decanoate and haloperidol decanoate in schizophrenic patients. Psychopharmacology (Berl) 1994;114:24–30.

Frankenburg FR. Choices in antipsychotic therapy in schizophrenia. Harv Rev Psychiatry 1999;6:241–9.

Lieberman JA, Stroup TS, McEvoy JP, et al. Effectiveness of antipsychotic drugs in patients with chronic schizophrenia. N Engl J Med 2005;353(12):1209–23.

Quraishi S, David A. Depot perphenazine decanoate and enanthate for schizophrenia. Cochrane Database Syst Rev 2000;(2):CD001717.

THERAPEUTICS

Brands • Nardil
• Nardelzine

see index for additional brand names

Generic? Yes

Class

- Neuroscience-based Nomenclature: serotonin, norepinephrine, dopamine enzyme inhibitor (SN-EI)
- Monoamine oxidase inhibitor (MAOI)

Commonly Prescribed for

(bold for FDA approved)

- **Depressed patients characterized as "atypical," "nonendogenous," or "neurotic"**
- Treatment-resistant depression
- Treatment-resistant panic disorder
- Treatment-resistant social anxiety disorder

How the Drug Works

- Irreversibly blocks monoamine oxidase (MAO) from breaking down norepinephrine, serotonin, and dopamine
- This presumably boosts noradrenergic, serotonergic, and dopaminergic neurotransmission

How Long Until It Works

- Onset of therapeutic actions usually not immediate, but often delayed 2–4 weeks
- If it is not working within 6–8 weeks, it may require a dosage increase or it may not work at all
- May continue to work for many years to prevent relapse of symptoms

If It Works

- The goal of treatment is complete remission of current symptoms as well as prevention of future relapses
- Treatment most often reduces or even eliminates symptoms, but not a cure since symptoms can recur after medicine stopped
- Continue treatment until all symptoms are gone (remission)
- Once symptoms gone, continue treating for 1 year for the first episode of depression
- For second and subsequent episodes of depression, treatment may need to be indefinite
- Use in anxiety disorders may also need to be indefinite

If It Doesn't Work

- Many patients have only a partial response where some symptoms are improved but others persist (especially insomnia, fatigue, and problems concentrating)
- Other patients may be nonresponders, sometimes called treatment-resistant or treatment-refractory
- Some patients who have an initial response may relapse even though they continue treatment, sometimes called "poop-out"
- Consider increasing dose, switching to another agent, or adding an appropriate augmenting agent
- Consider psychotherapy
- Consider evaluation for another diagnosis or for a comorbid condition (e.g., medical illness, substance abuse, etc.)
- Some patients may experience apparent lack of consistent efficacy due to activation of latent or underlying bipolar disorder, and require antidepressant discontinuation and a switch to a mood stabilizer

Best Augmenting Combos for Partial Response or Treatment Resistance

✽ Augmentation of MAOIs has not been systematically studied, and this is something for the expert, to be done with caution and with careful monitoring

✽ A stimulant such as d-amphetamine or methylphenidate (with caution; may activate bipolar disorder and suicidal ideation; may elevate blood pressure)

- Lithium
- Mood-stabilizing anticonvulsants
- Atypical antipsychotics (with special caution for those agents with monoamine reuptake blocking properties, such as ziprasidone and zotepine)

Tests

- Patients should be monitored for changes in blood pressure
- Patients receiving high doses or long-term treatment should have hepatic function evaluated periodically

✽ Since MAOIs are frequently associated with weight gain, before starting treatment, weigh all patients and determine if

the patient is already overweight (BMI 25.0–29.9) or obese (BMI ≥30)
- Before giving a drug that can cause weight gain to an overweight or obese patient, consider determining whether the patient already has pre-diabetes (fasting plasma glucose 100–125 mg/dL), diabetes (fasting plasma glucose >126 mg/dL), or dyslipidemia (increased total cholesterol, LDL cholesterol, and triglycerides; decreased HDL cholesterol), and treat or refer such patients for treatment, including nutrition and weight management, physical activity counseling, smoking cessation, and medical management

✻ Monitor weight and BMI during treatment

✻ While giving a drug to a patient who has gained >5% of initial weight, consider evaluating for the presence of pre-diabetes, diabetes, or dyslipidemia, or consider switching to a different antidepressant

SIDE EFFECTS

How Drug Causes Side Effects
- Theoretically due to increases in monoamines in parts of the brain and body and at receptors other than those that cause therapeutic actions (e.g., unwanted actions of serotonin in sleep centers causing insomnia, unwanted actions of norepinephrine on vascular smooth muscle causing changes in blood pressure, etc.)
- Side effects are generally immediate, but immediate side effects often disappear in time

Notable Side Effects
- Dizziness, sedation, headache, sleep disturbances, fatigue, weakness, tremor, movement problems, blurred vision, increased sweating
- Constipation, dry mouth, nausea, change in appetite, weight gain
- Sexual dysfunction
- Orthostatic hypotension (dose-related); syncope may develop at high doses

Life-Threatening or Dangerous Side Effects
- Hypertensive crisis (especially when MAOIs are used with certain tyramine-containing foods or prohibited drugs)
- Induction of mania
- Rare activation of suicidal ideation and behavior (suicidality) (short-term studies did not show an increase in the risk of suicidality with antidepressants compared to placebo beyond age 24)
- Seizures
- Hepatotoxicity

Weight Gain
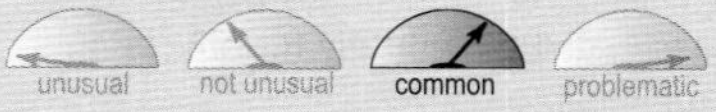

- Many experience and/or can be significant in amount

Sedation
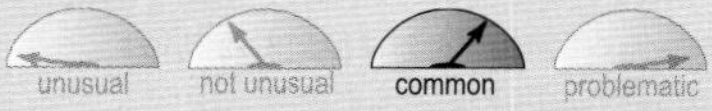

- Many experience and/or can be significant in amount
- Can also cause activation

What to Do About Side Effects
- Wait
- Wait
- Wait
- Lower the dose
- Take at night if daytime sedation
- Switch after appropriate washout to an SSRI or newer antidepressant

Best Augmenting Agents for Side Effects
- Trazodone (with caution) for insomnia
- Benzodiazepines for insomnia

✻ Single oral or sublingual dose of a calcium channel blocker (e.g., nifedipine) for urgent treatment of hypertension due to drug interaction or dietary tyramine
- Many side effects cannot be improved with an augmenting agent

DOSING AND USE

Usual Dosage Range
- 45–75 mg/day

Dosage Forms
- Tablet 15 mg

How to Dose
- Initial 45 mg/day in 3 divided doses; increase to 60–90 mg/day; after desired therapeutic effect is achieved lower dose as far as possible

Dosing Tips

- Once dosing is stabilized, some patients may tolerate once or twice daily dosing rather than 3-times-a-day dosing
- Orthostatic hypotension, especially at high doses, may require splitting into 4 daily doses
- Patients receiving high doses may need to be evaluated periodically for effects on the liver
- Little evidence to support efficacy of phenelzine below doses of 45 mg/day

Overdose

- Death may occur; dizziness, ataxia, sedation, headache, insomnia, restlessness, anxiety, irritability, cardiovascular effects, confusion, respiratory depression, coma

Long-Term Use

- May require periodic evaluation of hepatic function
- MAOIs may lose efficacy long-term

Habit Forming

- Some patients have developed dependence to MAOIs

How to Stop

- Generally no need to taper, as the drug wears off slowly over 2–3 weeks

Pharmacokinetics

- Clinical duration of action may be up to 14 days due to irreversible enzyme inhibition

Drug Interactions

- Tramadol may increase the risk of seizures in patients taking an MAOI
- Can cause a fatal "serotonin syndrome" when combined with drugs that block serotonin reuptake, so do not use with a serotonin reuptake inhibitor or for 5 half-lives after stopping the serotonin reuptake inhibitor (see Table 1 after Pearls)
- Hypertensive crisis with headache, intracranial bleeding, and death may result from combining MAOIs with sympathomimetic drugs (e.g., amphetamines, methylphenidate, cocaine, dopamine, epinephrine, norepinephrine, and related compounds methyldopa, levodopa, L-tryptophan, L-tyrosine, and phenylalanine)
- Do not combine with another MAOI, alcohol, or guanethidine
- Adverse drug reactions can result from combining MAOIs with tricyclic/tetracyclic antidepressants and related compounds, including carbamazepine, cyclobenzaprine, and mirtazapine, and should be avoided except by experts to treat difficult cases
- MAOIs in combination with spinal anesthesia may cause combined hypotensive effects
- Combination of MAOIs and CNS depressants may enhance sedation and hypotension

Other Warnings/ Precautions

- Use requires low tyramine diet (see Table 2 after Pearls)
- Patient and prescriber must be vigilant to potential interactions with any drug, including antihypertensives and over-the-counter cough/cold preparations
- Over-the-counter medications to avoid include cough and cold preparations, including those containing dextromethorphan, nasal decongestants (tablets, drops, or spray), hay-fever medications, sinus medications, asthma inhalant medications, anti-appetite medications, weight reducing preparations, "pep" pills (see Table 3 after Pearls)
- Hypoglycemia may occur in diabetic patients receiving insulin or oral antidiabetic agents
- Use cautiously in patients receiving reserpine, anesthetics, disulfiram, metrizamide, anticholinergic agents
- Phenelzine is not recommended for use in patients who cannot be monitored closely
- When treating children, carefully weigh the risks and benefits of pharmacological treatment against the risks and benefits of nontreatment with antidepressants and make sure to document this in the patient's chart
- Distribute the brochures provided by the FDA and the drug companies
- Warn patients and their caregivers about the possibility of activating side effects and advise them to report such symptoms immediately

- Monitor patients for activation of suicidal ideation, especially children and adolescents

Do Not Use

- If patient is taking meperidine (pethidine)
- If patient is taking a sympathomimetic agent or taking guanethidine
- If patient is taking another MAOI
- If patient is taking any agent that can inhibit serotonin reuptake (e.g., SSRIs, sibutramine, tramadol, milnacipran, duloxetine, venlafaxine, clomipramine, etc.)
- If patient is taking diuretics, dextromethorphan
- If patient has pheochromocytoma
- If patient has cardiovascular or cerebrovascular disease
- If patient has frequent or severe headaches
- If patient is undergoing elective surgery and requires general anesthesia
- If patient has a history of liver disease or abnormal liver function tests
- If patient is taking a prohibited drug
- If patient is not compliant with a low-tyramine diet
- If there is a proven allergy to phenelzine

SPECIAL POPULATIONS

Renal Impairment

- Use with caution – drug may accumulate in plasma
- May require lower than usual adult dose

Hepatic Impairment

- Phenelzine should not be used

Cardiac Impairment

- Contraindicated in patients with congestive heart failure or hypertension
- Any other cardiac impairment may require lower than usual adult dose
- Patients with angina pectoris or coronary artery disease should limit their exertion

Elderly

- Initial dose 7.5 mg/day; increase every few days by 7.5–15 mg/day
- Elderly patients may have greater sensitivity to adverse effects
- Reduction in the risk of suicidality with antidepressants compared to placebo in adults age 65 and older

Children and Adolescents

- Not recommended for use under age 16
- Carefully weigh the risks and benefits of pharmacological treatment against the risks and benefits of nontreatment with antidepressants and make sure to document this in the patient's chart
- Monitor patients face-to-face regularly, particularly during the first several weeks of treatment
- Use with caution, observing for activation of known or unknown bipolar disorder and/or suicidal ideation, and inform parents or guardians of this risk so they can help observe child or adolescent patients

Pregnancy

- Effective June 30, 2015, the US FDA requires changes to the content and format of pregnancy and lactation information in prescription drug labels, including the elimination of the pregnancy letter categories; the Pregnancy and Lactation Labeling Rule (PLLR or final rule) applies only to prescription drugs and will be phased in gradually for drugs approved on or after June 30, 2001
- Controlled studies have not been conducted in pregnant women
- Not generally recommended for use during pregnancy, especially during first trimester
- Possible increased incidence of fetal malformations if phenelzine is taken during the first trimester
- Should evaluate patient for treatment with an antidepressant with a better risk/benefit ratio

Breast Feeding

- Some drug is found in mother's breast milk
- If child becomes irritable or sedated, breast feeding or drug may need to be discontinued
- Immediate postpartum period is a high-risk time for depression, especially in women who have had prior depressive episodes, so drug may need to be reinstituted late in the third trimester or shortly after childbirth to prevent a recurrence during the postpartum period
- Should evaluate patient for treatment with an antidepressant with a better risk/benefit ratio

THE ART OF PSYCHOPHARMACOLOGY

Potential Advantages

- Atypical depression
- Severe depression
- Treatment-resistant depression or anxiety disorders

Potential Disadvantages

- Requires compliance to dietary restrictions, concomitant drug restrictions
- Patients with cardiac problems or hypertension
- Multiple daily doses

Primary Target Symptoms

- Depressed mood
- Somatic symptoms
- Sleep and eating disturbances
- Psychomotor retardation
- Morbid preoccupation

Pearls

- MAOIs are generally reserved for second-line use after SSRIs, SNRIs, and combinations of newer antidepressants have failed
- Patient should be advised not to take any prescription or over-the-counter drugs without consulting their doctor because of possible drug interactions with the MAOI
- Headache is often the first symptom of hypertensive crisis
- The rigid dietary restrictions may reduce compliance (see Table 2 after Pearls)
- Mood disorders can be associated with eating disorders (especially in adolescent females), and phenelzine can be used to treat both depression and bulimia
- MAOIs are a viable second-line treatment option in depression, but are not frequently used

✻ Myths about the danger of dietary tyramine can be exaggerated, but prohibitions against concomitant drugs often not followed closely enough
- Orthostatic hypotension, insomnia, and sexual dysfunction are often the most troublesome common side effects

✻ MAOIs should be for the expert, especially if combining with agents of potential risk (e.g., stimulants, trazodone, TCAs)

✻ MAOIs should not be neglected as therapeutic agents for the treatment-resistant
- Although generally prohibited, a heroic but potentially dangerous treatment for severely treatment-resistant patients is for an expert to give a tricyclic/tetracyclic antidepressant other than clomipramine simultaneously with an MAOI for patients who fail to respond to numerous other antidepressants
- Use of MAOIs with clomipramine is always prohibited because of the risk of serotonin syndrome and death
- Amoxapine may be the preferred trycyclic/tetracyclic antidepressant to combine with an MAOI in heroic cases due to its theoretically protective 5HT2A antagonist properties
- If this option is elected, start the MAOI with the tricyclic/tetracyclic antidepressant simultaneously at low doses after appropriate drug washout, then alternately increase doses of these agents every few days to a week as tolerated
- Although very strict dietary and concomitant drug restrictions must be observed to prevent hypertensive crises and serotonin syndrome, the most common side effects of MAOI and tricyclic/tetracyclic combinations may be weight gain and orthostatic hypotension

Table 1. Drugs contraindicated due to risk of serotonin syndrome/toxicity

Do Not Use:			
Antidepressants	**Drugs of Abuse**	**Opioids**	**Other**
SSRIs	MDMA (ecstasy)	Meperidine	Non-subcutaneous sumatriptan
SNRIs	Cocaine	Tramadol	Chlorpheniramine
Clomipramine	Methamphetamine	Methadone	Brompheniramine
St. John's wort	High-dose or injected amphetamine	Fentanyl	Dextromethorphan
			Procarbazine?

Table 2. Dietary guidelines for patients taking MAOIs

Foods to avoid*	**Foods allowed**
Dried, aged, smoked, fermented, spoiled, or improperly stored meat, poultry, and fish	Fresh or processed meat, poultry, and fish; properly stored pickled or smoked fish
Broad bean pods	All other vegetables
Aged cheeses	Processed cheese slices, cottage cheese, ricotta cheese, yogurt, cream cheese
Tap and unpasteurized beer	Canned or bottled beer and alcohol
Marmite	Brewer's and baker's yeast
Sauerkraut, kimchee	
Soy products/tofu	Peanuts
Banana peel	Bananas, avocados, raspberries
Tyramine-containing nutritional supplement	

*Not necessary for 6-mg transdermal or low-dose oral selegiline

Table 3. Drugs that boost norepinephrine: should only be used with caution with MAOIs

Use With Caution:			
Decongestants	**Stimulants**	**Antidepressants with norepinephrine reuptake inhibition**	**Other**
Phenylephrine	Amphetamines	Most tricyclics	Phentermine
Pseudoephedrine	Methylphenidate	NRIs	Local anesthetics containing vasoconstrictors
	Cocaine	NDRIs	
	Methamphetamine		
	Modafinil		Tapentadol
	Armodafinil		

Suggested Reading

Kennedy SH. Continuation and maintenance treatments in major depression: the neglected role of monoamine oxidase inhibitors. J Psychiatry Neurosci 1997;22:127–31.

Lippman SB, Nash K. Monoamine oxidase inhibitor update. Potential adverse food and drug interactions. Drug Saf 1990;5:195–204.

Parsons B, Quitkin FM, McGrath PJ, et al. Phenelzine, imipramine, and placebo in borderline patients meeting criteria for atypical depression. Psychopharmacol Bull 1989;25:524–34.

PHENTERMINE-TOPIRAMATE

THERAPEUTICS

Brands • Qsymia

see index for additional brand names

Generic? No

Class

- Norepinephrine and dopamine reuptake inhibitor (phentermine) combined with a voltage-sensitive sodium channel modulator (topiramate); weight management medication

Commonly Prescribed for

(bold for FDA approved)

- **Chronic weight management (adjunct to reduced-calorie diet and increased physical activity) in adults with an initial BMI of at least 30 kg/m^2 (obese) or at least 27 kg/m^2 (overweight) in the presence of at least 1 weight-related comorbid condition**

How the Drug Works

- Phentermine increases dopamine and norepinephrine by blocking both the dopamine and the norepinephrine transporters. In the hypothalamus, these 2 neurotransmitters activate POMC neurons, causing the release of POMC. POMC is then broken down into α-melanocyte-stimulating hormone, which binds to melanocortin 4 receptors to suppress appetite. However, stimulation of POMC neurons also activates an endogenous opioid-mediated negative feedback loop, which mitigates the appetite-suppressing effects.
- Theoretically, through modulation of voltage-sensitive sodium channels topiramate may reduce glutamatergic stimulation and increase GABAergic inhibition in the appetite-stimulating pathway, resulting in net inhibition of this pathway. Such an action would synergize with simultaneous activation of the appetite-suppressing pathway by phentermine. This results in more robust and long-lasting appetite suppression than with either drug alone.

How Long Until It Works

- At least 3% weight loss is generally achieved after 14 weeks; at least 5% weight loss is generally achieved after an additional 12 weeks on maximum daily dose

If It Works

- Patients may achieve 5–10% reduction from baseline in body weight

If It Doesn't Work

- Discontinue if 5% weight loss is not achieved after 12 weeks on maximum daily dose

Best Augmenting Combos for Partial Response or Treatment Resistance

- Phentermine-topiramate itself should be administered in conjunction with reduced-calorie diet and increased physical activity
- Often best to try another strategy prior to resorting to augmentation

Tests

- Women of childbearing potential should have a negative pregnancy test before starting phentermine-topiramate and monthly during treatment
- Regular measurement of resting heart rate, especially for patients with cardiac or cerebrovascular disease or when initiating or increasing the dose of phentermine-topiramate
- Obtain a blood chemistry profile that includes bicarbonate, creatinine, potassium, and glucose at baseline and periodically during treatment
- Measurement of blood pressure prior to starting phentermine-topiramate and during phentermine-topiramate treatment is recommended in patients being treated for hypertension

SIDE EFFECTS

How Drug Causes Side Effects

- CNS side effects theoretically due to excessive actions at voltage-sensitive sodium channels or excessive actions on norepinephrine and dopamine
- Weak inhibition of carbonic anhydrase may lead to kidney stones and paresthesias

- Inhibition of carbonic anhydrase may also lead to metabolic acidosis

Notable Side Effects

- Constipation, dry mouth
- Paresthesia, dizziness, dysgeusia, insomnia
- Cognitive impairment (may be more likely with rapid titration or high initial doses)

Life-Threatening or Dangerous Side Effects

- Hypoglycemia
- Increased heart rate
- Metabolic acidosis
- Kidney stones
- Secondary angle-closure glaucoma
- Oligohidrosis and hyperthermia (more common in children)
- Sudden unexplained deaths have occurred in epilepsy (unknown if related to topiramate use)
- Rare activation of suicidal ideation and behavior (suicidality)

Weight Gain

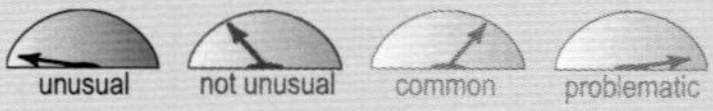

- Reported but not expected

Sedation

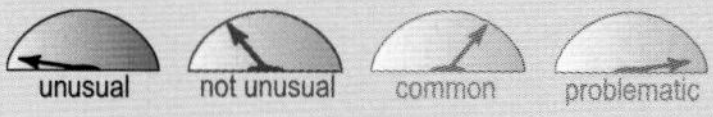

- Reported but not expected

What to Do About Side Effects

- Wait
- Avoid dosing in evening due to the possibility of insomnia
- In a few weeks, switch to another agent

Best Augmenting Agents for Side Effects

- Often best to try another treatment prior to resorting to augmentation strategies to treat side effects

DOSING AND USE

Usual Dosage Range

- 7.5 mg/46 mg per day up to 15 mg/92 mg per day

Dosage Forms

- Capsule (phentermine mg/topiramate mg extended-release) 3.75 mg/23 mg, 7.5 mg/46 mg, 11.25 mg/69 mg, 15 mg/92 mg

How to Dose

- Initial 3.75 mg/23 mg per day; after 14 days increase to 7.5 mg/46 mg per day
- If at least 3% weight loss is not achieved after 12 weeks on 7.5 mg/46 mg per day, can increase to 11.25 mg/69 mg per day; after 14 days increase to 15 mg/92 mg per day
- Discontinue if at least 5% weight loss is not achieved after 12 weeks on 15 mg/92 mg per day

Dosing Tips

- Can be taken with or without food
- Side effects tend to abate with time but may recur again briefly with dose increases

Overdose

- Phentermine: restlessness, tremor, hyperreflexia, rapid respiration, confusion, aggression, hallucinations, panic
- Topiramate: severe metabolic acidosis, convulsions, sedation, speech disturbance, blurred or double vision, impaired coordination, hypotension, abdominal pain, agitation, dizziness

Long-Term Use

- Has been evaluated in controlled studies up to 1 year

Habit Forming

- Phentermine is a Schedule IV drug
- Topiramate is not controlled in the Controlled Substances Act

How to Stop

- For patients taking 15 mg/92 mg per day, take a dose every other day for at least 1 week prior to discontinuing treatment, due to the possibility of precipitating a seizure

Pharmacokinetics

- Phentermine mean terminal half-life approximately 20 hours
- Topiramate mean terminal half-life approximately 65 hours
- Neither phentermine nor topiramate is extensively metabolized

Drug Interactions

- May cause irregular bleeding in patients taking oral contraceptives, but does not increase risk of pregnancy; patients should be advised not to discontinue oral contraceptives if spotting occurs
- May increase effects of CNS depressants
- May potentiate hypokalemia in patients taking non-potassium-sparing diuretic agents
- Weight loss associated with phentermine-topiramate may increase the risk of hypotension in patients taking antihypertensive medications
- Carbamazepine, phenytoin, and valproate may increase the clearance of topiramate, and thus decrease topiramate levels, possibly requiring a higher dose of topiramate
- Topiramate may increase the clearance of phenytoin and thus decrease phenytoin levels, possibly requiring a higher dose of phenytoin
- Topiramate may increase the clearance of valproate and thus decrease valproate levels, possibly requiring a higher dose of valproate
- Topiramate may increase plasma levels of metformin; also, metformin may reduce clearance of topiramate and increase topiramate levels
- Topiramate may interact with carbonic anhydrase inhibitors to increase the risk of kidney stones
- Reports of hyperammonemia with or without encephalopthay in patients taking topiramate combined with valproate, though this is not due to a pharmacokinetic interaction; in patients who develop unexplained lethargy, vomiting, or change in mental status, an ammonia level should be measured
- Phentermine is contraindicated with MAOIs due to risk of hypertensive crisis

Other Warnings/ Precautions

- Phentermine-topiramate can cause fetal toxicity; women of childbearing potential should obtain a negative pregnancy test before treatment and monthly thereafter and use effective contraception
- If a patient develops a sustained increase in resting heart rate while taking phentermine/ topiramate, the dose should be reduced or the medication should be discontinued
- May cause an increase in serum creatinine; if persistent elevations in creatinine occur during phentermine-topiramate treatment, the dose should be reduced or the medication should be discontinued
- Phentermine-topiramate has not been studied in combination with insulin; weight loss may increase the risk of hypoglycemia in patients with type 2 diabetes mellitus treated with insulin and/ or insulin secretagogues, and medication adjustments may be necessary
- Warn patients and their caregivers about the possibility of activation of suicidal ideation and advise them to report such side effects immediately

Do Not Use

- If patient is pregnant
- If patient has glaucoma
- If patient has hyperthyroidism
- If patient is taking an MAOI
- If there is a proven allergy to phentermine or topiramate

SPECIAL POPULATIONS

Renal Impairment

- Maximum dose is 7.5 mg/46 mg per day in patients with moderate to severe impairment
- Not studied or recommended for use in patients with end-stage renal disease

Hepatic Impairment

- Maximum dose is 7.5 mg/46 mg per day in patients with moderate impairment
- Not recommended for use in patients with severe impairment

Cardiac Impairment

- Not systematically evaluated in patients with cardiac impairment
- Not recommended for patients with recent or unstable cardiac or cerebrovascular disease

Elderly

- Some patients may tolerate lower doses better

Children and Adolescents

- Safety and efficacy have not been established
- Not recommended for use in children or adolescents

Pregnancy

- Contraindicated
- Effective June 30, 2015, the US FDA requires changes to the content and format of pregnancy and lactation information in prescription drug labels, including the elimination of the pregnancy letter categories; the Pregnancy and Lactation Labeling Rule (PLLR or final rule) applies only to prescription drugs and will be phased in gradually for drugs approved on or after June 30, 2001
- There is an increased risk of cleft lip/palate with topiramate

Breast Feeding

- Some drug is found in mother's breast milk
- Recommended to discontinue drug or bottle feed

THE ART OF PSYCHOPHARMACOLOGY

Potential Advantages

- Patients who have had past weight loss on either active compound alone may experience a more robust weight loss effect and better tolerability on the combination of phentermine with topiramate than with administration of either drug alone

Potential Disadvantages

- Patients with a history of kidney stones or risks for metabolic acidosis
- Women who are pregnant or wish to become pregnant
- Patients with a history of past stimulant abuse

Primary Target Symptoms

- Excess weight

Pearls

- Has perhaps the largest effect size on weight loss of drugs available for the treatment of obesity
- Could theoretically be effective in binge-eating disorder
- Because of the teratogenic risk with phentermine-topiramate, it is available only through a Risk Evaluation and Mitigation Strategy (REMS) program; only certified pharmacies may distribute it

Suggested Reading

Colman E, Golden J, Roberts M, et al. The FDA's assessment of two drugs for chronic weight management. N Engl J Med 2012;367(17):1577–9.

Cosentino G, Conrad AO, Uwaifo GI. Phentermine and topiramate for the management of obesity: a review. Drug Des Devel Ther 2011;7:267–87.

Holes-Lewis KA, Malcolm R, O'Neil PM. Pharmacotherapy of obesity: clinical treatments and considerations. Am J Med Sci 2013;345(4):284–8.

Shin JH, Gadde KM. Clinical utility of phentermine/topiramate (QsymiaTM) combination for the treatment of obesity. Diabetes Metab Syndr Obes 2013;6:1319.

PIMAVANSERIN

THERAPEUTICS

Brands • Nuplazid

see index for additional brand names

Generic? No

Class

- Atypical antipsychotic; serotonin 2A/2C antagonist/inverse agonist

Commonly Prescribed for

(bold for FDA approved)

- **Hallucinations and delusions associated with Parkinson's disease psychosis**

How the Drug Works

✻ Antagonism/inverse agonism at 5HT2A receptors

- Pimavanserin is also an antagonist/inverse agonist at 5HT2C receptors (activity is very low compared to that at 5HT2A receptors)

How Long Until It Works

- In clinical trials psychotic symptom improvement reached significance within 1 month

If It Works

- Most often reduces hallucinations and delusions without worsening parkinsonism

If It Doesn't Work

- Try reducing the dose of antiparkinsonian dopaminergic therapies
- Try low-dose quetiapine
- Try low-dose clozapine
- Do not try any other atypical or conventional antipsychotic

Best Augmenting Combos for Partial Response or Treatment Resistance

- None known
- Theoretically, might be possible to combine with low-dose quetiapine, especially during prolonged cross-titration when switching from one to the other

Tests

- None

SIDE EFFECTS

How Drug Causes Side Effects

- Mechanism of peripheral edema, confusional state, and nausea unknown

Notable Side Effects

- Peripheral edema
- Confusional state
- Nausea

Life Threatening or Dangerous Side Effects

- QTc prolongation
- Increased risk of death and cerebrovascular events in elderly patients with dementia-related psychosis has occurred with antipsychotic use

Weight Gain

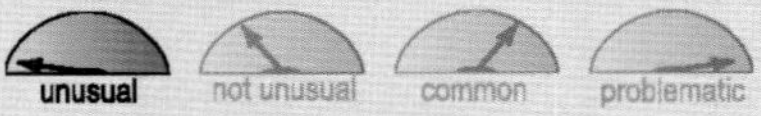

- Reported but not expected

Sedation

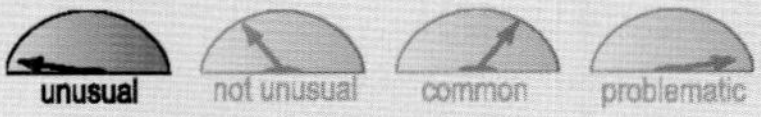

- Reported but not expected

What to Do About Side Effects

- Wait
- Wait
- Wait
- Discontinue if side effects are intolerable

Best Augmenting Agents for Side Effects

- Many side effects cannot be improved with an augmenting agent

DOSING AND USE

Usual Dosage Range

- 34 mg once daily

Dosage Forms

- Tablet 17 mg

How to Dose

- 34 mg/day taken once daily; no titration required

Dosing Tips
- Can be taken with or without food
- No dose adjustment of carbidopa/levodopa is required

Overdose
- Limited experience

Long-Term Use
- Not studied, but long-term maintenance treatment is often necessary for Parkinson's disease psychosis

Habit Forming
- No

How to Stop
- The long half-life suggests that it may be possible to stop pimavanserin abruptly
- Rapid discontinuation could theoretically lead to rebound psychosis and worsening of symptoms, but less likely with pimavanserin due to its long half-life

Pharmacokinetics
- Mean half-life 57 hours (pimavanserin) and 200 hours (active metabolite N-desmethylated metabolite)
- Metabolized primarily by CYP450 3A4 and CYP450 3A5

Drug Interactions
- In the presence of strong/moderate CYP450 3A4 inhibitors (e.g., ketaconazole), reduce pimavanserin dose by half
- Strong CYP450 3A4 inducers (e.g., carbamazepine) may reduce pimavanserin levels and a dosage increase may be necessary
- May enhance QTc prolongation of other drugs capable of prolonging QTc interval

Other Warnings/ Precautions
- Pimavanserin can cause prolongation of the QTc interval

Do Not Use
- If there is a proven allergy to pimavanserin

SPECIAL POPULATIONS

Renal Impairment
- Dose adjustment not necessary in patients with mild-to-moderate impairment
- Not studied in patients with severe impairment; not recommended in patients with severe renal impairment (creatine clearance<30 mL/min)

Hepatic Impairment
- Not studied; not recommend in patients with hepatic impairment

Cardiac Impairment
- Pimavanserin can cause QTc prolongation and should be avoided in patients with known QT prolongation or in combination with drugs that are known to prolong QT interval
- Pimavanserin should be avoided in patients with a history of cardiac arrhythmias, symptomatic bradycardia, hypokalemia or hypomagnesemia, or presence of congenital prolongation of the QT interval

Elderly
- Dose adjustment not necessary
- Pimavanserin is not approved for the treatment of dementia-related psychosis UNRELATED to the hallucinations and delusions associated with Parkinson's disease psychosis, such as the behavioral symptoms of comorbid Alzheimer dementia
- However, pimavanserin is not contraindicated for patients with dementia RELATED to Parkinson's disease who have hallucinations and delusions of Parkinson's disease psychosis

Children and Adolescents
- Safety and efficacy have not been established

Pregnancy
- Effective June 30, 2015, the US FDA requires changes to the content and format of pregnancy and lactation information in prescription drug labels, including the elimination of the pregnancy letter categories; the Pregnancy and Lactation Labeling Rule (PLLR or final rule) applies

only to prescription drugs and will be phased in gradually for drugs approved on or after June 30, 2001
- Controlled studies have not been conducted in pregnant women
- In rat and rabbit studies, pimavanserin did not demonstrate teratogenicity at doses up to 10 times the maximum recommended human dose
- In rat studies, doses 2 times the maximum recommended daily dose in humans based on area under the curve (AUC) resulted in maternal toxicity, including mortality and reduced body weight and food consumption, with corresponding decreases in pup survival, reduced litter size, and reduced pup body weight

Breast Feeding
- Unknown if pimavanserin is secreted in human breast milk, but all psychotropics assumed to be secreted in breast milk
- ❊ Recommended to either discontinue drug or bottle feed unless the potential benefit to the mother justifies the potential risk to the child
- Infants of women who choose to breast feed while on pimavanserin should be monitored for possible adverse effects

THE ART OF PSYCHOPHARMACOLOGY

Potential Advantages
- Does not worsen motor symptoms of Parkinson's disease
- Not associated with the metabolic side effects of quetiapine and clozapine, including weight gain, dyslipidemia, and diabetes mellitus
- Not associated with the sedation sometimes caused by quetiapine and clozapine
- Does not require dose reduction of antiparkinsonian dopaminergic therapy given concomitantly

Potential Disadvantages
- Expensive

Primary Target Symptoms
- Hallucinations and delusions associated with Parkinson's disease

Pearls
- Trials are underway for the use of pimavanserin to treat Alzheimer's disease psychosis
- Theoretically should be effective for the hallucinations associated with Lewy Body psychosis
- Enhances slow wave sleep and may have hypnotic properties
- May enhance the antipsychotic action of atypical antipsychotics in patients with schizophrenia
- May be effective in other types of psychosis but based on theory and not on large randomized trials

Suggested Reading

Cummings J, Isaacson S, Mills R, et al. Pimavanserin for patients with Parkinson's disease psychosis: a randomized, placebo-controlled phase 3 trial. Lancet 2014;383(9916):533–40.

Hacksell U, Burstein ES, McFarland K, Mills RG, Williams H. On the discovery and development of pimavanserin: a novel drug candidate for Parkinson's psychosis. Neurochem Res 2014 Oct;39(10):2008–17.

Hermanowicz S, Hermanowicz N. The safety, tolerability and efficacy of pimavanserin tartrate in the treatment of psychosis in Parkinson's disease. Expert Rev Neurother 2016;16(6):625–33.

Howland RJ. Pimavanserin: an inverse agonist antipsychotic drug. J Psychosoc Nurs Ment Health Serv 2016;54(6):21–4.

Stahl SM. Mechanism of action of pimavanserin in Parkinson's disease psychosis: targeting serotonin 5HT2A and 5HT2C receptors. CNS Spectr 2016;21(4):271–5.

PIMOZIDE

THERAPEUTICS

Brands • Orap

see index for additional brand names

Generic? Not in USA

Class

- Neuroscience-based Nomenclature: dopamine receptor antagonist (D-RAn)
- Tourette's syndrome/tic suppressant; conventional antipsychotic (neuroleptic, dopamine 2 antagonist)

Commonly Prescribed for

(bold for FDA approved)

- **Suppression of motor and phonic tics in patients with Tourette syndrome who have failed to respond satisfactorily to standard treatment**
- Psychotic disorders in patients who have failed to respond satisfactorily to standard treatment

How the Drug Works

- Blocks dopamine 2 receptors in the nigrostriatal dopamine pathway, reducing tics in Tourette's syndrome
- When used for psychosis, can block dopamine 2 receptors in the mesolimbic dopamine pathway, reducing positive symptoms of psychosis

How Long Until It Works

- Relief from tics may occur more rapidly than antipsychotic actions
- Psychotic symptoms can improve within 1 week, but it may take several weeks for full effect on behavior

If It Works

✽ Is a second-line treatment option for Tourette's syndrome

✽ Is a secondary or tertiary treatment option for psychosis or other behavioral disorders

- Should evaluate for switching to an antipsychotic with a better/risk benefit ratio

If It Doesn't Work

- Consider trying one of the first-line atypical antipsychotics (risperidone, olanzapine, quetiapine, ziprasidone, aripiprazole, paliperidone, amisulpride, asenapine, iloperidone, lurasidone)
- Consider trying another conventional antipsychotic
- If 2 or more antipsychotic monotherapies do not work, consider clozapine

Best Augmenting Combos for Partial Response or Treatment Resistance

✽ Augmentation of pimozide has not been systematically studied and can be dangerous, especially with drugs that can either prolong QTc interval or raise pimozide plasma levels

Tests

✽ Baseline EKG and serum potassium levels should be determined

✽ Periodic evaluation of EKG and serum potassium levels, especially during dose titration

- Serum magnesium levels may also need to be monitored

✽ Since conventional antipsychotics are frequently associated with weight gain, before starting treatment, weigh all patients and determine if the patient is already overweight (BMI 25.0–29.9) or obese (BMI ≥30)

- Before giving a drug that can cause weight gain to an overweight or obese patient, consider determining whether the patient already has pre-diabetes (fasting plasma glucose 100–125 mg/dL), diabetes (fasting plasma glucose >126 mg/dL), or dyslipidemia (increased total cholesterol, LDL cholesterol, and triglycerides; decreased HDL cholesterol), and treat or refer such patients for treatment, including nutrition and weight management, physical activity counseling, smoking cessation, and medical management

✽ Monitor weight and BMI during treatment

✽ Consider monitoring fasting triglycerides monthly for several months in patients at high risk for metabolic complications and when initiating or switching antipsychotics

✽ While giving a drug to a patient who has gained >5% of initial weight, consider evaluating for the presence of pre-diabetes, diabetes, or dyslipidemia, or consider switching to a different antipsychotic

- Should check blood pressure in the elderly before starting and for the first few weeks of treatment
- Monitoring elevated prolactin levels of dubious clinical benefit

- Patients with low white blood cell count (WBC) or history of drug-induced leucopenia/neutropenia should have complete blood count (CBC) monitored frequently during the first few months and pimozide should be discontinued at the first sign of decline of WBC in the absence of other causative factors

SIDE EFFECTS

How Drug Causes Side Effects

- By blocking dopamine 2 receptors in the striatum, it can cause motor side effects
- By blocking dopamine 2 receptors in the pituitary, it can cause elevations in prolactin
- By blocking dopamine 2 receptors excessively in the mesocortical and mesolimbic dopamine pathways, especially at high doses, it can cause worsening of negative and cognitive symptoms (neuroleptic-induced deficit syndrome)
- Anticholinergic actions may cause sedation, blurred vision, constipation, dry mouth
- Antihistaminic actions may cause sedation, weight gain
- By blocking alpha 1 adrenergic receptors, it can cause dizziness, sedation, and hypotension
- Mechanism of weight gain and any possible increased incidence of diabetes or dyslipidemia with conventional antipsychotics is unknown

✱ Mechanism of potentially dangerous QTc prolongation may be related to actions at ion channels

Notable Side Effects

✱ Neuroleptic-induced deficit syndrome
✱ Akathisia
✱ Extrapyramidal symptoms, parkinsonism, tardive dyskinesia
✱ Hypotension

- Sedation, akinesia
- Galactorrhea, amenorrhea
- Dry mouth, constipation, blurred vision
- Sexual dysfunction

✱ Weight gain

Life-Threatening or Dangerous Side Effects

- Rare neuroleptic malignant syndrome
- Rare seizures

✱ Dose-dependent QTc prolongation

- Ventricular arrhythmias and sudden death
- Increased risk of death and cerebrovascular events in elderly patients with dementia-related psychosis

Weight Gain

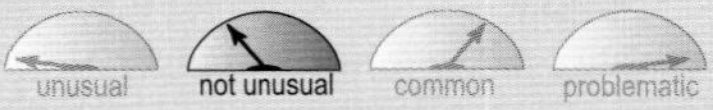

- Occurs in significant minority

Sedation

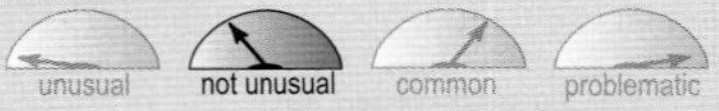

- Occurs in significant minority

What to Do About Side Effects

- Wait
- Wait
- Wait
- For motor symptoms, add an anticholinergic agent
- Reduce the dose
- For sedation, give at night
- Switch to an atypical antipsychotic
- Weight loss, exercise programs, and medical management for high BMIs, diabetes, dyslipidemia

Best Augmenting Agents for Side Effects

✱ Augmentation of pimozide has not been systematically studied and can be dangerous, especially with drugs that can either prolong QTc interval or raise pimozide plasma levels

DOSING AND USE

Usual Dosage Range

- Less than 10 mg/day

Dosage Forms

- Tablet 1 mg scored, 2 mg scored

How to Dose

- Initial 1–2 mg/day in divided doses; can increase dose every other day; maximum 10 mg/day or 0.2 mg/kg per day
- Children: initial 0.05 mg/kg per day at night; can increase every 3 days; maximum 10 mg/day or 0.2 mg/kg per day

Dosing Tips

- ✻ The effects of pimozide on the QTc interval are dose-dependent, so start low and go slow while carefully monitoring QTc interval
- Treatment should be suspended if absolute neutrophil count falls below 1,000/mm^3

Overdose

- Deaths have occurred; extrapyramidal symptoms, EKG changes, hypotension, respiratory depression, coma

Long-Term Use

- Some side effects may be irreversible (e.g., tardive dyskinesia)

Habit Forming

- No

How to Stop

- Slow down-titration (over 6 to 8 weeks), especially when simultaneously beginning a new antipsychotic while switching (i.e., cross-titration)
- Rapid discontinuation may lead to rebound psychosis and worsening of symptoms
- If antiparkinson agents are being used, they should be continued for a few weeks after pimozide is discontinued

Pharmacokinetics

- Metabolized by CYP450 3A and to a lesser extent by CYP450 1A2
- Mean elimination half-life approximately 55 hours

Drug Interactions

- May decrease the effects of levodopa, dopamine agonists
- May enhance QTc prolongation of other drugs capable of prolonging QTc interval
- May increase the effects of antihypertensive drugs
- ✻ Use with CYP450 3A4 inhibitors (e.g., drugs such as fluoxetine, sertraline, fluvoxamine, and nefazodone; foods such as grapefruit juice) can raise pimozide levels and increase the risks of dangerous arrhythmias
- Use of pimozide and fluoxetine may lead to bradycardia
- Additive effects may occur if used with CNS depressants
- Some patients taking a neuroleptic and lithium have developed an encephalopathic syndrome similar to neuroleptic malignant syndrome
- Combined use with epinephrine may lower blood pressure

Other Warnings/ Precautions

- If signs of neuroleptic malignant syndrome develop, treatment should be immediately discontinued
- Use cautiously in patients with alcohol withdrawal or convulsive disorders because of possible lowering of seizure threshold
- Antiemetic effect can mask signs of other disorders or overdose
- Do not use epinephrine in event of overdose as interaction with some pressor agents may lower blood pressure
- Use only with caution if at all in Parkinson's disease or Lewy body dementia
- Because pimozide may dose-dependently prolong QTc interval, use with caution in patients who have bradycardia or who are taking drugs that can induce bradycardia (e.g., beta blockers, calcium channel blockers, clonidine, digitalis)
- Because pimozide may dose-dependently prolong QTc interval, use with caution in patients who have hypokalemia and/ or hypomagnesemia or who are taking drugs that can induce hypokalemia and/ or magnesemia (e.g., diuretics, stimulant laxatives, intravenous amphotericin B, glucocorticoids, tetracosactide)
- Pimozide can increase tumors in mice (dose-related effect)
- ✻ Pimozide can increase the QTc interval and potentially cause arrhythmia or sudden death, especially in combination with drugs that raise its levels

Do Not Use

- If patient is in a comatose state or has CNS depression
- ✻ If patient is taking an agent capable of significanty prolonging QTc interval (e.g., thioridazine, selected antiarrhythmics, moxifoxacin, and sparfloxacin)
- ✻ If there is a history of QTc prolongation or cardiac arrhythmia, recent acute

myocardial infarction, uncompensated heart failure
- If patient is taking drugs that can cause tics
- ✻ If patient is taking drugs that inhibit pimozide metabolism, such as macrolide antibiotics, azole antifungal agents (ketoconazole, itraconazole), protease inhibitors, nefazodone, fluvoxamine, fluoxetine, sertaline, etc.
- If there is a proven allergy to pimozide
- If there is a known sensitivity to other antipsychotics

SPECIAL POPULATIONS

Renal Impairment
- Use with caution

Hepatic Impairment
- Use with caution

Cardiac Impairment
- Pimozide produces a dose-dependent prolongation of QTc interval, which may be enhanced by the existence of bradycardia, hypokalemia, congenital or acquired long QTc interval, which should be evaluated prior to administering pimozide
- Use with caution if treating concomitantly with a medication likely to produce prolonged bradycardia, hypokalemia, slowing of intracardiac conduction, or prolongation of the QTc interval
- Avoid pimozide in patients with a known history of QTc prolongation, recent acute myocardial infarction, and uncompensated heart failure

Elderly
- Some patients may tolerate lower doses better
- Although conventional antipsychotics are commonly used for behavioral disturbances in dementia, no agent has been approved for treatment of elderly patients with dementia-related psychosis
- Elderly patients with dementia-related psychosis treated with antipsychotics are at an increased risk of death compared to placebo, and also have an increased risk of cerebrovascular events

Children and Adolescents
- Safety and efficacy established for patients over age 12
- Preliminary data show similar safety for patients age 2–12 as for patients over 12
- Generally use second-line after atypical antipsychotics and other conventional antipsychotics

Pregnancy
- Effective June 30, 2015, the US FDA requires changes to the content and format of pregnancy and lactation information in prescription drug labels, including the elimination of the pregnancy letter categories; the Pregnancy and Lactation Labeling Rule (PLLR or final rule) applies only to prescription drugs and will be phased in gradually for drugs approved on or after June 30, 2001
- Controlled studies have not been conducted in pregnant women
- Renal papillary abnormalities have been seen in rats during pregnancy
- There is a risk of abnormal muscle movements and withdrawal symptoms in newborns whose mothers took an antipsychotic during the third trimester; symptoms may include agitation, abnormally increased or decreased muscle tone, tremor, sleepiness, severe difficulty breathing, and difficulty feeding
- Psychotic symptoms may worsen during pregnancy and some form of treatment may be necessary
- Atypical antipsychotics may be preferable to conventional antipsychotics or anticonvulsant mood stabilizers if treatment is required during pregnancy
- Should evaluate for an antipsychotic with a better risk/benefit ratio if treatment required during pregnancy

Breast Feeding
- Unknown if pimozide is secreted in human breast milk, but all psychotropics assumed to be secreted in breast milk
- Not recommended for use because of potential for tumorigenicity or cardiovascular effects on infant
- ✻ Recommended either to discontinue drug or bottle feed

THE ART OF PSYCHOPHARMACOLOGY

Potential Advantages

- Only for patients who respond to this agent and not to other antipsychotics

Potential Disadvantages

- Vulnerable populations such as children and elderly
- Patients on other drugs

Primary Target Symptoms

- Vocal and motor tics in patients who fail to respond to treatment with other antipsychotics
- Psychotic symptoms in patients who fail to respond to treatment with other antipsychotics

Pearls

* In the past, was a first-line choice for Tourette's syndrome and for certain behavioral disorders, including monosymptomatic hypochondriasis; however, it is now recognized that the benefits of pimozide generally do not outweigh its risks in most patients
* Because of its effects on the QTc interval, pimozide is not intended for use unless other options for tic disorders (or psychotic disorders) have failed

Suggested Reading

Pringsheim T, Marras C. Pimozide for tics in Tourette's syndrome. Cochrane Database Syst Rev 2009;15(2):CD006996.

Rathbone J, McMonagle T. Pimozide for schizophrenia or related psychoses. Cochrane Database Syst Rev 2007;18(3):CD001949.

THERAPEUTICS

Brands • Piportil

see index for additional brand names

Generic? No

Class

- Neuroscience-based Nomenclature: dopamine receptor antagonist (D-RAn)
- Conventional antipsychotic (neuroleptic, phenothiazine, dopamine 2 antagonist)

Commonly Prescribed for

(bold for FDA approved)

- Maintenance treatment of schizophrenia
- Other psychotic disorders
- Bipolar disorder

How the Drug Works

- Blocks dopamine 2 receptors, reducing positive symptoms of psychosis

How Long Until It Works

- Psychotic symptoms can improve within 1 week, but it may take several weeks for full effect on behavior

If It Works

- Most often reduces positive symptoms in schizophrenia but does not eliminate them
- Most schizophrenic patients do not have a total remission of symptoms but rather a reduction of symptoms by about a third
- Continue treatment in schizophrenia until reaching a plateau of improvement
- After reaching a satisfactory plateau, continue treatment for at least a year after first episode of psychosis in schizophrenia
- For second and subsequent episodes of psychosis in schizophrenia, treatment may need to be indefinite
- Reduces symptoms of acute psychotic mania but not proven as a mood stabilizer or as an effective maintenance treatment in bipolar disorder
- After reducing acute psychotic symptoms in mania, switch to a mood stabilizer and/ or an atypical antipsychotic for mood stabilization and maintenance

If It Doesn't Work

- Consider trying one of the first-line atypical antipsychotics (risperidone, olanzapine, quetiapine, ziprasidone, aripiprazole, paliperidone, amisulpride, asenapine, iloperidone, lurasidone)
- Consider trying another conventional antipsychotic
- If 2 or more antipsychotic monotherapies do not work, consider clozapine

Best Augmenting Combos for Partial Response or Treatment Resistance

- Augmentation of conventional antipsychotics has not been systematically studied
- Addition of a mood-stabilizing anticonvulsant such as valproate, carbamazepine, or lamotrigine may be helpful in both schizophrenia and bipolar mania
- Augmentation with lithium in bipolar mania may be helpful
- Addition of a benzodiazepine, especially short-term for agitation

Tests

- ✻ Since conventional antipsychotics are frequently associated with weight gain, before starting treatment, weigh all patients and determine if the patient is already overweight (BMI 25.0–29.9) or obese (BMI ≥30)
- Before giving a drug that can cause weight gain to an overweight or obese patient, consider determining whether the patient already has pre-diabetes (fasting plasma glucose 100–125 mg/dL), diabetes (fasting plasma glucose >126 mg/dL), or dyslipidemia (increased total cholesterol, LDL cholesterol, and triglycerides; decreased HDL cholesterol), and treat or refer such patients for treatment, including nutrition and weight management, physical activity counseling, smoking cessation, and medical management
- ✻ Monitor weight and BMI during treatment
- ✻ Consider monitoring fasting triglycerides monthly for several months in patients at high risk for metabolic complications and when initiating or switching antipsychotics
- ✻ While giving a drug to a patient who has gained >5% of initial weight, consider evaluating for the presence of pre-diabetes, diabetes, or dyslipidemia, or consider switching to a different antipsychotic
- Should check blood pressure in the elderly before starting and for the first few weeks
- Monitoring elevated prolactin levels of dubious clinical benefit

- Phenothiazines may cause false-positive phenylketonuria results
- Patients with low white blood cell count (WBC) or history of drug-induced leucopenia/neutropenia should have complete blood count (CBC) monitored frequently during the first few months and pipothiazine should be discontinued at the first sign of decline of WBC in the absence of other causative factors

SIDE EFFECTS

How Drug Causes Side Effects

- By blocking dopamine 2 receptors in the striatum, it can cause motor side effects
- By blocking dopamine 2 receptors in the pituitary, it can cause elevations in prolactin
- By blocking dopamine 2 receptors excessively in the mesocortical and mesolimbic dopamine pathways, especially at high doses, it can cause worsening of negative and cognitive symptoms (neuroleptic-induced deficit syndrome)
- Anticholinergic actions may cause sedation, blurred vision, constipation, dry mouth
- Antihistaminic actions may cause sedation, weight gain
- By blocking alpha 1 adrenergic receptors, it can cause dizziness, sedation, and hypotension
- Mechanism of weight gain and any possible increased incidence of diabetes or dyslipidemia with conventional antipsychotics is unknown

Notable Side Effects

✻ Excitement, insomnia, restlessness
✻ Rare tardive dyskinesia (risk increases with duration of treatment and with dose)
✻ Galactorrhea, amenorrhea

- Dry mouth, nausea, blurred vision, sweating, appetite change
- Sexual dysfunction (impotence)
- Hypotension, arrhythmia, tachycardia
- Weight gain
- Rare rash

Life-Threatening or Dangerous Side Effects

- Rare neuroleptic malignant syndrome
- Jaundice, leucopenia
- Rare seizures
- Increased risk of death and cerebrovascular events in elderly patients with dementia-related psychosis

Weight Gain

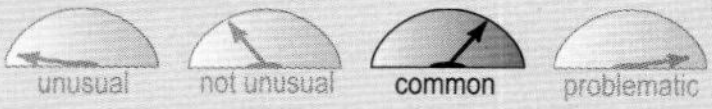

- Many experience and/or can be significant in amount

Sedation

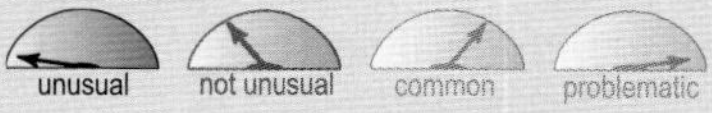

- Reported but not expected

What to Do About Side Effects

- Wait
- Wait
- Wait
- For motor symptoms, add an anticholinergic agent
- Reduce the dose
- For sedation, take at night
- Switch to an atypical antipsychotic
- Weight loss, exercise programs, and medical management for high BMIs, diabetes, dyslipidemia

Best Augmenting Agents for Side Effects

- Benztropine or trihexyphenidyl for motor side effects
- Sometimes amantadine can be helpful for motor side effects
- Benzodiazepines may be helpful for akathisia
- Many side effects cannot be improved with an augmenting agent

DOSING AND USE

Usual Dosage Range

- 50–100 mg once a month

Dosage Forms

- Injection 50 mg/mL

How to Dose

- Initial 25 mg; can be increased by 25–50 mg; maximum 200 mg once a month
- Drug should be administerd intramuscularly in the gluteal region

Dosing Tips

- ✻ Only available as long-acting intramuscular formulation and not as oral formulation
- The peak of action generally occurs after 9–10 days
- May need to treat with an oral antipsychotic for 1–2 weeks when initiating treatment
- One of the few conventional antipsychotics available in a depot formulation lasting for up to a month
- Treatment should be suspended if absolute neutrophil count falls below 1,000/mm^3

Overdose

- Sedation, tachycardia, extrapyramidal symptoms, arrhythmia, hypothermia, EKG changes, hypotension

Long-Term Use

- Some side effects may be irreversible (e.g., tardive dyskinesia)

Habit Forming

- No

How to Stop

- If antiparkinson agents are being used, they should be continued for a few weeks after pipothiazine is discontinued

Pharmacokinetics

- Onset of action of palmitic ester formulation within 2–3 days
- Duration of action of palmitic ester formulation 3–6 weeks

Drug Interactions

- Use with TCAs may increase risk of cardiac symptoms
- CNS effects may be increased if used with other CNS depressants
- May increase the effects of antihypertensive agents
- May decrease the effects of amphetamines, levodopa, dopamine agonists, clonidine, guanethidine, adrenaline
- Effects may be reduced by anticholinergic agents
- Antacids, antiparkinson drugs, and lithium may reduce pipothiazine absorption
- Combined use with epinephrine may lower blood pressure
- Some patients taking a neuroleptic and lithium have developed an encephalopathic syndrome similar to neuroleptic malignant syndrome

Other Warnings/ Precautions

- Patients may be more sensitive to extreme temperatures
- Use with caution in patients with Parkinson's disease, Lewy body dementia, or extrapyramidal symptoms with previous treatments
- Avoid undue exposure to sunlight
- Use with caution in patients with respiratory disease, Lewy body dementia, angle-closure glaucoma (including family history), alcohol withdrawal syndrome, brain damage, epilepsy, hypothyroidism, myaesthenia gravis, prostatic hypertrophy, thyrotoxicosis
- Contact with skin can cause rash
- Antiemetic effect can mask signs of other disorders or overdose
- Do not use epinephrine in event of overdose as interaction with some pressor agents may lower blood pressure

Do Not Use

- If patient is comatose
- If there is cerebral atherosclerosis
- If patient has phaeochromocytoma
- If patient has renal or liver failure, blood dyscrasias
- If patient has severe cardiac impairment
- If patient has subcortical brain damage
- If there is a proven allergy to pipothiazine
- If there is a known sensitivity to any phenothiazine

SPECIAL POPULATIONS

Renal Impairment

- Use with caution

Hepatic Impairment

- Use with caution

Cardiac Impairment

- Use with caution

Elderly

- Elderly patients do not metabolize the drug as quickly
- Dose should be reduced
- Recommended starting dose 5–10 mg
- Although conventional antipsychotics are commonly used for behavioral disturbances in dementia, no agent has been approved for treatment of elderly patients with dementia-related psychosis
- Elderly patients with dementia-related psychosis treated with antipsychotics are at an increased risk of death compared to placebo, and also have an increased risk of cerebrovascular events

Children and Adolescents

- Not recommended for use in children

Pregnancy

- There is a risk of abnormal muscle movements and withdrawal symptoms in newborns whose mothers took an antipsychotic during the third trimester; symptoms may include agitation, abnormally increased or decreased muscle tone, tremor, sleepiness, severe difficulty breathing, and difficulty feeding
- Reports of extrapyramidal symptoms, jaundice, hyperreflexia, hyporeflexia in infants whose mothers took a phenothiazine during pregnancy
- Not recommended unless absolutely necessary
- Psychotic symptoms may worsen during pregnancy and some form of treatment may be necessary
- Atypical antipsychotics may be preferable to conventional antipsychotics or anticonvulsant mood stabilizers if treatment is required during pregnancy

Breast Feeding

- Unknown if pipothiazine is secreted in human breast milk, but all psychotropics assumed to be secreted in breast milk

✻ Recommended either to discontinue drug or bottle feed

THE ART OF PSYCHOPHARMACOLOGY

Potential Advantages

- Noncompliant patients

Potential Disadvantages

- Patients who need immediate onset of antipsychotic actions

Primary Target Symptoms

- Positive symptoms of psychosis
- Negative symptoms of psychosis
- Aggressive symptoms

Pearls

- Pipothiazine is a higher potency phenothiazine
- Less risk of sedation and orthostatic hypotension but greater risk of extrapyramidal symptoms than with low potency phenothiazines

✻ Only available in long-acting parenteral formulation

- Generally, patients must be stabilized on an oral antipsychotic prior to switching to parenteral long-acting pipothiazine
- Patients have very similar antipsychotic responses to any conventional antipsychotic, which is different from atypical antipsychotics where antipsychotic responses of individual patients can occasionally vary greatly from one atypical antipsychotic to another
- Patients with inadequate responses to atypical antipsychotics may benefit from a trial of augmentation with a conventional antipsychotic such as pipothiazine or from switching to a conventional antipsychotic such as pipothiazine
- However, long-term polypharmacy with a combination of a conventional antipsychotic with an atypical antipsychotic such as pipothiazine may combine their side effects without clearly augmenting the efficacy of either
- Although a frequent practice by some prescribers, adding 2 conventional antipsychotics together has little rationale and may reduce tolerability without clearly enhancing efficacy
- For treatment-resistant patients, especially those with impulsivity, aggression, violence, and self-harm, long-term polypharmacy

with 2 atypical antipsychotics or with 1 atypical antipsychotic and 1 conventional antipsychotic may be useful or even necessary while closely monitoring

- In such cases, it may be beneficial to combine 1 depot antipsychotic with 1 oral antipsychotic

Suggested Reading

Leong OK, Wong KE, Tay WK, Gill RC. A comparative study of pipothiazine palmitate and fluphenazine decanoate in the maintenance of remission of schizophrenia. Singapore Med J 1989;30(5):436–40.

Quraishi S, David A. Depot pipothiazine palmitate and undecylenate for schizophrenia. Cochrane Database Syst Rev 2001;(3): CD001720.

Schmidt K. Pipothiazine palmitate: a versatile, sustained-action neuroleptic in psychiatric practice. Curr Med Res Opin 1986;10(5): 326–9.

PRAZOSIN

THERAPEUTICS

Brands • Minipress

see index for additional brand names

Generic? Yes

Class

- Alpha 1 adrenergic blocker

Commonly Prescribed for

(bold for FDA approved)

- **Hypertension**
- Nightmares associated with PTSD
- Blood circulation disorders
- Problems urinating due to enlarged prostate
- Passing of kidney stones

How the Drug Works

- Blocks alpha 1 adrenergic receptors to reduce noradrenergic hyperactivation
- Stimulation of central noradrenergic receptors during sleep may activate traumatic memories, so blocking this activation may reduce nightmares

How Long Until It Works

- Within a few days to a few weeks

If It Works

- Reduces the severity and frequency of nightmares associated with PTSD

If It Doesn't Work

- Increase dose
- Switch to another agent

Best Augmenting Combos for Partial Response or Treatment Resistance

- Prazosin is itself an adjunct agent for the treatment of nightmares associated with PTSD

Tests

- None for healthy individuals.
- False positive results may occur in screening tests for pheochromocytoma in patients who are being treated with prazosin; if an elevated urinary VMA is found, prazosin should be discontinued and the patient retested after a month.

SIDE EFFECTS

How Drug Causes Side Effects

- Excessive blockade of alpha 1 peripheral noradrenergic receptors

Notable Side Effects

- Dizziness, lightheadedness, headache, fatigue, blurred vision
- Nausea

Life-Threatening or Dangerous Side Effects

- Syncope with sudden loss of consciousness

Weight Gain

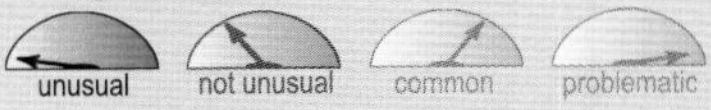

- Reported but not expected

Sedation

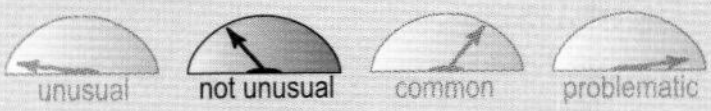

- Occurs in significant minority

What to Do About Side Effects

- Lower the dose
- Wait
- Wait
- Wait
- In a few weeks, switch to another agent

Best Augmenting Agents for Side Effects

- Often best to try another treatment prior to resorting to augmentation strategies to treat side effects

DOSING AND USE

Usual Dosage Range

- 1–16 mg/day, generally in divided doses

Dosage Forms

- Capsule 1 mg, 2 mg, 5 mg

How to Dose

- Formal dosing recommendations for treating nightmares have not been established
- Initial 1 mg at bedtime; increase dose (divided) until the nightmares resolve or an intolerable side effect occurs

Dosing Tips
- Dosing may be extremely individualized, with as little as 2 mg/day helpful for some patients and as much as 40 mg/day necessary for other patients
- Therapeutic dose does not correlate with blood levels
- Divided dosing may be preferable; in particular, giving a smaller dose during the day may be beneficial if the patient has persistent hyperarousal and re-experiencing symptoms during the day
- Risk of syncope can be decreased by limiting the initial dose to 1 mg and using slow dose titration

Overdose
- No fatalities have been reported; sedation, depressive reflexes, hypotension

Long-Term Use
- Has not been evaluated in controlled studies
- Nightmares may return if prazosin is stopped

Habit Forming
- No

How to Stop
- Taper to avoid hypertension

Pharmacokinetics
- Elimination half-life 2–3 hours

Drug Interactions
- Concomitant use with a phosphodiesterase-5 inhibitor (PDE-5) can have additive effects on blood pressure, potentially leading to hypotension; thus, a PDE-5 inhibitor should be initiated at the lowest possible dose
- Concomitant use with a beta blocker (e.g., propranolol) can have additive effects on blood pressure
- Concomitant use with other alpha 1 blockers, which include many psychotropic agents, can have additive effects leading to hypotension

Other Warnings/ Precautions
- Prazosin can cause syncope with sudden loss of consciousness, most often in association with rapid dose increases or the introduction of another antihypertensive drug
- Intraoperative floppy iris syndrome (IFIS) has been observed during cataract surgery in some patients treated with alpha 1 adrenergic blockers, which may require modifications to the surgical technique; however, there does not appear to be a benefit of stopping the alpha 1 adrenergic blocker prior to cataract surgery
- Avoid situations that can cause orthostatic hypotension, such as extensive periods of standing, prolonged or intense exercise, and exposure to heat

Do Not Use
- If there is a proven allergy to quinazolines or prazosin

SPECIAL POPULATIONS

Renal Impairment
- Use with caution in patients with severe impairment
- May require lower dose

Hepatic Impairment
- Use with caution

Cardiac Impairment
- Use with caution in patients who are predisposed to hypotensive or syncopal episodes

Elderly
- Some patients may tolerate lower doses better
- Higher risk of orthostatic hypotension and syncope

Children and Adolescents
- Safety and efficacy have not been established

Pregnancy

- Effective June 30, 2015, the US FDA requires changes to the content and format of pregnancy and lactation information in prescription drug labels, including the elimination of the pregnancy letter categories; the Pregnancy and Lactation Labeling Rule (PLLR or final rule) applies only to prescription drugs and will be phased in gradually for drugs approved on or after June 30, 2001
- Controlled studies have not been conducted in pregnant women
- Prazosin has been used alone or in combination with other hypotensive agents in severe hypertension of pregnancy, with no fetal or neonatal abnormalities reported
- Prazosin should be used during pregnancy only if the potential benefits justify the potential risks to the mother and fetus

Breast Feeding

- Some drug is present in breast milk
- If child becomes irritable or sedated, breast feeding or drug may need to be discontinued
- Must weigh benefits of breast feeding with risks and benefits of treatment versus nontreatment to both the infant and the mother

THE ART OF PSYCHOPHARMACOLOGY

Potential Advantages

- For patients with PTSD who do not respond to SSRIs/SNRIs or exposure therapy
- Specifically for nightmares and other symptoms of autonomic arousal

Potential Disadvantages

- Patients with cardiovascular disease
- Patients taking concomitant psychotropic drugs with alpha 1 antagonist properties

Primary Target Symptoms

- Nightmares

Pearls

- The evidence base for using prazosin to treat nightmares associated with PTSD is limited but positive, and prazosin is recommended by the Department of Veterans Affairs as an adjunct treatment for this purpose
- Initiate treatment early in the onset of nightmares following exposure to trauma
- May also be useful for nightmares and symptoms of autonomic arousal in other trauma and stress-related disorders in addition to PTSD

Suggested Reading

Kung S, Espinel Z, Lapid MI. Treatment of nightmares with prazosin: a systematic review. Mayo Clin Proc 2012;87(9):890–900.

Schoenfeld FB, Deviva JC, Manber R. Treatment of sleep disturbances in posttraumatic stress disorder: a review. J Rehabil Res Dev 2012;49(5):729–52.

Van Berkel VM, Bevelander SE, Mommersteeg PM. Placebo-controlled comparison of prazosin and cognitive-behavioral treatments for sleep disturbances in US Military Veterans. J Psychosom Res 2012;73(2):153.

THERAPEUTICS

Brands • Lyrica

see index for additional brand names

Generic? Yes

Class

- Neuroscience-based Nomenclature: glutamate voltage-gated calcium channel blocker (Glu-CB)
- Anticonvulsant, antineuralgic for chronic pain, alpha 2 delta ligand at voltage-sensitive calcium channels

Commonly Prescribed for

(bold for FDA approved)

- **Diabetic peripheral neuropathy**
- **Postherpetic neuralgia**
- **Fibromyalgia**
- **Neuropathic pain associated with spinal cord injury**
- **Partial seizures in adults (adjunctive)**
- Peripheral neuropathic pain
- Generalized anxiety disorder (GAD)
- Panic disorder
- Social anxiety disorder

How the Drug Works

- Is a leucine analogue and is transported both into the blood from the gut and also across the blood-brain barrier into the brain from the blood by the system L transport system (a sodium independent transporter) as well as by additional sodium-dependent amino acid transporter systems
- ✻ Binds to the alpha 2 delta subunit of voltage-sensitive calcium channels
- This closes N and P/Q presynaptic calcium channels, diminishing excessive neuronal activity and neurotransmitter release
- Although structurally related to gamma-aminobutyric acid (GABA), no known direct actions on GABA or its receptors

How Long Until It Works

- Can reduce neuropathic pain and anxiety within a week
- Should reduce seizures by 2 weeks
- If it is not producing clinical benefits within 6–8 weeks, it may require a dosage increase or it may not work at all

If It Works

- The goal of treatment of neuropathic pain, seizures, and anxiety disorders is to reduce symptoms as much as possible, and if necessary in combination with other treatments
- Treatment of neuropathic pain most often reduces but does not eliminate all symptoms and is not a cure since symptoms usually recur after medicine stopped
- Continue treatment until all symptoms are gone or until improvement is stable and then continue treating indefinitely as long as improvement persists

If It Doesn't Work (for neuropathic pain)

- Many patients have only a partial response where some symptoms are improved but others persist
- Other patients may be nonresponders, sometimes called treatment-resistant or treatment-refractory
- Consider increasing dose, switching to another agent or adding an appropriate augmenting agent
- Consider biofeedback or hypnosis for pain
- Consider psychotherapy for anxiety
- Consider the presence of noncompliance and counsel patient
- Consider evaluation for another diagnosis or for a comorbid condition (e.g., medical illness, substance abuse, etc.)

Best Augmenting Combos for Partial Response or Treatment Resistance

- ✻ In addition to being a first-line treatment for neuropathic pain and anxiety disorders, pregabalin is itself an augmenting agent to numerous other anticonvulsants in treating epilepsy
- For postherpetic neuralgia, pregabalin can decrease concomitant opiate use
- ✻ For neuropathic pain, TCAs and SNRIs as well as tiagabine, other anticonvulsants, and even opiates can augment pregabalin if done by experts while carefully monitoring in difficult cases
- For anxiety, SSRIs, SNRIs, or benzodiazepines can augment pregabalin

Tests

- None for healthy individuals

SIDE EFFECTS

How Drug Causes Side Effects

- CNS side effects may be due to excessive blockade of voltage-sensitive calcium channels

Notable Side Effects

✽ Sedation, dizziness
- Ataxia, fatigue, tremor, dysarthria, paresthesia, memory impairment, coordination abnormal, impaired attention, confusion, euphoric mood, irritability
- Vomiting, dry mouth, constipation, weight gain, increased appetite, flatulence
- Blurred vision, diplopia
- Peripheral edema
- Libido decreased, erectile dysfunction

Life-Threatening or Dangerous Side Effects

- Rare activation of suicidal ideation and behavior (suicidality)

Weight Gain

unusual | **not unusual** | common | problematic

- Occurs in significant minority

Sedation

unusual | not unusual | **common** | problematic

- Many experience and/or can be significant in amount
- Dose-related
- Can wear off with time

What to Do About Side Effects

- Wait
- Wait
- Wait
- Take more of the dose at night to reduce daytime sedation
- Lower the dose
- Switch to another agent

Best Augmenting Agents for Side Effects

- Many side effects cannot be improved with an augmenting agent

DOSING AND USE

Usual Dosage Range

- 150–600 mg/day in 2–3 doses

Dosage Forms

- Capsule 25 mg, 50 mg, 75 mg, 100 mg, 150 mg, 200 mg, 225 mg, 300 mg

How to Dose

- Neuropathic pain: initial 150 mg/day in 2–3 doses; can increase to 300 mg/day in 2–3 doses after 7 days; can increase to 600 mg/day in 2–3 doses after 7 more days; maximum dose generally 600 mg/day (may be lower for diabetic peripheral neuropathy and fibromyalgia)
- Seizures: initial 150 mg/day in 2–3 doses; can increase to 300 mg/day in 2–3 doses after 7 days; can increase to 600 mg/day in 2–3 doses after 7 more days; maximum dose generally 600 mg/day

Dosing Tips

✽ Generally given in one-third to one-sixth the dose of gabapentin
- If pregabalin is added to a second sedating agent, such as another anticonvulsant, a benzodiazepine, or an opiate, the titration period should be at least a week to improve tolerance to sedation
- Most patients need to take pregabalin only twice daily
- At the high end of the dosing range, tolerability may be enhanced by splitting dose into 3 or more divided doses
- For intolerable sedation, can give most of the dose at night and less during the day
- To improve slow-wave sleep, may only need to take pregabalin at bedtime
- May be taken with or without food

Overdose

- No fatalities

Long-Term Use

- Safe

Habit Forming

- No

How to Stop

- Taper over a minimum of 1 week

- Epilepsy patients may seize upon withdrawal, especially if withdrawal is abrupt
- Discontinuation symptoms uncommon

Pharmacokinetics

- Pregabalin is not metabolized but excreted intact renally
- Elimination half-life approximately 5–7 hours

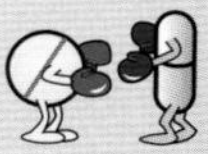

Drug Interactions

- Pregabalin has not been shown to have significant pharmacokinetic drug interactions
- Because pregabalin is excreted unchanged, it is unlikely to have significant pharmacokinetic drug interactions
- May add to or potentiate the sedative effects of oxycodone, lorazepam, and alcohol

Other Warnings/ Precautions

- Dizziness and sedation could increase the chances of accidental injury (falls) in the elderly
- Increased incidence of hemangiosarcoma at high doses in mice involves platelet changes and associated endothelial cell proliferation not present in rats or humans; no evidence to suggest an associated risk for humans
- Warn patients and their caregivers about the possibility of activation of suicidal ideation and advise them to report such side effects immediately

Do Not Use

- If there is a proven allergy to pregabalin or gabapentin
- If patient has a problem of galactose intolerance, the Lapp lactase deficiency, or glucose-galactose malabsorption

SPECIAL POPULATIONS

Renal Impairment

- Pregabalin is renally excreted, so the dose may need to be lowered
- Dosing can be adjusted according to creatinine clearance, such that patients with clearance below 15 mL/min should receive 25–75 mg/day in 1 dose, patients with clearance between 15–29 mL/min should receive 25–150 mg/day in 1–2 doses, and patients with clearance between 30–59 mL/min should receive 75–300 mg/day in 2–3 doses
- Starting dose should be at the bottom of the range; titrate as usual up to maximum dose
- Can be removed by hemodialysis; patients receiving hemodialysis may require a supplemental dose of pregabalin following hemodialysis (25–100 mg)

Hepatic Impairment

- Dose adjustment not necessary

Cardiac Impairment

- No specific recommendations

Elderly

- Some patients may tolerate lower doses better
- Elderly patients may be more susceptible to adverse effects

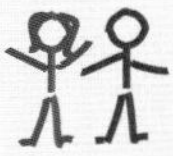

Children and Adolescents

- Safety and efficacy have not been established
- Use should be reserved for the expert

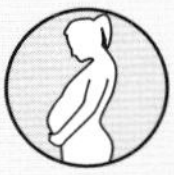

Pregnancy

- Effective June 30, 2015, the US FDA requires changes to the content and format of pregnancy and lactation information in prescription drug labels, including the elimination of the pregnancy letter categories; the Pregnancy and Lactation Labeling Rule (PLLR or final rule) applies only to prescription drugs and will be phased in gradually for drugs approved on or after June 30, 2001
- Controlled studies have not been conducted in pregnant women
- Use in women of childbearing potential requires weighing potential benefits to the mother against the risks to the fetus
- Antiepileptic Drug Pregnancy Registry: (888) 233–2334
- Taper drug if discontinuing
- Seizures, even mild seizures, may cause harm to the embryo/fetus

Breast Feeding

- Unknown if pregabalin is secreted in human breast milk, but all psychotropics assumed to be secreted in breast milk
- ✻ Recommended either to discontinue drug or bottle feed
- If drug is continued while breast feeding, infant should be monitored for possible adverse effects
- If infant becomes irritable or sedated, breast feeding or drug may need to be discontinued

THE ART OF PSYCHOPHARMACOLOGY

Potential Advantages

- First-line for diabetic peripheral neuropathy
- Fibromyalgia
- Anxiety disorders
- Sleep
- Has relatively mild side effect profile
- Has few pharmacokinetic drug interactions
- More potent and probably better tolerated than gabapentin

Potential Disadvantages

- Requires 2–3 times a day dosing
- Not approved for anxiety disorders in the USA
- Not approved for fibromyalgia in Europe

Primary Target Symptoms

- Seizures
- Pain
- Anxiety

Pearls

- ✻ First treatment approved for fibromyalgia
- ✻ One of the first treatments approved for neuropathic pain associated with diabetic peripheral neuropathy
- Also approved in postherpetic neuralgia
- Improves sleep disruption as well as pain in patients with painful diabetic peripheral neuropathy or postherpetic neuralgia
- Improves sleep disruption as well as pain associated with fibromyalgia
- Well studied in epilepsy, peripheral neuropathic pain, and GAD, and actually approved for GAD in Europe
- ✻ Off-label use for GAD, panic disorder, and social anxiety disorder may be justified in the USA
- May have uniquely robust therapeutic actions for both the somatic and the psychic symptoms of GAD
- ✻ Off-label use as an adjunct for bipolar disorder may not be justified
- ✻ One of the few agents that enhances slow-wave delta sleep, which may be helpful in chronic neuropathic pain syndromes
- Pregabalin is generally well tolerated, with only mild adverse effects
- ✻ Although no head-to-head studies, appears to be better tolerated and more consistently efficacious at high doses than gabapentin
- ✻ Drug absorption and clinical efficacy may be more consistent at high doses for pregabalin compared to gabapentin because of the higher potency of pregabalin and the fact that, unlike gabapentin, it is transported by more than one transport system

Suggested Reading

Lauria-Horner BA, Pohl RB. Pregabalin: a new anxiolytic. Expert Opin Investig Drugs 2003;12:663–72.

Moore RA, Straube S, Wiffen PJ, Derry S, McQuay HJ. Pregabalin for acute and chronic pain in adults. Cochrane Database Syst Rev 2009;8(3):CD007076.

Stahl SM. Anticonvulsants and the relief of chronic pain: pregabalin and gabapentin as alpha(2)delta ligands at voltage-gated calcium channels. J Clin Psychiatry 2004;65:596–7.

Stahl SM. Anticonvulsants as anxiolytics, part 2: Pregabalin and gabapentin as alpha(2)delta ligands at voltage-gated calcium channels. J Clin Psychiatry 2004;65:460–1.

Stahl SM, Eisenach JC, Taylor CP, et al. The diverse therapeutic actions of pregabalin: is a single mechanism responsible for several pharmacologic activities. Trends Pharmacological Sci 2013;34(6):332–9.

PROPRANOLOL

THERAPEUTICS

Brands
- Inderal
- Inderal LA
- InnoPran XL

see index for additional brand names

Generic? Yes

Class
- Beta blocker, antihypertensive

Commonly Prescribed for
(bold for FDA approved)
- **Migraine prophylaxis**
- **Essential tremor**
- **Hypertension**
- **Angina pectoris due to coronary atherosclerosis**
- **Cardiac arrhythmias (including supraventricular arrhythmias, ventricular tachycardia, digitalis intoxication)**
- **Myocardial infarction**
- **Hypertrophic subaortic stenosis**
- **Pheochromocytoma**
- Akathisia (antipsychotic induced)
- Parkinsonian tremor
- Violence, aggression
- PTSD, prophylactic
- Generalized anxiety disorder (GAD)
- Prevention of variceal bleeding
- Congestive heart failure
- Tetralogy of Fallot
- Hyperthyroidism (adjunctive)

How the Drug Works
- For migraine, proposed mechanisms include inhibition of the adrenergic pathway, interaction with the serotonin system and receptors, inhibition of nitric oxide synthesis, and normalization of contingent negative variation
- For tremor, antagonism of peripheral beta 2 receptors is the proposed mechanism
- For PTSD, blockade of beta 1 adrenergic receptors may theoretically prevent fear conditioning and reconsolidation of fear
- For violence/aggression, the mechanism is poorly established; presumed to be related to central actions at beta adrenergic and serotonin receptors

How Long Until It Works
- For migraine, can begin to work within 2 weeks, but may take up to 3 months on a stable dose to see full effect
- For tremor, can begin to work within days

If It Works
- For migraine, the goal is a 50% or greater decrease in migraine frequency or severity; consider tapering or stopping if headaches remit for more than 6 months
- For tremor, can cause reduction in the severity of tremor, allowing greater functioning with daily activities and clearer speech
- For PTSD, may theoretically block the effects of stress from prior traumatic experiences
- For aggression, may reduce aggression, agitation, or uncooperativeness

If It Doesn't Work
- Increase to highest tolerated dose
- For migraine, address other issues such as medication overuse or other coexisting medical disorders; consider changing to another drug or adding a second drug
- For tremor, coadministration with primidone up to 250 mg/day can augment response; second-line medications include benzodiazepines, gabapentin, topiramate, methazolamide, nadolol, and botulinum toxin (useful for voice and hand tremor); alternative treatments include caffeine and hand weights
- For patients with truly refractory tremor, thalamotomy or deep brain stimulation of the ventral intermediate nucleus of the thalamus is an option
- For PTSD, consider initiating first-line pharmacotherapy (SSRI, SNRI) and psychotherapy
- For violence/aggression, switch to another agent, e.g., valproate or an antipsychotic

Best Augmenting Combos for Partial Response or Treatment Resistance
- Migraine: for some patients, low-dose polytherapy with 2 or more drugs may be better tolerated and more effective than high-dose monotherapy; may use propranolol in combination with anticonvulsants, antidepressants, natural products, and non-pharmacologic

treatments, such as biofeedback, to improve headache control
- For tremor, can combine with primidone or second-line medications
- For aggression and violence, can combine with valproate and/or antipsychotics

Tests
- None for healthy individuals

SIDE EFFECTS

How Drug Causes Side Effects
- By blocking beta adrenergic receptors, it can cause dizziness, bradycardia, and hypotension

Notable Side Effects
- Bradycardia, hypotension, hyper- or hypoglycemia, weight gain
- Bronchospasm, cold/flu symptoms, sinusitis, pneumonias
- Dizziness, vertigo, fatigue/tiredness, depression, sleep disturbances
- Sexual dysfunction, decreased libido, dysuria, urinary retention, joint pain
- Exacerbation of symptoms in peripheral vascular disease and Raynaud's syndrome

Life-Threatening or Dangerous Side Effects
- In acute congestive heart failure, may further depress myocardial contractility
- Can blunt premonitory symptoms of hypoglycemia in diabetes and mask clinical signs of hyperthyroidism
- Non-selective beta blockers such as propranolol can inhibit bronchodilation, making them contraindicated in asthma, severe COPD
- Do not use in pheochromocytoma unless alpha blockers are already being used
- Risk of excessive myocardial depression in general anesthesia

Weight Gain
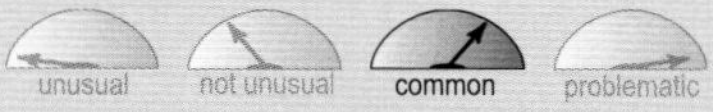

- Many experience and/or can be significant in amount

Sedation
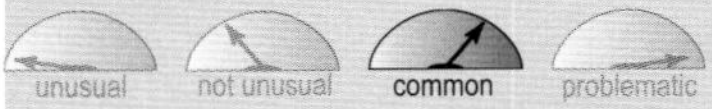

- Many experience and/or can be significant in amount

What to Do About Side Effects
- Lower dose, change to an extended-release formulation, or switch to another agent

Best Augmenting Agents for Side Effects
- When patients have significant benefit from beta blocker therapy but hypotension limits treatment, consider alpha agonists (midodrine) or volume expanders (fludrocortisones) for symptomatic relief
- Many side effects cannot be improved with an augmenting agent

DOSING AND USE

Usual Dosage Range
- 40–400 mg/day

Dosage Forms
- Tablet 10 mg, 20 mg, 40 mg, 60 mg, 80 mg, 90 mg
- Extended-release capsule 60 mg, 80 mg, 120 mg, 160 mg
- Oral solution 4 mg/mL, 8 mg/mL
- Injection 1 mg/mL

How to Dose
- Migraine: initial dose 40 mg/day in divided doses or once daily in extended-release preparations; gradually increase over days to weeks until effective dose is reached; maximum dose 400 mg/day
- Tremor: initial dose 40 mg twice per day; dosage may be gradually increased as needed to 120–320 mg/day in 2 to 3 divided doses
- PTSD: effective dose varies greatly; up to 240 mg/day have been used
- Aggression: same as migraine; up to 400 mg/day if tolerated and effective

Dosing Tips
- For extended-release capsules, give once daily at bedtime consistently, with or without food

- Doses above 120 mg had no additional antihypertensive effect in clinical trials
- High doses may be effective in some patients with tremor, migraine, or aggression/violence

Overdose

- Bradycardia, hypotension, low-output heart failure, shock, seizures, coma, hypoglycemia, apnea, cyanosis, respiratory depression, and broncospasm

Long-Term Use

- Safe

Habit Forming

- No

How to Stop

- Should not be discontinued abruptly; instead gradually reduce dosage over 1–2 weeks
- May exacerbate angina, and there are reports of tachyarrhythmias or myocardial infarction with rapid discontinuation in patients with cardiac disease

Pharmacokinetics

- Half-life 3–5 hours (immediate-release) or 8–11 hours (extended-release)

Drug Interactions

- Cimetidine, oral contraceptives, ciprofloxacin, hydralazine, hydroxychloroquine, loop diuretics, certain SSRIs (with CYP 2D6 metabolism), and phenothiazines can increase levels and/or effects of propranolol
- Use with calcium channel blockers can be synergistic or additive, use with caution
- Barbiturates, penicillins, rifampin, calcium and aluminum salts, thyroid hormones, and cholestyramine can decrease effects of beta blockers
- NSAIDs, sulfinpyrazone, and salicyclates inhibit prostaglandin synthesis and may inhibit the antihypertensive activity of beta blockers
- Propranolol can increase adverse effects of gabapentin and benzodiazapines
- Propranolol can increase levels of lidocaine, resulting in toxicity, and increase the anticoagulant effect of warfarin
- Increased postural hypotension with prazosin and peripheral ischemia with ergot alkaloids
- Sudden discontinuation of clonidine while on beta blockers or when stopping together can cause life-threatening increases in blood pressure

Other Warnings/ Precautions

- May elevate blood urea, serum transaminases, alkaline phosphatase, and lactate dehydrogenase (LDH)
- Rare development of antinuclear antibodies (ANAs)
- May worsen symptoms of myasthenia gravis
- Can lower intraocular pressure, interfering with glaucoma screening test

Do Not Use

- If patient has bradycardia, greater than first-degree heart block, or cardiogenic shock
- If patient has bronchial asthma or severe COPD
- If there is a proven allergy to propranolol

SPECIAL POPULATIONS

Renal Impairment

- No dose adjustment necessary

Hepatic Impairment

- Use with caution with severe impairment; dose reduction may be necessary

Cardiac Impairment

- Do not use in acute shock, myocardial infarction, hypotension, and greater than first-degree heart block, but indicated in clinically stable patients post-myocardial infarction to reduce risk of re-infarction starting 1–4 weeks after event

Elderly

- Use with caution
- May increase risk of stroke

Children and Adolescents

- Usual dose in children is 2–4 mg/kg in 2 divided doses; maximum 16 mg/kg/day
- Clinical trials for migraine prophylaxis did not include children

Pregnancy

- Effective June 30, 2015, the US FDA requires changes to the content and format of pregnancy and lactation information in prescription drug labels, including the elimination of the pregnancy letter categories; the Pregnancy and Lactation Labeling Rule (PLLR or final rule) applies only to prescription drugs and will be phased in gradually for drugs approved on or after June 30, 2001
- Controlled studies have not been conducted in pregnant women
- May reduce perfusion of the placenta
- Use only if potential benefits outweigh the potential risks to the fetus

Breast Feeding

- Some drug is found in mother's breast milk
- Due to high lipid solubility, propranolol is found in breast milk more than many other beta blockers

❋ Recommended either to discontinue drug or bottle feed unless the potential benefit to the mother justifies the potential risk to the child

THE ART OF PSYCHOPHARMACOLOGY

Potential Advantages

- Patients who do not respond to or tolerate other options
- Patients with autonomic hyperactivity

Potential Disadvantages

- Multiple potential undesirable adverse effects, including bradycardia, hypotension, and fatigue

Primary Target Symptoms

- Migraine frequency and severity
- Tremor
- Effects of stress from prior traumatic experience
- Aggression, agitation

Pearls

- Often used in combination with other drugs in migraine, which may allow patients to better tolerate medications that cause tremor, such as valproate
- May worsen depression, but helpful for anxiety
- 50–70% of patients with essential tremor receive some relief, usually with about 50% improvement or greater
- Propranolol may theoretically block the effects of stress from prior traumatic experiences, but this is unproven and data thus far are mixed

Suggested Reading

Brunet A, Poundja J, Tremblay J, et al. Trauma reactivation under the influence of propranolol decreases posttraumatic stress symptoms and disorders: 3 open-label trials. J Clin Psychopharmacol 2011;31(4):547–50.

Cohen H, Kaplan Z, Koresh O, et al. Early post-stressor intervention with propranolol is ineffective in preventing posttraumatic stress responses in an animal model for PTSD. Eur Neuropsychopharmacol 2011;21(3):230–40.

Fleminger S, Greenwood RJ, Oliver DL. Pharmacological management for agitation and aggression in people with acquired brain injury. Cochrane Database Syst Rev 2003;(1):CD003299.

Lyons KE, Pahwa R. Pharmacotherapy of essential tremor: an overview of existing and upcoming agents. CNS Drugs 2008;22(12):1037–45.

Silberstein SD. Preventive migraine treatment. Neurol Clin 2009;27(2):429–43.

PROTRIPTYLINE

THERAPEUTICS

Brands • Triptil
• Vivactil

see index for additional brand names

Generic? Yes

Class

- Neuroscience-based Nomenclature: serotonin, norepinephrine reuptake inhibitor
- Tricyclic antidepressant (TCA)
- Predominantly a norepinephrine/ noradrenaline reuptake inhibitor

Commonly Prescribed for

(bold for FDA approved)

- **Mental depression**
- Treatment-resistant depression

How the Drug Works

- Boosts neurotransmitter norepinephrine/ noradrenaline
- Blocks norepinephrine reuptake pump (norepinephrine transporter), presumably increasing noradrenergic neurotransmission
- Since dopamine is inactivated by norepinephrine reuptake in frontal cortex, which largely lacks dopamine transporters, protriptyline can increase dopamine neurotransmission in this part of the brain
- A more potent inhibitor of norepinephrine reuptake pump than serotonin reuptake pump (serotonin transporter)
- At high doses may also boost neurotransmitter serotonin and presumably increase serotonergic neurotransmission

How Long Until It Works

✽ Some evidence it may have an early onset of action with improvement in activity and energy as early as 1 week
- Onset of therapeutic actions usually not immediate, but often delayed 2 to 4 weeks
- If it is not working within 6 to 8 weeks for depression, it may require a dosage increase or it may not work at all
- May continue to work for many years to prevent relapse of symptoms

If It Works

- The goal of treatment is complete remission of current symptoms as well as prevention of future relapses
- Treatment most often reduces or even eliminates symptoms, but not a cure since symptoms can recur after medicine stopped
- Continue treatment until all symptoms are gone (remission)
- Once symptoms gone, continue treating for 1 year for the first episode of depression
- For second and subsequent episodes of depression, treatment may need to be indefinite
- Use in anxiety disorders may also need to be indefinite

If It Doesn't Work

- Many patients have only a partial response where some symptoms are improved but others persist (especially insomnia, fatigue, and problems concentrating)
- Other patients may be nonresponders, sometimes called treatment-resistant or treatment-refractory
- Consider increasing dose, switching to another agent or adding an appropriate augmenting agent
- Consider psychotherapy
- Consider evaluation for another diagnosis or for a comorbid condition (e.g., medical illness, substance abuse, etc.)
- Some patients may experience apparent lack of consistent efficacy due to activation of latent or underlying bipolar disorder, and require antidepressant discontinuation and a switch to a mood stabilizer

Best Augmenting Combos for Partial Response or Treatment Resistance

- Lithium, buspirone, thyroid hormone

Tests

- Baseline ECG is recommended for patients over age 50

✽ Since tricyclic and tetracyclic antidepressants are frequently associated with weight gain, before starting treatment, weigh all patients and determine if the patient is already overweight (BMI 25.0–29.9) or obese (BMI ≥30)
- Before giving a drug that can cause weight gain to an overweight or obese

patient, consider determining whether the patient already has pre-diabetes (fasting plasma glucose 100–125 mg/dL), diabetes (fasting plasma glucose >126 mg/dL), or dyslipidemia (increased total cholesterol, LDL cholesterol, and triglycerides; decreased HDL cholesterol), and treat or refer such patients for treatment, including nutrition and weight management, physical activity counseling, smoking cessation, and medical management

- ❄ Monitor weight and BMI during treatment
- ❄ While giving a drug to a patient who has gained >5% of initial weight, consider evaluating for the presence of pre-diabetes, diabetes, or dyslipidemia, or consider switching to a different antidepressant
- EKGs may be useful for selected patients (e.g., those with personal or family history of QTc prolongation; cardiac arrhythmia; recent myocardial infarction; uncompensated heart failure; or taking agents that prolong QTc interval such as pimozide, thioridazine, selected antiarrhythmics, moxifloxacin, sparfloxacin, etc.)
- Patients at risk for electrolyte disturbances (e.g., patients on diuretic therapy) should have baseline and periodic serum potassium and magnesium measurements

SIDE EFFECTS

How Drug Causes Side Effects

- ❄ Anticholinergic activity for protriptyline may be more potent than for some other TCAs and may explain sedative effects, dry mouth, constipation, blurred vision, tachycardia, and hypotension
- Sedative effects and weight gain may be due to antihistamine properties
- Blockade of alpha 1 adrenergic receptors may explain dizziness, sedation, and hypotension
- Cardiac arrhythmias, especially in overdose, may be caused by blockade of ion channels

Notable Side Effects

- Blurred vision, constipation, urinary retention, increased appetite, dry mouth, nausea, diarrhea, heartburn, unusual taste in mouth, weight gain
- Fatigue, weakness, dizziness, sedation, headache, anxiety, nervousness, restlessness
- Sexual dysfunction (impotence, change in libido)
- Sweating, rash, itching

Life-Threatening or Dangerous Side Effects

- Paralytic ileus, hyperthermia (TCAs + anticholinergic agents)
- Lowered seizure threshold and rare seizures
- Orthostatic hypotension, sudden death, arrhythmias, tachycardia
- QTc prolongation
- Hepatic failure, extrapyramidal symptoms
- Increased intraocular pressure
- Rare induction of mania
- Rare activation of suicidal ideation and behavior (suicidality) (short-term studies did not show an increase in the risk of suicidality with antidepressants compared to placebo beyond age 24)

Weight Gain

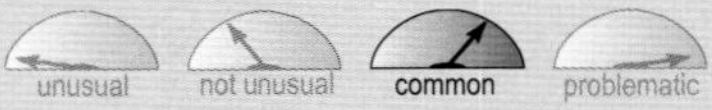

- Many experience and/or can be significant in amount
- Can increase appetite and carbohydrate craving

Sedation

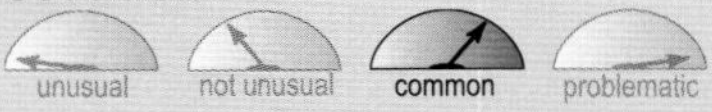

- Many experience and/or can be significant in amount
- ❄ Not as sedating as other TCAs; more likely to be activating than other TCAs

What to Do About Side Effects

- Wait
- Wait
- Wait
- Lower the dose
- Switch to an SSRI or newer antidepressant

Best Augmenting Agents for Side Effects

- Trazodone or a hypnotic for insomnia
- Benzodiazepines for agitation and anxiety
- Many side effects cannot be improved with an augmenting agent

DOSING AND USE

Usual Dosage Range
- 15–40 mg/day in 3–4 divided doses

Dosage Forms
- Tablets 5 mg, 10 mg

How to Dose
- Initial 15 mg/day in divided doses; increase morning dose as needed; maximum dose 60 mg/day

Dosing Tips
✻ Be aware that among this class of agents (tricyclic/tetracyclic antidepressants), protriptyline has uniquely low dosing (15–40 mg/day for protriptyline compared to 75–300 mg/day for most other tricyclic/tetracyclic antidepressants)

✻ Be aware that among this class of agents (tricyclic/tetracyclic antidepressants), protriptyline has uniquely frequent dosing (3–4 times a day compared to once daily for most other tricyclic/tetracyclic antidepressants)

- If intolerable anxiety, insomnia, agitation, akathisia, or activation occur either upon dosing initiation or discontinuation, consider the possibility of activated bipolar disorder, and switch to a mood stabilizer or an atypical antipsychotic

Overdose
- Death may occur; CNS depression, convulsions, cardiac dysrhythmias, severe hypotension, EKG changes, coma

Long-Term Use
- Safe

Habit Forming
- No

How to Stop
- Taper to avoid withdrawal effects
- Even with gradual dose reduction some withdrawal symptoms may appear within the first 2 weeks
- Many patients tolerate 50% dose reduction for 3 days, then another 50% reduction for 3 days, then discontinuation
- If withdrawal symptoms emerge during discontinuation, raise dose to stop symptoms and then restart withdrawal much more slowly

Pharmacokinetics
- Substrate for CYP450 2D6
- Half-life approximately 74 hours

Drug Interactions
- Tramadol increases the risk of seizures in patients taking TCAs
- Use of TCAs with anticholinergic drugs may result in paralytic ileus or hyperthermia
- Fluoxetine, paroxetine, bupropion, duloxetine, and other 2D6 inhibitors may increase TCA concentrations
- Cimetidine may increase plasma concentrations of TCAs and cause anti-cholinergic symptoms
- Phenothiazines or haloperidol may raise TCA blood concentrations
- May alter effects of antihypertensive drugs; may inhibit hypotensive effects of clonidine
- Use with sympathomimetic agents may increase sympathetic activity
- Methylphenidate may inhibit metabolism of TCAs
- Activation and agitation, especially following switching or adding antidepressants, may represent the induction of a bipolar state, especially a mixed dysphoric bipolar II condition sometimes associated with suicidal ideation, and require the addition of lithium, a mood stabilizer or an atypical antipsychotic, and/or discontinuation of protriptyline

Other Warnings/ Precautions
- Add or initiate other antidepressants with caution for up to 2 weeks after discontinuing protriptyline
- Generally, do not use with MAOIs, including 14 days after MAOIs are stopped; do not start an MAOI for at least 5 half-lives (5 to 7 days for most drugs) after discontinuing protriptyline
- Use with caution in patients with history of seizures, urinary retention, angle-closure glaucoma, hyperthyroidism
- TCAs can increase QTc interval, especially at toxic doses, which can be attained not

only by overdose but also by combining with drugs that inhibit TCA metabolism via CYP450 2D6, potentially causing torsade de pointes-type arrhythmia or sudden death
- Because TCAs can prolong QTc interval, use with caution in patients who have bradycardia or who are taking drugs that can induce bradycardia (e.g., beta blockers, calcium channel blockers, clonidine, digitalis)
- Because TCAs can prolong QTc interval, use with caution in patients who have hypokalemia and/or hypomagnesemia or who are taking drugs that can induce hypokalemia and/or magnesemia (e.g., diuretics, stimulant laxatives, intravenous amphotericin B, glucocorticoids, tetracosactide)
- When treating children, carefully weigh the risks and benefits of pharmacological treatment against the risks and benefits of nontreatment with antidepressants and make sure to document this in the patient's chart
- Distribute the brochures provided by the FDA and the drug companies
- Warn patients and their caregivers about the possibility of activating side effects and advise them to report such symptoms immediately
- Monitor patients for activation of suicidal ideation, especially children and adolescents

Do Not Use

- If patient is recovering from myocardial infarction
- If patient is taking agents capable of significantly prolonging QTc interval (e.g., pimozide, thioridazine, selected antiarrhythmics, moxifloxacin, sparfloxacin)
- If there is a history of QTc prolongation or cardiac arrhythmia, recent acute myocardial infarction, uncompensated heart failure
- If patient is taking drugs that inhibit TCA metabolism, including CYP450 2D6 inhibitors, except by an expert
- If there is reduced CYP450 2D6 function, such as patients who are poor 2D6 metabolizers, except by an expert and at low doses
- If there is a proven allergy to protriptyline

SPECIAL POPULATIONS

Renal Impairment

- Use with caution; may need to lower dose
- Patient may need to be monitored closely

Hepatic Impairment

- Use with caution; may need to lower dose
- Patient may need to be monitored closely

Cardiac Impairment

- Baseline ECG is recommended
- TCAs have been reported to cause arrhythmias, prolongation of conduction time, orthostatic hypotension, sinus tachycardia, and heart failure, especially in the diseased heart
- Myocardial infarction and stroke have been reported with TCAs
- TCAs produce QTc prolongation, which may be enhanced by the existence of bradycardia, hypokalemia, congenital or acquired long QTc interval, which should be evaluated prior to administering protriptyline
- Use with caution if treating concomitantly with a medication likely to produce prolonged bradycardia, hypokalemia, slowing of intracardiac conduction, or prolongation of the QTc interval
- Avoid TCAs in patients with a known history of QTc prolongation, recent acute myocardial infarction, and uncompensated heart failure
- TCAs may cause a sustained increase in heart rate in patients with ischemic heart disease and may worsen (decrease) heart rate variability, an independent risk of mortality in cardiac populations
- Since SSRIs may improve (increase) heart rate variability in patients following a myocardial infarct and may improve survival as well as mood in patients with acute angina or following a myocardial infarction, these are more appropriate agents for cardiac population than tricyclic/tetracyclic antidepressants

✽ Risk/benefit ratio may not justify use of TCAs in cardiac impairment

Elderly

- Baseline ECG is recommended for patients over age 50
- May be more sensitive to anticholinergic, cardiovascular, hypotensive, and sedative effects

- Recommended dose is between 15–20 mg/day; doses >20 mg/day require close monitoring of patient
- Reduction in the risk of suicidality with antidepressants compared to placebo in adults age 65 and older

Children and Adolescents

- Carefully weigh the risks and benefits of pharmacological treatment against the risks and benefits of nontreatment with antidepressants and make sure to document this in the patient's chart
- Monitor patients face-to-face regularly, particularly during the first several weeks of treatment
- Use with caution, observing for activation of known or unknown bipolar disorder and/or suicidal ideation, and inform parents or guardians of this risk so they can help observe child or adolescent patients
- Not recommended for use under age 12
- Not intended for use under age 6
- Several studies show lack of efficacy of TCAs for depression
- Some cases of sudden death have occurred in children taking TCAs
- Recommended dose: 15–20 mg/day

Pregnancy

- Effective June 30, 2015, the US FDA requires changes to the content and format of pregnancy and lactation information in prescription drug labels, including the elimination of the pregnancy letter categories; the Pregnancy and Lactation Labeling Rule (PLLR or final rule) applies only to prescription drugs and will be phased in gradually for drugs approved on or after June 30, 2001
- Controlled studies have not been conducted in pregnant women
- Crosses the placenta
- Adverse effects have been reported in infants whose mothers took a TCA (lethargy, withdrawal symptoms, fetal malformations)
- Must weigh the risk of treatment (first trimester fetal development, third trimester newborn delivery) to the child against the risk of no treatment (recurrence of depression, maternal health, infant bonding) to the mother and child
- For many patients this may mean continuing treatment during pregnancy

Breast Feeding

- Some drug is found in mother's breast milk

✻ Recommended either to discontinue drug or bottle feed

- Immediate postpartum period is a high-risk time for depression, especially in women who have had prior depressive episodes, so drug may need to be reinstituted late in the third trimester or shortly after childbirth to prevent a recurrence during the postpartum period
- Must weigh benefits of breast feeding with risks and benefits of antidepressant treatment versus nontreatment to both the infant and the mother
- For many patients this may mean continuing treatment during breast feeding

THE ART OF PSYCHOPHARMACOLOGY

Potential Advantages

- Severe or treatment-resistant depression
- Withdrawn, anergic patients

Potential Disadvantages

- Pediatric, geriatric, and cardiac patients
- Patients concerned with weight gain
- Patients noncompliant with 3–4 times daily dosing

Primary Target Symptoms

- Depressed mood

Pearls

- TCAs are no longer generally considered a first-line treatment option for depression because of their side effect profile
- TCAs continue to be useful for severe or treatment-resistant depression

✻ Has some potential advantages for withdrawn, anergic patients

✻ May have a more rapid onset of action than some other TCAs

✻ May aggravate agitation and anxiety more than some other TCAs

* May have more anticholinergic side effects, hypotension, and tachycardia than some other TCAs
- Noradrenergic reuptake inhibitors such as protriptyline can be used as a second-line treatment for smoking cessation, cocaine dependence, and attention deficit disorder
- TCAs may aggravate psychotic symptoms
- Alcohol should be avoided because of additive CNS effects
- Underweight patients may be more susceptible to adverse cardiovascular effects
- Children, patients with inadequate hydration, and patients with cardiac disease may be more susceptible to TCA-induced cardiotoxicity than healthy adults
- For the expert only: a heroic treatment (but potentially dangerous) for severely treatment-resistant patients is to give simultaneously with MAOIs for patients who fail to respond to numerous other antidepressants, but generally recommend a different TCA than protriptyline for this use
- If this option is elected, start the MAOI with the tricyclic/tetracyclic antidepressant simultaneously at low doses after appropriate drug washout, then alternately increase doses of these agents every few days to a week as tolerated
- Although very strict dietary and concomitant drug restrictions must be observed to prevent hypertensive crises and serotonin syndrome, the most common side effects of MAOI and tricyclic/tetracyclic antidepressant combinations may be weight gain and orthostatic hypotension
- Patients on TCAs should be aware that they may experience symptoms such as photosensitivity or blue-green urine
- SSRIs may be more effective than TCAs in women, and TCAs may be more effective than SSRIs in men
- Since tricyclic/tetracyclic antidepressants are substrates for CYP450 2D6, and 7% of the population (especially Caucasians) may have a genetic variant leading to reduced activity of 2D6, such patients may not safely tolerate normal doses of tricyclic/tetracyclic antidepressants and may require dose reduction
- Phenotypic testing may be necessary to detect this genetic variant prior to dosing with a tricyclic/tetracyclic antidepressant, especially in vulnerable populations such as children, elderly, cardiac populations, and those on concomitant medications
- Patients who seem to have extraordinarily severe side effects at normal or low doses may have this phenotypic CYP450 2D6 variant and require low doses or switching to another antidepressant not metabolized by 2D6

Suggested Reading

Anderson IM. Meta-analytical studies on new antidepressants. Br Med Bull 2001;57:161–78.

Anderson IM. Selective serotonin reuptake inhibitors versus tricyclic antidepressants: a meta-analysis of efficacy and tolerability. J Aff Disorders 2000;58:19–36.

Rudorfer MV, Potter WZ. Metabolism of tricyclic antidepressants. Cell Mol Neurobiol 1999;19(3):373–409.

QUAZEPAM

THERAPEUTICS

Brands
• Doral

see index for additional brand names

Generic? No

Class
- Neuroscience-based Nomenclature: GABA positive allosteric modulator (GABA-PAM)
- Benzodiazepine (hypnotic)

Commonly Prescribed for
(bold for FDA approved)
- **Short-term treatment of insomnia**
- Catatonia

How the Drug Works
- Binds to benzodiazepine receptors at the GABA-A ligand-gated chloride channel complex
- Enhances the inhibitory effects of GABA
- Boosts chloride conductance through GABA-regulated channels
- Inhibitory actions in sleep centers may provide sedative hypnotic effects

How Long Until It Works
- Generally takes effect in less than an hour

If It Works
- Improves quality of sleep
- Effects on total wake-time and number of nighttime awakenings may be decreased over time

If It Doesn't Work
- If insomnia does not improve after 7–10 days, it may be a manifestation of a primary psychiatric or physical illness such as obstructive sleep apnea or restless leg syndrome, which requires independent evaluation
- Increase the dose
- Improve sleep hygiene
- Switch to another agent

Best Augmenting Combos for Partial Response or Treatment Resistance
- Generally, best to switch to another agent
- Trazodone
- Agents with antihistamine actions (e.g., diphenhydramine, TCAs)

Tests
- In patients with seizure disorders, concomitant medical illness, and/or those with multiple concomitant long-term medications, periodic liver tests and blood counts may be prudent

SIDE EFFECTS

How Drug Causes Side Effects
- Same mechanism for side effects as for therapeutic effects – namely due to excessive actions at benzodiazepine receptors
- Actions at benzodiazepine receptors that carry over to the next day can cause daytime sedation, amnesia, and ataxia
- Long-term adaptations in benzodiazepine receptors may explain the development of dependence, tolerance, and withdrawal

Notable Side Effects
- ✻ Sedation, fatigue, depression
- ✻ Dizziness, ataxia, slurred speech, weakness
- ✻ Forgetfulness, confusion
- ✻ Hyperexcitability, nervousness
- Rare hallucinations, mania
- Rare hypotension
- Hypersalivation, dry mouth
- Rebound insomnia when withdrawing from long-term treatment

Life-Threatening or Dangerous Side Effects
- Respiratory depression, especially when taken with CNS depressants in overdose
- Rare hepatic dysfunction, renal dysfunction, blood dyscrasias

Weight Gain

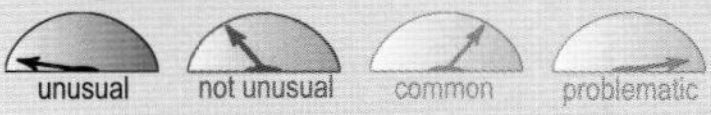

- Reported but not expected

Sedation

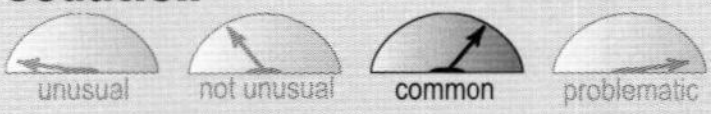

- Many experience and/or can be significant in amount

What to Do About Side Effects
- Wait

- To avoid problems with memory, only take quazepam if planning to have a full night's sleep
- Lower the dose
- Switch to a shorter-acting sedative hypnotic
- Switch to a non-benzodiazepine hypnotic
- Administer flumazenil if side effects are severe or life-threatening

Best Augmenting Agents for Side Effects
- Many side effects cannot be improved with an augmenting agent

DOSING AND USE

Usual Dosage Range
- 15 mg/day at bedtime

Dosage Forms
- Tablet 7.5 mg, 15 mg

How to Dose
- 15 mg/day at bedtime; increase to 30 mg/day if ineffective; maximum dose 30 mg/day

Dosing Tips
- Use lowest possible effective dose and assess need for continued treatment regularly
- Quazepam should generally not be prescribed in quantities greater than a 1-month supply
- Patients with lower body weights may require lower doses
- Risk of dependence may increase with dose and duration of treatment

Overdose
- No death reported in monotherapy; sedation, respiratory depression, poor coordination, confusion, coma

Long-Term Use
- Not generally intended for use beyond 4 weeks

✻ Because of its relatively longer half-life, quazepam may cause some daytime sedation and/or impaired motor/cognitive function, and may do so progressively over time

Habit Forming
- Quazepam is a Schedule IV drug
- Some patients may develop dependence and/or tolerance; risk may be greater with higher doses
- History of drug addiction may increase risk of dependence

How to Stop
- If taken for more than a few weeks, taper to reduce chances of withdrawal effects
- Patients with seizure history may seize upon sudden withdrawal
- Rebound insomnia may occur the first 1–2 nights after stopping
- For patients with severe problems discontinuing a benzodiazepine, dosing may need to be tapered over many months (i.e., reduce dose by 1% every 3 days by crushing tablet and suspending or dissolving in 100 mL of fruit juice and then disposing of 1 mL while drinking the rest; 3–7 days later, dispose of 2 mL, and so on). This is both a form of very slow biological tapering and a form of behavioral desensitization

Pharmacokinetics
- Half life 25–41 hours
- Active metabolite
- Metabolized in part by CYP450 3A4

Drug Interactions
- Increased depressive effects when taken with other CNS depressants (see Warnings below)
- Effects of quazepam may be increased by CYP450 3A4 inhibitors such as nefazodone or fluvoxamine

Other Warnings/ Precautions
- Boxed warning regarding the increased risk of CNS depressant effects when benzodiazepines and opioid medications are used together, including specifically the risk of slowed or difficulty breathing and death
- If alternatives to the combined use of benzodiazepines and opioids are not available, clinicians should limit the dosage and duration of each drug to the minimum possible while still achieving therapeutic efficacy

- Patients and their caregivers should be warned to seek medical attention if unusual dizziness, lightheadedness, sedation, slowed or difficulty breathing, or unresponsiveness occur
- Insomnia may be a symptom of a primary disorder, rather than a primary disorder itself
- Some patients may exhibit abnormal thinking or behavioral changes similar to those caused by other CNS depressants (i.e., either depressant actions or disinhibiting actions)
- Some depressed patients may experience a worsening of suicidal ideation
- Use only with extreme caution in patients with impaired respiratory function or obstructive sleep apnea
- Quazepam should be administered only at bedtime

Do Not Use

- If patient is pregnant
- If patient has angle-closure glaucoma
- If there is a proven allergy to quazepam or any benzodiazepine

SPECIAL POPULATIONS

Renal Impairment

- Recommended dose: 7.5 mg/day

Hepatic Impairment

- Recommended dose: 7.5 mg/day

Cardiac Impairment

- Benzodiazepines have been used to treat insomnia associated with acute myocardial infarction

Elderly

- Recommended dose: 7.5 mg/day
- If 15 mg/day is given initially, try to reduce the dose to 7.5 mg/day after the first 1–2 nights

Children and Adolescents

- Safety and efficacy have not been established
- Long-term effects of quazepam in children/adolescents are unknown
- Should generally receive lower doses and be more closely monitored

Pregnancy

- Contraindicated for use in pregnancy
- Effective June 30, 2015, the US FDA requires changes to the content and format of pregnancy and lactation information in prescription drug labels, including the elimination of the pregnancy letter categories; the Pregnancy and Lactation Labeling Rule (PLLR or final rule) applies only to prescription drugs and will be phased in gradually for drugs approved on or after June 30, 2001
- Infants whose mothers received a benzodiazepine late in pregnancy may experience withdrawal effects
- Neonatal flaccidity has been reported in infants whose mothers took a benzodiazepine during pregnancy

Breast Feeding

- Some drug is found in mother's breast milk
- ✻ Recommended either to discontinue drug or bottle feed
- Effects on infant have been observed and include feeding difficulties, sedation, and weight loss

THE ART OF PSYCHOPHARMACOLOGY

Potential Advantages

- Transient insomnia

Potential Disadvantages

- Chronic nightly insomnia

Primary Target Symptoms

- Time to sleep onset
- Total night sleep
- Nighttime awakening

Pearls

- ✻ Because quazepam tends to accumulate over time, perhaps not the best hypnotic for chronic nightly use
- If tolerance develops, it may result in increased anxiety during the day and/or increased wakefulness during the latter part of the night

- Quazepam has a longer half-life than some other sedative hypnotics, so it may be less likely to cause rebound insomnia on discontinuation
- ✻ Long-term accumulation of quazepam and its active metabolites may cause insidious onset of confusion or falls, especially in the elderly
- Though not systematically studied, benzodiazepines have been used effectively to treat catatonia and are the initial recommended treatment

Suggested Reading

Ankier SI, Goa KL. Quazepam. A preliminary review of its pharmacodynamic and pharmacokinetic properties, and therapeutic efficacy in insomnia. Drugs 1988;35:42–62.

Hilbert JM, Battista D. Quazepam and flurazepam: differential pharmacokinetic and pharmacodynamic characteristics. J Clin Psychiatry 1991;52(Suppl):S21–6.

Kales A. Quazepam: hypnotic efficacy and side effects. Pharmacotherapy 1990;10:1–10.

Kirkwood CK. Management of insomnia. J Am Pharm Assoc (Wash) 1999;39:688–96.

Roth T, Roehrs TA. A review of the safety profiles of benzodiazepine hypnotics. J Clin Psychiatry 1991;52(Suppl):S38–41.

THERAPEUTICS

Brands • Seroquel
• Seroquel XR

see index for additional brand names

Generic? Yes

Class

- Neuroscience-based Nomenclature: dopamine, serotonin multimodal (DS-MM)
- Atypical antipsychotic (serotonin-dopamine antagonist; second-generation antipsychotic; also a mood stabilizer)

Commonly Prescribed for

(bold for FDA approved)

- **Acute schizophrenia in adults (quetiapine, quetiapine XR) and ages 13–17 (quetiapine)**
- **Schizophrenia maintenance (quetiapine XR)**
- **Acute mania in adults (quetiapine and quetiapine XR, monotherapy and adjunct to lithium or valproate) and ages 10–17 (quetiapine, monotherapy and adjunct to lithium or valproate)**
- **Bipolar maintenance (quetiapine, quetiapine XR)**
- **Bipolar depression (quetiapine, quetiapine XR)**
- **Depression (quetiapine XR, adjunct)**
- Other psychotic disorders
- Mixed mania
- Behavioral disturbances in dementias
- Behavioral disturbances in Parkinson's disease and Lewy body dementia
- Psychosis associated with levodopa treatment in Parkinson's disease
- Behavioral disturbances in children and adolescents
- Disorders associated with problems with impulse control
- Severe treatment-resistant anxiety

How the Drug Works

- Blocks dopamine 2 receptors, reducing positive symptoms of psychosis and stabilizing affective symptoms
- Blocks serotonin 2A receptors, causing enhancement of dopamine release in certain brain regions and thus reducing motor side effects and possibly improving cognitive and affective symptoms

* Interactions at a myriad of other neurotransmitter receptors may contribute to quetiapine's efficacy in treatment-resistant depression or bipolar depression, especially 5HT1A partial agonist action, norepinephrine reuptake blockade and 5HT2C antagonist and 5HT7 antagonist properties
* Specifically, actions at 5HT1A receptors may contribute to efficacy for cognitive and affective symptoms in some patients, especially at moderate to high doses

How Long Until It Works

- Psychotic and manic symptoms can improve within 1 week, but it may take several weeks for full effect on behavior as well as on cognition and affective stabilization
- Classically recommended to wait at least 4–6 weeks to determine efficacy of drug, but in practice some patients require up to 16–20 weeks to show a good response, especially on cognitive symptoms

If It Works

- Most often reduces positive symptoms in schizophrenia but does not eliminate them
- Can improve negative symptoms, as well as aggressive, cognitive, and affective symptoms in schizophrenia
- Most schizophrenic patients do not have a total remission of symptoms but rather a reduction of symptoms by about a third
- Perhaps 5–15% of schizophrenic patients can experience an overall improvement of greater than 50–60%, especially when receiving stable treatment for more than a year
- Such patients are considered super-responders or "awakeners" since they may be well enough to be employed, live independently, and sustain long-term relationships
- Many bipolar patients may experience a reduction of symptoms by half or more
- Continue treatment until reaching a plateau of improvement
- After reaching a satisfactory plateau, continue treatment for at least a year after first episode of psychosis
- For second and subsequent episodes of psychosis, treatment may need to be indefinite

- Even for first episodes of psychosis, it may be preferable to continue treatment indefinitely to avoid subsequent episodes
- Treatment may not only reduce mania but also prevent recurrences of mania in bipolar disorder

If It Doesn't Work

- Try one of the other atypical antipsychotics (risperidone, olanzapine, ziprasidone, aripiprazole, paliperidone, amisulpride, asenapine, iloperidone, lurasidone)
- If 2 or more antipsychotic monotherapies do not work, consider clozapine
- Some patients may require treatment with a conventional antipsychotic
- If no first-line atypical antipsychotic is effective, consider higher doses or augmentation with valproate or lamotrigine
- Consider noncompliance and switch to another antipsychotic with fewer side effects or to an antipsychotic that can be given by depot injection
- Consider initiating rehabilitation and psychotherapy such as coginitive remediation
- Consider presence of concomitant drug abuse

Best Augmenting Combos for Partial Response or Treatment Resistance

- Valproic acid (valproate, divalproex, divalproex ER)
- Other mood-stabilizing anticonvulsants (carbamazepine, oxcarbazepine, lamotrigine)
- Lithium
- Benzodiazepines

Tests

Before starting an atypical antipsychotic

✽ Weigh all patients and track BMI during treatment

- Get baseline personal and family history of diabetes, obesity, dyslipidemia, hypertension, and cardiovascular disease

✽ Get waist circumference (at umbilicus), blood pressure, fasting plasma glucose, and fasting lipid profile

- Determine if the patient is
  - overweight (BMI 25.0–29.9)
  - obese (BMI ≥30)
  - has pre-diabetes (fasting plasma glucose 100–125 mg/dL)
  - has diabetes (fasting plasma glucose >126 mg/dL)
  - has hypertension (BP >140/90 mm Hg)
  - has dyslipidemia (increased total cholesterol, LDL cholesterol, and triglycerides; decreased HDL cholesterol)
- Treat or refer such patients for treatment, including nutrition and weight management, physical activity counseling, smoking cessation, and medical management

Monitoring after starting an atypical antipsychotic

✽ BMI monthly for 3 months, then quarterly

✽ Consider monitoring fasting triglycerides monthly for several months in patients at high risk for metabolic complications and when initiating or switching antipsychotics

✽ Blood pressure, fasting plasma glucose, fasting lipids within 3 months and then annually, but earlier and more frequently for patients with diabetes or who have gained >5% of initial weight

- Treat or refer for treatment and consider switching to another atypical antipsychotic for patients who become overweight, obese, pre-diabetic, diabetic, hypertensive, or dyslipidemic while receiving an atypical antipsychotic

✽ Even in patients without known diabetes, be vigilant for the rare but life-threatening onset of diabetic ketoacidosis, which always requires immediate treatment, by monitoring for the rapid onset of polyuria, polydipsia, weight loss, nausea, vomiting, dehydration, rapid respiration, weakness, and clouding of sensorium, even coma

- Although US manufacturer recommends 6-month eye checks for cataracts, clinical experience suggests this may be unnecessary
- Patients with low white blood cell count (WBC) or history of drug-induced leucopenia/neutropenia should have complete blood count (CBC) monitored frequently during the first few months and quetiapine should be discontinued at the first sign of decline of WBC in the absence of other causative factors

SIDE EFFECTS

How Drug Causes Side Effects
- By blocking histamine 1 receptors in the brain, it can cause sedation and possibly weight gain
- By blocking alpha 1 adrenergic receptors, it can cause dizziness, sedation, and hypotension
- By blocking muscarinic 1 receptors, it can cause dry mouth, constipation, and sedation
- By blocking dopamine 2 receptors in the striatum, it can cause motor side effects (rare)
- Mechanism of weight gain and increased incidence of diabetes and dyslipidemia with atypical antipsychotics is unknown

Notable Side Effects
- Dose-dependent weight gain
- ✻ May increase risk for diabetes and dyslipidemia
- ✻ Dizziness, sedation
- Dry mouth, constipation
- Dyspepsia, abdominal pain
- Tachycardia
- Orthostatic hypotension, usually during initial dose titration
- Theoretical risk of tardive dyskinesia

Life-Threatening or Dangerous Side Effects
- Hyperglycemia, in some cases extreme and associated with ketoacidosis or hyperosmolar coma or death, has been reported in patients taking atypical antipsychotics
- Rare neuroleptic malignant syndrome (much reduced risk compared to conventional antipsychotics)
- Rare seizures
- Increased risk of death and cerebrovascular events in elderly patients with dementia-related psychosis

Weight Gain
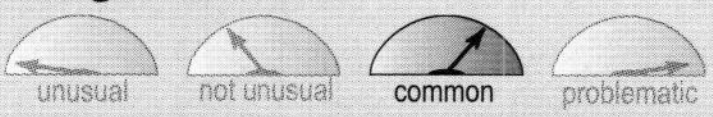

- Many patients experience and/or can be significant in amount at effective antipsychotic doses
- Can become a health problem in some
- May be less than for some antipsychotics, more than for others

Sedation
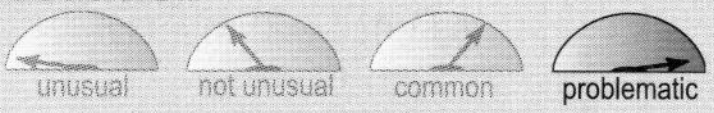

- Frequent and can be significant in amount
- Some patients may not tolerate it
- More than for some other antipsychotics, but never say always as not a problem in everyone
- Can wear off over time
- Can reemerge as dose increases and then wear off again over time
- Not necessarily increased as dose is raised

What to Do About Side Effects
- Wait
- Wait
- Wait
- Usually dosed twice daily, so take more of the total daily dose at bedtime to help reduce daytime sedation
- Start dosing low and increase slowly as side effects wear off at each dosing increment
- Weight loss, exercise programs, and medical management for high BMIs, diabetes, dyslipidemia
- Switch to another atypical antipsychotic

Best Augmenting Agents for Side Effects
- Many side effects cannot be improved with an augmenting agent

DOSING AND USE

Usual Dosage Range
- 400–800 mg/day in 1 (quetiapine XR) or 2 (quetiapine) doses for schizophrenia
- 400–800 mg/day in 1 (quetiapine XR) or 2 (quetiapine) doses for bipolar mania
- 300 mg once daily for bipolar depression

Dosage Forms
- Tablets 25 mg, 50 mg, 100 mg, 200 mg, 300 mg, 400 mg
- Extended-release tablets 50 mg, 150 mg 200 mg, 300 mg, 400 mg

How to Dose
- (According to manufacturer for quetiapine in schizophrenia): initial 25 mg/day twice a day; increase by 25–50 mg twice a day

each day until desired efficacy is reached; maximum approved dose 800 mg/day
- In practice, can start adults with schizophrenia under age 65 with same doses as recommended for acute bipolar mania
- (According to manufacturer for quetiapine in acute bipolar mania): initiate in twice daily doses, totaling 100 mg/day on day 1, increasing to 400 mg/day on day 4 in increments of up to 100 mg/day; further dosage adjustments up to 800 mg/day by day 6 should be in increments of no greater than 200 mg/day
- Bipolar depression for quetiapine and quetiapine XR: once daily at bedtime; titrate as needed to reach 300 mg/day by day 4
- Quetiapine XR in schizophrenia and acute mania: initial 300 mg once daily, preferably in the evening; can increase by 300 mg/day each day until desired efficacy is reached; maximum approved dose 800 mg/day
- See also The Art of Switching section, after Pearls

Dosing Tips

❇ **More may be much more:** clinical practice suggests quetiapine often underdosed, then switched prior to adequate trials
- Clinical practice suggests that at low doses it may be a sedative hypnotic, possibly due to potent H1 antihistamine actions, but this can risk numerous antipsychotic-related side effects and there are many other options

❇ Initial target dose of 400–800 mg/day should be reached in most cases to optimize the chances of success in treating acute psychosis and acute mania, but many patients are not adequately dosed in clinical practice
- Many patients do well with immediate-release as a single daily oral dose, usually at bedtime
- Recommended titration to 400 mg/day by the fourth day can often be achieved when necessary to control acute symptoms
- Rapid dose escalation in manic or psychotic patients may lessen sedative side effects

❇ Higher doses generally achieve greater response for manic or psychotic symptoms
- In contrast, some patients with bipolar depression may respond well to doses less than 300 mg/day and as little as 25 mg/day
- Dosing in major depression may be even lower than in bipolar depression, and dosing may be even lower still in GAD

❇ Occasional patients may require more than 800–1,200 mg/day for psychosis or mania
- Rather than raise the dose above these levels in acutely agitated patients requiring acute antipsychotic actions, consider augmentation with a benzodiazepine or conventional antipsychotic, either orally or intramuscularly
- Rather than raise the dose above these levels in partial responders, consider augmentation with a mood-stabilizing anticonvulsant such as valproate or lamotrigine
- Children and elderly should generally be dosed at the lower end of the dosage spectrum
- Quetiapine XR is controlled-release and therefore should not be chewed or crushed but rather should be swallowed whole
- Quetiapine XL may theoretically generate increased concentrations of active metabolite norquetiapine, with theoretically improved profile for affective and anxiety disorders
- Treatment should be suspended if absolute neutrophil count falls below 1,000/mm^3

Overdose
- Rarely lethal in monotherapy overdose; sedation, slurred speech, hypotension

Long-Term Use
- Approved for long-term maintenance in schizophrenia and bipolar disorder, and often used for long-term maintenance in various behavioral disorders

Habit Forming
- No

How to Stop
- See also the Switching section of individual agents for how to stop quetiapine
- Rapid discontinuation may lead to rebound psychosis and worsening of symptoms

Pharmacokinetics
- Parent drug has 6–7 hour half-life
- Substrate for CYP450 3A4
- Food may slightly increase absorption

Drug Interactions

- CYP450 3A inhibitors and CYP450 2D6 inhibitors may reduce clearance of quetiapine and thus raise quetiapine plasma levels, but dosage reduction of quetiapine usually not necessary
- May increase effect of anti-hypertensive agents
- There are case reports of increased international normalized ratio (INR) (used to monitor the degree of anticoagulation) when quetiapine is coadministered with warfarin, which is also a substrate of CYP450 3A4

Other Warnings/ Precautions

- In the USA, manufacturer recommends examination for cataracts before and every 6 months after initiating quetiapine, but this does not seem to be necessary in clinical practice
- Quetiapine should be used cautiously in patients at risk for aspiration pneumonia, as dysphagia has been reported
- Priapism has been reported
- Use with caution in patients with known cardiovascular disease, cerebrovascular disease
- Use with caution in patients with conditions that predispose to hypotension (dehydration, overheating)
- Monitor patients for activation of suicidal ideation, especially children and adolescents
- Avoid use with drugs that increase the QT interval and in patients with risk factors for prolonged QT interval

Do Not Use

- If there is a proven allergy to quetiapine

SPECIAL POPULATIONS

Renal Impairment

- No dose adjustment required

Hepatic Impairment

- Downward dose adjustment may be necessary

Cardiac Impairment

- Drug should be used with caution because of risk of orthostatic hypotension

Elderly

- Lower dose is generally used (e.g., 25–100 mg twice a day), although higher doses may be used if tolerated
- Although atypical antipsychotics are commonly used for behavioral disturbances in dementia, no agent has been approved for treatment of elderly patients with dementia-related psychosis
- Elderly patients with dementia-related psychosis treated with atypical antipsychotics are at an increased risk of death compared to placebo, and also have an increased risk of cerebrovascular events

Children and Adolescents

- Approved for use in schizophrenia (ages 13 and older) and manic/mixed episodes (ages 10 and older)
- Clinical experience and early data suggest quetiapine may be safe and effective for behavioral disturbances in children and adolescents
- Children and adolescents using quetiapine may need to be monitored more often than adults
- Use with caution, observing for activation of suicidal ideation, and inform parents or guardians of this risk so they can help observe child or adolescent patients
- May tolerate lower doses better

Pregnancy

- Effective June 30, 2015, the US FDA requires changes to the content and format of pregnancy and lactation information in prescription drug labels, including the elimination of the pregnancy letter categories; the Pregnancy and Lactation Labeling Rule (PLLR or final rule) applies only to prescription drugs and will be phased in gradually for drugs approved on or after June 30, 2001
- Controlled studies have not been conducted in pregnant women
- There is a risk of abnormal muscle movements and withdrawal symptoms

in newborns whose mothers took an antipsychotic during the third trimester; symptoms may include agitation, abnormally increased or decreased muscle tone, tremor, sleepiness, severe difficulty breathing, and difficulty feeding
- Psychotic symptoms may worsen during pregnancy and some form of treatment may be necessary
- Quetiapine may be preferable to anticonvulsant mood stabilizers if treatment is required during pregnancy
- National Pregnancy Registry for Atypical Antipsychotics: 1-866-961-2388 or http://womensmentalhealth.org/clinical-and-research-programs/pregnancyregistry/

Breast Feeding
- Unknown if quetiapine is secreted in human breast milk, but all psychotropics assumed to be secreted in breast milk
- Recommended either to discontinue drug or bottle feed
- Infants of women who choose to breast feed while on quetiapine should be monitored for possible adverse effects

THE ART OF PSYCHOPHARMACOLOGY

Potential Advantages
- Bipolar depression
- Some cases of psychosis and bipolar disorder refractory to treatment with other antipsychotics
- ✻ Patients with Parkinson's disease who need an antipsychotic or mood stabilizer
- ✻ Patients with Lewy body dementia who need an antipsychotic or mood stabilizer

Potential Disadvantages
- Patients requiring rapid onset of action
- Patients who have difficulty tolerating sedation

Primary Target Symptoms
- Positive symptoms of psychosis
- Negative symptoms of psychosis
- Cognitive symptoms
- Unstable mood (both depression and mania)
- Aggressive symptoms
- Insomnia and anxiety

Pearls
- ✻ May be the preferred antipsychotic for psychosis in Parkinson's disease and Lewy body dementia
- Anecdotal reports of efficacy in treatment-refractory cases and positive symptoms of psychoses other than schizophrenia
- ✻ Efficacy may be underestimated for psychosis and mania since quetiapine is often under-dosed in clinical practice
- ✻ Approved in bipolar depression
- The active metabolite of quetiapine, norquetiapine, has the additional properties of norepinephrine reuptake inhibition and antagonism of 5HT2C receptors, which may contribute to therapeutic effects for mood and cognition
- Dosing differs depending on the indication, with high-dose mechanisms including robust blockade of D2 receptors above 60% occupancy and equal or greater 5HT2A blockade; medium-dose mechanisms including moderate amounts of NET inhibition combined with 5HT2C antagonism and 5HT1A partial agonism; and low-dose mechanisms including H1 antagonism and 5HT1A partial agonism and, to a lesser extent, NET inhibition and 5HT2C antagonism
- More sedation than some other antipsychotics, which may be of benefit in acutely manic or psychotic patients but not for stabilized patients in long-term maintenance
- ✻ Essentially no motor side effects or prolactin elevation
- May have less weight gain than some antipsychotics, more than others
- ✻ Controversial as to whether quetiapine has more or less risk of diabetes and dyslipidemia than some other antipsychotics
- Commonly used at low doses to augment other atypical antipsychotics, but such antipsychotic polypharmacy has not been systematically studied and can be quite expensive
- Anecdotal reports of efficacy in PTSD, including symptoms of sleep disturbance and anxiety
- Patients with inadequate responses to atypical antipsychotics may benefit from determination of plasma drug levels and,

if low, a dosage increase even beyond the usual prescribing limits
- For treatment-resistant patients, especially those with impulsivity, aggression, violence, and self-harm, long-term polypharmacy with 2 atypical antipsychotics or with 1 atypical antipsychotic and 1 conventional antipsychotic may be useful or even necessary while closely monitoring
- In such cases, it may be beneficial to combine 1 depot antipsychotic with 1 oral antipsychotic

THE ART OF SWITCHING

Switching from Oral Antipsychotics to Quetiapine

- With aripiprazole, amisulpride, and paliperidone ER, immediate stop is possible; begin quetiapine at middle dose
- With risperidone, ziprasidone, iloperidone, and lurasidone, it is generally advisable to begin quetiapine gradually, titrating over at least 2 weeks to allow patients to become tolerant to the sedating effect
- For more convenient dosing, patients who are currently being treated with divided doses of immediate-release tablets may be switched to extended-release quetiapine at the equivalent total daily dose taken once daily

*May need to taper clozapine slowly over 4 weeks or longer

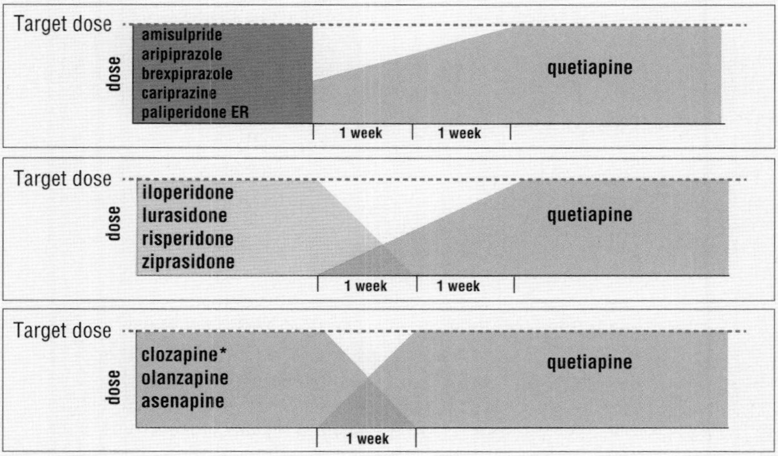

Suggested Reading

Citrome L. Adjunctive aripiprazole, olanzapine, or quetiapine for major depressive disorder: an analysis of number needed to treat, number needed to harm, and likelihood to be helped or harmed. Postgrad Med 2010;122(4):39–48.

Keating GM, Robinson DM. Quetiapine: a review of its use in the treatment of bipolar depression. Drugs 2007;67(7):1077–95.

Komossa K, Rummel-Kluge C, Schmid F, et al. Quetiapine versus other atypical antipsychotics for schizophrenia. Cochrane Database Syst Rev 2010;20(1):CD006625.

Lieberman JA, Stroup TS, McEvoy JP. Effectiveness of antipsychotics drugs in patients with chronic schizophrenia. N Engl J Med 2005;353(12):1209–23.

Nasrallah HA. Atypical antipsychotic-induced metabolic side effects: insights from receptor-binding profiles. Mol Psychiatry 2008;13(1):27–35.

Smith LA, Cornelius V, Warnock A, Tacchi MJ, Taylor D. Pharmacological interventions for acute bipolar mania: a systematic review of randomized placebo-controlled trials. Bipolar Disord 2007;9(6):551–60.

THERAPEUTICS

Brands • Rozerem

see index for additional brand names

Generic? No

Class
- Neuroscience-based Nomenclature: melatonin receptor agonist (Mel-RA)
- Melatonin 1 and 2 receptor agonist

Commonly Prescribed for
(bold for FDA approved)
- **Insomnia (difficulty with sleep onset)**
- Primary insomnia
- Chronic insomnia
- Transient insomnia
- Insomnia associated with shift work, jet lag, or circadian rhythm disturbances

How the Drug Works
- Binds selectively to melatonin 1 and melatonin 2 receptors as a full agonist

How Long Until It Works
- Generally takes effect in less than an hour

If It Works
- Reduces time to sleep onset
- Increases total sleep time
- May improve quality of sleep

If It Doesn't Work
- If insomnia does not improve after 7–10 days, it may be a manifestation of a primary psychiatric or physical illness such as obstructive sleep apnea or restless leg syndrome, which requires independent evaluation
- Increase the dose
- Improve sleep hygiene
- Switch to another agent

Best Augmenting Combos for Partial Response or Treatment Resistance
- Generally, best to switch to another agent
- Eszopiclone, zolpidem
- Trazodone
- Agents with antihistamine actions (e.g., diphenhydramine, TCAs)

Tests
- None for healthy individuals
- For patients presenting with unexplained amenorrhea, galactorrhea, decreased libido, or problems with fertility, could consider measuring prolactin and testosterone levels

SIDE EFFECTS

How Drug Causes Side Effects
- Actions at melatonin receptors that carry over to the next day could theoretically cause daytime sedation, fatigue, and sluggishness, but this is not common

Notable Side Effects
- * Sedation
- * Dizziness
- * Fatigue
- * Headache

Life-Threatening or Dangerous Side Effects
- Respiratory depression, especially when taken with other CNS depressants in overdose
- Rare angioedema

Weight Gain
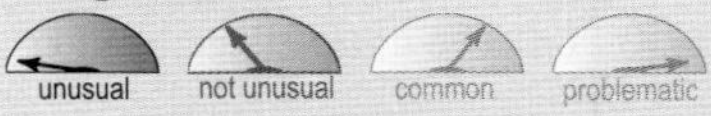

- Reported but not expected

Sedation
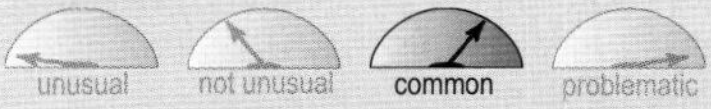

- Many experience and/or can be significant in amount
- May experience sedation or sleepiness immediately after dosing, but not commonly after awakening from a night's sleep

What to Do About Side Effects
- Wait
- To avoid problems with memory, only take ramelteon if planning to have a full night's sleep
- Lower the dose
- Switch to a non-benzodiazepine sedative hypnotic

Best Augmenting Agents for Side Effects
- Many side effects cannot be improved with an augmenting agent

DOSING AND USE

Usual Dosage Range
- 8 mg at bedtime

Dosage Forms
- Tablet 8 mg

How to Dose
- No titration, take dose at bedtime

Dosing Tips
- Unusual lack of apparent dose response curve
- Doses between 4 mg and 64 mg may have similar effects on sleep and similar side effects
- Doses up to 160 mg were studied without apparent abuse liability
- Suggests therapeutic effects may be mediated by an "on-off" type of therapeutic effect on a sleep switch that works at any dose over a certain threshold
- Since ramelteon has very low oral bioavailability and thus highly variable absorption, a substantial dose range may be required to generate sufficient absorption in various patients
- Thus, "one size does not fit all" despite approval at only one dose without titration (i.e., 8 mg)
- Suggest increasing dose before concluding lack of efficacy
- Do not administer with or immediately after a high-fat meal as this may delay its onset of action or diminish its efficacy

Overdose
- No reports of ramelteon overdose
- No safety or tolerability concerns in studies up to 160 mg

Long-Term Use
- No reports of dependence, tolerance, or abuse liability
- Not restricted to short-term use but few long-term studies

Habit Forming
- No

How to Stop
- No evidence of rebound insomnia the first night after stopping
- No need to taper dose

Pharmacokinetics
- Metabolized predominantly by CYP450 1A2
- CYP450 3A4 and 2C are also involved in metabolism of ramelteon
- Mean elimination half-life of parent drug 1–2.6 hours
- Mean elimination half-life of major metabolite, M-II, is 2–5 hours

Drug Interactions
- Inhibitors of CYP450 1A2, such as fluvoxamine, could increase plasma levels of ramelteon
- Inducers of CYP450, such as rifampin, could decrease plasma levels of ramelteon
- Inhibitors of CYP450 3A4, such as ketoconazole, could increase plasma levels of ramelteon
- Inhibitors of CYP450 2C9, such as fluconazole, could increase plasma levels of ramelteon
- Exercise caution if combining with alcohol
- No interaction with fluoxetine (CYP450 2D6 inhibitor)

Other Warnings/ Precautions
- Insomnia may be a symptom of a primary disorder, rather than a primary disorder itself
- Use only with extreme caution in patients with impaired respiratory function or obstructive sleep apnea
- Ramelteon should only be administered at bedtime
- May decrease testosterone levels or increase prolactin levels, but the clinical significance of this is unknown
- Patients who develop angioedema after treatment with ramelteon should not be rechallenged

Do Not Use
- With fluvoxamine
- In patients with severe hepatic impairment
- If there is a proven allergy to ramelteon

SPECIAL POPULATIONS

Renal Impairment
- Dose adjustment not generally necessary

Hepatic Impairment
- Use with caution in patients with moderate hepatic impairment
- Not recommended for use in patients with severe impairment

Cardiac Impairment
- Dosage adjustment may not be necessary

Elderly
- No adjustment necessary
- Greater absorption and higher plasma drug concentrations but no increase in side effects

Children and Adolescents
- Safety and efficacy have not been established

Pregnancy
- Effective June 30, 2015, the US FDA requires changes to the content and format of pregnancy and lactation information in prescription drug labels, including the elimination of the pregnancy letter categories; the Pregnancy and Lactation Labeling Rule (PLLR or final rule) applies only to prescription drugs and will be phased in gradually for drugs approved on or after June 30, 2001
- Controlled studies have not been conducted in pregnant women

Breast Feeding
- Unknown if ramelteon is secreted in human breast milk, but all psychotropics assumed to be secreted in breast milk
- ✽ Recommended either to discontinue drug or bottle feed

THE ART OF PSYCHOPHARMACOLOGY

Potential Advantages
- Those who require long-term treatment
- Those who need a hypnotic but have a past history of substance abuse
- Possibly for circadian rhythm disturbances

Potential Disadvantages
- More expensive than some other hypnotics
- For patients who require sedation

Primary Target Symptoms
- Time to sleep onset

Pearls
- First in a new class of agents, chronohypnotics, that act upon circadian rhythms by stimulating melatonin receptors in the brain's "pacemaker," namely the suprachiasmatic nucleus
- Theoretically, stimulation of melatonin 1 receptors mediates the suppressive effects of melatonin on the suprachiasmatic nucleus
- Theoretically, stimulation of melatonin 2 receptors mediates the phase shifting effect of melatonin
- Ramelteon may act by promoting the proper maintenance of circadian rhythms underlying a normal sleep-wake cycle
- Thus, ramelteon may also prove effective for treatment of circadian rhythm disturbances such as shift work sleep disorder and jet lag
- Lack of actions on GABA systems, which may be related to lack of apparent abuse liability
- Only approved hypnotic agent that is not scheduled and is considered to have no abuse liability
- No evidence that ramelteon worsens apnea/hypopnea index in COPD or in obstructive sleep apnea, but not recommended in severe cases
- ✽ May be preferred over benzodiazepines because of its rapid onset of action, short duration of effect, and safety profile
- Rebound insomnia does not appear to be common
- May have fewer carryover side effects than some other sedative hypnotics

Suggested Reading

Erman M, Seiden D, Zammit G, Sainati S, Zhang J. An efficacy, safety, and dose-response study of Ramelteon in patients with chronic primary insomnia. Sleep Med 2006;7(1):17–24.

Kato K, Hirai K, Nishiyama K, et al. Neurochemical properties of ramelteon (TAK-375), a selective MT1/MT2 receptor agonist. Neuropharmacology 2005;48(2):301–10.

McGechan A, Wellington K. Ramelteon. CNS Drugs 2005;19(12):1057–65.

Pandi-Perumal SR, Zisapel N, Srinivasan V, Cardinali DP. Melatonin and sleep in aging population. Exp Gerontol 2005;40(12):911–25.

THERAPEUTICS

Brands • Norebox
• Edronax

see index for additional brand names

Generic? No

Class

- Neuroscience-based Nomenclature: norepinephrine reuptake inhibitor (N-RI)
- Selective norepinephrine reuptake inhibitor (NRI); antidepressant

Commonly Prescribed for

(bold for FDA approved)

- Major depressive disorder
- Dysthymia
- Panic disorder
- Attention deficit hyperactivity disorder (ADHD)

How the Drug Works

- Boosts neurotransmitter norepinephrine/noradrenaline and may also increase dopamine in prefrontal cortex
- Blocks norepinephrine reuptake pump (norepinephrine transporter)
- Presumably, this increases noradrenergic neurotransmission
- Since dopamine is inactivated by norepinephrine reuptake in frontal cortex which largely lacks dopamine transporters, reboxetine can increase dopamine neurotransmission in this part of the brain

How Long Until It Works

- Onset of therapeutic actions usually not immediate, but often delayed 2–4 weeks
- If it is not working within 6–8 weeks for depression, it may require a dosage increase or it may not work at all
- May continue to work for many years to prevent relapse of symptoms

If It Works

- The goal of treatment is complete remission of current symptoms as well as prevention of future relapses
- Treatment most often reduces or even eliminates symptoms, but not a cure since symptoms can recur after medicine stopped
- Continue treatment until all symptoms are gone (remission)
- Once symptoms gone, continue treating for 1 year for the first episode of depression
- For second and subsequent episodes of depression, treatment may need to be indefinite

If It Doesn't Work

- Many patients have only a partial response where some symptoms are improved but others persist (especially insomnia, fatigue, and problems concentrating)
- Other patients may be nonresponders, sometimes called treatment-resistant or treatment-refractory
- Consider increasing dose, switching to another agent or adding an appropriate augmenting agent
- Consider psychotherapy
- Consider evaluation for another diagnosis or for a comorbid condition (e.g., medical illness, substance abuse, etc.)
- Some patients may experience apparent lack of consistent efficacy due to activation of latent or underlying bipolar disorder, and require antidepressant discontinuation and a switch to a mood stabilizer

Best Augmenting Combos for Partial Response or Treatment Resistance

- Trazodone, especially for insomnia
- SSRIs, SNRIs, mirtazapine (use combinations of antidepressants with caution as this may activate bipolar disorder and suicidal ideation)
- Modafinil, especially for fatigue, sleepiness, and lack of concentration
- Mood stabilizers or atypical antipsychotics for bipolar depression, psychotic depression or treatment-resistant depression
- Benzodiazepines for anxiety
- Hypnotics for insomnia
- Classically, lithium, buspirone, or thyroid hormone

Tests

- None for healthy individuals

SIDE EFFECTS

How Drug Causes Side Effects

- Norepinephrine increases in parts of the brain and body and at receptors other than those that cause therapeutic actions

(e.g., unwanted actions of norepinephrine on acetylcholine release causing constipation and dry mouth, etc.)
- Most side effects are immediate but often go away with time

Notable Side Effects
- Insomnia, dizziness, anxiety, agitation
- Dry mouth, constipation
- Urinary hesitancy, urinary retention
- Sexual dysfunction (impotence)
- Dose-dependent hypotension

Life-Threatening or Dangerous Side Effects
- Rare seizures
- Rare induction of mania
- Rare activation of suicidal ideation and behavior (suicidality) (short-term studies did not show an increase in the risk of suicidality with antidepressants compared to placebo beyond age 24)

Weight Gain
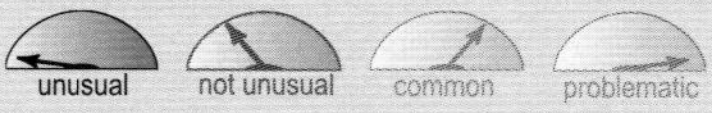

- Reported but not expected

Sedation
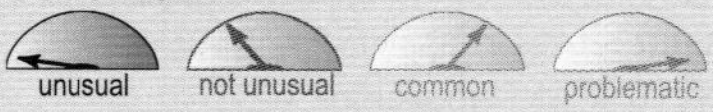

- Reported but not expected

What to Do About Side Effects
- Wait
- Wait
- Wait
- Lower the dose
- In a few weeks, switch or add other drugs

Best Augmenting Agents for Side Effects
- For urinary hesitancy, give an alpha 1 blocker such as tamsulosin
- Often best to try another antidepressant monotherapy prior to resorting to augmentation strategies to treat side effects
- Trazodone or a hypnotic for drug-induced insomnia
- Benzodiazepines for drug-induced anxiety and activation
- Mirtazapine for drug-induced insomnia or anxiety
- Many side effects are dose-dependent (i.e., they increase as dose increases, or they reemerge until tolerance redevelops)
- Many side effects are time-dependent (i.e., they start immediately upon dosing and upon each dose increase, but go away with time)
- Activation and agitation may represent the induction of a bipolar state, especially a mixed dysphoric bipolar II condition sometimes associated with suicidal ideation, and require the addition of lithium, a mood stabilizer or an atypical antipsychotic, and/or discontinuation of reboxetine

DOSING AND USE

Usual Dosage Range
- 8 mg/day in 2 doses (10 mg usual maximum daily dose)

Dosage Forms
- Tablet 2 mg, 4 mg scored

How to Dose
- Initial 2 mg/day twice a day for 1 week, 4 mg/day twice a day for second week

Dosing Tips
- When switching from another antidepressant or adding to another antidepressant, dosing may need to be lower and titration slower to prevent activating side effects (e.g., 2 mg in the daytime for 2–3 days, then 2 mg bid for 1–2 weeks)
- Give second daily dose in late afternoon rather than at bedtime to avoid undesired activation or insomnia in the evening
- May not need full dose of 8 mg/day when given in conjunction with another antidepressant
- Some patients may need 10 mg/day or more if well tolerated without orthostatic hypotension and if additional efficacy is seen at high doses in difficult cases
- Early dosing in patients with panic and anxiety may need to be lower and titration slower, perhaps with the use of concomitant short-term benzodiazepines to increase tolerability

Overdose
- Postural hypotension, anxiety, hypertension

Long-Term Use
- Safe

Habit Forming
- No

How to Stop
- Taper not necessary

Pharmacokinetics
- Metabolized by CYP450 3A4
- Inhibits CYP450 2D6 and 3A4 at high doses
- Elimination half-life approximately 13 hours

Drug Interactions
- Tramadol increases the risk of seizures in patients taking an antidepressant
- May need to reduce reboxetine dose or avoid concomitant use with inhibitors of CYP450 3A4, such as azole and antifungals, macrolide antibiotics, fluvoxamine, nefazodone, fluoxetine, sertraline, etc.
- Via CYP450 2D6 inhibition, reboxetine could theoretically interfere with the analgesic actions of codeine, and increase the plasma levels of some beta blockers and of atomoxetine and TCAs
- Via CYP450 2D6 inhibition, reboxetine could theoretically increase concentrations of thioridazine and cause dangerous cardiac arrhythmias
- Via CYP450 3A4 inhibition, reboxetine may increase the levels of alprazolam, buspirone, and triazolam
- Via CYP450 3A4 inhibition, reboxetine could theoretically increase concentrations of certain cholesterol lowering HMG CoA reductase inhibitors, especially simvastatin, atorvastatin, and lovastatin, but not pravastatin or fluvastatin, which would increase the risk of rhabdomyolysis; thus, coadministration of reboxetine with certain HMG CoA reductase inhibitors should proceed with caution
- Via CYP450 3A4 inhibition, reboxetine could theoretically increase the concentrations of pimozide, and cause QTc prolongation and dangerous cardiac arrhythmias
- Use with ergotamine may increase blood pressure
- Hypokalemia may occur if reboxetine is used with diuretics
- Use with caution with MAO inhibitors, including 14 days after MAOIs are stopped

Other Warnings/ Precautions
- Use with caution in patients with bipolar disorder unless treated with concomitant mood-stabilizing agent
- Use with caution in patients with urinary retention, benign prostatic hyperplasia, glaucoma, epilepsy
- Use with caution with drugs that lower blood pressure
- When treating children, carefully weigh the risks and benefits of pharmacological treatment against the risks and benefits of nontreatment with antidepressants and make sure to document this in the patient's chart
- Distribute the brochures provided by the FDA and the drug companies
- Warn patients and their caregivers about the possibility of activating side effects and advise them to report such symptoms immediately
- Monitor patients for activation of suicidal ideation, especially children and adolescents

Do Not Use
- If patient has angle-closure glaucoma
- If patient is taking an MAOI (except as noted under drug interactions)
- If patient is taking pimozide or thioridazine
- If there is a proven allergy to reboxetine

SPECIAL POPULATIONS

Renal Impairment
- Plasma concentrations are increased
- May need to lower dose

Hepatic Impairment
- Plasma concentrations are increased
- May need to lower dose

Cardiac Impairment
- Use with caution

Elderly

- Lower dose is recommended (4–6 mg/day)
- Reduction in the risk of suicidality with antidepressants compared to placebo in adults age 65 and older

Children and Adolescents

- Carefully weigh the risks and benefits of pharmacological treatment against the risks and benefits of nontreatment with antidepressants and make sure to document this in the patient's chart
- Monitor patients face-to-face regularly, particularly during the first several weeks of treatment
- Use with caution, observing for activation of known or unknown bipolar disorder and/or suicidal ideation, and inform parents or guardians of this risk so they can help observe child or adolescent patients
- No guidelines for children; safety and efficacy have not been established

Pregnancy

- No controlled studies in humans
- Not generally recommended for use during pregnancy, especially during first trimester
- Must weigh the risk of treatment (first trimester fetal development, third trimester newborn delivery) to the child against the risk of no treatment (recurrence of depression, maternal health, infant bonding) to the mother and child
- For many patients this may mean continuing treatment during pregnancy

Breast Feeding

- Some drug is found in mother's breast milk
- Immediate postpartum period is a high-risk time for depression, especially in women who have had prior depressive episodes, so drug may need to be reinstituted late in the third trimester or shortly after childbirth to prevent a recurrence during the postpartum period
- Must weigh benefits of breast feeding with risks and benefits of antidepressant treatment versus nontreatment to both the infant and the mother
- For many patients, this may mean continuing treatment during breast feeding

THE ART OF PSYCHOPHARMACOLOGY

Potential Advantages

- Tired, unmotivated patients
- Patients with cognitive disturbances
- Patients with psychomotor retardation

Potential Disadvantages

- Patients unable to comply with twice daily dosing
- Patients unable to tolerate activation

Primary Target Symptoms

- Depressed mood
- Energy, motivation, and interest
- Suicidal ideation
- Cognitive disturbance
- Psychomotor retardation

Pearls

- May be effective if SSRIs have failed or for SSRI "poop-out"

✻ May be more likely than SSRIs to improve social and work functioning

- Reboxetine is a mixture of an active and an inactive enantiomer, and the active enantiomer may be developed in future clinical testing

✻ Side effects may appear "anticholinergic," but reboxetine does not directly block muscarinic receptors

- Constipation, dry mouth, and urinary retention are noradrenergic, due in part to peripheral alpha 1 receptor stimulation causing decreased acetylcholine release

✻ Thus, antidotes for these side effects can be alpha 1 antagonists such as tamsulosin, especially for urinary retention in men over 50 with borderline urine flow

- Novel use of reboxetine may be for attention deficit disorder, analogous to the actions of another norepinephrine selective reuptake inhibitor, atomoxetine, but few controlled studies
- Another novel use may be for neuropathic pain, alone or in combination with other antidepressants, but few controlled studies
- Some studies suggest efficacy in panic disorder

Suggested Reading

Eyding D, Lelgemann M, Grouven U, et al. Reboxetine for acute treatment of major depression: systematic review and meta-analysis of published and unpublished placebo and selective serotonin reuptake inhibitor controlled trials. BMJ 2010;341:c4737.

Fleishaker JC. Clinical pharmacokinetics of reboxetine, a selective norepinephrine reuptake inhibitor for the treatment of patients with depression. Clin Pharmacokinet 2000;39(6):413–27.

Kasper S, el Giamal N, Hilger E. Reboxetine: the first selective noradrenaline re-uptake inhibitor. Expert Opin Pharmacother 2000;1(4):771–82.

Keller M. Role of serotonin and noradrenaline in social dysfunction: a review of data on reboxetine and the Social Adaptation Self-evaluation Scale (SASS). Gen Hosp Psychiatry 2001;23(1):15–19.

Tanum L. Reboxetine: tolerability and safety profile in patients with major depression. Acta Psychiatr Scand Suppl 2000;402:37–40.

RISPERIDONE

THERAPEUTICS

Brands • Risperdal
• CONSTA

see index for additional brand names

Generic? Yes

Class

- Neuroscience-based Nomenclature: dopamine, serotonin, norepinephrine receptor antagonist (DSN-RAn)
- Atypical antipsychotic (serotonin-dopamine antagonist; second generation antipsychotic; also a mood stabilizer)

Commonly Prescribed for

(bold for FDA approved)

- **Schizophrenia, ages 13 and older (oral, long-acting microspheres intramuscularly)**
- **Delaying relapse in schizophrenia (oral)**
- **Other psychotic disorders (oral)**
- **Acute mania/mixed mania, ages 10 and older (oral, monotherapy and adjunct to lithium or valproate)**
- **Autism-related irritability in children ages 5–16**
- **Bipolar maintenance (long-acting microspheres intramuscularly, monotherapy and adjunct to lithium or valproate)**
- Bipolar depression
- Behavioral disturbances in dementias
- Behavioral disturbances in children and adolescents
- Disorders associated with problems with impulse control

How the Drug Works

- Blocks dopamine 2 receptors, reducing positive symptoms of psychosis and stabilizing affective symptoms
- Blocks serotonin 2A receptors, causing enhancement of dopamine release in certain brain regions and thus reducing motor side effects and possibly improving cognitive and affective symptoms
- Interactions at a myriad of other neurotransmitter receptors may contribute to risperidone's efficacy

✻ Specifically, 5HT7 antagonist properties may contribute to antidepressant actions

How Long Until It Works

- Psychotic and manic symptoms can improve within 1 week, but it may take several weeks for full effect on behavior as well as on cognition and affective stabilization
- Classically recommended to wait at least 4–6 weeks to determine efficacy of drug, but in practice some patients require up to 16–20 weeks to show a good response, especially on cognitive symptoms

If It Works

- Most often reduces positive symptoms in schizophrenia but does not eliminate them
- Can improve negative symptoms, as well as aggressive, cognitive, and affective symptoms in schizophrenia
- Most schizophrenic patients do not have a total remission of symptoms but rather a reduction of symptoms by about a third
- Perhaps 5–15% of schizophrenic patients can experience an overall improvement of greater than 50–60%, especially when receiving stable treatment for more than a year
- Such patients are considered super-responders or "awakeners" since they may be well enough to be employed, live independently, and sustain long-term relationships
- Many bipolar patients may experience a reduction of symptoms by half or more
- Continue treatment until reaching a plateau of improvement
- After reaching a satisfactory plateau, continue treatment for at least a year after first episode of psychosis
- For second and subsequent episodes of psychosis, treatment may need to be indefinite
- Even for first episodes of psychosis, it may be preferable to continue treatment indefinitely to avoid subsequent episodes
- Treatment may not only reduce mania but also prevent recurrences of mania in bipolar disorder

If It Doesn't Work

- Try one of the other atypical antipsychotics (olanzapine, quetiapine, ziprasidone, aripiprazole, paliperidone, amisulpride, asenapine, iloperidone, lurasidone)
- If 2 or more antipsychotic monotherapies do not work, consider clozapine

- Some patients may require treatment with a conventional antipsychotic
- If no first-line atypical antipsychotic is effective, consider higher doses or augmentation with valproate or lamotrigine
- Consider noncompliance and switch to another antipsychotic with fewer side effects or to an antipsychotic that can be given by depot injection
- Consider initiating rehabilitation and psychotherapy such as cognitive remediation
- Consider presence of concomitant drug abuse

Best Augmenting Combos for Partial Response or Treatment Resistance

- Valproic acid (valproate, divalproex, divalproex ER)
- Other mood-stabilizing anticonvulsants (carbamazepine, oxcarbazepine, lamotrigine)
- Lithium
- Benzodiazepines

Tests

Before starting an atypical antipsychotic

✽ Weigh all patients and track BMI during treatment

- Get baseline personal and family history of diabetes, obesity, dyslipidemia, hypertension, and cardiovascular disease

✽ Get waist circumference (at umbilicus), blood pressure, fasting plasma glucose, and fasting lipid profile

- Determine if the patient is
  - overweight (BMI 25.0–29.9)
  - obese (BMI ≥30)
  - has pre-diabetes (fasting plasma glucose 100–125 mg/dL)
  - has diabetes (fasting plasma glucose >126 mg/dL)
  - has hypertension (BP >140/90 mm Hg)
  - has dyslipidemia (increased total cholesterol, LDL cholesterol, and triglycerides; decreased HDL cholesterol)
- Treat or refer such patients for treatment, including nutrition and weight management, physical activity counseling, smoking cessation, and medical management

Monitoring after starting an atypical antipsychotic

✽ BMI monthly for 3 months, then quarterly

✽ Consider monitoring fasting triglycerides monthly for several months in patients at high risk for metabolic complications and when initiating or switching antipsychotics

✽ Blood pressure, fasting plasma glucose, fasting lipids within 3 months and then annually, but earlier and more frequently for patients with diabetes or who have gained >5% of initial weight

- Treat or refer for treatment and consider switching to another atypical antipsychotic for patients who become overweight, obese, pre-diabetic, diabetic, hypertensive, or dyslipidemic while receiving an atypical antipsychotic

✽ Even in patients without known diabetes, be vigilant for the rare but life-threatening onset of diabetic ketoacidosis, which always requires immediate treatment, by monitoring for the rapid onset of polyuria, polydipsia, weight loss, nausea, vomiting, dehydration, rapid respiration, weakness, and clouding of sensorium, even coma

- Should check blood pressure in the elderly before starting and for the first few weeks of treatment
- Monitoring elevated prolactin levels of dubious clinical benefit
- Patients with low white blood cell count (WBC) or history of drug-induced leucopenia/neutropenia should have complete blood count (CBC) monitored frequently during the first few months and risperidone should be discontinued at the first sign of decline of WBC in the absence of other causative factors

SIDE EFFECTS

How Drug Causes Side Effects

- By blocking alpha 1 adrenergic receptors, it can cause dizziness, sedation, and hypotension
- By blocking dopamine 2 receptors in the striatum, it can cause motor side effects, especially at high doses
- By blocking dopamine 2 receptors in the pituitary, it can cause elevations in prolactin
- Mechanism of weight gain and increased incidence of diabetes and dyslipidemia with atypical antipsychotics is unknown

Notable Side Effects

✽ May increase risk for diabetes and dyslipidemia
✽ Dose-dependent extrapyramidal symptoms
✽ Dose-related hyperprolactinemia
✽ Dose-dependent dizziness, insomnia, anxiety, sedation
- Nausea, constipation, abdominal pain, weight gain
- Tachycardia, dose-dependent sexual dysfunction
- Rare tardive dyskinesia (much reduced risk compared to conventional antipsychotics)
- Rare orthostatic hypotension, usually during initial dose titration

Life-Threatening or Dangerous Side Effects

- Hyperglycemia, in some cases extreme and associated with ketoacidosis or hyperosmolar coma or death, has been reported in patients taking atypical antipsychotics
- Increased risk of death and cerebrovascular events in elderly patients with dementia-related psychosis
- Rare neuroleptic malignant syndrome (much reduced risk compared to conventional antipsychotics)
- Rare seizures

Weight Gain

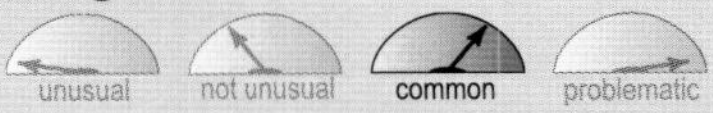

- Many patients experience and/or can be significant in amount
- Can become a health problem in some
- May be less than for some antipsychotics, more than for others

Sedation

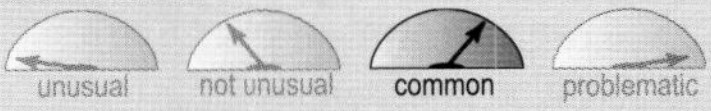

- Many patients experience and/or can be significant in amount
- Usually transient
- May be less than for some antipsychotics, more than for others

What to Do About Side Effects

- Wait
- Wait
- Wait
- Take at bedtime to help reduce daytime sedation
- Anticholinergics may reduce motor side effects when present
- Weight loss, exercise programs, and medical management for high BMIs, diabetes, dyslipidemia
- Switch to another atypical antipsychotic

Best Augmenting Agents for Side Effects

- Benztropine or trihexyphenidyl for motor side effects
- Many side effects cannot be improved with an augmenting agent

DOSING AND USE

Usual Dosage Range

- 2–8 mg/day orally for acute psychosis and bipolar disorder
- 0.5–2.0 mg/day orally for children and elderly
- 12.5–50 mg depot intramuscularly every 2 weeks (see Risperidone Microspheres section after Pearls for dosing and use)

Dosage Forms

- Tablets 0.25 mg, 0.5 mg, 1 mg, 2 mg, 3 mg, 4 mg, 6 mg
- Orally disintegrating tablets 0.5 mg, 1 mg, 2 mg
- Liquid 1 mg/mL – 30 mL bottle
- Risperidone long-acting depot microspheres formulation for deep intramuscular administration
  12.5 mg vial/kit, 25 mg vial/kit, 37.5 mg vial/kit, 50 mg vial/kit

How to Dose

- In adults with psychosis in nonemergent settings, initial dosage recommendation is 1 mg/day orally in 2 divided doses
- Increase each day by 1 mg/day orally until desired efficacy is reached
- Maximum generally 16 mg/day orally
- Typically maximum effect is seen at 4–8 mg/day orally
- See also the Switching section, after Pearls
- Can be administered on a once daily schedule as well as twice daily orally

Dosing Tips – Oral Formulation

- ✻ **Less may be more:** lowering the dose in some patients with stable efficacy but side effects may reduce side effects without loss of efficacy, especially for doses over 6 mg/day orally
- ✻ Target doses for best efficacy/best tolerability in many adults with psychosis or bipolar disorder may be 2–6 mg/day (average 4.5 mg/day) orally
- Low doses may not be adequate in difficult patients
- Rather than raise the dose above these levels in acutely agitated patients requiring acute antipsychotic actions, consider augmentation with a benzodiazepine or conventional antipsychotic, either orally or intramuscularly
- Rather than raise the dose above these levels in partial responders, consider augmentation with a mood-stabilizing anticonvulsant, such as valproate or lamotrigine
- Approved for use up to 16 mg/day orally, but data suggest that risk of extrapyramidal symptoms is increased above 6 mg/day
- Risperidone oral solution is not compatible with cola or tea
- Children and elderly may need to have oral twice daily dosing during initiation and titration of drug dosing and then can switch to oral once daily when maintenance dose is reached
- Children and elderly should generally be dosed at the lower end of the dosage spectrum
- Treatment should be suspended if absolute neutrophil count falls below 1,000/mm^3

Overdose

- Rarely lethal in monotherapy overdose; sedation, rapid heartbeat, convulsions, low blood pressure, difficulty breathing

Long-Term Use

- Approved to delay relapse in long-term treatment of schizophrenia
- Often used for long-term maintenance in bipolar disorder and various behavioral disorders

Habit Forming

- No

How to Stop

- See Switching section of individual agents for how to stop risperidone
- Rapid oral discontinuation may lead to rebound psychosis and worsening of symptoms

Pharmacokinetics

- Metabolites are active
- Metabolized by CYP450 2D6
- Parent drug of oral formulation has 20–24 hour half-life
- Long-acting risperidone has 3–6 day half-life
- Long-acting risperidone has elimination phase of approximately 7–8 weeks after last injection
- Food does not affect absorption

Drug Interactions

- May increase effect of antihypertensive agents
- May antagonize levodopa, dopamine agonists
- Clearance of risperidone may be reduced and thus plasma levels increased by clozapine; dosing adjustment usually not necessary
- Coadministration with carbamazepine may decrease plasma levels of risperidone
- Coadministration with fluoxetine and paroxetine may increase plasma levels of risperidone
- Since risperidone is metabolized by CYP450 2D6, any agent that inhibits this enzyme could theoretically raise risperidone plasma levels; however, dose reduction of risperidone is usually not necessary when such combinations are used

Other Warnings/ Precautions

- Use with caution in patients with conditions that predispose to hypotension (dehydration, overheating)
- Risperidone should be used cautiously in patients at risk for aspiration pneumonia, as dysphagia has been reported
- Priapism has been reported

Do Not Use

- If there is a proven allergy to risperidone or paliperidone

SPECIAL POPULATIONS

Renal Impairment

- Initial 0.5 mg orally twice a day for first week; increase to 1 mg twice a day during second week; dosage increases above 1.5 mg twice a day should occur at least 1 week apart
- LAI risperidone should not be administered unless patient has demonstrated tolerability of at least 2 mg/day orally
- LAI risperidone should be dosed at 25 mg every 2 weeks; oral administration should be continued for 3 weeks after the first injection

Hepatic Impairment

- Initial 0.5 mg orally twice a day for first week; increase to 1 mg twice a day during second week
- LAI risperidone should not be administered unless patient has demonstrated tolerability of at least 2 mg/day orally
- LAI risperidone should be dosed at 25 mg every 2 weeks; oral administration should be continued for 3 weeks after the first injection

Cardiac Impairment

- Drug should be used with caution because of risk of orthostatic hypotension

✽ When administered to elderly patients with atrial fibrillation, may increase the chances of stroke

Elderly

- Initial 0.5 mg orally twice a day; increase by 0.5 mg twice a day; titrate once a week for doses above 1.5 mg twice a day
- Recommended dose of long-acting risperidone is 25 mg every 2 weeks; oral administration should be continued for 3 weeks after the first injection
- Although atypical antipsychotics are commonly used for behavioral disturbances in dementia, no agent has been approved for treatment of elderly patients with dementia-related psychosis
- Elderly patients with dementia-related psychosis treated with atypical antipsychotics are at an increased risk of death compared to placebo, and also have an increased risk of cerebrovascular events

Children and Adolescents

✽ Approved for use in schizophrenia (ages 13 and older), mania/mixed episodes (ages 10 and older), and irritability associated with autism (ages 5–16)

✽ Risperidone is the most frequently used atypical antipsychotic in children and adolescents

- Clinical experience and early data suggest risperidone is safe and effective for behavioral disturbances in children and adolescents
- Children and adolescents using risperidone may need to be monitored more often than adults

Pregnancy

- Effective June 30, 2015, the US FDA requires changes to the content and format of pregnancy and lactation information in prescription drug labels, including the elimination of the pregnancy letter categories; the Pregnancy and Lactation Labeling Rule (PLLR or final rule) applies only to prescription drugs and will be phased in gradually for drugs approved on or after June 30, 2001
- Controlled studies have not been conducted in pregnant women
- There is a risk of abnormal muscle movements and withdrawal symptoms in newborns whose mothers took an antipsychotic during the third trimester; symptoms may include agitation, abnormally increased or decreased muscle tone, tremor, sleepiness, severe difficulty breathing, and difficulty feeding
- Psychotic symptoms may worsen during pregnancy and some form of treatment may be necessary
- Early findings of infants exposed to risperidone in utero do not show adverse consequences
- Risperidone may be preferable to anticonvulsant mood stabilizers if treatment is required during pregnancy
- Effects of hyperprolactinemia on the fetus are unknown
- National Pregnancy Registry for Atypical Antipsychotics: 1-866-961-2388 or http://

womensmentalhealth.org/clinical-and-research-programs/pregnancyregistry/

Breast Feeding

- Some drug is found in mother's breast milk
- ✱ Recommended either to discontinue drug or bottle feed
- Infants of women who choose to breast feed while on risperidone should be monitored for possible adverse effects

THE ART OF PSYCHOPHARMACOLOGY

Potential Advantages

- Some cases of psychosis and bipolar disorder refractory to treatment with other antipsychotics
- ✱ Often a preferred treatment for dementia with aggressive features
- ✱ Often a preferred atypical antipsychotic for children with behavioral disturbances of multiple causations
- ✱ Noncompliant patients (LAI risperidone)
- ✱ Long-term outcomes may be enhanced when compliance is enhanced (LAI risperidone)

Potential Disadvantages

- Patients for whom elevated prolactin may not be desired (e.g., possibly pregnant patients; pubescent girls with amenorrhea; postmenopausal women with low estrogen who do not take estrogen replacement therapy)

Primary Target Symptoms

- Positive symptoms of psychosis
- Negative symptoms of psychosis
- Cognitive functioning
- Unstable mood (both depression and mania)
- Aggressive symptoms

Pearls

- ✱ Well accepted for treatment of behavioral symptoms in children and adolescents, but may have more sedation and weight gain in pediatric populations than in adult populations
- ✱ Well accepted for treatment of agitation and aggression in elderly demented patients
- Many anecdotal reports of utility in treatment-refractory cases and for positive symptoms of psychosis in disorders other than schizophrenia
- Hyperprolactinemia in women with low estrogen may accelerate osteoporosis
- Less weight gain than some antipsychotics, more than others
- Less sedation than some antipsychotics, more than others
- Increased risk of stroke may be most relevant in the elderly with atrial fibrillation
- May cause more motor side effects than some other atypical antipsychotics, especially when administered to patients with Parkinson's disease or Lewy body dementia
- Patients with inadequate responses to atypical antipsychotics may benefit from determination of plasma drug levels and, if low, a dosage increase even beyond the usual prescribing limits
- Patients with inadequate responses to atypical antipsychotics may also benefit from a trial of augmentation with a conventional antipsychotic or switching to a conventional antipsychotic
- However, long-term polypharmacy with a combination of a conventional antipsychotic with an atypical antipsychotic may combine their side effects without clearly augmenting the efficacy of either
- For treatment-resistant patients, especially those with impulsivity, aggression, violence, and self-harm, long-term polypharmacy with 2 atypical antipsychotics or with 1 atypical antipsychotic and 1 conventional antipsychotic may be useful or even necessary while closely monitoring
- In such cases, it may be beneficial to combine 1 depot antipsychotic with 1 oral antipsychotic
- Although a frequent practice by some prescribers, adding 2 conventional antipsychotics together has little rationale and may reduce tolerability without clearly enhancing efficacy

MICROSPHERES

Vehicle	Water
Tmax	21 days
T1/2 with multiple dosing	3–6 days
Time to reach steady state	6 weeks (4 injections)
Able to be loaded	No
Dosing schedule (maintenance)	2 weeks
Injection site	Intramuscular
Needle gauge	20 or 21
Dosage Forms	12.5 mg, 25 mg, 37.5 mg, 50 mg
Injection volume	2 mL

Usual Dosage Range

- 12.5–50 mg/2 weeks

How to Dose

- Not recommended for patients who have not first demonstrated tolerability to oral risperidone (in clinical trials, 2 oral or short-acting IM doses are generally used to establish tolerability)
- Conversion from oral: oral coverage is required for 3–4 weeks; 2 mg oral risperidone is approximately 25 mg LAI every 2 weeks

Dosing Tips

- With LAIs, the absorption rate constant is slower than the elimination rate constant, thus resulting in "flip-flop" kinetics; i.e., time to steady-state is a function of absorption rate, while concentration at steady-state is a function of elimination rate
- The rate-limiting step for plasma drug levels for LAIs is not drug metabolism, but rather slow absorption from the injection site
- In general, 5 half-lives of any medication are needed to achieve 97% of steady-state levels
- The long half-lives of depot antipsychotics mean that one must either adequately load the dose (if possible) or provide oral supplementation
- The failure to adequately load the dose leads either to prolonged cross-titration from oral antipsychotic or to sub-therapeutic antipsychotic plasma levels for weeks or months in patients who are not receiving (or adhering to) oral supplementation
- Because plasma antipsychotic levels increase gradually over time, dose requirements may ultimately decrease from initial; obtaining periodic plasma levels can be beneficial to prevent unnecessary plasma level creep
- The time to get a blood level for patients receiving LAI is the morning of the day they will receive their next injection
- Advantages: also indicated for bipolar I maintenance (adjunct); pharmacokinetics are linear and stable over time
- Disadvantages: Tmax is long (21 days) and loading is not possible, thus necessitating oral coverage for 3–4 weeks; split doses are not possible since drug is not in a solution (i.e., half a syringe is not necessarily half the drug dose); vials require refrigeration storage
- Response threshold is generally 20 ng/mL; the tolerability threshold is poorly defined
- Changes in blood levels due to dosage changes (or missed dose) are not apparent for 3–4 weeks, so titration should occur at intervals of no less than 4 weeks
- Two different dosage strengths of LAI risperidone should not be combined in a single administration
- Missed dose: if dose is 2 or more weeks late, oral coverage for 3 weeks while reinitiating injections may be necessary
- Steady-state plasma concentrations are maintained for 4–6 weeks after the last injection

SWITCHING FROM ORAL ANTIPSYCHOTICS TO RISPERIDONE MICROSPHERES

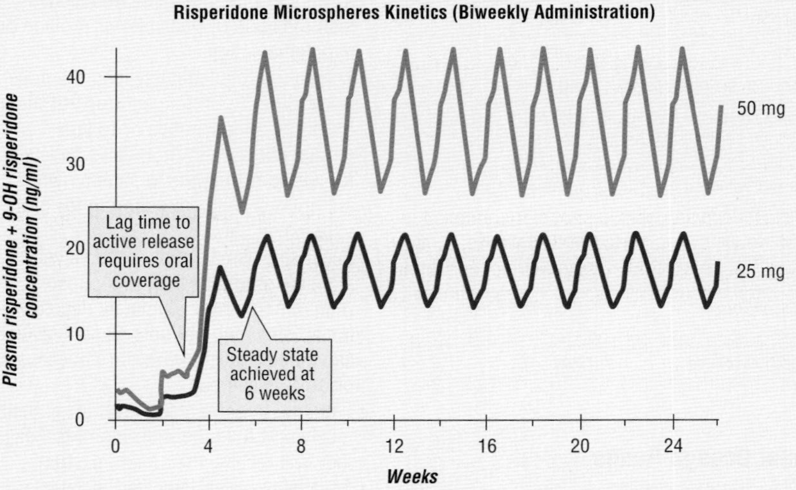

- Discontinuation of oral antipsychotic can begin following a 3–4 week oral coverage period
- How to discontinue oral formulations
  - Down-titration is not required for: amisulpride, aripiprazole, brexpiprazole, cariprazine, paliperidone ER
  - 1-week down-titration is required for: iloperidone, lurasidone, risperidone, ziprasidone
  - 3–4-week down-titration is required for: asenapine, olanzapine, quetiapine
  - 4+-week down-titration is required for: clozapine
  - For patients taking benzodiazepine or anticholinergic medication, this can be continued during cross-titration to help alleviate side effects such as insomnia, agitation, and/or psychosis. Once the patient is stable on LAI, these can be tapered one at a time as appropriate.

THE ART OF SWITCHING

Switching from Oral Antipsychotics to Risperidone

- With aripiprazole, amisulpride, and paliperidone ER, immediate stop is possible; begin risperidone at an intermediate dose
- Concomitant use with paliperidone ER is not recommended; paliperidone ER is the active metabolite of risperidone, and the combination of the 2 may lead to additive active antipsychotic fraction exposure
- Clinical experience has shown that quetiapine, olanzapine, and asenapine should be tapered off slowly over a period of 3–4 weeks, to allow patients to readapt to the withdrawal of blocking cholinergic, histaminergic, and alpha 1 receptors
- Clozapine should always be tapered off slowly, over a period of 4 weeks or more

* Benzodiazepine or anticholinergic medication can be administered during cross-titration to help alleviate side effects such as insomnia, agitation, and/or psychosis

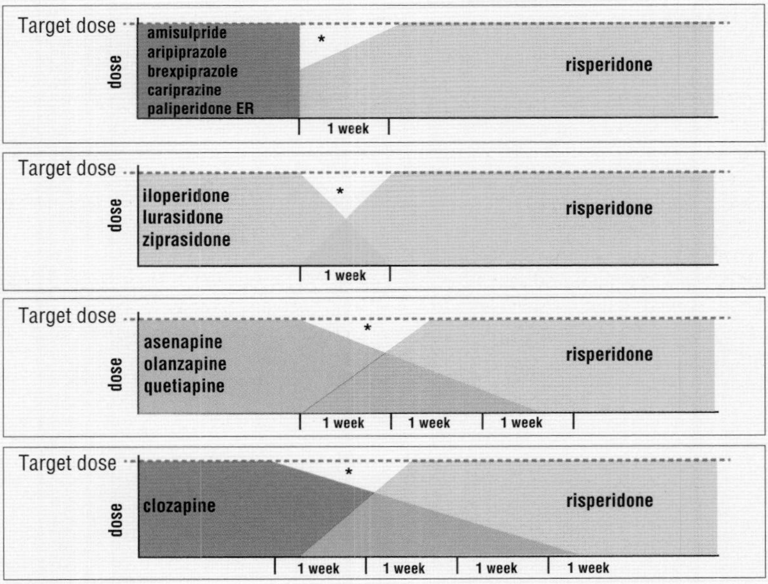

Suggested Reading

Komossa K, Rummel-Kluge C, Schwarz S, et al. Risperidone versus other atypical antipsychotics for schizophrenia. Cochrane Database Syst Rev 2011;19(1):CD006626.

Lieberman JA, Stroup TS, McEvoy JP. Effectiveness of antipsychotic drugs in patients with chronic schizophrenia. N Engl J Med 2005;353(12):1209–23.

Moller HJ. Long-acting injectable risperidone for the treatment of schizophrenia: clinical perspectives. Drugs 2007;67(11):1541–66.

Nasrallah HA. Atypical antipsychotic-induced metabolic side effects: insights from receptor-binding profiles. Mol Psychiatry 2008;13(1):27–35.

Scott LJ, Dhillon S. Risperidone: a review of its use in the treatment of irritability associated with autistic disorder in children and adolescents. Paediatr Drs 2007;9(5):343–54.

Smith LA, Cornelius V, Warnock A, Tacchi MJ, Taylor D. Pharmacological interventions for acute bipolar mania: a systematic review of randomized placebo-controlled trials. Bipolar Disord 2007;9(6):551–60.

Wilson WH. A visual guide to expected blood levels of long-acting injectable risperidone in clinical practice. J Psychiatr Pract 2004;10:393–401.

THERAPEUTICS

Brands • Exelon

see index for additional brand names

Generic? Yes

Class

- Neuroscience-based Nomenclature: Acetylcholine enzyme inhibitor (ACh-EI)
- Cholinesterase inhibitor (acetylcholinesterase inhibitor and butyrylcholinesterase inhibitor); cognitive enhancer

Commonly Prescribed for

(bold for FDA approved)

- **Alzheimer disease (mild to moderate)**
- **Parkinson's disease dementia (mild to moderate)**
- Memory disorders in other conditions
- Mild cognitive impairment

How the Drug Works

✻ Pseudoirreversibly inhibits centrally active acetylcholinesterase (AChE), making more acetylcholine available

- Increased availability of acetylcholine compensates in part for degenerating cholinergic neurons in neocortex that regulate memory

✻ Inhibits butyrylcholinesterase (BuChE)

- May release growth factors or interfere with amyloid deposition

How Long Until It Works

- May take up to 6 weeks before any improvement in baseline memory or behavior is evident
- May take months before any stabilization in degenerative course is evident

If It Works

- May improve symptoms and slow progression of disease, but does not reverse the degenerative process

If It Doesn't Work

- Consider adjusting dose, switching to a different cholinesterase inhibitor or adding an appropriate augmenting agent
- Reconsider diagnosis and rule out other conditions such as depression or a dementia other than Alzheimer disease

Best Augmenting Combos for Partial Response or Treatment Resistance

✻ Atypical antipsychotics to reduce behavioral disturbances

✻ Antidepressants if concomitant depression, apathy, or lack of interest

✻ Memantine for moderate to severe Alzheimer disease

- Divalproex, carbamazepine, or oxcarbazepine for behavioral disturbances

Tests

- None for healthy individuals

SIDE EFFECTS

How Drug Causes Side Effects

- Peripheral inhibition of acetylcholinesterase can cause gastrointestinal side effects
- Peripheral inhibition of butyrylcholinesterase can cause gastrointestinal side effects
- Central inhibition of acetylcholinesterase may contribute to nausea, vomiting, weight loss, and sleep disturbances

Notable Side Effects

✻ Nausea, diarrhea, vomiting, appetite loss, weight loss, dyspepsia, increased gastric acid secretion

- Headache, dizziness
- Fatigue, asthenia, sweating

Life-Threatening or Dangerous Side Effects

- Rare seizures
- Rare syncope

Weight Gain

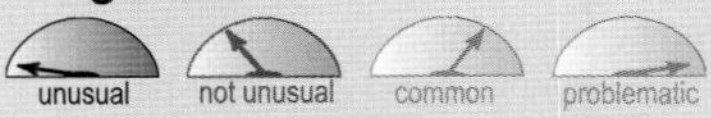

- Reported but not expected
- Some patients may experience weight loss

Sedation

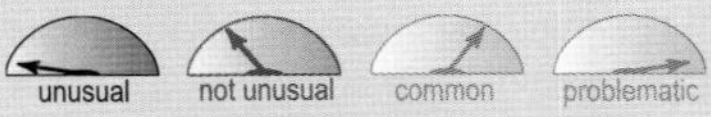

- Reported but not expected

What to Do About Side Effects

- Wait

- Wait
- Wait
- Use slower dose titration
- Consider lowering dose, switching to a different agent or adding an appropriate augmenting agent

Best Augmenting Agents for Side Effects

- Many side effects cannot be improved with an augmenting agent

DOSING AND USE

Usual Dosage Range

- Oral: 6–12 mg/day in 2 doses
- Transdermal: 9.5 mg/24 hours once daily

Dosage Forms

- Capsule 1.5 mg, 3 mg, 4.5 mg, 6 mg
- Liquid 2 mg/mL – 120 mL bottle
- Transdermal 9 mg/5 cm^2 (4.6 mg/24 hours), 18 mg/10 cm^2 (9.5 mg/24 hours), 27 mg/15 cm^2 (13.3 mg/24 hours)

How to Dose

- Oral: initial 1.5 mg twice daily; increase by 3 mg every 2 weeks; titrate to tolerability; maximum dose generally 6 mg twice daily
- Transdermal: initial 4.6 mg/24 hours; after 4 weeks increase to 9.5 mg/24 hours; maximum recommended dose 13.3 mg/24 hours

Dosing Tips

- Incidence of nausea is generally higher during the titration phase than during maintenance treatment

❋ If restarting treatment after a lapse of several days or more, dose titration should occur as when starting drug for the first time

- Oral doses between 6–12 mg/day have been shown to be more effective than doses between 1–4 mg/day
- Recommended to take oral rivastigmine with food
- Rapid dose titration increases the incidence of gastrointestinal side effects
- For transdermal formulation, dose increases should occur after a minimum of 4 weeks at the previous dose and only if the previous dose was well tolerated
- Transdermal patch should only be applied to dry, intact skin on the upper torso or another area unlikely to rub against tight clothing
- Plasma exposure with transdermal rivastigmine is 20–30% lower when applied to the abdomen or thigh as compared to the upper back, chest, or upper arm
- New application site should be selected for each day; patch should be applied at approximately the same time every day; only one patch should be applied at a time; patches should not be cut; new patch should not be applied to the same spot for at least 14 days
- Avoid touching the exposed (sticky) side of the patch, and after application, wash hands with soap and water; do not touch eyes until after hands have been washed
- Switching from oral formulation to transdermal formulation: patients receiving oral rivastigmine <6 mg/day can switch to 4.6 mg/24 hours transdermal; patients receiving oral rivastigmine 6–12 mg/day can switch to 9.5 mg/24 hours transdermal; apply the first patch on the day following the last oral dose
- Probably best to utilize highest tolerated dose within the usual dosage range

❋ When switching to another cholinesterase inhibitor, probably best to cross-titrate from one to the other to prevent precipitous decline in function if the patient washes out of one drug entirely

Overdose

- Can be lethal; nausea, vomiting, excess salivation, sweating, hypotension, bradycardia, collapse, convulsions, muscle weakness (weakness of respiratory muscles can lead to death)

Long-Term Use

- Drug may lose effectiveness in slowing degenerative course of Alzheimer disease after 6 months
- Can be effective in many patients for several years

Habit Forming

- No

How to Stop

- Taper not necessary

- Discontinuation may lead to notable deterioration in memory and behavior, which may not be restored when drug is restarted or another cholinesterase inhibitor is initiated

Pharmacokinetics

- Elimination half-life 1–2 hours
- Not hepatically metabolized; no CYP450-mediated pharmacokinetic drug interactions

Drug Interactions

- Rivastigmine may increase the effects of anesthetics and should be discontinued prior to surgery
- Rivastigmine may interact with anticholinergic agents and the combination may decrease the efficacy of both
- Clearance of rivastigmine may be increased by nicotine
- May have synergistic effect if administered with cholinomimetics (e.g., bethanechol)
- Bradycardia may occur if combined with beta blockers
- Theoretically, could reduce the efficacy of levodopa in Parkinson's disease
- Not recommended in combination with metoclopramide due to risk of additive extrapyramidal effects
- Not rational to combine with another cholinesterase inhibitor

Other Warnings/ Precautions

- May exacerbate asthma or other pulmonary disease
- Increased gastric acid secretion may increase the risk of ulcers
- Bradycardia or heart block may occur in patients with or without cardiac impairment

✻ Severe vomiting with esophageal rupture may occur if rivastigmine therapy is resumed without retitrating the drug to full dosing

- Individuals with low body weight may be at greater risk for adverse effects
- Certain transdermal patches containing even small traces of aluminum or other metals in the adhesive backing can cause skin burns if worn during MRI, so warn patients taking the transdermal formulation about this possibility and advise them to disclose this information if they need an MRI

Do Not Use

- If there is a proven allergy to rivastigmine or other carbamates

SPECIAL POPULATIONS

Renal Impairment

- Dose adjustment not necessary; titrate to point of tolerability

Hepatic Impairment

- Dose adjustment not necessary; titrate to point of tolerability

Cardiac Impairment

- Should be used with caution
- Syncopal episodes have been reported with the use of rivastigmine

Elderly

- Some patients may tolerate lower doses better
- Use of cholinesterase inhibitors may be associated with increased rates of syncope, bradycardia, pacemaker insertion, and hip fracture in older adults with dementia

Children and Adolescents

- Safety and efficacy have not been established

Pregnancy

- Effective June 30, 2015, the US FDA requires changes to the content and format of pregnancy and lactation information in prescription drug labels, including the elimination of the pregnancy letter categories; the Pregnancy and Lactation Labeling Rule (PLLR or final rule) applies only to prescription drugs and will be phased in gradually for drugs approved on or after June 30, 2001
- Controlled studies have not been conducted in pregnant women
- Animal studies do not show adverse effects

✻ Not recommended for use in pregnant women or women of childbearing potential

Breast Feeding

- Unknown if rivastigmine is secreted in human breast milk, but all psychotropics assumed to be secreted in breast milk
- ✻ Recommended either to discontinue drug or bottle feed
- Rivastigmine is not recommended for use in nursing women

THE ART OF PSYCHOPHARMACOLOGY

Potential Advantages

- Theoretically, butyrylcholinesterase inhibition centrally could enhance therapeutic efficacy
- May be useful in some patients who do not respond to or do not tolerate other cholinesterase inhibitors
- Later stages or rapidly progressive Alzheimer disease

Potential Disadvantages

- Theoretically, butyrylcholinesterase inhibition peripherally could enhance side effects

Primary Target Symptoms

- Memory loss in Alzheimer disease
- Behavioral symptoms in Alzheimer disease
- Memory loss in other dementias

Pearls

- Dramatic reversal of symptoms of Alzheimer disease is not generally seen with cholinesterase inhibitors
- Can lead to therapeutic nihilism among prescribers and lack of an appropriate trial of a cholinesterase inhibitor
- ✻ Perhaps only 50% of Alzheimer patients are diagnosed, and only 50% of those diagnosed are treated, and only 50% of those treated are given a cholinesterase inhibitor, and then only for 200 days in a disease that lasts 7–10 years
- Must evaluate lack of efficacy and loss of efficacy over months, not weeks
- ✻ Treats behavioral and psychological symptoms of Alzheimer dementia as well as cognitive symptoms (i.e., especially apathy, disinhibition, delusions, anxiety, lack of cooperation, pacing)
- Patients who themselves complain of memory problems may have depression, whereas patients whose spouses or children complain of the patient's memory problems may have Alzheimer disease
- Treat the patient but ask the caregiver about efficacy
- What you see may depend upon how early you treat
- The first symptoms of Alzheimer disease are generally mood changes; thus, Alzheimer disease may initially be diagnosed as depression
- Women may experience cognitive symptoms in perimenopause as a result of hormonal changes that are not a sign of dementia or Alzheimer disease
- Aggressively treat concomitant symptoms with augmentation (e.g., atypical antipsychotics for agitation, antidepressants for depression)
- If treatment with antidepressants fails to improve apathy and depressed mood in the elderly, it is possible that this represents early Alzheimer disease and a cholinesterase inhibitor like rivastigmine may be helpful
- What to expect from a cholinesterase inhibitor:
    - Patients do not generally improve dramatically although this can be observed in a significant minority of patients
    - Onset of behavioral problems and nursing home placement can be delayed
    - Functional outcomes, including activities of daily living, can be preserved
    - Caregiver burden and stress can be reduced
- Delay in progression in Alzheimer disease is not evidence of disease-modifying actions of cholinesterase inhibition
- Cholinesterase inhibitors like rivastigmine depend upon the presence of intact targets for acetylcholine for maximum effectiveness and thus may be most effective in the early stages of Alzheimer disease
- The most prominent side effects of rivastigmine are gastrointestinal effects, which are usually mild and transient
- ✻ May cause more gastrointestinal side effects than some other cholinesterase inhibitors, especially if not slowly titrated
- At recommended doses, transdermal formulation may have lower incidence

of gastrointestinal side effects than oral formulation
- Use with caution in underweight or frail patients
- Weight loss can be a problem in Alzheimer patients with debilitation and muscle wasting
- Women over 85, particularly with low body weights, may experience more adverse effects
- For patients with intolerable side effects, generally allow a washout period with resolution of side effects prior to switching to another cholinesterase inhibitor
- Cognitive improvement may be linked to substantial (>65%) inhibition of acetylcholinesterase
- Rivastigmine may be more selective for the form of acetylcholinesterase in hippocampus (G1)

✻ More potent inhibitor of the G1 form of acetylcholinesterase enzyme, found in high concentrations in Alzheimer patient's brains, than the G4 form of the enzyme
- Butyrylcholinesterase action in the brain may not be relevant in individuals without Alzheimer disease or in early Alzheimer disease; in the later stages of the disease, enzyme actively increases as gliosis occurs
- Rivastigmine's effects on butyrylcholinesterase may be more relevant in later stages of Alzheimer disease, when gliosis is occurring

✻ May be more useful for later stages or for more rapidly progressive forms of Alzheimer disease, when gliosis increases butyrlylcholinesterase

✻ Butyrylcholinesterase actively could interfere with amyloid plaque formation, which contains this enzyme
- Some Alzheimer patients who fail to respond to another cholinesterase inhibitor may respond when switched to rivastigmine
- Some Alzheimer patients who fail to respond to rivastigmine may respond to another cholinesterase inhibitor
- To prevent potential clinical deterioration, generally switch from long-term treatment with one cholinesterase inhibitor to another without a washout period

✻ May slow the progression of mild cognitive impairment to Alzheimer disease

✻ May be useful for dementia with Lewy bodies (DLB, constituted by early loss of attentiveness and visual perception with possible hallucinations, Parkinson-like movement problems, fluctuating cognition such as daytime drowsiness and lethargy, staring into space for long periods, episodes of disorganized speech)
- May decrease delusion, apathy, agitation, and hallucinations in dementia with Lewy bodies

✻ May be useful for vascular dementia (e.g., acute onset with slow stepwise progression that has plateaus, often with gait abnormalities, focal signs, imbalance, and urinary incontinence)
- May be helpful for dementia in Down's syndrome
- Suggestions of utility in some cases of treatment-resistant bipolar disorder
- Theoretically, may be useful for ADHD, but not yet proven
- Theoretically, could be useful in any memory condition characterized by cholinergic deficiency (e.g., some cases of brain injury, cancer chemotherapy-induced cognitive changes, etc.)

Suggested Reading

Bentue-Ferrer D, Tribut O, Polard E, Allain H. Clinically significant drug interactions with cholinesterase inhibitors: a guide for neurologists. CNS Drugs 2003;17:947–63.

Birks J, Grimley Evans J, Iakovidou V, Tsolaki M, Holt FE. Rivastigmine for Alzheimer's disease. Cochrane Database Syst Rev 2009;15(2):CD001191.

Dhillon S. Rivastigmine transdermal patch: a review of its use in the management of dementia of the Alzheimer's type. Drugs 2011;71(9):1209–31.

Jones RW. Have cholinergic therapies reached their clinical boundary in Alzheimer's disease? Int J Geriatr Psychiatry 2003;18(Suppl 1): S7–13.

THERAPEUTICS

Brands • EMSAM
• Eldepryl

see index for additional brand names

Generic? Yes (oral only)

Class

- Neuroscience-based Nomenclature: dopamine, serotonin, norepinephrine enzyme inhibitor (DSM-EI)
- Transdermal: tissue selective monoamine oxidase (MAO) inhibitor (MAO-A and MAO-B inhibitor in brain and relatively selective MAO-B inhibitor in gut)
- Oral: selective MAO-B inhibitor

Commonly Prescribed for

(bold for FDA approved)

- **Major depressive disorder (transdermal)**
- **Oral: Parkinson's disease or symptomatic parkinsonism (adjunctive)**
- Treatment-resistant depression
- Panic disorder (transdermal)
- Social anxiety disorder (transdermal)
- Treatment-resistant anxiety disorders (transdermal)
- Alzheimer disease and other dementias (oral)

How the Drug Works

- Transdermal selegiline (recommended doses): in the brain, irreversibly inhibits both MAO-A and MAO-B from breaking down norepinephrine, serotonin, and dopamine, which presumably boosts noradrenergic, serotonergic, and dopaminergic neurotransmission
- Transdermal selegiline (recommended doses): in the gut, is a relatively selective irreversible inhibitor of MAO-B (intestine and liver), reducing the chances of dietary interactions with the MAO-A substrate tyramine
- Oral: at recommended doses, selectively and irreversibly blocks MAO-B, which presumably boosts dopaminergic neurotransmission
- Oral: above recommended doses, irreversibly blocks both MAO-A and MAO-B from breaking down norepinephrine, serotonin, and dopamine while simultaneously blocking metabolism of tyramine in the gut
- Thus, high dose oral administration is not tissue selective and is not MAO-A sparing in the gut, and may interact with tyramine-containing foods to cause hypertension

How Long Until It Works

- Onset of therapeutic actions in depression with transdermal administration is usually not immediate, but often delayed 2–4 weeks or longer
- If it is not working for depression within 6–8 weeks, it may require a dosage increase or it may not work at all
- May continue to work in depression for many years to prevent relapse of symptoms
- Can enhance the actions of levodopa in Parkinson's disease within a few weeks of initiating oral dosing
- Theoretical slowing of functional loss in both Parkinson's disease and Alzheimer disease is a provocative possibility under investigation and would take many months or more than a year to observe

If It Works

- The goal of treatment in depression is complete remission of current symptoms as well as prevention of future relapses
- Treatment of depression most often reduces or even eliminates symptoms, but not a cure since symptoms can recur after medicine stopped
- Continue treatment of depression until all symptoms of depression are gone (remission)
- Once symptoms of depression are gone, continue treating for 1 year for the first episode of depression
- For second and subsequent episodes of depression, treatment may need to be indefinite
- Continue use in Parkinson's disease as long as there is evidence that selegiline is favorably enhancing the actions of levodopa
- Use of selegiline to slow functional loss in Parkinson's disease or Alzheimer disease would be long-term if proven effective for this use

If It Doesn't Work

- Many depressed patients have only a partial response where some symptoms

are improved but others persist (especially insomnia, fatigue, and problems concentrating)
- Other depressed patients may be nonresponders, sometimes called treatment-resistant or treatment-refractory
- Some depressed patients who have an initial response may relapse even though they continue treatment, sometimes called "poop out"
- For depression, consider increasing dose, switching to another agent or adding an appropriate augmenting agent, psychotherapy, and evaluation for another diagnosis or for a comorbid condition (e.g., medical illness, substance abuse, etc.)
- Some patients may experience apparent lack of consistent efficacy due to activation of latent or underlying bipolar disorder, and require antidepressant discontinuation and a switch to a mood stabilizer
- Use alternate treatments for Parkinson's disease or Alzheimer disease

Best Augmenting Combos for Partial Response or Treatment Resistance

✽ Augmentation of selegiline has not been systematically studied in depression, and this is something for the expert, to be done with caution and with careful monitoring
- A stimulant such as d-amphetamine or methylphenidate (with caution and by experts only as use of stimulants with selegiline is listed as a warning; may activate bipolar disorder and suicidal ideation; may elevate blood pressure)
- Lithium
- Mood-stabilizing anticonvulsants
- Atypical antipsychotics (with special caution for those agents with monoamine reuptake blocking properties, such as ziprasidone and zotepine)
- Carbidopa-levodopa (for Parkinson's disease)

Tests

- Patients should be monitored for changes in blood pressure
- Although preliminary evidence from clinical trials suggests little or no weight gain, nonselective MAOIs are frequently associated with weight gain. Thus, before starting treatment for depression with high doses of selegiline, weigh all patients and determine if the patient is already overweight (BMI 25.0–29.9) or obese (BMI ≥30)
- Before giving a drug that can cause weight gain to an overweight or obese patient, consider determining whether the patient already has pre-diabetes (fasting plasma glucose 100–125 mg/dL), diabetes (fasting plasma glucose >126 mg/dL), or dyslipidemia (increased total cholesterol, LDL cholesterol, and triglycerides; decreased HDL cholesterol), and treat or refer such patients for treatment including nutrition and weight management, physical activity counseling, smoking cessation, and medical management

✽ Monitor weight and BMI during treatment

✽ While giving a drug to a patient who has gained >5% of initial weight, consider evaluating for the presence of pre-diabetes, diabetes, or dyslipidemia, or consider switching to a different antidepressant

SIDE EFFECTS

How Drug Causes Side Effects

- At recommended transdermal doses, norepinephrine, serotonin, and dopamine increase in parts of the brain and at receptors other than those that cause therapeutic actions
- At high transdermal doses, loss of tissue selectivity and loss of MAO-A sparing actions in the gut may enhance the possibility of dietary tyramine interactions if MAO-B inhibition occurs in the gut
- At recommended oral doses, dopamine increases in parts of the brain and body and at receptors other than those that cause therapeutic actions
- Side effects are generally immediate, but immediate side effects often disappear in time

Notable Side Effects

- Transdermal: application site reactions, headache, insomnia, diarrhea, dry mouth
- Oral: exacerbation of levodopa side effects, especially nausea, dizziness, abdominal pain, dry mouth, headache, dyskinesia, confusion, hallucinations, vivid dreams

Life-Threatening or Dangerous Side Effects

- Transdermal: hypertensive crisis was not observed with preliminary experience in clinical trials, even in patients who were not following a low tyramine diet
- Oral: hypertensive crisis (especially when MAOIs are used with certain tryamine-containing foods or prohibited drugs) – reduced risk at low oral doses compared to nonselective MAOIs
- Theoretically, when used at high doses may induce seizures and mania as do nonselective MAOIs
- Rare activation of suicidal ideation and behavior (suicidality) (short-term studies did not show an increase in the risk of suicidality with antidepressants compared to placebo beyond age 24)

Weight Gain

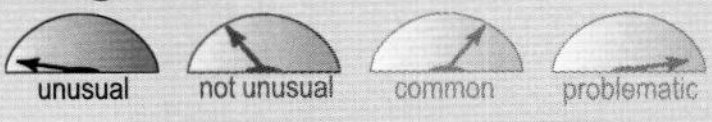

- Transdermal: reported but not expected; some patients may experience weight loss
- Oral: occurs in significant minority

Sedation

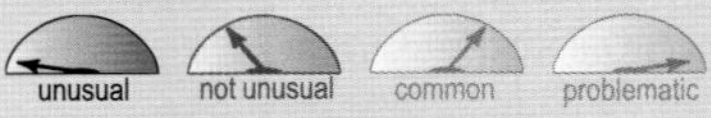

- Reported but not expected
- Can be activating in some patients

What to Do About Side Effects

- Wait
- Wait
- Wait
- Lower the dose
- Switch after appropriate washout to an SSRI or newer antidepressant (depression)
- Switch to other antiparkinsonian therapies (Parkinson's disease)

Best Augmenting Agents for Side Effects

- Trazodone (with caution) for insomnia in depression
- Benzodiazepines for insomnia in depression
- Single oral or sublingual dose of a calcium channel blocker (e.g., nifedipine) for urgent treatment of hypertension due to drug interaction or dietary tyramine
- Many side effects cannot be improved with an augmenting agent, especially at lower doses

DOSING AND USE

Usual Dosage Range

- Depression (transdermal): 6 mg/24 hours–12 mg/24 hours
- Depression (oral): 30–60 mg/day
- Parkinson's disease/Alzheimer disease: 5–10 mg/day

Dosage Forms

- Transdermal patch 20 mg/20 cm^2 (6 mg/24 hours), 30 mg/30 cm^2 (9 mg/24 hours), 40 mg/40cm^2 (12 mg/24 hours)
- Capsule 5 mg
- Tablet 5 mg scored
- Orally disintegrating tablet 1.25 mg

How to Dose

- Depression (transdermal): initial 6 mg/24 hours; can increase by 3 mg/24 hours every 2 weeks; maximum dose generally 12 mg/24 hours
- Parkinson's disease: initial 2.5 mg/day twice daily; increase to 5 mg twice daily; reduce dose of levodopa after 2–3 days

Dosing Tips

- Transdermal patch contains 1 mg of selegiline per 1 cm^2 and delivers approximately 0.3 mg of selegiline per cm^2 over 24 hours
- Patch is available in three sizes – 20 mg/20 cm^2, 30 mg/30 cm^2, and 40 mg/40 cm^2 – that deliver doses of approximately 6 mg, 9 mg, and 12 mg, respectively, over 24 hours
- At 6 mg/24 hours (transdermal) dietary adjustments are not generally required
- Dietary modifications to restrict tyramine intake from foods are recommended for doses above 6 mg/24 hours (transdermal)
- Transdermal patch should only be applied to dry, intact skin on the upper torso, upper thigh, or outer surface of the upper arm
- New application site should be selected for each day; patch should be applied at approximately the same time every day; only one patch should be applied at a time; patches should not be cut

- Avoid touching the exposed (sticky) side of the patch, and after application, wash hands with soap and water; do not touch eyes until after hands have been washed
- Heat could theoretically increase the amount of selegiline absorbed from the transdermal patch, so patients should avoid exposing the application site to external sources of direct heat (e.g., heating pads, prolonged direct sunlight)
- Although there is theoretically a 3-day reservoir of drug in each patch, multiday administration from a single patch is generally not recommended and has not been tested; because of residual drug in the patch after 24 hours of administration, discard used patches in a manner that prevents accidental application or ingestion by children, pets, or others
- For Parkinson's disease, oral dosage above 10 mg/day generally not recommended
- Dosage of carbidopa-levodopa can at times be reduced by 10–30% after 2–3 days of administering oral selegiline 5–10 mg/day in Parkinson's disease
- At doses above 10 mg/day (oral), selegiline may become nonselective and inhibit both MAO-A and MAO-B
- At doses above 30 mg/day (oral), selegiline may have antidepressant properties
- Patients receiving high oral doses may need to be evaluated periodically for effects on the liver
- Doses above 10 mg/day (oral) may increase the risk of hypertensive crisis, tyramine interactions, and drug interactions similar to those of phenelzine and tranylcypromine

Overdose

- Overdose with the transdermal formulation is likely to produce substantial amounts of MAO-A inhibition as well as MAO-B inhibition, and should be treated the same as overdose with a nonselective oral MAOI
- Dizziness, anxiety, ataxia, insomnia, sedation, irritability, headache; cardiovascular effects, confusion, respiratory depression, coma

Long-Term Use

- Long-term use has not been systematically studied although generally recommended for chronic use as for other antidepressants

Habit Forming

- Lack of evidence for abuse potential with transdermal selegiline despite its metabolism to l-amphetamine and l-methamphetamine
- Some patients have developed dependence to other MAOIs

How to Stop

- Transdermal: MAOI slowly recovers over 2–3 weeks after patch removed
- Oral: generally no need to taper, as the drug wears off slowly over 2–3 weeks

Pharmacokinetics

- Clinical duration of action may be up to 14 days due to irreversible enzyme inhibition
- Major metabolite of selegiline is desmethylselegiline; other metabolites are l-methamphetamine and l-amphetamine
- Because first-pass metabolism is not extensive with transdermal dosing, this results in notably higher exposure to selegiline and lower exposure to metabolites as compared to oral dosing
- With transdermal selegiline, 25–30% of selegiline content is delivered systemically over 24 hours from each patch
- Mean half-life of transdermal selegiline is approximately 18–25 hours
- Steady-state mean elimination half-life of oral selegiline is approximately 10 hours

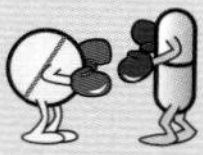

Drug Interactions

- Many misunderstandings about what drugs can be combined with MAOIs
- Theoretically and especially at high doses, selegiline could cause a fatal "serotonin syndrome" when combined with drugs that block serotonin reuptake, so do not use with a serotonin reuptake inhibitor for up to 5 half-lives after stopping the serotonin reuptake inhibitor (i.e., "wash-in" of selegiline should be about 1 week after discontinuing most agents [except 5 weeks or more after discontinuing fluoxetine because of its long half-life and that of its active metabolite]) (see Table 1 after Pearls)

- When discontinuing selegiline ("wash-out" period), wait 2 weeks before starting another antidepressant in order to allow enough time for the body to regenerate MAO enzyme
- Transdermal: no pharmacokinetic drug interactions present in studies with alprazolam, ibuprofen, levothyroxine, olanzapine, risperidone, and warfarin
- Tramadol may increase the risk of seizures in patients taking an MAOI
- Hypertensive crisis with headache, intracranial bleeding, and death may result from combining nonselective MAOIs with sympathomimetic drugs (e.g., amphetamines, methylphenidate, cocaine, dopamine, epinephrine, nonepinephrine, and related compounds methyldopa, levodopa, L-tryptophan, L-tyrosine, and phenylalanine)
- Do not combine with another MAOI, alcohol, or guanethidine
- Adverse drug reactions can result from combining MAOIs with tricyclic/tetracyclic antidepressants and related compounds, including carbamazepine, cyclobenzaprine, and mirtazapine, and should be avoided except by experts to treat difficult cases
- Carbamazepine increases plasma levels of selegiline and is contraindicated with MAOIs
- MAOIs in combination with spinal anesthesia may cause combined hypotensive effects
- Combination of MAOIs and CNS depressants may enhance sedation and hypotension

Other Warnings/ Precautions

- Ingestion of a "high tyramine meal" is generally defined as 40 mg or more of tyramine in the fasted state
- Studies show that 200–400 mg of tyramine in the fasted state (and even more ingestion of tyramine in the fed state) may be required for a hypertensive response with administration of the low-dose transdermal patch (6 mg/24 hours); thus, no dietary precautions are required at this dose
- Tyramine sensitivity of the low-dose transdermal patch (6 mg/24 hours) may be comparable to that of low-dose oral selegiline (10 mg) with neither causing a hypertensive reaction to high tyramine meals
- Tyramine sensitivity and hypertensive responses to the high-dose transdermal patch (12 mg/24 hours) may occur with administration of 70–100 mg of tyramine in the fasted state, so dietary restrictions may also not be necessary at 9 mg/24 hours or 12 mg/24 hours of transdermal administration of selegiline
- However, insufficient studies have been performed to be sure of the safety of transdermal administration at 9 mg/24 hours or 12 mg/24 hours, so dietary restrictions of tyramine are still recommended at these higher doses
- Oral administration of nonselective irreversible MAOIs generally requires adherence to a low tyramine diet (see Table 2 after Pearls)
- Ingestion of a "high tyramine meal" defined as 40 mg or more of tyramine in the fasted state or as little as ingestion of 10 mg of tyramine in the fasted state can cause hypertensive reactions in patients taking a nonselective irreversible MAOI orally
- Food restrictions (see Table 2 after Pearls) are generally recommended for patients taking the higher doses of transdermal selegiline (9 mg/24 hours or 12 mg/24 hours) but not for the lower doses of transdermal selegiline (6 mg/24 hours) or for the low dose orally (10 mg)
- Transdermal: studies of low-dose transdermal administration of selegiline (6 mg/24 hours) failed to show changes in systolic or diastolic blood pressure or pulse when administered to normal volunteers taking either pseudoephedrine 60 mg three times a day for 2 days or 25 mg of phenylpropanolamine (no longer commercially available in the USA) every 4 hours for 1 day
- However, sufficient safety information is not available to recommend administration of pseudoephedrine without a precaution; blood pressure should be monitored if low-dose transdermal selegiline is given at all with pseudoephedrine
- Pseudoephedrine may need to be avoided when administering transdermal selegiline,

particularly at higher doses of selegiline or in vulnerable patients with hypertension
- Although risk may be reduced with transdermal administration of selegiline, patient and prescriber must be vigilant to potential interactions with any drug, including antihypertensives and over-the-counter cough/cold preparations
- Over-the-counter medications to avoid or use with caution under the care of an expert include cough and cold preparations, including those containing dextromethorphan, nasal decongestants (tablets, drops, or spray), hay-fever medications, sinus medications, asthma inhalant medications, anti-appetite medications, weight reducing preparations, "pep" pills (see Table 3 after Pearls)
- Certain transdermal patches containing even small traces of aluminum or other metals in the adhesive backing can cause skin burns if worn during MRI, so warn patients taking the transdermal formulation about this possibility and advise them to disclose this information if they need an MRI
- Hypoglycemia may occur in diabetic patients receiving insulin or oral antidiabetic agents
- Use cautiously in patients receiving reserpine, anesthetics, disulfiram, metrizamide, anticholinergic agents
- Selegiline is not recommended for use in patients who cannot be monitored closely
- Only use sympathomimetic agents or guanethidine with oral doses of selegiline below 10 mg/day
- When treating children, carefully weigh the risks and benefits of pharmacological treatment against the risks and benefits of nontreatment with antidepressants and make sure to document this in the patient's chart
- Distribute the brochures provided by the FDA and the drug companies
- Warn patients and their caregivers about the possibility of activating side effects and advise them to report such symptoms immediately
- Monitor patients for activation of suicidal ideation, especially children and adolescents

Do Not Use
- If patient is taking meperidine (pethidine)
- If patient is taking a sympathomimetic agent or taking guanethidine
- If patient is taking another MAOI
- If patient is taking any agent that can inhibit serotonin reuptake (e.g., SSRIs, sibutramine, tramadol, milnacipran, duloxetine, venlafaxine, clomipramine, etc.)
- If patient is taking diuretics, dextromethorphan
- If patient is taking St. John's wort, cyclobenzaprine, methadone, propoxyphene
- If patient has pheochromocytoma
- If patient is undergoing elective surgery and requires general anesthesia
- If there is a proven allergy to selegiline

SPECIAL POPULATIONS

Renal Impairment
- No dose adjustment necessary for transdermal administration in patients with mild to moderate renal impairment
- Use oral administration with caution – drug may accumulate in plasma in patients with renal impairment
- Oral administration may require lower than usual adult dose

Hepatic Impairment
- No dose adjustment necessary for transdermal administration in patients with mild to moderate hepatic impairment
- Oral administration may require lower than usual adult dose

Cardiac Impairment
- May require lower than usual adult dose
- Observe closely for orthostatic hypotension

Elderly
- Recommended dose for patients over 65 years old is 20 mg oral and 6 mg/day transdermal
- Dose increases in the elderly should be made with caution and patients should be observed for postural changes in blood pressure throughout treatment
- Reduction in the risk of suicidality with antidepressants compared to placebo in adults age 65 and older

Children and Adolescents
- Not recommended for use in children under 18
- Use with caution, observing for activation of known or unknown bipolar disorder and/or suicidal ideation, and inform parents or guardians of this risk so they can help observe child or adolescent patients
- Carefully weigh the risks and benefits of pharmacological treatment against the risks and benefits of nontreatment with antidepressants and make sure to document this in the patient's chart
- Monitor patients face-to-face regularly, particularly during the first several weeks of treatment

Pregnancy
- Effective June 30, 2015, the US FDA requires changes to the content and format of pregnancy and lactation information in prescription drug labels, including the elimination of the pregnancy letter categories; the Pregnancy and Lactation Labeling Rule (PLLR or final rule) applies only to prescription drugs and will be phased in gradually for drugs approved on or after June 30, 2001
- Controlled studies have not been conducted in pregnant women
- Not generally recommended for use during pregnancy, especially during first trimester
- Should evaluate patient for treatment with an antidepressant with a better risk/benefit ratio

Breast Feeding
- Some drug is found in mother's breast milk
- Immediate postpartum period is a high-risk time for depression, especially in women who have had prior depressive episodes, so drug may need to be reinstituted late in the third trimester or shortly after childbirth to prevent a recurrence during the postpartum period
- Should evaluate patient for treatment with an antidepressant with a better risk/benefit ratio

THE ART OF PSYCHOPHARMACOLOGY

Potential Advantages
- Treatment-resistant depression
- Patients with atypical depression (hypersomnia, hyperphagia)
- Patients who wish to avoid weight gain and sexual dysfunction
- Parkinson's patients inadequately responsive to levodopa

Potential Disadvantages
- Noncompliant patients
- Patients with motor complications and fluctuations on levodopa treatment
- Patients with cardiac problems or hypertension

Primary Target Symptoms
- Depressed mood (depression)
- Somatic symptoms (depression)
- Sleep and eating disturbances (depression)
- Psychomotor disturbances (depression)
- Motor symptoms (Parkinson's disease)

Pearls
- Transdermal administration may allow freedom from dietary restrictions
- Transdermal selegiline theoretically appealing as a triple action agent (serotonin, norepinephrine, and dopamine) for treatment-refractory and difficult cases of depression
- Transdermal selegiline may have low risk of weight gain and sexual dysfunction, and may be useful for cognitive dysfunction in attention deficit disorder and other cognitive disorders, as it increases dopamine and is metabolized to l-amphetamine and l-methamphetamine
- Low-dose oral administration generally used as an adjunctive treatment for Parkinson's disease after other drugs have lost efficacy
- At oral doses used for Parkinson's disease, virtually no risk of interactions with food
- Neuroprotective effects are possible but unproved

✻ Enhancement of levodopa action can occur for Parkinson's patients at low oral doses, but antidepressant actions probably require high oral doses that do not have the potential tissue selectivity and lack

of dietary restrictions of the low-dose transdermal formulation
❋ High doses may lose safety features
- MAOIs are generally reserved for second-line use after SSRIs, SNRIs, and combinations of newer antidepressants have failed
- Patient should be advised not to take any prescription or over-the-counter drugs without consulting their doctor because of possible drug interactions
- Headache is often the first symptom of hypertensive crisis
- Myths about the danger of dietary tyramine can be exaggerated, but prohibitions against concomitant drugs often not followed closely enough

❋ Combining multiple psychotropic agents with MAOIs should be for the expert, especially if combining with agents of potential risk (e.g., stimulants, trazodone, TCAs)
❋ MAOIs should not be neglected as therapeutic agents for the treatment-resistant

Table 1. Drugs contraindicated due to risk of serotonin syndrome/toxicity

Do Not Use:			
Antidepressants	**Drugs of Abuse**	**Opioids**	**Other**
SSRIs	MDMA (ecstasy)	Meperidine	Non-subcutaneous sumatriptan
SNRIs	Cocaine	Tramadol	Chlorpheniramine
Clomipramine	Methamphetamine	Methadone	Brompheniramine
St. John's wort	High-dose or injected amphetamine	Fentanyl	Dextromethorphan
			Procarbazine?

Table 2. Dietary guidelines for patients taking MAOIs

Foods to avoid*	**Foods allowed**
Dried, aged, smoked, fermented, spoiled, or improperly stored meat, poultry, and fish	Fresh or processed meat, poultry, and fish; properly stored pickled or smoked fish
Broad bean pods	All other vegetables
Aged cheeses	Processed cheese slices, cottage cheese, ricotta cheese, yogurt, cream cheese
Tap and unpasteurized beer	Canned or bottled beer and alcohol
Marmite	Brewer's and baker's yeast
Sauerkraut, kimchee	
Soy products/tofu	Peanuts
Banana peel	Bananas, avocados, raspberries
Tyramine-containing nutritional supplement	

*Not necessary for 6-mg transdermal or low-dose oral selegiline

Table 3. Drugs that boost norepinephrine: should only be used with caution with MAOIs

Use With Caution:			
Decongestants	**Stimulants**	**Antidepressants with norepinephrine reuptake inhibition**	**Other**
Phenylephrine	Amphetamines	Most tricyclics	Phentermine
Pseudoephedrine	Methylphenidate	NRIs	Local anesthetics containing vasoconstrictors
	Cocaine	NDRIs	
	Methamphetamine		
	Modafinil		Tapentadol
	Armodafinil		

Suggested Reading

Bodkin JA, Amsterdam JD. Transdermal selegiline in major depression: a double-blind, placebo-controlled, parallel-group study in outpatients. Am J Psychiatry 2002;159(11):1869–75.

Kennedy SH. Continuation and maintenance treatments in major depression: the neglected role of monoamine oxidase inhibitors. J Psychiatry Neurosci 1997;22:127–31.

Shulman KI, Walker SE. A reevaluation of dietary restrictions for irreversible monoamine oxidase inhibitors. Psychiatr Ann 2001;31:378–84.

SERTINDOLE

THERAPEUTICS

Brands • SERDOLECT

see index for additional brand names

Generic? No

Class

- Neuroscience-based Nomenclature: dopamine and serotonin receptor antagonist (DS-RAn)
- Atypical antipsychotic (serotonin-dopamine antagonist; second-generation antipsychotics; also a mood stabilizer)

Commonly Prescribed for

(bold for FDA approved)

- Schizophrenia (for patients intolerant to at least one other antipsychotic)
- Acute mania/mixed mania
- Other psychotic disorders
- Bipolar maintenance
- Bipolar depression
- Treatment-resistant depression

How the Drug Works

- Blocks dopamine 2 receptors, reducing positive symptoms of psychosis and stabilizing affective symptoms
- Blocks serotonin 2A receptors, causing enhancement of dopamine release in certain brain regions and thus reducing motor side effects and possibly improving cognitive and affective symptoms

✻ Serotonin 2C properties may contribute to antidepressant actions

How Long Until It Works

- Psychotic symptoms can improve within 1 week, but it may take several weeks for full effect on behavior as well as on cognition
- Classically recommended to wait at least 4–6 weeks to determine efficacy of drug, but in practice some patients may require up to 16–20 weeks to show a good response, especially on cognitive symptoms

If It Works

- Most often reduces positive symptoms but does not eliminate them
- Can improve negative symptoms, as well as aggressive, cognitive, and affective symptoms in schizophrenia
- Most schizophrenia patients do not have a total remission of symptoms but rather a reduction of symptoms by about a third
- Perhaps 5–15% of schizophrenia patients can experience an overall improvement of greater than 50–60%, especially when receiving stable treatment for more than a year
- Such patients are considered super-responders or "awakeners" since they may be well enough to be employed, live independently, and sustain long-term relationships
- Continue treatment until reaching a plateau of improvement
- After reaching a satisfactory plateau, continue treatment for at least a year after first episode of psychosis
- For second and subsequent episodes of psychosis, treatment may need to be indefinite
- Even for first episodes of psychosis, it may be preferable to continue treatment

If It Doesn't Work

- Try one of the other atypical antipsychotics (risperidone, olanzapine, quetiapine, ziprasidone, aripiprazole, paliperidone, iloperidone, asenapine, amisulpride, lurasidone)
- If 2 or more antipsychotic monotherapies do not work, consider clozapine
- Some patients may require treatment with a conventional antipsychotic
- If no first-line atypical antipsychotic is effective, consider higher doses or augmentation with valproate or lamotrigine
- Consider noncompliance and switch to another antipsychotic with fewer side effects or to an antipsychotic that can be given by depot injection
- Consider initiating rehabilitation and psychotherapy such as cognitive remediation
- Consider presence of concomitant drug abuse

Best Augmenting Combos for Partial Response or Treatment Resistance

- Valproic acid (valproate, divalproex, divalproex ER)
- Other mood-stabilizing anticonvulsants (carbamazepine, oxcarbazepine, lamotrigine)
- Lithium
- Benzodiazepines

Tests

- Baseline EKG, serum potassium, and serum magnesium measurements
- EKG should be repeated upon reaching steady state about 3 weeks after treatment initiation or upon reaching 16 mg/day, at 3 months, and then every 3 months for the duration of treatment
- EKG is recommended prior to and after any dose increase as well as after addition of any drug that can change sertindole concentration (e.g., CYP450 2D6 or 3A4 inhibitors)

Before starting an atypical antipsychotic

✽ Weigh all patients and track BMI during treatment

- Get baseline personal and family history of diabetes, obesity, dyslipidemia, hypertension, and cardiovascular disease

✽ Get waist circumference (at umbilicus), blood pressure, fasting plasma glucose, and fasting lipid profile

- Determine if the patient is
  - overweight (BMI 25.0–29.9)
  - obese (BMI >30)
  - has pre-diabetes (fasting plasma glucose 100–125 mg/dL)
  - has diabetes (fasting plasma glucose >126 mg/dL)
  - has hypertension (BP >140/90 mm Hg)
  - has dyslipidemia (increased total cholesterol, LDL cholesterol, and triglycerides; decreased HDL cholesterol)
- Treat or refer such patients for treatment, including nutrition and weight management, physical activity counseling, smoking cessation, and medical management

Monitoring after starting an atypical antipsychotic

✽ BMI monthly for 3 months, then quarterly

✽ Consider monitoring fasting triglycerides monthly for several months in patients at high risk for metabolic complications and when initiating or switching antipsychotics

✽ Blood pressure, fasting plasma glucose, fasting lipids within 3 months and then annually, but earlier and more frequently for patients with diabetes or who have gained >5% of initial weight

- Treat or refer for treatment and consider switching to another atypical antipsychotic for patients who become overweight, obese, pre-diabetic, diabetic, hypertensive, or dyslipidemic while receiving an atypical antipsychotic

✽ Even in patients without known diabetes, be vigilant for the rare but life-threatening onset of diabetic ketoacidosis, which always requires immediate treatment, by monitoring for the rapid onset of polyuria, polydipsia, weight loss, nausea, vomiting, dehydration, rapid respiration, weakness, and clouding of sensorium, even coma

- Should check blood pressure during titration and early maintenance treatment

SIDE EFFECTS

How Drug Causes Side Effects

- By blocking alpha 1 adrenergic receptors, it can cause dizziness, sedation, and hypotension
- By blocking dopamine 2 receptors in the striatum, it can cause motor side effects
- By blocking dopamine 2 receptors in the pituitary, it can cause elevations in prolactin
- Mechanism of weight gain and increased incidence of diabetes and dyslipidemia with atypical antipsychotics is unknown

Notable Side Effects

✽ Orthostatic hypotension

- Dizziness, dry mouth, nasal congestion
- Weight gain, peripheral edema, decreased ejaculatory volume

✽ May increase risk for diabetes and dyslipidemia

- Rare tardive dyskinesia (much reduced risk compared to conventional antipsychotics)

Life-Threatening or Dangerous Side Effects

- Hyperglycemia, in some cases extreme and associated with ketoacidosis or hyperosmolar coma or death, has been reported in patients taking atypical antipsychotics
- Increased risk of death and cerebrovascular events in elderly patients with dementia-related psychosis
- Rare neuroleptic malignant syndrome (much reduced risk compared to conventional antipsychotics)
- Rare seizures

Weight Gain

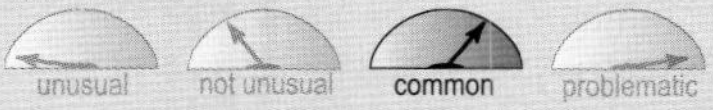

- Many experience and/or can be significant in amount
- May be less than for some antipsychotics, more than for others

Sedation

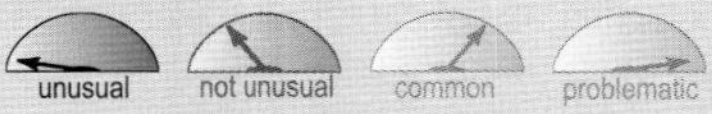

- Reported but not expected

What to Do About Side Effects

- Wait
- Wait
- Wait
- Anticholinergics may reduce motor side effects when present
- Weight loss, exercise programs, and medical management for high BMIs, diabetes, dyslipidemia
- Switch to another atypical antipsychotic

Best Augmenting Agents for Side Effects

- Benztropine or trihexyphenidyl for motor side effects
- Many side effects cannot be improved with an augmenting agent

DOSING AND USE

Usual Dosage Range

- 12–20 mg/day

Dosage Forms

- Tablet 4 mg, 12 mg, 16 mg, 20 mg

How to Dose

- Initial 4 mg/day; increase by 4 mg every 4–5 days; maximum dose generally 24 mg/day

Dosing Tips

- A starting dose of 8 mg or a rapid increase in dose significantly increase risk of orthostatic hypotension
- Sertindole should be discontinued if QTc interval of more than 500 msec is observed during treatment

Overdose

- Fatalities have been reported; sedation, slurred speech, tachycardia, hypotension, transient QTc prolongation; torsade de pointes

Long-Term Use

- Not studied, but long-term maintenance treatment is often necessary for schizophrenia

Habit Forming

- No

How to Stop

- Down-titration, especially when simultaneously beginning a new antipsychotic while switching (i.e., cross-titration)
- Rapid discontinuation could theoretically lead to rebound psychosis and worsening of symptoms

Pharmacokinetics

- Terminal half-life approximately 3 days
- Extensively metabolized by CYP450 2D6 and 3A

Drug Interactions

- May increase effects of antihypertensive agents
- May antagonize levodopa, dopamine agonists
- May enhance QTc prolongation of other drugs capable of prolonging QTc interval
- Inhibitors of CYP450 2D6 (e.g., paroxetine, fluoxetine, duloxetine, quinidine) may significantly increase plasma levels of sertindole and require a dosage reduction of sertindole
- Inhibitors of CYP450 3A (e.g., nefazodone, fluvoxamine, fluoxetine, ketoconazole) can increase plasma levels of sertindole and concomitant use of these agents with sertindole is contraindicated

Other Warnings/ Precautions

- Use with caution in patients with conditions that predispose to hypotension (dehydration, overheating)
- Dysphagia has been associated with antipsychotic use, and sertindole should

be used cautiously in patients at risk for aspiration pneumonia
- Sertindole prolongs QTc interval more than some other antipsychotics

Do Not Use
- If patient is taking agents capable of significantly prolonging QTc interval (e.g., pimozide, thioridazine, selected antiarrhythmics, moxifloxacin, sparfloxacin)
- If there is a personal or family history of QTc prolongation
- If there is a history of significant cardiovascular illness, including congestive heart failure, cardiac hypertrophy, arrhythmia, bradycardia, or congential prolonged QT syndrome
- If patient has hypokalemia, hypomagnesemia, or QTc greater than 450 msec (males) or 470 msec (females)
- If patient is taking a CYP450 3A inhibitor
- If patient has severe hepatic impairment
- If patient has galactose intolerance, Lapp lactase deficiency, or glucose-galactose malabsorption
- If there is a proven allergy to sertindole

SPECIAL POPULATIONS

Renal Impairment
- Dose adjustment not generally necessary

Hepatic Impairment
- For mild to moderate impairment, use slower titration and lower maintenance dose
- Contraindicated in patients with severe hepatic impairment

Cardiac Impairment
- Drug should be used with caution because of risk of orthostatic hypotension
- Not recommended for patients with significant cardiovascular illness, including congestive heart failure, cardiac hypertrophy, arrhythmia, bradycardia, or congential prolonged QT syndrome

Elderly
- Use cautiously and only after thorough cardiovascular examination
- Some patients may tolerate lower doses better
- Although atypical antipsychotics are commonly used for behavioral disturbances in dementia, no agent has been approved for treatment of elderly patients with dementia-related psychosis
- Elderly patients with dementia-related psychosis treated with atypical antipsychotics are at an increased risk of death compared to placebo, and also have an increased risk of cerebrovascular events

Children and Adolescents
- Safety and efficacy have not been established
- Children and adolescents using sertindole may need to be monitored more often than adults

Pregnancy
- Some animal studies show adverse effects; no controlled studies in humans
- There is a risk of abnormal muscle movements and withdrawal symptoms in newborns whose mothers took an antipsychotic during the third trimester; symptoms may include agitation, abnormally increased or decreased muscle tone, tremor, sleepiness, severe difficulty breathing, and difficulty feeding
- Psychotic symptoms may worsen during pregnancy and some form of treatment may be necessary

Breast Feeding
- Unknown if sertindole is secreted in human breast milk, but all psychotropics assumed to be secreted in breast milk

* Recommended either to discontinue drug or bottle feed

- Infants of women who choose to breast feed while on sertindole should be monitored for possible adverse effects

THE ART OF PSYCHOPHARMACOLOGY

Potential Advantages
- Some cases of psychosis and bipolar disorder refractory to treatment with other antipsychotics

Potential Disadvantages

- Patients requiring rapid onset of antipsychotic action without dosage titration

Primary Target Symptoms

- Positive symptoms of psychosis
- Negative symptoms of psychosis
- Cognitive symptoms
- Unstable mood (both depression and mania)
- Aggressive symptoms

Pearls

- Aimed at patients intolerant to at least one other antipsychotic and when potential benefits outweigh potential risks
- Not approved for mania, but all atypical antipsychotics approved for acute schizophrenia are generally also useful for acute bipolar mania
- Not approved for depression, but binding properties suggest potential use in treatment-resistant and bipolar depression, though probably not as a first- or second-line agent given the need to accumulate more real-world clinical experience of any actual risks of sertindole

Suggested Reading

Komossa K, Rummel-Kluge C, Hunger H, et al. Sertindole versus other atypical antipsychotics for schizophrenia. Cochrane Database Syst Rev 2009;2:CD006752.

Lindstrom E, Farde L, Eberhard L, Haverkamp W. QTc interval prolongation and antipsychotic drug treatments: focus on sertindole. Int J Neuropsychopharmacol 2005;8:615–29.

Spina E, Zoccali R. Sertindole: pharmacological and clinical profile and role in the treatment of schizophrenia. Expert Opin Drug Metab Toxicol 2008;4:629–38.

SERTRALINE

THERAPEUTICS

Brands • Zoloft

see index for additional brand names

Generic? Yes

Class

- Neuroscience-based Nomenclature: serotonin reuptake inhibitor (S-RI)
- SSRI (selective serotonin reuptake inhibitor); often classified as an antidepressant, but it is not just an antidepressant

Commonly Prescribed for

(bold for FDA approved)

- **Major depressive disorder**
- **Premenstrual dysphoric disorder (PMDD)**
- **Panic disorder**
- **Posttraumatic stress disorder (PTSD)**
- **Social anxiety disorder (social phobia)**
- **Obsessive-compulsive disorder (OCD)**
- Generalized anxiety disorder (GAD)

How the Drug Works

- Boosts neurotransmitter serotonin
- Blocks serotonin reuptake pump (serotonin transporter)
- Desensitizes serotonin receptors, especially serotonin 1A receptors
- Presumably increases serotonergic neurotransmission

✽ Sertraline also has some ability to block dopamine reuptake pump (dopamine transporter), which could increase dopamine neurotransmission and contribute to its therapeutic actions

- Sertraline also binds at sigma 1 receptors

How Long Until It Works

✽ Some patients may experience increased energy or activation early after initiation of treatment

- Onset of therapeutic actions usually not immediate, but often delayed 2–4 weeks
- If it is not working within 6–8 weeks, it may require a dosage increase or it may not work at all
- May continue to work for many years to prevent relapse of symptoms

If It Works

- The goal of treatment is complete remission of current symptoms as well as prevention of future relapses
- Treatment most often reduces or even eliminates symptoms, but not a cure since symptoms can recur after medicine stopped
- Continue treatment until all symptoms are gone (remission) or significantly reduced (e.g., OCD, PTSD)
- Once symptoms are gone, continue treating for 1 year for the first episode of depression
- For second and subsequent episodes of depression, treatment may need to be indefinite
- Use in anxiety disorders may also need to be indefinite

If It Doesn't Work

- Many patients have only a partial response where some symptoms are improved but others persist (especially insomnia, fatigue, and problems concentrating in depression)
- Other patients may be nonresponders, sometimes called treatment-resistant or treatment-refractory
- Some patients who have an initial response may relapse even though they continue treatment, sometimes called "poop-out"
- Consider increasing dose, switching to another agent or adding an appropriate augmenting agent
- Consider psychotherapy
- Consider evaluation for another diagnosis or for a comorbid condition (e.g., medical illness, substance abuse, etc.)
- Some patients may experience apparent lack of consistent efficacy due to activation of latent or underlying bipolar disorder, and require antidepressant discontinuation and a switch to a mood stabilizer

Best Augmenting Combos for Partial Response or Treatment Resistance

- Trazodone, especially for insomnia
- In the USA, sertraline (Zoloft) is commonly augmented with bupropion (Wellbutrin) with good results in a combination anecdotally called "Well-loft" (use combinations of antidepressants with caution as this may activate bipolar disorder and suicidal ideation)

- Mirtazapine, reboxetine, or atomoxetine (add with caution and at lower doses since sertraline could theoretically raise atomoxetine levels); use combinations of antidepressants with caution as this may activate bipolar disorder and suicidal ideation
- Modafinil, especially for fatigue, sleepiness, and lack of concentration
- Mood stabilizers or atypical antipsychotics for bipolar depression, psychotic depression, treatment-resistant depression, or treatment-resistant anxiety disorders
- Benzodiazepines
- If all else fails for anxiety disorders, consider gabapentin or tiagabine
- Hypnotics for insomnia
- Classically, lithium, buspirone, or thyroid hormone

Tests

- None for healthy individuals

SIDE EFFECTS

How Drug Causes Side Effects

- Theoretically due to increases in serotonin concentrations at serotonin receptors in parts of the brain and body other than those that cause therapeutic actions (e.g., unwanted actions of serotonin in sleep centers causing insomnia, unwanted actions of serotonin in the gut causing diarrhea, etc.)
- * Increasing serotonin can cause diminished dopamine release and might contribute to emotional flattening, cognitive slowing, and apathy in some patients, although this could theoretically be diminished in some patients by sertraline's dopamine reuptake blocking properties
- Most side effects are immediate but often go away with time, in contrast to most therapeutic effects which are delayed and are enhanced over time
- Sertraline's possible dopamine reuptake blocking properties could contribute to agitation, anxiety, and undesirable activation, especially early in dosing

Notable Side Effects

- Sexual dysfunction (dose-dependent; men: delayed ejaculation, erectile dysfunction; men and women: decreased sexual desire, anorgasmia)
- Gastrointestinal (decreased appetite, nausea, diarrhea, constipation, dry mouth)
- Mostly CNS (insomnia but also sedation, agitation, tremors, headache, dizziness)
- Note: patients with diagnosed or undiagnosed bipolar or psychotic disorders may be more vulnerable to CNS-activating actions of SSRIs
- Autonomic (sweating)
- Bruising and rare bleeding
- Rare hyponatremia (mostly in elderly patients and generally reversible on discontinuation of sertraline)
- Rare hypotension
- SIADH (syndrome of inappropriate antidiuretic hormone secretion)

Life-Threatening or Dangerous Side Effects

- Rare seizures
- Rare induction of mania
- Rare activation of suicidal ideation and behavior (suicidality) (short-term studies did not show an increase in the risk of suicidality with antidepressants compared to placebo beyond age 24)

Weight Gain

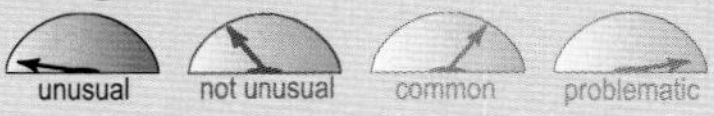

- Reported but not expected
- Some patients may actually experience weight loss

Sedation

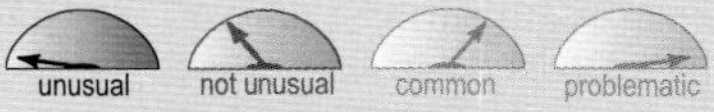

- Reported but not expected
- Possibly activating in some patients

What to Do About Side Effects

- Wait
- Wait
- Wait
- If sertraline is activating, take in the morning to help reduce insomnia
- Reduce dose to 25 mg or even 12.5 mg until side effects abate, then increase dose as tolerated, usually to at least 50 mg/day
- In a few weeks, switch or add other drugs

Best Augmenting Agents for Side Effects
- Often best to try another SSRI or another antidepressant monotherapy prior to resorting to augmentation strategies to treat side effects
- Trazodone or a hypnotic for insomnia
- Bupropion, sildenafil, vardenafil, or tadalafil for sexual dysfunction
- Bupropion for emotional flattening, cognitive slowing, or apathy
- Mirtazapine for insomnia, agitation, and gastrointestinal side effects
- Benzodiazepines for jitteriness and anxiety, especially at initiation of treatment and especially for anxious patients
- Many side effects are dose-dependent (i.e., they increase as dose increases, or they reemerge until tolerance redevelops)
- Many side effects are time-dependent (i.e., they start immediately upon dosing and upon each dose increase, but go away with time)
- Activation and agitation may represent the induction of a bipolar state, especially a mixed dysphoric bipolar II condition sometimes associated with suicidal ideation, and require the addition of lithium, a mood stabilizer or an atypical antipsychotic, and/or discontinuation of sertraline

DOSING AND USE

Usual Dosage Range
- 50–200 mg/day

Dosage Forms
- Tablets 25 mg scored, 50 mg scored, 100 mg
- Oral solution 20 mg/mL

How to Dose
- Depression and OCD: initial 50 mg/day; usually wait a few weeks to assess drug effects before increasing dose, but can increase once a week; maximum generally 200 mg/day; single dose
- Panic, PTSD, and social anxiety: initial 25 mg/day; increase to 50 mg/day after 1 week thereafter, usually wait a few weeks to assess drug effects before increasing dose; maximum generally 200 mg/day; single dose
- PMDD: initial 50 mg/day; can dose daily through the menstrual cycle or limit to the luteal phase
- Oral solution: mix with 4 oz of water, ginger ale, lemon/lime soda, lemonade, or orange juice only; drink immediately after mixing

Dosing Tips
- All tablets are scored, so to save costs, give 50 mg as half of 100-mg tablet, since 100-mg and 50-mg tablets cost about the same in many markets
- Give once daily, often in the mornings to reduce chances of insomnia
- Many patients ultimately require more than 50 mg dose per day
- Some patients are dosed above 200 mg
- Evidence that some treatment-resistant OCD patients may respond safely to doses up to 400 mg/day, but this is for experts and use with caution
- The more anxious and agitated the patient, the lower the starting dose, the slower the titration, and the more likely the need for a concomitant agent such as trazodone or a benzodiazepine
- If intolerable anxiety, insomnia, agitation, akathisia, or activation occur either upon dosing initiation or discontinuation, consider the possibility of activated bipolar disorder and switch to a mood stabilizer or atypical antipsychotic
- Utilize half a 25-mg tablet (12.5 mg) when initiating treatment in patients with a history of intolerance to previous antidepressants

Overdose
- Rarely lethal in monotherapy overdose; vomiting, sedation, heart rhythm disturbances, dilated pupils, agitation; fatalities have been reported in sertraline overdose combined with other drugs or alcohol

Long-Term Use
- Safe

Habit Forming
- No

How to Stop

- Taper to avoid withdrawal effects (dizziness, nausea, stomach cramps, sweating, tingling, dysesthesias)
- Many patients tolerate 50% dose reduction for 3 days, then another 50% reduction for 3 days, then discontinuation
- If withdrawal symptoms emerge during discontinuation, raise dose to stop symptoms and then restart withdrawal much more slowly

Pharmacokinetics

- Parent drug has 22–36 hour half-life
- Metabolite half-life 62–104 hours
- Inhibits CYP450 2D6 (weakly at low doses)
- Inhibits CYP450 3A4 (weakly at low doses)

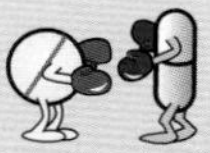

Drug Interactions

- Tramadol increases the risk of seizures in patients taking an antidepressant
- Can increase TCA levels; use with caution with TCAs or when switching from a TCA to sertraline
- Can cause a fatal "serotonin syndrome" when combined with MAOIs, so do not use with MAOIs or for at least 14 days after MAOIs are stopped
- Do not start an MAOI for at least 5 half-lives (5 to 7 days for most drugs) after discontinuing sertraline
- May displace highly protein bound drugs (e.g., warfarin)
- Can rarely cause weakness, hyperreflexia, and incoordination when combined with sumatriptan or possibly with other triptans, requiring careful monitoring of patient
- Possible increased risk of bleeding, especially when combined with anticoagulants (e.g., warfarin, NSAIDs)
- NSAIDs may impair effectiveness of SSRIs
- Via CYP450 2D6 inhibition, sertraline could theoretically interfere with the analgesic actions of codeine, and increase the plasma levels of some beta blockers and of atomoxetine
- Via CYP450 2D6 inhibition sertraline could theoretically increase concentrations of thioridazine and cause dangerous cardiac arrhythmias
- Via CYP450 3A4 inhibition, sertraline may increase the levels of alprazolam, buspirone, and triazolam
- Via CYP450 3A4 inhibition, sertraline could theoretically increase concentrations of certain cholesterol lowering HMG CoA reductase inhibitors, especially simvastatin, atorvastatin, and lovastatin, but not pravastatin or fluvastatin, which would increase the risk of rhabdomyolysis; thus, coadministration of sertraline with certain HMG CoA reductase inhibitors should proceed with caution
- Via CYP450 3A4 inhibition, sertraline could theoretically increase the concentrations of pimozide, and cause QTc prolongation and dangerous cardiac arrhythmias
- Via CYP450 3A4 inhibition, sertraline could theoretically increase the concentrations of pimozide, and cause QTc prolongation and dangerous cardiac arrhythmias
- False-positive urine immunoassay screening tests for benzodiazepine have been reported in patients taking sertraline due to a lack of specificity of the screening tests. False-positive results may be expected for several days following discontinuation of sertraline

Other Warnings/ Precautions

- Add or initiate other antidepressants with caution for up to 2 weeks after discontinuing sertraline
- Use with caution in patients with history of seizures
- Use with caution in patients with bipolar disorder unless treated with concomitant mood-stabilizing agent
- When treating children, carefully weigh the risks and benefits of pharmacological treatment against the risks and benefits of nontreatment with antidepressants and make sure to document this in the patient's chart
- Distribute the brochures provided by the FDA and the drug companies
- Warn patients and their caregivers about the possibility of activating side effects and advise them to report such symptoms immediately
- Monitor patients for activation of suicidal ideation, especially children and adolescents

Do Not Use

- If patient is taking an MAOI
- If patient is taking pimozide
- If patient is taking thioridazine
- Use of sertraline oral concentrate is contraindicated with disulfiram due to the alcohol content of the concentrate
- If there is a proven allergy to sertraline

SPECIAL POPULATIONS

Renal Impairment

- No dose adjustment
- Not removed by hemodialysis

Hepatic Impairment

- Lower dose or give less frequently, perhaps by half

Cardiac Impairment

- Proven cardiovascular safety in depressed patients with recent myocardial infarction or angina
- Treating depression with SSRIs in patients with acute angina or following myocardial infarction may reduce cardiac events and improve survival as well as mood

Elderly

- Some patients may tolerate lower doses and/or slower titration better
- Risk of SIADH with SSRIs is higher in the elderly
- Reduction in the risk of suicidality with antidepressants compared to placebo in adults age 65 and older

Children and Adolescents

- Carefully weigh the risks and benefits of pharmacological treatment against the risks and benefits of nontreatment with antidepressants and make sure to document this in the patient's chart
- Monitor patients face-to-face regularly, particularly during the first several weeks of treatment
- Use with caution, observing for activation of known or unknown bipolar disorder and/or suicidal ideation, and inform parents or guardians of this risk so they can help observe child or adolescent patients
- Approved for use in OCD
- Ages 6–12: initial dose 25 mg/day
- Ages 13 and up: adult dosing
- Long-term effects, particularly on growth, have not been studied

Pregnancy

- Effective June 30, 2015, the US FDA requires changes to the content and format of pregnancy and lactation information in prescription drug labels, including the elimination of the pregnancy letter categories; the Pregnancy and Lactation Labeling Rule (PLLR or final rule) applies only to prescription drugs and will be phased in gradually for drugs approved on or after June 30, 2001
- Controlled studies have not been conducted in pregnant women
- Not generally recommended for use during pregnancy, especially during first trimester
- Nonetheless, continuous treatment during pregnancy may be necessary and has not been proven to be harmful to the fetus
- At delivery there may be more bleeding in the mother and transient irritability or sedation in the newborn
- Must weigh the risk of treatment (first trimester fetal development, third trimester newborn delivery) to the child against the risk of no treatment (recurrence of depression, maternal health, infant bonding) to the mother and child
- For many patients this may mean continuing treatment during pregnancy
- Exposure to SSRIs early in pregnancy may be associated with increased risk of septal heart defects (absolute risk is small)
- SSRI use beyond the 20th week of pregnancy may be associated with increased risk of pulmonary hypertension in newborns, although this is not proven
- Exposure to SSRIs late in pregnancy may be associated with increased risk of gestational hypertension and preeclampsia
- Neonates exposed to SSRIs or SNRIs late in the third trimester have developed complications requiring prolonged hospitalization, respiratory support, and tube feeding; reported symptoms are consistent with either a direct toxic effect of SSRIs and SNRIs or, possibly, a drug discontinuation syndrome, and

include respiratory distress, cyanosis, apnea, seizures, temperature instability, feeding difficulty, vomiting, hypoglycemia, hypotonia, hypertonia, hyperreflexia, tremor, jitteriness, irritability, and constant crying

Breast Feeding

- Some drug is found in mother's breast milk
- Trace amounts may be present in nursing children whose mothers are on sertraline
- Sertraline has shown efficacy in treating postpartum depression
- If child becomes irritable or sedated, breast feeding or drug may need to be discontinued
- Immediate postpartum period is a high-risk time for depression, especially in women who have had prior depressive episodes, so drug may need to be reinstituted late in the third trimester or shortly after childbirth to prevent a recurrence during the postpartum period
- Must weigh benefits of breast feeding with risks and benefits of antidepressant treatment versus nontreatment to both the infant and the mother
- For many patients, this may mean continuing treatment during breast feeding

THE ART OF PSYCHOPHARMACOLOGY

Potential Advantages

- Patients with atypical depression (hypersomnia, increased appetite)
- Patients with fatigue and low energy
- Patients who wish to avoid hyperprolactinemia (e.g., pubescent children, girls and women with galactorrhea, girls and women with unexplained amenorrhea, postmenopausal women who are not taking estrogen replacement therapy)
- Patients who are sensitive to the prolactin-elevating properties of other SSRIs (sertraline is the one SSRI that generally does not elevate prolactin)

Potential Disadvantages

- Initiating treatment in anxious patients with some insomnia
- Patients with comorbid irritable bowel syndrome
- Can require dosage titration

Primary Target Symptoms

- Depressed mood
- Anxiety
- Sleep disturbance, both insomnia and hypersomnia (eventually, but may actually cause insomnia, especially short-term)
- Panic attacks, avoidant behavior, re-experiencing, hyperarousal

Pearls

✻ May be a type of "dual action" agent with both potent serotonin reuptake inhibition and less potent dopamine reuptake inhibition, but the clinical significance of this is unknown

- Cognitive and affective "flattening" may theoretically be diminished in some patients by sertraline's dopamine reuptake blocking properties

✻ May be a first-line choice for atypical depression (e.g., hypersomnia, hyperphagia, low energy, mood reactivity)

- Best documented cardiovascular safety of any antidepressant, proven safe for depressed patients with recent myocardial infarction or angina
- May bind to sigma 1 receptors, enhancing sertraline's anxiolytic actions
- Can have more gastrointestinal effects, particularly diarrhea, than some other antidepressants
- May be more effective treatment for women with PTSD or depression than for men with PTSD or depression, but the clinical significance of this is unknown
- SSRIs may be less effective in women over 50, especially if they are not taking estrogen
- SSRIs may be useful for hot flushes in perimenopausal women
- For sexual dysfunction, can augment with bupropion, sildenafil, vardenafil, tadalafil, or switch to a non-SSRI such as bupropion or mirtazapine
- Some postmenopausal women's depression will respond better to sertraline plus estrogen augmentation than to sertraline alone
- Nonresponse to sertraline in elderly may require consideration of mild cognitive impairment or Alzheimer disease
- Not as well tolerated as some SSRIs for panic, especially when dosing is initiated,

unless given with co-therapies such as benzodiazepines or trazodone
- Relative lack of effect on prolactin may make it a preferred agent for some children, adolescents, and women

- Some evidence suggests that sertraline treatment during only the luteal phase may be more effective than continuous treatment for patients with PMDD

Suggested Reading

Cipriani A, La Ferla T, Furukawa TA, et al. Sertraline versus other antidepressive agents for depression. Cochrane Database Syst Rev 2010;14(4):CD006117.

DeVane CL, Liston HL, Markowitz JS. Clinical pharmacokinetics of sertraline. Clin Pharmacokinet 2002;41:1247–66.

Flament MF, Lane RM, Zhu R, Ying Z. Predictors of an acute antidepressant response to fluoxetine and sertraline. Int Clin Psychopharmacol 1999;14:259–75.

Khouzam HR, Emes R, Gill T, Raroque R. The antidepressant sertraline: a review of its uses in a range of psychiatric and medical conditions. Compr Ther 2003;29:47–53.

McRae AL, Brady KT. Review of sertraline and its clinical applications in psychiatric disorders. Expert Opin Pharmacother 2001;2:883–92.

SODIUM OXYBATE

THERAPEUTICS

Brands • Xyrem

see index for additional brand names

Generic? No

Class

- Neuroscience-based Nomenclature: GABA receptor agonist
- CNS depressant; GABA-B receptor partial agonist

Commonly Prescribed for

(bold for FDA approved)

- **Reducing excessive sleepiness in patients with narcolepsy**
- **Cataplexy in patients with narcolepsy**
- Fibromyalgia
- Chronic pain/neuropathic pain

How the Drug Works

- Gamma hydroxybutyrate (GHB) is an endogenous putative neurotransmitter synthesized from its parent compound, GABA; sodium oxybate is the sodium salt of GHB and is administered exogenously
- Has agonist actions at GHB receptors and partial agonist actions at GABA-B receptors
- Improves slow-wave sleep at night, presumably leaving patients better rested and more alert during the day

How Long Until It Works

- Can immediately reduce daytime sleepiness
- Can take several days to optimize dosing and clinical improvement

If It Works

- Improves daytime sleepiness and may improve fatigue in patients with narcolepsy
- Reduces frequency of cataplexy attacks
- May improve sleep physiology and subjective experience of pain and fatigue in patients with fibromyalgia and other chronic pain conditions

If It Doesn't Work

- Increase dose
- Consider an alternative treatment

Best Augmenting Combos for Partial Response or Treatment Resistance

- ✻ Sodium oxybate is itself often used as an augmenting therapy to stimulants, modafinil, or armodafinil for excessive sleepiness in narcolepsy
- ✻ The majority of patients taking sodium oxybate in clinical trials for narcolepsy and cataplexy were taking a concomitant stimulant
- Often used as an augmenting agent for fibromyalgia with SNRIs (e.g., duloxetine, milnacipran) and alpha 2 delta ligands (e.g., gabapentin, pregabalin), but has not been well studied in combination with these agents

Tests

- None for healthy individuals

SIDE EFFECTS

How Drug Causes Side Effects

- Unknown
- CNS side effects presumably due to excessive CNS actions on various neurotransmitter systems

Notable Side Effects

- Headache, dizziness, sedation
- Nausea, vomiting
- Enuresis

Life-Threatening or Dangerous Side Effects

- Respiratory depression, especially when taken in overdose
- Neuropsychiatric events (psychosis, depression, paranoia, agitation)
- Confusion and wandering at night (unclear if this is true somnambulism)

Weight Gain

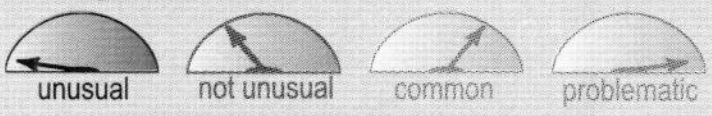

- Reported but not expected
- May cause weight loss

Sedation

unusual | **not unusual** | common | problematic

- Occurs in significant minority

What to Do About Side Effects

- Wait
- Lower the dose
- If unacceptable side effects persist, discontinue use
- Discontinue concomitant medications that might be contributing to sedation

Best Augmenting Agents for Side Effects

- Many side effects cannot be improved with an augmenting agent

DOSING AND USE

Usual Dosage Range

- 6–9 g/night in 2 doses, 2.5–4 hours apart

Dosage Forms

- Oral solution 500 mg/mL

How to Dose

- Initial 2.25 g at bedtime and while seated in bed; second dose of 2.25 g should be taken 2.5–4 hours later, also while seated in bed; dosing can be increased by 1.5 g/night every 1–2 weeks; maximum recommended dose 9 g/night

Dosing Tips

- ✻ Both nightly doses of sodium oxybate should be prepared prior to bedtime, and the prepared second dose should be placed in close proximity to the patient's bed before the first dose is ingested
- Each dose must be diluted with 2 ounces of water in a child-resistant cup that is supplied by the pharmacist
- The patient will probably need to set an alarm clock in order to wake up for the second dose
- Once prepared, the solution containing sodium oxybate should be consumed within 24 hours in order to minimize bacterial growth and contamination
- Food significantly reduces the bioavailability of sodium oxybate, so the patient should wait at least 2 hours after eating before taking the first dose of sodium oxybate
- It is best to minimize variability in the timing of dosing in relation to meals
- Once-nightly dosing has been studied and found effective in fibromyalgia

Overdose

- Fatalities have been reported; headache, psychomotor impairment, diaphoresis, vomiting (even when obtunded), confusion, agitation, aggression, ataxia, seizures, coma, death

Long-Term Use

- Long-term use has not been studied
- The need for continued treatment should be reevaluated periodically

Habit Forming

- Medical use of sodium oxybate is classified under Schedule III
- Non-medical use of sodium oxybate is classified under Schedule I
- Some patients may develop dependence and/or tolerance; risk may be greater with higher doses
- History of drug addiction may increase risk of dependence

How to Stop

- Taper may not be necessary when used at therapeutic doses; however, it is possible that some patients could develop withdrawal syndrome

Pharmacokinetics

- Metabolized by the liver
- Elimination half-life approximately 30–60 minutes
- Absorption is delayed and decreased by high-fat meals

Drug Interactions

- Should not be used in combination with CNS depressants or sedative hypnotics

Other Warnings/Precautions

- ✻ Because of the rapid onset of CNS depressant effects, sodium oxybate should only be ingested at bedtime and while in bed

- Sodium oxybate should not be used with alcohol or other CNS depressants, including opiates
- Use only with extreme caution in patients with impaired respiratory function or obstructive sleep apnea
- Patients with history of drug abuse should be monitored closely
- Sodium oxybate may cause CNS effects similar to those caused by other CNS agents (e.g., confusion, psychosis, paranoia, agitation, depression, and suicidality)

Do Not Use

- In patients taking sedative hypnotics
- In patients with succinic semialdehyde dehydrogenase deficiency
- If there is a proven allergy to sodium oxybate (gamma hydroxybutyrate)

SPECIAL POPULATIONS

Renal Impairment

- Dose adjustment is not necessary
- Not excreted renally
- Because sodium oxybate has sodium content, this may need to be considered in patients with renal impairment

Hepatic Impairment

- Reduce dose by one-half and monitor patients closely

Cardiac Impairment

- Not studied
- Because sodium oxybate has sodium content, this may need to be considered in patients with hypertension or heart failure

Elderly

- Safety and efficacy have not been established
- Patients should be monitored closely

Children and Adolescents

- Safety and efficacy have not been established

Pregnancy

- Effective June 30, 2015, the US FDA requires changes to the content and format of pregnancy and lactation information in prescription drug labels, including the elimination of the pregnancy letter categories; the Pregnancy and Lactation Labeling Rule (PLLR or final rule) applies only to prescription drugs and will be phased in gradually for drugs approved on or after June 30, 2001
- Controlled studies have not been conducted in pregnant women
- Animal studies do not show adverse effects
- Use in women of childbearing potential requires weighing potential benefits to the mother against potential risks to the fetus

* Generally, sodium oxybate should be discontinued prior to anticipated pregnancies

Breast Feeding

- Unknown if sodium oxybate is secreted in human breast milk, but all psychotropics assumed to be secreted in breast milk

* Recommended either to discontinue drug or bottle feed

THE ART OF PSYCHOPHARMACOLOGY

Potential Advantages

- Less activating than stimulants
- For narcolepsy, may help patients insufficiently responsive to stimulants
- Has the biggest effect size on pain, fatigue, and sleep in fibromyalgia

Potential Disadvantages

- Has abuse potential
- Requires a second dose in the middle of the night
- Potentially more dangerous than other treatments, especially for fibromyalgia or chronic pain, and especially if taken with sedative hypnotics and/or opiates

Primary Target Symptoms

- Sleepiness, fatigue
- Cataplexy

- Painful physical symptoms
- Lack of nonrestorative sleep in fibromyalgia and chronic pain

Pearls

- Sodium oxybate increases slow-wave sleep, thereby improving sleep quality at night and allowing individuals to feel more rested during the day
- Sodium oxybate also increases growth hormone, which is one of the reasons that it has been abused by athletes

* There are positive trials for efficacy in fibromyalgia, with improvement in sleep, pain, and fatigue, but an FDA advisory committee voted it down because of safety concerns and the drug is not officially approved for this indication

Suggested Reading

Carter LP, Pardi D, Gorsline J, Griffiths RR. Illicit gamma-hydroxybutyrate (GHB) and pharmaceutical sodium oxybate (Xyrem): differences in characteristics and misuse. Drug Alcohol Depend 2009;104(1–2):1–10.

Moldofsky H, Inhaber NH, Guinta DR, Alvarez-Horine SB. Effects of sodium oxybate on sleep physiology and sleep/wake-related symptoms in patients with fibromyalgia syndrome: a double-blind, randomized, placebo-controlled study. J Rheumatol 2010;37(10):2156–66.

Owen RT. Sodium oxybate: efficacy, safety and tolerability in the treatment of narcolepsy with or without cataplexy. Drugs Today (Barc) 2008;44(3):197–204.

Russell IJ, Perkins AT, Michalek JE, et al. Sodium oxybate relieves pain and improves function in fibromyalgia syndrome: a randomized, double-blind, placebo-controlled, multicenter clinical trial. Arthritis Rheum 2009;60(1):299–309.

Wang YG, Swich TJ, Carter LP, Thorpy MJ, Benowitz NL. Safety overview of postmarketing and clinical experience of sodium oxybate (Xyrem): abuse, misuse, dependence, and diversion. J Clin Sleep Med 2009;15(4):365–71.

THERAPEUTICS

Brands • Dolmatil
see index for additional brand names

Generic? Yes

Class

- Neuroscience-based Nomenclature: dopamine receptor antagonist (D-RAn)
- Conventional antipsychotic (neuroleptic, benzamide, dopamine 2 antagonist)

Commonly Prescribed for

(bold for FDA approved)

- Schizophrenia
- Depression

How the Drug Works

- Blocks dopamine 2 receptors, reducing positive symptoms of psychosis
- Blocks dopamine 3 and 4 receptors, which may contribute to sulpiride's actions
- ✽ Possibly blocks presynaptic dopamine 2 autoreceptors more potently at low doses, which could theoretically contribute to improving negative symptoms of schizophrenia as well as depression

How Long Until It Works

- Psychotic symptoms can improve within 1 week, but it may take several weeks for full effect on behavior

If It Works

- Most often reduces positive symptoms in schizophrenia but does not eliminate them
- Most schizophrenic patients do not have a total remission of symptoms but rather a reduction of symptoms by about a third
- Continue treatment in schizophrenia until reaching a plateau of improvement
- After reaching a satisfactory plateau, continue treatment for at least a year after first episode of psychosis in schizophrenia
- For second and subsequent episodes of psychosis in schizophrenia, treatment may need to be indefinite

If It Doesn't Work

- Consider trying one of the first-line atypical antipsychotics (risperidone, olanzapine, quetiapine, ziprasidone, aripiprazole, paliperidone, amisulpride, asenapine, iloperidone, lurasidone)
- Consider trying another conventional antipsychotic
- If 2 or more antipsychotic monotherapies do not work, consider clozapine

Best Augmenting Combos for Partial Response or Treatment Resistance

- Augmentation of conventional antipsychotics has not been systematically studied
- Addition of a mood-stabilizing anticonvulsant such as valproate, carbamazepine, or lamotrigine may be helpful in both schizophrenia and bipolar mania
- Augmentation with lithium in bipolar mania may be helpful
- Addition of a benzodiazepine, especially short-term for agitation

Tests

- ✽ Since conventional antipsychotics are frequently associated with weight gain, before starting treatment, weigh all patients and determine if the patient is already overweight (BMI 25.0–29.9) or obese (BMI ≥30)
- Before giving a drug that can cause weight gain to an overweight or obese patient, consider determining whether the patient already has pre-diabetes (fasting plasma glucose 100–125 mg/dL), diabetes (fasting plasma glucose >126 mg/dL), or dyslipidemia (increased total cholesterol, LDL cholesterol, and triglycerides; decreased HDL cholesterol), and treat or refer such patients for treatment, including nutrition and weight management, physical activity counseling, smoking cessation, and medical management
- ✽ Consider monitoring fasting triglycerides monthly for several months in patients at high risk for metabolic complications and when initiating or switching antipsychotics
- ✽ Monitor weight and BMI during treatment
- ✽ While giving a drug to a patient who has gained >5% of initial weight, consider evaluating for the presence of pre-diabetes, diabetes, or dyslipidemia, or consider switching to a different antipsychotic
- Monitoring elevated prolactin levels of dubious clinical benefit
- Patients with low white blood cell count (WBC) or history of drug-induced

leucopenia/neutropenia should have complete blood count (CBC) monitored frequently during the first few months and sulpiride should be discontinued at the first sign of decline of WBC in the absence of other causative factors

SIDE EFFECTS

How Drug Causes Side Effects

- By blocking dopamine 2 receptors in the striatum, it can cause motor side effects
- By blocking dopamine 2 receptors in the pituitary, it can cause elevations in prolactin
- By blocking dopamine 2 receptors excessively in the mesocortical and mesolimbic dopamine pathways, especially at high doses, it can cause worsening of negative and cognitive symptoms (neuroleptic-induced deficit syndrome)
- Anticholinergic actions may cause sedation, blurred vision, constipation, dry mouth
- Antihistaminic actions may cause sedation, weight gain
- By blocking alpha 1 adrenergic receptors, it can cause dizziness, sedation, and hypotension
- Mechanism of weight gain and any possible increased incidence of diabetes or dyslipidemia with conventional antipsychotics is unknown

Notable Side Effects

✻ Extrapyramidal symptoms, akathisia
✻ Prolactin elevation, galactorrhea, amenorrhea

- Sedation, dizziness, sleep disturbance, headache, impaired concentration
- Dry mouth, nausea, vomiting, constipation, anorexia
- Impotence
- Rare tardive dyskinesia
- Rare hypomania
- Palpitations, hypertension
- Weight gain

Life-Threatening or Dangerous Side Effects

- Rare neuroleptic malignant syndrome
- Rare seizures
- Increased risk of death and cerebrovascular events in elderly patients with dementia-related psychosis

Weight Gain

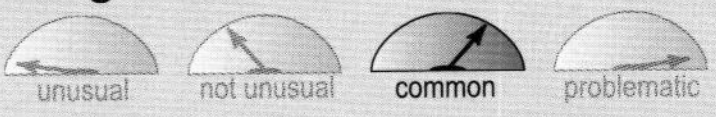

- Many experience and/or can be significant in amount

Sedation

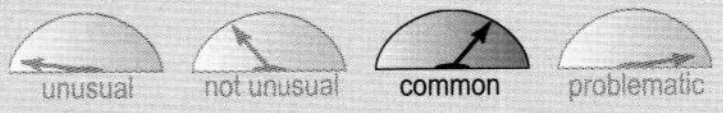

- Many experience and/or can be significant in amount, especially at high doses

What to Do About Side Effects

- Wait
- Wait
- Wait
- For motor symptoms, add an anticholinergic agent
- Reduce the dose
- For sedation, give at night
- Switch to an atypical antipsychotic
- Weight loss, exercise programs, and medical management for high BMIs, diabetes, dyslipidemia

Best Augmenting Agents for Side Effects

- Benztropine or trihexyphenidyl for motor side effects
- Sometimes amantadine can be helpful for motor side effects
- Benzodiazepines may be helpful for akathisia
- Many side effects cannot be improved with an augmenting agent

DOSING AND USE

Usual Dosage Range

- Schizophrenia: 400–800 mg/day in 2 doses (oral)
- Predominantly negative symptoms: 50–300 mg/day (oral)
- Intramuscular injection: 600–800 mg/day
- Depression: 150–300 mg/day (oral)

Dosage Forms

- Different formulations may be available in different markets

- Tablet 200 mg, 400 mg, 500 mg
- Intramuscular injection 50 mg/mL, 100 mg/mL

How to Dose
- Initial 400–800 mg/day in 1–2 doses; may need to increase dose to control positive symptoms; maximum generally 2,400 mg/day

Dosing Tips
✻ Low doses of sulpiride may be more effective at reducing negative symptoms than positive symptoms in schizophrenia; high doses may be equally effective at reducing both symptom dimensions

✻ Lower doses are more likely to be activating; higher doses are more likely to be sedating

- Some patients receive more than 2,400 mg/day
- Treatment should be suspended if absolute neutrophil count falls below 1,000/mm^3

Overdose
- Can be fatal; vomiting, agitation, hypotension, hallucinations, CNS depression, sinus tachycardia, arrhythmia, dystonia, dysarthria, hyperreflexia

Long-Term Use
- Apparently safe, but not well studied

Habit Forming
- No

How to Stop
- Recommended to reduce dose over a week
- Slow down-titration (over 6–8 weeks), especially when simultaneously beginning a new antipsychotic while switching (i.e., cross-titration)
- Rapid discontinuation may lead to rebound psychosis and worsening of symptoms
- If antiparkinson agents are being used, they should be continued for a few weeks after sulpiride is discontinued

Pharmacokinetics
- Elimination half-life approximately 6–8 hours
- Excreted largely unchanged

Drug Interactions
- Sulpiride may increase the effects of antihypertensive drugs
- CNS effects may be increased if sulpiride is used with other CNS depressants
- May decrease the effects of levodopa, dopamine agonists
- Antacids or sucralfate may reduce the absorption of sulpiride

Other Warnings/ Precautions
- If signs of neuroleptic malignant syndrome develop, treatment should be immediately discontinued
- Use cautiously in patients with alcohol withdrawal or convulsive disorders because of possible lowering of seizure threshold
- Antiemetic effect of sulpiride may mask signs of other disorders or overdose; suppression of cough reflex may cause asphyxia
- Use with caution in patients with hypertension, cardiovascular disease, pulmonary disease, hyperthyroidism, urinary retention, glaucoma
- May exacerbate symptoms of mania or hypomania
- Use only with caution if at all in Parkinson's disease or Lewy body dementia

Do Not Use
- If patient has pheochromocytoma
- If patient has prolactin-dependent tumor
- If patient is pregnant or nursing
- In children under age 15
- If there is a proven allergy to sulpiride

SPECIAL POPULATIONS

Renal Impairment
- Use with caution; drug may accumulate
- Sulpiride is eliminated by the renal route; in cases of severe renal insufficiency, the dose should be decreased and intermittent treatment or switching to another antipsychotic should be considered

Heptic Impairment
- Use with caution

Cardiac Impairment
- Use with caution

Elderly
- Some patients may tolerate lower doses better
- Although conventional antipsychotics are commonly used for behavioral disturbances in dementia, no agent has been approved for treatment of elderly patients with dementia-related psychosis
- Elderly patients with dementia-related psychosis treated with antipsychotics are at an increased risk of death compared to placebo, and also have an increased risk of cerebrovascular events

Children and Adolescents
- Not recommended for use in children under age 15
- 14 and older: recommended 3–5 mg/kg per day

Pregnancy
- There is a risk of abnormal muscle movements and withdrawal symptoms in newborns whose mothers took an antipsychotic during the third trimester; symptoms may include agitation, abnormally increased or decreased muscle tone, tremor, sleepiness, severe difficulty breathing, and difficulty feeding
- Potential risks should be weighed against the potential benefits, and sulpiride should be used only if deemed necessary
- Psychotic symptoms may worsen during pregnancy and some form of treatment may be necessary
- Atypical antipsychotics may be preferable to conventional antipsychotics or anticonvulsant mood stabilizers if treatment is required during pregnancy

Breast Feeding
- Some drug is found in mother's breast milk

✽ Recommended either to discontinue drug or bottle feed

- Immediate postpartum period is a high-risk time for relapse of psychosis

THE ART OF PSYCHOPHARMACOLOGY

Potential Advantages
- For negative symptoms in some patients

Potential Disadvantages
- Patients who cannot tolerate sedation at high doses
- Patients with severe renal impairment

Primary Target Symptoms
- Positive symptoms of psychosis
- Negative symptoms of psychosis
- Cognitive functioning
- Depressive symptoms
- Aggressive symptoms

Pearls

✽ There is some controversy over whether sulpiride is more effective than older conventionals at treating negative symptoms

- Sulpiride has been used to treat migraine associated with hormonal changes

✽ Some patients with inadequate response to clozapine may benefit from augmentation with sulpiride

- Sulpiride is poorly absorbed from the gastrointestinal tract and penetrates the blood-brain barrier poorly, which can lead to highly variable clinical responses, especially at lower doses
- Small studies and clinical anecdotes suggest efficacy in depression and anxiety disorders ("neuroses") at low doses
- Patients have very similar antipsychotic responses to any conventional antipsychotic, which is different from atypical antipsychotics where antipsychotic responses of individual patients can occasionally vary greatly from one atypical antipsychotic to another
- Patients with inadequate responses to atypical antipsychotics may benefit from a trial of augmentation with a conventional antipsychotic such as sulpiride or from switching to a conventional antipsychotic such as sulpiride
- However, long-term polypharmacy with a combination of a conventional antipsychotic with an atypical antipsychotic may combine their side effects without clearly augmenting the efficacy of either

- For treatment-resistant patients, especially those with impulsivity, aggression, violence, and self-harm, long-term polypharmacy with 2 atypical antipsychotics or with 1 atypical antipsychotic and 1 conventional antipsychotic may be useful or even necessary while closely monitoring
- In such cases, it may be beneficial to combine 1 depot antipsychotic with 1 oral antipsychotic
- Although a frequent practice by some prescribers, adding 2 conventional antipsychotics together has little rationale and may reduce tolerability without clearly enhancing efficacy

Suggested Reading

Caley CF, Weber SS. Sulpiride: an antipsychotic with selective dopaminergic antagonist properties. Ann Pharmacother 1995;29(2): 152–60.

Mauri MC, Bravin S, Bitetto A, Rudelli R, Invernizzi G. A risk-benefit assessment of sulpiride in the treatment of schizophrenia. Drug Saf 1996;14(5):288–98.

O'Connor SE, Brown RA. The pharmacology of sulpiride – a dopamine receptor antagonist. Gen Pharmacol 1982;13(3):185–93.

Omori IM, Wang J. Sulpiride versus placebo for schizophrenia. Cochrane Database Syst Rev 2009;15(2):CD007811.

Wang J, Omori IM, Fenton M, Soares B. Sulpiride augmentation for schizophrenia. Cochrane Database Syst Rev 2010;20(1):CD008125.

SUVOREXANT

THERAPEUTICS

Brands • Belsomra

Generic? No

Class
• Orexin receptor antagonist; hypnotic

Commonly Prescribed for
(bold for FDA approved)
• **Insomnia (problems with sleep onset and/or sleep maintenance)**

How the Drug Works
• Orexin serves to stabilize and promote wakefulness; suvorexant binds to orexin 1 and orexin 2 receptors, blocking orexin from binding there and thus preventing it from promoting wakefulness

How Long Until It Works
• Generally takes effect in less than an hour

If It Works
• Improves quality of sleep
• Effects on total wake-time and number of nighttime awakenings could theoretically be decreased over time

If It Doesn't Work
• If insomnia does not improve after 7–10 days, it may be a manifestation of a primary psychiatric or physical illness such as obstructive sleep apnea or restless leg syndrome, which requires independent evaluation
• Increase the dose
• Improve sleep hygiene
• Switch to another agent

Best Augmenting Combos for Partial Response or Treatment Resistance
• No controlled trials of combinations with other hypnotics or psychotropic drugs
• Generally, best to switch to another agent

Tests
• None for healthy individuals

SIDE EFFECTS

How Drug Causes Side Effects
• Theoretically due to downstream effects of blocking orexin receptors

Notable Side Effects
• Sedation, headache, dizziness, abnormal dreams

Life-Threatening or Dangerous Side Effects
• Sleep paralysis and hypnagogic/hypnopompic hallucinations (rare)
• Dose-dependent symptoms similar to mild cataplexy (rare)

Weight Gain
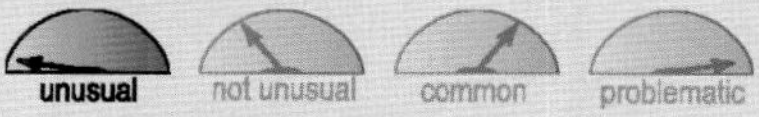

• Reported but not expected

Sedation
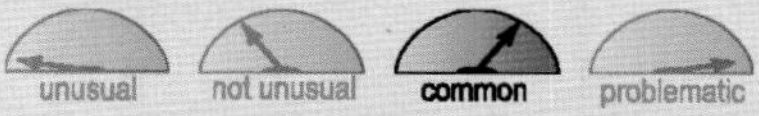

• Many experience and/or can be significant in amount

What to Do About Side Effects
• Wait
• To avoid problems with memory, take suvorexant only if planning to have a full night's sleep
• Lower the dose
• Switch to a different hypnotic

Best Augmenting Agents for Side Effects
• Many side effects cannot be improved with an augmenting agent

DOSING AND USE

Usual Dosage Range
• 10 mg/night

Dosage Forms
• Tablet 5 mg, 10 mg, 15 mg, 20 mg

How to Dose
• Starting dose is 10 mg, no more than once per night and within 30 minutes of bedtime

- Should not take unless there are at least 7 hours remaining of sleep time

Dosing Tips
- Patients who tolerate but do not respond to 10 mg may receive 15 mg or 20 mg doses; 20 mg is the maximum recommended dose
- Use the lowest dose effective for the patient
- Taking suvorexant with or soon after a meal can delay the time to effect
- Not restricted to short-term use

Overdose
- Limited data; sedation

Long-Term Use
- Has been evaluated and found effective in trials up to 1 year

Habit Forming
- Suvorexant is a Schedule IV drug
- There was no evidence of physiological dependence or withdrawal symptoms with prolonged use of suvorexant

How to Stop
- Taper not necessary

Pharmacokinetics
- Metabolized by CYP450 3A4
- Mean terminal half-life approximately 12 hours

Drug Interactions
- Not recommended in patients taking concomitant strong CYP450 3A4 inhibitors
- Patients taking moderate CYP3A4 inhibitors should receive a 5-mg dose; dose can be increased to 10 mg if needed
- Patients taking CYP3A4 inducers may experience reduced efficacy of suvorexant

Other Warnings/Precautions
- Insomnia may be a symptom of a primary disorder, rather than a primary disorder itself
- Some patients may exhibit abnormal thinking or behavioral changes similar to those caused by other CNS depressants (i.e., either depressant actions or disinhibiting actions)
- Some depressed patients may experience a worsening of suicidal ideation
- Use only with caution in patients with impaired respiratory function or obstructive sleep apnea
- Suvorexant should only be administered at bedtime
- Label contains warning for risk of next-day impaired alertness and motor coordination

Do Not Use
- If patient has narcolepsy
- If patient is taking strong CYP450 3A4 inhibitors
- If there is a proven allergy to suvorexant

SPECIAL POPULATIONS

Renal Impairment
- Dose adjustment not necessary

Hepatic Impairment
- Dose adjustment not necessary in mild to moderate hepatic impairment
- Not recommended in patients with severe hepatic impairment

Cardiac Impairment
- Not studied in patients with cardiac impairment

Elderly
- Some patients may tolerate lower doses better

Children and Adolescents
- Safety and efficacy have not been established

Pregnancy
- Effective June 30, 2015, the US FDA requires changes to the content and format of pregnancy and lactation information in prescription drug labels, including the elimination of the pregnancy letter categories; the Pregnancy and Lactation Labeling Rule (PLLR or final rule) applies only to prescription drugs and will be phased in gradually for drugs approved on or after June 30, 2001
- Controlled studies have not been conducted in pregnant women

Breast Feeding
- Unknown if suvorexant is secreted in human breast milk, but all psychotropics assumed to be secreted in breast milk
- Recommended to either discontinue drug or bottle feed

THE ART OF PSYCHOPHARMACOLOGY

Potential Advantages
- Primary insomnia
- Chronic insomnia
- Those who require long-term treatment
- Those with depression whose insomnia does not resolve with antidepressant treatment

Potential Disadvantages
- More expensive than some other sedative hypnotics

Primary Target Symptoms
- Time to sleep onset
- Nighttime awakenings
- Total sleep time

Pearls
- Targeting insomnia may prevent the onset of major depressive disorder or GAD and help maintain remission after recovery from major depressive disorder or GAD
- Rebound insomnia does not appear to be common
- Suvorexant may be safe for long-term use, with little or no suggestion of tolerance, dependence, or abuse
- May even be safe to consider in patients with a past history of substance abuse who require treatment with a hypnotic
- May be effective in patients with insomnia unresponsive to medications with other mechanisms of action (e.g., Z-drug hypnotics, benzodiazepines)

Suggested Reading

Citrome L. Suvorexant for insomnia: a systematic review of the efficacy and safety profile for this newly approved hypnotic – what is the number needed to treat, number needed to harm and likelihood to be helped or harmed? Int J Clin Pract 2014;68(12):1429–41.

Michelson D, Snyder E, Paradis E, et al. Safety and efficacy of suvorexant during 1-year treatment of insomnia with subsequent abrupt treatment discontinuation: a phase 3 randomised, double-blind, placebo-controlled trial. Lancet Neurol 2014;13(5):461–71.

TASIMELTEON

THERAPEUTICS

Brands • Hetlioz

Generic? No

Class
• Melatonin 1 and 2 receptor agonist

Commonly Prescribed for
(bold for FDA approved)
- **Non-24-Hour Sleep-Wake Disorder (Non-24)**
- Insomnia associated with shift work, jet lag, or circadian rhythm disturbances

How the Drug Works
- Binds selectively to melatonin 1 and melatonin 2 receptors as a full agonist, with greater affinity for melatonin 2 receptors than for melatonin 1 receptors

How Long Until It Works
- Because of individual differences in circadian rhythms, daily use for several weeks or months may be necessary before efficacy is observed

If It Works
- Causes circadian entrainment
- Increases nighttime sleep time
- Reduces daytime nap time

If It Doesn't Work
- Switch to another agent

Best Augmenting Combos for Partial Response or Treatment Resistance
- No controlled trials of combinations with other hypnotics or psychotropic drugs
- Generally, best to switch to another agent

Tests
- None for healthy individuals

SIDE EFFECTS

How Drug Causes Side Effects
- Actions at melatonin receptors that carry over to the next day could theoretically cause daytime sedation, fatigue, and sluggishness, but this is not common

Notable Side Effects
- Headache, nightmares or unusual dreams
- Increased alanine aminotransferase
- Upper respiratory, infection, urinary infection

Life-Threatening or Dangerous Side Effects
- None reported

Weight Gain
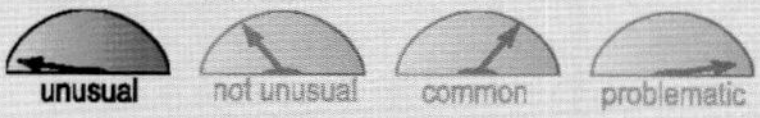

- Reported but not expected

Sedation
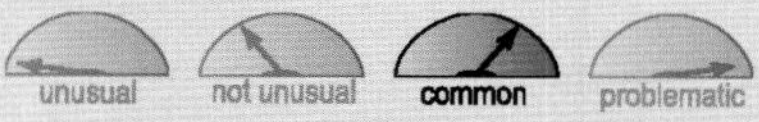

- Many experience, and/or can be significant in amount

What to Do About Side Effects
- Wait
- To avoid problems with memory, take tasimelteon only if planning to have a full night's sleep
- Switch to a different hypnotic

Best Augmenting Agents for Side Effects
- Over-the-counter pain medication for headache
- Many side effects cannot be improved with an augmenting agent

DOSING AND USE

Usual Dosage Range
- 20 mg at bedtime

Dosage Forms
- Capsule 20 mg

How to Dose
- Should be taken at the same time every night
- Should be taken without food

Dosing Tips
- If tasimelteon cannot be taken at its usual time on a given night, the dose for that night should be skipped
- Capsule should be swallowed whole

Overdose
- Limited experience

Long-Term Use
- Not restricted to short-term use
- Continued use is necessary to maintain circadian entrainment
- Has been studied and found safe in a small number of patients for up to 1 year

Habit Forming
- No

How to Stop
- Taper not necessary

Pharmacokinetics
- Mean elimination half-life 1.3 hours
- Metabolized by CYP450 1A2 and CYP 450 3A4

Drug Interactions
- Inhibitors of CYP450 1A2, such as fluvoxamine, could increase plasma levels of tasimelteon, so combination of tasimelteon with fluvoxamine or other strong CYP450 1A2 inhibitors should be avoided
- Inducers of CYP450 3A4, such as rifampin, could decrease plasma levels of tasimelteon, so combination of tasimelteon with CYP450 3A4 inducers should be avoided
- Efficacy may be reduced if given in conjunction with CYP450 1A2 inducers (e.g., cigarette smoke)
- Inhibitors of CYP450 3A4, such as ketoconazole, could increase plasma levels of tasimelteon

Other Warnings/ Precautions
- Tasimelteon should only be administered at bedtime

Do Not Use
- In patients with severe hepatic impairment
- If there is a proven allergy to tasimelteon

SPECIAL POPULATIONS

Renal Impairment
- Dose adjustment not necessary

Hepatic Impairment
- Dose adjustment not necessary for mild to moderate impairment
- Not recommended for patients with severe impairment

Cardiac Impairment
- Not studied

Elderly
- Exposure to tasimelteon is increased by approximately 2-fold

Children and Adolescents
- Safety and efficacy have not been established

Pregnancy
- Effective June 30, 2015, the US FDA requires changes to the content and format of pregnancy and lactation information in prescription drug labels, including the elimination of the pregnancy letter categories; the Pregnancy and Lactation Labeling Rule (PLLR or final rule) applies only to prescription drugs and will be phased in gradually for drugs approved on or after June 30, 2001
- Controlled studies have not been conducted in pregnant women
- In animal studies, administration of tasimelteon during pregnancy resulted in developmental toxicity (embryofetal mortality, neurobehavioral impairment, decreased growth and development in offspring)

Breast Feeding
- Unknown if tasimelteon is secreted in human breast milk, but all psychotropics assumed to be secreted in breast milk
- Use caution if patient is breast feeding

THE ART OF PSYCHOPHARMACOLOGY

Potential Advantages
- Those who require long-term treatment
- Circadian rhythm disorders

Potential Disadvantages
- Expensive

Primary Target Symptoms
- Total nighttime sleep time

Pearls
- Tasimelteon acts upon circadian rhythms by stimulating melatonin receptors in the brain's "pacemaker," namely the suprachiasmatic nucleus
- Theoretically, stimulation of melatonin 1 receptors mediates the suppressive effects of melatonin on the suprachiasmatic nucleus
- Theoretically, stimulation of melatonin 2 receptors mediates the phase shifting effect of melatonin
- Tasimelteon may act by promoting the proper entrainment of circadian rhythms underlying a normal sleep-wake cycle; this is supported by biomarker data involving both melatonin and cortisol
- Thus, tasimelteon may also prove effective for treatment of circadian rhythm disturbances such as shift work sleep disorder and jet lag, and studies in jet lag are currently under way; however, this would be an expensive alternative
- Theoretically could boost the effects of an antidepressant in blind individuals with depression or anxiety, but this has not been properly studied and augmentation studies in depression are not positive
- Lack of actions on GABA systems, which may be related to lack of apparent abuse liability

Suggested Reading

Leger D, Quera-Salva MA, Vecchierini MF, et al. Safety profile of tasimelteon, a melatonin MT1 and MT2 receptor agonist: pooled safety analyses from six clinical studies. Expert Opin Drug Saf 2015;14(11):1673–85.

Lockley SW, Dressman MA, Licamele L, et al. Tasimelteon for non-24-hour sleep-wake disorder in totally blind people (SET and RESET): two multicentre, randomised, double-masked, placebo-controlled phase 3 trials. Lancet 2015;386(10005):1754–64.

Stahl SM. Mechanism of action of tasimelteon in non-24 sleep-wake syndrome: treatment for a circadian rhythm disorder in blind patients. CNS Spectr 2014;19(6):475–8.

TEMAZEPAM

THERAPEUTICS

Brands • Restoril

see index for additional brand names

Generic? Yes

Class

- Neuroscience-based Nomenclature: GABA positive allosteric modulator (GABA-PAM)
- Benzodiazepine (hypnotic)

Commonly Prescribed for

(bold for FDA approved)

- **Short-term treatment of insomnia**
- Catatonia

How the Drug Works

- Binds to benzodiazepine receptors at the GABA-A ligand-gated chloride channel complex
- Enhances the inhibitory effects of GABA
- Boosts chloride conductance through GABA-regulated channels
- Inhibitory actions in sleep centers may provide sedative hypnotic effects

How Long Until It Works

- Generally takes effect in less than an hour, but can take longer in some patients

If It Works

- Improves quality of sleep
- Effects on total wake-time and number of nighttime awakenings may be decreased over time

If It Doesn't Work

- If insomnia does not improve after 7–10 days, it may be a manifestation of a primary psychiatric or physical illness such as obstructive sleep apnea or restless leg syndrome, which requires independent evaluation
- Increase the dose
- Improve sleep hygiene
- Switch to another agent

Best Augmenting Combos for Partial Response or Treatment Resistance

- Generally, best to switch to another agent
- Trazodone
- Agents with antihistamine actions (e.g., diphenhydramine, TCAs)

Tests

- In patients with seizure disorders, concomitant medical illness, and/or those with multiple concomitant long-term medications, periodic liver tests and blood counts may be prudent

SIDE EFFECTS

How Drug Causes Side Effects

- Same mechanism for side effects as for therapeutic effects – namely due to excessive actions at benzodiazepine receptors
- Actions at benzodiazepine receptors that carry over to the next day can cause daytime sedation, amnesia, and ataxia
- Long-term adaptations in benzodiazepine receptors may explain the development of dependence, tolerance, and withdrawal

Notable Side Effects

- ✱ Sedation, fatigue, depression
- ✱ Dizziness, ataxia, slurred speech, weakness
- ✱ Forgetfulness, confusion
- ✱ Hyperexcitability, nervousness
- Rare hallucinations, mania
- Rare hypotension
- Hypersalivation, dry mouth
- Rebound insomnia when withdrawing from long-term treatment

Life-Threatening or Dangerous Side Effects

- Respiratory depression, especially when taken with CNS depressants in overdose
- Rare hepatic dysfunction, renal dysfunction, blood dyscrasias

Weight Gain

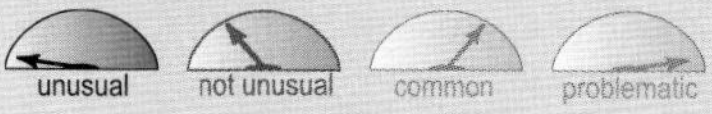

- Reported but not expected

Sedation

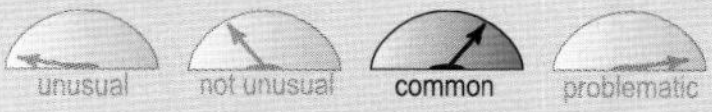

- Many experience and/or can be significant in amount

What to Do About Side Effects
- Wait
- To avoid problems with memory, only take temazepam if planning to have a full night's sleep
- Lower the dose
- Switch to a shorter-acting sedative hypnotic
- Switch to a non-benzodiazepine hypnotic
- Administer flumazenil if side effects are severe or life-threatening

Best Augmenting Agents for Side Effects
- Many side effects cannot be improved with an augmenting agent

DOSING AND USE

Usual Dosage Range
- 15 mg/day at bedtime

Dosage Forms
- Capsule 7.5 mg, 15 mg, 30 mg

How to Dose
- 15 mg/day at bedtime; may increase to 30 mg/day at bedtime if ineffective

Dosing Tips
- Use lowest possible effective dose and assess need for continued treatment regularly
- Temazepam should generally not be prescribed in quantities greater than a 1-month supply
- Patients with lower body weights may require lower doses
- ✽ Because temazepam is slowly absorbed, administering the dose 1–2 hours before bedtime may improve onset of action and shorter sleep latency
- Risk of dependence may increase with dose and duration of treatment

Overdose
- Can be fatal in monotherapy; slurred speech, poor coordination, respiratory depression, sedation, confusion, coma

Long-Term Use
- Not generally intended for long-term use

Habit Forming
- Temazepam is a Schedule IV drug
- Some patients may develop dependence and/or tolerance; risk may be greater with higher doses
- History of drug addiction may increase risk of dependence

How to Stop
- If taken for more than a few weeks, taper to reduce chances of withdrawal effects
- Patients with history of seizure may seize upon sudden withdrawal
- Rebound insomnia may occur the first 1–2 nights after stopping
- For patients with severe problems discontinuing a benzodiazepine, dosing may need to be tapered over many months (i.e., reduce dose by 1% every 3 days by crushing tablet and suspending or dissolving in 100 mL of fruit juice and then disposing of 1 mL while drinking the rest; 3–7 days later, dispose of 2 mL, and so on). This is both a form of very slow biological tapering and a form of behavioral desensitization

Pharmacokinetics
- No active metabolites
- Half-life approximately 8–15 hours

Drug Interactions
- Increased depressive effects when taken with other CNS depressants (see Warnings below)
- If temazepam is used with kava, clearance of either drug may be affected

Other Warnings/ Precautions
- Boxed warning regarding the increased risk of CNS depressant effects when benzodiazepines and opioid medications are used together, including specifically the risk of slowed or difficulty breathing and death
- If alternatives to the combined use of benzodiazepines and opioids are not available, clinicians should limit the dosage and duration of each drug to the minimum

possible while still achieving therapeutic efficacy
- Patients and their caregivers should be warned to seek medical attention if unusual dizziness, lightheadedness, sedation, slowed or difficulty breathing, or unresponsiveness occur
- Insomnia may be a symptom of a primary disorder, rather than a primary disorder itself
- Some patients may exhibit abnormal thinking or behavioral changes similar to those caused by other CNS depressants (i.e., either depressant actions or disinhibiting actions)
- Some depressed patients may experience a worsening of suicidal ideation
- Use only with extreme caution in patients with impaired respiratory function or obstructive sleep apnea
- Temazepam should only be administered at bedtime

Do Not Use
- If patient is pregnant
- If patient has angle-closure glaucoma
- If there is a proven allergy to temazepam or any benzodiazepine

SPECIAL POPULATIONS

Renal Impairment
- Recommended dose: 7.5 mg/day

Hepatic Impairment
- Recommended dose: 7.5 mg/day

Cardiac Impairment
- Dosage adjustment may not be necessary
- Benzodiazepines have been used to treat insomnia associated with acute myocardial infarction

Elderly
- Recommended dose: 7.5 mg/day

Children and Adolescents
- Safety and efficacy have not been established
- Long-term effects of temazepam in children/adolescents are unknown
- Should generally receive lower doses and be more closely monitored

Pregnancy
- Contraindicated for use in pregnancy
- Effective June 30, 2015, the US FDA requires changes to the content and format of pregnancy and lactation information in prescription drug labels, including the elimination of the pregnancy letter categories; the Pregnancy and Lactation Labeling Rule (PLLR or final rule) applies only to prescription drugs and will be phased in gradually for drugs approved on or after June 30, 2001
- Infants whose mothers received a benzodiazepine late in pregnancy may experience withdrawal effects
- Neonatal flaccidity has been reported in infants whose mothers took a benzodiazepine during pregnancy

Breast Feeding
- Unknown if temazepam is secreted in human breast milk, but all psychotropics assumed to be secreted in breast milk
- * Recommended either to discontinue drug or bottle feed
- Effects on infant have been observed and include feeding difficulties, sedation, and weight loss

THE ART OF PSYCHOPHARMACOLOGY

Potential Advantages
- Patients with middle insomnia (nocturnal awakening)

Potential Disadvantages
- Patients with early insomnia (problems falling asleep)

Primary Target Symptoms
- Time to sleep onset
- Total sleep time
- Nighttime awakenings

Pearls
- If tolerance develops, it may result in increased anxiety during the day and/or increased wakefulness during the latter part of the night

❋ Slow gastrointestinal absorption compared to other sedative benzodiazepines, so may be more effective for nocturnal awakening than for initial insomnia unless dosed 1–2 hours prior to bedtime

❋ Notable for delayed onset of action compared to some other sedative hypnotics

- Though not systematically studied, benzodiazepines have been used effectively to treat catatonia and are the initial recommended treatment

Suggested Reading

Ashton H. Guidelines for the rational use of benzodiazepines. When and what to use. Drugs 1994;48:25–40.

Fraschini F, Stankov B. Temazepam: pharmacological profile of a benzodiazepine and new trends in its clinical application. Pharmacol Res 1993;27:97–113.

Heel RC, Brogden RN, Speight TM, Avery GS. Temazepam: a review of its pharmacological properties and therapeutic efficacy as an hypnotic. Drugs 1981;21:321–40.

McElnay JC, Jones ME, Alexander B. Temazepam (Restoril, Sandoz Pharmaceuticals). Drug Intell Clin Pharm 1982;16:650–6.

THERAPEUTICS

Brands • Mellaril

see index for additional brand names

Generic? Yes

Class

- Neuroscience-based Nomenclature: dopamine and serotonin receptor antagonist (DS-RAn)
- Conventional antipsychotic (neuroleptic, phenothiazine, dopamine 2 antagonist)

Commonly Prescribed for

(bold for FDA approved)

- **Schizophrenic patients who fail to respond to treatment with other antipsychotic drugs**

How the Drug Works

- Blocks dopamine 2 receptors, reducing positive symptoms of psychosis

How Long Until It Works

- Psychotic symptoms can improve within 1 week, but it may take several weeks for full effect on behavior

If It Works

- Is a second-line treatment option

✽ Should evaluate for switching to an antipsychotic with a better risk/benefit ratio

If It Doesn't Work

- Consider trying one of the first-line atypical antipsychotics (risperidone, olanzapine, quetiapine, ziprasidone, aripiprazole, paliperidone, amisulpride, asenapine, iloperidone, lurasidone)
- Consider trying another conventional antipsychotic
- If 2 or more antipsychotic monotherapies do not work, consider clozapine

Best Augmenting Combos for Partial Response or Treatment Resistance

✽ Augmentation of thioridazine has not been systematically studied and can be dangerous, especially with drugs that can either prolong QTc interval or raise thioridazine plasma levels

Tests

✽ Baseline EKG and serum potassium levels should be determined

✽ Periodic evaluation of EKG and serum potassium levels

- Serum magnesium levels may also need to be monitored

✽ Since conventional antipsychotics are frequently associated with weight gain, before starting treatment, weigh all patients and determine if the patient is already overweight (BMI 25.0–29.9) or obese (BMI ≥30)

- Before giving a drug that can cause weight gain to an overweight or obese patient, consider determining whether the patient already has pre-diabetes (fasting plasma glucose 100–125 mg/dL), diabetes (fasting plasma glucose >126 mg/dL), or dyslipidemia (increased total cholesterol, LDL cholesterol, and triglycerides; decreased HDL cholesterol), and treat or refer such patients for treatment, including nutrition and weight management, physical activity counseling, smoking cessation, and medical management

✽ Monitor weight and BMI during treatment

✽ Consider monitoring fasting triglycerides monthly for several months in patients at high risk for metabolic complications and when initiating or switching antipsychotics

✽ While giving a drug to a patient who has gained >5% of initial weight, consider evaluating for the presence of pre-diabetes, diabetes, or dyslipidemia, or consider switching to a different antipsychotic

- Should check blood pressure in the elderly before starting and for the first few weeks of treatment
- Monitoring elevated prolactin levels of dubious clinical benefit
- Phenothiazines may cause false-positive phenylketonuria results
- Patients with low white blood cell count (WBC) or history of drug-induced leucopenia/neutropenia should have complete blood count (CBC) monitored frequently during the first few months and thioridazine should be discontinued at the first sign of decline of WBC in the absence of other causative factors

SIDE EFFECTS

How Drug Causes Side Effects

- By blocking dopamine 2 receptors in the striatum, it can cause motor side effects

- By blocking dopamine 2 receptors in the pituitary, it can cause elevations in prolactin
- By blocking dopamine 2 receptors excessively in the mesocortical and mesolimbic dopamine pathways, especially at high doses, it can cause worsening of negative and cognitive symptoms (neuroleptic-induced deficit syndrome)
- Anticholinergic actions may cause sedation, blurred vision, constipation, dry mouth
- Antihistaminic actions may cause sedation, weight gain
- By blocking alpha 1 adrenergic receptors, it can cause dizziness, sedation, and hypotension
- Mechanism of weight gain and any possible increased incidence of diabetes or dyslipidemia with conventional antipsychotics is unknown

✻ Mechanism of potentially dangerous QTc prolongation may be related to actions at ion channels

Notable Side Effects

✻ Neuroleptic-induced deficit syndrome
✻ Akathisia
✻ Priapism
✻ Extrapyramidal symptoms, parkinsonism, tardive dyskinesia
✻ Galactorrhea, amenorrhea
✻ Pigmentary retinopathy at high doses

- Dizziness, sedation
- Dry mouth, constipation, blurred vision
- Decreased sweating
- Sexual dysfunction
- Hypotension
- Weight gain

Life-Threatening or Dangerous Side Effects

- Rare neuroleptic malignant syndrome
- Rare jaundice, agranulocytosis
- Rare seizures

✻ Dose-dependent QTc prolongation

- Ventricular arrhythmias and sudden death
- Increased risk of death and cerebrovascular events in elderly patients with dementia-related psychosis

Weight Gain

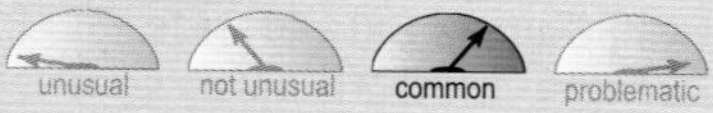

- Many experience and/or can be significant in amount

Sedation

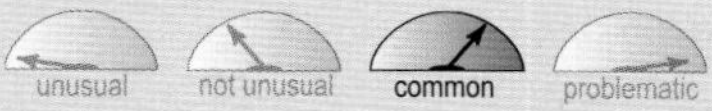

- Many experience and/or can be significant in amount
- Sedation is usually transient

What to Do About Side Effects

- Wait
- Wait
- Wait
- For motor symptoms, add an anticholinergic agent
- Reduce the dose
- For sedation, give at night
- Switch to an atypical antipsychotic
- Weight loss, exercise programs, and medical management for high BMIs, diabetes, dyslipidemia

Best Augmenting Agents for Side Effects

✻ Augmentation of thioridazine has not been systematically studied and can be dangerous

DOSING AND USE

Usual Dosage Range

- 200–800 mg/day in divided doses

Dosage Forms

- Tablet 10 mg, 15 mg, 25 mg, 50 mg, 100 mg, 150 mg, 200 mg
- Liquid 30 mg/mL, 100 mg/mL
- Suspension 5 mg/mL, 20 mg/mL

How to Dose

- 50–100 mg 3 times a day; increase gradually; maximum 800 mg/day in divided doses

Dosing Tips

✻ Prolongation of the QTc interval is dose-dependent, so start low and go slow while carefully monitoring QTc interval

- Pigmentary retinopathy has been reported in patients taking doses exceeding the recommended range
- Treatment should be suspended if absolute neutrophil count falls below 1,000/mm^3

Overdose
- Sedation, confusion, respiratory depression, cardiac disturbance, hypotension, seizure, coma

Long-Term Use
- Some side effects may be irreversible (e.g., tardive dyskinesia)

Habit Forming
- No

How to Stop
- Slow down-titration (over 6–8 weeks), especially when simultaneously beginning a new antipsychotic while switching (i.e., cross-titration)
- Rapid discontinuation may lead to rebound psychosis and worsening of symptoms
- If antiparkinson agents are being used, they should be continued for a few weeks after thioridazine is discontinued

Pharmacokinetics
- Metabolized by CYP450 2D6

Drug Interactions
- May decrease the effects of levodopa, dopamine agonists
- May increase the effects of antihypertensive drugs
- May enhance QTc prolongation of other drugs capable of prolonging QTc interval

✽ CYP450 2D6 inhibitors including paroxetine, fluoxetine, duloxetine, bupropion, sertraline, citalopram, and others can raise thioridazine to dangerous levels

✽ Fluvoxamine, propranolol, and pindolol also inhibit thioridazine metabolism and can raise thioridazine to dangerous levels

- Respiratory depression/arrest may occur if used with a barbiturate
- Additive effects may occur if used with CNS depressants
- Alcohol and diuretics may increase the risk of hypotension; epinephrine may lower blood pressure
- Some patients taking a neuroleptic and lithium have developed an encephalopathic syndrome similar to neuroleptic malignant syndrome

Other Warnings/Precautions
- If signs of neuroleptic malignant syndrome develop, treatment should be immediately discontinued

✽ Thioridazine can increase the QTc interval and potentially cause torsades de pointes-type arrhythmia or sudden death, especially in combination with drugs that raise its levels

- Use cautiously in patients with respiratory disorders, glaucoma, or urinary retention
- Avoid extreme heat exposure
- Antiemetic effect can mask signs of other disorders or overdose
- Use cautiously in patients with alcohol withdrawal or convulsive disorders because of possible lowering of seizure threshold
- Do not use epinephrine in event of overdose, as interaction with some pressor agents may lower blood pressure
- Use only with caution if at all in Parkinson's disease or Lewy body dementia
- Observe for signs of pigmentary retinopathy, especially at higher doses
- Because thioridazine may dose-dependently prolong QTc interval, use with caution in patients who have bradycardia or who are taking drugs that can induce bradycardia (e.g., beta blockers, calcium channel blockers, clonidine, digitalis)
- Because thioridazine may dose-dependently prolong QTc interval, use with caution in patients who have hypokalemia and/or hypomagnesemia or who are taking drugs that can induce hypokalemia and/or magnesemia (e.g., diuretics, stimulant laxatives, intravenous amphotericin B, glucocorticoids, tetracosactide)

Do Not Use
- If patient is in a comatose state or has CNS depression
- If patient suffers from extreme hypertension/hypotension

✽ If QTc interval greater than 450 msec or if taking an agent capable of significantly prolonging QTc interval (e.g., pimozide,

selected antiarrhythmics, moxifoxacin, and sparfloxacin)
* If there is a history of QTc prolongation or cardiac arrhythmia, recent acute myocardial infarction, uncompensated heart failure
* If patient is taking drugs that inhibit thioridazine metabolism, including CYP450 inhibitors
* If there is reduced CYP450 2D6 function, such as in patients who are 2D6 poor metabolizers
- If there is a proven allergy to thioridazine
- If there is a known sensitivity to any phenothiazine

SPECIAL POPULATIONS

Renal Impairment
- Use with caution

Hepatic Impairment
- Use with caution

Cardiac Impairment
- Thioridazine produces a dose-dependent prolongation of QTc interval, which may be enhanced by the existence of bradycardia, hypokalemia, congenital or acquired long QTc interval, which should be evaluated prior to administering thioridazine
- Use with caution if treating concomitantly with a medication likely to produce prolonged bradycardia, hypokalemia slowing of intracardiac conduction, or prolongation of the QTc interval
- Avoid thioridazine in patients with a known history of QTc prolongation, recent acute myocardial infarction, and uncompensated heart failure
* Risk/benefit ratio may not justify use in cardiac impairment

Elderly
- Some patients may tolerate lower doses better
- Elderly patients may be more sensitive to adverse effects, including agranulocytosis and leukopenia
- Although conventional antipsychotics are commonly used for behavioral disturbances in dementia, no agent has been approved for treatment of elderly patients with dementia-related psychosis
- Elderly patients with dementia-related psychosis treated with antipsychotics are at an increased risk of death compared to placebo, and also have an increased risk of cerebrovascular events

Children and Adolescents
- Safety and efficacy not established in children under age 2
- Dose: initial 0.5 mg/kg per day in divided doses; increase gradually; maximum 3 mg/kg per day
- Risk/benefit ratio may not justify use in children or adolescents

Pregnancy
- Effective June 30, 2015, the US FDA requires changes to the content and format of pregnancy and lactation information in prescription drug labels, including the elimination of the pregnancy letter categories; the Pregnancy and Lactation Labeling Rule (PLLR or final rule) applies only to prescription drugs and will be phased in gradually for drugs approved on or after June 30, 2001
- Controlled studies have not been conducted in pregnant women
- There is a risk of abnormal muscle movements and withdrawal symptoms in newborns whose mothers took an antipsychotic during the third trimester; symptoms may include agitation, abnormally increased or decreased muscle tone, tremor, sleepiness, severe difficulty breathing, and difficulty feeding
- Reports of extrapyramidal symptoms, jaundice, hyperreflexia, hyporeflexia in infants whose mothers took a phenothiazine during pregnancy
- Psychotic symptoms may worsen during pregnancy and some form of treatment may be necessary
- Atypical antipsychotic may be preferable to conventional antipsychotics or anticonvulsant mood stabilizers if treatment is required during pregnancy

- Should evaluate for an antipsychotic with a better risk/benefit ratio if treatment is required during pregnancy

Breast Feeding

- Unknown if thioridazine is secreted in human breast milk, but all psychotropics assumed to be secreted in breast milk

❋ Recommended either to discontinue drug or bottle feed

THE ART OF PSYCHOPHARMACOLOGY

Potential Advantages

- Only for patients who respond to this agent and not other antipsychotics

Potential Disadvantages

- Children
- Elderly
- Patients on other drugs
- Those with low CYP450 2D6 metabolism

Primary Target Symptoms

- Positive symptoms of psychosis in patients who fail to respond to treatment with other antipsychotics
- Motor and autonomic hyperactivity in patients who fail to respond to treatment with other antipsychotics
- Violent or aggressive behavior in patients who fail to respond to treatment with other antipsychotics

Pearls

❋ Generally, the benefits of thioridazine do not outweigh its risks for most patients

❋ Because of its effects on the QTc interval, thioridazine is not intended for use unless other options (at least 2 antipsychotics) have failed

- Thioridazine has not been systematically studied in treatment-refractory schizophrenia

❋ Phenotypic testing may be necessary in order to detect the 7% of the Caucasian population for whom thioridazine is contraindicated due to a genetic variant leading to reduced activity of CYP450 2D6

- Conventional antipsychotics are much less expensive than atypical antipsychotics
- Thioridazine causes less extrapyramidal symptoms than some other conventional antipsychotics

❋ Was once a preferred antipsychotic for children and the elderly, and for those whose symptoms benefited from a sedating low potency phenothiazine with a lower incidence of extrapyramidal symptoms

❋ However, now it is recognized that the dangers of cardiac arrhythmias and drug interactions outweigh the benefits of thioridazine, and it is now considered a second-line treatment if it is considered at all

Suggested Reading

Fenton M, Rathbone J, Reilly J, Sultana A. Thioridazine for schizophrenia. Cochrane Database Syst Rev 2007;18(3):CD001944.

Frankenburg FR. Choices in antipsychotic therapy in schizophrenia. Harv Rev Psychiatry 1999;6:241–9.

Gardos G, Tecce JJ, Hartmann E, Bowers P, Cole JO. Treatment with mesoridazine and thioridazine in chronic schizophrenia: II. Potential predictors of drug response. Compr Psychiatry 1978;19:527–32.

Leucht S, Wahlbeck K, Hamann J, Kissling W. New generation antipsychotics versus low-potency conventional antipsychotics: a systematic review and meta-analysis. The Lancet 2003;361:1581–9.

THERAPEUTICS

Brands • Navane

see index for additional brand names

Generic? Yes

Class

- Conventional antipsychotic (neuroleptic, thioxanthene, dopamine 2 antagonist)

Commonly Prescribed for

(bold for FDA approved)

- **Schizophrenia**
- Other psychotic disorders
- Bipolar disorder

How the Drug Works

- Blocks dopamine 2 receptors, reducing positive symptoms of psychosis

How Long Until It Works

- Psychotic symptoms can improve within 1 week, but it may take several weeks for full effect on behavior

If It Works

- Most often reduces positive symptoms in schizophrenia but does not eliminate them
- Most schizophrenic patients do not have a total remission of symptoms but rather a reduction of symptoms by about a third
- Continue treatment in schizophrenia until reaching a plateau of improvement
- After reaching a satisfactory plateau, continue treatment for at least a year after first episode of psychosis in schizophrenia
- For second and subsequent episodes of psychosis in schizophrenia, treatment may need to be indefinite
- Reduces symptoms of acute psychotic mania but not proven as a mood stabilizer or as an effective maintenance treatment in bipolar disorder
- After reducing acute psychotic symptoms in mania, switch to a mood stabilizer and/or an atypical antipsychotic for mood stabilization and maintenance

If It Doesn't Work

- Consider trying one of the first-line atypical antipsychotics (risperidone, olanzapine, quetiapine, ziprasidone, aripiprazole, paliperidone, amisulpride, asenapine, iloperidone, lurasidone)
- Consider trying another conventional antipsychotic
- If 2 or more antipsychotic monotherapies do not work, consider clozapine

Best Augmenting Combos for Partial Response or Treatment Resistance

- Augmentation of conventional antipsychotics has not been systematically studied
- Addition of a mood-stabilizing anticonvulsant such as valproate, carbamazepine, or lamotrigine may be helpful in both schizophrenia and bipolar mania
- Augmentation with lithium in bipolar mania may be helpful
- Addition of a benzodiazepine, especially short-term for agitation

Tests

❋ Since conventional antipsychotics are frequently associated with weight gain, before starting treatment, weigh all patients and determine if the patient is already overweight (BMI 25.0–29.9) or obese (BMI ≥30)

- Before giving a drug that can cause weight gain to an overweight or obese patient, consider determining whether the patient already has pre-diabetes (fasting plasma glucose 100–125 mg/dL), diabetes (fasting plasma glucose >126 mg/dL), or dyslipidemia (increased total cholesterol, LDL cholesterol, and triglycerides; decreased HDL cholesterol), and treat or refer such patients for treatment, including nutrition and weight management, physical activity counseling, smoking cessation, and medical management

❋ Monitor weight and BMI during treatment

❋ Consider monitoring fasting triglycerides monthly for several months in patients at high risk for metabolic complications and when initiating or switching antipsychotics

❋ While giving a drug to a patient who has gained >5% of initial weight, consider evaluating for the presence of pre-diabetes, diabetes, or dyslipidemia, or consider switching to a different antipsychotic

- Monitoring elevated prolactin levels of dubious clinical benefit
- Patients with low white blood cell count (WBC) or history of drug-induced

leucopenia/neutropenia should have complete blood count (CBC) monitored frequently during the first few months and thiothixene should be discontinued at the first sign of decline of WBC in the absence of other causative factors

SIDE EFFECTS

How Drug Causes Side Effects

- By blocking dopamine 2 receptors in the striatum, it can cause motor side effects
- By blocking dopamine 2 receptors in the pituitary, it can cause elevations in prolactin
- By blocking dopamine 2 receptors excessively in the mesocortical and mesolimbic dopamine pathways, especially at high doses, it can cause worsening of negative and cognitive symptoms (neuroleptic-induced deficit syndrome)
- Anticholinergic actions may cause sedation, blurred vision, constipation, dry mouth
- Antihistaminic actions may cause sedation, weight gain
- By blocking alpha 1 adrenergic receptors, it can cause dizziness, sedation, and hypotension
- Mechanism of weight gain and any possible increased incidence of diabetes or dyslipidemia with conventional antipsychotics is unknown

Notable Side Effects

✻ Neuroleptic-induced deficit syndrome
✻ Akathisia
✻ Extrapyramidal symptoms, parkinsonism, tardive dyskinesia
✻ Galactorrhea, amenorrhea
- Sedation
- Dry mouth, constipation, vision disturbance, urninary retention
- Hypotension, tachycardia
- Rare fine lenticular pigmentation

Life-Threatening or Dangerous Side Effects

- Rare neuroleptic malignant syndrome
- Rare seizures
- Rare blood dyscrasias
- Rare hepatic toxicity
- Increased risk of death and cerebrovascular events in elderly patients with dementia-related psychosis

Weight Gain

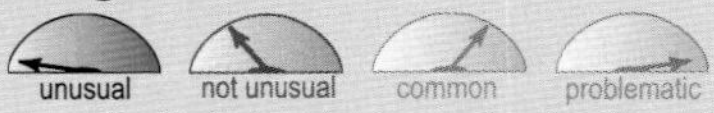

✻ Reported but not expected

Sedation

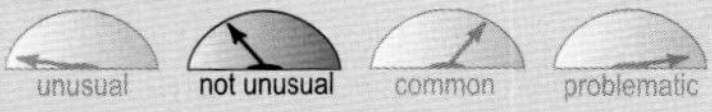

- Occurs in significant minority

What to Do About Side Effects

- Wait
- Wait
- Wait
- For motor symptoms, add an anticholinergic agent
- For sedation, take at night
- Reduce the dose
- Switch to an atypical antipsychotic
- Weight loss, exercise programs, and medical management for high BMIs, diabetes, dyslipidemia

Best Augmenting Agents for Side Effects

- Benztropine or trihexyphenidyl for motor side effects
- Sometimes amantadine can be helpful for motor side effects
- Benzodiazepines may be helpful for akathisia
- Many side effects cannot be improved with an augmenting agent

DOSING AND USE

Usual Dosage Range

- 15–30 mg/day

Dosage Forms

- Capsule 2 mg, 5 mg, 10 mg

How To Dose

- Initial 5–10 mg/day; maximum dose generally 60 mg/day; higher doses may be given in divided doses

Dosing Tips

- When thiothixene is dosed too high, it can induce or worsen negative symptoms of schizophrenia

- Lower doses may provide the best benefit with fewest side effects in patients who respond to low doses
- Treatment should be suspended if absolute neutrophil count falls below 1,000/mm^3

Overdose
- Muscle twitching, sedation, dizziness, CNS depression, rigidity, weakness, torticollis, dysphagia, hypotension, coma

Long-Term Use
- Some side effects may be irreversible (e.g., tardive dyskinesia)

Habit Forming
- No

How to Stop
- Slow down-titration (over 6–8 weeks), especially when simultaneously beginning a new antipsychotic while switching (i.e., cross-titration)
- Rapid discontinuation may lead to rebound psychosis and worsening of symptoms
- If antiparkinson agents are being used, they should be continued for a few weeks after thiothixene is discontinued

Pharmacokinetics
- Initial elimination half-life approximately 3.4 hours
- Terminal elimination half-life approximately 34 hours

Drug Interactions
- Respiratory depression may occur when thiothixene is combined with lorazepam
- Additive effects may occur if used with CNS depressants
- May decrease the effects of levodopa, dopamine agonists
- Some patients taking a neuroleptic and lithium have developed an encephalopathic syndrome similar to neuroleptic malignant syndrome
- Combined use with epinephrine may lower blood pressure
- May increase the effects of antihypertensive drugs except for guanethidine, whose antihypertensive actions thiothixene may antagonize

Other Warnings/ Precautions
- If signs of neuroleptic malignant syndrome develop, treatment should be immediately discontinued
- Use cautiously in patients with alcohol withdrawal or convulsive disorders because of possible lowering of seizure threshold
- Antiemetic effect can mask signs of other disorders or overdose
- Do not use epinephrine in event of overdose, as interaction with some pressor agents may lower blood pressure
- Use cautiously in patients with glaucoma, urinary retention
- Observe for signs of ocular toxicity (pigmentary retinopathy, lenticular pigmentation)
- Avoid extreme heat exposure
- Use only with caution if at all in Parkinson's disease or Lewy body dementia

Do Not Use
- If patient has CNS depression, is in a comatose state, has circulatory collapse, or there is presence of blood dyscrasias
- If there is a proven allergy to thiothixene

SPECIAL POPULATIONS

Renal Impairment
- Use with caution

Hepatic Impairment
- Use with caution

Cardiac Impairment
- Thiothixene may cause or aggravate EKG changes

Elderly
- Some patients may tolerate lower doses better
- Although conventional antipsychotics are commonly used for behavioral disturbances in dementia, no agent has been approved for treatment of elderly patients with dementia-related psychosis
- Elderly patients with dementia-related psychosis treated with antipsychotics are at an increased risk of death compared to placebo, and also have an increased risk of cerebrovascular events

Children and Adolescents

- Safety and efficacy have not been established in children under age 12
- Generally consider second-line after atypical antipsychotics

Pregnancy

- Controlled studies have not been conducted in pregnant women
- There is a risk of abnormal muscle movements and withdrawal symptoms in newborns whose mothers took an antipsychotic during the third trimester; symptoms may include agitation, abnormally increased or decreased muscle tone, tremor, sleepiness, severe difficulty breathing, and difficulty feeding
- Reports of extrapyramidal symptoms, jaundice, hyperreflexia, hyporeflexia in infants whose mothers took a phenothiazine during pregnancy
- Psychotic symptoms may worsen during pregnancy and some form of treatment may be necessary
- Atypical antipsychotics may be preferable to conventional antipsychotics or anticonvulsant mood stabilizers if treatment is required during pregnancy
- Thiothixene should generally not be used during the first trimester
- Thiothixene should be used during pregnancy only if clearly needed

Breast Feeding

- Unknown if thiothixene is secreted in human breast milk, but all psychotropics assumed to be secreted in breast milk

✻ Recommended either to discontinue drug or bottle feed

THE ART OF PSYCHOPHARMACOLOGY

Potential Advantages

- For patients who do not respond to other antipsychotics

Potential Disadvantages

- Patients with tardive dyskinesia
- Children
- Elderly

Primary Target Symptoms

- Positive symptoms of psychosis
- Negative symptoms of psychosis

Pearls

✻ Although not systematically studied, may cause less weight gain than other antipsychotics

- Conventional antipsychotics are less expensive than atypical antipsychotics
- Patients have very similar antipsychotic responses to any conventional antipsychotic, which is different from atypical antipsychotics where antipsychotic responses of individual patients can occasionally vary greatly from one atypical antipsychotic to another
- Patients with inadequate responses to atypical antipsychotics may benefit from a trial of augmentation with a conventional antipsychotic such as thiothixene or from switching to a conventional antipsychotic such as thiothixene
- However, long-term polypharmacy with a combination of a conventional antipsychotic such as thiothixene with an atypical antipsychotic may combine their side effects without clearly augmenting the efficacy of either
- For treatment-resistant patients, especially those with impulsivity, aggression, violence, and self-harm, long-term polypharmacy with 2 atypical antipsychotics or with 1 atypical antipsychotic and 1 conventional antipsychotic may be useful or even necessary while closely monitoring
- In such cases, it may be beneficial to combine 1 depot antipsychotic with 1 oral antipsychotic
- Although a frequent practice by some prescribers, adding 2 conventional antipsychotics together has little rationale and may reduce tolerability without clearly enhancing efficacy

Suggested Reading

Huang CC, Gerhardstein RP, Kim DY, Hollister L. Treatment-resistant schizophrenia: controlled study of moderate- and high-dose thiothixene. Int Clin Psychopharmacol 1987;2:69–75.

Sterlin C, Ban TA, Jarrold L. The place of thiothixene among the thioxanthenes. Curr Ther Res Clin Exp 1972;14:205–14.

THERAPEUTICS

Brands • Gabitril

see index for additional brand names

Generic? Yes

Class
- Anticonvulsant; selective GABA reuptake inhibitor (SGRI)

Commonly Prescribed for
(bold for FDA approved)
- **Partial seizures (adjunctive; adults and children 12 years and older)**
- Anxiety disorders
- Neuropathic pain/chronic pain

How the Drug Works
- Selectively blocks reuptake of gamma-aminobutyric acid (GABA) by presynaptic and glial GABA transporters

How Long Until It Works
- Should reduce seizures by 2 weeks
- Not clear that it works in anxiety disorders or chronic pain but some patients may respond, and if they do, therapeutic actions can be seen by 2 weeks

If It Works
- The goal of treatment is complete remission of symptoms (e.g., seizures, anxiety)
- The goal of treatment of chronic neuropathic pain is to reduce symptoms as much as possible, especially in combination with other treatments
- Treatment of chronic neuropathic pain most often reduces but does not eliminate symptoms and is not a cure since symptoms usually recur after medicine stopped
- Continue treatment until all symptoms are gone or until improvement is stable and then continue treating indefinitely as long as improvement persists

If It Doesn't Work (for neuropathic pain or anxiety disorders)
- Many patients have only a partial response where some symptoms are improved but others persist
- Other patients may be nonresponders, sometimes called treatment-resistant or treatment-refractory
- May only be effective in a subset of patients with neuropathic pain or anxiety disorders, in some patients who fail to respond to other treatments, or it may not work at all
- Consider increasing dose, switching to another agent or adding an appropriate augmenting agent
- Consider biofeedback or hypnosis for pain
- Consider evaluation for another diagnosis or for a comorbid condition (e.g., medical illness, substance abuse, etc.)
- Switch to another agent with fewer side effects

Best Augmenting Combos for Partial Response or Treatment Resistance
- Tiagabine is itself an augmenting agent for numerous other anticonvulsants in treating epilepsy

✽ For neuropathic pain, tiagabine can augment TCAs and SNRIs as well as gabapentin, other anticonvulsants, and even opiates if done by experts while carefully monitoring in difficult cases

- For anxiety, tiagabine is a second-line treatment to augment SSRIs, SNRIs, or benzodiazepines

Tests
- None for healthy individuals
- Tiagabine may bind to tissue that contains melanin, so for long-term treatment opthalmological checks may be considered

SIDE EFFECTS

How Drug Causes Side Effects
- CNS side effects may be due to excessive actions of GABA

Notable Side Effects
✽ Sedation, dizziness, asthenia, nervousness, difficulty concentrating, speech/language problems, confusion, tremor

- Diarrhea, vomiting, nausea
- Ecchymosis, depression

Life-Threatening or Dangerous Side Effects

- Exacerbation of EEG abnormalities in epilepsy
- Status epilepticus in epilepsy (unknown if associated with tiagabine use)
- Sudden unexplained deaths have occurred in epilepsy (unknown if related to tiagabine use)
- New onset seizures and status epilepticus have been reported in patients without epilepsy
- Rare activation of suicidal ideation and behavior (suicidality)

Weight Gain

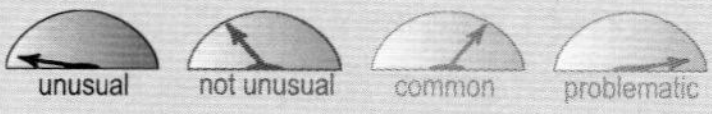

- Reported but not expected
- Some patients experience increased appetite

Sedation

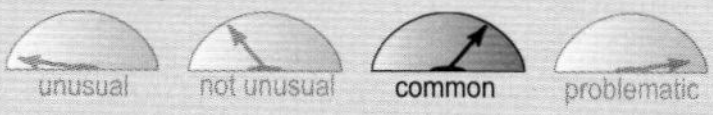

- Many experience and/or can be significant in amount

What To do About Side Effects

- Wait
- Wait
- Wait
- Take more of the dose at night or all of the dose at night to reduce daytime sedation
- Lower the dose
- Switch to another agent

Best Augmenting Agents for Side Effects

- Many side effects cannot be improved with an augmenting agent

DOSING AND USE

Usual Dosage Range

- 32–56 mg/day in 2–4 divided doses for adjunctive treatment of epilepsy
- 2–12 mg/day for adjunctive treatment of chronic pain and anxiety disorders

Dosage Forms

- Tablet 2 mg, 4 mg, 12 mg, 16 mg, 20 mg

How To Dose

- Adjunct to enzyme-inducing antiepileptic drugs: initial 4 mg once daily; after 1 week can increase dose by 4–8 mg/day each week; maximum dose generally 56 mg/day in 2–4 divided doses
- Dosing for chronic pain or anxiety disorders not well established, but start as low as 2 mg at night, increasing by 2 mg increments every few days as tolerated to 8–12 mg/day
- Exercise particular caution when prescribing in uninduced patients

Dosing Tips

- Usually administered as adjunctive medication to other anticonvulsants in the treatment of epilepsy
- ✻ Dosing recommendations are based on studies of adjunctive use with enzyme-inducing antiepileptic drugs, which lower plasma levels of tiagabine by half; thus, when tiagabine is used without enzyme-inducing antiepileptic drugs the dose may need to be significantly reduced and may require a much slower titration rate
- ✻ Also administered as adjunctive medication to benzodiazepines, SSRIs, and/or SNRIs in the treatment of anxiety disorders; and to SNRIs, gabapentin, other anticonvulsants, and even opiates in the treatment of chronic pain
- ✻ Dosing varies considerably among individual patients but is definitely at the lower end of the dosing spectrum for patients with chronic neuropathic pain or anxiety disorders (i.e., 2–12 mg either as a split dose or all at night)
- ✻ Patients with chronic neuropathic pain and anxiety disorders are far less tolerant of CNS side effects, so they require a much slower dosage titration as well as a lower maintenance dose
- Gastrointestinal absorption is markedly slowed by the concomitant intake of food, which also lessens the peak plasma concentrations
- ✻ Thus, for improved tolerability and consistent clinical actions, instruct patients to always take with food
- Side effects may increase with dose

Overdose

- No fatalities have been reported; sedation, agitation, confusion, speech difficulty, hostility, depression, weakness, myoclonus, seizures, status epilepticus

Long-Term Use

- Safe

Habit Forming

- No

How to Stop

- Taper
- Epilepsy patients may seize upon withdrawal, especially if withdrawal is abrupt
- Discontinuation symptoms uncommon

Pharmacokinetics

- Primarily metabolized by CYP450 3A4
- Steady-state concentrations tend to be lower in the evening than in the morning
- Half-life approximately 7–9 hours
- Renally excreted

Drug Interactions

- Clearance of tiagabine may be reduced and thus plasma levels increased if taken with a non-enzyme-inducing antiepileptic drug (e.g., valproate, gabapentin, lamotrigine), so tiagabine dose may need to be reduced
- CYP450 3A4 inducers such as carbamazepine can lower the plasma levels of tiagabine
- CYP450 3A4 inhibitors such as nefazodone, fluvoxamine, and fluoxetine could theoretically increase the plasma levels of tiagabine
- Clearance of tiagabine is increased if taken with an enzyme-inducing antiepileptic drug (e.g., carbamazepine, phenobarbital, phenytoin, primidone) and thus plasma levels are reduced; however, no dose adjustments are necessary for treatment of epilepsy as the dosing recommendations for epilepsy are based on adjunctive treatment with an enzyme-inducing antiepileptic drug
- Despite common actions upon GABA, no pharmacodynamic or pharmacokinetic interations have been shown when tiagabine is combined with the benzodiazepine triazolam or with alcohol
- However, sedating actions of any two sedative drugs given in combination can be additive

Other Warnings/ Precautions

- Seizures have occurred in individuals without epilepsy who took tiagabine
- Risk of seizure may be dose-related; when tiagabine is used in the absence of enzyme-inducing antiepileptic drugs, which lower plasma levels of tiagabine, the dose may need to be reduced
- Depressive effects may be increased by other CNS depressants (alcohol, MAOIs, other anticonvulsants, etc.)
- Tiagabine may bind to melanin, raising the possibility of long-term ophthalmologic effects
- Warn patients and their caregivers about the possibility of activation of suicidal ideation and advise them to report such side effects immediately

Do Not Use

- If there is a proven allergy to tiagabine

SPECIAL POPULATIONS

Renal Impairment

- Although tiagabine is renally excreted, the pharmacokinetics of tiagabine in healthy patients and in those with impaired renal function are similar and no dose adjustment is recommended

Hepatic Impairment

- Clearance is decreased
- May require lower dose

Cardiac Impairment

- No dose adjustment recommended

Elderly

- Some patients may tolerate lower doses better

Children and Adolescents

- Safety and efficacy not established in children under age 12
- Maximum recommended dose generally 32 mg/day in 2–4 divided doses

Pregnancy

- Effective June 30, 2015, the US FDA requires changes to the content and format of pregnancy and lactation information in prescription drug labels, including the elimination of the pregnancy letter categories; the Pregnancy and Lactation Labeling Rule (PLLR or final rule) applies only to prescription drugs and will be phased in gradually for drugs approved on or after June 30, 2001
- Controlled studies have not been conducted in pregnant women
- Use in women of childbearing potential requires weighing potential benefits to the mother against the risks to the fetus
- Antiepileptic Drug Pregnancy Registry: (888) 233–2334
- Taper drug if discontinuing
- Seizures, even mild seizures, may cause harm to the embryo/fetus

✻ Lack of definitive evidence of efficacy for chronic neuropathic pain or anxiety disorders suggests risk/benefit ratio is in favor of discontinuing tiagabine during pregnancy for those indications

Breast Feeding

- Some drug is found in mother's breast milk

✻ Recommended either to discontinue drug or bottle feed

- If drug is continued while breast feeding, infant should be monitored for possible adverse effects
- If infant shows signs of irritability or sedation, drug may need to be discontinued

THE ART OF PSYCHOPHARMACOLOGY

Potential Advantages

- Treatment-resistant chronic neuropathic pain
- Treatment-resistant anxiety disorders

Potential Disadvantages

- May require 2–4 times a day dosing
- Needs to be taken with food

Primary Target Symptoms

- Incidence of seizures
- Pain
- Anxiety

Pearls

- Well studied in epilepsy
- Much use is off label

✻ Off-label use second-line and as an augmenting agent may be justified for treatment-resistant anxiety disorders and neuropathic pain and also for fibromyalgia

✻ Off-label use for bipolar disorder may <u>not</u> be justified

✻ One of the few agents that enhances slow-wave delta sleep, which may be helpful in chronic neuropathic pain syndromes

- Can be difficult to dose in patients who are not taking enzyme-inducing anticonvulsant drugs as the doses in uninduced patients have not been well studied, are generally much lower, and titration is much slower than in induced patients
- Can cause seizures even in patients without epilepsy, especially in patients taking other agents (antidepressants, antipsychotics, stimulants, narcotics) that are thought to lower the seizure threshold

Suggested Reading

Backonja NM. Use of anticonvulsants for treatment of neuropathic pain. Neurology 2002 10;59(Suppl 2):S14–17.

Carta MG, Hardoy MC, Grunze H, Carpiniello B. The use of tiagabine in affective disorders. Pharmacopsychiatry 2002;35:33–4.

Evans EA. Efficacy of newer anticonvulsant medications in bipolar spectrum mood disorders. J Clin Psychiatry 2003;64 (Suppl 8):S9–14.

Lydiard RB. The role of GABA in anxiety disorders. J Clin Psychiatry 2003;64 (Suppl 3):S21–7.

Schmidt D, Gram L, Brodie M, et al. Tiagabine in the treatment of epilepsy – a clinical review with a guide for the prescribing physician. Epilepsy Res 2000;41:245–51.

Stahl SM. Anticonvulsants as anxiolytics, part 1: tiagabine and other anticonvulsants with actions on GABA. J Clin Psychiatry 2004;65:291–2.

Stahl SM. Psychopharmacology of anticonvulsants: do all anticonvulsants have the same mechanism of action? J Clin Psychiatry 2004;65:149–50.

TIANEPTINE

THERAPEUTICS

Brands
- Coaxil
- Stablon
- Tatinol

see index for additional brand names

Generic? Yes

Class
- Neuroscience-based Nomenclature: glutamate; yet to be determined (Glu)
- Glutamatergic modulator
- Often classified as a tricyclic antidepressant, but pharmacologically distinct

Commonly Prescribed for
(bold for FDA approved)
- Major depressive disorder
- Dysthymia
- Anxiety associated with depression

How the Drug Works
✽ Modulates glutamatergic neurotransmission, perhaps through potentiation of AMPA (alpha-amino-3-hydroxy-5-methyl-4-isoxazolepropioninc acid) receptor function

How Long Until It Works
- Onset of therapeutic actions usually not immediate, but often delayed 2–4 weeks
- If it is not working within 6–8 weeks for depression, it may require a dosage increase or it may not work at all
- May continue to work for many years to prevent relapse of symptoms

If It Works
- The goal of treatment is complete remission of current symptoms as well as prevention of future relapses
- Treatment most often reduces or even eliminates symptoms, but not a cure since symptoms can recur after medicine stopped
- Continue treatment until all symptoms are gone (remission)
- Once symptoms gone, continue treating for 1 year for the first episode of depression
- For second and subsequent episodes of depression, treatment may need to be indefinite

If It Doesn't Work
- Many patients have only a partial response where some symptoms are improved but others persist (especially insomnia, fatigue, and problems concentrating)
- Other patients may be nonresponders, sometimes called treatment-resistant or treatment-refractory
- Consider increasing dose, switching to another agent, or adding an appropriate augmenting agent
- Consider psychotherapy
- Consider evaluation for another diagnosis or for a comorbid condition (e.g., medical illness, substance abuse, etc.)

Best Augmenting Combos for Partial Response or Treatment Resistance
- Augmentation has not been systematically studied with tianeptine

Tests
- None recommended for healthy individuals

SIDE EFFECTS

How Drug Causes Side Effects
✽ Mild anticholinergic activity (less than some TCAs) could possibly lead to sedative effects, dry mouth, constipation, and blurred vision
- Most side effects are immediate but often go away with time

✽ Pharmacologic studies do not indicate tianeptine to be a potent alpha 1 antagonist or H1 antihistamine

Notable Side Effects
- Headache, dizziness, insomnia, sedation
- Nausea, constipation, abdominal pain, dry mouth
- Abnormal dreams
- Increased transaminases
- Tachycardia

Life-Threatening or Dangerous Side Effects

- Theoretically, rare induction of mania and activation of suicidal ideation or behavior
- Cases of activation of suicidal ideation and behavior (suicidality) (short-term did not show an increase in the risk of suicidality with antidepressants compared to placebo beyond age 24)
- Hepatitis that can, in exceptional cases, be severe
- Dermatitis bulbous in exceptional cases

Weight Gain

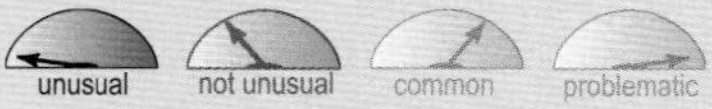

- Not well studied

Sedation

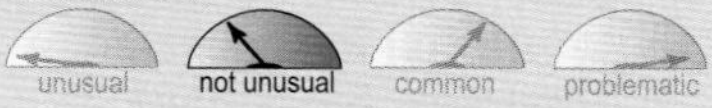

- Occurs in significant minority

What to Do About Side Effects

- Wait
- Wait
- Wait
- Lower the dose
- In a few weeks, switch or add other drugs
- For skin reactions, stop treatment

Best Augmenting Agents for Side Effects

- Augmentation for side effects of tianeptine has not been systematically studied

DOSING AND USE

Usual Dosage Range

- 37.5 mg/day

Dosage Forms

- Tablet 12.5 mg

How to Dose

- 12.5 mg 3 times/day

Dosing Tips

- Tianeptine's rapid elimination necessitates strict adherence to the dosing schedule

✻ Short half-life means multiple daily doses

Overdose

- Effects are generally mild and nonfatal; unlikely to cause cardiovascular effects

Long-Term Use

- Safe

Habit Forming

- Abuse and dependence may occur, in particular in patients under 50 years of age with a history of drug or alcohol dependence

How to Stop

- Many patients tolerate 50% dose reduction for 3 days, then another 50% reduction for 3 days, then discontinuation
- If withdrawal symptoms emerge during discontinuation, raise dose to stop symptoms and then restart withdrawal much more slowly

Pharmacokinetics

- Not primarily metabolized by CYP 450 enzyme system
- Tianeptine is rapidly eliminated
- Half-life approximately 2.5 hours

Drug Interactions

- Activation and agitation, especially following switching or adding antidepressants, may represent the induction of a bipolar state, especially a mixed dysphoric bipolar II condition sometimes associated with suicidal ideation, and require the addition of lithium, a mood stabilizer or an atypical antipsychotic, and/or discontinuation of tianeptine
- Other drug interactions not well studied

Other Warnings/ Precautions

- For elective surgery, tianeptine should be stopped 24–48 hours before general anesthesia is administered
- Generally, use only with extreme caution with MAOIs; do not use until 14 days after MAOIs are stopped; do not start an MAOI for at least 5 half-lives (5 to 7 days for most drugs) after discontinuing tianeptine

- Warn patients and their caregivers about the possibility of activating side effects and advise them to report such symptoms immediately
- Monitor patients for activation of suicidal ideation, especially children and adolescents
- Warn doctors to pay attention to patients with history of drug dependencies

Do Not Use
- If patient is taking an MAOI
- If patient is pregnant or nursing
- If there is a proven allergy to tianeptine

SPECIAL POPULATIONS

Renal Impairment
- Dose should be reduced for severe impairment to 25 mg/day

Hepatic Impairment
- In patients with severe cirrhosis (class C, Child Plugh's Scale), the dosage should be restricted to 25 mg/day

Cardiac Impairment
- Baseline ECG is recommended

Elderly
- Baseline ECG is recommended for patients over age 50
- Dose should be reduced to 25 mg/day
- Reduction in the risk of suicidality with antidepressants compared to placebo in adults age 65 and older

Children and Adolescents
- Tianeptine is not recommended for use in children or adolescents under 18
- Carefully weigh the risks and benefits of pharmacological treatment against the risks and benefits of nontreatment with antidepressants and make sure to document this in the patient's chart
- Monitor patients face-to-face regularly, particularly during the first several weeks of treatment
- Use with caution, observing for activation of known or unknown bipolar disorder and/or suicidal ideation, and inform parents or guardians of this risk so they can help observe child or adolescent patients

Pregnancy
- Not recommended for use during pregnancy

Breast Feeding
- Some drug is found in mother's breast milk

✻ Not recommended for use during pregnancy

- Immediate postpartum period is a high-risk time for depression, especially in women who have had prior depressive episodes, so drug may need to be reinstituted late in the third trimester or shortly after childbirth to prevent a recurrence during the postpartum period
- Must weigh benefits of breast feeding with risks and benefits of antidepressant treatment versus nontreatment to both the infant and the mother
- For many patients, this may mean continuing treatment during breast feeding

THE ART OF PSYCHOPHARMACOLOGY

Potential Advantages
- Elderly patients

Potential Disadvantages
- Patients who have difficulty being compliant with multiple daily dosing

Primary Target Symptoms
- Depressed mood
- Symptoms of anxiety

Pearls

✻ Possibly a unique mechanism of action as a glutamatergic antidepressant

- It is not metabolized by CYP450; therefore, the risk of pharmacokinetic drug–drug interactions is minimized

Suggested Reading

Kasper S, McEwen BS. Neurobiological and clinical effects of the antidepressant tianeptine. CNS Drugs 2008;22(1):15–26.

Kasper S, Olie JP. A meta-analysis of randomized controlled trials of tianeptine versus SSRI in the short-term treatment of depression. Eur Psychiatry 2002;17(suppl 3):331–40.

McEwen BS, Chattarji S, Diamond DM, et al. The neurobiological properties of tianeptine (Stablon): from monoamine hypothesis to glutamatergic modulation. Mol Psychiatry 2010;15:237–49.

Svenningsson P, Bateup H, Qi H, et al. Involvement of AMPA receptor phosphorylation in antidepressant actions with special reference to tianeptine. Eur J Neuorsci 2007;26:3509–17.

Wagstaff AJ, Ormrod D, Spencer CM. Tianeptine: a review of its use in depressive disorders. CNS Drugs 2001;15(3):231–59.

THERAPEUTICS

Brands
- Topamax
- Epitomax
- Topamac
- Topimax
- Trokendi XR
- Qsymia

see index for additional brand names

Generic? Yes (not for Qsymia)

Class

- Anticonvulsant, voltage-sensitive sodium channel modulator

Commonly Prescribed for

(bold for FDA approved)

- **Partial onset seizures (for immediate-release: adjunctive for adults and pediatric patients 2–16 years of age; for extended-release: monotherapy for patients 10 years and older, adjunctive for patients 6 years and older)**
- **Primary generalized tonic-clonic seizures (adjunctive; adults and pediatric patients 2–16 years of age)**
- **Seizures associated with Lennox-Gastaut Syndrome (2 years of age or older for immediate-release, 6 years of age and older for extended-release (adjunct))**
- **Migraine prophylaxis**
- **Chronic weight management (adjunct to reduced calorie diet and increased physical activity) in adults with an initial body mass index (BMI) of at least 30 kg/m^2 (obese) or at least 27 kg/m^2 (overweight) in the presence of at least one weight-related comorbid condition [in combination with phentermine (Qsymia)]**
- Bipolar disorder (adjunctive; no longer in development)
- Psychotropic drug-induced weight gain
- Binge eating disorder

How the Drug Works

* Blocks voltage-sensitive sodium channels by an unknown mechanism
- Inhibits release of glutamate
- Potentiates activity of gamma-aminobutyric acid (GABA)
- Carbonic anhydrase inhibitor

How Long Until It Works

- Should reduce seizures by 2 weeks
- Not clear that it has mood-stabilizing properties, but some bipolar patients may respond and if so, it may take several weeks to months to optimize an effect on mood stabilization

If It Works

- The goal of treatment is complete remission of symptoms (e.g., mania, seizures, migraine)
- Continue treatment until all symptoms are gone or until improvement is stable and then continue treating indefinitely as long as improvement persists
- Continue treatment indefinitely to avoid recurrence of mania, seizures, and headaches

If It Doesn't Work (for bipolar disorder)

* May be effective only in a subset of bipolar patients, in some patients who fail to respond to other mood stabilizers, or it may not work at all
* Consider increasing dose or switching to another agent with better demonstrated efficacy in bipolar disorder

Best Augmenting Combos for Partial Response or Treatment Resistance

- Topiramate is itself a second-line augmenting agent for numerous other anticonvulsants, lithium, and antipsychotics in treating bipolar disorder

Tests

* Baseline and periodic serum bicarbonate levels to monitor for hyperchloremic, non-anion gap metabolic acidosis (i.e., decreased serum bicarbonate below the normal reference range in the absence of chronic respiratory alkalosis)

SIDE EFFECTS

How Drug Causes Side Effects

- CNS side effects theoretically due to excessive actions at voltage-sensitive sodium channels
- Weak inhibition of carbonic anhydrase may lead to kidney stones and paresthesias

- Inhibition of carbonic anhydrase may also lead to metabolic acidosis

Notable Side Effects

✽ Sedation, asthenia, dizziness, ataxia, parasthesia, nervousness, nystagmus, tremor
✽ Nausea, appetite loss, weight loss
- Blurred or double vision, mood problems, problems concentrating, confusion, memory problems, psychomotor retardation, language problems, speech problems, fatigue, taste perversion

Life-Threatening or Dangerous Side Effects

✽ Metabolic acidosis
✽ Kidney stones
- Secondary angle-closure glaucoma
- Oligohidrosis and hyperthermia (more common in children)
- Sudden unexplained deaths have occurred in epilepsy (unknown if related to topiramate use)
- Rare activation of suicidal ideation and behavior(suicidality)

Weight Gain

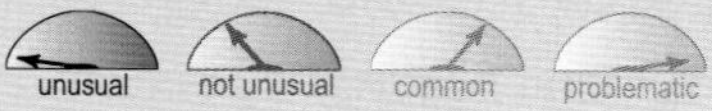

- Reported but not expected

✽ Patients may experience weight loss

Sedation

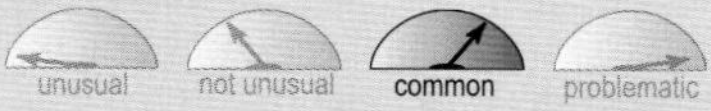

- Many experience and/or can be significant in amount

What to Do About Side Effects

- Wait
- Wait
- Wait
- Take at night to reduce daytime sedation
- Increase fluid intake to reduce the risk of kidney stones
- Switch to another agent

Best Augmenting Agents for Side Effects

- Many side effects cannot be improved with an augmenting agent

DOSING AND USE

Usual Dosage Range

- Adults, immediate-release: 200–400 mg/day in 2 divided doses for epilepsy; 50–300 mg/day for adjunctive treatment of bipolar disorder
- Adults, extended-release: 200–400 mg/day as adjunct for partial onset seizures seizures; 400 mg/day as adjunct for primary generalized tonic clonic seizures; 400 mg/day as monotherapy for seizures

Dosage Forms

- Tablet 25 mg, 100 mg, 200 mg
- Sprinkle capsule 15 mg, 25 mg
- Extended-release capsule 25 mg, 50 mg, 100 mg, 200 mg

How to Dose

- Adults (immediate-release): initial 25–50 mg/day; increase each week by 50 mg/day; administer in 2 divided doses; maximum dose generally 1,600 mg/day
- Adults (extended-release, adjunct for seizures): initial 25–50 mg once daily; increase weekly by 25–50 mg
- Seizures (extended-release, monotherapy, patients ages 10 and older): initial 50 mg once daily; increase by 50 mg weekly for 4 weeks, increase by 100 mg weekly for weeks 5 and 6; recommended dose 400 mg/day
- Seizures (immediate-release, ages 2–16): see Children and Adolescents

Dosing Tips

- Adverse effects may increase as dose increases
- Topiramate is available in a sprinkle capsule formulation, which can be swallowed whole or sprinkled over approximately a teaspoon of soft food (e.g., applesauce); the mixture should be consumed immediately
- Bipolar patients are generally administered doses at the lower end of the dosing range
- Slow upward titration from doses as low as 25 mg/day can reduce the incidence of unacceptable sedation
- Many bipolar patients do not tolerate more than 200 mg/day

✽ Weight loss is dose-related but most patients treated for weight gain receive doses at the lower end of the dosing range

Overdose
- No fatalities have been reported in monotherapy; convulsions, sedation, speech disturbance, blurred or double vision, metabolic acidosis, impaired coordination, hypotension, abdominal pain, agitation, dizziness

Long-Term Use
- Probably safe
- Periodic monitoring of serum bicarbonate levels may be required

Habit Forming
- No

How to Stop
- Taper
- Epilepsy patients may seize upon withdrawal, especially if withdrawal is abrupt

✻ Rapid discontinuation may increase the risk of relapse in bipolar patients

✻ Discontinuation symptoms uncommon

Pharmacokinetics
- Elimination half-life approximately 21 hours
- Renally excreted

Drug Interactions
- Carbamazepine, phenytoin, and valproate may increase the clearance of topiramate, and thus decrease topiramate levels, possibly requiring a higher dose of topiramate
- Topiramate may increase the clearance of phenytoin and thus decrease phenytoin levels, possibly requiring a higher dose of phenytoin
- Topiramate may increase the clearance of valproate and thus decrease valproate levels, possibly requiring a higher dose of valproate
- Topiramate may increase plasma levels of metformin; also, metformin may reduce clearance of topiramate and increase topiramate levels
- Topiramate may interact with carbonic anhydrase inhibitors to increase the risk of kidney stones
- Topiramate may reduce the effectiveness of oral contraceptives
- Reports of hyperammonemia with or without encephalopthay in patients taking topiramate combined with valproate, though this is not due to a pharmacokinetic interaction; in patients who develop unexplained lethargy, vomiting, or change in mental status, an ammonia level should be measured

Other Warnings/ Precautions

✻ If symptoms of metabolic acidosis develop (hyperventilation, fatigue, anorexia, cardiac arrhythmias, stupor), then dose may need to be reduced or treatment may need to be discontinued

- Depressive effects may be increased by other CNS depressants (alcohol, MAOIs, other anticonvulsants, etc.)
- Use with caution when combining with other drugs that predispose patients to heat-related disorders, including carbonic anhydrase inhibitors and anticholinergics
- Warn patients and their caregivers about the possibility of activation of suicidal ideation and advise them to report such side effects immediately

Do Not Use
- Within 6 hours prior to and 6 hours after alcohol use (extended-release)
- In patients with metabolic acidosis who are taking metformin (extended-release)
- If there is a proven allergy to topiramate

SPECIAL POPULATIONS

Renal Impairment
- Topiramate is renally excreted, so the dose should be lowered by half
- Can be removed by hemodialysis; patients receiving hemodialysis may require supplemental doses of topiramate

Hepatic Impairment
- Drug should be used with caution

Cardiac Impairment
- Drug should be used with caution

Elderly
- Elderly patients may be more susceptible to adverse effects

Children and Adolescents
- Approved for use in children age 2 and older (immediate-release) for treatment of seizures
- Clearance is increased in pediatric patients
- Seizures (immediate-release, ages 2–16): initial 1–3 mg/kg per day at night; after 1 week increase by 1–3 mg/kg per day every 1–2 weeks with total daily dose administered in 2 divided doses; recommended dose generally 5–9 mg/kg per day in 2 divided doses
- Effectiveness was not demonstrated in infants/toddlers 1 to 24 months of age with refractory partial onset seizures; some adverse effects/toxicities not observed in older patients did occur
- Seizures (extended-release, adjunct): initial 25 mg once nightly (1–3 mg/kg/night) for first week; increase at 1- or 2-week intervals by increments of 1–3 mg/kg/night; recommended dose 5–9 mg/kg/night

Pregnancy
- Effective June 30, 2015, the US FDA requires changes to the content and format of pregnancy and lactation information in prescription drug labels, including the elimination of the pregnancy letter categories; the Pregnancy and Lactation Labeling Rule (PLLR or final rule) applies only to prescription drugs and will be phased in gradually for drugs approved on or after June 30, 2001
- Increased risk of cleft lip/palate
- Use in women of childbearing potential requires weighing potential benefits to the mother against the risks to the fetus
- Hypospadia has occurred in some male infants whose mothers took topiramate during pregnancy

✱ Lack of convincing efficacy for treatment of bipolar disorder suggests risk/benefit ratio is in favor of discontinuing topiramate in bipolar patients during pregnancy

✱ For bipolar patients, topiramate should generally be discontinued before anticipated pregnancies
- Antiepileptic Drug Pregnancy Registry: (888) 233-2334
- Taper drug if discontinuing

✱ For bipolar patients, given the risk of relapse in the postpartum period, mood stabilizer treatment, especially with agents with better evidence of efficacy than topiramate, should generally be restarted immediately after delivery if patient is unmedicated during pregnancy

✱ Atypical antipsychotics may be preferable to topiramate if treatment of bipolar disorder is required during pregnancy
- Bipolar symptoms may recur or worsen during pregnancy and some form of treatment may be necessary
- Seizures, even mild seizures, may cause harm to the embryo/fetus

Breast Feeding
- Some drug is found in mother's breast milk

✱ Recommended either to discontinue drug or bottle feed
- If drug is continued while breast feeding, infant should be monitored for possible adverse effects
- If infant shows signs of irritability or sedation, drug may need to be discontinued

✱ Bipolar disorder may recur during the postpartum period, particularly if there is a history of prior postpartum episodes of either depression or psychosis

✱ Relapse rates may be lower in women who receive prophylactic treatment for postpartum episodes of bipolar disorder
- Atypical antipsychotics and anticonvulsants such as valproate may be safer and more effective than topiramate during the postpartum period when treating nursing mother with bipolar disorder

THE ART OF PSYCHOPHARMACOLOGY

Potential Advantages
- Treatment-resistant bipolar disorder
- Patients who wish to avoid weight gain

Potential Disadvantages
- Efficacy in bipolar disorder uncertain

- Patients with a history of kidney stones or risks for metabolic acidosis

Primary Target Symptoms

- Incidence of seizures
- Unstable mood

Pearls

- Side effects may actually occur less often in pediatric patients
- Has been studied in a wide range of psychiatric disorders, including bipolar disorder, PTSD, binge eating disorder, obesity, and others
- Some anecdotes, case series, and open-label studies have been published and are widely known suggesting efficacy in bipolar disorder
- ✽ However, randomized clinical trials do not suggest efficacy in bipolar disorder; unfortunately these important studies have not been published by the manufacturer, who has dropped topiramate from further development as a mood stabilizer, though this is not widely known
- ✽ Misperceptions about topiramate's efficacy in bipolar disorder have led to its use in more patients than other agents with proven efficacy, such as lamotrigine
- ✽ Due to reported weight loss in some patients in trials with epilepsy, topiramate is commonly used to treat weight gain, especially in patients with psychotropic drug-induced weight gain
- ✽ Weight loss in epilepsy patients is dose-related with more weight loss at high doses (mean 6.5 kg or 7.3% decline) and less weight loss at lower doses (mean 1.6 kg or 2.2% decline)
- ✽ Changes in weight were greatest in epilepsy patients who weighed the most at baseline (>100 kg), with mean loss of 9.6 kg or 8.4% decline, while those weighing <60 kg had only a mean loss of 1.3 kg or 2.5% decline
- ✽ Long-term studies demonstrate that weight losses in epilepsy patients were seen within the first 3 months of treatment and peaked at a mean of 6 kg after 12–18 months of treatment; however, weight tended to return to pretreatment levels after 18 months
- ✽ Some patients with psychotropic drug-induced weight gain may experience significant weight loss (>7% of body weight) with topiramate up to 200 mg/day for 3 months, but this is not typical, is not often sustained, and has not been systemically studied
- Early studies suggest potential efficacy in binge eating disorder
- The combination of topiramate and phentermine is approved as a treatment for obesity (see phentermine-topiramate); the combination is also being studied in diabetes and sleep apnea

Suggested Reading

Johnson BA, Ait-Daoud N. Topiramate in the new generation of drugs: efficacy in the treatment of alcoholic patients. Curr Pharm Des 2010;16(19):2103–12.

Kramer CK, Leitao CB, Pinto LC, et al. Efficacy and safety of topiramate on weight loss: a meta-analysis of randomized controlled trials. Obes Rev 2011;12(5):e338–47.

Ormrod D, McClellan K. Topiramate: a review of its use in childhood epilepsy. Paediatr Drugs 2001;3:293–319.

Shank RP, Gardocki JF, Streeter AJ, Maryanoff BE. An overview of the preclinical aspects of topiramate: pharmacology, pharmacokinetics, and mechanism of action. Epilepsia 2000;41(Suppl 1):S3–9.

Suppes T. Review of the use of topiramate for treatment of bipolar disorders. J Clin Psychopharmacol 2002;22:599–609.

THERAPEUTICS

Brands • Parnate

see index for additional brand names

Generic? Yes

Class

- Neuroscience-based Nomenclature: serotonin, norepinephrine, dopamine multi-modal enzyme inhibitor (SN-MM)
- Monoamine oxidase inhibitor (MAOI)

Commonly Prescribed for

(bold for FDA approved)

- **Major depressive episode without melancholia**
- Treatment-resistant depression
- Treatment-resistant panic disorder
- Treatment-resistant social anxiety disorder

How the Drug Works

- Irreversibly blocks monoamine oxidase (MAO) from breaking down norepinephrine, serotonin, and dopamine
- This presumably boosts noradrenergic, serotonergic, and dopaminergic neurotransmission

✻ As the drug is structurally related to amphetamine, it may have some stimulant-like actions due to monoamine release and reuptake inhibition

How Long Until It Works

- Some patients may experience stimulant-like actions early in dosing
- Onset of therapeutic actions usually not immediate, but often delayed 2–4 weeks
- If it is not working within 6–8 weeks, it may require a dosage increase or it may not work at all
- May continue to work for many years to prevent relapse of symptoms

If It Works

- The goal of treatment is complete remission of current symptoms as well as prevention of future relapses
- Treatment most often reduces or even eliminates symptoms, but not a cure since symptoms can recur after medicine stopped
- Continue treatment until all symptoms are gone (remission)
- Once symptoms gone, continue treating for 1 year for the first episode of depression
- For second and subsequent episodes of depression, treatment may need to be indefinite
- Use in anxiety disorders may also need to be indefinite

If It Doesn't Work

- Many patients have only a partial response where some symptoms are improved but others persist (especially insomnia, fatigue, and problems concentrating)
- Other patients may be nonresponders, sometimes called treatment-resistant or treatment-refractory
- Some patients who have an initial response may relapse even though they continue treatment, sometimes called "poop-out"
- Consider increasing dose, switching to another agent, or adding an appropriate augmenting agent
- Consider psychotherapy
- Consider evaluation for another diagnosis or for a comorbid condition (e.g., medical illness, substance abuse, etc.)
- Some patients may experience apparent lack of consistent efficacy due to activation of latent or underlying bipolar disorder, and require antidepressant discontinuation and a switch to a mood stabilizer

Best Augmenting Combos for Partial Response or Treatment Resistance

✻ Augmentation of MAOIs has not been systematically studied, and this is something for the expert, to be done with caution and with careful monitoring

✻ A stimulant such as d-amphetamine or methylphenidate (with caution; may activate bipolar disorder and suicidal ideation; may elevate blood pressure)

- Lithium
- Mood-stabilizing anticonvulsants
- Atypical antipsychotics (with special caution for those agents with monoamine reuptake blocking properties, such as ziprasidone and zotepine)

Tests

- Patients should be monitored for changes in blood pressure
- Patients receiving high doses or long-term treatment should have hepatic function evaluated periodically

SIDE EFFECTS

How Drug Causes Side Effects

- Theoretically due to increases in monoamines in parts of the brain and body and at receptors other than those that cause therapeutic actions (e.g., unwanted actions of serotonin in sleep centers causing insomnia, unwanted actions of norepinephrine on vascular smooth muscle causing hypertension, etc.)
- Side effects are generally immediate, but immediate side effects often disappear in time

Notable Side Effects

- Agitation, anxiety, insomnia, weakness, sedation, dizziness
- Constipation, dry mouth, nausea, diarrhea, change in appetite, weight gain
- Sexual dysfunction
- Orthostatic hypotension (dose-related); syncope may develop at high doses

Life-Threatening or Dangerous Side Effects

- Hypertensive crisis (especially when MAOIs are used with certain tyramine-containing foods or prohibited drugs)
- Induction of mania
- Rare activation of suicidal ideation and behavior (suicidality) (short-term studies did not show an increase in the risk of suicidality with antidepressants compared to placebo beyond age 24)
- Seizures
- Hepatotoxicity

Weight Gain

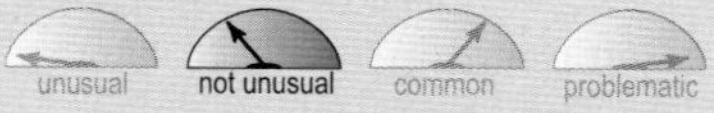

- Occurs in significant minority

Sedation

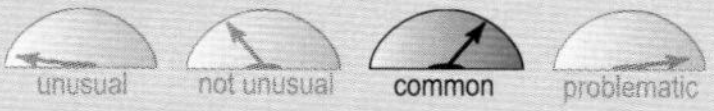

- Many experience and/or can be significant in amount
- Can also cause activation

What to Do About Side Effects

- Wait
- Wait
- Wait
- Lower the dose
- Take at night if daytime sedation; take in daytime if overstimulated at night
- Switch after appropriate washout to an SSRI or newer antidepressant

Best Augmenting Agents for Side Effects

- Trazodone (with caution) for insomnia
- Benzodiazepines for insomnia
- ✻ Single oral or sublingual dose of a calcium channel blocker (e.g., nifedipine) for urgent treatment of hypertension due to drug interaction or dietary tyramine
- Many side effects cannot be improved with an augmenting agent

DOSING AND USE

Usual Dosage Range

- 30 mg/day in divided doses

Dosage Forms

- Tablet 10 mg

How to Dose

- Initial 30 mg/day in divided doses; after 2 weeks increase by 10 mg/day each 1–3 weeks; maximum 60 mg/day

Dosing Tips

- Orthostatic hypotension, especially at high doses, may require splitting into 3–4 daily doses
- Patients receiving high doses may need to be evaluated periodically for effects on the liver

Overdose

- Dizziness, sedation, ataxia, headache, insomnia, restlessness, anxiety, irritability; cardiovascular effects, confusion, respiratory depression, or coma may also occur

Long-Term Use

- May require periodic evaluation of hepatic function
- MAOIs may lose efficacy long-term

Habit Forming

- Some patients have developed dependence to MAOIs

How to Stop

- Generally no need to taper, as the drug wears off slowly over 2–3 weeks

Pharmacokinetics

- Clinical duration of action may be up to 14 days due to irreversible enzyme inhibition

Drug Interactions

- Tramadol may increase the risk of seizures in patients taking an MAOI
- Can cause a fatal "serotonin syndrome" when combined with drugs that block serotonin reuptake, so do not use with a serotonin reuptake inhibitor or for 5 half-lives after stopping the serotonin reuptake inhibitor (see Table 1 after Pearls)
- Hypertensive crisis with headache, intracranial bleeding, and death may result from combining MAOIs with sympathomimetic drugs (e.g., amphetamines, methylphenidate, cocaine, dopamine, epinephrine, norepinephrine, and related compounds methyldopa, levodopa, L-tryptophan, L-tyrosine, and phenylalanine
- Do not combine with another MAOI, alcohol, or guanethidine
- Adverse drug reactions can result from combining MAOIs with tricyclic/tetracyclic antidepressants and related compounds, including carbamazepine, cyclobenzaprine, and mirtazapine, and should be avoided except by experts to treat difficult cases
- MAOIs in combination with spinal anesthesia may cause combined hypotensive effects
- Combination of MAOIs and CNS depressants may enhance sedation and hypotension

Other Warnings/ Precautions

- Use requires low tyramine diet (see Table 2 after Pearls)
- Patient and prescriber must be vigilant to potential interactions with any drug, including antihypertensives and over-the-counter cough/cold preparations
- Over-the-counter medications to avoid include cough and cold preparations, including those containing dextromethorphan, nasal decongestants (tablets, drops, or spray), hay-fever medications, sinus medications, asthma inhalant medications, anti-appetite medications, weight reducing preparations, "pep" pills (see Table 3 after Pearls)
- Hypoglycemia may occur in diabetic patients receiving insulin or oral antidiabetic agents
- Use cautiously in patients receiving reserpine, anesthetics, disulfiram, metrizamide, anticholinergic agents
- Tranylcypromine is not recommended for use in patients who cannot be monitored closely
- When treating children, carefully weigh the risks and benefits of pharmacological treatment against the risks and benefits of nontreatment with antidepressants and make sure to document this in the patient's chart
- Distribute the brochures provided by the FDA and the drug companies
- Warn patients and their caregivers about the possibility of activating side effects and advise them to report such symptoms immediately
- Monitor patients for activation of suicidal ideation, especially children and adolescents

Do Not Use

- If patient is taking meperidine (pethidine)
- If patient is taking a sympathomimetic agent or taking guanethidine
- If patient is taking another MAOI
- If patient is taking any agent that can inhibit serotonin reuptake (e.g., SSRIs, sibutramine, tramadol, milnacipran, duloxetine, venlafaxine, clomipramine, etc.)
- If patient is taking diuretics, dextromethorphan
- If patient has pheochromocytoma
- If patient has cardiovascular or cerebrovascular disease
- If patient has frequent or severe headaches
- If patient is undergoing elective surgery and requires general anesthesia
- If patient has a history of liver disease or abnormal liver function tests
- If patient is taking a prohibited drug
- If patient is not compliant with a low-tyramine diet
- If there is a proven allergy to tranylcypromine

SPECIAL POPULATIONS

Renal Impairment
- Use with caution – drug may accumulate in plasma
- May require lower than usual adult dose

Hepatic Impairment
- Tranylcypromine should not be used in patients with history of hepatic impairment or in patients with abnormal liver function tests

Cardiac Impairment
- Contraindicated in patients with any cardiac impairment

Elderly
- Initial dose lower than usual adult dose
- Elderly patients may have greater sensitivity to adverse effects
- Reduction in the risk of suicidality with antidepressants compared to placebo in adults age 65 and older

Children and Adolescents
- Not generally recommended for use in children under age 18
- Carefully weigh the risks and benefits of pharmacological treatment against the risks and benefits of nontreatment with antidepressants and make sure to document this in the patient's chart
- Monitor patients face-to-face regularly, particularly during the first several weeks of treatment
- Use with caution, observing for activation of known or unknown bipolar disorder and/or suicidal ideation, and inform parents or guardians of this risk so they can help observe child or adolescent patients

Pregnancy
- Effective June 30, 2015, the US FDA requires changes to the content and format of pregnancy and lactation information in prescription drug labels, including the elimination of the pregnancy letter categories; the Pregnancy and Lactation Labeling Rule (PLLR or final rule) applies only to prescription drugs and will be phased in gradually for drugs approved on or after June 30, 2001
- Controlled studies have not been conducted in pregnant women
- Not generally recommended for use during pregnancy, especially during first trimester
- Should evaluate patient for treatment with an antidepressant with a better risk/benefit ratio

Breast Feeding
- Some drug is found in mother's breast milk
- Effects on infant unknown
- Immediate postpartum period is a high-risk time for depression, especially in women who have had prior depressive episodes, so drug may need to be reinstituted late in the third trimester or shortly after childbirth to prevent a recurrence during the postpartum period
- Should evaluate patient for treatment with an antidepressant with a better risk/benefit ratio

THE ART OF PSYCHOPHARMACOLOGY

Potential Advantages
- Atypical depression
- Severe depression
- Treatment-resistant depression or anxiety disorders

Potential Disadvantages
- Requires compliance to dietary restrictions, concomitant drug restrictions
- Patients with cardiac problems or hypertension
- Multiple daily doses

Primary Target Symptoms
- Depressed mood
- Somatic symptoms
- Sleep and eating disturbances
- Psychomotor retardation
- Morbid preoccupation

Pearls
- MAOIs are generally reserved for second-line use after SSRIs, SNRIs, and combinations of newer antidepressants have failed

- Patient should be advised not to take any prescription or over-the-counter drugs without consulting their doctor because of possible drug interactions with the MAOI
- Headache is often the first symptom of hypertensive crisis
- The rigid dietary restrictions may reduce compliance (see Table 2 after Pearls)
- Mood disorders can be associated with eating disorders (especially in adolescent females), and tranylcypromine can be used to treat both depression and bulimia
- MAOIs are a viable second-line treatment option in depression, but are not frequently used

✻ Myths about the danger of dietary tyramine can be exaggerated, but prohibitions against concomitant drugs often not followed closely enough

- Orthostatic hypotension, insomnia, and sexual dysfunction are often the most troublesome common side effects

✻ MAOIs should be for the expert, especially if combining with agents of potential risk (e.g., stimulants, trazodone, TCAs)

✻ MAOIs should not be neglected as therapeutic agents for the treatment-resistant

- Although generally prohibited, a heroic but potentially dangerous treatment for severely treatment-resistant patients is for an expert to give a tricyclic/tetracyclic antidepressant other than clomipramine simultaneously with an MAOI for patients who fail to respond to numerous other antidepressants
- Use of MAOIs with clomipramine is always prohibited because of the risk of serotonin syndrome and death
- Amoxapine may be the preferred trycyclic/tetracyclic antidepressant to combine with an MAOI in heroic cases due to its theoretically protective 5HT2A antagonist properties
- If this option is elected, start the MAOI with the tricyclic/tetracyclic antidepressant simultaneously at low doses after appropriate drug washout, then alternately increase doses of these agents every few days to a week as tolerated
- Although very strict dietary and concomitant drug restrictions must be observed to prevent hypertensive crises and serotonin syndrome, the most common side effects of MAOI and tricyclic/tetracyclic combinations may be weight gain and orthostatic hypotension

Table 1. Drugs contraindicated due to risk of serotonin syndrome/toxicity

Do Not Use:			
Antidepressants	**Drugs of Abuse**	**Opioids**	**Other**
SSRIs	MDMA (ecstasy)	Meperidine	Non-subcutaneous sumatriptan
SNRIs	Cocaine	Tramadol	Chlorpheniramine
Clomipramine	Methamphetamine	Methadone	Brompheniramine
St. John's wort	High-dose or injected amphetamine	Fentanyl	Dextromethorphan
			Procarbazine?

Table 2. Dietary guidelines for patients taking MAOIs

Foods to avoid*	**Foods allowed**
Dried, aged, smoked, fermented, spoiled, or improperly stored meat, poultry, and fish	Fresh or processed meat, poultry, and fish; properly stored pickled or smoked fish
Broad bean pods	All other vegetables
Aged cheeses	Processed cheese slices, cottage cheese, ricotta cheese, yogurt, cream cheese
Tap and unpasteurized beer	Canned or bottled beer and alcohol
Marmite	Brewer's and baker's yeast
Sauerkraut, kimchee	
Soy products/tofu	Peanuts
Banana peel	Bananas, avocados, raspberries
Tyramine-containing nutritional supplement	

*Not necessary for 6-mg transdermal or low-dose oral selegiline

Table 3. Drugs that boost norepinephrine: should only be used with caution with MAOIs

Use With Caution:			
Decongestants	**Stimulants**	**Antidepressants with norepinephrine reuptake inhibition**	**Other**
Phenylephrine	Amphetamines	Most tricyclics	Phentermine
Pseudoephedrine	Methylphenidate	NRIs	Local anesthetics containing vasoconstrictors
	Cocaine	NDRIs	
	Methamphetamine		
	Modafinil		Tapentadol
	Armodafinil		

Suggested Reading

Baker GB, Coutts RT, McKenna KF, Sherry-McKenna RL. Insights into the mechanisms of action of the MAO inhibitors phenelzine and tranylcypromine: a review. J Psychiatry Neurosci 1992;17:206–14.

Kennedy SH. Continuation and maintenance treatments in major depression: the neglected role of monoamine oxidase inhibitors. J Psychiatry Neurosci 1997;22:127–31.

Lippman SB, Nash K. Monoamine oxidase inhibitor update. Potential adverse food and drug interactions. Drug Saf 1990;5:195–204.

Thase ME, Triyedi MH, Rush AJ. MAOIs in the contemporary treatment of depression. Neuropsychopharmacology 1995;12:185–219.

TRAZODONE

THERAPEUTICS

Brands • Desyrel
• Oleptro

see index for additional brand names

Generic? Yes

Class

- Neuroscience-based Nomenclature: serotonin receptor antagonist (S-MM)
- SARI (serotonin 2 antagonist/reuptake inhibitor); antidepressant; hypnotic

Commonly Prescribed for

(bold for FDA approved)

- **Depression**
- Insomnia (primary and secondary)
- Anxiety

How the Drug Works

- Blocks serotonin 2A receptors potently
- Blocks serotonin reuptake pump (serotonin transporter) less potently

How Long Until It Works

✽ Onset of therapeutic actions in insomnia are immediate if dosing is correct
- Onset of therapeutic actions in depression usually not immediate, but often delayed 2–4 weeks whether given as an adjunct to another antidepressant or as a monotherapy
- If it is not working within 6–8 weeks for depression, it may require a dosage increase or it may not work at all
- May continue to work for many years to prevent relapse of symptoms in depression and to reduce symptoms of chronic insomnia

If It Works

✽ For insomnia, use possibly can be indefinite as there is no reliable evidence of tolerance, dependence, or withdrawal, but few long-term studies
- For secondary insomnia, if underlying condition (e.g., depression, anxiety disorder) is in remission, trazodone treatment may be discontinued if insomnia does not reemerge
- The goal of treatment for depression is complete remission of current symptoms of depression as well as prevention of future relapses
- Treatment most often reduces or even eliminates symptoms of depression, but is not a cure since symptoms can recur after medicine stopped
- Continue treatment until all symptoms of depression are gone (remission)
- Once symptoms of depression are gone, continue treating for 1 year for the first episode of depression
- For second and subsequent episodes of depression, treatment may need to be indefinite

If It Doesn't Work

- For insomnia, try escalating doses or switch to another agent
- Many patients have only a partial antidepressant response where some symptoms are improved but others persist (especially insomnia, fatigue, and problems concentrating)
- Other patients may be nonresponders, sometimes called treatment-resistant or treatment-refractory
- Consider increasing dose, switching to another agent or adding an appropriate augmenting agent for treatment of depression
- Consider psychotherapy
- Consider evaluation for another diagnosis or for a comorbid condition (e.g., medical illness, substance abuse, etc.)
- Some patients may experience apparent lack of consistent efficacy due to activation of latent or underlying bipolar disorder, and require antidepressant discontinuation and a switch to a mood stabilizer

Best Augmenting Combos for Partial Response or Treatment Resistance

- Trazodone is not frequently used as a monotherapy for insomnia, but can be combined with sedative hypnotic benzodiazepines in difficult cases
- Trazodone is most frequently used in depression as an augmenting agent to numerous psychotropic drugs
- Trazodone can not only improve insomnia in depressed patients treated with antidepressants, but can also be an effective booster of antidepressant actions of other antidepressants (use combinations of antidepressants with caution as this

may activate bipolar disorder and suicidal ideation)
- Trazodone can also improve insomnia in numerous other psychiatric conditions (e.g., bipolar disorder, schizophrenia, alcohol withdrawal) and be added to numerous other psychotropic drugs (e.g., lithium, mood stabilizers, antipsychotics)

Tests
- None for healthy individuals

SIDE EFFECTS

How Drug Causes Side Effects
- Sedative effects may be due to antihistamine properties
- Blockade of alpha adrenergic 1 receptors may explain dizziness, sedation, and hypotension
- Most side effects are immediate but often go away with time

Notable Side Effects
- Nausea, vomiting, edema, blurred vision, constipation, dry mouth
- Dizziness, sedation, fatigue, headache, incoordination, tremor
- Hypotension, syncope
- Occasional sinus bradycardia (long-term)
- Rare rash

Life-Threatening or Dangerous Side Effects
- Rare priapism
- Rare seizures
- Rare induction of mania
- Rare activation of suicidal ideation and behavior (suicidality) (short-term studies did not show an increase in the risk of suicidality with antidepressants compared to placebo beyond age 24)

Weight Gain

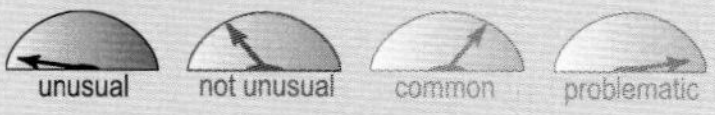

- Reported but not expected

Sedation

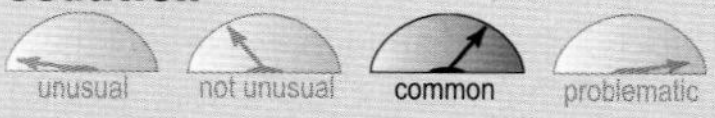

- Many experience and/or can be significant in amount

What to Do About Side Effects
- Wait
- Wait
- Wait
- Take larger dose at night to prevent daytime sedation
- Switch to another agent

Best Augmenting Agents for Side Effects
- Most side effects cannot be improved with an augmenting agent
- Activation and agitation may represent the induction of a bipolar state, especially a mixed dysphoric bipolar II condition sometimes associated with suicidal ideation, and require the addition of lithium, a mood stabilizer or an atypical antipsychotic, and/or discontinuation of trazodone

DOSING AND USE

Usual Dosage Range
- 150–600 mg/day
- 150–375 mg/day (extended-release)

Dosage Forms
- Tablet 50 mg scored, 100 mg scored, 150 mg, 150 mg with povidone scored, 300 mg with povidone scored
- Extended-release tablet 150 mg scored, 300 mg scored

How to Dose
- Depression as a monotherapy: initial 150 mg/day in divided doses; can increase every 3–4 days by 50 mg/day as needed; maximum 400 mg/day (outpatient) or 600 mg/day (inpatient), split into 2 daily doses
- Insomnia: initial 25–50 mg at bedtime; increase as tolerated, usually to 50–100 mg/day, but some patients may require up to full antidepressant dose range
- Augmentation of other antidepressants in the treatment of depression: dose as recommended for insomnia
- Extended-release: initial 150 mg once daily; may be increased by 75 mg/day every 3 days; maximum dose generally 375 mg/day

Dosing Tips
- Start low and go slow

✻ Patients can have carryover sedation, ataxia, and intoxicated-like feeling if dosed too aggressively, particularly when initiating dosing

✻ Do not discontinue trials if ineffective at low doses (<50 mg) as many patients with difficult cases may respond to higher doses (150–300 mg, even up to 600 mg in some cases)

- For relief of daytime anxiety, can give part of the dose in the daytime if not too sedating
- Although use as a monotherapy for depression is usually in divided doses due to its short half-life, use as an adjunct is often effective and best tolerated once daily at bedtime

Overdose
- Rarely lethal; sedation, vomiting, priapism, respiratory arrest, seizure, EKG changes

Long-Term Use
- Safe

Habit Forming
- No

How to Stop
- Taper is prudent to avoid withdrawal effects, but tolerance, dependence, and withdrawal effects have not been reliably demonstrated

Pharmacokinetics
- Metabolized by CYP450 3A4
- Half-life is biphasic; first phase is approximately 3–6 hours; second phase is approximately 5–9 hours

Drug Interactions
- Tramadol increases the risk of seizures in patients taking an antidepressant
- Fluoxetine and other SSRIs may raise trazodone plasma levels
- Trazodone may block the hypotensive effects of some antihypertensive drugs
- Trazodone may increase digoxin or phenytoin concentrations
- Trazodone may interfere with the antihypertensive effects of clonidine
- Generally, do not use with MAOIs, including 14 days after MAOIs are stopped
- Reports of increased and decreased prothrombin time in patients taking warfarin and trazodone

Other Warnings/ Precautions
- Possibility of additive effects if trazodone is used with other CNS depressants
- Treatment should be discontinued if prolonged penile erection occurs because of the risk of permanent erectile dysfunction
- Advise patients to seek medical attention immediately if painful erections occur lasting more than 1 hour
- Generally, priapism reverses spontaneously, while penile blood flow and other signs being monitored, but in urgent cases, local phenylephrine injections or even surgery may be indicated
- Use with caution in patients with history of seizures
- Use with caution in patients with bipolar disorder unless treated with concomitant mood-stabilizing agent
- When treating children, carefully weigh the risks and benefits of pharmacological treatment against the risks and benefits of nontreatment with antidepressants and make sure to document this in the patient's chart
- Distribute the brochures provided by the FDA and the drug companies
- Warn patients and their caregivers about the possibility of activating side effects and advise them to report such symptoms immediately
- Monitor patients for activation of suicidal ideation, especially children and adolescents

Do Not Use
- If patient is taking an MAOI, but see Pearls
- If there is a proven allergy to trazodone

SPECIAL POPULATIONS

Renal Impairment
- No dose adjustment necessary

Hepatic Impairment
- Drug should be used with caution

Cardiac Impairment
- Trazodone may be arrhythmogenic
- Monitor patients closely
- Not recommended for use during recovery from myocardial infarction

Elderly
- Elderly patients may be more sensitive to adverse effects and may require lower doses
- Reduction in the risk of suicidality with antidepressants compared to placebo in adults age 65 and older

Children and Adolescents
- Carefully weigh the risks and benefits of pharmacological treatment against the risks and benefits of nontreatment with antidepressants and make sure to document this in the patient's chart
- Monitor patients face-to-face regularly, particularly during the first several weeks of treatment
- Use with caution, observing for activation of known or unknown bipolar disorder and/or suicidal ideation, and inform parents or guardians of this risk so they can help observe child or adolescent patients
- Safety and efficacy have not been established, but trazodone has been used for behavioral disturbances, depression, and night terrors
- Children require lower initial dose and slow titration
- Boys may be even more sensitive to having prolonged erections than adult men

Pregnancy
- Effective June 30, 2015, the US FDA requires changes to the content and format of pregnancy and lactation information in prescription drug labels, including the elimination of the pregnancy letter categories; the Pregnancy and Lactation Labeling Rule (PLLR or final rule) applies only to prescription drugs and will be phased in gradually for drugs approved on or after June 30, 2001
- Controlled studies have not been conducted in pregnant women
- Avoid use during first trimester
- Must weigh the risk of treatment (first trimester fetal development, third trimester newborn delivery) to the child against the risk of no treatment (recurrence of depression, maternal health, infant bonding) to the mother and child
- For many patients this may mean continuing treatment during pregnancy

Breast Feeding
- Some drug is found in mother's breast milk
- If child becomes irritable or sedated, breast feeding or drug may need to be discontinued
- Immediate postpartum period is a high-risk time for depression, especially in women who have had prior depressive episodes, so drug may need to be reinstituted late in the third trimester or shortly after childbirth to prevent a recurrence during the postpartum period
- Must weigh benefits of breast feeding with risks and benefits of antidepressant treatment versus nontreatment to both the infant and the mother
- For many patients, this may mean continuing treatment during breast feeding

THE ART OF PSYCHOPHARMACOLOGY

Potential Advantages
- For insomnia when it is preferred to avoid the use of dependence-forming agents
- As an adjunct to the treatment of residual anxiety and insomnia with other antidepressants
- Depressed patients with anxiety
- Patients concerned about sexual side effects or weight gain

Potential Disadvantages
- For patients with fatigue, hypersomnia
- For patients intolerant to sedating effects

Primary Target Symptoms
- Depression
- Anxiety
- Sleep disturbances

Pearls
- May be less likely than some antidepressants to precipitate hypomania or mania

- Preliminary data suggest that trazodone may be effective treatment for drug-induced dyskinesias, perhaps in part because it reduces accompanying anxiety
- Trazodone may have some efficacy in treating agitation and aggression associated with dementia
- ✻ May cause sexual dysfunction only infrequently
- Can cause carryover sedation, sometimes severe, if dosed too high
- Often not tolerated as a monotherapy for moderate to severe cases of depression, as many patients cannot tolerate high doses (>150 mg)
- Do not forget to try at high doses, up to 600 mg/day, if lower doses well tolerated but ineffective
- ✻ For the expert psychopharmacologist, trazodone can be used cautiously for insomnia associated with MAOIs, despite the warning – must be attempted only if patients closely monitored and by experts experienced in the use of MAOIs
- Priapism may occur in 1 in 8,000 men
- Early indications of impending priapism may be slow penile detumescence when awakening from REM sleep
- When using to treat insomnia, remember that insomnia may be a symptom of some other primary disorder, and not a primary disorder itself, and thus warrant evaluation for comorbid psychiatric and/or medical conditions
- Rarely, patients may complain of visual "trails" or after-images on trazodone

Suggested Reading

DeVane CL. Differential pharmacology of newer antidepressants. J Clin Psychiatry 1998;59 (Suppl 20):S85–93.

Haria M, Fitton A, McTavish D. Trazodone. A review of its pharmacology, therapeutic use in depression and therapeutic potential in other disorders. Drugs Aging 1994;4:331–55.

Rotzinger S, Bourin M, Akimoto Y, Coutts RT, Baker GB. Metabolism of some "second"- and "fourth"-generation antidepressants: iprindole, viloxazine, bupropion, mianserin, maprotiline, trazodone, nefazodone, and venlafaxine. Cell Mol Neurobiol 1999;19:427–42.

Stahl SM. Mechanism of action of trazodone: a multifunctional drug. CNS Spectr 2009;14(10):536–46.

THERAPEUTICS

Brands • Halcion
see index for additional brand names

Generic? Yes

Class
- Neuroscience-based Nomenclature: GABA positive allosteric modulator (GABA-PAM)
- Benzodiazepine (hypnotic)

Commonly Prescribed for
(bold for FDA approved)
- **Short-term treatment of insomnia**
- Catatonia

How the Drug Works
- Binds to benzodiazepine receptors at the GABA-A ligand-gated chloride channel complex
- Enhances the inhibitory effects of GABA
- Boosts chloride conductance through GABA-regulated channels
- Inhibitory actions in sleep centers may provide sedative hypnotic effects

How Long Until It Works
- Generally takes effect in less than an hour

If It Works
- Improves quality of sleep
- Effects on total wake-time and number of nighttime awakenings may be decreased over time

If It Doesn't Work
- If insomnia does not improve after 7–10 days, it may be a manifestation of a primary psychiatric or physical illness such as obstructive sleep apnea or restless leg syndrome, which requires independent evaluation
- Increase the dose
- Improve sleep hygiene
- Switch to another agent

Best Augmenting Combos for Partial Response or Treatment Resistance
- Generally, best to switch to another agent
- Trazodone
- Agents with antihistamine actions (e.g., diphenhydramine, TCAs)

Tests
- In patients with seizure disorders, concomitant medical illness, and/or those with multiple concomitant long-term medications, periodic liver tests and blood counts may be prudent

SIDE EFFECTS

How Drug Causes Side Effects
- Same mechanism for side effects as for therapeutic effects – namely due to excessive actions at benzodiazepine receptors
- Actions at benzodiazepine receptors that carry over to the next day can cause daytime sedation, amnesia, and ataxia
- Long-term adaptations in benzodiazepine receptors may explain the development of dependence, tolerance, and withdrawal

Notable Side Effects
- ✻ Sedation, fatigue, depression
- ✻ Dizziness, ataxia, slurred speech, weakness
- ✻ Forgetfulness, confusion
- ✻ Hyperexcitability, nervousness
- ✻ Anterograde amnesia
- Rare hallucinations, mania
- Rare hypotension
- Hypersalivation, dry mouth
- Rebound insomnia when withdrawing from long-term treatment

Life-Threatening or Dangerous Side Effects
- Respiratory depression, especially when taken with CNS depressants in overdose
- Rare hepatic dysfunction, renal dysfunction, blood dyscrasias

Weight Gain

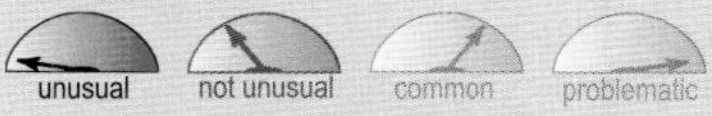

- Reported but not expected

Sedation

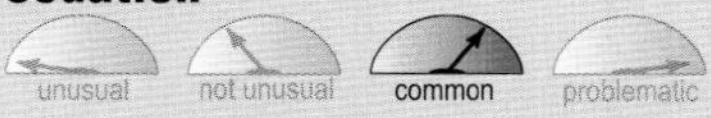

- Many experience and/or can be significant in amount

What to Do About Side Effects
- Wait
- To avoid problems with memory, take triazolam only if planning to have a full night's sleep
- Lower the dose
- Switch to a shorter-acting sedative hypnotic
- Switch to a non-benzodiazepine hypnotic
- Administer flumazenil if side effects are severe or life-threatening

Best Augmenting Agents for Side Effects
- Many side effects cannot be improved with an augmenting agent

DOSING AND USE

Usual Dosage Range
- 0.125–0.25 mg/day at bedtime for 7–10 days

Dosage Forms
- Tablet 0.125 mg, 0.25 mg

How to Dose
- Initial 0.125 or 0.25 mg/day at bedtime; may increase cautiously to 0.5 mg/day if ineffective; maximum dose generally 0.5 mg/day

Dosing Tips
- Use lowest possible effective dose and assess need for continued treatment regularly

✻ Many patients cannot tolerate 0.5 mg dose (e.g., developing anterograde amnesia)

- Triazolam should generally not be prescribed in quantities greater than a 1-month supply
- Some side effects (sedation, dizziness, lightheadedness, amnesia) seem to increase with dose
- Patients with lower weights may require only a 0.125 mg dose
- Risk of dependence may increase with dose and duration of treatment

✻ Higher doses associated with more behavioral problems and anterograde amnesia

Overdose
- Can be fatal in monotherapy; poor coordination, confusion, seizure, slurred speech, sedation, coma, respiratory depression

Long-Term Use
- Not generally intended for long-term use
- Increased wakefulness during the latter part of night (wearing off) or an increase in daytime anxiety (rebound) may occur because of short half-life

Habit Forming
- Triazolam is a Schedule IV drug
- Some patients may develop dependence and/or tolerance; risk may be greater with higher doses
- History of drug addiction may increase risk of dependence

How to Stop
- If taken for more than a few weeks, taper to reduce chances of withdrawal effects
- Patients with seizure history may seize upon sudden withdrawal
- Rebound insomnia may occur the first 1–2 nights after stopping
- For patients with severe problems discontinuing a benzodiazepine, dosing may need to be tapered over many months (i.e., reduce dose by 1% every 3 days by crushing tablet and suspending or dissolving in 100 mL of fruit juice and then disposing of 1 mL while drinking the rest; 3–7 days later, dispose of 2 mL, and so on). This is both a form of very slow biological tapering and a form of behavioral desensitization

Pharmacokinetics
- Half-life 1.5–5.5 hours
- Inactive metabolites

Drug Interactions
- CYP450 3A inhibitors such as nefazodone, fluoxetine, and fluvoxamine may decrease clearance of triazolam and raise triazolam levels significantly
- Ranitidine may increase plasma concentrations of triazolam
- Increased depressive effects when taken with other CNS depressants (see Warnings below)

Other Warnings/ Precautions

- Boxed warning regarding the increased risk of CNS depressant effects when benzodiazepines and opioid medications are used together, including specifically the risk of slowed or difficulty breathing and death
- If alternatives to the combined use of benzodiazepines and opioids are not available, clinicians should limit the dosage and duration of each drug to the minimum possible while still achieving therapeutic efficacy
- Patients and their caregivers should be warned to seek medical attention if unusual dizziness, lightheadedness, sedation, slowed or difficulty breathing, or unresponsiveness occur
- Insomnia may be a symptom of a primary disorder, rather than a primary disorder itself
- Some patients may exhibit abnormal thinking or behavioral changes similar to those caused by other CNS depressants (i.e., either depressant actions or disinhibiting actions)
- Some depressed patients may experience a worsening of suicidal ideation
- Use only with extreme caution in patients with impaired respiratory function or obstructive sleep apnea
- Triazolam should be administered only at bedtime
- Grapefruit juice could increase triazolam levels

Do Not Use

- If patient is pregnant
- If patient has angle-closure glaucoma
- If patient is taking ketoconazole, itraconazole, nefazodone, or other potent CYP450 3A4 inhibitors
- If there is a proven allergy to triazolam or any benzodiazepine

SPECIAL POPULATIONS

Renal Impairment

- Drug should be used with caution

Hepatic Impairment

- Drug should be used with caution

Cardiac Impairment

- Benzodiazepines have been used to treat insomnia associated with acute myocardial infarction

Elderly

- Recommended initial dose: 0.125 mg
- May be more sensitive to adverse effects

Children and Adolescents

- Safety and efficacy have not been established
- Long-term effects of triazolam in children/ adolescents are unknown
- Should generally receive lower doses and be more closely monitored

Pregnancy

- Contraindicated for use in pregnancy
- Effective June 30, 2015, the US FDA requires changes to the content and format of pregnancy and lactation information in prescription drug labels, including the elimination of the pregnancy letter categories; the Pregnancy and Lactation Labeling Rule (PLLR or final rule) applies only to prescription drugs and will be phased in gradually for drugs approved on or after June 30, 2001
- Infants whose mothers received a benzodiazepine late in pregnancy may experience withdrawal effects
- Neonatal flaccidity has been reported in infants whose mothers took a benzodiazepine during pregnancy

Breast Feeding

- Unknown if triazolam is secreted in human breast milk, but all psychotropics assumed to be secreted in breast milk

* Recommended either to discontinue drug or bottle feed

- Effects on infant have been observed and include feeding difficulties, sedation, and weight loss

THE ART OF PSYCHOPHARMACOLOGY

Potential Advantages
- Short-acting

Potential Disadvantages
- Patients on concomitant CYP450 3A4 inhibitors
- Patients with terminal insomnia (early morning awakenings)

Primary Target Symptoms
- Time to sleep onset
- Total sleep time
- Nighttime awakenings

Pearls
✻ The shorter half-life should prevent impairments in cognitive and motor performance during the day as well as daytime sedation

✻ If tolerance develops, the short half-life of elimination may result in increased anxiety during the day and/or increased wakefulness during the latter part of the night

- The short half-life may minimize the risk of drug interactions with agents taken during the day (e.g., alcohol)

✻ However, the risk of drug interactions with alcohol taken at night may be greater than for some other sedative hypnotics, especially for anterograde amnesia

✻ Anterograde amnesia may be more likely with triazolam than with other sedative benzodiazepines

- Because of its short half-life and inactive metabolites, triazolam may be preferred over some benzodiazepines for patients with liver disease

✻ The risk of unusual behaviors or hallucinations may be greater with triazolam than with other sedative benzodiazepines

- Clearance of triazolam may be slightly faster in women than in men
- Women taking oral progesterone may be more sensitive to the effects of triazolam
- Though not systematically studied, benzodiazepines have been used effectively to treat catatonia and are the initial recommended treatment

Suggested Reading

Jonas JM, Coleman BS, Sheridan AQ, Kalinske RW. Comparative clinical profiles of triazolam versus other shorter-acting hypnotics. J Clin Psychiatry 1992;53(Suppl):S19–31.

Lobo BL, Greene WL. Zolpidem: distinct from triazolam? Ann Pharmacother 1997;31:625–32.

Rothschild AJ. Disinhibition, amnestic reactions, and other adverse reactions secondary to triazolam: a review of the literature. J Clin Psychiatry 1992;53(Suppl):S69–79.

Yuan R, Flockhart DA, Balian JD. Pharmacokinetic and pharmacodynamic consequences of metabolism-based drug interactions with alprazolam, midazolam, and triazolam. J Clin Pharmacol 1999;39:1109–25.

THERAPEUTICS

Brands • Stelazine

see index for additional brand names

Generic? Yes

Class

- Neuroscience-based Nomenclature: dopamine receptor antagonist (D-RAn)
- Conventional antipsychotic (neuroleptic, phenothiazine, dopamine 2 antagonist)

Commonly Prescribed for

(bold for FDA approved)

- **Schizophrenia (oral, intramuscular)**
- **Nonpsychotic anxiety (short-term, second-line)**
- Other psychotic disorders
- Bipolar disorder

How the Drug Works

- Blocks dopamine 2 receptors, reducing positive symptoms of psychosis

How Long Until It Works

- Psychotic symptoms can improve within 1 week, but it may take several weeks for full effect on behavior

If It Works

- Most often reduces positive symptoms in schizophrenia but does not eliminate them
- Most schizophrenic patients do not have a total remission of symptoms but rather a reduction of symptoms by about a third
- Continue treatment in schizophrenia until reaching a plateau of improvement
- After reaching a satisfactory plateau, continue treatment for at least a year after first episode of psychosis in schizophrenia
- For second and subsequent episodes of psychosis in schizophrenia, treatment may need to be indefinite
- Reduces symptoms of acute psychotic mania but not proven as a mood stabilizer or as an effective maintenance treatment in bipolar disorder
- After reducing acute psychotic symptoms in mania, switch to a mood stabilizer and/or an atypical antipsychotic for mood stabilization and maintenance

If It Doesn't Work

- Consider trying one of the first-line atypical antipsychotics (risperidone, olanzapine, quetiapine, ziprasidone, aripiprazole, paliperidone, amisulpride, asenapine, iloperidone, lurasidone)
- Consider trying another conventional antipsychotic
- If 2 or more antipsychotic monotherapies do not work, consider clozapine

Best Augmenting Combos for Partial Response or Treatment Resistance

- Augmentation of conventional antipsychotics has not been systematically studied
- Addition of a mood-stabilizing anticonvulsant such as valproate, carbamazepine, or lamotrigine may be helpful in both schizophrenia and bipolar mania
- Augmentation with lithium in bipolar mania may be helpful
- Addition of a benzodiazepine, especially short-term for agitation

Tests

❋ Since conventional antipsychotics are frequently associated with weight gain, before starting treatment, weigh all patients and determine if the patient is already overweight (BMI 25.0–29.9) or obese (BMI ≥30)

- Before giving a drug that can cause weight gain to an overweight or obese patient, consider determining whether the patient already has pre-diabetes (fasting plasma glucose 100–125 mg/dL), diabetes (fasting plasma glucose >126 mg/dL), or dyslipidemia (increased total cholesterol, LDL cholesterol, and triglycerides; decreased HDL cholesterol), and treat or refer such patients for treatment, including nutrition and weight management, physical activity counseling, smoking cessation, and medical management

❋ Monitor weight and BMI during treatment

❋ Consider monitoring fasting triglycerides monthly for several months in patients at high risk for metabolic complications and when initiating or switching antipsychotics

❋ While giving a drug to a patient who has gained >5% of initial weight, consider

evaluating for the presence of pre-diabetes, diabetes, or dyslipidemia, or consider switching to a different antipsychotic
- Should check blood pressure in the elderly before starting and for the first few weeks of treatment
- Monitoring elevated prolactin levels of dubious clinical benefit
- Phenothiazines may cause false-positive phenylketonuria results
- Patients with low white blood cell count (WBC) or history of drug-induced leucopenia/neutropenia should have complete blood count (CBC) monitored frequently during the first few months and trifluoperazine should be discontinued at the first sign of decline of WBC in the absence of other causative factors

SIDE EFFECTS

How Drug Causes Side Effects
- By blocking dopamine 2 receptors in the striatum, it can cause motor side effects
- By blocking dopamine 2 receptors in the pituitary, it can cause elevations in prolactin
- By blocking dopamine 2 receptors excessively in the mesocortical and mesolimbic dopamine pathways, especially at high doses, it can cause worsening of negative and cognitive symptoms (neuroleptic-induced deficit syndrome)
- Anticholinergic actions may cause sedation, blurred vision, constipation, dry mouth
- Antihistaminic actions may cause sedation, weight gain
- By blocking alpha 1 adrenergic receptors, it can cause dizziness, sedation, and hypotension
- Mechanism of weight gain and any possible increased incidence of diabetes or dyslipidemia with conventional antipsychotics is unknown

Notable Side Effects
✽ Neuroleptic-induced deficit syndrome
✽ Akathisia
✽ Rash
✽ Priapism
✽ Extrapyramidal symptoms, parkinsonism, tardive dyskinesia, tardive dystonia
✽ Galactorrhea, amenorrhea
- Dizziness, sedation
- Dry mouth, constipation, blurred vision, urinary retention
- Decreased sweating
- Sexual dysfunction
- Hypotension

Life-Threatening or Dangerous Side Effects
- Rare neuroleptic malignant syndrome
- Rare jaundice, agranulocytosis
- Rare seizures
- Increased risk of death and cerebrovascular events in elderly patients with dementia-related psychosis

Weight Gain
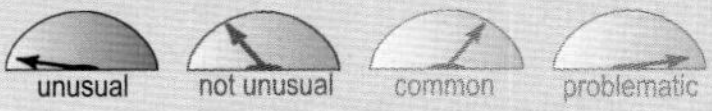

✽ Reported but not expected

Sedation
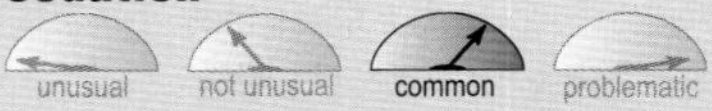

- Many experience and/or can be significant in amount
- Sedation is usually transient

What to Do About Side Effects
- Wait
- Wait
- Wait
- For motor symptoms, add an anticholinergic agent
- Reduce the dose
- For sedation, give at night
- Switch to an atypical antipsychotic
- Weight loss, exercise programs, and medical management for high BMIs, diabetes, dyslipidemia

Best Augmenting Agents for Side Effects
- Benztropine or trihexyphenidyl for motor side effects
- Sometimes amantadine can be helpful for motor side effects
- Benzodiazepines may be helpful for akathisia
- Many side effects cannot be improved with an augmenting agent

DOSING AND USE

Usual Dosage Range
- Oral: psychosis: 15–20 mg/day

Dosage Forms
- Tablet 1 mg, 2 mg, 5 mg, 10 mg
- Vial 2 mg/mL
- Concentrate 10 mg/mL

How to Dose
- Psychosis: oral: initial 2–5 mg twice a day; increase gradually over 2–3 weeks
- Psychosis: intramuscular: 1–2 mg every 4–6 hours; generally do not exceed 6 mg/day
- Anxiety: initial 1–2 mg/day; maximum 6 mg/day

Dosing Tips
- ✻ Use only low doses and short-term for anxiety because trifluoperazine is now a second-line treatment and has the risk of tardive dyskinesia
- Concentrate contains sulfites that may cause allergic reactions, particularly in patients with asthma
- Many patients can be dosed once a day
- Treatment should be suspended if absolute neutrophil count falls below 1,000/mm^3

Overdose
- Extrapyramidal symptoms, sedation, seizures, coma, hypotension, respiratory depression

Long-Term Use
- Some side effects may be irreversible (e.g., tardive dyskinesia)
- Not intended to treat anxiety long-term (i.e., longer than 12 weeks)

Habit Forming
- No

How to Stop
- Slow down-titration of oral formulation (over 6–8 weeks), especially when simultaneously beginning a new antipsychotic while switching (i.e., cross-titration)
- Rapid oral discontinuation may lead to rebound psychosis and worsening of symptoms
- If antiparkinson agents are being used, they should be continued for a few weeks after trifluoperazine is discontinued

Pharmacokinetics
- Mean elimination half-life approximately 12.5 hours

Drug Interactions
- May decrease the effects of levodopa, dopamine agonists
- May increase the effects of antihypertensive drugs except for guanethidine, whose antihypertensive actions trifluoperazine may antagonize
- Additive effects may occur if used with CNS depressants
- Alcohol and diuretics may increase the risk of hypotension; epinephrine may lower blood pressure
- Phenothiazines may reduce effects of anticoagulants
- Some patients taking a neuroleptic and lithium have developed an encephalopathic syndrome similar to neuroleptic malignant syndrome
- If used with propranolol, plasma levels of both drugs may rise

Other Warnings/ Precautions
- If signs of neuroleptic malignant syndrome develop, treatment should be immediately discontinued
- Use cautiously in patients with alcohol withdrawal or convulsive disorders because of possible lowering of seizure threshold
- Use with caution in patients with respiratory disorders, glaucoma, or urinary retention
- Avoid undue exposure to sunlight
- Avoid extreme heat exposure
- Antiemetic effect may mask signs of other disorders or overdose; suppression of cough reflex may cause asphyxia
- Do not use epinephrine in event of overdose as interaction with some pressor agents may lower blood pressure
- Use only with caution if at all in Parkinson's disease or Lewy body dementia

Do Not Use
- If patient is in a comatose state or has CNS depression
- If there is the presence of blood dyscrasias, bone marrow depression, or liver disease

- If there is a proven allergy to trifluoperazine
- If there is a known sensitivity to any phenothiazine

SPECIAL POPULATIONS

Renal Impairment
- Use with caution

Hepatic Impairment
- Not recommended for use

Cardiac Impairment
- Dose should be lowered
- Do not use parenteral administration unless necessary

Elderly
- Lower doses should be used and patient should be monitored closely
- Although conventional antipsychotics are commonly used for behavioral disturbances in dementia, no agent has been approved for treatment of elderly patients with dementia-related psychosis
- Elderly patients with dementia-related psychosis treated with antipsychotics are at an increased risk of death compared to placebo, and also have an increased risk of cerebrovascular events

Children and Adolescents
- Not recommended for use in children under age 6
- Children should be closely monitored when taking trifluoperazine
- Oral: initial 1 mg; increase gradually; maximum 15 mg/day except in older children with severe symptoms
- Intramuscular: 1 mg once or twice a day
- Generally consider second-line after atypical antipsychotics

Pregnancy
- Effective June 30, 2015, the US FDA requires changes to the content and format of pregnancy and lactation information in prescription drug labels, including the elimination of the pregnancy letter categories; the Pregnancy and Lactation Labeling Rule (PLLR or final rule) applies only to prescription drugs and will be phased in gradually for drugs approved on or after June 30, 2001
- Controlled studies have not been conducted in pregnant women
- There is a risk of abnormal muscle movements and withdrawal symptoms in newborns whose mothers took an antipsychotic during the third trimester; symptoms may include agitation, abnormally increased or decreased muscle tone, tremor, sleepiness, severe difficulty breathing, and difficulty feeding
- Reports of extrapyramidal symptoms, jaundice, hyperreflexia, hyporeflexia in infants whose mothers took a phenothiazine during pregnancy
- Trifluoperazine should only be used during pregnancy if clearly needed
- Psychotic symptoms may worsen during pregnancy and some form of treatment may be necessary
- Atypical antipsychotics may be preferable to conventional antipsychotics or anticonvulsant mood stabilizers if treatment is required during pregnancy

Breast Feeding
- Some drug is found in mother's breast milk

✽ Recommended either to discontinue drug or bottle feed

THE ART OF PSYCHOPHARMACOLOGY

Potential Advantages
- Intramuscular formulation for emergency use

Potential Disadvantages
- Patients with tardive dyskinesia
- Children
- Elderly

Primary Target Symptoms
- Positive symptoms of psychosis
- Motor and autonomic hyperactivity
- Violent or aggressive behavior

Pearls
- Trifluoperazine is a higher potency phenothiazine

- ✻ Although not systematically studied, may cause less weight gain than other antipsychotics
- Less risk of sedation and orthostatic hypotension but greater extrapyramidal symptoms than with low potency phenothiazines
- Patients have very similar antipsychotic responses to any conventional antipsychotic, which is different from atypical antipsychotics where antipsychotic responses of individual patients can occasionally vary greatly from one atypical antipsychotic to another
- Patients with inadequate responses to atypical antipsychotics may benefit from a trial of augmentation with a conventional antipsychotic such as trifluoperazine or from switching to a conventional antipsychotic such as trifluoperazine
- However, long-term polypharmacy with a combination of a conventional antipsychotic such as trifluoperazine with an atypical antipsychotic may combine their side effects without clearly augmenting the efficacy of either
- For treatment-resistant patients, especially those with impulsivity, aggression, violence, and self-harm, long-term polypharmacy with 2 atypical antipsychotics or with 1 atypical antipsychotic and 1 conventional antipsychotic may be useful or even necessary while closely monitoring
- In such cases, it may be beneficial to combine 1 depot antipsychotic with 1 oral antipsychotic
- Although a frequent practice by some prescribers, adding 2 conventional antipsychotics together has little rationale and may reduce tolerability without clearly enhancing efficacy

Suggested Reading

Doongaji DR, Satoskar RS, Sheth AS, et al. Centbutindole vs trifluoperazine: a double-blind controlled clinical study in acute schizophrenia. J Postgrad Med 1989;35:3–8.

Frankenburg FR. Choices in antipsychotic therapy in schizophrenia. Harv Rev Psychiatry 1999;6:241–9.

Kiloh LG, Williams SE, Grant DA, Whetton PS. A double-blind comparative trial of loxapine and trifluoperazine in acute and chronic schizophrenic patients. J Int Med Res 1976;4:441–8.

Marques LO, Lima MS, Soares BG. Trifluoperazine for schizophrenia. Cochrane Database Syst Rev 2004;(1):CD003545.

TRIHEXYPHENIDYL

THERAPEUTICS

Brands • Artane
see index for additional brand names

Generic? Yes

Class
• Antiparkinson agent; anticholinergic

Commonly Prescribed for
(bold for FDA approved)
• **Extrapyramidal disorders**
• **Parkinsonism**
• Idiopathic generalized dystonia
• Focal dystonias
• Dopa-responsive dystonia

How the Drug Works
• Diminishes the excess acetylcholine activity caused by removal of dopamine inhibition when dopamine receptors are blocked
• May also inhibit the reuptake and storage of dopamine at central dopamine receptors, prolonging dopamine action

How Long Until It Works
• For extrapyramidal disorders and parkinsonism, onset of action can be within minutes or hours

If It Works
• Reduces motor side effects
• Does not lessen the ability of antipsychotics to cause tardive dyskinesia

If It Doesn't Work
• For extrapyramidal disorders, increase to highest tolerated dose
• Consider switching to benztropine, diphenhydramine, or a benzodiazepine
• Disorders that develop after prolonged antipsychotic use may not respond to treatment
• Consider discontinuing the agent that precipitated the EPS

Best Augmenting Combos for Partial Response or Treatment Resistance
• If ineffective, switch to another agent rather than augment
• Trihexyphenidyl itself is an augmenting agent to antipsychotics

Tests
• None for healthy individuals

SIDE EFFECTS

How Drug Causes Side Effects
• Prevents the action of acetylcholine on muscarinic receptors

Notable Side Effects
• Dry mouth, blurred vision, diplopia
• Confusion, hallucinations
• Constipation, nausea, vomiting
• Dilation of colon
• Erectile dysfunction

Life-Threatening or Dangerous Side Effects
• Angle-closure glaucoma
• Heat stroke, especially in elderly patients
• Tachycardia, cardiac arrhythmias, hypotension
• Urinary retention
• Anticholinergic agents such as trihexyphenidyl can exacerbate or unmask tardive dyskinesia

Weight Gain
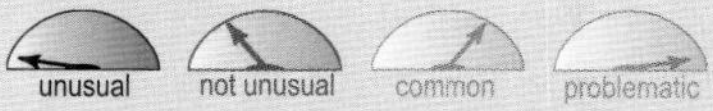

• Reported but not expected

Sedation
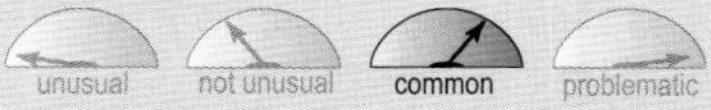

• Many experience and/or can be significant in amount

What to Do About Side Effects
• For confusion or hallucinations, discontinue use
• For sedation, lower the dose and/or take the entire dose at night
• For dry mouth, chew gum or drink water
• For urinary retention, obtain a urological evaluation; may need to discontinue use

Best Augmenting Agents for Side Effects
- Many side effects cannot be improved with an augmenting agent

DOSING AND USE

Usual Dosage Range
- Extrapyramidal disorders: 5–15 mg/day
- Parkinsonism: 6–15 mg/day

Dosage Forms
- Tablet 2 mg, 5 mg
- Injection 2 mg/5 mL

How to Dose
- Extrapyramidal disorders: 5–15 mg/day; assess effect and increase dose empirically as tolerated; total daily dose varies from patient to patient
- Parkinsonism (oral): initial 1 mg/day; after 3 days can increase the dose in 2 mg increments every 3–5 days as tolerated until clinical effect is reached; total daily dose should be divided into 3 doses and given with meals

Dosing Tips
- If drug-induced EPS occur soon after initiation of a neuroleptic drug, they are likely to be transient; thus, attempt to withdraw trihexyphenidyl after 1–2 weeks to determine if still needed
- To achieve more rapid relief, temporarily lower the dose of the offending agent (phenothiazine, thioxanthene, or butyrophenone) when starting trihexyphenidyl
- Taking trihexyphenidyl with meals can reduce side effects
- In Parkinson's disease, the usual dose is 6–10 mg/day (divided into 3 doses) for idiopathic Parkinson's disease and 12–15 mg/day (divided into 3 or 4 doses) for post-encephalitic Parkinson's disease

Overdose
- Circulatory collapse, cardiac arrest, respiratory depression or arrest, CNS depression or stimulation, psychosis, shock, coma, seizure, ataxia, combativeness, anhidrosis and hyperthermia, fever, dysphagia, decreased bowel sounds, sluggish pupils

Long-Term Use
- Safe
- Effectiveness may decrease over time (years) and side effects such as sedation and cognitive impairment may worsen

Habit Forming
- No

How to Stop
- Taper not necessary

Pharmacokinetics
- Half-life 6–10 hours; time to peak effect is 1–1.3 hours
- Metabolism is not well understood

Drug Interactions
- Use with amantadine may increase side effects
- Trihexyphenidyl and all other anticholinergic agents may increase serum levels and effects of digoxin
- Can lower concentration of haloperidol and other phenothiazines, causing worsening of schizophrenia symptoms
- Can decrease gastric motility, resulting in increased gastric deactivation of levodopa and reduction in efficacy

Other Warnings/ Precautions
- Use with caution in hot weather, as trihexyphenidyl may increase susceptibility to heat stroke
- Anticholinergic agents have additive effects when used with drugs of abuse such as cannabinoids, barbiturates, opioids, and alcohol

Do Not Use
- In patients with glaucoma, particularly angle-closure glaucoma
- In patients with pyloric or duodenal obstruction, stenosing peptic ulcers, prostate hypertrophy or bladder neck obstructions, achalasia, or megacolon
- If there is a proven allergy to trihexyphenidyl

SPECIAL POPULATIONS

Renal Impairment
- No known effects, but use with caution

Hepatic Impairment
- No known effects, but use with caution

Cardiac Impairment
- Use with caution in patients with known arrhythmias, especially tachycardia

Elderly
- Use with caution
- Elderly patients may be more susceptible to side effects

Children and Adolescents
- Do not use in children ages 3 and younger
- Generalized dystonias may respond to anticholinergic treatment and young patients usually tolerate the medication better than the elderly
- Usual dose is 0.05 mg/kg once or twice daily

Pregnancy
- Effective June 30, 2015, the US FDA requires changes to the content and format of pregnancy and lactation information in prescription drug labels, including the elimination of the pregnancy letter categories; the Pregnancy and Lactation Labeling Rule (PLLR or final rule) applies only to prescription drugs and will be phased in gradually for drugs approved on or after June 30, 2001
- Controlled studies have not been conducted in pregnant women

Breast Feeding
- Unknown if trihexyphenidyl is secreted in human breast milk, but all psychotropics assumed to be secreted in breast milk
- ✻ Recommended either to discontinue drug or bottle feed unless the potential benefit to the mother justifies the potential risk to the child
- Infants of women who choose to breast feed while on trihexyphenidyl should be monitored for possible adverse effects

THE ART OF PSYCHOPHARMACOLOGY

Potential Advantages
- Extrapyramidal disorders related to antipsychotic use
- Generalized dystonias (well tolerated in younger age groups)

Potential Disadvantages
- Patients with long-standing extrapyramidal disorders may not respond to treatment
- Multiple dose-dependent side effects may limit use

Primary Target Symptoms
- Tremor, akinesia, rigidity, drooling, dystonia

Pearls
- Often abused in correctional settings for its euphoric and sedative/hypnotic action, especially at high doses
- Although any anticholinergic agent is potentially abusable, especially in a correctional setting, trihexyphenidyl may be more abusable than others, presumably due to its dopamine-enhancing actions
- Useful adjunct in younger Parkinson's patients with tremor
- Useful in the treatment of post-encephalitic Parkinson's disease and for extrapyramidal reactions, other than tardive dyskinesias
- Post-encephalitic Parkinson's patients usually tolerate higher doses better than idiopathic Parkinson's patients
- Generalized dystonias are more likely to benefit from anticholinergic therapy than focal dystonias; trihexyphenidyl is used more commonly than benztropine
- Sedation limits use, especially in older patients
- Patients with mental impairment do poorly
- Dystonias related to cerebral palsy, head injuries, and stroke may improve with trihexyphenidyl, especially in younger, cognitively normal patients
- Schizophrenia patients may abuse trihexyphenidyl and other anticholinergic medications to relieve negative symptoms, for a stimulant effect or to improve symptoms of drug-induced parkinsonism
- Can cause cognitive side effects with chronic use, so periodic trials of discontinuation may be useful to justify continuous use, especially in institutional settings as adjunct to antipsychotics

Suggested Reading

Brocks DR. Anticholinergic drugs used in Parkinson's disease: an overlooked class of drugs from a pharmacokinetic perspective. J Pharm Pharm Sci 1999;2(2):39–46.

Colosimo C, Gori MC, Inghilleri M. Postencephalitic tremor and delayed-onset parkinsonism. Parkinsonism Relat Disord 1999;5(3):123–4.

Costa J, Espírito-Santo C, Borges A, et al. Botulinum toxin type A versus anticholinergics for cervical dystonia. Cochrane Database Syst Rev 2005;(1):CD004312.

Sanger TD, Bastian A, Brunstrom J, et al. Prospective open-label clinical trial of trihexyphenidyl in children with secondary dystonia due to cerebral palsy. J Child Neurol 2007;22(5):530–7.

Zemishlany Z, Aizenberg D, Weiner Z, Weizman A. Trihexyphenidyl (Artane) abuse in schizophrenic patients. Int Clin Psychopharmacol 1996;11(3):199–202.

THERAPEUTICS

Brands • Cytomel

see index for additional brand names

Generic? Yes

Class

- Synthetic hormone; antidepressant adjunct

Commonly Prescribed for

(bold for FDA approved)

- **Replacement or supplemental therapy in patients with hypothyroidism (except transient hypothyroidism during the recovery phase of subacute thyroiditis)**
- **Pituitary thyroid-stimulating hormone (TSH) suppressant in the treatment or prevention of various types of euthyroid goiters**
- Major depressive disorder (adjunct)

How the Drug Works

- Hypothetically boosts monoamine actions in the CNS
- May work synergistically with traditional antidepressants

How Long Until It Works (for depression)

- Can work within days, but therapeutic effects may be delayed for up to 8 weeks

If It Works (for depression)

- The goal of treatment is complete remission of current symptoms as well as prevention of future relapses
- Treatment most often reduces or even eliminates symptoms, but not a cure since symptoms can recur after medicine stopped
- Continue treatment until all symptoms are gone (remission) or significantly reduced
- Once symptoms gone, continue treating for 1 year for the first episode of depression
- For second and subsequent episodes of depression, treatment may need to be indefinite

If It Doesn't Work (for depression)

- Many patients only have a partial response where some symptoms are improved but others persist (especially insomnia, fatigue, and problems concentrating)
- Other patients may be nonresponders, sometimes called treatment-resistant or treatment-refractory
- Some patients who have an initial response may relapse even though they continue treatment, sometimes called "poop-out"
- Consider switching to another antidepressant or adding a different augmenting agent
- Consider psychotherapy
- Consider evaluation for another diagnosis or for a comorbid condition (e.g., medical illness, substance abuse, etc.)
- Some patients may experience apparent lack of consistent efficacy due to activation of latent or underlying bipolar disorder, and require antidepressant discontinuation and switch to a mood stabilizer

Best Augmenting Combos for Partial Response or Treatment Resistance

- Triiodothyronine is itself an augmenting agent for partial response in depression

Tests

- Periodic assessment of thyroid status
- Administration of triiodothyronine may lead to mild hyperthyroidism with reduced levels of TSH

SIDE EFFECTS

How Drug Causes Side Effects

- Increases in thyroid hormone concentrations

Notable Side Effects

- Hyperthyroidism (headache, irritability, nervousness, sweating, arrhythmia, increased bowel motility, menstrual irregularities)
- Possible acceleration of bone demineralization, especially in postmenopausal women (controversial)

Life-Threatening or Dangerous Side Effects

- Angina pectoris, congestive heart failure
- Shock

Weight Gain

unusual · not unusual · common · problematic

- Reported but not expected
- May cause weight loss

Sedation

unusual · not unusual · common · problematic

- Reported but not expected

What to Do About Side Effects

- Wait
- Wait
- Wait
- In a few weeks, switch to another agent

Best Augmenting Agents for Side Effects

- Often best to try another treatment prior to resorting to augmentation strategies to treat side effects

DOSING AND USE

Usual Dosage Range

- 25–50 mcg/day

Dosage Forms

- Tablet 5 mcg, 25 mcg, 50 mcg

How to Dose

- Initial 25 mcg/day; if no response can increase to 50 mcg/day after 2–4 weeks

Dosing Tips

- Monitor TSH levels to determine efficacy or thyroid actions in the periphery and to guide dosing
- If no effects on depressed mood, may want to discontinue in 8–12 weeks
- To assess efficacy in stabilizing mood in combination with other mood stabilizers, may need to monitor for a few months

Overdose

- Chest pain, increased pulse rate, palpitations, excessive sweating, heat intolerance, nervousness

Long-Term Use

- Has not been evaluated in controlled studies, but long-term treatment of major depressive disorder is generally necessary

Habit Forming

- No

How to Stop

- Taper not necessary

Pharmacokinetics

- Half-life approximately 2.5 days

Drug Interactions

- Thyroid hormones appear to increase catabolism of vitamin K-dependent clotting factors; patients stabilized on oral anticoagulants who are treated with triiodothyronine should be watched very closely when triiodothyronine is started and may require dose reduction of the oral anticoagulant
- Initiating thyroid replacement therapy may cause increases in insulin or oral hypoglycemic requirements; patients receiving insulin or oral hypoglycemics should be closely watched during initiation of triiodothyronine
- Cholestyramine binds both T4 and T3 in the intestine, thus impairing absorption of these thyroid hormones; therefore, 4 to 5 hours should elapse between administration of cholestyramine and thyroid hormones
- Use of thyroid products with imipramine and other TCAs may increase receptor sensitivity and enhance antidepressant activity; transient cardiac arrhythmias have been observed; thyroid hormone activity may also be enhanced
- Thyroid preparations may potentiate the toxic effects of digitalis
- Use with caution with ketamine; may cause hypertension and tachycardia
- Use with catecholamines may increase their adrenergic effects; careful observation is required

Other Warnings/ Precautions

- Use of thyroid hormones in the therapy of obesity, alone or in combination, is not

effective at doses within the range of daily hormonal requirements; larger doses may produce serious or even life-threatening manifestations of toxicity, particularly when given in association with sympathomimetic amines
- Use of thyroid hormones is not justified for the treatment of male or female infertility unless accompanied by hypothyroidism
- Use with caution in patients in whom the integrity of the cardiovascular system is suspected, including elderly patients or those with angina pectoris
- Thyroid hormone therapy in patients with concomitant diabetes mellitus or insipidus or adrenal cortical insufficiency aggravates the intensity of their symptoms

Do Not Use
- If patient has uncorrected adrenal cortical insufficiency
- If patient has untreated thyrotoxicosis
- If there is a proven allergy to triiodothyronine

SPECIAL POPULATIONS

Renal Impairment
- No dose adjustment necessary

Hepatic Impairment
- No dose adjustment necessary

Cardiac Impairment
- Use with caution
- Requires dose reduction: initial 5 mcg; increase by no more than 5 mcg at 2-week intervals; reduce dose if cardiovascular disease is aggravated

Elderly
- Some patients may tolerate lower doses better

Children and Adolescents
- Thyroid hormone is used safely in infants, children, and adolescents for hypothyroidism
- Not studied for use as adjunct in depression

Pregnancy
- Effective June 30, 2015, the US FDA requires changes to the content and format of pregnancy and lactation information in prescription drug labels, including the elimination of the pregnancy letter categories; the Pregnancy and Lactation Labeling Rule (PLLR or final rule) applies only to prescription drugs and will be phased in gradually for drugs approved on or after June 30, 2001
- Adequate, well-controlled studies in pregnant women have failed to demonstrate risk to the fetus
- Thyroid hormones do not readily cross the placental barrier, and the clinical experience to date does not indicate any adverse effect on fetuses when thyroid hormones are administered to pregnant women

Breast Feeding
- Some drug is found in mother's breast milk
- No known adverse effects but use should be cautious
- Must weigh benefits of breast feeding with risks and benefits of treatment versus nontreatment to both the infant and the mother
- For many patients, this may mean continuing treatment during breast feeding

THE ART OF PSYCHOPHARMACOLOGY

Potential Advantages
- Patients with lethargy and fatigue
- Patients with unstable or rapidly fluctuating mood

Potential Disadvantages
- Patients with osteoporosis
- Patients already taking thyroid replacement

Primary Target Symptoms
- Depressed mood

Pearls
- Have periodic monitoring by primary care physician, including neck examination and thyroid palpation

- Generally well tolerated, especially compared to other augmentation options for depression

- May be useful in stabilizing fluctuating mood states as well as improving depressed mood

Suggested Reading

Aronson R, Offman HJ, Joffe RT, et al. Triiodothyronine augmentation in the treatment of refractory depression: a meta-analysis. Arch Gen Psychiatry 1996;53:842–8.

Connolly KR, Thase ME. If at first you don't succeed: a review of the evidence for antidepressant augmentation, combination and switching strategies. Drugs 2011;71(1):43–64.

Garlow SJ, Dunlop BW, Ninan PT, Nemeroff CB. The combination of triiodothyronine (T3) and sertraline is not superior to sertraline monotherapy in the treatment of major depressive disorder. J Psychiatr Res 2012;46(11):1406–13.

Hage MP, Azar ST. The link between thyroid function and depression. J Thyroid Res 2012;2012:590648.

Nierenberg AA, Fava M, Trivedi MH, et al. A comparison of lithium and T(3) augmentation following two failed medication treatments for depression: a STAR*D report. Am J Psychiatry 2006;163:1519–30.

TRIMIPRAMINE

THERAPEUTICS

Brands • Surmontil

see index for additional brand names

Generic? Yes

Class

- Neuroscience-based Nomenclature: dopamine and serotonin receptor antagonist (DS-RAn)
- Tricyclic antidepressant (TCA)
- Serotonin and norepinephrine/noradrenaline reuptake inhibitor

Commonly Prescribed for

(bold for FDA approved)

- **Depression**
- **Endogenous depression**
- Anxiety
- Insomnia
- Neuropathic pain/chronic pain
- Treatment-resistant depression

How the Drug Works

- Boosts neurotransmitters serotonin and norepinephrine/noradrenaline
- Blocks serotonin reuptake pump (serotonin transporter), presumably increasing serotonergic neurotransmission
- Blocks norepinephrine reuptake pump (norepinephrine transporter), presumably increasing noradrenergic neurotransmission
- Presumably desensitizes both serotonin 1A receptors and beta adrenergic receptors
- Since dopamine is inactivated by norepinephrine reuptake in frontal cortex, which largely lacks dopamine transporters, trimipramine can increase dopamine neurotransmission in this part of the brain

How Long Until It Works

- May have immediate effects in treating insomnia, agitation, or anxiety
- Onset of therapeutic actions usually not immediate, but often delayed 2–4 weeks
- If it is not working within 6–8 weeks for depression, it may require a dosage increase or it may not work at all
- May continue to work for many years to prevent relapse of symptoms

If It Works

- The goal of treatment of depression is complete remission of current symptoms as well as prevention of future relapses
- The goal of treatment of chronic neuropathic pain is to reduce symptoms as much as possible, especially in combination with other treatments
- Treatment of depression most often reduces or even eliminates symptoms, but not a cure since symptoms can recur after medicine stopped
- Treatment of chronic neuropathic pain may reduce symptoms, but rarely eliminates them completely, and is not a cure since symptoms can recur after medicine is stopped
- Continue treatment of depression until all symptoms are gone (remission)
- Once symptoms of depression are gone, continue treating for 1 year for the first episode of depression
- For second and subsequent episodes of depression, treatment may need to be indefinite
- Use in anxiety disorders and chronic pain may also need to be indefinite, but long-term treatment is not well studied in these conditions

If It Doesn't Work

- Many depressed patients have only a partial response where some symptoms are improved but others persist (especially insomnia, fatigue, and problems concentrating)
- Other depressed patients may be nonresponders, sometimes called treatment-resistant or treatment-refractory
- Consider increasing dose, switching to another agent or adding an appropriate augmenting agent
- Consider psychotherapy
- Consider evaluation for another diagnosis or for a comorbid condition (e.g., medical illness, substance abuse, etc.)
- Some patients may experience apparent lack of consistent efficacy due to activation of latent or underlying bipolar disorder, and require antidepressant discontinuation and a switch to a mood stabilizer

Best Augmenting Combos for Partial Response or Treatment Resistance

- Lithium, buspirone, thyroid hormone (for depression)
- Gabapentin, tiagabine, other anticonvulsants, even opiates if done by experts while monitoring carefully in difficult cases (for chronic pain)

Tests

- Baseline ECG is recommended for patients over age 50
- ❊ Since tricyclic and tetracyclic antidepressants are frequently associated with weight gain, before starting treatment, weigh all patients and determine if the patient is already overweight (BMI 25.0–29.9) or obese (BMI ≥30)
- Before giving a drug that can cause weight gain to an overweight or obese patient, consider determining whether the patient already has pre-diabetes (fasting plasma glucose 100–125 mg/dL), diabetes (fasting plasma glucose >126 mg/dL), or dyslipidemia (increased total cholesterol, LDL cholesterol, and triglycerides; decreased HDL cholesterol), and treat or refer such patients for treatment, including nutrition and weight management, physical activity counseling, smoking cessation, and medical management
- ❊ Monitor weight and BMI during treatment
- ❊ While giving a drug to a patient who has gained >5% of initial weight, consider evaluating for the presence of pre-diabetes, diabetes, or dyslipidemia, or consider switching to a different antipsychotic
- EKGs may be useful for selected patients (e.g., those with personal or family history of QTc prolongation; cardiac arrhythmia; recent myocardial infarction; uncompensated heart failure; or taking agents that prolong QTc interval such as pimozide, thioridazine, selected antiarrhythmics, moxifloxacin, sparfloxacin, etc.)
- Patients at risk for electrolyte disturbances (e.g., patients on diuretic therapy) should have baseline and periodic serum potassium and magnesium measurements

SIDE EFFECTS

How Drug Causes Side Effects

- Anticholinergic activity may explain sedative effects, dry mouth, constipation, and blurred vision
- Sedative effects and weight gain may be due to antihistamine properties
- Blockade of alpha adrenergic 1 receptors may explain dizziness, sedation, and hypotension
- Cardiac arrhythmias and seizures, especially in overdose, may be caused by blockade of ion channels

Notable Side Effects

- Blurred vision, constipation, urinary retention, increased appetite, dry mouth, nausea, diarrhea, heartburn, unusual taste in mouth, weight gain
- Fatigue, weakness, dizziness, sedation, headache, anxiety, nervousness, restlessness
- Sexual dysfunction (impotence, change in libido)
- Sweating, rash, itching

Life-Threatening or Dangerous Side Effects

- Paralytic ileus, hyperthermia (TCAs + anticholinergic agents)
- Lowered seizure threshold and rare seizures
- Orthostatic hypotension, sudden death, arrhythmias, tachycardia
- QTc prolongation
- Hepatic failure, extrapyramidal symptoms
- Increased intraocular pressure
- Rare induction of mania
- Rare activation of suicidal ideation and behavior (suicidality) (short-term studies did not show an increase in the risk of suicidality with antidepressants compared to placebo beyond age 24)

Weight Gain

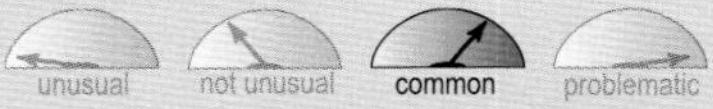

- Many experience and/or can be significant in amount
- Can increase appetite and carbohydrate craving

Sedation

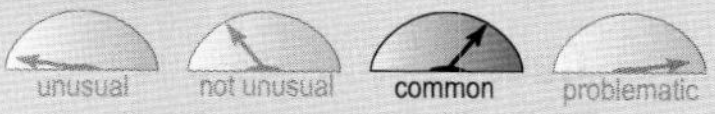

- Many experience and/or can be significant in amount
- Tolerance to sedative effects may develop with long-term use

What to Do About Side Effects

- Wait
- Wait
- Wait
- Lower the dose
- Switch to an SSRI or newer antidepressant

Best Augmenting Agents for Side Effects

- Many side effects cannot be improved with an augmenting agent

DOSING AND USE

Usual Dosage Range

- 50–150 mg/day

Dosage Forms

- Capsule 25 mg, 50 mg, 100 mg

How to Dose

- Initial 25 mg/day at bedtime; increase by 75 mg every 3–7 days
- 75 mg/day in divided doses; increase to 150 mg/day; maximum 200 mg/day; hospitalized patients may receive doses up to 300 mg/day

Dosing Tips

- If given in a single dose, should generally be administered at bedtime because of its sedative properties
- If given in split doses, largest dose should generally be given at bedtime because of its sedative properties
- If patients experience nightmares, split dose and do not give large dose at bedtime
- Patients treated for chronic pain may only require lower doses
- If intolerable anxiety, insomnia, agitation, akathisia, or activation occur either upon dosing initiation or discontinuation, consider the possibility of activated bipolar disorder, and switch to a mood stabilizer or an atypical antipsychotic

Overdose

- Death may occur; CNS depression, convulsions, cardiac dysrhythmias, severe hypotension, EKG changes, coma

Long-Term Use

- Safe

Habit Forming

- No

How to Stop

- Taper to avoid withdrawal effects
- Even with gradual dose reduction some withdrawal symptoms may appear within the first 2 weeks
- Many patients tolerate 50% dose reduction for 3 days, then another 50% reduction for 3 days, then discontinuation
- If withdrawal symptoms emerge during discontinuation, raise dose to stop symptoms and then restart withdrawal much more slowly

Pharmacokinetics

- Substrate for CYP450 2D6, 2C19, and 2C9
- Half-life approximately 7–23 hours

Drug Interactions

- Tramadol increases the risk of seizures in patients taking TCAs
- Use of TCAs with anticholinergic drugs may result in paralytic ileus or hyperthermia
- Fluoxetine, paroxetine, bupropion, duloxetine, and other CYP450 2D6 inhibitors may increase TCA concentrations
- Cimetidine may increase plasma concentrations of TCAs and cause anticholinergic symptoms
- Phenothiazines or haloperidol may raise TCA blood concentrations
- May alter effects of antihypertensive drugs; may inhibit hypotensive effects of clonidine
- Use with sympathomimetic agents may increase sympathetic activity
- Methylphenidate may inhibit metabolism of TCAs
- Activation and agitation, especially following switching or adding antidepressants, may represent the

induction of a bipolar state, especially a mixed dysphoric bipolar II condition sometimes associated with suicidal ideation, and require the addition of lithium, a mood stabilizer or an atypical antipsychotic, and/or discontinuation of trimipramine

Other Warnings/ Precautions

- Add or initiate other antidepressants with caution for up to 2 weeks after discontinuing trimipramine
- Generally, do not use with MAOIs, including 14 days after MAOIs are stopped; do not start an MAOI for at least 5 half-lives (5 to 7 days for most drugs) after discontinuing trimipramine, but see Pearls
- Use with caution in patients with history of seizures, urinary retention, angle-closure glaucoma, hyperthyroidism
- TCAs can increase QTc interval, especially at toxic doses, which can be attained not only by overdose but also by combining with drugs that inhibit TCA metabolism via CYP450 2D6, potentially causing torsade de pointes-type arrhythmia or sudden death
- Because TCAs can prolong QTc interval, use with caution in patients who have bradycardia or who are taking drugs that can induce bradycardia (e.g., beta blockers, calcium channel blockers, clonidine, digitalis)
- Because TCAs can prolong QTc interval, use with caution in patients who have hypokalemia and/or hypomagnesemia or who are taking drugs that can induce hypokalemia and/or magnesemia (e.g., diuretics, stimulant laxatives, intravenous amphotericin B, glucocorticoids, tetracosactide)
- When treating children, carefully weigh the risks and benefits of pharmacological treatment against the risks and benefits of nontreatment with antidepressants and make sure to document this in the patient's chart
- Distribute the brochures provided by the FDA and the drug companies
- Warn patients and their caregivers about the possibility of activating side effects and advise them to report such symptoms immediately
- Monitor patients for activation of suicidal ideation, especially children and adolescents

Do Not Use

- If patient is recovering from myocardial infarction
- If patient is taking agents capable of significantly prolonging QTc interval (e.g., pimozide, thioridazine, selected antiarrhythmics, moxifloxacin, sparfloxacin)
- If there is a history of QTc prolongation or cardiac arrhythmia, recent acute myocardial infarction, uncompensated heart failure
- If patient is taking drugs that inhibit TCA metabolism, including CYP450 2D6 inhibitors, except by an expert
- If there is reduced CYP450 2D6 function, such as patients who are poor 2D6 metabolizers, except by an expert and at low doses
- If there is a proven allergy to trimipramine

SPECIAL POPULATIONS

Renal Impairment

- Use with caution; may need to lower dose

Hepatic Impairment

- Use with caution; may need to lower dose

Cardiac Impairment

- Baseline ECG is recommended
- TCAs have been reported to cause arrhythmias, prolongation of conduction time, orthostatic hypotension, sinus tachycardia, and heart failure, especially in the diseased heart
- Myocardial infarction and stroke have been reported with TCAs
- TCAs produce QTc prolongation, which may be enhanced by the existence of bradycardia, hypokalemia, congenital or acquired long QTc interval, which should be evaluated prior to administering trimipramine
- Use with caution if treating concomitantly with a medication likely to produce prolonged bradycardia, hypokalemia, slowing of intracardiac conduction, or prolongation of the QTc interval
- Avoid TCAs in patients with a known history of QTc prolongation, recent acute

myocardial infarction, and uncompensated heart failure
- TCAs may cause a sustained increase in heart rate in patients with ischemic heart disease and may worsen (decrease) heart rate variability, an independent risk of mortality in cardiac populations
- Since SSRIs may improve (increase) heart rate variability in patients following a myocardial infarct and may improve survival as well as mood in patients with acute angina or following a myocardial infarction, these are more appropriate agents for cardiac population than tricyclic/tetracyclic antidepressants

✻ Risk/benefit ratio may not justify use of TCAs in cardiac impairment

Elderly

- Baseline ECG is recommended for patients over age 50
- May be more sensitive to anticholinergic, cardiovascular, hypotensive, and sedative effects
- Initial dose 50 mg/day; increase gradually up to 100 mg/day
- Reduction in the risk of suicidality with antidepressants compared to placebo in adults age 65 and older

Children and Adolescents

- Carefully weigh the risks and benefits of pharmacological treatment against the risks and benefits of nontreatment with antidepressants and make sure to document this in the patient's chart
- Monitor patients face-to-face regularly, particularly during the first several weeks of treatment
- Use with caution, observing for activation of known or unknown bipolar disorder and/or suicidal ideation, and inform parents or guardians of this risk so they can help observe child or adolescent patients
- Not recommended for use in children under age 12
- Several studies show lack of efficacy of TCAs for depression
- May be used to treat enuresis or hyperactive/impulsive behaviors
- Some cases of sudden death have occurred in children taking TCAs
- Adolescents: initial dose 50 mg/day; increase gradually up to 100 mg/day

Pregnancy

- Effective June 30, 2015, the US FDA requires changes to the content and format of pregnancy and lactation information in prescription drug labels, including the elimination of the pregnancy letter categories; the Pregnancy and Lactation Labeling Rule (PLLR or final rule) applies only to prescription drugs and will be phased in gradually for drugs approved on or after June 30, 2001
- Controlled studies have not been conducted in pregnant women
- Crosses the placenta
- Adverse effects have been reported in infants whose mothers took a TCA (lethargy, withdrawal symptoms, fetal malformations)
- Must weigh the risk of treatment (first trimester fetal development, third trimester newborn delivery) to the child against the risk of no treatment (recurrence of depression, maternal health, infant bonding) to the mother and child
- For many patients this may mean continuing treatment during pregnancy

Breast Feeding

- Some drug is found in mother's breast milk

✻ Recommended either to discontinue drug or bottle feed

- Immediate postpartum period is a high-risk time for depression, especially in women who have had prior depressive episodes, so drug may need to be reinstituted late in the third trimester or shortly after childbirth to prevent a recurrence during the postpartum period
- Must weigh the risk of treatment (first trimester fetal development, third trimester newborn delivery) to the child against the risk of no treatment (recurrence of depression, maternal health, infant bonding) to the mother and child
- For many patients this may mean continuing treatment during breast feeding

THE ART OF PSYCHOPHARMACOLOGY

Potential Advantages

- Patients with insomnia, anxiety
- Severe or treatment-resistant depression

Potential Disadvantages

- Pediatric and geriatric patients
- Patients concerned with weight gain and sedation

Primary Target Symptoms

- Depressed mood
- Symptoms of anxiety
- Somatic symptoms

Pearls

❋ May be more useful than some other TCAs for patients with anxiety, sleep disturbance, and depression with physical illness

❋ May be more sedating than some other TCAs

- TCAs are often a first-line treatment option for chronic pain
- TCAs are no longer generally considered a first-line option for depression because of their side effect profile
- TCAs continue to be useful for severe or treatment-resistant depression
- TCAs may aggravate psychotic symptoms
- Alcohol should be avoided because of additive CNS effects
- Underweight patients may be more susceptible to adverse cardiovascular effects
- Children, patients with inadequate hydration, and patients with cardiac disease may be more susceptible to TCA-induced cardiotoxicity than healthy adults
- For the expert only: although generally prohibited, a heroic but potentially dangerous treatment for severely treatment-resistant patients is for an expert to give a tricyclic/tetracyclic antidepressant other than clomipramine simultaneously with an MAOI for patients who fail to respond to numerous other antidepressants
- If this option is elected, start the MAOI with the tricyclic/tetracyclic antidepressant simultaneously at low doses after appropriate drug washout, then alternately increase doses of these agents every few days to a week as tolerated
- Although very strict dietary and concomitant drug restrictions must be observed to prevent hypertensive crises and serotonin syndrome, the most common side effects of MAOI and tricyclic/tetracyclic antidepressant combinations may be weight gain and orthostatic hypotension
- Patients on tricyclics should be aware that they may experience symptoms such as photosensitivity or blue-green urine
- SSRIs may be more effective than TCAs in women, and TCAs may be more effective than SSRIs in men
- Since tricyclic/tetracyclic antidepressants are substrates for CYP450 2D6, and 7% of the population (especially Caucasians) may have a genetic variant leading to reduced activity of 2D6, such patients may not safely tolerate normal doses of tricyclic/tetracyclic antidepressants and may require dose reduction
- Phenotypic testing may be necessary to detect this genetic variant prior to dosing with a tricyclic/tetracyclic antidepressant, especially in vulnerable populations such as children, elderly, cardiac populations, and those on concomitant medications
- Patients who seem to have extraordinarily severe side effects at normal or low doses may have this phenotypic CYP450 2D6 variant and require low doses or switching to another antidepressant not metabolized by 2D6

Suggested Reading

Anderson IM. Meta-analytical studies on new antidepressants. Br Med Bull 2001;57:161–78.

Anderson IM. Selective serotonin reuptake inhibitors versus tricyclic antidepressants: a meta-analysis of efficacy and tolerability. J Aff Disorders 2000;58:19–36.

Berger M, Gastpar M. Trimipramine: a challenge to current concepts on antidepressives. Eur Arch Psychiatry Clin Neurosci 1996;246:235–9.

Lapierre YD. A review of trimipramine. 30 years of clinical use. Drugs 1989;38(Suppl 1):S17–24; discussion S49–50.

THERAPEUTICS

Brands
- Depakene
- Depacon
- Depakote, Depakote ER
- Stavzor

see index for additional brand names

Generic? Yes

Class
- Neuroscience-based Nomenclature: glutamate (Glu); yet to be determined
- Anticonvulsant, mood stabilizer, migraine prophylaxis, voltage-sensitive sodium channel modulator

Commonly Prescribed for
(bold for FDA approved)
- **Acute mania (divalproex) and mixed episodes (divalproex, divalproex ER, valproic acid delayed-release)**
- **Complex partial seizures that occur either in isolation or in association with other types of seizures (monotherapy and adjunctive)**
- **Simple and complex absence seizures (monotherapy and adjunctive)**
- **Multiple seizure types, which include absence seizures (adjunctive)**
- **Migraine prophylaxis (divalproex, divalproex ER, valproic acid delayed-release)**
- Maintenance treatment of bipolar disorder
- Bipolar depression
- Psychosis, schizophrenia (adjunctive)

How the Drug Works
✻ Blocks voltage-sensitive sodium channels by an unknown mechanism
- Increases brain concentrations of gamma-aminobutyric acid (GABA) by an unknown mechanism

How Long Until It Works
- For acute mania, effects should occur within a few days depending on the formulation of the drug
- May take several weeks to months to optimize an effect on mood stabilization
- Should also reduce seizures and improve migraine within a few weeks

If It Works
- The goal of treatment is complete remission of symptoms (e.g., mania, seizures, migraine)
- Continue treatment until all symptoms are gone or until improvement is stable and then continue treating indefinitely as long as improvement persists
- Continue treatment indefinitely to avoid recurrence of mania, depression, seizures, and headaches

If It Doesn't Work (for bipolar disorder)
✻ Many patients have only a partial response where some symptoms are improved but others persist or continue to wax and wane without stabilization of mood
- Other patients may be nonresponders, sometimes called treatment-resistant or treatment-refractory
- Consider checking plasma drug level, increasing dose, switching to another agent or adding an appropriate augmenting agent
- Consider adding psychotherapy
- Consider the presence of noncompliance and counsel patient
- Switch to another mood stabilizer with fewer side effects
- Consider evaluation for another diagnosis or for a comorbid condition (e.g., medical illness, substance abuse, etc.)

Best Augmenting Combos for Partial Response or Treatment Resistance (for bipolar disorder)
- Lithium
- Atypical antipsychotics (especially risperidone, olanzapine, quetiapine, ziprasidone, and aripiprazole)

✻ Lamotrigine (with caution and at half the dose in the presence of valproate because valproate can double lamotrigine levels)

✻ Antidepressants (with caution because antidepressants can destabilize mood in some patients, including induction of rapid cycling or suicidal ideation; in particular consider bupropion; also SSRIs, SNRIs, others; generally avoid TCAs, MAOIs)

Tests
✻ Before starting treatment, complete blood counts, coagulation tests, and liver function tests

- Consider coagulation tests prior to planned surgery or if there is a history of bleeding
- During the first few months of treatment, regular liver function tests and platelet counts; this can be shifted to once or twice a year for the remainder of treatment
- Plasma drug levels can assist monitoring of efficacy, side effects, and compliance

✽ Since valproate is frequently associated with weight gain, before starting treatment, weigh all patients and determine if the patient is already overweight (BMI 25.0–29.9) or obese (BMI ≥30)

- Before giving a drug that can cause weight gain to an overweight or obese patient, consider determining whether the patient already has pre-diabetes (fasting plasma glucose 100–125 mg/dL), diabetes (fasting plasma glucose >126 mg/dL), or dyslipidemia (increased total cholesterol, LDL cholesterol, and triglycerides; decreased HDL cholesterol), and treat or refer such patients for treatment, including nutrition and weight management, physical activity counseling, smoking cessation, and medical management

✽ Monitor weight and BMI during treatment

✽ While giving a drug to a patient who has gained >5% of initial weight, consider evaluating for the presence of pre-diabetes, diabetes, or dyslipidemia, or consider switching to a different agent

SIDE EFFECTS

How Drug Causes Side Effects

- CNS side effects theoretically due to excessive actions at voltage-sensitive sodium channels

Notable Side Effects

✽ Sedation, dose-dependent tremor, dizziness, ataxia, asthenia, headache

✽ Abdominal pain, nausea, vomiting, diarrhea, reduced appetite, constipation, dyspepsia, weight gain

✽ Alopecia (unusual)

- Polycystic ovaries (controversial)
- Hyperandrogenism, hyperinsulinemia, lipid dysregulation (controversial)
- Decreased bone mineral density (controversial)

Life-Threatening or Dangerous Side Effects

- Can cause tachycardia or bradycardia
- Rare hepatotoxicity with liver failure sometimes severe and fatal, particularly in children under 2 years old
- Rare pancreatitis, sometimes fatal
- Rare but serious skin condition known as Drug Reaction with Eosinophilia (DRESS)
- Rare activation of suicidal ideation and behavior (suicidality)

Weight Gain

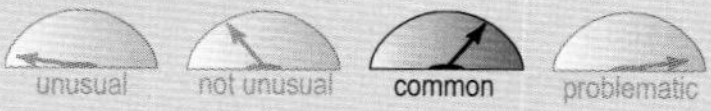

- Many experience and/or can be significant in amount
- Can become a health problem in some

Sedation

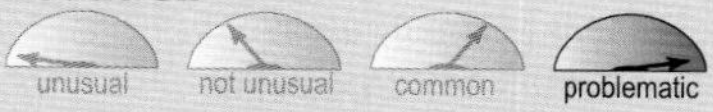

- Frequent and can be significant in amount
- Some patients may not tolerate it
- Can wear off over time
- Can reemerge as dose increases and then wear off again over time

What to Do About Side Effects

- Wait
- Wait
- Wait
- Take at night to reduce daytime sedation, especially with divalproex ER
- Lower the dose
- Switch to another agent

Best Augmenting Agents for Side Effects

✽ Propranolol 20–30 mg 2–3 times/day may reduce tremor

✽ Multivitamins fortified with zinc and selenium may help reduce alopecia

- Many side effects cannot be improved with an augmenting agent

DOSING AND USE

Usual Dosage Range

- Mania: 1,200–1,500 mg/day
- Migraine: 500–1,000 mg/day
- Epilepsy: 10–60 mg/kg per day

Dosage Forms

- Tablet [delayed-release, as divalproex sodium (Depakote)] 125 mg, 250 mg, 500 mg
- Tablet [extended-release, as divalproex sodium (Depakote ER)] 250 mg, 500 mg
- Capsule [sprinkle, as divalproex sodium (Depakote Sprinkle)] 125 mg
- Capsule [as valproic acid (Depakene)] 250 mg
- Capsule [delayed-release, as valproic acid (Stavzor)] 125 mg, 250 mg, 500 mg
- Injection [as sodium valproate (Depacon)] 100 mg/mL (5 mL)
- Syrup [as sodium valproate (Depakene)] 250 mg/5mL

How to Dose

- Usual starting dose for mania or epilepsy is 15 mg/kg in 2 divided doses (once daily for extended-release valproate)
- Acute mania (adults): initial 1,000 mg/day; increase dose rapidly; maximum dose generally 60 mg/kg per day
- For less acute mania, may begin at 250–500 mg the first day, and then titrate upward as tolerated
- Migraine (adults): initial 500 mg/day; maximum recommended dose 1,000 mg/day
- Epilepsy (adults): initial 10–15 mg/kg per day; increase by 5–10 mg/kg per week; maximum dose generally 60 mg/kg per day

Dosing Tips

* Oral loading with 20–30 mg/kg per day may reduce onset of action to 5 days or less and may be especially useful for treatment of acute mania in inpatient settings
- Given the half-life of immediate-release valproate (e.g., Depakene, Depakote), twice daily dosing is probably ideal
- Extended-release valproate (e.g., Depakote ER) can be given once daily
- However, extended-release valproate is only about 80% as bioavailable as immediate-release valproate, producing plasma drug levels 10–20% lower than with immediate-release valproate
* Thus, extended-release valproate is dosed approximately 8–20% higher when converting patients to the ER formulation
- Depakote (divalproex sodium) is an enteric-coated stable compound containing both valproic acid and sodium valproate
* Divalproex immediate-release formulation reduces gastrointestinal side effects compared to generic valproate
* Divalproex ER improves gastrointestinal side effects and alopecia compared to immediate-release divalproex or generic valproate
- The amide of valproic acid is available in Europe [valpromide (Depamide)]
- Trough plasma drug levels >45 μg/mL may be required for either antimanic effects or anticonvulsant actions
- Trough plasma drug levels up to 100 μg/mL are generally well tolerated
- Trough plasma drug levels up to 125 μg/mL may be required in some acutely manic patients
- Dosages to achieve therapeutic plasma levels vary widely, often between 750–3,000 mg/day

Overdose

- Fatalities have been reported; coma, restlessness, hallucinations, sedation, heart block

Long-Term Use

- Requires regular liver function tests and platelet counts

Habit Forming

- No

How to Stop

- Taper; may need to adjust dosage of concurrent medications as valproate is being discontinued
- Patients may seize upon withdrawal, especially if withdrawal is abrupt
* Rapid discontinuation increases the risk of relapse in bipolar disorder
- Discontinuation symptoms uncommon

Pharmacokinetics

- Mean terminal half-life 9–16 hours
- Metabolized primarily by the liver, approximately 25% dependent upon CYP450 system (CYP450 2C9 and 2C19)
- Inhibits CYP450 2C9
- Food slows rate but not extent of absorption

Drug Interactions

* Lamotrigine dose should be reduced by perhaps 50% if used with valproate,

as valproate inhibits metabolism of lamotrigine and raises lamotrigine plasma levels, theoretically increasing the risk of rash
- Plasma levels of valproate may be lowered by carbamazepine, phenytoin, ethosuximide, phenobarbital, rifampin
- Aspirin may inhibit metabolism of valproate and increase valproate plasma levels
- Plasma levels of valproate may also be increased by felbamate, chlorpromazine, fluoxetine, fluvoxamine, topiramate, cimetidine, erythromycin, and ibuprofen
- Valproate inhibits metabolism of ethosuximide, phenobarbital, and phenytoin, and can thus increase their plasma levels
- No likely pharmacokinetic interactions of valproate with lithium or atypical antipsychotics
- Use of valproate with clonazepam may cause absence status
- Reports of hyperammonemia with or without encephalopthay in patients taking topiramate combined with valproate, though this is not due to a pharmacokinetic interaction; in patients who develop unexplained lethargy, vomiting, or change in mental status, an ammonia level should be measured

Other Warnings/ Precautions

✻ Be alert to the following symptoms of hepatotoxicity that require immediate attention: malaise, weakness, lethargy, facial edema, anorexia, vomiting, yellowing of the skin and eyes

✻ Be alert to the following symptoms of pancreatitis that require immediate attention: abdominal pain, nausea, vomiting, anorexia

✻ Teratogenic effects in developing fetuses such as neural tube defects may occur with valproate use

✻ Somnolence may be more common in the elderly and may be associated with dehydration, reduced nutritional intake, and weight loss, requiring slower dosage increases, lower doses, and monitoring of fluid and nutritional intake

- Use in patients with thrombocytopenia is not recommended; patients should report easy bruising or bleeding
- Evaluate for urea cycle disorders, as hyperammonemic encephalopathy, sometimes fatal, has been associated with valproate administration in these uncommon disorders; urea cycle disorders, such as ormithine transcarbamylase deficiency, are associated with unexplained encephalopathy, mental retardation, elevated plasma ammonia, cyclical vomiting, and lethargy
- Valproate is associated with a rare but serious skin condition known as Drug Reaction with Eosinophilia (DRESS). DRESS may begin as a rash but can progress to others parts of the body and can include symptoms such as fever, swollen lymph nodes, inflammation of organs, and an increase in white blood cells known as eosinophilia. In some cases, DRESS can lead to death.
- Warn patients and their caregivers about the possibility of activation of suicidal ideation and advise them to report such side effects immediately

Do Not Use

- If patient has pancreatitis
- If patient has serious liver disease
- If patient has urea cycle disorder
- If there is a proven allergy to valproic acid, valproate, or divalproex

SPECIAL POPULATIONS

Renal Impairment

- No dose adjustment necessary

Hepatic Impairment

- Contraindicated

Cardiac Impairment

- No dose adjustment necessary

Elderly

- Reduce starting dose and titrate slowly; dosing is generally lower than in healthy adults

✻ Sedation in the elderly may be more common and associated with dehydration, reduced nutritional intake, and weight loss

- Monitor fluid and nutritional intake
- 1 in 3 elderly patients in long-term care who receive valproate may ultimately develop thrombocytopenia

Children and Adolescents

✽ Not generally recommended for use in children under age 10 for bipolar disorder except by experts and when other options have been considered
- Children under age 2 have significantly increased risk of hepatotoxicity, as they have a markedly decreased ability to eliminate valproate compared to older children and adults
- Use requires close medical supervision

Pregnancy

- Effective June 30, 2015, the US FDA requires changes to the content and format of pregnancy and lactation information in prescription drug labels, including the elimination of the pregnancy letter categories; the Pregnancy and Lactation Labeling Rule (PLLR or final rule) applies only to prescription drugs and will be phased in gradually for drugs approved on or after June 30, 2001

✽ Use during first trimester may raise risk of neural tube defects (e.g., spina bifida) or other congenital anomalies
- Cases of developmental delay in the absence of teratogenicity associated with fetal exposure have been identified
- Increased risk of lower cognitive test scores in children whose mothers took valproate during pregnancy
- Use in women of childbearing potential requires weighing potential benefits to the mother against the risks to the fetus

✽ If drug is continued, monitor clotting parameters and perform tests to detect birth defects

✽ If drug is continued, start on folate 1 mg/day early in pregnancy to reduce risk of neural tube defects

✽ If drug is continued, consider vitamin K during the last 6 weeks of pregnancy to reduce risks of bleeding
- Antiepileptic Drug Pregnancy Registry: (888) 233–2334
- Taper drug if discontinuing
- Seizures, even mild seizures, may cause harm to the embryo/fetus

✽ For bipolar patients, valproate should generally be discontinued before anticipated pregnancies
- Recurrent bipolar illness during pregnancy can be quite disruptive

✽ For bipolar patients, given the risk of relapse in the postpartum period, mood stabilizer treatment such as valproate should generally be restarted immediately after delivery if patient is unmedicated during pregnancy

✽ Atypical antipsychotics may be preferable to lithium or anticonvulsants such as valproate if treatment of bipolar disorder is required during pregnancy
- Bipolar symptoms may recur or worsen during pregnancy and some form of treatment may be necessary

Breast Feeding

- Some drug is found in mother's breast milk

✽ Generally considered safe to breast feed while taking valproate
- If drug is continued while breast feeding, infant should be monitored for possible adverse effects
- If infant shows signs of irritability or sedation, drug may need to be discontinued

✽ Bipolar disorder may recur during the postpartum period, particularly if there is a history of prior postpartum episodes of either depression or psychosis

✽ Relapse rates may be lower in women who receive prophylactic treatment for postpartum episodes of bipolar disorder
- Atypical antipsychotics and anticonvulsants such as valproate may be safer than lithium during the postpartum period when breast feeding

THE ART OF PSYCHOPHARMACOLOGY

Potential Advantages

- Manic phase of bipolar disorder
- Works well in combination with lithium and/or atypical antipsychotics
- Patients for whom therapeutic drug monitoring is desirable

Potential Disadvantages

- Depressed phase of bipolar disorder
- Patients unable to tolerate sedation or weight gain

- Multiple drug interactions
- Multiple side effect risks
- Pregnant patients

Primary Target Symptoms

- Unstable mood
- Incidence of migraine
- Incidence of partial complex seizures

Pearls (for bipolar disorder)

* ✻ Valproate is a first-line treatment option that may be best for patients with mixed states of bipolar disorder or for patients with rapid-cycling bipolar disorder
* ✻ Seems to be more effective in treating manic episodes than depressive episodes in bipolar disorder (treats from above better than it treats from below)
* ✻ May also be more effective in preventing manic relapses than in preventing depressive episodes (stabilizes from above better than it stabilizes from below)
* Only a third of bipolar patients experience adequate relief with a monotherapy, so most patients need multiple medications for best control
* Useful in combination with atypical antipsychotics and/or lithium for acute mania
* ✻ May also be useful for bipolar disorder in combination with lamotrigine, but must reduce lamotrigine dose by half when combined with valproate
* Usefulness for bipolar disorder in combination with anticonvulsants other than lamotrigine is not well demonstrated; such combinations can be expensive and are possibly ineffective or even irrational
* ✻ May be useful as an adjunct to atypical antipsychotics for rapid onset of action in schizophrenia
* ✻ Used to treat aggression, agitation, and impulsivity not only in bipolar disorder and schizophrenia but also in many other disorders, including dementia, personality disorders, and brain injury
* Patients with acute mania tend to tolerate side effects better than patients with hypomania or depression
* Multivitamins fortified with zinc and selenium may help reduce alopecia
* Association of valproate with polycystic ovaries is controversial and may be related to weight gain, obesity, or epilepsy
* Nevertheless, may wish to be cautious in administering valproate to women of childbearing potential, especially adolescent female bipolar patients, and carefully monitor weight, endocrine status, and ovarian size and function
* ✻ In women of childbearing potential who are or are likely to become sexually active, should inform about risk of harm to the fetus and monitor contraceptive status
* Association of valproate with decreased bone mass is controversial and may be related to activity levels, exposure to sunlight, and epilepsy, and might be prevented by supplemental vitamin D 2,000 IU/day and calcium 600–1,000 mg/day
* New delayed-release capsule of valproic acid (Stavzor) may be easier to swallow than other formulations
* A prodrug of valproic acid, valpromide, is available in several European countries
* Although valpromide is rapidly transformed to valproic acid, it has some unique characteristics that can affect drug interactions
* In particular, valpromide is a potent inhibitor of liver microsomal epoxide hydrolase and thus causes clinically significant increases in the plasma levels of carbamazepine-10,11-epoxide (the active metabolite of carbamazepine)

Suggested Reading

Bowden CL. Valproate. Bipolar Disorders 2003;5:189–202.

Gill D, Derry S, Wiffen PJ, Moore RA. Valproic acid and sodium valproate for neuropathic pain and fibromyalgia in adults. Cochrane Database Syst Rev 2011;(10):CD009183.

Landy SH, McGinnis J. Divalproex sodium – review of prophylactic migraine efficacy, safety and dosage, with recommendations. Tenn Med 1999;92:135–6.

Macritchie KA, Geddes JR, Scott J, Haslam DR, Goodwin GM. Valproic acid, valproate and divalproex in the maintenance treatment of bipolar disorder. Cochrane Database Syst Rev 2001;(3):CD003196.

Smith LA, Cornelius V, Warnock A, Tacchi MJ, Taylor D. Pharmacological interventions for acute bipolar mania: a systematic review of randomized placebo-controlled trials. Bipolar Disord 2007;9(6):551–60.

VARENICLINE

THERAPEUTICS

Brands • Chantix
• Champix

see index for additional brand names

Generic? No

Class
- Neuroscience-based Nomenclature: Acetylcholine receptor partial agonist (ACh-RPA)
- Smoking cessation treatment; alpha 4 beta 2 partial agonist at nicotinic acetylcholine receptors

Commonly Prescribed for
(bold for FDA approved)
- **Nicotine addiction/dependence**

How the Drug Works
- Causes sustained but small amounts of dopamine release (less than with nicotine)
- Specifically, as a partial agonist at alpha 4 beta 2 nicotinic acetylcholine receptors, varenicline activates these receptors to a lesser extent than the full agonist nicotine and also prevents nicotine from binding to these receptors
- Most prominent actions are on mesolimbic dopaminergic neurons in the ventral tegmental area

How Long Until It Works
- Recommended initial treatment trial is 12 weeks; an additional 12-week trial in individuals who stop smoking after 12 weeks may increase likelihood of long-term abstinence

If It Works
- Reduces withdrawal symptoms and the urge to smoke; increases abstinence

If It Doesn't Work
- Evaluate for and address contributing factors, then reattempt treatment
- Consider switching to another agent

Best Augmenting Combos for Partial Response or Treatment Resistance
- Best to attempt other monotherapies

Tests
- None for healthy individuals

SIDE EFFECTS

How Drug Causes Side Effects
- Theoretically due to increases in dopamine concentrations at receptors in parts of the brain and body other than those that cause therapeutic actions

Notable Side Effects
- Dose-dependent nausea, vomiting, constipation, flatulence
- Insomnia, headache, abnormal dreams

Life-Threatening or Dangerous Side Effects
- Rare activation of agitation, depressed mood, suicidal ideation, suicidal behavior
- Rare seizures

Weight Gain
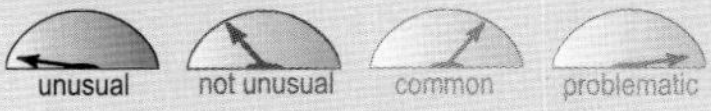

- Reported but not expected
- Some patients report weight loss

Sedation
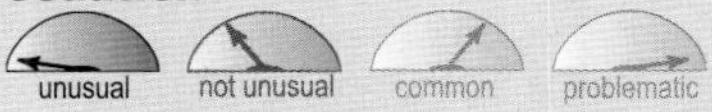

- Reported but not expected
- Some patients report activation and insomnia

What to Do About Side Effects
- Wait
- Adjust dose
- If side effects persist, discontinue use

Best Augmenting Agents for Side Effects
- Dose reduction or switching to another agent may be more effective since most side effects cannot be improved with an augmenting agent

DOSING AND USE

Usual Dosage Range
- 1 mg twice daily

Dosage Forms
- Tablet 0.5 mg, 1 mg

How to Dose
- Patient should either set a quit date and then begin taking varenicline 1 week before the quit date or start varenicline and then quit smoking between days 8 and 35 of treatment
- Initial 0.5 mg/day; after 3 days increase to 1 mg/day in two divided doses; after 4 days can increase to 2 mg/day in two divided doses

Dosing Tips
- Varenicline should be taken following a meal and with a full glass of water
- Providing educational materials and counseling in combination with varenicline treatment can increase the chances of success
- Initial recommended treatment duration is 12 weeks; for individuals who have stopped smoking after 12 weeks continued treatment for an additional 12 weeks can increase the likelihood of long-term abstinence
- For patients who are unsuccessful in their attempt to quit following 12 weeks of treatment or those who relapse following treatment, it is best to attempt to address factors contributing to the failed attempt and then reintroduce treatment

Overdose
- Limited available data

Long-Term Use
- Treatment for up to 24 weeks has been found effective

Habit Forming
- No

How to Stop
- Taper to avoid withdrawal effects, but no well-documented tolerance, dependence, or withdrawal reactions

Pharmacokinetics
- Elimination half-life 24 hours

Drug Interactions
- Does not inhibit hepatic enzymes or renal transport proteins, and thus is unlikely to affect plasma concentrations of other drugs
- Is not hepatically metabolized and thus is unlikely to be affected by other drugs
- Side effects may be increased if varenicline is taken with nicotine replacement therapy
- Varenicline may alter one's reaction to alcohol, with case reports showing decreased tolerance to alcohol, increased drunkenness, unusual or aggressive behavior, or no memory of things that happened

Other Warnings/ Precautions
- Monitor patients for changes in behavior, agitation, depressed mood, worsening of preexisting psychiatric illness, and suicidality
- Use cautiously in individuals with known psychiatric illness
- Use cautiously in patients with a history of seizures or other factors that can lower the seizure threshold
- Discontinuing smoking may lead to pharmacokinetic or pharmacodynamic changes in other drugs the patient is taking, which could potentially require dose adjustment

Do Not Use
- If there is a proven allergy to varenicline

SPECIAL POPULATIONS

Renal Impairment
- For severe impairment, maximum recommended dose is 0.5 mg twice per day
- For patients with end-stage renal disease undergoing hemodialysis, maximum recommended dose is 0.5 mg once per day
- Removed by hemodialysis

Hepatic Impairment
- Dose adjustment not generally necessary

Cardiac Impairment

- Effective in patients with cardiovascular disease; small increased risk of certain cardiovascular adverse effects in these patients

Elderly

- Some patients may tolerate lower doses better

Children and Adolescents

- Safety and efficacy have not been established

Pregnancy

- Effective June 30, 2015, the US FDA requires changes to the content and format of pregnancy and lactation information in prescription drug labels, including the elimination of the pregnancy letter categories; the Pregnancy and Lactation Labeling Rule (PLLR or final rule) applies only to prescription drugs and will be phased in gradually for drugs approved on or after June 30, 2001
- Controlled studies have not been conducted in pregnant women
- Pregnant women wishing to stop smoking may consider behavioral therapy before pharmacotherapy
- Not generally recommended for use during pregnancy, especially during first trimester

Breast Feeding

- Unknown if varenicline is secreted in human breast milk, but all psychotropics assumed to be secreted in breast milk
- Recommended either to discontinue drug or bottle feed

THE ART OF PSYCHOPHARMACOLOGY

Potential Advantages

- More effective than other pharmacotherapies for smoking cessation

Potential Disadvantages

- Not well studied in patients with comorbid psychiatric disorders

Primary Target Symptoms

- Cravings associated with nicotine withdrawal

Pearls

- More effective than nicotine or bupropion
- Unlike nicotine or bupropion, the patient cannot "smoke over" varenicline since varenicline, but not the others, will block the effects of additional smoked nicotine if the patient decides to smoke during treatment
- Although tested in the general population excluding psychiatric patients, where smoking rates in the USA are about 20–25%, there is great unmet need for smoking cessation treatments in patients with psychiatric disorders, especially attention deficit hyperactivity disorder and schizophrenia, which have smoking rates in the USA as high as 50–75%
- Smoking cessation treatment in patients with comorbid psychiatric disorders is not well studied
- Preliminary results suggest that varenicline is not associated with worsening of psychiatric symptoms in stable patients with schizophrenia, schizoaffective disorder, or depression
- Patients with comorbid psychiatric disorders should be closely monitored in terms of their psychiatric symptoms, especially suicidality
- In a large multinational study requested by the FDA, there was no significant increase in moderate-to-severe neuropsychiatric adverse events with varenicline relative to nicotine patch or placebo in participants with or without history of psychiatric disorder

Suggested Reading

Anthenelli RM, Benowitz N, West R, et al. Neuropsychiatric safety and efficacy of varenicline, bupropion, and nicotine patch in smokers with and without psychiatric disorders (EAGLES): a double-blind, randomised, placebo-controlled clinical trial. The Lancet 2016;387(10037):2507–20.

Cerimele JM, Durango A. Does varenicline worsen psychiatric symptoms in patients with schizophrenia or schizoaffective disorder? A review of published studies. J Clin Psychiatry 2012;73(8):e1039–47.

Jorenby DE, Hays JT, Rigotti NA. Efficacy of varenicline, an alpha4beta2 nicotinic acetylcholine receptor partial agonist, vs placebo or sustained-release bupropion for smoking cessation: a randomized controlled trial. JAMA 2006;296(1):56–63.

Meszaros ZS, Abdul-Malak Y, Dimmock JA, et al. Varenicline treatment of concurrent alcohol and nicotine dependence in schizophrenia: a randomized, placebo-controlled pilot trial. J Clin Psychopharmacol 2013;33(2):243–7.

Rollema H, Coe JW, Chambers LK, et al. Rationale, pharmacology and clinical efficacy of partial agonists of alpha4beta2 nACh receptors for smoking cessation. Trends Pharmacol Sci 2007;28(7):316–25.

Wu P, Wilson K, Dimoulas P, Mills EJ. Effectiveness of smoking cessation therapies: a systematic review and meta-analysis. BMC Public Health 2006;6:300.

VENLAFAXINE

THERAPEUTICS

Brands
- Effexor
- Effexor XR

see index for additional brand names

Generic? Yes

Class
- Neuroscience-based Nomenclature: Serotonin and norepinephrine reuptake inhibitor (SN-RI)
- SNRI (dual serotonin and norepinephrine reuptake inhibitor); often classified as an antidepressant, but it is not just an antidepressant

Commonly Prescribed for
(bold for FDA approved)
- **Depression**
- **Generalized anxiety disorder (GAD)**
- **Social anxiety disorder (social phobia)**
- **Panic disorder**
- Posttraumatic stress disorder (PTSD)
- Premenstrual dysphoric disorder (PMDD)

How the Drug Works
- Boosts neurotransmitters serotonin, norepinephrine/noradrenaline, and dopamine
- Blocks serotonin reuptake pump (serotonin transporter), presumably increasing serotonergic neurotransmission
- Blocks norepinephrine reuptake pump (norepinephrine transporter), presumably increasing noradrenergic neurotransmission
- Presumably desensitizes both serotonin 1A receptors and beta adrenergic receptors
- Since dopamine is inactivated by norepinephrine reuptake in frontal cortex, which largely lacks dopamine transporters, venlafaxine can increase dopamine neurotransmission in this part of the brain
- Weakly blocks dopamine reuptake pump (dopamine transporter), and may increase dopamine neurotransmission

How Long Until It Works
- Onset of therapeutic actions usually not immediate, but often delayed 2–4 weeks
- If it is not working within 6–8 weeks for depression, it may require a dosage increase or it may not work at all
- By contrast, for generalized anxiety, onset of response and increases in remission rates may still occur after 8 weeks, and for up to 6 months after initiating dosing
- May continue to work for many years to prevent relapse of symptoms

If It Works
- The goal of treatment is complete remission of current symptoms as well as prevention of future relapses
- Treatment most often reduces or even eliminates symptoms, but not a cure since symptoms can recur after medicine stopped
- Continue treatment until all symptoms are gone (remission), especially in depression and whenever possible in anxiety disorders
- Once symptoms gone, continue treating for 1 year for the first episode of depression
- For second and subsequent episodes of depression, treatment may need to be indefinite
- Use in anxiety disorders may also need to be indefinite

If It Doesn't Work
- Many patients have only a partial response where some symptoms are improved but others persist (especially insomnia, fatigue, and problems concentrating)
- Other patients may be nonresponders, sometimes called treatment-resistant or treatment-refractory
- Some patients who have an initial response may relapse even though they continue treatment, sometimes called "poop-out"
- Consider increasing dose, switching to another agent or adding an appropriate augmenting agent
- Consider psychotherapy
- Consider evaluation for another diagnosis or for a comorbid condition (e.g., medical illness, substance abuse, etc.)
- Some patients may experience apparent lack of consistent efficacy due to activation of latent or underlying bipolar disorder, and require antidepressant discontinuation and a switch to a mood stabilizer

Best Augmenting Combos for Partial Response or Treatment Resistance
✻ Mirtazapine ("California rocket fuel"; a potentially powerful dual serotonin and

norepinephrine combination, but observe for activation of bipolar disorder and suicidal ideation)
- Bupropion, reboxetine, nortriptyline, desipramine, maprotiline, atomoxetine (all potentially powerful enhancers of noradrenergic action, but observe for activation of bipolar disorder and suicidal ideation)
- Modafinil, especially for fatigue, sleepiness, and lack of concentration
- Mood stabilizers or atypical antipsychotics for bipolar depression, psychotic depression, or treatment-resistant depression
- Benzodiazepines
- If all else fails for anxiety disorders, consider gabapentin or tiagabine
- Hypnotics or trazodone for insomnia
- Classically, lithium, buspirone, or thyroid hormone

Tests
- Check blood pressure before initiating treatment and regularly during treatment

SIDE EFFECTS

How Drug Causes Side Effects
- Theoretically due to increases in serotonin and norepinephrine concentrations at receptors in parts of the brain and body other than those that cause therapeutic actions (e.g., unwanted actions of serotonin in sleep centers causing insomnia, unwanted actions of norepinephrine on acetylcholine release causing constipation and dry mouth, etc.)
- Most side effects are immediate but often go away with time

Notable Side Effects
- Most side effects increase with higher doses, at least transiently
- Headache, nervousness, insomnia, sedation
- Nausea, diarrhea, decreased appetite
- Sexual dysfunction (abnormal ejaculation/ orgasm, impotence)
- Asthenia, sweating
- SIADH (syndrome of inappropriate antidiuretic hormone secretion)
- Hyponatremia
- Dose-dependent increase in blood pressure

Life-Threatening or Dangerous Side Effects
- Rare seizures
- Rare induction of hypomania
- Rare activation of suicidal ideation and behavior (suicidality) (short-term studies did not show an increase in the risk of suicidality with antidepressants compared to placebo beyond age 24)

Weight Gain

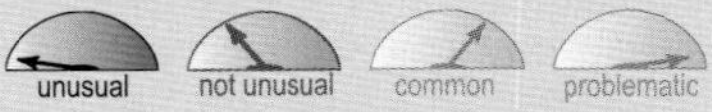

- Reported but not expected
- Possible weight loss, especially short-term

Sedation

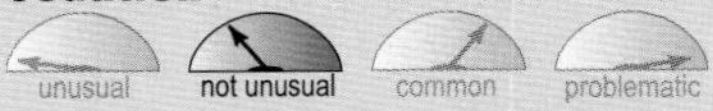

- Occurs in significant minority
- May also be activating in some patients

What to Do About Side Effects
- Wait
- Wait
- Wait
- Lower the dose
- In a few weeks, switch or add other drugs

Best Augmenting Agents for Side Effects
- Often best to try another antidepressant monotherapy prior to resorting to augmentation strategies to treat side effects
- Trazodone or a hypnotic for insomnia
- Bupropion, sildenafil, vardenafil, or tadalafil for sexual dysfunction
- Benzodiazepines for jitteriness and anxiety, especially at initiation of treatment and especially for anxious patients
- Mirtazapine for insomnia, agitation, and gastrointestinal side effects
- Many side effects are dose-dependent (i.e., they increase as dose increases, or they reemerge until tolerance redevelops)
- Many side effects are time-dependent (i.e., they start immediately upon dosing and upon each dose increase, but go away with time)
- Activation and agitation may represent the induction of a bipolar state, especially a mixed dysphoric bipolar II condition

sometimes associated with suicidal ideation, and require the addition of lithium, a mood stabilizer or an atypical antipsychotic, and/or discontinuation of venlafaxine

DOSING AND USE

Usual Dosage Range

- Depression: 75–225 mg/day, once daily (extended-release) or divided into 2–3 doses (immediate-release)
- GAD: 150–225 mg/day

Dosage Forms

- Capsule (extended-release) 37.5 mg, 75 mg, 150 mg
- Tablet (extended-release) 37.5 mg, 75 mg, 150 mg, 225 mg
- Tablet 25 mg scored, 37.5 mg scored, 50 mg scored, 75 mg scored, 100 mg scored

How to Dose

- Initial dose 37.5 mg once daily (extended-release) or 25–50 mg divided into 2–3 doses (immediate-release) for a week, if tolerated; increase daily dose generally no faster than 75 mg every 4 days until desired efficacy is reached; maximum dose generally 375 mg/day
- Usually try doses at 75 mg increments for a few weeks prior to incrementing by an additional 75 mg

Dosing Tips

- At all doses, potent serotonin reuptake blockade
- 75–225 mg/day may be predominantly serotonergic in some patients, and dual serotonin and norepinephrine acting in other patients
- 225–375 mg/day is dual serotonin and norepinephrine acting in most patients

✽ Thus, nonresponders at lower doses should try higher doses to be assured of the benefits of dual SNRI action

- At very high doses (e.g., >375 mg/day), dopamine reuptake blocked as well in some patients
- Up to 600 mg/day has been given for heroic cases
- Venlafaxine has an active metabolite O-desmethylvenlafaxine (ODV), which is formed as the result of CYP450 2D6
- Thus, CYP450 2D6 inhibition reduces the formation of ODV, but this is of uncertain clinical significance

✽ Consider checking plasma levels of ODV and venlafaxine in nonresponders who tolerate high doses, and if plasma levels are low, experts can prudently prescribe doses above 375 mg/day while monitoring closely

- Do not break or chew venlafaxine XR capsules, as this will alter controlled-release properties

✽ For patients with severe problems discontinuing venlafaxine, dosing may need to be tapered over many months (i.e., reduce dose by 1% every 3 days by crushing tablet and suspending or dissolving in 100 mL of fruit juice, and then disposing of 1 mL while drinking the rest; 3–7 days later, dispose of 2 mL, and so on). This is both a form of very slow biological tapering and a form of behavioral desensitization (not for XR)

- For some patients with severe problems discontinuing venlafaxine, it may be useful to add an SSRI with a long half-life, especially fluoxetine, prior to taper of venlafaxine; while maintaining fluoxetine dosing, first slowly taper venlafaxine and then taper fluoxetine
- Be sure to differentiate between reemergence of symptoms requiring reinstitution of treatment and withdrawal symptoms

Overdose

- Can be lethal; may cause no symptoms; possible symptoms include sedation, convulsions, rapid heartbeat
- Fatal toxicity index data from the UK suggest a higher rate of deaths from overdose with venlafaxine than with SSRIs
- Unknown whether this is related to differences in patients who receive venlafaxine or to potential cardiovascular toxicity of venlafaxine

Long-Term Use

- See doctor regularly to monitor blood pressure, especially at doses >225 mg/day

Habit Forming

- No

How to Stop

- Taper to avoid withdrawal effects (dizziness, nausea, stomach cramps, sweating, tingling, dysesthesias)
- Many patients tolerate 50% dose reduction for 3 days, then another 50% reduction for 3 days, then discontinuation
- If withdrawal symptoms emerge during discontinuation, raise dose to stop symptoms and then restart withdrawal much more slowly

✱ Withdrawal effects can be more common or more severe with venlafaxine than with some other antidepressants

Pharmacokinetics

- Parent drug has 3–7 hour half-life
- Active metabolite has 9–13 hour half-life
- Food does not affect absorption

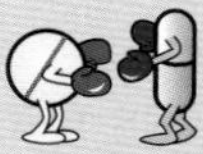

Drug Interactions

- Tramadol increases the risk of seizures in patients taking an antidepressant
- Can cause a fatal "serotonin syndrome" when combined with MAOIs, so do not use with MAOIs or for at least 14 days after MAOIs are stopped
- Do not start an MAOI for at least 5 half-lives (5 to 7 days for most drugs) after discontinuing venlafaxine
- Possible increased risk of bleeding, especially when combined with anticoagulants (e.g., warfarin, NSAIDs)
- Concomitant use with cimetidine may reduce clearance of venlafaxine and raise venlafaxine levels
- Could theoretically interfere with the analgesic actions of codeine or possibly with other triptans
- Few known adverse drug interactions

Other Warnings/ Precautions

- Use with caution in patients with history of seizures
- Use with caution in patients with heart disease
- Use with caution in patients with bipolar disorder unless treated with concomitant mood-stabilizing agent
- When treating children, carefully weigh the risks and benefits of pharmacological treatment against the risks and benefits of nontreatment with antidepressants and make sure to document this in the patient's chart
- Distribute the brochures provided by the FDA and the drug companies
- Warn patients and their caregivers about the possibility of activating side effects and advise them to report such symptoms immediately
- Monitor patients for activation of suicidal ideation, especially children and adolescents

Do Not Use

- If patient has uncontrolled angle-closure glaucoma
- If patient is taking an MAOI
- If there is a proven allergy to venlafaxine

SPECIAL POPULATIONS

Renal Impairment

- Lower dose by 25–50%
- Patients on dialysis should not receive subsequent dose until dialysis is completed

Hepatic Impairment

- Lower dose by 50%

Cardiac Impairment

- Drug should be used with caution
- Hypertension should be controlled prior to initiation of venlafaxine and should be monitored regularly during treatment
- Venlafaxine has a dose-dependent effect on increasing blood pressure
- Venlafaxine is contraindicated in patients with heart disease in the UK
- Venlafaxine can block cardiac ion channels in vitro
- Venlafaxine worsens (i.e., reduces) heart rate variability in depression, perhaps due to norepinephrine reuptake inhibition

Elderly

- Some patients may tolerate lower doses better
- Risk of SIADH with SSRIs is higher in the elderly
- Reduction in the risk of suicidality with antidepressants compared to placebo in adults age 65 and older

Children and Adolescents

- Carefully weigh the risks and benefits of pharmacological treatment against the risks and benefits of nontreatment with antidepressants and make sure to document this in the patient's chart
- Monitor patients face-to-face regularly, particularly during the first several weeks of treatment
- Use with caution, observing for activation of known or unknown bipolar disorder and/or suicidal ideation, and inform parents or guardians of this risk so they can help observe child or adolescent patients
- Not specifically approved, but preliminary data suggest that venlafaxine is effective in children and adolescents with depression, anxiety disorders, and ADHD

Pregnancy

- Effective June 30, 2015, the US FDA requires changes to the content and format of pregnancy and lactation information in prescription drug labels, including the elimination of the pregnancy letter categories; the Pregnancy and Lactation Labeling Rule (PLLR or final rule) applies only to prescription drugs and will be phased in gradually for drugs approved on or after June 30, 2001
- Controlled studies have not been conducted in pregnant women
- Not generally recommended for use during pregnancy, especially during first trimester
- Nonetheless, continuous treatment during pregnancy may be necessary and has not been proven to be harmful to the fetus
- Must weigh the risk of treatment (first trimester fetal development, third trimester newborn delivery) to the child against the risk of no treatment (recurrence of depression, maternal health, infant bonding) to the mother and child
- For many patients this may mean continuing treatment during pregnancy
- Neonates exposed to SSRIs or SNRIs late in the third trimester have developed complications requiring prolonged hospitalization, respiratory support, and tube feeding; reported symptoms are consistent with either a direct toxic effect of SSRIs and SNRIs or, possibly, a drug discontinuation syndrome, and include respiratory distress, cyanosis, apnea, seizures, temperature instability, feeding difficulty, vomiting, hypoglycemia, hypotonia, hypertonia, hyperreflexia, tremor, jitteriness, irritability, and constant crying

Breast Feeding

- Some drug is found in mother's breast milk
- Trace amounts may be present in nursing children whose mothers are on venlafaxine
- If child becomes irritable or sedated, breast feeding or drug may need to be discontinued
- Immediate postpartum period is a high-risk time for depression, especially in women who have had prior depressive episodes, so drug may need to be reinstituted late in the third trimester or shortly after childbirth to prevent a recurrence during the postpartum period
- Must weigh benefits of breast feeding with risks and benefits of antidepressant treatment versus nontreatment to both the infant and the mother
- For many patients, this may mean continuing treatment during breast feeding

THE ART OF PSYCHOPHARMACOLOGY

Potential Advantages

- Patients with retarded depression
- Patients with atypical depression
- Patients with comorbid anxiety
- Patients with depression may have higher remission rates on SNRIs than on SSRIs
- Depressed patients with somatic symptoms, fatigue, and pain
- Patients who do not respond or remit on treatment with SSRIs

Potential Disadvantages

- Patients sensitive to nausea
- Patients with borderline or uncontrolled hypertension
- Patients with cardiac disease

Primary Target Symptoms

- Depressed mood
- Energy, motivation, and interest
- Sleep disturbance
- Anxiety

Pearls

- ✻ May be effective in patients who fail to respond to SSRIs, and may be one of the preferred treatments for treatment-resistant depression
- ✻ May be used in combination with other antidepressants for treatment-refractory cases
- XR formulation improves tolerability, reduces nausea, and requires only once daily dosing
- May be effective in a broad array of anxiety disorders
- May be effective in adult ADHD
- Not studied in stress urinary incontinence
- ✻ Has greater potency for serotonin reuptake blockade than for norepinephrine reuptake blockade, but this is of unclear clinical significance as a differentiating feature from other SNRIs
- ✻ In vitro binding studies tend to underestimate in vivo potency for reuptake blockade, as they do not factor in the presence of high concentrations of an active metabolite, higher oral mg dosing, or the lower protein binding which can increase functional drug levels at receptor sites
- Effective dose range is broad (i.e., 75–375 mg in many difficult cases, and up to 600 mg or more in heroic cases)
- ✻ Preliminary studies in neuropathic pain and fibromyalgia suggest potential efficacy
- Efficacy as well as side effects (especially nausea and increased blood pressure) are dose-dependent
- Blood pressure increases rare for XR formulation in doses up to 225 mg
- More withdrawal reactions reported upon discontinuation than for some other antidepressants
- May be helpful for hot flushes in perimenopausal women
- May be associated with higher depression remission rates than SSRIs
- ✻ Because of recent studies from the UK that suggest a higher rate of deaths from overdose with venlafaxine than with SSRIs, and because of its potential to affect heart function, venlafaxine can only be prescribed in the UK by specialist doctors and is contraindicated there in patients with heart disease
- Overdose data are from fatal toxicity index studies, which do not take into account patient characteristics or whether drug use was first- or second-line
- Venlafaxine's toxicity in overdose is less than that for TCAs

Suggested Reading

Buckley NA, McManus PR. Fatal toxicity of serotonergic and other antidepressant drugs: analysis of United Kingdom mortality data. BMJ 2002;325:1332–3.

Cheeta S, Schifano F, Oyefeso A, Webb L, Ghodse AH. Antidepressant-related deaths and antidepressant prescriptions in England and Wales, 1998–2000. Br J Psychiatry 2004;184:41–7.

Davidson J, Watkins L, Owens M, et al. Effects of paroxetine and venlafaxine XR on heart rate variability in depression. J Clin Psychopharmacol 2005;25:480–4.

Hackett D. Venlafaxine XR in the treatment of anxiety. Acta Psychiatrica Scand 2000;406(Suppl):S30–5.

Sheehan DV. Attaining remission in generalized anxiety disorder: venlafaxine extended-release comparative data. J Clin Psychiatry 2001;62 (Suppl 19):S26–31.

Smith D, Dempster C, Glanville J, Freemantle N, Anderson I. Efficacy and tolerability of venlafaxine compared with selective serotonin reuptake inhibitors and other antidepressants: a meta-analysis. Br J Psychiatry 2002;180:396–404.

Wellington K, Perry CM. Venlafaxine extended-release: a review of its use in the management of major depression. CNS Drugs 2001;15:643–9.

THERAPEUTICS

Brands • Viibryd

see index for additional brand names

Generic? No

Class

- Neuroscience-based Nomenclature: serotonin multimodal (S-MM)
- SPARI (serotonin partial agonist reuptake inhibitor)
- Dual-acting serotonin reuptake inhibitor plus 5HT1A partial agonist

Commonly Prescribed for

(bold for FDA approved)

- **Major depressive disorder**
- Anxiety
- Obsessive compulsive disorder

How the Drug Works

- Boosts neurotransmitter serotonin
- Blocks serotonin reuptake pump (serotonin transporter)
- Desensitizes serotonin receptors, especially serotonin 1A autoreceptors
- Presumably increases serotonergic neurotransmission
- Partial agonist actions at presynaptic somatodendritic serotonin 1A autoreceptors may theoretically enhance serotonergic activity and contribute to antidepressant actions
- Partial agonist actions at postsynaptic serotonin 1A receptors may theoretically diminish sexual dysfunction caused by serotonin reuptake inhibition

How Long Until It Works

- Onset of therapeutic actions may be sooner than with other SSRIs due to vilazodone's actions at serotonin 1A receptors, with current data suggesting onset of efficacy as early as week 1, despite the fact that standard titration does not arrive at full therapeutic dose of 40 mg until the third week
- If it is not working within 6 or 8 weeks, it may require a dosage increase (off label) or it may not work at all
- May continue to work for many years to prevent relapse of symptoms

If It Works

- The goal of treatment is complete remission of current symptoms as well as prevention of future relapses
- Treatment most often reduces or even eliminates symptoms, but not a cure since symptoms can recur after medicine stopped
- Continue treatment until all symptoms are gone (remission) or significantly reduced
- Once symptoms gone, continue treating for 1 year for the first episode of depression
- For second and subsequent episodes of depression, treatment may need to be indefinite
- Use in anxiety disorders may also need to be indefinite

If It Doesn't Work

- Many patients have only a partial response where some symptoms are improved but others persist (especially insomnia, fatigue, and problems concentrating)
- Other patients may be nonresponders, sometimes called treatment-resistant or treatment-refractory
- Some patients who have an initial response may relapse even though they continue treatment, sometimes called "poop-out"
- Consider increasing dose to 50–80 mg/day "off label" over several weeks if tolerated
- Consider switching to another agent or adding an appropriate augmenting agent
- Consider psychotherapy
- Consider evaluation for another diagnosis or for a comorbid condition (e.g., medical illness, substance abuse, etc.)
- Some patients may experience apparent lack of consistent efficacy due to activation of latent or underlying bipolar disorder, and require antidepressant discontinuation and switch to a mood stabilizer

Best Augmenting Combos for Partial Response or Treatment Resistance

- Trazodone, especially for insomnia
- Bupropion, mirtazapine, reboxetine, or atomoxetine (use combinations of antidepressants with caution as this may activate bipolar disorder and suicidal ideation)
- Modafinil, especially for fatigue, sleepiness, and lack of concentration

- Mood stabilizers or atypical antipsychotics for bipolar depression, psychotic depression, treatment-resistant depression, or treatment-resistant anxiety disorders
- Benzodiazepines
- If all else fails for anxiety disorders, consider gabapentin, pregabalin, or tiagabine
- Hypnotics for insomnia
- Classically, lithium, buspirone, or thyroid hormone

Tests

- None for healthy individuals

SIDE EFFECTS

How Drug Causes Side Effects

- Theoretically due to increases in serotonin concentrations at serotonin receptors in parts of the brain and body other than those that cause therapeutic actions (e.g., unwanted actions of serotonin in sleep centers causing insomnia, unwanted actions of serotonin in the gut causing diarrhea, etc.)
- Increasing serotonin can cause diminished dopamine release and might contribute to emotional flattening, cognitive slowing, and apathy in some patients
- Most side effects are immediate but often go away with time, in contrast to most therapeutic effects, which are delayed and are enhanced over time

Notable Side Effects

- Nausea, diarrhea, vomiting
- Insomnia, dizziness
- Note: patients with diagnosed or undiagnosed bipolar or psychotic disorders may be more vulnerable to CNS-activating actions of serotonergic antidepressants
- Bruising and rare bleeding
- Rare hyponatremia (mostly in elderly patients and generally reversible on discontinuation of vilazodone)
- Sexual dysfunction (men: delayed ejaculation; men and women: decreased sexual desire, anorgasmia) slightly greater than placebo and generally less than for SSRIs/SNRIs, but no head-to-head studies
- SIADH (syndrome of inappropriate antidiuretic hormone secretion)

Life-Threatening or Dangerous Side Effects

- Rare seizures
- Rare induction of mania and activation of suicidal ideation

Weight Gain

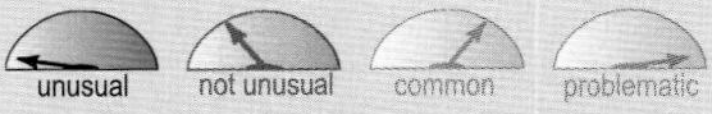

- Reported but not expected

Sedation

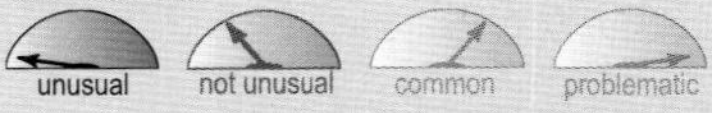

- Reported but not expected

What to Do About Side Effects

- Wait
- Wait
- Wait
- In a few weeks, switch to another agent or add other drugs

Best Augmenting Agents for Side Effects

- Often best to try another antidepressant monotherapy prior to resorting to augmentation strategies to treat side effects
- Trazodone or a hypnotic for insomnia
- Bupropion, sildenafil, vardenafil, or tadalafil for sexual dysfunction
- Bupropion for emotional flattening, cognitive slowing, or apathy
- Mirtazapine for insomnia, agitation, and gastrointestinal side effects
- Benzodiazepines for jitteriness and anxiety, especially at initiation of treatment and especially for anxious patients
- Many side effects are dose-dependent (i.e., they increase as dose increases, or they reemerge until tolerance redevelops)
- Many side effects are time-dependent (i.e., they start immediately upon dosing and upon each dose increase, but go away with time)
- Activation and agitation may represent the induction of a bipolar state, especially a mixed dysphoric bipolar II condition sometimes associated with suicidal ideation, and require the addition of lithium, a mood stabilizer or an atypical antipsychotic, and/or discontinuation of vilazodone

DOSING AND USE

Usual Dosage Range
- 20–40 mg/day

Dosage Forms
- Tablets 10 mg, 20 mg, 40 mg

How To Dose
- Initial 10 mg/day; increase to 20 mg/day after one week; can increase to 40 mg/day after one more week; should be taken with food

Dosing Tips
- Given once daily, any time of day tolerated but must be administered with food, because taking on an empty stomach may reduce absorption of vilazodone by 50%
- If intolerable anxiety, insomnia, agitation, akathisia, or activation occur either upon dosing initiation or discontinuation, consider the possibility of activating a bipolar disorder and switch to a mood stabilizer or an atypical antipsychotic
- No minimally effective dose has been established, so theoretically possible that doses lower than 40 mg daily may be effective in some patients
- Doses higher than 40 mg daily have not been well studied, but theoretically possible that slow titration to doses higher than 40 mg may be effective in some patients, particularly those with treatment-resistant depression who fail to respond adequately to 40 mg daily

Overdose
- Few reports of vilazodone overdose
- No fatalities; serotonin syndrome, lethargy, restlessness, hallucinations, disorientation

Long-Term Use
- Has not been evaluated in controlled studies, but long-term treatment of major depressive disorder is generally necessary

Habit Forming
- No

How to Stop
- Tapering to avoid potential withdrawal reactions generally prudent
- Many patients tolerate 50% dose reduction for 3 days, then another 50% reduction for 3 days, then discontinuation
- If withdrawal symptoms emerge during discontinuation, raise dose to stop symptoms and then restart withdrawal much more slowly

Pharmacokinetics
- Mean terminal half-life 25 hours
- Metabolized by CYP450 3A4
- Absorption and bioavailability are reduced by half when taken on an empty stomach

Drug Interactions
- Tramadol increases the risk of seizures in patients taking an antidepressant
- Can cause a fatal "serotonin syndrome" when combined with MAOIs, so do not use with MAOIs or for at least 14 days after MAOIs are stopped
- Do not start an MAOI for at least 5 half-lives (5 to 7 days for most drugs) after discontinuing vilazodone
- Inhibitors of CYP450 3A4, such as nefazodone, fluoxetine, fluvoxamine, and even grapefruit juice, may decrease the clearance of vilazodone and thereby raise its plasma levels, so dose should be reduced to 20 mg when coadminstered with strong CYP3A4 inhibitors
- Inducers of CYP450 3A4, such as carbamazepine, may increase clearance of vilazodone and thus lower its plasma levels and possibly reduce therapeutic effects
- Could theoretically cause weakness, hyperreflexia, and incoordination when combined with sumatriptan or possibly other triptans, requiring careful monitoring of patient
- Possible increased risk of bleeding, especially when combined with anticoagulants (e.g., warfarin, NSAIDs)

Other Warnings/ Precautions
- Use with caution in patients with history of seizure
- Use with caution in patients with bipolar disorder unless treated with concomitant mood-stabilizing agent
- Not approved in children, so when treating children off label, carefully weigh the risks and benefits of pharmacological treatment against the risks and benefits of nontreatment with antidepressants and

make sure to document this in the patient's chart
- Distribute the brochures provided by the FDA and the drug companies
- Warn patients and their caregivers about the possibility of activating side effects and advise them to report such symptoms immediately
- Monitor patients for activation of suicidal ideation, especially children and adolescents

Do Not Use
- If patient is taking an MAOI
- If there is a proven allergy to vilazodone

SPECIAL POPULATIONS

Renal Impairment
- No dose adjustment necessary

Hepatic Impairment
- No dose adjustment necessary for mild to moderate impairment
- Has not been studied in patients with severe hepatic impairment

Cardiac Impairment
- Not systematically evaluated in patients with cardiac impairment
- Vilazodone has not shown any significant effect on blood pressure, heart rate, or QT interval in placebo-controlled trials
- Treating depression with SSRIs in patients with acute angina or following myocardial infarction may reduce cardiac events and improve survival as well as mood

Elderly
- No dose adjustment necessary
- Some patients may tolerate lower doses better
- Risk of SIADH with SSRIs is higher in the elderly
- Reduction in the risk of suicidality with antidepressants compared to placebo in adults age 65 and older

Children and Adolescents
- Safety and efficacy have not been established
- Use with caution, observing for activation of known or unknown bipolar disorder and/or suicidal ideation, and strongly consider informing parents or guardians of this risk so they can help observe child or adolescent patients

Pregnancy
- Effective June 30, 2015, the US FDA requires changes to the content and format of pregnancy and lactation information in prescription drug labels, including the elimination of the pregnancy letter categories; the Pregnancy and Lactation Labeling Rule (PLLR or final rule) applies only to prescription drugs and will be phased in gradually for drugs approved on or after June 30, 2001
- Controlled studies have not been conducted in pregnant women
- Not generally recommended for use during pregnancy, especially during first trimester
- Nonetheless, continuous treatment during pregnancy may be necessary and has not been proven to be harmful to the fetus
- At delivery there may be more bleeding in the mother and transient irritability or sedation in the newborn
- Must weigh the risk of treatment (first trimester fetal development, third trimester newborn delivery) to the child against the risk of no treatment (recurrence of depression, maternal health, infant bonding) to the mother and child
- For many patients, this may mean continuing treatment during pregnancy
- Exposure to serotonin reuptake inhibitors early in pregnancy may be associated with increased risk of septal heart defects (absolute risk is small)
- Serotonin reuptake inhibitor use beyond the 20th week of pregnancy may be associated with increased risk of pulmonary hypertension in newborns, although this is not proven
- Exposure to serotonin reuptake inhibitors late in pregnancy may be associated with increased risk of gestational hypertension and preeclampsia
- Neonates exposed to SSRIs or SNRIs late in the third trimester have developed complications requiring prolonged

hospitalization, respiratory support, and tube feeding; reported symptoms are consistent with either a direct toxic effect of SSRIs and SNRIs or, possibly, a drug discontinuation syndrome, and include respiratory distress, cyanosis, apnea, seizures, temperature instability, feeding difficulty, vomiting, hypoglycemia, hypotonia, hypertonia, hyperreflexia, tremor, jitteriness, irritability, and constant crying

Breast Feeding

- Unknown if vilazodone is secreted in human breast milk, but all psychotropics assumed to be secreted in breast milk
- Trace amounts may be present in nursing children whose mothers are on vilazodone
- If child becomes irritable or sedated, breast feeding or drug may need to be discontinued
- Immediate postpartum period is a high-risk time for depression, especially in women who have had prior depressive episodes, so drug may need to be reinstituted late in the third trimester or shortly after childbirth to prevent a recurrence during the postpartum period
- Must weigh benefits of breast feeding with risks and benefits of antidepressant treatment versus nontreatment to both the infant and the mother
- For many patients, this may mean continuing treatment during breast feeding

THE ART OF PSYCHOPHARMACOLOGY

Potential Advantages

- Patients with sexual dysfunction on an SSRI/SNRI or who wish to avoid sexual dysfunction on an antidepressant
- Patients with weight gain on another antidepressant or who wish to avoid weight gain on an antidepressant
- Patients with mixed anxiety and depression

Potential Disadvantages

- Patients who cannot take medication reliably with food
- Patients sensitive to gastrointestinal side effects such as diarrhea and nausea

Primary Target Symptoms

- Depressed mood
- Anxiety

Pearls

- Serotonin 1A partial agonist property is a relatively unique mechanism of action among approved antidepressants (also vortioxetine and atypical antipsychotic augmenting agents such as quetiapine, aripiprazole, brexpiprazole, and others)
- First member of a new antidepressant class, SPARIs, or serotonin partial agonist reuptake inhibitors
- Relative lack of sexual dysfunction and weight gain compared to many other antidepressants that block serotonin reuptake may be due to the serotonin 1A partial agonist properties of vilazodone
- High doses would theoretically raise brain serotonin levels more robustly than the standard dose, and may improve efficacy in some patients but reduce tolerability in some patients
- Consider doses of 50–80 mg daily if effective and well tolerated for patients with treatment-resistant depression or treatment-resistant OCD and other anxiety disorders
- Consider for patients with comorbid anxiety disorders plus depression
- Nonresponse to vilazodone in elderly may require consideration of mild cognitive impairment or Alzheimer disease

Suggested Reading

Citrome L. Vilazodone for major depressive disorder: a systematic review of the efficacy and safety profile for this newly approved antidepressant – what is the number needed to treat, number needed to harm and likelihood to be helped or harmed? Int J Clin Pract 2012;66(4):356–68.

Dawson LA, Watson JM. Vilazodone: a 5HT1A receptor agonist/serotonin transporter inhibitor for the treatment of affective disorders. CNS Neurosci Therapeutics 2009;15:107–17.

Laughren TP, Gobburu J, Temple RJ, et al. Vilazodone: clinical basis for the US Food and Drug Administration's approval of a new antidepressant. J Clin Psychiatry 2011;72(9):1166–73.

Rickels K, Athanasiou M, Robinson D, et al. Evidence for efficacy and tolerability of vilazodone in the treatment of major depressive disorder: a randomized, double-blind, placebo-controlled trial. J Clin Psychiatry 2009;e1–e8.

THERAPEUTICS

Brands • Trintellix (formerly Brintellix)
see index for additional brand names

Generic? No

Class

- Neuroscience-based Nomenclature: serotonin multimodal (S-MM)
- Multimodal antidepressant

Commonly Prescribed for

(bold for FDA approved)

- **Major depressive disorder**
- Generalized anxiety disorder (GAD)
- Cognitive symptoms associated with depression
- Geriatric depression

How the Drug Works

- Increases release of several different neurotransmitters (serotonin, norepinephrine, dopamine, glutamate, acetylcholine, and histamine) and reduces the release of GABA through 3 different modes of action
- Mode 1: blocks serotonin reuptake pump (serotonin transporter)
- Mode 2: binds to G protein-linked receptors (full agonist at serotonin 1A receptors, partial agonist at serotonin 1B receptors, antagonist at serotonin 1D and serotonin 7 receptors)
- Mode 3: binds to ion channel-linked receptors (antagonist at serotonin 3 receptors)
- Full agonist actions at presynaptic somatodendritic serotonin 1A autoreceptors may theoretically enhance serotonergic activity and contribute to antidepressant actions
- Full agonist actions at postsynaptic serotonin 1A receptors may theoretically diminish sexual dysfunction caused by serotonin reuptake inhibition
- Antagonist actions at serotonin 3 receptors may theoretically enhance noradrenergic, acetylcholinergic, and glutamatergic activity and contribute to antidepressant and pro-cognitive actions
- Antagonist actions at serotonin 3 receptors may theoretically reduce nausea and vomiting caused by serotonin reuptake inhibition
- Antagonist actions at serotonin 7 receptors may theoretically contribute to antidepressant and pro-cognitive actions as well as reduce insomnia caused by serotonin reuptake inhibition
- Partial agonist actions at serotonin 1B receptors may enhance not only serotonin release, but also acetylcholine and histamine release
- Antagonist actions at serotonin 1D receptors may enhance serotonin release and may also theoretically enhance the release of pro-cognitive neurotransmitters and thereby enhance pro-cognitive actions

How Long Until It Works

- Onset of therapeutic actions is usually not immediate, but often delayed 2–4 weeks
- However, vortioxetine has a specific claim of onset of action at week 2
- If it is not working within 6 or 8 weeks, it may require a dosage increase or it may not work at all
- May continue to work for many years to prevent relapse of symptoms

If It Works

- The goal of treatment is complete remission of current symptoms as well as prevention of future relapses
- Treatment most often reduces or even eliminates symptoms, but not a cure since symptoms can recur after medicine stopped
- Continue treatment until all symptoms are gone (remission) or significantly reduced
- Once symptoms gone, continue treating for 1 year for the first episode of depression
- For second and subsequent episodes of depression, treatment may need to be indefinite
- Use in anxiety disorders may also need to be indefinite

If It Doesn't Work

- Many patients only have a partial response where some symptoms are improved but others persist (especially insomnia, fatigue, and problems concentrating)

- Other patients may be nonresponders, sometimes called treatment-resistant or treatment-refractory
- Some patients who have an initial response may relapse even though they continue treatment, sometimes called "poop-out"
- Consider switching to another agent or adding an appropriate augmenting agent
- Consider psychotherapy
- Consider evaluation for another diagnosis or for a comorbid condition (e.g., medical illness, substance abuse, etc.)
- Some patients may experience apparent lack of consistent efficacy due to activation of latent or underlying bipolar disorder, and require antidepressant discontinuation and switch to a mood stabilizer

Best Augmenting Combos for Partial Response or Treatment Resistance

- Augmentation experience is limited compared to other antidepressants
- Trazodone, especially for insomnia
- Bupropion, mirtazapine, reboxetine, or atomoxetine (use combinations of antidepressants with caution as this may activate bipolar disorder and suicidal ideation)
- Use with caution with antidepressants that are CYP450 2D6 inhibitors (e.g., bupropion, duloxetine, fluoxetine, paroxetine), as these agents will increase vortioxetine levels and may require a dose reduction of vortioxetine
- Modafinil, especially for fatigue, sleepiness, and lack of concentration
- Mood stabilizers or atypical antipsychotics for bipolar depression, psychotic depression, treatment-resistant depression, or treatment-resistant anxiety disorders
- Benzodiazepines
- If all else fails for anxiety disorders, consider gabapentin, pregabalin, or tiagabine
- Hypnotics for insomnia
- Classically, lithium, buspirone, or thyroid hormone

Tests

- None for healthy individuals

SIDE EFFECTS

How Drug Causes Side Effects

- Theoretically due to increases in serotonin concentrations at serotonin receptors in parts of the brain and body other than those that cause therapeutic actions (e.g., unwanted actions of serotonin at central serotonin 1A receptors causing nausea, unwanted actions of serotonin in the CNS causing sexual dysfunction, etc.)
- Most side effects are immediate but often go away with time, in contrast to most therapeutic effects, which are delayed and are enhanced over time

Notable Side Effects

- Nausea, vomiting, constipation
- Sexual dysfunction

Life-Threatening or Dangerous Side Effects

- Rare seizures
- Rare induction of mania and activation of suicidal ideation

Weight Gain

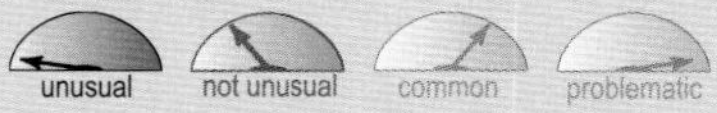

- Reported but not expected

Sedation

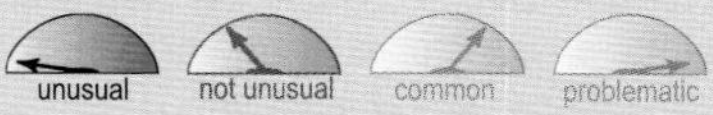

- Reported but not expected

What to Do About Side Effects

- Wait
- Wait
- Wait
- In a few weeks, switch to another agent or add other drugs

Best Augmenting Agents for Side Effects

- Often best to try another antidepressant monotherapy prior to resorting to augmentation strategies to treat side effects
- Trazodone or a hypnotic for insomnia

- Sildenafil, vardenafil, or tadalafil for sexual dysfunction
- Bupropion for emotional flattening, cognitive slowing, apathy, or sexual dysfunction (with caution, as bupropion can raise vortioxetine levels via CYP450 2D6 inhibition)
- Mirtazapine for insomnia, agitation, and gastrointestinal side effects
- Benzodiazepines for jitteriness and anxiety, especially at initiation of treatment and especially for anxious patients
- Many side effects are dose-dependent (i.e., they increase as dose increases, or they reemerge until tolerance redevelops)
- Many side effects are time-dependent (i.e., they start immediately upon dosing and upon each dose increase, but go away with time)
- Activation and agitation may represent the induction of a bipolar state, especially a mixed dysphoric bipolar II condition sometimes associated with suicidal ideation, and require the addition of lithium, a mood stabilizer, or an atypical antipsychotic, and/or discontinuation of vortioxetine

DOSING AND USE

Usual Dosage Range
- 5–20 mg/day

Dosage Forms
- Tablet 5 mg, 10 mg, 15 mg, 20 mg

How to Dose
- Initial 10 mg once daily; can decrease to 5 mg once daily or increase to 20 mg once daily depending on patient response; maximum recommended dose generally 20 mg once daily

Dosing Tips
- Can be taken with or without food
- Tablet should not be divided, crushed, or dissolved
- If intolerable anxiety, insomnia, agitation, akathisia, or activation occur either upon dosing initiation or discontinuation, consider the possibility of activating a bipolar disorder and switch to a mood stabilizer or an atypical antipsychotic

Overdose
- No fatalities have been reported; nausea, dizziness, diarrhea, abdominal discomfort, generalized pruritus, somnolence, flushing

Long-Term Use
- Long-term treatment of major depressive disorder is generally necessary

Habit Forming
- No

How to Stop
- Taper not necessary with recommended doses

Pharmacokinetics
- Metabolized by CYP450 2D6, 3A4/5, 2C19, 2C9, 2A6, 2C8, and 2B6
- Mean terminal half-life approximately 66 hours

Drug Interactions
- Tramadol increases the risk of seizures in patients taking an antidepressant
- Can cause a fatal “serotonin syndrome” when combined with MAOIs, so do not use with MAOIs or for at least 14–21 days after MAOIs are stopped
- Do not start an MAOI for at least 5 half-lives (about 14 days for vortioxetine with a half-life of 66 hours) after discontinuing vortioxetine
- Strong CYP450 2D6 inhibitors can increase plasma levels of vortioxetine, possibly requiring its dose to be decreased
- Broad CYP450 2D6 inducers can decrease plasma levels of vortioxetine, possibly requiring its dose to be increased
- Could theoretically cause weakness, hyperreflexia, and incoordination when combined with sumatriptan or possibly other triptans, requiring careful monitoring of patient
- Possible increased risk of bleeding, especially when combined with anticoagulants (e.g., warfarin, NSAIDs)

Other Warnings/ Precautions

- Use with caution in patients with history of seizures
- Use with caution in patients with bipolar disorder unless treated with concomitant mood-stabilizing agent
- Possible risk of hyponatremia related to SIADH (syndrome of inappropriate antidiuretic hormone secretion) with serotonergic drugs
- Not approved in children, so when treating children off label, carefully weigh the risks and benefits of pharmacological treatment against the risks and benefits of non-treatment with antidepressants and make sure to document this in the patient's chart
- Distribute the brochures provided by the FDA and the drug companies
- Warn patients and their caregivers about the possibility of activating side effects and advise them to report such symptoms immediately
- Monitor patients for activation of suicidal ideation, especially children and adolescents

Do Not Use

- If patient is taking an MAOI
- If there is a proven allergy to vortioxetine

SPECIAL POPULATIONS

Renal Impairment

- No dose adjustment necessary

Hepatic Impairment

- No dose adjustment necessary for mild to moderate impairment
- Has not been studied in patients with severe hepatic impairment

Cardiac Impairment

- Not systematically evaluated in patients with cardiac impairment
- Treating depression with SSRIs in patients with acute angina or following myocardial infarction may reduce cardiac events and improve survival as well as mood; not known for vortioxetine

Elderly

- No dose adjustment necessary
- Some patients may tolerate lower doses better
- Risk of SIADH with SSRIs is higher in the elderly
- Reduction in risk of suicidality with antidepressants compared to placebo in adults age 65 and older

Children and Adolescents

- Safety and efficacy have not been established
- Carefully weigh the risks and benefits of pharmacological treatment against the risks and benefits of nontreatment with antidepressants and make sure to document this in the patient's chart
- Monitor patients face-to-face regularly, particularly during the first several weeks of treatment
- Use with caution, observing for activation of known or unknown bipolar disorder and/or suicidal ideation, and strongly consider informing parents or guardian of this risk so they can help observe child or adolescent patients

Pregnancy

- Effective June 30, 2015, the US FDA requires changes to the content and format of pregnancy and lactation information in prescription drug labels, including the elimination of the pregnancy letter categories; the Pregnancy and Lactation Labeling Rule (PLLR or final rule) applies only to prescription drugs and will be phased in gradually for drugs approved on or after June 30, 2001
- Controlled studies have not been conducted in pregnant women
- Not generally recommended for use during pregnancy, especially during first trimester
- Nonetheless, continuous treatment during pregnancy may be necessary and has not been proven to be harmful to the fetus
- At delivery there may be more bleeding in the mother and transient irritability or sedation in the newborn
- Must weigh the risk of treatment (first trimester fetal development, third trimester

newborn delivery) to the child against the risk of no treatment (recurrence of depression, maternal health, infant bonding) to the mother and child
- For many patients, this may mean continuing treatment during pregnancy
- Exposure to serotonin reuptake inhibitors early in pregnancy may be associated with increased risk of septal heart defects (absolute risk is small)
- Use of serotonin reuptake inhibitors beyond the 20th week of pregnancy may be associated with increased risk of pulmonary hypertension in newborns, although this is not proven
- Exposure to serotonin reuptake inhibitors late in pregnancy may be associated with increased risk of gestational hypertension and preeclampsia
- Neonates exposed to SSRIs or SNRIs late in the third trimester have developed complications requiring prolonged hospitalization, respiratory support, and tube feeding; reported symptoms are consistent with either a direct toxic effect of SSRIs and SNRIs or, possibly, a drug discontinuation syndrome, and include respiratory distress, cyanosis, apnea, seizures, temperature instability, feeding difficulty, vomiting, hypoglycemia, hypotonia, hypertonia, hyperreflexia, tremor, jitteriness, irritability, and constant crying

Breast Feeding
- Unknown if vortioxetine is secreted in human breast milk, but all psychotropics assumed to be secreted in breast milk
- If child becomes irritable or sedated, breast feeding or drug may need to be discontinued
- Immediate postpartum period is a high-risk time for depression, especially in women who have had prior depressive episodes, so drug may need to be reinstituted late in the third trimester or shortly after childbirth to prevent a recurrence during the postpartum period
- Must weigh benefits of breast feeding with risks and benefits of antidepressant treatment versus nontreatment to both the infant and the mother
- For many patients, this may mean continuing treatment during breast feeding

THE ART OF PSYCHOPHARMACOLOGY

Potential Advantages
- Patients with sexual dysfunction
- Patients with cognitive symptoms of depression
- Patients with residual cognitive symptoms after treatment with another antidepressant
- Elderly patients
- Patients who have not responded to other antidepressants
- Patients who do not want weight gain

Potential Disadvantages
- Cost

Primary Target Symptoms
- Depressed mood
- Cognitive symptoms
- Anxiety

Pearls
- In May 2016 the US FDA approved a brand name change from Brintellix to Trintellix in order to decrease prescribing and dispensing errors due to name confusion with the anti-platelet medication Brilinta (ticagrelor)
- May have less sexual dysfunction than SSRIs
- Multiple studies show pro-cognitive effects greater than a comparator antidepressant in patients with major depressive episodes
- Patients who do not respond to antidepressants with other mechanisms of action may respond to vortioxetine
- Shown effective specifically in elderly patients with depression, with a positive trial in geriatric depression with improvement of cognition as well as mood
- Has a unique claim of preventing recurrences in major depression
- No weight gain in clinical trials
- Long half-life means vortioxetine can generally be abruptly discontinued, although some caution may be necessary when stopping higher doses (i.e., 15 or 20 mg/day)
- Despite serotonin 3 antagonist actions, nausea is common, presumably due to full agonist actions at serotonin 1A receptors
- Dose response for efficacy in depression: higher doses are more effective
- Vortioxetine has a unique multimodal mechanism of action
- Nonresponse to vortioxetine in elderly may require consideration of mild cognitive impairment or Alzheimer disease

Suggested Reading

Bang-Anderson B, Ruhland T, Jorgensen M, et al. Discovery of 1-[2-(2,4-dimethylphenylsulfanyl) phenyl]piperazine (Lu AA21004): a novel multimodal compound for the treatment of major depressive disorder. J Med Chem 2011;54(9):3206–21.

Mork A, Montezinho LP, Miller S, et al. Vortioxetine (LU AA21004), a novel multimodal antidepressant, enhanced memory in rats. Pharmacol Biochem Behav 2013;105:41–50.

Stahl SM, Lee-Zimmerman C, Cartwright S, Morrissette DA. Serotonergic drugs for depression and beyond. Curr Drug Targets 2013;14(5):578–85.

Westrich I, Pehrson A, Zhong H, et al. In vitro and in vivo effects of the multimodal antidepressant vortioxetine (Lu AA21004) at human and rat targets. Int J Psychiatry Clin Pract 2012;5(Suppl 1):S47.

THERAPEUTICS

Brands • Sonata

see index for additional brand names

Generic? Yes

Class

- Neuroscience-based Nomenclature: GABA positive allosteric modulator (GABA-PAM)
- Non-benzodiazepine hypnotic; alpha 1 isoform agonist of GABA-A/benzodiazepine receptors

Commonly Prescribed for

(bold for FDA approved)

- **Short-term treatment of insomnia**

How the Drug Works

- Binds selectively to a subtype of the benzodiazepine receptor, the alpha 1 isoform
- May enhance GABA inhibitory actions that provide sedative hypnotic effects more selectively than other actions of GABA
- Boosts chloride conductance through GABA-regulated channels
- Inhibitory actions in sleep centers may provide sedative hypnotic effects

How Long Until It Works

- Generally takes effect in less than an hour

If It Works

- Improves quality of sleep
- Effects on total wake-time and number of nighttime awakenings may be decreased over time

If It Doesn't Work

- If insomnia does not improve after 7–10 days, it may be a manifestation of a primary psychiatric or physical illness such as obstructive sleep apnea or restless leg syndrome, which requires independent evaluation
- Increase the dose
- Improve sleep hygiene
- Switch to another agent

Best Augmenting Combos for Partial Response or Treatment Resistance

- Generally, best to switch to another agent
- Trazodone
- Agents with antihistamine actions (e.g., diphenhydramine, TCAs)

Tests

- None for healthy individuals

SIDE EFFECTS

How Drug Causes Side Effects

- Actions at benzodiazepine receptors that carry over to the next day can cause daytime sedation, amnesia, and ataxia
- Long-term adaptations of zaleplon not well studied, but chronic studies of other alpha 1 selective non-benzodiazepine hypnotics suggest lack of notable tolerance or dependence developing over time

Notable Side Effects

- ✻ Sedation
- ✻ Dizziness, ataxia
- ✻ Dose-dependent amnesia
- ✻ Hyperexcitability, nervousness
- Rare hallucinations
- Headache
- Decreased appetite

Life-Threatening or Dangerous Side Effects

- Respiratory depression, especially when taken with other CNS depressants in overdose
- Rare angioedema

Weight Gain

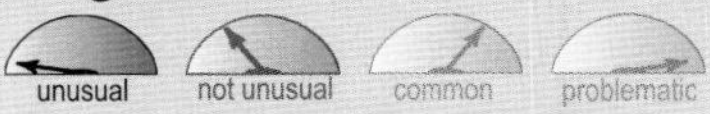

- Reported but not expected

Sedation

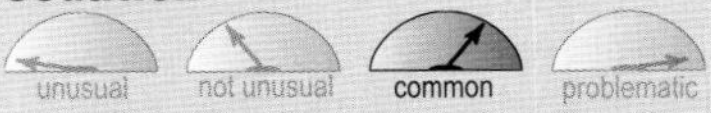

- Many experience and/or can be significant in amount

What to Do About Side Effects

- Wait
- To avoid problems with memory, do not take zaleplon if planning to sleep for less than 4 hours
- Lower the dose
- Administer flumazenil if side effects are severe or life-threatening

Best Augmenting Agents for Side Effects

- Many side effects cannot be improved with an augmenting agent

DOSING AND USE

Usual Dosage Range

- 10 mg/day at bedtime for 7–10 days

Dosage Forms

- Capsule 5 mg, 10 mg

How to Dose

- Initial 10 mg/day at bedtime; may increase to 20 mg/day at bedtime if ineffective; maximum dose generally 20 mg/day

Dosing Tips

- Patients with lower body weights may require only a 5-mg dose
- Zaleplon should generally not be prescribed in quantities greater than a 1-month supply
- Risk of dependence may increase with dose and duration of treatment

✽ However, treatment with alpha 1 selective non-benzodiazepine hypnotics may cause less tolerance or dependence than benzodiazepine hypnotics

Overdose

- No fatalities reported with zaleplon; fatalities have occurred with other sedative hypnotics; sedation, confusion, ataxia, hypotension, respiratory depression, coma

Long-Term Use

- Not generally intended for long-term use
- Increased wakefulness during the latter part of night (wearing off) or an increase in daytime anxiety (rebound) may occur because of short half-life

Habit Forming

- Zaleplon is a Schedule IV drug
- Some patients may develop dependence and/or tolerance; risk may be greater with higher doses
- History of drug addiction may increase risk of dependence

How to Stop

- Rebound insomnia may occur the first night after stopping
- If taken for more than a few weeks, taper to reduce chances of withdrawal effects

Pharmacokinetics

- Terminal phase elimination half-life approximately 1 hour (ultra-short half-life)

Drug Interactions

- Increased depressive effects when taken with other CNS depressants
- Cimetidine may increase plasma concentrations of zaleplon, requiring a lower initial dose of zaleplon (5 mg/day)
- CYP450 3A4 inducers such as carbamazepine may reduce the effectiveness of zaleplon

Other Warnings/ Precautions

- Insomnia may be a symptom of a primary disorder, rather than a primary disorder itself
- Some patients may exhibit abnormal thinking or behavioral changes similar to those caused by other CNS depressants (i.e., either depressant actions or disinhibiting actions)
- Some depressed patients may experience a worsening of suicidal ideation
- Use only with extreme caution in patients with impaired respiratory function or obstructive sleep apnea
- Zaleplon should be administered only at bedtime
- Rare angioedema has occurred with sedative hypnotic use and could potentially cause fatal airway obstruction if it involves the throat, glottis, or larynx; thus if angioedema occurs treatment should be discontinued
- Sleep driving and other complex behaviors, such as eating and preparing food and making phone calls, have been reported in patients taking sedative hypnotics

Do Not Use

- If there is a proven allergy to zaleplon

SPECIAL POPULATIONS

Renal Impairment
- No dose adjustment necessary
- Use with caution in patients with severe impairment

Hepatic Impairment
- Mild to moderate impairment: recommended dose 5 mg
- Not recommended for use in patients with severe impairment

Cardiac Impairment
- Zaleplon has not been studied in patients with cardiac impairment, but dose adjustment may not be necessary

Elderly
- Recommended dose: 5 mg

Children and Adolescents
- Safety and efficacy have not been established
- Long-term effects of zaleplon in children/ adolescents are unknown
- Should generally receive lower doses and be more closely monitored

Pregnancy
- Effective June 30, 2015, the US FDA requires changes to the content and format of pregnancy and lactation information in prescription drug labels, including the elimination of the pregnancy letter categories; the Pregnancy and Lactation Labeling Rule (PLLR or final rule) applies only to prescription drugs and will be phased in gradually for drugs approved on or after June 30, 2001
- Controlled studies have not been conducted in pregnant women
- Infants whose mothers took sedative hypnotics during pregnancy may experience some withdrawal symptoms
- Neonatal flaccidity has been reported in infants whose mothers took sedative hypnotics during pregnancy

Breast Feeding
- Some drug is found in mother's breast milk

✻ Recommended either to discontinue drug or bottle feed

THE ART OF PSYCHOPHARMACOLOGY

Potential Advantages
- Those needing short duration of action

Potential Disadvantages
- Those needing longer duration of action
- More expensive than some other sedative hypnotics

Primary Target Symptoms
- Time to sleep onset
- Total sleep time
- Nighttime awakenings

Pearls
- Zaleplon has not been shown to increase the total time asleep or to decrease the number of awakenings

✻ May be preferred over benzodiazepines because of its rapid onset of action, short duration of effect, and safety profile

✻ Popular for uses requiring short half-life (e.g., dosing in the middle of the night, sleeping on airplanes, jet lag)

✻ May not be ideal for patients who desire immediate hypnotic onset and eat just prior to bedtime

- Not a benzodiazepine itself, but binds to benzodiazepine receptors
- May have fewer carryover side effects than some other sedative hypnotics
- May not have sufficient efficacy in patients with severe chronic insomnia resistant to some other sedative hypnotics
- May cause less dependence than some other sedative hypnotics, especially in those without a history of substance abuse

✻ Zaleplon is not absorbed as quickly if taken with high-fat foods, which may reduce onset of action

Suggested Reading

Dooley M, Plosker GL. Zaleplon: a review of its use in the treatment of insomnia. Drugs 2000;60:413–45.

Heydorn WE. Zaleplon – a review of a novel sedative hypnotic used in the treatment of insomnia. Expert Opin Invest Drugs 2000;9:841–58.

Mangano RM. Efficacy and safety of zaleplon at peak plasma levels. Int J Clin Pract Suppl 2001;116:9–13.

Weitzel KW, Wickman JM, Augustin SG, Strom JG. Zaleplon: a pyrazolopyrimidine sedative-hypnotic agent for the treatment of insomnia. Clin Ther 2000;22:1254–67.

ZIPRASIDONE

THERAPEUTICS

Brands • Geodon

see index for additional brand names

Generic? Yes

Class

- Neuroscience-based Nomenclature: dopamine and serotonin receptor antagonist (DS_RAn)
- Atypical antipsychotic (serotonin-dopamine antagonist; second-generation antipsychotic; also a mood stabilizer)

Commonly Prescribed for

(bold for FDA approved)

- **Schizophrenia**
- **Delaying relapse in schizophrenia**
- **Acute agitation in schizophrenia (intramuscular)**
- **Acute mania/mixed mania**
- **Bipolar maintenance**
- Other psychotic disorders
- Bipolar depression
- Behavioral disturbances in dementias
- Behavioral disturbances in children and adolescents
- Disorders associated with problems with impulse control

How the Drug Works

- Blocks dopamine 2 receptors, reducing positive symptoms of psychosis and stabilizing affective symptoms
- Blocks serotonin 2A receptors, causing enhancement of dopamine release in certain brain regions and thus reducing motor side effects and possibly improving cognitive and affective symptoms
- Interactions at a myriad of other neurotransmitter receptors may contribute to ziprasidone's efficacy

✻ Specifically, interactions at 5HT2C and 5HT1A receptors may contribute to efficacy for cognitive and affective symptoms in some patients

✻ Specifically, interactions at 5HT1D and 5HT7 receptors and at serotonin and norepinephrine transporters (especially at high doses) may contribute to efficacy for affective symptoms in some patients

How Long Until It Works

- Psychotic and manic symptoms can improve within 1 week, but it may take several weeks for full effect on behavior as well as on cognition and affective stabilization
- Classically recommended to wait at least 4–6 weeks to determine efficacy of drug, but in practice some patients require up to 16–20 weeks to show a good response, especially on cognitive symptoms
- IM formulation can reduce agitation in 15 minutes

If It Works

- Most often reduces positive symptoms in schizophrenia but does not eliminate them
- Can improve negative symptoms, as well as aggressive, cognitive, and affective symptoms in schizophrenia
- Most schizophrenic patients do not have a total remission of symptoms but rather a reduction of symptoms by about a third
- Perhaps 5–15% of schizophrenic patients can experience an overall improvement of greater than 50–60%, especially when receiving stable treatment for more than a year
- Such patients are considered super-responders or "awakeners" since they may be well enough to be employed, live independently, and sustain long-term relationships
- Many bipolar patients may experience a reduction of symptoms by half or more
- Continue treatment until reaching a plateau of improvement
- After reaching a satisfactory plateau, continue treatment for at least a year after first episode of psychosis
- For second and subsequent episodes of psychosis, treatment may need to be indefinite
- Even for first episodes of psychosis, it may be preferable to continue treatment indefinitely to avoid subsequent episodes
- Treatment may not only reduce mania but also prevent recurrences of mania in bipolar disorder

If It Doesn't Work

- Try one of the other atypical antipsychotics (risperidone, olanzapine, quetiapine, aripiprazole, paliperidone, amisulpride, asenapine, iloperidone, lurasidone)
- If 2 or more antipsychotic monotherapies do not work, consider clozapine

- Some patients may require treatment with a conventional antipsychotic
- If no first-line atypical antipsychotic is effective, consider higher doses or augmentation with valproate or lamotrigine
- Consider noncompliance and switch to another antipsychotic with fewer side effects or to an antipsychotic that can be given by depot injection
- Consider initiating rehabilitation and psychotherapy such as cognitive remediation
- Consider presence of concomitant drug abuse

Best Augmenting Combos for Partial Response or Treatment Resistance

- Valproic acid (valproate, divalproex, divalproex ER)
- Other mood-stabilizing anticonvulsants (carbamazepine, oxcarbazepine, lamotrigine)
- Lithium
- Benzodiazepines

Tests

Before starting an atypical antipsychotic

✽ Weigh all patients and track BMI during treatment
- Get baseline personal and family history of diabetes, obesity, dyslipidemia, hypertension, and cardiovascular disease

✽ Get waist circumference (at umbilicus), blood pressure, fasting plasma glucose, and fasting lipid profile
- Determine if the patient is
  - overweight (BMI 25.0–29.9)
  - obese (BMI ≥30)
  - has pre-diabetes (fasting plasma glucose 100–125 mg/dL)
  - has diabetes (fasting plasma glucose >126 mg/dL)
  - has hypertension (BP >140/90 mm Hg)
  - has dyslipidemia (increased total cholesterol, LDL cholesterol, and triglycerides; decreased HDL cholesterol)
- Treat or refer such patients for treatment, including nutrition and weight management, physical activity counseling, smoking cessation, and medical management

Monitoring after starting an atypical antipsychotic

✽ BMI monthly for 3 months, then quarterly

✽ Consider monitoring fasting triglycerides monthly for several months in patients at high risk for metabolic complications and when initiating or switching antipsychotics

✽ Blood pressure, fasting plasma glucose, fasting lipids within 3 months and then annually, but earlier and more frequently for patients with diabetes or who have gained >5% of initial weight
- Treat or refer for treatment and consider switching to another atypical antipsychotic for patients who become overweight, obese, pre-diabetic, diabetic, hypertensive, or dyslipidemic while receiving an atypical antipsychotic

✽ Even in patients without known diabetes, be vigilant for the rare but life-threatening onset of diabetic ketoacidosis, which always requires immediate treatment, by monitoring for the rapid onset of polyuria, polydipsia, weight loss, nausea, vomiting, dehydration, rapid respiration, weakness, and clouding of sensorium, even coma
- Routine EKGs for screening or monitoring of dubious clinical value
- EKGs may be useful for selected patients (e.g., those with personal or family history of QTc prolongation; cardiac arrhythmia; recent myocardial infarction; uncompensated heart failure; or those taking agents that prolong QTc interval such as pimozide, thioridazine, selected antiarrhythmics, moxifloxacin, sparfloxacin, etc.)
- Patients at risk for electrolyte disturbances (e.g., patients on diuretic therapy) should have baseline and periodic serum potassium and magnesium measurements
- Patients with low white blood cell count (WBC) or history of drug-induced leucopenia/neutropenia should have complete blood count (CBC) monitored frequently during the first few months and ziprasidone should be discontinued at the first sign of decline of WBC in the absence of other causative factors

SIDE EFFECTS

How Drug Causes Side Effects

- By blocking alpha 1 adrenergic receptors, it can cause dizziness, sedation, and hypotension, especially at high doses

- By blocking dopamine 2 receptors in the striatum, it can cause motor side effects (unusual)

✻ Mechanism of any possible weight gain is unknown; weight gain is not common with ziprasidone and may thus have a different mechanism from atypical antipsychotics for which weight gain is common or problematic

✻ Mechanism of any possible increased incidence of diabetes or dyslipidemia is unknown; early experience suggests these complications are not clearly associated with ziprasidone and if present may therefore have a different mechanism from that of atypical antipsychotics associated with an increased incidence of diabetes and dyslipidemia

Notable Side Effects

✻ Activation (at very low to low doses)

- Dizziness, extrapyramidal symptoms, sedation (dose-dependent), dystonia at high doses
- Nausea, dry mouth (dose-dependent)
- Asthenia, skin rash
- Orthostatic hypotension (dose-dependent)

Life-Threatening or Dangerous Side Effects

- Rare but serious skin condition known as Drug Reaction with Eosinophilia (DRESS)
- Rare neuroleptic malignant syndrome (much reduced risk compared to conventional antipsychotics)
- Rare tardive dyskinesia (much reduced risk compared to conventional antipsychotics)
- Rare seizures
- Increased risk of death and cerebrovascular events in elderly patients with dementia-related psychosis

Weight Gain

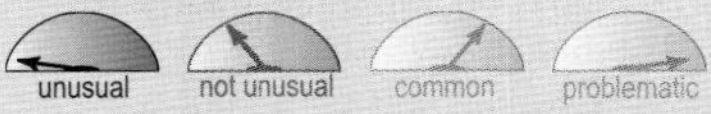

- Reported in a few patients, especially those with low BMIs, but not expected
- Less frequent and less severe than for most other antipsychotics

Sedation

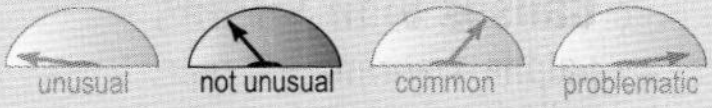

- Some patients experience, especially at high doses
- May be less than for some antipsychotics, more than for others
- Usually transient and at higher doses
- Can be activating at low doses

What to Do About Side Effects

- Wait
- Wait
- Wait
- Usually dosed twice daily, so take more of the total daily dose at bedtime to help reduce daytime sedation
- Anticholinergics may reduce motor side effects when present
- Weight loss, exercise programs, and medical management for high BMIs, diabetes, dyslipidemia

✻ For activating side effects at low doses, raise the dose

✻ For sedating side effects at high doses, lower the dose

- Switch to another atypical antipsychotic

Best Augmenting Agents for Side Effects

- Benztropine or trihexyphenidyl for motor side effects
- Many side effects cannot be improved with an augmenting agent

DOSING AND USE

Usual Dosage Range

- Schizophrenia: 40–200 mg/day (in divided doses) orally
- Bipolar disorder: 80–160 mg/day (in divided doses) orally
- 10–20 mg intramuscularly

Dosage Forms

- Capsules 20 mg, 40 mg, 60 mg, 80 mg
- Injection 20 mg/mL

How to Dose

- Schizophrenia (according to manufacturer): initial oral dose 20 mg twice a day; however, 40 mg twice a day or 60 mg twice a day may be better tolerated in many patients (less activation); maximum approved dose 100 mg twice a day
- Bipolar disorder (according to manufacturer): initial oral dose 40 mg twice a day; on day 2 increase to 60 or 80 mg twice a day

- For intramuscular formulation, recommended dose is 10–20 mg given as required; doses of 10 mg may be administered every 2 hours; doses of 20 mg may be administered every 4 hours; maximum daily dose 40 mg intramuscularly; should not be administered for more than 3 consecutive days
- See also The Art of Switching section, after Pearls

Dosing Tips

✻ **More may be much more:** clinical practice suggests ziprasidone often under-dosed, then switched prior to adequate trials, perhaps due to unjustified fears of QTc prolongation

✻ Dosing many patients at 20–40 mg twice a day is too low and in fact activating, perhaps due to potent 5HT2C antagonist properties

✻ Paradoxically, such activation is often reduced by increasing the dose to 60–80 mg twice a day, perhaps due to increasing amounts of dopamine 2 receptor antagonism

✻ Best efficacy in schizophrenia and bipolar disorder is at doses >120 mg/day, but only a minority of patients are adequately dosed in clinical practice

✻ Recommended to be taken with food because food can double bioavailability by increasing absorption and thus increasing plasma drug levels

- Meals of a few hundred calories (e.g., turkey sandwich and a piece of fruit) or more are necessary to enhance the absorption of ziprasidone
- Some patients respond better to doses >160 mg/day and up to 320 mg/day in 2 divided doses (i.e., 80–160 mg twice a day)
- Many patients do well with a single daily oral dose, usually at bedtime
- QTc prolongation at 320 mg/day not significantly greater than at 160 mg/day
- Rather than raise the dose above these levels in acutely agitated patients requiring acute antipsychotic actions, consider augmentation with a benzodiazepine or conventional antipsychotic, either orally or intramuscularly
- Rather than raise the dose above these levels in partial responders, consider augmentation with a mood-stabilizing anticonvulsant, such as valproate or lamotrigine
- Children and elderly should generally be dosed at the lower end of the dosage spectrum
- Ziprasidone intramuscular can be given short-term, both to initiate dosing with oral ziprasidone or another oral antipsychotic and to treat breakthrough agitation in patients maintained on oral antipsychotics
- QTc prolongation of intramuscular ziprasidone is the same or less than with intramuscular haloperidol
- Treatment should be suspended if absolute neutrophil count falls below 1,000/mm^3

Overdose

- Rarely lethal in monotherapy overdose; sedation, slurred speech, transitory hypertension

Long-Term Use

- Approved to delay relapse in long-term treatment of schizophrenia
- Often used for long-term maintenance in bipolar disorder and various behavioral disorders

Habit Forming

- No

How to Stop

- See Switching section of individual agents for how to stop ziprasidone
- Rapid oral discontinuation may lead to rebound psychosis and worsening of symptoms

Pharmacokinetics

- Mean half-life 6.6 hours
- Protein binding >99%
- Metabolized by CYP450 3A4
- Absorption is approximately doubled if taken with food

Drug Interactions

- Neither CYP450 3A4 nor CYP450 2D6 inhibitors significantly affect ziprasidone plasma levels
- Little potential to affect metabolism of drugs cleared by CYP450 enzymes
- May enhance the effects of antihypertensive drugs

- May antagonize levodopa, dopamine agonists
- May enhance QTc prolongation of other drugs capable of prolonging QTc interval

Other Warnings/ Precautions

- Ziprasidone prolongs QTc interval more than some other antipsychotics
- Ziprasidone is associated with a rare but serious skin condition known as Drug Reaction with Eosinophilia (DRESS). DRESS may begin as a rash but can progress to others parts of the body and can include symptoms such as fever, swollen lymph nodes, swollen face, inflammation of organs, and an increase in white blood cells known as eosinophilia. In some cases, DRESS can lead to death. Clinicians prescribing ziprasidone should inform patients about the risk of DRESS; patients who develop a fever with rash and swollen lymph nodes or swollen face should seek medical care. Patients are not advised to stop their medication without consulting their prescribing clinician.
- Use with caution in patients with conditions that predispose to hypotension (dehydration, overheating)
- Priapism has been reported
- Dysphagia has been associated with antipsychotic use, and ziprasidone should be used cautiously in patients at risk for aspiration pneumonia

Do Not Use

- If patient is taking agents capable of significantly prolonging QTc interval (e.g., pimozide, thioridazine, selected antiarrhythmics, moxifloxacin, sparfloxacin)
- If there is a history of QTc prolongation or cardiac arrhythmia, recent acute myocardial infarction, uncompensated heart failure
- If there is a proven allergy to ziprasidone

SPECIAL POPULATIONS

Renal Impairment

- No dose adjustment necessary
- Not removed by hemodialysis
- Intramuscular formulation should be used with caution

Hepatic Impairment

- No dose adjustment necessary

Cardiac Impairment

- Ziprasidone is contraindicated in patients with a known history of QTc prolongation, recent acute myocardial infarction, and uncompensated heart failure
- Should be used with caution in other cases of cardiac impairment because of risk of orthostatic hypotension

Elderly

- Some patients may tolerate lower doses better
- Although atypical antipsychotics are commonly used for behavioral disturbances in dementia, no agent has been approved for treatment of elderly patients with dementia-related psychosis
- Elderly patients with dementia-related psychosis treated with atypical antipsychotics are at an increased risk of death compared to placebo, and also have an increased risk of cerebrovascular events

Children and Adolescents

- Not officially recommended for patients under age 18
- Clinical experience and early data suggest ziprasidone may be safe and effective for behavioral disturbances in children and adolescents
- Children and adolescents using ziprasidone may need to be monitored more often than adults and may tolerate lower doses better

Pregnancy

- Effective June 30, 2015, the US FDA requires changes to the content and format of pregnancy and lactation information in prescription drug labels, including the elimination of the pregnancy letter categories; the Pregnancy and Lactation Labeling Rule (PLLR or final rule) applies only to prescription drugs and will be phased in gradually for drugs approved on or after June 30, 2001
- Controlled studies have not been conducted in pregnant women

- There is a risk of abnormal muscle movements and withdrawal symptoms in newborns whose mothers took an antipsychotic during the third trimester; symptoms may include agitation, abnormally increased or decreased muscle tone, tremor, sleepiness, severe difficulty breathing, and difficulty feeding
- Psychotic symptoms may worsen during pregnancy and some form of treatment may be necessary
- Ziprasidone may be preferable to anticonvulsant mood stabilizers if treatment is required during pregnancy
- National Pregnancy Registry for Atypical Antipsychotics: 1-866-961-2388 or http://womensmentalhealth.org/clinical-and-research-programs/pregnancyregistry/

Breast Feeding

- Unknown if ziprasidone is secreted in human breast milk, but all psychotropics assumed to be secreted in breast milk

✽ Recommended either to discontinue drug or bottle feed

- Infants of women who choose to breast feed while on ziprasidone should be monitored for possible adverse effects

THE ART OF PSYCHOPHARMACOLOGY

Potential Advantages

- Some cases of psychosis and bipolar disorder refractory to treatment with other antipsychotics

✽ Patients concerned about gaining weight and patients who are already obese or overweight

✽ Patients with diabetes

✽ Patients with dyslipidemia (especially elevated triglycerides)

- Patients requiring rapid relief of symptoms (intramuscular injection)
- Patients switching from intramuscular ziprasidone to an oral preparation

Potential Disadvantages

- Patients noncompliant with twice daily dosing

✽ Patients noncompliant with dosing with food

Primary Target Symptoms

- Positive symptoms of psychosis
- Negative symptoms of psychosis
- Cognitive symptoms
- Unstable mood (both depression and mania)
- Aggressive symptoms

Pearls

- Recent landmark head-to-head study in schizophrenia suggests lower metabolic side effects and comparable efficacy compared to some other atypical and conventional antipsychotics

✽ When given to patients with obesity and dyslipidemia associated with prior treatment with another atypical antipsychotic, many experience weight loss and decrease in fasting triglycerides

✽ QTc prolongation fears are often exaggerated and not justified since QTc prolongation with ziprasidone is not dose-related and few drugs have any potential to increase ziprasidone's plasma levels

✽ Efficacy may be underestimated since ziprasidone is mostly under-dosed (<120 mg/day) in clinical practice

✽ Well accepted in clinical practice when wanting to avoid weight gain because less weight gain than most other atypical antipsychotics

✽ May not have diabetes or dyslipidemia risk, but monitoring is still indicated

- Less sedation than some antipsychotics, more than others (at moderate to high doses)

✽ More activating than some other antipsychotics at low doses

- Anecdotal reports of utility in treatment-resistant cases, especially when adequately dosed

✽ A short-acting intramuscular dosage formulation is available

- Approved for mania in children ages 10–17
- Patients with inadequate responses to atypical antipsychotics may benefit from determination of plasma drug levels and, if low, a dosage increase even beyond the usual prescribing limits
- For treatment-resistant patients, especially those with impulsivity,

aggression, violence, and self-harm, long-term polypharmacy with 2 atypical antipsychotics or with 1 atypical antipsychotic and 1 conventional antipsychotic may be useful or even necessary while closely monitoring

- In such cases, it may be beneficial to combine 1 depot antipsychotic with 1 oral antipsychotic

THE ART OF SWITCHING

Switching from Oral Antipsychotics to Ziprasidone

- With aripiprazole, amisulpride, and paliperidone ER, immediate stop is possible; begin ziprasidone at an intermediate dose
- Clinical experience has shown that quetiapine, olanzapine, and asenapine should be tapered off slowly over a period of 3–4 weeks, to allow patients to readapt to the withdrawal of blocking cholinergic, histaminergic, and alpha 1 receptors
- Clozapine should always be tapered off slowly, over a period of 4 weeks or more

* Benzodiazepine or anticholinergic medication can be administered during cross-titration to help alleviate side effects such as insomnia, agitation, and/or psychosis

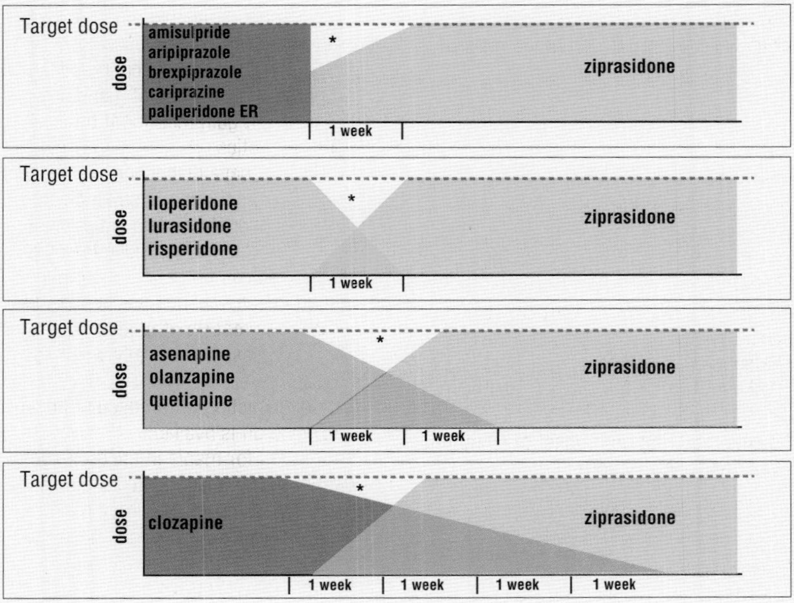

Suggested Reading

Komossa K, Rummel-Kluge C, Hunger H, et al. Ziprasidone versus other atypical antipsychotics for schizophrenia. Cochrane Database Syst Rev 2009;7(4):CD006627.

Lieberman JA, Stroup TS, McEvoy JP, et al. Effectiveness of antipsychotic drugs in patients with chronic schizophrenia. N Engl J Med 2005;353(12):1209–23.

Nasrallah HA Jr. Atypical antipsychotic-induced metabolic side effects: insights from receptor-binding profiles. Mol Psychiatry 2008;13(1):27–35.

Smith LA, Cornelius V, Warnock A, Tacchi MJ, Taylor D. Pharmacological interventions for acute bipolar mania: a systematic review of randomized placebo-controlled trials. Bipolar Disord 2007;9(6):551–60.

Taylor D. Ziprasidone in the management of schizophrenia: the QT interval issue in context. CNS Drugs 2003;17:423–30.

ZOLPIDEM

THERAPEUTICS

Brands • Ambien, Ambien CR
• Intermezzo

see index for additional brand names

Generic? Yes

Class

• Neuroscience-based Nomenclature: GABA positive allosteric modulator (GABA-PAM)
• Non-benzodiazepine hypnotic; alpha 1 isoform selective agonist of GABA-A/benzodiazepine receptors

Commonly Prescribed for

(bold for FDA approved)

• **Short-term treatment of insomnia (controlled-release indication is not restricted to short-term)**
• **As needed for the treatment of insomnia when a middle-of-the-night awakening is followed by difficulty returning to sleep and there are at least 4 hours of bedtime remaining before the planned time of wakening (Intermezzo)**

How the Drug Works

• Binds selectively to a subtype of the benzodiazepine receptor, the alpha 1 isoform
• May enhance GABA inhibitory actions that provide sedative hypnotic effects more selectively than other actions of GABA
• Boosts chloride conductance through GABA-regulated channels
• Inhibitory actions in sleep centers may provide sedative hypnotic effects
• CR formulation may allow sufficient drug to persist at receptors to improve total sleep time and to prevent early morning awakenings that can be associated with the immediate-release formulation of zolpidem

How Long Until It Works

• Generally takes effect in less than an hour

If It Works

• Improves quality of sleep
• Effects on total wake-time and number of nighttime awakenings may be decreased over time

If It Doesn't Work

• If insomnia does not improve after 7–10 days, it may be a manifestation of a primary psychiatric or physical illness such as obstructive sleep apnea or restless leg syndrome, which requires independent evaluation
• Increase the dose
• Improve sleep hygiene
• Switch to another agent

Best Augmenting Combos for Partial Response or Treatment Resistance

• Generally, best to switch to another agent
• Trazodone
• Agents with antihistamine actions (e.g., diphenhydramine, TCAs)

Tests

• None for healthy individuals

SIDE EFFECTS

How Drug Causes Side Effects

• Actions at benzodiazepine receptors that carry over to the next day can cause daytime sedation, amnesia, and ataxia
• Long-term adaptations of zolpidem immediate-release not well studied, but chronic studies of zolpidem CR and other alpha 1 selective non-benzodiazepine hypnotics suggest lack of notable tolerance or dependence developing over time

Notable Side Effects

✻ Sedation
✻ Dizziness, ataxia
✻ Dose-dependent amnesia
✻ Hyperexcitability, nervousness
• Rare hallucinations
• Diarrhea, nausea
• Headache

Life-Threatening or Dangerous Side Effects

• Respiratory depression, especially when taken with other CNS depressants in overdose
• Rare angioedema

Weight Gain

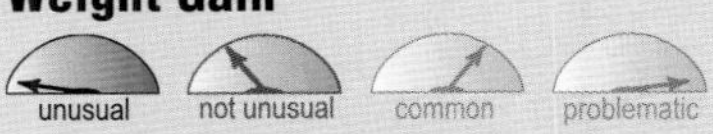

• Reported but not expected

Sedation

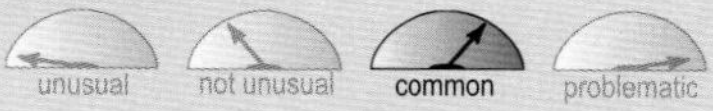

- Many experience and/or can be significant in amount

What to Do About Side Effects

- Wait
- To avoid problems with memory, only take zolpidem or zolpidem CR if planning to have a full night's sleep
- Lower the dose
- Switch to a shorter-acting sedative hypnotic
- Administer flumazenil if side effects are severe or life-threatening

Best Augmenting Agents for Side Effects

- Many side effects cannot be improved with an augmenting agent

DOSING AND USE

Usual Dosage Range

- 10 mg/day at bedtime for 7–10 days (immediate-release)
- 12.5 mg/day at bedtime (controlled-release)

Dosage Forms

- Immediate-release tablet 5 mg
- Controlled-release tablet 6.25 mg, 12.5 mg
- Sublingual tablet 1.75 mg, 3.5 mg, 5 mg, 10 mg
- Oral spray 5 mg

How to Dose

- Men: 10 mg at bedtime for 7–10 days (immediate-release); 12.5 mg at bedtime for 7–10 days (controlled-release); 3.5 mg sublingually in the middle of the night if more than 4 hours of bedtime remain (Intermezzo)
- Women: 5 mg at bedtime for 7–10 days (immediate-release); 6.25 mg at bedtime for 7–10 days (controlled-release); 1.75 mg sublingually in the middle of the night if more than 4 hours of bedtime remain (Intermezzo)
- Intermezzo formulation is administered sublingually in the middle of the night; it should be placed under the tongue and allowed to dissolve completely before swallowing
- Intermezzo formulation should not be taken more than once per night

Dosing Tips

- ✻ Zolpidem is not absorbed as quickly if taken with food, which could reduce onset of action
- Patients with lower body weights may require only a 5-mg dose immediate-release or 6.25 mg controlled-release
- Zolpidem should generally not be prescribed in quantities greater than a 1-month supply; however, zolpidem CR is not restricted to short-term use
- Risk of dependence may increase with dose and duration of treatment
- ✻ However, treatment with alpha 1 selective non-benzodiazepine hypnotics may cause less tolerance or dependence than benzodiazepine hypnotics
- Controlled-release tablets should be swallowed whole and should not be divided, crushed, or chewed

Overdose

- No fatalities reported with zolpidem monotherapy; sedation, ataxia, confusion, hypotension, respiratory depression, coma

Long-Term Use

- Original studies with zolpidem immediate-release did not assess long-term use
- Zolpidem CR is not restricted to short-term use
- Increased wakefulness during the latter part of night (wearing off) or an increase in daytime anxiety (rebound) may occur with immediate-release and be less common with controlled-release

Habit Forming

- Zolpidem is a Schedule IV drug
- Some patients may develop dependence and/or tolerance; risk may be greater with higher doses
- History of drug addiction may increase risk of dependence

How to Stop

- Although rebound insomnia could occur, this effect has not generally been seen

with therapeutic doses of zolpidem or zolpidem CR
- If taken for more than a few weeks, taper to reduce chances of withdrawal effects

Pharmacokinetics
- Short elimination half-life (approximately 2.5 hours)

Drug Interactions
- Increased depressive effects when taken with other CNS depressants
- Sertraline may increase plasma levels of zolpidem
- Rifampin may decrease plasma levels of zolpidem
- Ketoconazole may increase plasma levels of zolpidem
- Use with imipramine or chlorpromazine may be associated with decreased alertness

Other Warnings/ Precautions
- Insomnia may be a symptom of a primary disorder, rather than a primary disorder itself
- Some patients may exhibit abnormal thinking or behavioral changes similar to those caused by other CNS depressants (i.e., either depressant actions or disinhibiting actions)
- Some depressed patients may experience a worsening of suicidal ideation
- Use only with extreme caution in patients with impaired respiratory function or obstructive sleep apnea
- Zolpidem and zolpidem CR should only be administered at bedtime
- Temporary memory loss may occur at doses above 10 mg/night
- Rare angioedema has occurred with sedative hypnotic use and could potentially cause fatal airway obstruction if it involves the throat, glottis, or larynx; thus if angioedema occurs treatment should be discontinued
- Sleep driving and other complex behaviors, such as eating and preparing food and making phone calls, have been reported in patients taking sedative hypnotics

Do Not Use
- If there is a proven allergy to zolpidem
- For Intermezzo, if the patient has fewer than 4 hours of bedtime remaining before the planned time of waking

SPECIAL POPULATIONS

Renal Impairment
- No dose adjustment necessary
- Patients should be monitored

Hepatic Impairment
- Recommended dose 5 mg (immediate-release), 6.25 mg (controlled-release), 1.75 mg (Intermezzo)
- Patients should be monitored

Cardiac Impairment
- No available data

Elderly
- Recommended initial dose: 5 mg (immediate-release), 6.25 mg (controlled-release), 1.75 mg (Intermezzo)
- Elderly may have increased risk for falls, confusion

Children and Adolescents
- Safety and efficacy have not been established
- Long-term effects of zolpidem or zolpidem CR in children/adolescents are unknown
- Should generally receive lower doses and be more closely monitored
- Hallucinations in children ages 6-17 have been reported

Pregnancy
- Effective June 30, 2015, the US FDA requires changes to the content and format of pregnancy and lactation information in prescription drug labels, including the elimination of the pregnancy letter categories; the Pregnancy and Lactation Labeling Rule (PLLR or final rule) applies only to prescription drugs and will be

phased in gradually for drugs approved on or after June 30, 2001
- Controlled studies have not been conducted in pregnant women
- Infants whose mothers took sedative hypnotics during pregnancy may experience some withdrawal symptoms
- Neonatal flaccidity has been reported in infants whose mothers took sedative hypnotics during pregnancy

Breast Feeding

- Some drug is found in mother's breast milk

✻ Recommended either to discontinue drug or bottle feed

THE ART OF PSYCHOPHARMACOLOGY

Potential Advantages

- Patients who require long-term treatment, especially CR formulation

Potential Disadvantages

- More expensive than some other sedative hypnotics

Primary Target Symptoms

- Time to sleep onset
- Total sleep time
- Nighttime awakenings

Pearls

✻ One of the most popular sedative hypnotic agents in psychopharmacology
- Zolpidem has been shown to increase the total time asleep and to reduce the amount of nighttime awakenings
- Zolpidem CR may be even more effective on these sleep parameters than immediate-release zolpidem due to prolonged drug delivery

✻ May be preferred over benzodiazepines because of its rapid onset of action, short duration of effect, and safety profile
- In some patients, zolpidem blood levels may be high enough the morning after use to impair activities that require alertness, including driving; this has prompted the US FDA to issue new dosing requirements
- Specifically, because clearance of zolpidem is slightly slower in women than in men, the FDA has required that the recommended dose be lowered for women
- The FDA also recommends that health-care professionals consider prescribing lower doses for men as well
- A low-dose zolpidem product is approved for middle-of-the-night awakenings by sublingual administration
- May not be ideal for patients who desire immediate hypnotic onset and eat just prior to bedtime
- Not a benzodiazepine itself, but binds to benzodiazepine receptors
- May have fewer carryover side effects than some other sedative hypnotics
- May cause less dependence than some other sedative hypnotics, especially in those without a history of substance abuse

Suggested Reading

Daley C, McNiel DE, Binder RL. "I did what?" Zolpidem and the courts. J Am Acad Psychiatry Law 2011;39(4):535–42.

Greenblatt DJ, Roth T. Zolpidem for insomnia. Expert Opin Pharmacother 2012;13(6):879–93.

Rush CR. Behavioral pharmacology of zolpidem relative to benzodiazepines: a review. Pharmacol Biochem Behav 1998;61:253–69.

Soyka M, Bottlender R, Moller HJ. Epidemiological evidence for a low abuse potential of zolpidem. Pharmacopsychiatry 2000;33:138–41.

Toner LC, Tsambiras BM, Catalano G, Catalano MC, Cooper DS. Central nervous system side effects associated with zolpidem treatment. Clin Neuropharmacol 2000;23:54–8.

THERAPEUTICS

Brands • Zonegran
• Excegran

see index for additional brand names

Generic? Yes

Class

• Anticonvulsant, voltage-sensitive sodium channel modulator; T-type calcium channel modulator; structurally a sulfonamide

Commonly Prescribed for

(bold for FDA approved)

• **Adjunct therapy for partial seizures in adults with epilepsy**
• Bipolar disorder
• Chronic neuropathic pain
• Migraine
• Parkinson's disease
• Psychotropic drug-induced weight gain
• Binge eating disorder

How the Drug Works

• Unknown
• Modulates voltage-sensitive sodium channels by an unknown mechanism
• Also modulates T-type calcium channels
• Facilitates dopamine and serotonin release
• Inhibits carbonic anhydrase

How Long Until It Works

• Should reduce seizures by 2 weeks
• Onset of action as well as convincing therapeutic efficacy have not been demonstrated for uses other than adjunctive treatment of partial seizures

If It Works

• The goal of treatment is complete remission of symptoms (e.g., seizures, pain, mania, migraine)
• Would currently only be expected to work in a subset of patients for conditions other than epilepsy as an adjunctive treatment to agents with better demonstration of efficacy

If It Doesn't Work (for conditions other than epilepsy)

• May be effective only in patients who fail to respond to agents with proven efficacy, or it may not work at all
• Consider increasing dose or switching to another agent with better demonstrated efficacy

Best Augmenting Combos for Partial Response or Treatment Resistance

• Zonisamide is itself a second-line augmenting agent to numerous other agents in treating conditions other than epilepsy, such as bipolar disorder, chronic neuropathic pain, and migraine

Tests

• Consider baseline and periodic monitoring of renal function

SIDE EFFECTS

How Drug Causes Side Effects

• CNS side effects theoretically due to excessive actions at voltage-sensitive ion channels
• Weak inhibition of carbonic anhydrase may lead to kidney stones
• Serious rash theoretically an allergic reaction

Notable Side Effects

✻ Sedation, depression, difficulty concentrating, agitation, irritability, psychomotor slowing, dizziness, ataxia
• Headache
• Nausea, anorexia, abdominal pain, vomiting
• Kidney stones
• Elevated serum creatinine and blood urea nitrogen

Life-Threatening or Dangerous Side Effects

• Rare serious rash (Stevens-Johnson syndrome, toxic epidermal necrolysis) (sulfonamide)
• Rare oligohidrosis and hyperthermia (pediatric patients)
• Rare blood dyscrasias (aplastic anemia; agranulocytosis)
• Sudden hepatic necrosis
• Sudden unexplained deaths have occurred (unknown if related to zonisamide use)
• Rare activation of suicidal ideation and behavior (suicidality)

Weight Gain

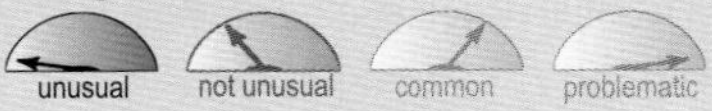

- Reported but not expected

✻ Patients may experience weight loss

Sedation

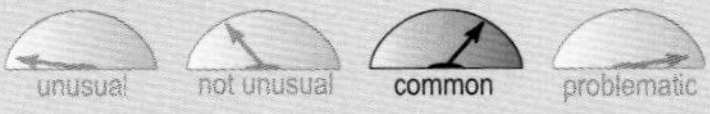

- Many experience and/or can be significant in amount
- Dose-related
- Can wear off with time but may not wear off at high doses

What to Do About Side Effects

- Wait
- Wait
- Wait
- Take more of the dose at night to reduce daytime sedation
- Lower the dose
- Switch to another agent

Best Augmenting Agents for Side Effects

- Many side effects cannot be improved with an augmenting agent

DOSING AND USE

Usual Dosage Range

- 100–600 mg/day in 1–2 doses

Dosage Forms

- Capsule 25 mg, 50 mg, 100 mg

How to Dose

- Initial 100 mg/day; after 2 weeks can increase to 200 mg/day; dose can be increased by 100 mg/day every 2 weeks if necessary and tolerated; maximum dose generally 600 mg/day; maintain stable dose for at least 2 weeks before increasing dose

Dosing Tips

✻ Most clinical experience is at doses up to 400 mg/day

- No evidence from controlled trials of increasing response over 400 mg/day
- However, some patients may tolerate and respond to doses up to 600 mg/day
- Little experience with doses greater than 600 mg/day
- Side effects may increase notably at doses greater than 300 mg/day
- For intolerable sedation, can give most of the dose at night and less during the day

Overdose

- Can cause bradycardia, hypotension, respiratory depression

Long-Term Use

- Safe
- Consider periodic monitoring of blood urea nitrogen and creatinine

Habit Forming

- No

How to Stop

- Taper
- Epilepsy patients may seize upon withdrawal, especially if withdrawal is abrupt
- Rapid discontinuation may increase the risk of relapse in bipolar patients
- Discontinuation symptoms uncommon

Pharmacokinetics

- Plasma elimination half-life approximately 63 hours
- Metabolized in part by CYP450 3A4
- Partially eliminated renally

Drug Interactions

- Agents that inhibit CYP450 3A4 (such as nefazodone, fluvoxamine, and fluoxetine) may decrease the clearance of zonisamide, and increase plasma zonisamide levels, possibly requiring lower doses of zonisamide
- Agents that induce CYP450 3A4 (such as carbamazepine) may increase the clearance of zonisamide and decrease plasma zonisamide levels, possibly requiring higher doses of zonisamide
- Enzyme-inducing antiepileptic drugs (carbamazepine, phenytoin, phenobarbital, and primidone) may decrease plasma levels of zonisamide
- Theoretically, zonisamide may interact with carbonic anhydrase inhibitors to increase the risk of kidney stones

Other Warnings/ Precautions

- Depressive effects may be increased by other CNS depressants (alcohol, MAOIs, other anticonvulsants, etc.)
- Use with caution when combining with other drugs that predispose patients to heat-related disorders, including carbonic anhydrase inhibitors and anticholinergics
- ✻ Life-threatening rashes have developed in association with zonisamide use; zonisamide should generally be discontinued at the first sign of serious rash
- Patient should be instructed to report any symptoms of hypersensitivity immediately (fever; flu-like symptoms; rash; blisters on skin or in eyes, mouth, ears, nose, or genital areas; swelling of eyelids, conjunctivitis, lymphadenopathy)
- Patients should be monitored for signs of unusual bleeding or bruising, mouth sores, infections, fever, and sore throat, as there may be an increased risk of aplastic anemia and agranulocytosis with zonisamide
- Warn patients and their caregivers about the possibility of activation of suicidal ideation and advise them to report such side effects immediately

Do Not Use

- If there is a proven allergy to zonisamide or sulfonamides

SPECIAL POPULATIONS

Renal Impairment

- Zonisamide is primarily renally excreted
- Use with caution
- May require slower titration

Hepatic Impairment

- Use with caution
- May require slower titration

Cardiac Impairment

- No specific recommendations

Elderly

- Some patients may tolerate lower doses better
- Elderly patients may be more susceptible to adverse effects

Children and Adolescents

- Cases of oligohidrosis and hyperthermia have been reported
- Not approved for use in children under age 16
- Use in children for the expert only, with close monitoring, after other options have failed

Pregnancy

- Effective June 30, 2015, the US FDA requires changes to the content and format of pregnancy and lactation information in prescription drug labels, including the elimination of the pregnancy letter categories; the Pregnancy and Lactation Labeling Rule (PLLR or final rule) applies only to prescription drugs and will be phased in gradually for drugs approved on or after June 30, 2001
- Controlled studies have not been conducted in pregnant women
- Use in women of childbearing potential requires weighing potential benefits to the mother against the risks to the fetus
- Antiepileptic Drug Pregnancy Registry: (888) 233–2334
- Taper drug if discontinuing
- Seizures, even mild seizures, may cause harm to the embryo/fetus
- Lack of convincing efficacy for treatment of conditions other than epilepsy suggests risk/benefit ratio is in favor of discontinuing zonisamide during pregnancy for these indications

Breast Feeding

- Unknown if zonisamide is secreted in human breast milk, but all psychotropics assumed to be secreted in breast milk
- ✻ Recommended either to discontinue drug or bottle feed
- If drug is continued while breast feeding, infant should be monitored for possible adverse effects
- If child becomes irritable or sedated, breast feeding or drug may need to be discontinued

THE ART OF PSYCHOPHARMACOLOGY

Potential Advantages
- Treatment-resistant conditions
- Patients who wish to avoid weight gain

Potential Disadvantages
- Poor documentation of efficacy for off-label uses
- Patients noncompliant with twice daily dosing

Primary Target Symptoms
- Seizures
- Numerous other symptoms for off-label uses
- Patients with a history of kidney stones

Pearls
- Well studied in epilepsy
- * Much off-label use is based upon theoretical considerations rather than clinical experience or compelling efficacy studies
- Early studies suggest efficacy in binge eating disorder
- Early studies suggest possible efficacy in migraine
- Early studies suggest possible utility in Parkinson's disease
- Early studies suggest possible utility in neuropathic pain
- Early studies suggest some therapeutic potential for mood stabilizing
- Chronic intake of caffeine may lower brain zonisamide concentrations and attenuate its anticonvulsant effects (based on animal studies)
- * Due to reported weight loss in some patients in trials with epilepsy, some patients with psychotropic-induced weight gain are treated with zonisamide
- Utility for this indication is not clear nor has it been systematically studied
- Phase II trials for the combination of zonisamide and bupropion as a treatment for obesity have been completed

Suggested Reading

Chadwick DW, Marson AG. Zonisamide add-on for drug-resistant partial epilepsy. Cochrane Database Syst Rev 2002;(2):CD001416.

Glauser TA, Pellock JM. Zonisamide in pediatric epilepsy: review of the Japanese experience. J Child Neurol 2002;17:87–96.

Jain KK. An assessment of zonisamide as an anti-epileptic drug. Expert Opin Pharmacother 2000;1:1245–60.

Leppik IE. Three new drugs for epilepsy: levetiracetam, oxcarbazepine, and zonisamide. J Child Neurol 2002;17(Suppl 1):S53–7.

THERAPEUTICS

Brands • Imovane

see index for additional brand names

Generic? No

Class

- Neuroscience-based Nomenclature: GABA positive allosteric modulator (GABA-PAM)
- Non-benzodiazepine hypnotic; alpha 1 isoform selective agonist of GABA-A/benzodiazepine receptors

Commonly Prescribed for

(bold for FDA approved)

- Short-term treatment of insomnia

How the Drug Works

- May bind selectively to a subtype of the benzodiazepine receptor, the alpha 1 isoform
- May enhance GABA inhibitory actions that provide sedative hypnotic effects more selectively than other actions of GABA
- Boosts chloride conductance through GABA-regulated channels
- Inhibitory actions in sleep centers may provide sedative hypnotic effects

How Long Until It Works

- Generally takes effect in less than an hour

If It Works

- Improves quality of sleep
- Effects on total wake-time and number of nighttime awakenings may be decreased over time

If It Doesn't Work

- If insomnia does not improve after 7–10 days, it may be a manifestation of a primary psychiatric or physical illness such as obstructive sleep apnea or restless leg syndrome, which requires independent evaluation
- Increase the dose
- Improve sleep hygiene
- Switch to another agent

Best Augmenting Combos for Partial Response or Treatment Resistance

- Generally, best to switch to another agent
- Trazodone
- Agents with antihistamine actions (e.g., diphenhydramine, TCAs)

Tests

- None for healthy individuals

SIDE EFFECTS

How Drug Causes Side Effects

- Actions at benzodiazepine receptors that carry over to the next day can cause daytime sedation, amnesia, and ataxia

✱ Long-term adaptations of zopiclone, a mixture of an active S enantiomer and an inactive R enantiomer, have not been well studied, but chronic studies of the active isomer eszopiclone suggest lack of notable tolerance or dependence developing over time

Notable Side Effects

✱ Sedation

✱ Dizziness, ataxia

✱ Dose-dependent amnesia

✱ Hyperexcitability, nervousness

- Dry mouth, loss of appetite, constipation, bitter taste
- Impaired vision

Life-Threatening or Dangerous Side Effects

- Respiratory depression, especially when taken with other CNS depressants in overdose
- Rare angioedema

Weight Gain

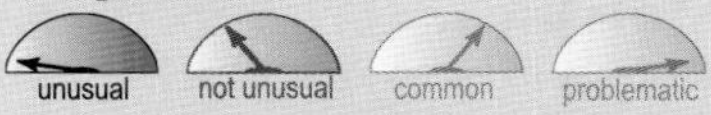

- Reported but not expected

Sedation

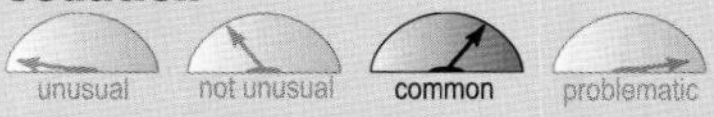

- Many experience and/or can be significant in amount

What to Do About Side Effects

- Wait
- To avoid problems with memory, only take zopiclone if planning to have a full night's sleep
- Lower the dose
- Switch to a shorter-acting sedative hypnotic

- Administer flumazenil if side effects are severe or life-threatening

Best Augmenting Agents for Side Effects
- Many side effects cannot be improved with an augmenting agent

DOSING AND USE

Usual Dosage Range
- 7.5 mg at bedtime

Dosage Forms
- Tablet 5 mg, 7.5 mg scored

How to Dose
- No titration, take dose at bedtime

Dosing Tips
- Zopiclone should generally not be prescribed in quantities greater than a 1-month supply
- Risk of dependence may increase with dose and duration of treatment
- However, chronic treatment with alpha 1 selective non-benzodiazepine hypnotics may cause less tolerance or dependence than benzodiazepine hypnotics

Overdose
- Can be fatal; clumsiness, mood changes, sedation, weakness, breathing trouble, unconsciousness

Long-Term Use
- Not generally intended for use past 4 weeks

Habit Forming
- Some patients may develop dependence and/or tolerance; risk may be greater with higher doses
- History of drug addiction may increase risk of dependence

How to Stop
- Rebound insomnia may occur the first night after stopping
- If taken for more than a few weeks, taper to reduce chances of withdrawal effects

Pharmacokinetics
- Metabolized by CYP450 3A4
- Terminal elimination half-life approximately 3.5–6.5 hours

Drug Interactions
- Increased depressive effects when taken with other CNS depressants
- Theoretically, inhibitors of CYP450 3A4, such as nefazodone and fluvoxamine, could increase plasma levels of zopiclone

Other Warnings/ Precautions
- Insomnia may be a symptom of a primary disorder, rather than a primary disorder itself
- Some patients may exhibit abnormal thinking or behavioral changes similar to those caused by other CNS depressants (i.e., either depressant actions or disinhibiting actions)
- Some depressed patients may experience a worsening of suicidal ideation
- Use only with extreme caution in patients with impaired respiratory function or obstructive sleep apnea
- Zopiclone should be administered only at bedtime
- Rare angioedema has occurred with sedative hypnotic use and could potentially cause fatal airway obstruction if it involves the throat, glottis, or larynx; thus if angioedema occurs treatment should be discontinued
- Sleep driving and other complex behaviors, such as eating and preparing food and making phone calls, have been reported in patients taking sedative hypnotics

Do Not Use
- If patient has myasthenia gravis
- If patient has severe respiratory impairment
- If patient has had a stroke
- If patient has severe hepatic insufficiency
- If there is a proven allergy to zopiclone

SPECIAL POPULATIONS

Renal Impairment
- Increased plasma levels
- May need to lower dose

Hepatic Impairment
- Increased plasma levels
- Recommended dose 3.75 mg
- Not recommended for use in patients with severe impairment

Cardiac Impairment
- Dosage adjustment may not be necessary

Elderly
- May be more susceptible to adverse effects
- Initial dose 3.75 mg at bedtime; can increase to usual adult dose if necessary and tolerated

Children and Adolescents
- Safety and efficacy have not been established
- Long-term effects of zopiclone in children/adolescents are unknown
- Should generally receive lower doses and be more closely monitored

Pregnancy
- Controlled studies have not been conducted in pregnant women
- Some animal studies show adverse effects
- Infants whose mothers took sedative hypnotics during pregnancy may experience some withdrawal symptoms
- Neonatal flaccidity has been reported in infants whose mothers took sedative hypnotics during pregnancy

Breast Feeding
- Some drug is found in mother's breast milk

❋ Recommended either to discontinue drug or bottle feed

THE ART OF PSYCHOPHARMACOLOGY

Potential Advantages
- Those who require long-term treatment

Potential Disadvantages
- More expensive than some other sedative hypnotics

Primary Target Symptoms
- Time to sleep onset
- Nighttime awakenings
- Total sleep time

Pearls

❋ May be preferred over benzodiazepines because of its rapid onset of action, short duration of effect, and safety profile

- Zopiclone does not appear to be a highly dependence-causing drug, at least not in patients with no history of drug abuse
- Rebound insomnia does not appear to be common
- Not a benzodiazepine itself, but binds to benzodiazepine receptors
- May have fewer carryover side effects than some other sedative hypnotics
- The active enantiomer of zopiclone, eszopiclone, has received an approvable letter from the US FDA

Suggested Reading

Fernandez C, Martin C, Gimenez F, Farinotti R. Clinical pharmacokinetics of zopiclone. Clin Pharmacokinet 1995;29:431–41.

Hajak G. A comparative assessment of the risks and benefits of zopiclone: a review of 15 years' clinical experience. Drug Saf 1999;21:457–69.

Noble S, Langtry HD, Lamb HM. Zopiclone. An update of its pharmacology, clinical efficacy and tolerability in the treatment of insomnia. Drugs 1998;55:277–302.

ZOTEPINE

THERAPEUTICS

Brands • Lodopin
• Zoleptil

see index for additional brand names

Generic? No

Class

- Neuroscience-based Nomenclature: dopamine and serotonin receptor antagonist (DS-RAn)
- Atypical antipsychotic (serotonin-dopamine antagonist)

Commonly Prescribed for

(bold for FDA approved)

- Schizophrenia
- Other psychotic disorders
- Mania

How the Drug Works

- Blocks dopamine 2 receptors, reducing positive symptoms of psychosis
- Blocks serotonin 2A receptors, causing enhancement of dopamine release in certain brain regions and thus reducing motor side effects and possibly improving cognitive and affective symptoms
- Interactions at a myriad of other neurotransmitter receptors may contribute to zotepine's efficacy

* Specifically inhibits norepinephrine uptake

How Long Until It Works

- Psychotic and manic symptoms can improve within 1 week, but it may take several weeks for full effect on behavior as well as on cognition and affective stabilization
- Classically recommended to wait at least 4–6 weeks to determine efficacy of drug, but in practice some patients require up to 16–20 weeks to show a good response, especially on cognitive symptoms

If It Works

- Most often reduces positive symptoms in schizophrenia but does not eliminate them
- Can improve negative symptoms, as well as aggressive, cognitive, and affective symptoms in schizophrenia
- Most schizophrenic patients do not have a total remission of symptoms but rather a reduction of symptoms by about a third
- Perhaps 5–15% of schizophrenic patients can experience an overall improvement of greater than 50–60%, especially when receiving stable treatment for more than a year
- Such patients are considered super-responders or "awakeners" since they may be well enough to be employed, live independently, and sustain long-term relationships
- Many bipolar patients may experience a reduction of symptoms by half or more
- Continue treatment until reaching a plateau of improvement
- After reaching a satisfactory plateau, continue treatment for at least a year after first episode of psychosis
- For second and subsequent episodes of psychosis, treatment may need to be indefinite
- Even for first episodes of psychosis, it may be preferable to continue treatment indefinitely to avoid subsequent episodes
- Treatment may not only reduce mania but also prevent recurrences of mania in bipolar disorder

If It Doesn't Work

- Consider trying one of the first-line atypical antipsychotics (risperidone, olanzapine, quetiapine, ziprasidone, aripiprazole, paliperidone, amisulpride, asenapine, iloperidone, lurasidone)
- If 2 or more antipsychotic monotherapies do not work, consider clozapine
- Some patients may require treatment with a conventional antipsychotic
- If no first-line atypical antipsychotic is effective, consider higher doses or augmentation with valproate or lamotrigine
- Consider noncompliance and switch to another antipsychotic with fewer side effects or to an antipsychotic that can be given by depot injection
- Consider initiating rehabilitation and psychotherapy such as cognitive remediation
- Consider presence of concomitant drug abuse

Best Augmenting Combos for Partial Response or Treatment Resistance

- Augmentation of zotepine has not been systematically studied

- Valproic acid (valproate, divalproex, divalproex ER)
- Other mood-stabilizing anticonvulsants (carbamazepine, oxcarbazepine, lamotrigine)
- Lithium
- Benzodiazepines

Tests

✻ Although risk of diabetes and dyslipidemia with zotepine has not been systematically studied, monitoring as for all other atypical antipsychotics is suggested

Before starting an atypical antipsychotic

✻ Weigh all patients and track BMI during treatment

- Get baseline personal and family history of diabetes, obesity, dyslipidemia, hypertension, and cardiovascular disease

✻ Get waist circumference (at umbilicus), blood pressure, fasting plasma glucose, and fasting lipid profile

- Determine if the patient is
  - overweight (BMI 25.0–29.9)
  - obese (BMI ≥30)
  - has pre-diabetes (fasting plasma glucose 100–125 mg/dL)
  - has diabetes (fasting plasma glucose >126 mg/dL)
  - has hypertension (BP >140/90 mm Hg)
  - has dyslipidemia (increased total cholesterol, LDL cholesterol, and triglycerides; decreased HDL cholesterol)
- Treat or refer such patients for treatment, including nutrition and weight management, physical activity counseling, smoking cessation, and medical management

Monitoring after starting an atypical antipsychotic

✻ BMI monthly for 3 months, then quarterly

✻ Consider monitoring fasting triglycerides monthly for several months in patients at high risk for metabolic complications and when initiating or switching antipsychotics

✻ Blood pressure, fasting plasma glucose, fasting lipids within 3 months and then annually, but earlier and more frequently for patients with diabetes or who have gained >5% of initial weight

- Treat or refer for treatment and consider switching to another atypical antipsychotic for patients who become overweight, obese, pre-diabetic, diabetic, hypertensive, or dyslipidemic while receiving an atypical antipsychotic

✻ Even in patients without known diabetes, be vigilant for the rare but life-threatening onset of diabetic ketoacidosis, which always requires immediate treatment, by monitoring for the rapid onset of polyuria, polydipsia, weight loss, nausea, vomiting, dehydration, rapid respiration, weakness, and clouding of sensorium, even coma

- EKGs may be useful for selected patients (e.g., those with personal or family history of QTc prolongation; cardiac arrhythmia; recent myocardial infarction; uncompensated heart failure; or those taking agents that prolong QTc interval such as pimozide, thioridazine, selected antiarrhythmics, moxifloxacin, sparfloxacin, etc.)
- Patients at risk for electrolyte disturbances (e.g., patients on diuretic therapy) should have baseline and periodic serum potassium and magnesium measurements
- Patients with suspected hematologic abnormalities may require a white blood cell count before initiating treatment
- Monitor liver function tests in patients with established liver disease
- Should check blood pressure in the elderly before starting and for the first few weeks of treatment
- Patients with low white blood cell count (WBC) or history of drug-induced leucopenia/neutropenia should have complete blood count (CBC) monitored frequently during the first few months and zotepine should be discontinued at the first sign of decline of WBC in the absence of other causative factors

SIDE EFFECTS

How Drug Causes Side Effects

- By blocking alpha 1 adrenergic receptors, it can cause dizziness, sedation, and hypotension
- By blocking histamine 1 receptors in the brain, it can cause sedation and weight gain
- By blocking dopamine 2 receptors in the striatum, it can cause motor side effects
- By blocking dopamine 2 receptors in the pituitary, it can cause elevations in prolactin

- Mechanism of weight gain and possible increased incidence of dyslipidemia and diabetes of atypical antipsychotics is unknown

Notable Side Effects

- Atypical antipsychotics may increase the risk for diabetes and dyslipidemia, although the specific risks associated with zotepine are unknown
- Agitation, anxiety, depression, asthenia, headache, insomnia, sedation, hypo/hyperthermia
- Constipation, dry mouth, dyspepsia, weight gain
- Tachycardia, hypotension, sweating, blurred vision
- Rare tardive dyskinesia
- Dose-related hyperprolactinemia

Life-Threatening or Dangerous Side Effects

- Rare neuroleptic malignant syndrome
- Rare seizures (risk increases with dose, especially over 300 mg/day)
- Blood dyscrasias
- Dose-dependent QTc prolongation
- Increased risk of death and cerebrovascular events in elderly patients with dementia-related psychosis

Weight Gain

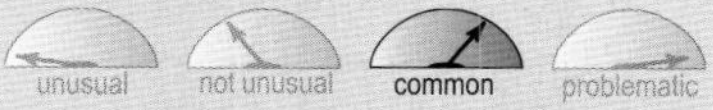

- Many experience and/or can be significant in amount

Sedation

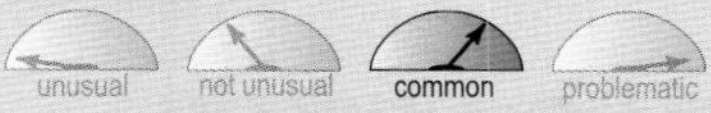

- Many experience and/or can be significant in amount

What to Do About Side Effects

- Wait
- Wait
- Wait
- For motor symptoms, add an anticholinergic agent
- Take more of the dose at bedtime to help reduce daytime sedation
- Weight loss, exercise programs, and medical management for high BMIs, diabetes, dyslipidemia
- Reduce the dose
- Switch to a first-line atypical antipsychotic

Best Augmenting Agents for Side Effects

- Benztropine or trihexyphenidyl for motor side effects
- Sometimes amantadine can be helpful for motor side effects
- Benzodiazepines may be helpful for akathisia
- Many side effects cannot be improved with an augmenting agent

DOSING AND USE

Usual Dosage Range

- 75–300 mg/day in 3 divided doses

Dosage Forms

- Tablet 25 mg, 50 mg, 100 mg

How to Dose

- Initial 75 mg/day in 3 doses; can increase every 4 days; maximum 300 mg/day in 3 doses

Dosing Tips

- Slow initial titration can minimize hypotension
- No formal studies, but some patients may do well on twice daily dosing rather than 3 times daily dosing
- * Dose-related QTc prolongation, so use with caution, especially at high doses
- Treatment should be suspended if absolute neutrophil count falls below 1,000/mm^3

Overdose

- Can be fatal, especially in mixed overdoses; seizures, coma

Long-Term Use

- Can be used to delay relapse in long-term treatment of schizophrenia

Habit Forming

- No

How to Stop

- Slow down-titration (over 6 to 8 weeks), especially when simultaneously beginning

a new antipsychotic while switching (i.e., cross-titration)
- Rapid discontinuation may lead to rebound psychosis and worsening of symptoms
- If antiparkinson agents are being used, they should be continued for a few weeks after zotepine is discontinued

Pharmacokinetics

- Metabolized by CYP450 3A4 and CYP450 1A2
- Active metabolite norzotepine

Drug Interactions

- Combined use with phenothiazines may increase risk of seizures
- Can decrease the effects of levodopa, dopamine agonists
- Epinephrine may lower blood pressure
- May interact with hypotensive agents due to alpha 1 adrenergic blockade
- May enhance QTc prolongation of other drugs capable of prolonging QTc interval
- Plasma concentrations increased by diazepam, fluoxetine
- Zotepine may increase plasma levels of phenytoin
- May increase risk of bleeding if used with anticoagulants
- Theoretically, dose may need to be raised if given in conjunction with CYP450 1A2 inducers (e.g., cigarette smoke)
- Theoretically, dose may need to be lowered if given in conjunction with CYP450 1A2 inhibitors (e.g., fluvoxamine) in order to prevent dangers of dose-dependent QTc prolongation
- Theoretically, dose may need to be lowered if given in conjunction with CYP450 3A4 inhibitors (e.g., fluvoxamine, nefazodone, fluoxetine) in order to prevent dangers of dose-dependent QTc prolongation

Other Warnings/ Precautions

- Not recommended for use with sibutramine
- Use cautiously in patients with alcohol withdrawal or convulsive disorders because of possible lowering of seizure threshold
- If signs of neuroleptic malignant syndrome develop, treatment should be immediately discontinued
- Because zotepine may dose-dependently prolong QTc interval, use with caution in patients who have bradycardia or who are taking drugs that can induce bradycardia (e.g., beta blockers, calcium channel blockers, clonidine, digitalis)
- Because zotepine may dose-dependently prolong QTc interval, use with caution in patients who have hypokalemia and or hypomagnesemia or who are taking drugs than can induce hypokalemia and/or magnesemia (e.g., diuretics, stimulant laxatives, intravenous amphotericin B, glucocorticoids, tetracosactide)
- Because zotepine dose-dependently prolongs QTc interval, use with caution in patients taking any agent capable of increasing zotepine plasma levels (e.g., diazepam, CYP450 1A2 inhibitors, and CYP450 3A4 inhibitors)

Do Not Use

- If patient has epilepsy or family history of epilepsy
- If patient has gout or history of nephrolithiasis
- If patient is taking other CNS depressants
- If patient is taking high doses of other antipsychotics
- If patient is taking agents capable of significantly prolonging QTc interval (e.g., pimozide; thioridazine; selected antiarrhythmics such as quinidine, disopyramide, amiodarone, and sotalol; selected antibiotics such as moxifloxacin and sparfloxacin)
- If there is a history of QTc prolongation or cardiac arrhythmia, recent acute myocardial infarction, uncompensated heart failure
- If patient is pregnant or breast feeding
- If there is a proven allergy to zotepine

SPECIAL POPULATIONS

Renal Impairment

- Recommended starting dose 25 mg twice a day; recommended maximum dose generally 75 mg twice a day

Hepatic Impairment

- Recommended starting dose 25 mg twice a day; recommended maximum dose generally 75 mg twice a day

- May require weekly monitoring of liver function during the first few months of treatment

Cardiac Impairment

- Drug should be used with caution
- Zotepine produces a dose-dependent prolongation of QTc interval, which may be enhanced by the existence of bradycardia, hypokalemia, congenital or acquired long QTc interval, which should be evaluated prior to administering zotepine
- Use with caution if treating concomitantly with a medication likely to produce prolonged bradycardia, hypokalemia, slowing of intracardiac conduction, or prolongation of the QTc interval
- Avoid zotepine in patients with a known history of QTc prolongation, recent acute myocardial infraction, and uncompensated heart failure

Elderly

- Recommended starting dose 25 mg twice a day; recommended maximum dose generally 75 mg twice a day
- Although atypical antipsychotics are commonly used for behavioral disturbances in dementia, no agent has been approved for treatment of elderly patients with dementia-related psychosis
- Elderly patients with dementia-related psychosis treated with atypical antipsychotics are at an increased risk of death compared to placebo, and also have an increased risk of cerebrovascular events

Children and Adolescents

- Not recommended for use in children under age 18

Pregnancy

- Insufficient data in humans to determine risk
- There is a risk of abnormal muscle movements and withdrawal symptoms in newborns whose mothers took an antipsychotic during the third trimester; symptoms may include agitation, abnormally increased or decreased muscle tone, tremor, sleepiness, severe difficulty breathing, and difficulty feeding
- Zotepine is not recommended during pregnancy

Breast Feeding

- Zotepine is not recommended during breast feeding
- Immediate postpartum period is a high-risk time for relapse of psychosis, so may consider treatment with another antipsychotic

THE ART OF PSYCHOPHARMACOLOGY

Potential Advantages

- Norepinephrine reuptake blocking actions have theoretical benefits for cognition (attention) and for depression

Potential Disadvantages

- Patients not compliant with 3 times daily dosing
- Patients requiring rapid onset of antipsychotic action
- Patients with uncontrolled seizures

Primary Target Symptoms

- Positive symptoms of psychosis
- Negative symptoms of psychosis
- Cognitive functioning
- Depressive symptoms

Pearls

* Zotepine inhibits norepinephrine reuptake, which may have implications for treatment of depression, as well as for cognitive symptoms of schizophrenia
- Risks of diabetes and dyslipidemia not well studied for zotepine, but known significant weight gain suggests the need for careful monitoring during zotepine treatment
- Not as well investigated in bipolar disorder, but its mechanism of action suggests efficacy in acute bipolar mania

Suggested Reading

Ackenheil M. [The biochemical effect profile of zotepine in comparison with other neuroleptics]. Fortschr Neurol Psychiatr 1991;59(Suppl 1):S2–9.

Fenton M, Morris S, De-Silva P, et al. Zotepine for schizophrenia. Cochrane Database Syst Rev 2000;(2):CD001948.

Stanniland C, Taylor D. Tolerability of atypical antipsychotics. Drug Saf 2000;22(3):195–214.

THERAPEUTICS

Brands • Clopixol
• Clopixol-Acuphase
see index for additional brand names

Generic? No

Class
- Neuroscience-based Nomenclature: dopamine receptor antagonist (D-RAn)
- Conventional antipsychotic (neuroleptic, thioxanthene, dopamine 2 antagonist)

Commonly Prescribed for
(bold for FDA approved)
- Acute schizophrenia (oral, acetate injection)
- Maintenance treatment of schizophrenia (oral, decanoate injection)
- Bipolar disorder
- Aggression

How the Drug Works
- Blocks dopamine 2 receptors, reducing positive symptoms of psychosis

How Long Until It Works
- For injection, psychotic symptoms can improve within a few days, but it may take 1–2 weeks for notable improvement
- For oral formulation, psychotic symptoms can improve within 1 week, but may take several weeks for full effect on behavior

If It Works
- Most often reduces positive symptoms in schizophrenia but does not eliminate them
- Most schizophrenic patients do not have a total remission of symptoms but rather a reduction of symptoms by about a third
- Continue treatment in schizophrenia until reaching a plateau of improvement
- After reaching a satisfactory plateau, continue treatment for at least a year after first episode of psychosis in schizophrenia
- For second and subsequent episodes of psychosis in schizophrenia, treatment may need to be indefinite
- Reduces symptoms of acute psychotic mania but not proven as a mood stabilizer or as an effective maintenance treatment in bipolar disorder
- After reducing acute psychotic symptoms in mania, switch to a mood stabilizer and/or an atypical antipsychotic for mood stabilization and maintenance

If It Doesn't Work
- Consider trying one of the first-line atypical antipsychotics (risperidone, olanzapine, quetiapine, ziprasidone, aripiprazole, paliperidone, amisulpride, asenapine, iloperidone, lurasidone)
- Consider trying another conventional antipsychotic
- If 2 or more antipsychotic monotherapies do not work, consider clozapine

Best Augmenting Combos for Partial Response or Treatment Resistance
- Augmentation of conventional antipsychotics has not been systematically studied
- Addition of a mood-stabilizing anticonvulsant such as valproate, carbamazepine, or lamotrigine may be helpful in both schizophrenia and bipolar mania
- Augmentation with lithium in bipolar mania may be helpful
- Addition of a benzodiazepine, especially short-term for agitation

Tests
- ✻ Since conventional antipsychotics are frequently associated with weight gain, before starting treatment, weigh all patients and determine if the patient is already overweight (BMI 25.0–29.9) or obese (BMI ≥30)
- Before giving a drug that can cause weight gain to an overweight or obese patient, consider determining whether the patient already has pre-diabetes (fasting plasma glucose 100–125 mg/dL), diabetes (fasting plasma glucose >126 mg/dL), or dyslipidemia (increased total cholesterol, LDL cholesterol, and triglycerides; decreased HDL cholesterol), and treat or refer such patients for treatment, including nutrition and weight management, physical activity counseling, smoking cessation, and medical management
- ✻ Monitor weight and BMI during treatment
- ✻ Consider monitoring fasting triglycerides monthly for several months in patients at high risk for metabolic complications and when initiating or switching antipsychotics
- ✻ While giving a drug to a patient who has gained >5% of initial weight, consider

evaluating for the presence of pre-diabetes, diabetes, or dyslipidemia, or consider switching to a different antipsychotic
- Should check blood pressure in the elderly before starting and for the first few weeks of treatment
- Monitoring elevated prolactin levels of dubious clinical benefit
- Patients with low white blood cell count (WBC) or history of drug-induced leucopenia/neutropenia should have complete blood count (CBC) monitored frequently during the first few months and zuclopenthixol should be discontinued at the first sign of decline of WBC in the absence of other causative factors

SIDE EFFECTS

How Drug Causes Side Effects
- By blocking dopamine 2 receptors in the striatum, it can cause motor side effects
- By blocking dopamine 2 receptors in the pituitary, it can cause elevations in prolactin
- By blocking dopamine 2 receptors excessively in the mesocortical and mesolimbic dopamine pathways, especially at high doses, it can cause worsening of negative and cognitive symptoms (neuroleptic-induced deficit syndrome)
- Anticholinergic actions may cause sedation, blurred vision, constipation, dry mouth
- Antihistaminic actions may cause sedation, weight gain
- By blocking alpha 1 adrenergic receptors, it can cause dizziness, sedation, and hypotension
- Mechanism of weight gain and any possible increased incidence of diabetes or dyslipidemia with conventional antipsychotics is unknown

Notable Side Effects
❋ Extrapyramidal symptoms
❋ Tardive dyskinesia (risk increases with duration of treatment and with dose)
❋ Priapism
❋ Galactorrhea, amenorrhea
- Rare lens opacity
- Sedation, dizziness
- Dry mouth, constipation, vision problems
- Hypotension
- Weight gain

Life-Threatening or Dangerous Side Effects
- Rare neuroleptic malignant syndrome
- Rare neutropenia
- Rare respiratory depression
- Rare agranulocytosis
- Rare seizures
- Increased risk of death and cerebrovascular events in elderly patients with dementia-related psychosis

Weight Gain
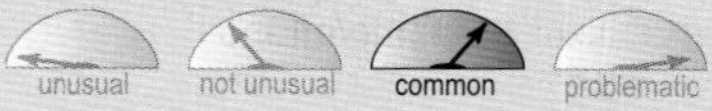

- Many experience and/or can be significant in amount
- Some people may lose weight

Sedation
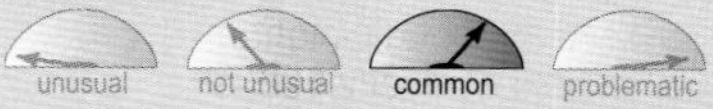

- Many experience and/or can be significant in amount
- Acetate formulation may be associated with an initial sedative response

What to Do About Side Effects
- Wait
- Wait
- Wait
- For motor symptoms, add an anticholinergic agent
- Reduce the dose
- For sedation, take at night
- Switch to an atypical antipsychotic
- Weight loss, exercise programs, and medical management for high BMIs, diabetes dyslipidemia

Best Augmenting Agents for Side Effects
- Benztropine or trihexyphenidyl for motor side effects
- Sometimes amantadine can be helpful for motor side effects
- Benzodiazepines may be helpful for akathisia
- Many side effects cannot be improved with an augmenting agent

DOSING AND USE

Usual Dosage Range
- Oral 20–60 mg/day
- Acetate 50–150 mg every 2–3 days
- Decanoate 150–300 mg every 2–4 weeks

Dosage Forms
- Tablet 10 mg, 25 mg, 40 mg
- Acetate 50 mg/mL (equivalent to zuclopenthixol 45.25 mg/mL), 100 mg/2 mL (equivalent to zuclopenthixol 45.25 mg/mL)
- Decanoate 200 mg/mL (equivalent to zuclopenthixol 144.4 mg/mL), 500 mg/mL (equivalent to zuclopenthixol 361.1 mg/mL)

How to Dose
- Oral: initial 10–15 mg/day in divided doses; can increase by 10–20 mg/day every 2–3 days; maintenance dose can be administered as a single nighttime dose; maximum dose generally 100 mg/day
- Injection should be administered intramuscularly in the gluteal region in the morning
- Acetate generally should be administered every 2–3 days; some patients may require a second dose 24–48 hours after the first injection; duration of treatment should not exceed 2 weeks; maximum cumulative dosage should not exceed 400 mg; maximum number of injections should not exceed 4
- Decanoate: initial dose 100 mg; after 1–4 weeks administer a second injection of 100–200 mg; maintenance treatment is generally 100–600 mg every 1–4 weeks

Dosing Tips
- Onset of action of the intramuscular acetate formulation following a single injection is generally 2–4 hours; duration of action is generally 2–3 days
- Zuclopenthixol acetate is not intended for long-term use, and should not generally be used for longer than 2 weeks; patients requiring treatment longer than 2 weeks should be switched to a depot or oral formulation of zuclopenthixol or another antipsychotic
- When changing from zuclopenthixol acetate to maintenance treatment with zuclopenthixol decanoate, administer the last injection of acetate concomitantly with the initial injection of decanoate
- The peak of action for the decanoate is usually 4–9 days, and doses generally have to be administered every 2–3 weeks
- Treatment should be suspended if absolute neutrophil count falls below 1,000/mm^3

Overdose
- Sedation, convulsions, extrapyramidal symptoms, coma, hypotension, shock, hypo/hyperthermia

Long-Term Use
- Zuclopenthixol decanoate is intended for maintenance treatment
- Some side effects may be irreversible (e.g., tardive dyskinesia)

Habit Forming
- No

How to Stop
- Slow down-titration of oral formulation (over 6–8 weeks), especially when simultaneously beginning a new antipsychotic while switching (i.e., cross-titration)
- Rapid oral discontinuation may lead to rebound psychosis and worsening of symptoms
- If antiparkinson agents are being used, they should be continued for a few weeks after zuclopenthixol is discontinued

Pharmacokinetics
- Metabolized by CYP450 2D6 and CYP450 3A4
- For oral formulation, elimination half-life approximately 20 hours
- For acetate, rate-limiting half-life approximately 32 hours
- For decanoate, rate-limiting half-life approximately 17–21 days with multiple doses

Drug Interactions
- Theoretically, concomitant use with CYP450 2D6 inhibitors (such as paroxetine and fluoxetine) or with CYP450 3A4 inhibitors (such as fluoxetine and ketoconazole) could raise zuclopenthixol plasma levels and require dosage reduction

- Theoretically, concomitant use with CYP450 3A4 inducers (such as carbamazepine) could lower zuclopenthixol plasma levels and require dosage increase
- CNS effects may be increased if used with other CNS depressants
- If used with anticholinergic agents, may potentiate their effects
- Combined use with epinephrine may lower blood pressure
- Zuclopenthixol may block the antihypertensive effects of drugs such as guanethidine, but may enhance the actions of other antihypertensive drugs
- Using zuclopenthixol with metoclopramide or piperazine may increase the risk of extrapyramidal symptoms
- Zuclopenthixol may antagonize the effects of levodopa and dopamine agonists
- Some patients taking a neuroleptic and lithium have developed an encephalopathic syndrome similar to neuroleptic malignant syndrome

Other Warnings/ Precautions

- If signs of neuroleptic malignant syndrome develop, treatment should be immediately discontinued
- Use with caution in patients with epilepsy, glaucoma, urinary retention
- Decanoate should not be used with clozapine because it cannot be withdrawn quickly in the event of serious adverse effects such as neutropenia
- Possible antiemetic effect of zuclopenthixol may mask signs of other disorders or overdose; suppression of cough reflex may cause asphyxia
- Use only with great caution if at all in Parkinson's disease or Lewy body dementia
- Observe for signs of ocular toxicity (pigmentary retinopathy and lenticular and corneal deposits)
- Avoid undue exposure to sunlight
- Avoid extreme heat exposure
- Do not use epinephrine in event of overdose as interaction with some pressor agents may lower blood pressure

Do Not Use

- If patient is taking a large concomitant dose of a sedative hypnotic
- If patient is taking guanethidine or a similar acting compound
- If patient has CNS depression, is comatose, or has subcortical brain damage
- If patient has acute alcohol, barbiturate, or opiate intoxication
- If patient has angle-closure glaucoma
- If patient has pheochromocytoma, circulatory collapse, or blood dyscrasias
- In case of pregnancy
- If there is a proven allergy to zuclopenthixol

SPECIAL POPULATIONS

Renal Impairment

- Use with caution

Hepatic Impairment

- Use with caution

Cardiac Impairment

- Use with caution

Elderly

- Some patients may tolerate lower doses better
- Maximum acetate dose 100 mg
- Although conventional antipsychotics are commonly used for behavioral disturbances in dementia, no agent has been approved for treatment of elderly patients with dementia-related psychosis
- Elderly patients with dementia-related psychosis treated with antipsychotics are at an increased risk of death compared to placebo, and also have an increased risk of cerebrovascular events

Children and Adolescents

- Safety and efficacy have not been established in children under age 18
- Preliminary open-label data show that oral zuclopenthixol may be effective in reducing aggression in mentally impaired children

Pregnancy

- Not recommended for use during pregnancy

- There is a risk of abnormal muscle movements and withdrawal symptoms in newborns whose mothers took an antipsychotic during the third trimester; symptoms may include agitation, abnormally increased or decreased muscle tone, tremor, sleepiness, severe difficulty breathing, and difficulty feeding
- Psychotic symptoms may worsen during pregnancy and some form of treatment may be necessary
- Atypical antipsychotics may be preferable to conventional antipsychotics or anticonvulsant mood stabilizers if treatment is required during pregnancy

Breast Feeding

- Some drug is found in mother's breast milk
- ✻ Recommended either to discontinue drug or bottle feed
- Infants of women who choose to breast feed should be monitored for possible adverse effects

THE ART OF PSYCHOPHARMACOLOGY

Potential Advantages

- Noncompliant patients (decanoate)
- Emergency use (acute injection)

Potential Disadvantages

- Children
- Elderly
- Patients with tardive dyskinesia

Primary Target Symptoms

- Positive symptoms of psychosis
- Negative symptoms of psychosis
- Aggressive symptoms

Pearls

- Zuclopenthixol depot may reduce risk of relapse more than some other depot conventional antipsychotics, but it may also be associated with more adverse effects
- Can combine acute injection with depot injection in the same syringe for rapid onset and long duration effects when initiating treatment
- Zuclopenthixol may have serotonin 2A antagonist properties, but these have never been systematically investigated for atypical antipsychotic properties at low doses
- Patients have very similar antipsychotic responses to any conventional antipsychotic, which is different from atypical antipsychotics where antipsychotic responses of individual patients can occasionally vary greatly from one atypical antipsychotic to another
- Patients with inadequate responses to atypical antipsychotics may benefit from a trial of augmentation with a conventional antipsychotic such as zuclopenthixol or from switching to a conventional antipsychotic such as zuclopenthixol
- However, long-term polypharmacy with a combination of a conventional antipsychotic such as zuclopenthixol with an atypical antipsychotic may combine their side effects without clearly augmenting the efficacy of either
- For treatment-resistant patients, especially those with impulsivity, aggression, violence, and self-harm, long-term polypharmacy with 2 atypical antipsychotics or with 1 atypical antipsychotic and 1 conventional antipsychotic may be useful or even necessary while closely monitoring
- In such cases, it may be beneficial to combine 1 depot antipsychotic with 1 oral antipsychotic
- Although a frequent practice by some prescribers, adding 2 conventional antipsychotics together has little rationale and may reduce tolerability without clearly enhancing efficacy

Suggested Reading

Coutinho E, Fenton M, Adams C, Campbell C. Zuclopenthixol acetate in psychiatric emergencies: looking for evidence from clinical trials. Schizophr Res 2000;46:111–18.

Coutinho E, Fenton M, Quraishi S. Zuclopenthixol decanoate for schizophrenia and other serious mental illnesses. Cochrane Database Syst Rev 2000;(2):CD001164.

Davies S, Westin A, Castberg I, et al. Characterisation of zuclopenthixol metabolism by in vitro and therapeutic drug monitoring studies. Acta Psychiatr Scand 2010;122(6):444–53.

Fenton M, Coutinho ES, Campbell C. Zuclopenthixol acetate in the treatment of acute schizophrenia and similar serious mental illnesses. Cochrane Database Syst Rev 2000;(2):CD000525.

Stahl SM. How to dose a psychotropic drug: beyond therapeutic drug monitoring to genotyping the patient. Acta Psychiatr Scand 2010;122(6):440–1.

Index by Drug Name

(trade names and generic names)

Index by Use

Commonly Prescribed For (bold for FDA approved)

Index by Class

Abbreviations

5HT	serotonin
ACh	acetylcholine
AChE	acetylcholinesterase
ADHD	attention deficit hyperactivity disorder
AE	adverse effect
ALPT	total serum alkaline phosphatase
ALT	alanine aminotransferase
AMPA	alpha-amino-3-hydroxy-5-methyl-4-isoxazolepropionic acid
ANA	antinuclear antibody
ANC	Absolute neutrophil count
AST	aspartate aminotransferase
BEN	benign ethnic neutropenia
BHB	beta-hydroxybutyric acid
bid	twice a day
BMI	body mass index
BP	blood pressure
BuChE	butyrylcholinesterase
CBC	complete blood count
CR	controlled-release
CRP	C-reactive protein
CSF	cerebrospinal fluid
CMI	clomipramine
CNS	central nervous system
COPD	chronic obstructive pulmonary disease
CPAP	continuous positive airway pressure
CYP450	cytochrome P450
DA	dopamine
De-CMI	desmethyl-clomipramine
dL	deciliter
DLB	dementia with Lewy bodies
ECG	electrocardiogram
EEG	electroencephalogram
EKG	electrocardiogram
EPS	extrapyramidal side effects
ER	extended-release
FDA	Food and Drug Administration
GABA	gamma-aminobutyric acid
GAD	generalized anxiety disorder

GFR	glomerular filtration rate
HDL	high-density lipoprotein
HMG CoA	beta-hydroxy-beta-methylglutaryl coenzyme A
IM	intramuscular
IR	immediate-release
IV	intravenous
LAI	long-acting injectable
lb	pound
LDH	lactate dehydrogenase
LDL	low-density lipoprotein
MAO	monoamine oxidase
MAOI	monoamine oxidase inhibitor
mCPP	meta-chloro-phenyl-piperazine
MDMA	3,4-methylenedioxymethamphetamine (ecstasy)
mg	milligram
mL	milliliter
mmHg	millimeters of mercury
MRI	magnetic resonance imaging
MRSA	methicillin-resistant *Staphylococcus aureus*
NE	norepinephrine
NET	norepinephrine transporter
NMDA	*N*-methyl-D-aspartate
NSAID	nonsteroidal anti-inflammatory drug
OCD	obsessive-compulsive disorder
ODT	oral disintegrating tablet
ODV	O-desmethylvenlafaxine
OSAHS	obstructive sleep apnea/hypopnea syndrome
PBA	pseudobulbar affect
PCP	phencyclidine
PET	positron emission tomography
PMDD	premenstrual dysphoric disorder
prn	as needed
PTSD	posttraumatic stress disorder
qd	once a day
qhs	once a day at bedtime
qid	4 times a day
RIMA	reversible inhibitor of monoamine oxidase A
SGRI	selective GABA reuptake inhibitor
SNRI	dual serotonin and norepinephrine reuptake inhibitor
SPARI	serotonin partial antagonist reuptake inhibitor
SR	sustained release

SSRI	selective serotonin reuptake inhibitor
TCA	tricyclic antidepressant
tid	3 times a day
TSH	thyroid-stimulating hormone
VMA	vanillylmandelic acid
WBC	white blood cell count

Stahl's Essential Psychopharmacology

Neuroscientific Basis and Practical Applications

Fourth Edition

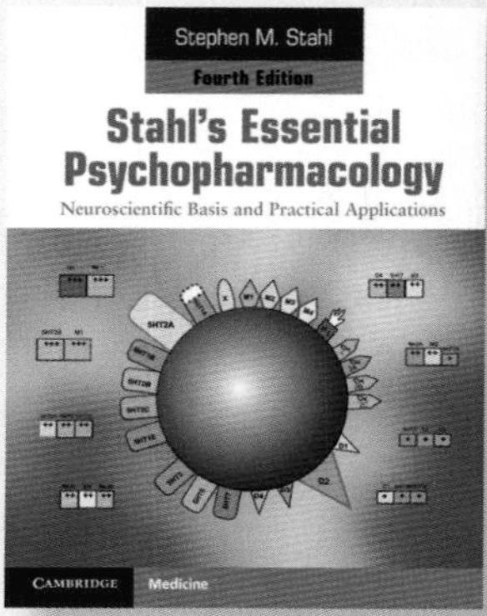

- Long established as the preeminent source in its field
- Features the author's highly-praised writing style with clear, easy-to-follow illustrations
- Thoroughly updated and extensively revised for the fourth edition, taking account of advances in neurobiology and recent clinical developments to explain the concepts underlying the drug treatment of psychiatric disorders with a sleek new look and feel, larger page size, and two-column layout
- Indispensable for all professionals and students in mental health

978-1-107-68646-5 | Pbk | 626 pp | 2013

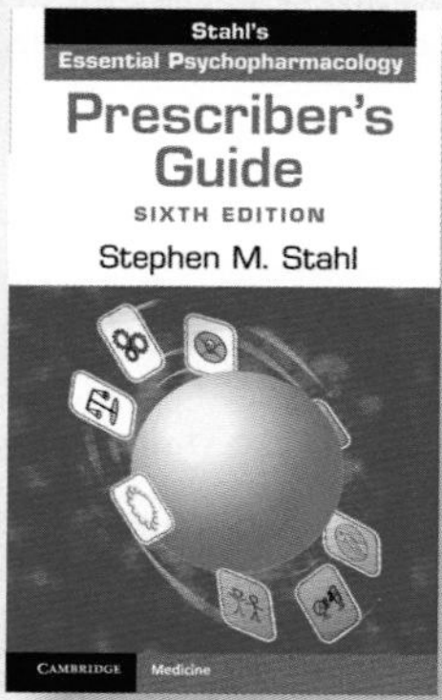

Prescriber's Guide

Sixth Edition

- Provides the most complete and up-to-date summary of the practical use of psychotropic drugs, including seven new drugs in this edition
- Presented in a templated format, fully indexed and cross-referenced for ease of navigation
- Written with the authority of evidence and the guidance of clinical wisdom

978-1-316-61813-4/978-1-108-40488-4 | Pbk/Spiral | 865 pp | 2017

Available on the App Store

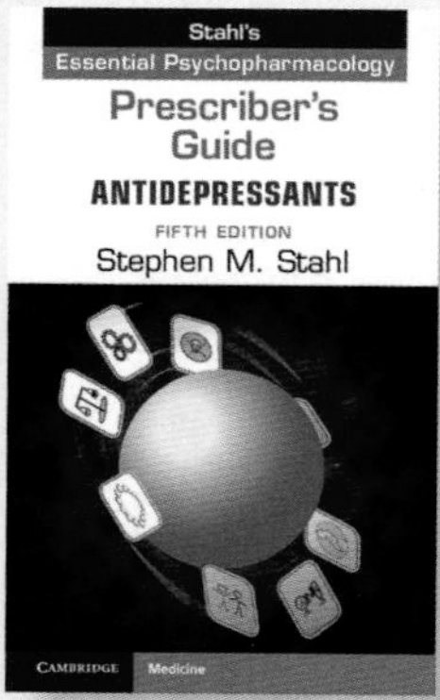

Prescriber's Guide

Antidepressants

Fifth Edition

- This spin-off from Stephen Stahl's new, completely revised, and fully updated fifth edition of the *Prescriber's Guide* covers the most important drugs in use today for treating depression

978-1-107-47617-2 | Pbk | 440 pp | 2014

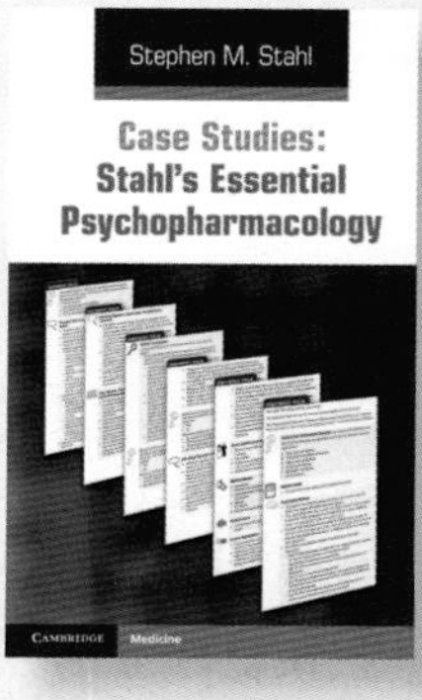

Case Studies

- Designed with the distinctive, user-friendly presentation that has been so popular in *Stahl's Essential Psychopharmacology* and The Prescriber's Guide
- Cases are followed through the complete clinical encounter, from start to resolution, acknowledging all the complications, issues, decisions, twists and turns along the way
- Psychiatry in real life!

978-0-521-18208-9 | Pbk | 500 pp | 2011

Case Studies

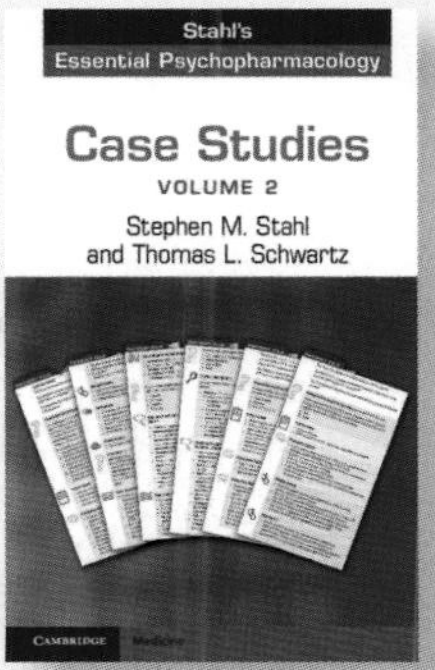

Volume 2

- Describes treatment options for a wide range of psychiatric disorders
- Explains what to try next if an intervention fails
- Highlights possible mistakes and pitfalls so that you don't have to make them

978-1-107-60733-0 | Pbk | 504 pp | 2016

Stahl's Self-Assessment Examination in Psychiatry

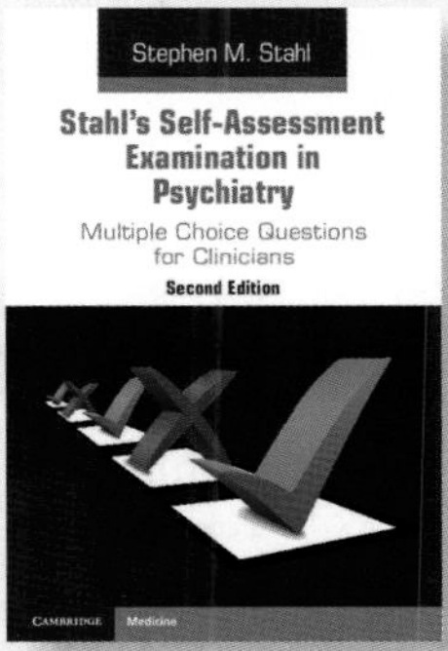

Second Edition

- All questions have been approved by the American Board of Psychiatry and Neurology as being pitched at an appropriate level for reaccreditation purposes
- Thorough explanations of the correct and incorrect answer choices for every question demystify complex principles and enable the user to build their knowledge and understanding
- The one hundred and fifty questions are divided into ten sections, reflecting the core areas of psychiatry and providing comprehensive self-assessment for American Board of Psychiatry and Neurology examinations

978-1-316-50249-5 | Pbk | 352 pp | 2017

Stahl's Illustrated Series

The books in the *Stahl's Illustrated Series* are designed to be fun. In full-color throughout, with illustrations in the style of his classic *Essential Psychopharmacology* and *Prescriber's Guide*, they provide a speedy way to learn or review specific concepts in psychopharmacology.

The visual learner will find that these books make psychopharmacology concepts easy to master, while the non-visual learner will enjoy a shortened text version of complex psychopharmacology concepts.

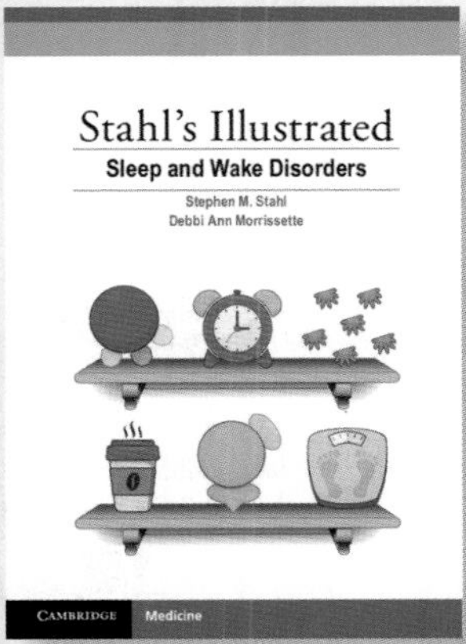

Stahl's Illustrated Sleep and Wake Disorders

978-1-107-56136-6

Pbk | 140 pp | 2016

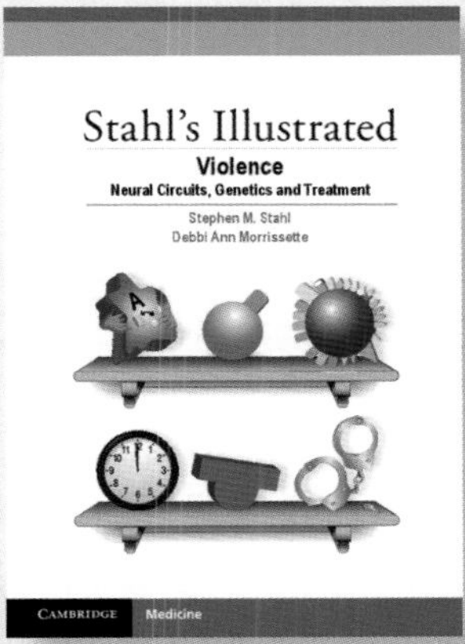

Stahl's Illustrated Violence: Neural Circuits, Genetics and Treatment

978-1-107-44160-6

Pbk | 120 pp | 2014

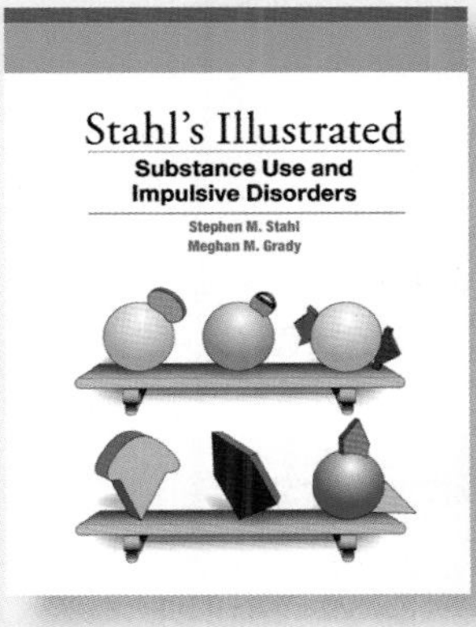

Substance Use and Impulsive Disorders

978-1-107-67453-0

Pbk | 183 pp | 2012

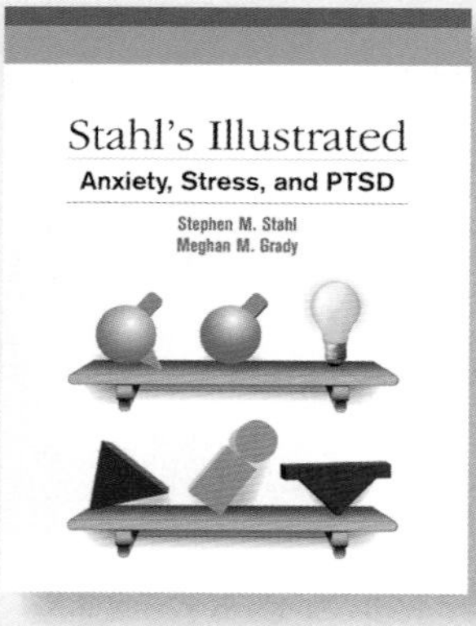

Anxiety, Stress, and PTSD

978-1-107-67453-0

Pbk | 183 pp | 2012

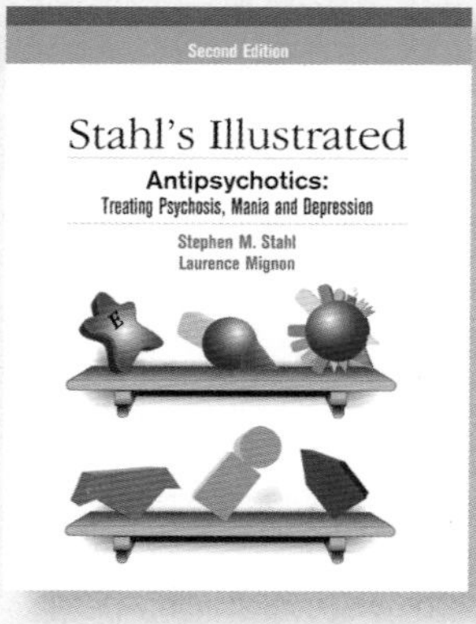

Antipsychotics: Treating Psychosis, Mania, and Depression

978-0-521-14905-1

Pbk | 200 pp | 2010

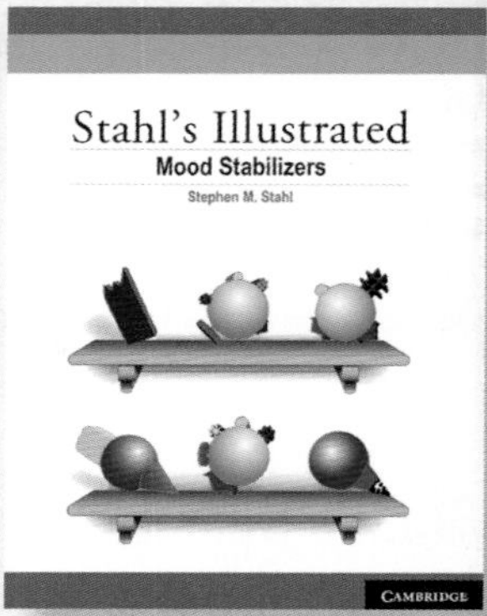

Mood Stabilizers

978-0-521-75849-9

Pbk | 176 pp | 2009

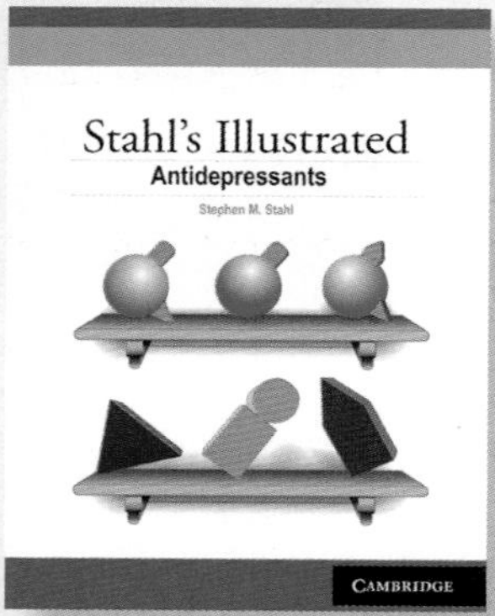

Antidepressants

978-0-521-75852-9

Pbk | 200 pp | 2009

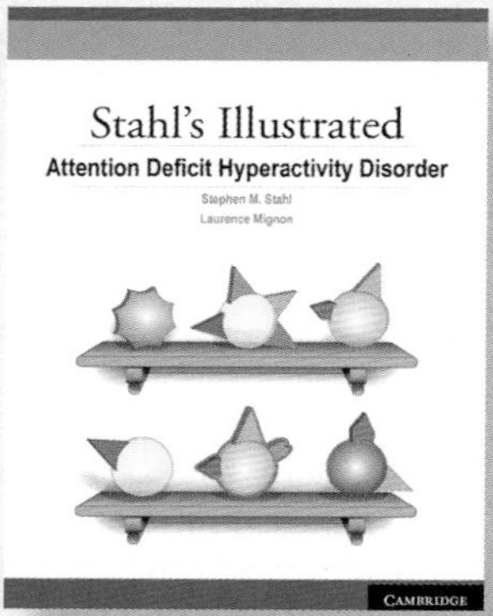

Attention Deficit Hyperactivity Disorder

978-0-521-13315-9

Pbk | 166 pp | 2009

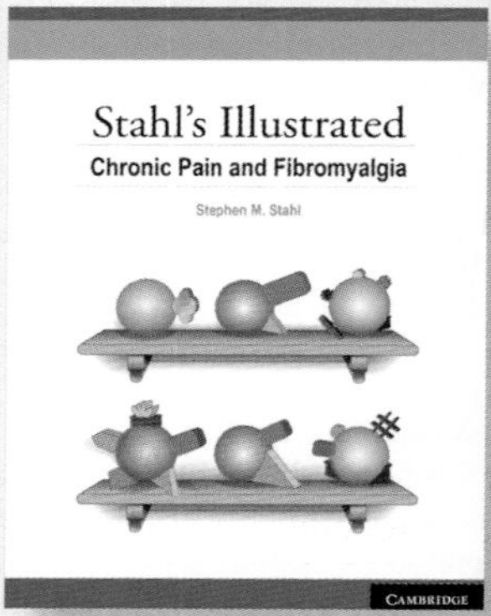

Chronic Pain and Fibromyalgia

978-0-521-13322-7

Pbk | 176 pp | 2009

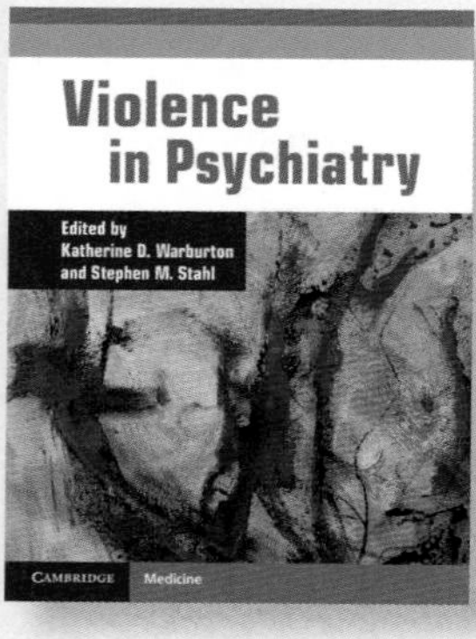

Violence in Psychiatry

Katherine D. Warburton, University of California, Davis, Stephen M. Stahl, University of California, San Diego

- Focuses on violence from assessment, through underlying neurobiology, to treatment and other recommendations for practice
- Reconceptualizes violence as a primary medical condition, not as the by-product of one
- Addresses new types of violence exhibited in inpatient environments to enhance a balance between safety and hospital treatment

978-1-107-09219-8 | Hbk | 360 pp | 2016

Next Generations Antidepressants

Moving Beyond Monoamines to Discover Novel Treatment Strategies for Mood Disorders

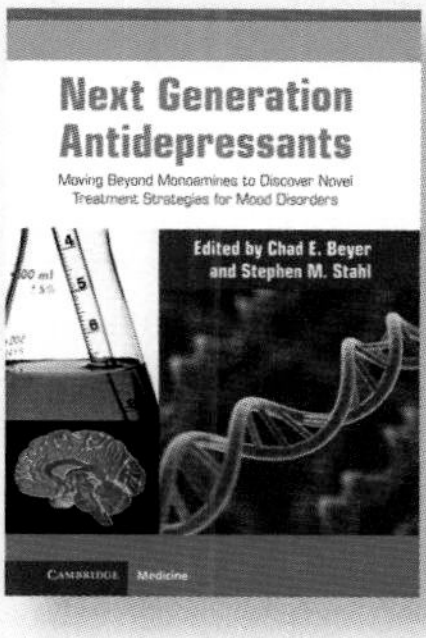

Chad E Beyer, MBA, University of Colorado School of Medicine, Aurora, Stephen M Stahl, MD, PhD, University of California, San Diego, USA, University of Cambridge, UK

- Looks at the future of mood-disorder research
- Essential reading for all those involved in psychopharmacologic drug development and mental health clinicians seeking a preview of discoveries soon to influence their practice

978-0-521-76058-4 | Hbk | 150 pp | 2010

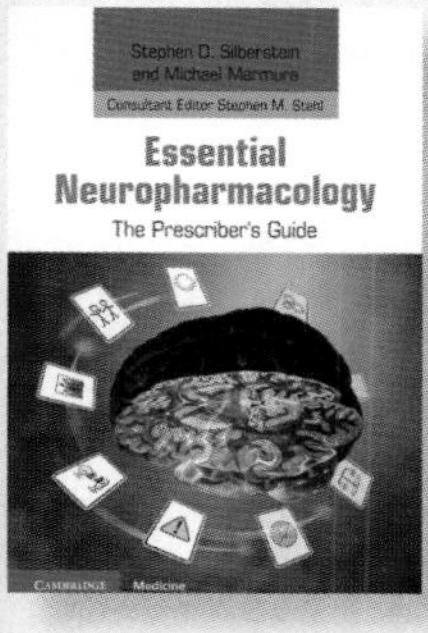

Essential Neuropharmacology

The Prescriber's Guide

Stephen D Silberstein, MD and Michael J Marmura, MD, Jefferson Medical College, Philadelphia, USA, Stephen M Stahl, MD, PhD, University of California, San Diego, USA, University of Cambridge, UK

- Expertly reviews the most important medications used by neurologists in their practice
- Evidence is taken from recent clinical trials, which helps the reader relate the content to everyday clinical practice
- Detailed descriptions of each medication enable user to make quick and informed decisions with confidence

978-0-521-13672-3 | Pbk | 415 pp | 2010

Essential Evidence-Based Psychopharmacology

Second Edition

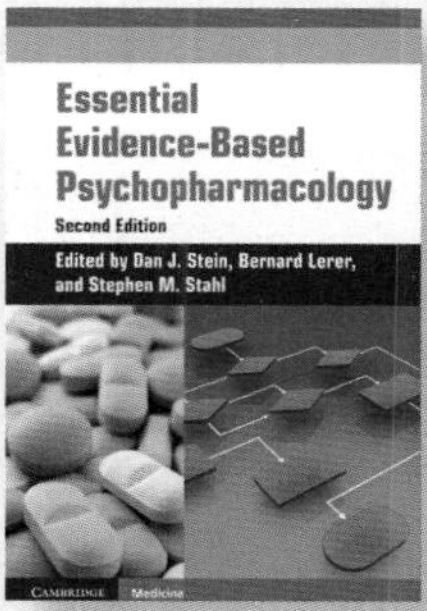

Prof Dan Stein, University of Cape Town, South Africa, Dr Bernard Lerer, Hadassah-Hebrew University Medical Center, Israel, Stephen M Stahl, MD, PhD, University of California, San Diego, USA, University of Cambridge, UK

- Fully updated, this volume summarizes the wealth of new developments in the field of psychopharmacology and sets them within context of day-to-day clinical practice
- Organized according to the DSM-V listing and covering all major conditions, this book is invaluable to all practicing and training clinicians in a mental health or less specialized environment

978-1-107-40010-8 | Pbk | 330 pp | 2012

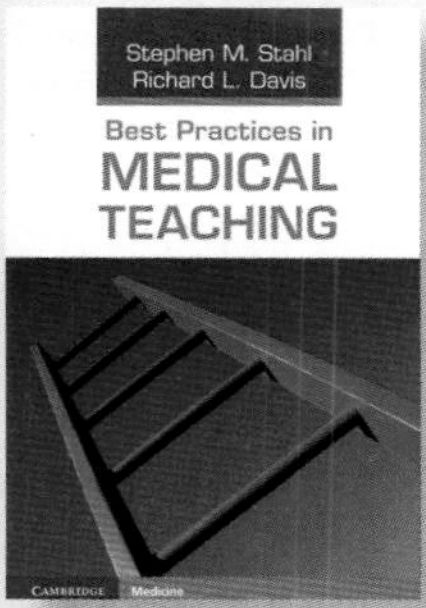

Best Practices in Medical Teaching

Stephen M Stahl, MD, PhD, University of California, San Diego, USA, University of Cambridge, UK, Richard L Davis, Arbor Scientia, Carlsbad, USA

- Written by two of the leading experts in medical communication, this book illustrates the general principles of effective medical presentation by applying the principles of adult learning
- Features examples of how to design a successful lecture, along with chapter summary, progress check, and performance self-assessment test to ensure that concepts are understood

978-0-521-15176-4 | Pbk | 192 pp | 2011